Please look for the following

Braid Your Own Hair

Tails

Headband

Circle

Single

Double

Junction

Classic

Teardrop

Fringe

Crown

Halo

Heart

Acknowledgments

Without my models I would not have this book. Photos are important and essential.

Many people were a part of this book. I extend my thanks to each person for their invaluable help.

Brain neuron art: Leslie Haubrick
Editors: Jerrid Wolflick and Samantha Gilman
Hairstylist: Raychel Emmons
Design and graphics: Raychel Emmons
Photography and photoshopping: Raychel Emmons

In the words of Mrs. E. R. Shepherd,

"The author of this book lays no claim to originality of subject-matter. She has nothing new to say. She does, however, claim originality upon one ground, that of making selections from the writings and teachings of others, and from observation and experience; that of culling here and there knowledge, facts, motives, ideas, and grouping them into practical form. Seeking to make the material for instruction as complete as possible, she has seized upon and appropriated anything, which could contribute to the general design." - 1882

This book is copyright 2013 Raychel Emmons

Dedication

I would like to dedicate this book to JoAnn Hoffman, who encouraged me when I needed it most.

She is also the lovely lady who first put a mini rope accent onto a braided hairstyle with the intent of creating a signature line of braids.

May you channel her ingenuity while your brain gets creative with braids.

Preface

I invite you to join me in my approach to hair braiding. It involves creating a hairstyle using three different components. Ways, Forms and Accents. In my glossary you will see words that look made up. That is because; I made up words to define what I am doing. I am also giving new definitions to old ideas.

I have gathered as much knowledge as I could find on braiding and put it in one place. I want this information handed down to future generations.

Factors that can determine a hairstyle are length and thickness of the hair, patience to sit still and the skill of the stylist.

Each hair type will have a favorite braid that it behaves for. I have been able to create hairstyles on as little as three inches of hair, using the techniques in this book. Applying the knowledge here gives you the opportunity to make thin hair look thicker, massive amounts of hair disappear into a tightly contained area, and short hair look intricately styled.

Practice makes perfect.
So do not give up, even if you feel it is too hard.

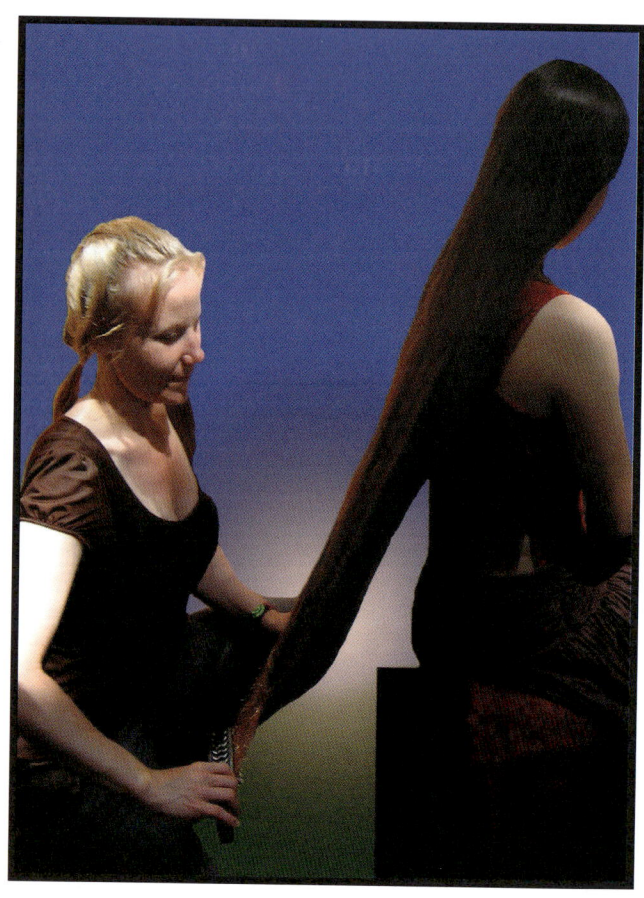
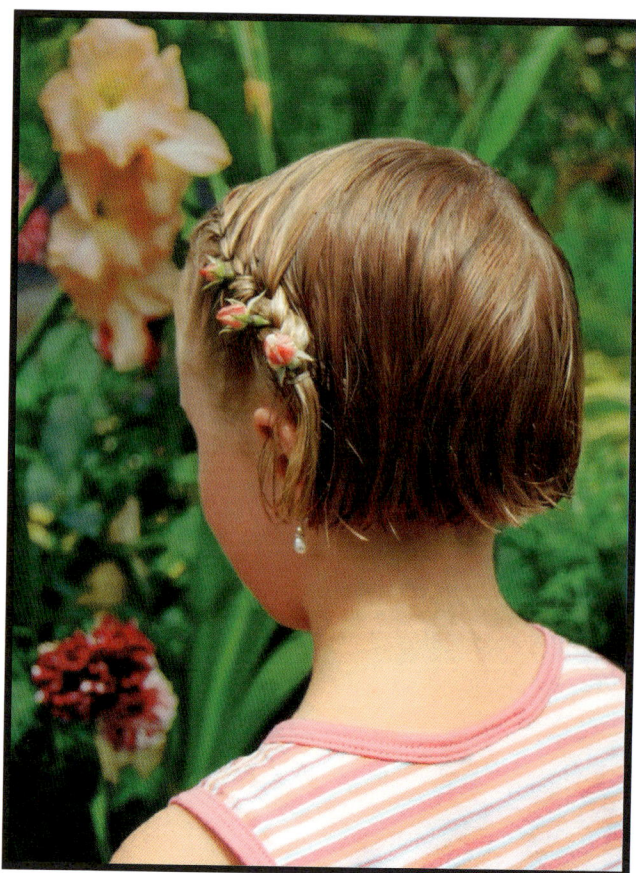

Author's Note

Our hair is an expression of ourselves. Some people color their hair. Others get mohawks.

This book is for braiders. I have created an innovative layout to inspire both beginner and advanced braiders. This book is truly a different approach to hairbraiding. It is my hope that you find what you need in here to do simple everyday hairsyles.

Special occasions will pop up in your life. The progression from basic to advanced techniques here is to provide you with the complicated hairstyles you need to add an air of sophistication to your prom dress or wedding gown.

Professionals who often lack resources for new and exciting ideas may feel stuck in a rut. I have provided a tool for download called a Braider Creator that will offer endless hair design possiblilities from one simple format.

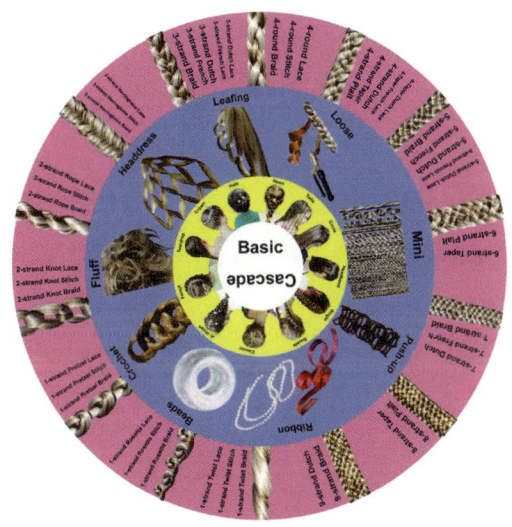

The Braider Creator is available for download on my website www.findingbraids.com. It is a device that points out hairstyles but it does not show the finished results. You must envision the final results. Each of you will come up with different versions of the same style.

The App created for this book is a place to see the finished hairstyles that the Braider Creator points out. If you are having a difficult time envisioning your own finished styles, dive into the app for ideas. This is also the best place to up load images of your creations. When you finish a style, take a well lit photograph and upload your image into the Finding Braids data base to help those of us who just want to see the finished results.

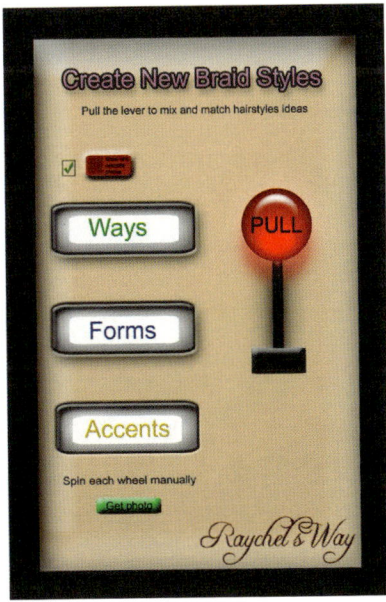

Braider Creator

"I don't believe her when she says I can use the Braider Creator to make 10,000 different hairstyles. That's impossible!"

So, let's take a look at that claim. It will require some interaction from you and a few of my friends. Grab your Braider Creator. Spin the layers until the arrow has Basic, Crown, Mini and Three-strand underneath it.

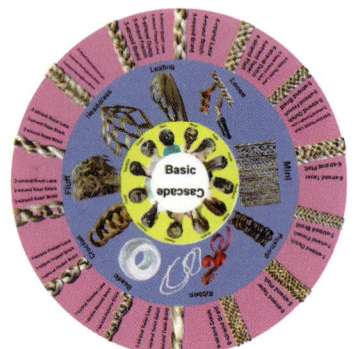
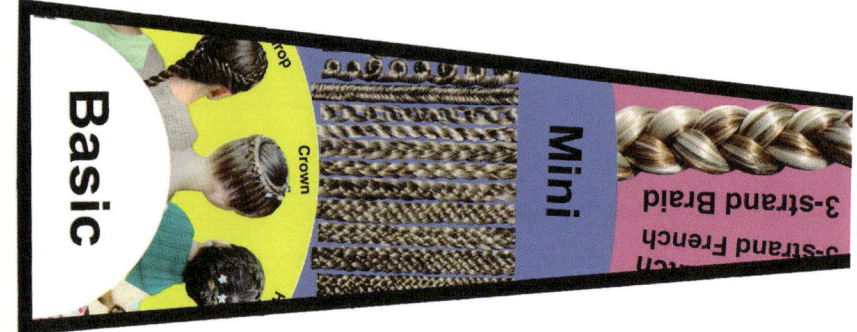

As a group we have to decide on one of the mini's. So, after much debate I chose the mini two-strand knot. You will be braiding with along with us. We are all going to do exactly what the Braider Creator is telling us to do. Let's make a basic crown using the three-strand technique and accent it with mini two-strand knot braids.

As you can see from the photos of our finished hairstyles below, it is your own imagination that truly decides what the Braider Creator is telling you to do. The Braider Creator only points out one style at a time. That one style looks so different in each person's imagination. So what does the Braider Creator really do? It points out 9,744 hairstyling ideas that lead to 10,000 plus hairstyles.

Please photograph your hairstyles and load them into the Finding Braids app.

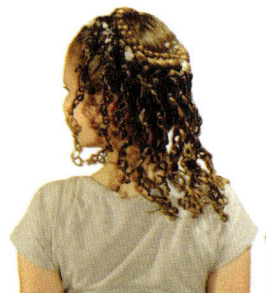
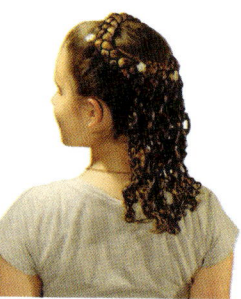
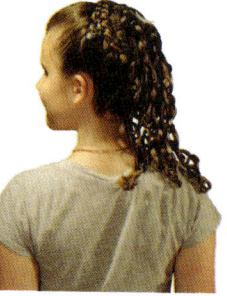
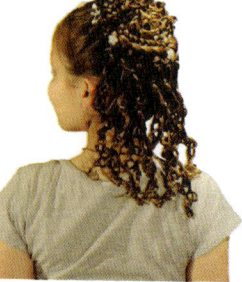
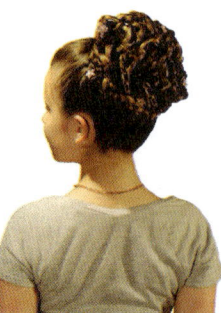

What Jen saw. What Kim saw. What Zoe saw. What Meg saw. What Eva saw.

Chapter One - Ways (Number of Strands)

One-strand Twist . . . . 28 - 41

One-strand Rosette . . . . 42 - 57

One-strand Pretzel . . . . 58 - 73

Two-strand Knot . . . . 74 - 89

Two-strand Rope . . . . 90 -105

Two-strand Herringbone . . . . 106 - 119

Three-strand . . . . 120 - 153

Four-strand Round . . . . 154 - 174

Four-strand Taper . . . . 176 - 211

Five-strand . . . . 212 - 243

Six-strand . . . . 244 - 259

Seven-strand . . . . 262 - 281

Eight-strand . . . . 282 - 297

Nine-strand . . . . 298 - 311

Chapter Two - Forms (Shapes)

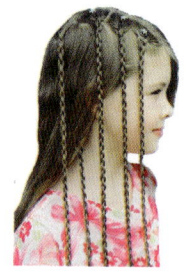 Tails . . . . 324 - 335

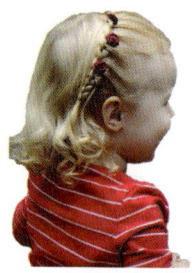 Headband . . . 336 - 347

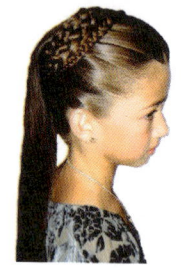 Circle . . . . . . 348 - 359

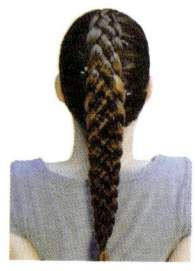 Single . . . . 360 - 371

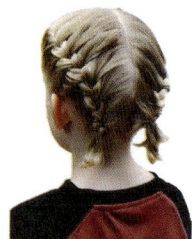 Double . . . . . . 372 - 383

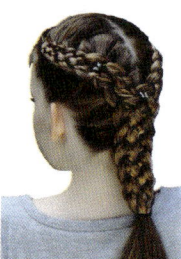 Junction . . . . 384 - 395

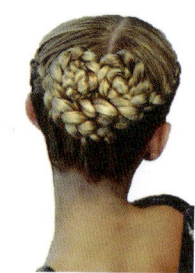 Classic . . . . . . 396 - 407

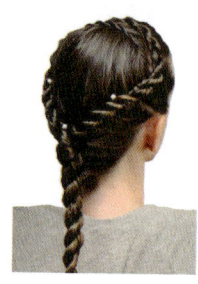 Teardrop . . . . 408 - 419

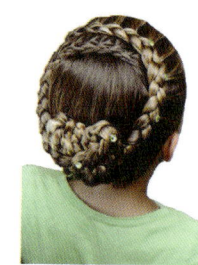 Fringe . . . . 420 - 431

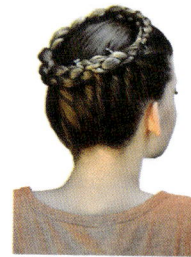 Crown . . . . . . 432 - 443

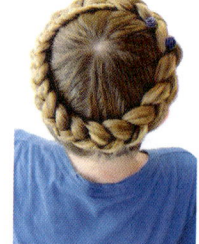 Halo . . . . 444 - 457

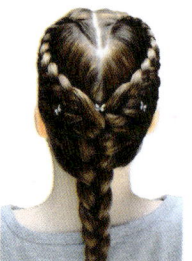 Heart . . . . 458 - 471

Chapter Three - Accents (Decorative Hair)

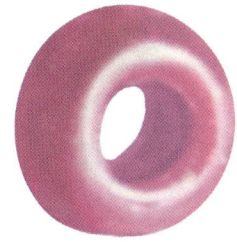 Beads . . . . . 480 - 481

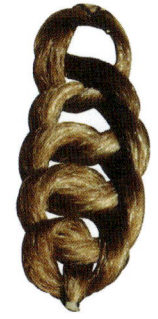 Crochet . . . 482 - 483

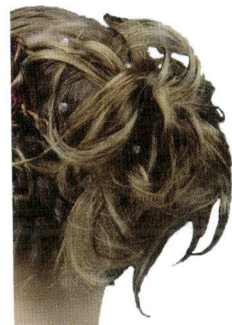 Fluff . . . . . . 484 - 485

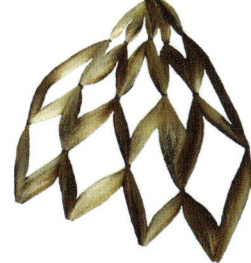 Headdress 486 - 487

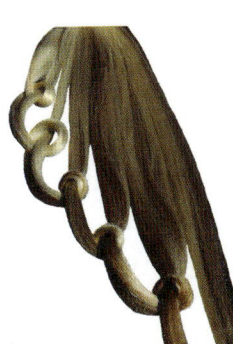 Leafing . . . . 488 - 489

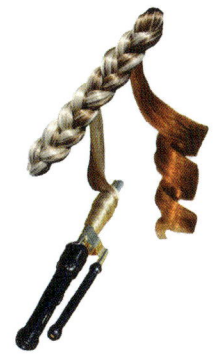 Loose . . . . 490 - 491

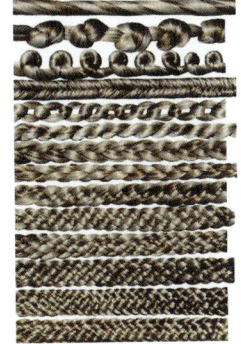 Mini . . . . . 492 - 493

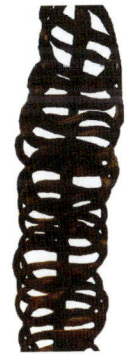 Push-up 494 - 495

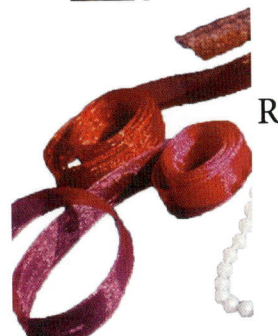 Ribbon . . . 496 - 497

The word <u>braid</u> typically conjures up an image of a cornrow or a french braid. What else comes to mind when you think of the word braid? The rope and herringbone? Yes, those are also two **ways** to braid.

Let's reshape how you think about braiding.

In this book, picking a **way** to braid involves choosing the number of strands you wish to work with and then deciding if you will braid with or without gathers. It is the first key to unlocking the mystery of braiding. Instead of thinking about braids in terms of three-strand braids with a few other options, I offer you the concept of *any number of strands* as a way to braid.

Pick a number, any number! Yes, when I say <u>any</u> I mean <u>any</u> number. Once you have chosen your number there are three options for braiding that number of strands.

1. **Braid** = no gathers. *Let's Braid it!*

   The braid icons indicate this. Do not add gathers into a braid. A braid is a free floating braid.

2. **Stitch** = gathers on both sides. *Let's Stitch it!*

   The stitch icons have arrows showing both sides being gathered into. So, gather into both sides.

3. **Lace** = gathers on one side. *Let's Lace it!*

   The lace icons show one side being gathered into. So, only gather into one side.

The *number of strands* you are braiding plus one of the options from above defines the WAY you are braiding.

Introduction to the Braid Icons

Let's Braid it!

Braid = no gathers.

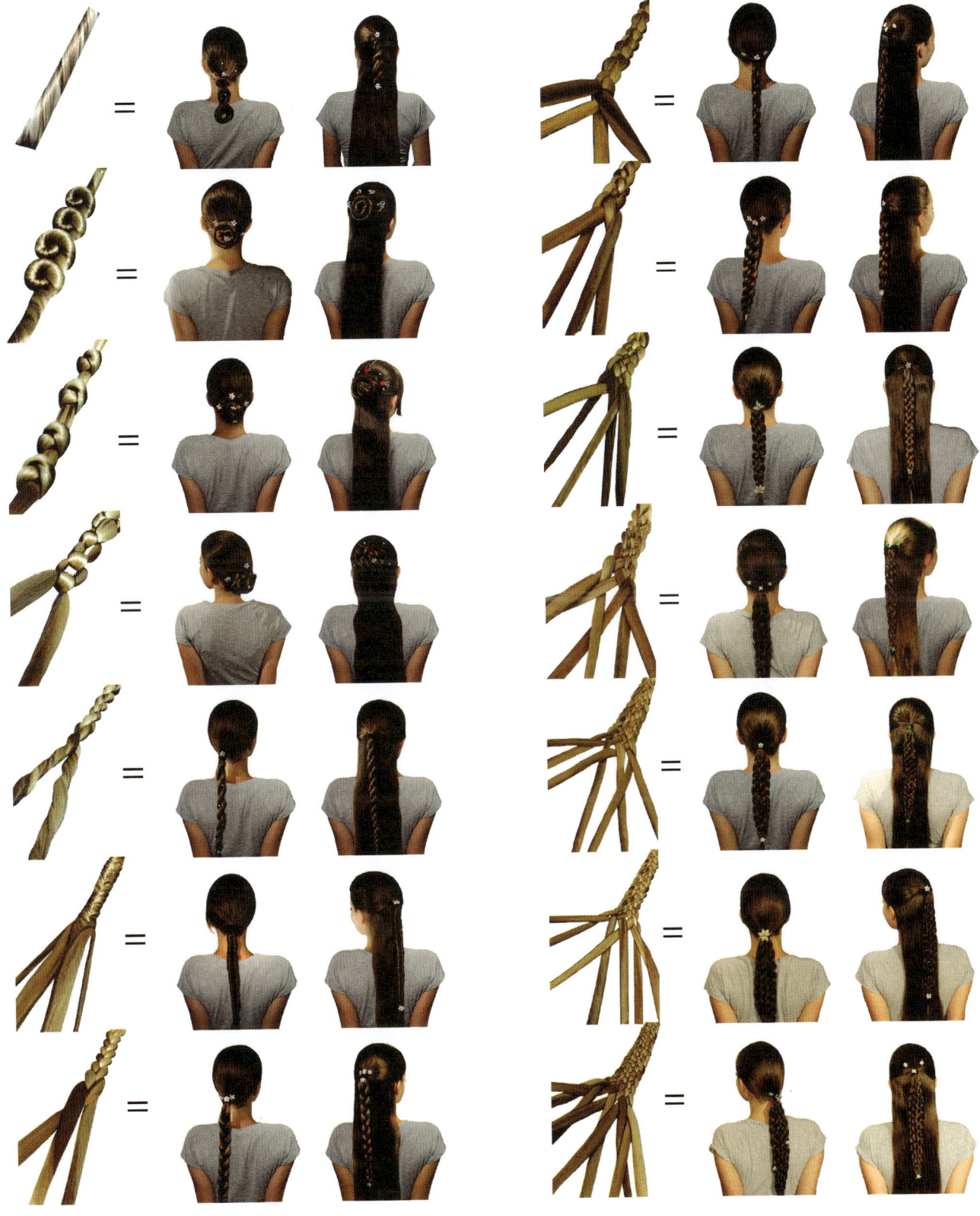

Introduction to the Stitch Icons

Let's Stitch it!

Stitch = gathers on both sides.

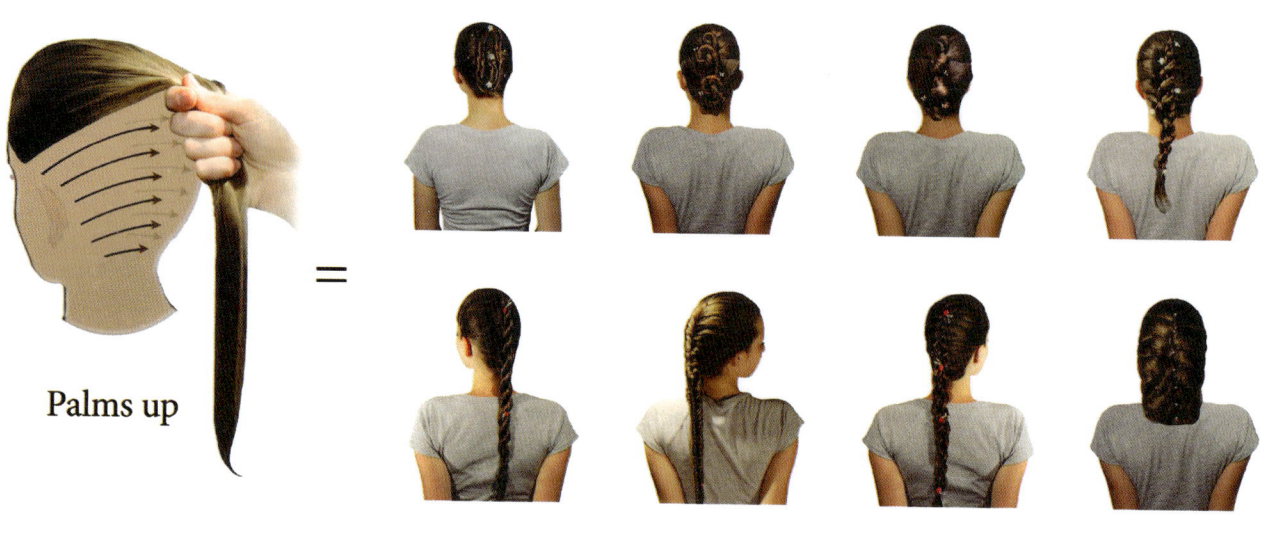

Palms up

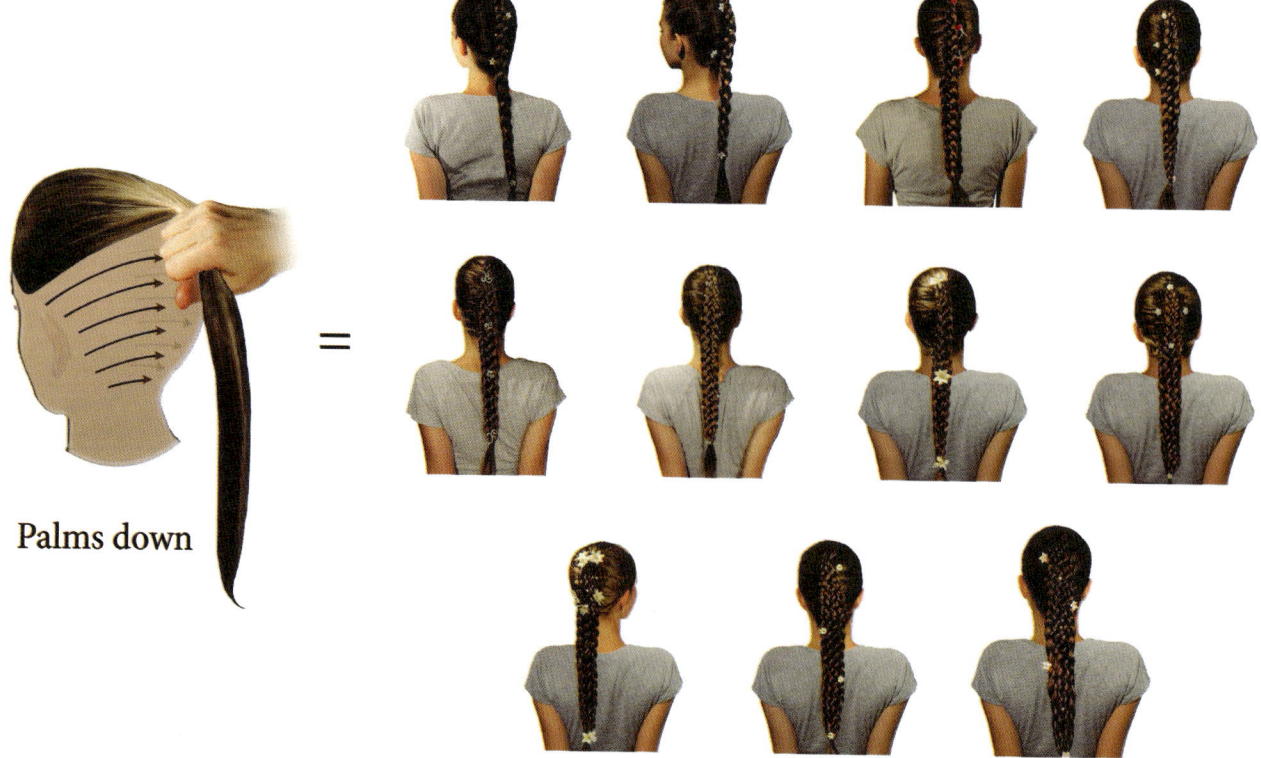

Palms down

Introduction to the Lace Icon

Let's Lace it!

Lace = gathers on one side.

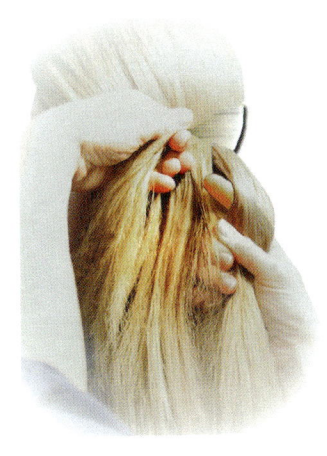

=

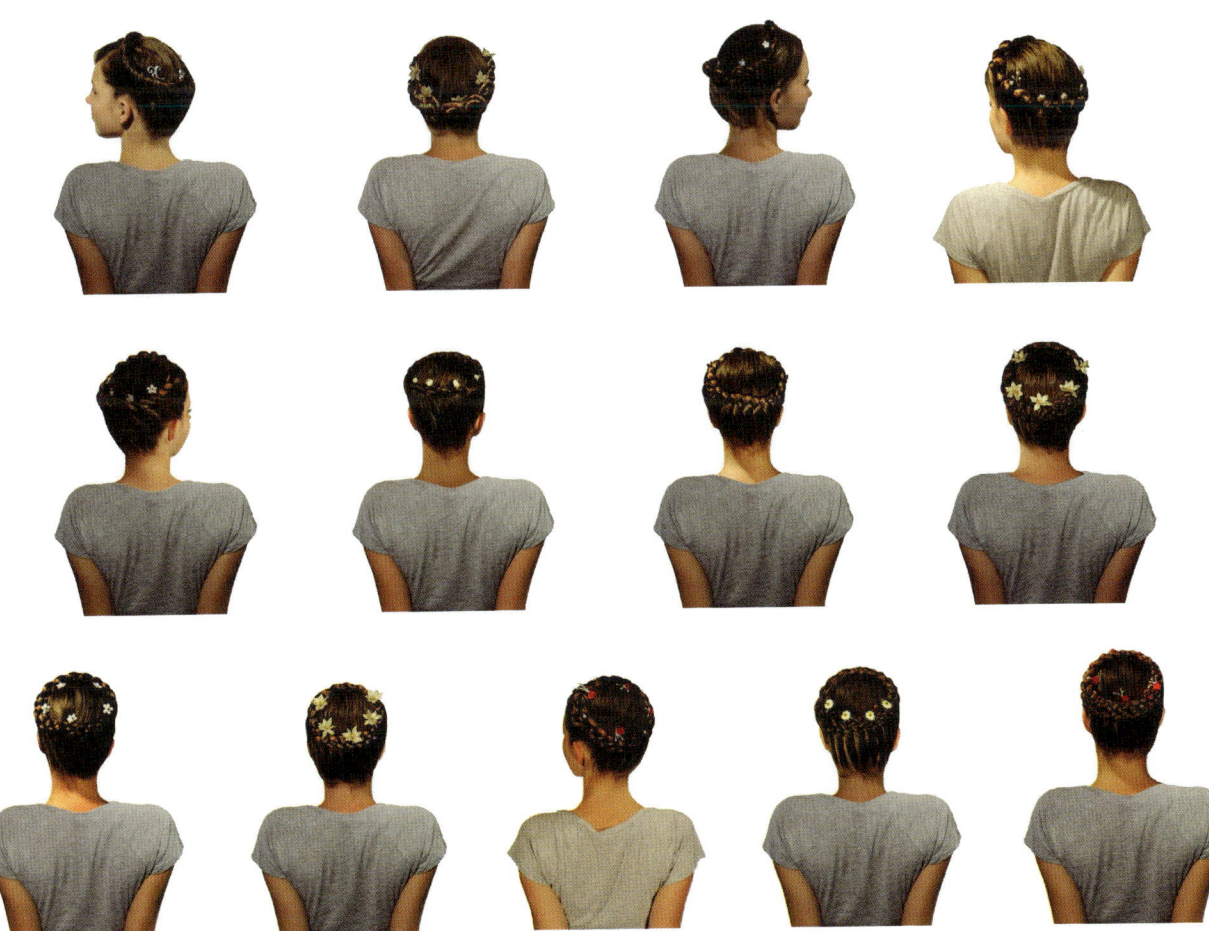

Introduction to Forms

The theory behind the options below stems from two types of people; those that like their hair all up and those who prefer the back half of their hair left down. (The forms shown in this book are just to simplify the teaching experience. This is an idea and concept to be put to use with many other forms not shown in this book.)

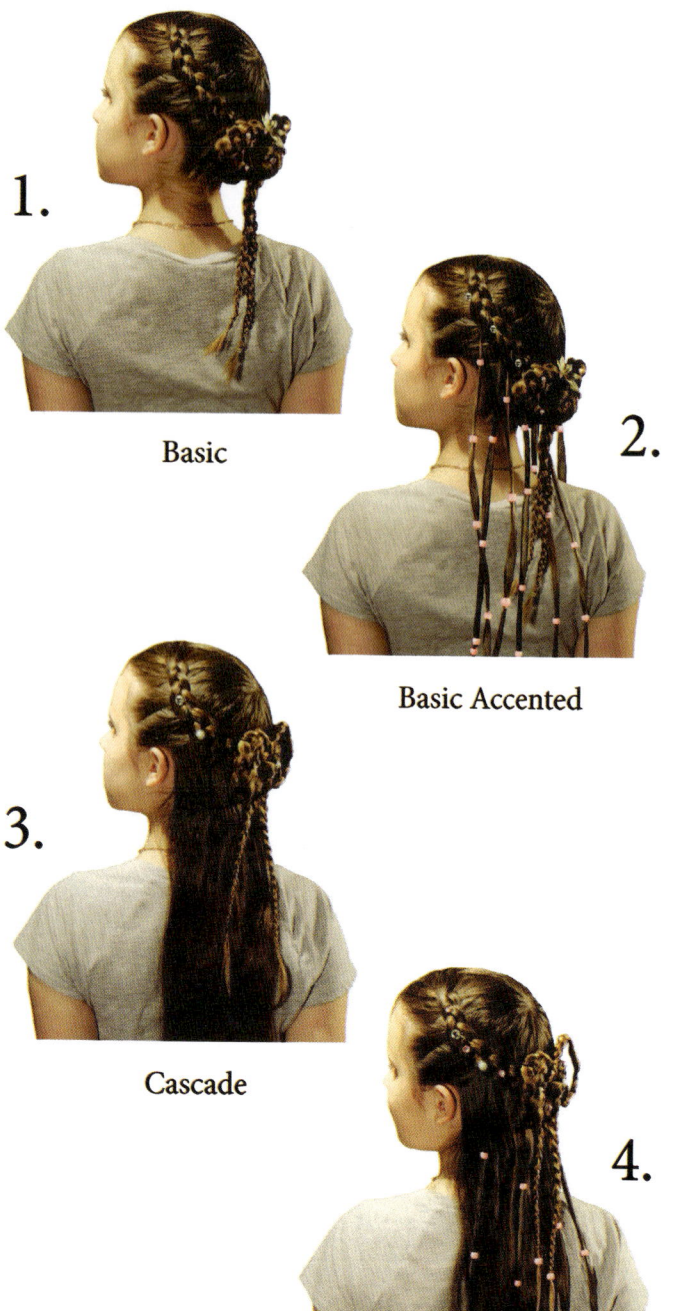

1. Basic

2. Basic Accented

The hair is up off the neck. It is all bound into the shape. The neck is visible and the shoulders are free of hair unless accents are added that hang down. These are more formal.

3. Cascade

4. Accented Cascade

The neck and shoulders are covered by hair left down in the back. This helps with warmth or showcasing the beauty of ones hair length. It softens the look of a hairstyle and is less formal.

The *shape you braid* plus one of the options from above defines the FORM you are braiding.

Introduction to the Form Icons

Each of the shapes below becomes a form when paired with an option on the previous page.

Watch for the icons in Chapter Two: Forms. There are two icons depicting each form. The first icon shows gather patterns and is meant to help teach the formation of the shape. The second marks the pages in the top corners.

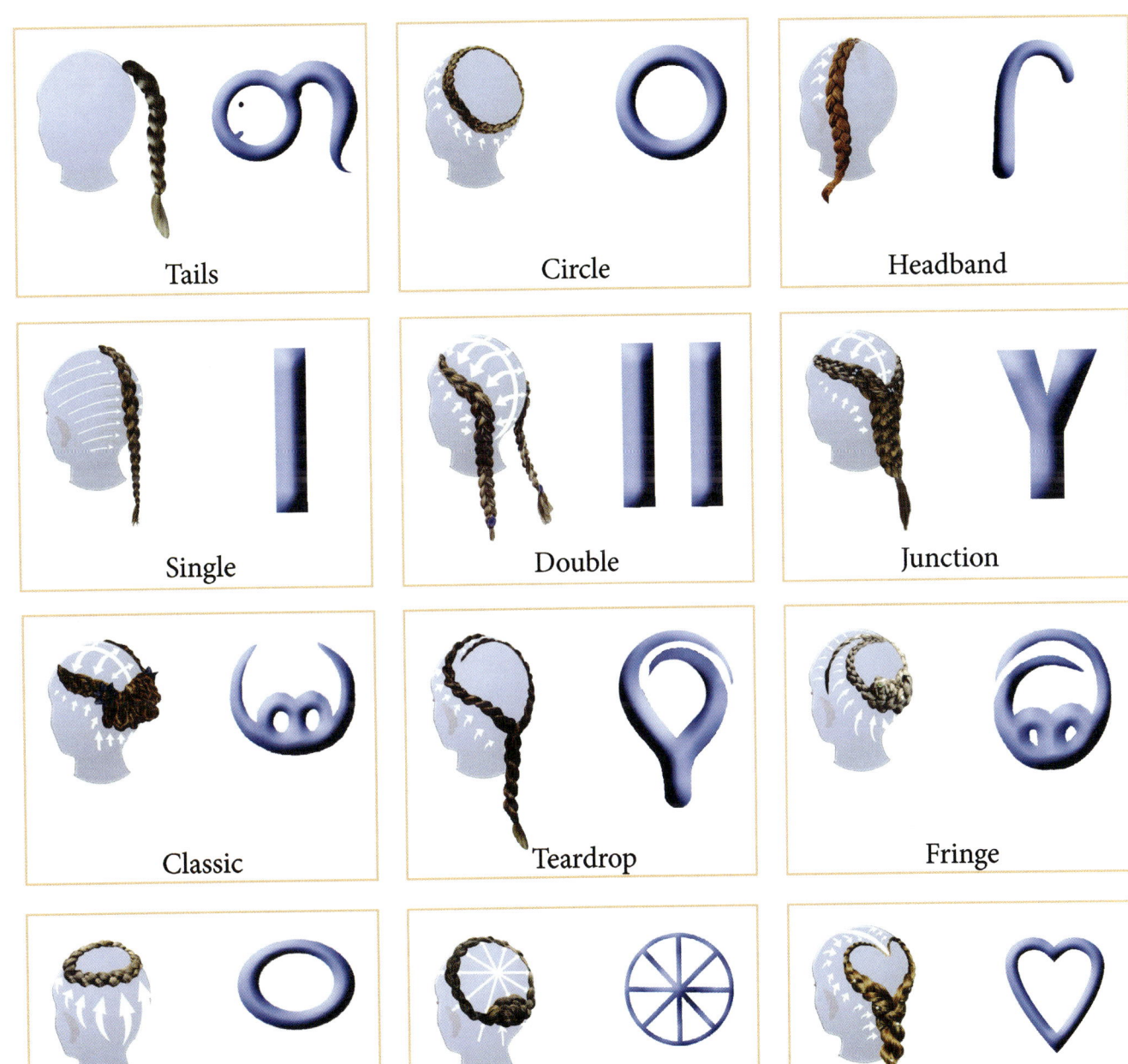

Combining Ways, Forms and Accents

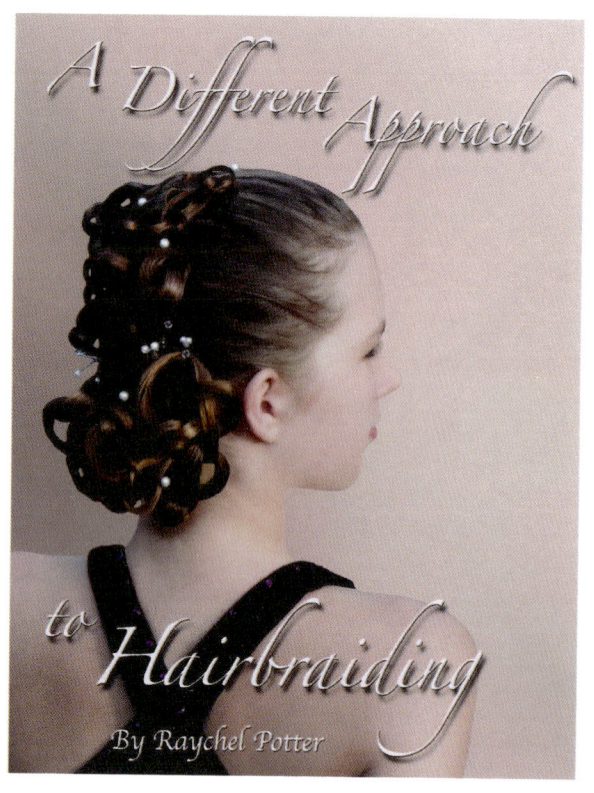

This book gives you the pieces to solve the puzzle to fabulous hairstyles.

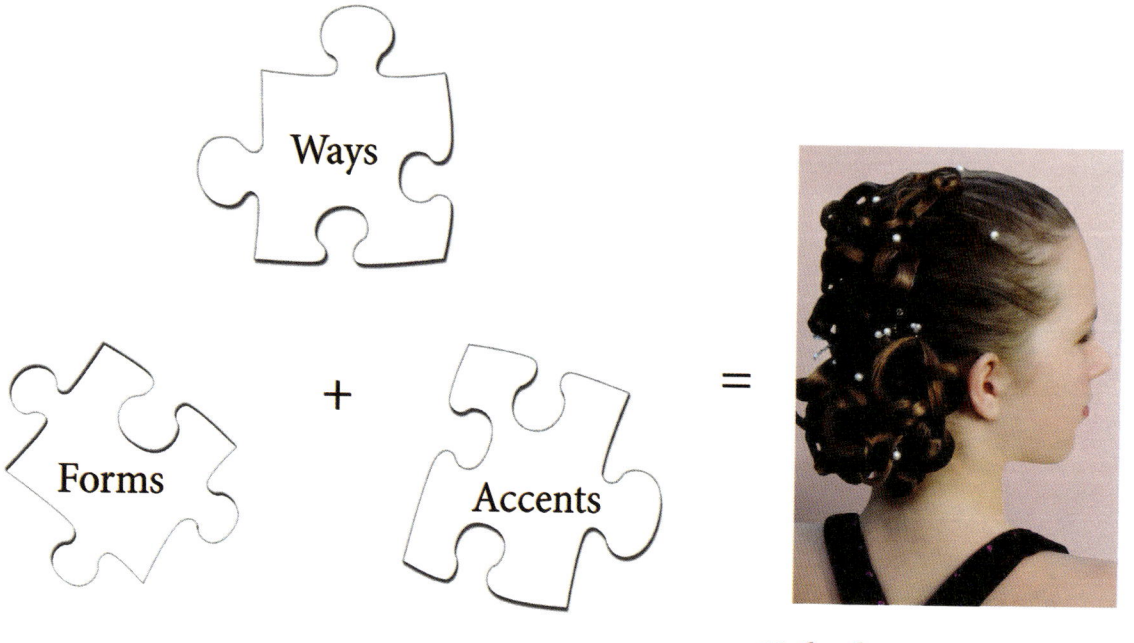

Fabulous Hairstyles

Braider Creator, Book and App

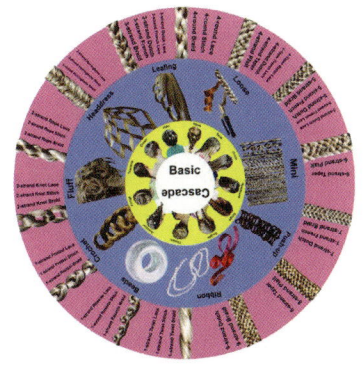

1. Line up the arrow on the Braider Creator.

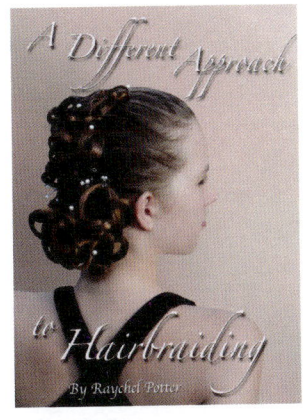

2. Use this book and your imagination to learn how to create hundreds of examples of that style.

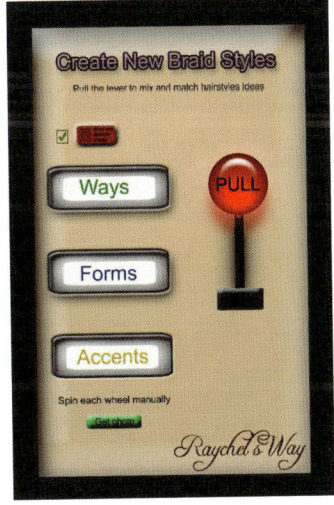

3. Take a well lit photo of each example you create and load it into the Finding Braids app database. Become a contributor to a worldwide database of braids.

Repeat! This is the essense of Raychel's Way.

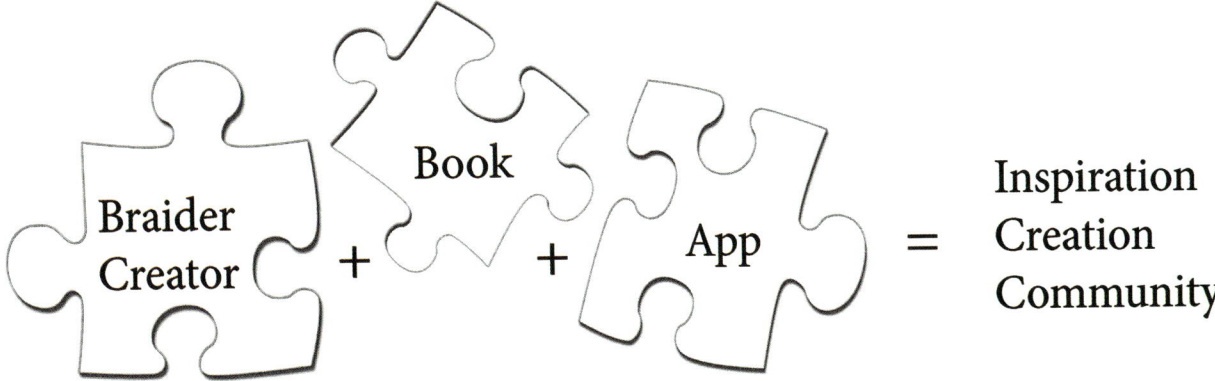

Products

Hair products can help you achieve the look you want, while preventing wisps.

This is a list of products starting with the simplest one available.
The type of hair you style will determine the product you will want to use.

Water: Use a spray bottle of water to mist the section of hair you are working with. This is the most basic way to control wisps while braiding. As you become more skilled, please consider the other alternatives to give your style a more sophisticated look.

Aloe Vera: Aloe Vera gives a "grip with slip" without making your grip slippery. Aloe Vera provides a protective coating for the hair and moisturizes both the hair and your hands. It is perfect for fine hair.

Oils: There are dozens of massage oil blends at your local health food store that work well on hair. Oils control wisps for the day while adding sheen. I caution you to use oil sparingly; only a few drops spread over your palms and fingers, run your hands through the hair, then braid. Oils are a natural product that works best on thick course hair.

Gel: Gel is similar to Aloe Vera in texture and feel. It is not natural but the hold is much better. Apply a pea-sized amount of gel to your palms and fingers. Run your hand over the section of hair being braided and comb the product through that section. Short, thick and/or course hair can be challenging. Use gel, palmade and hairspray during the braiding process with this type of hair.

Hairspray: Hairspray works best if it can coat the hair like a spider's web. The best way to achieve this is by spraying from a distance. Hold the hairspray 10"–15" away from the hair. Avoid holding the bottle too close to the hair while spraying. Soaking the hair makes it look congealed.

Many years ago, hairstyles were protected with toilet paper while sleeping. Fortunately, today you do not have to wrap your head in toilet paper. The most effective way to protect a hairstyle today, is to spray it with hairspray then wrap your head in a satin wrap while sleeping on a satin pillowcase. Satin on satin creates a non-friction surface preventing wisps.

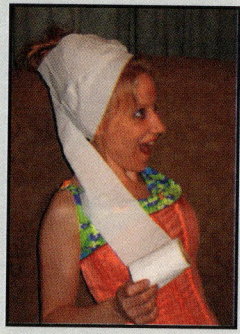

No matter what you achieve, somebody helps you. Behind the creation that we call our own, are the thoughts and efforts of many. – Althea Gibson

Tools

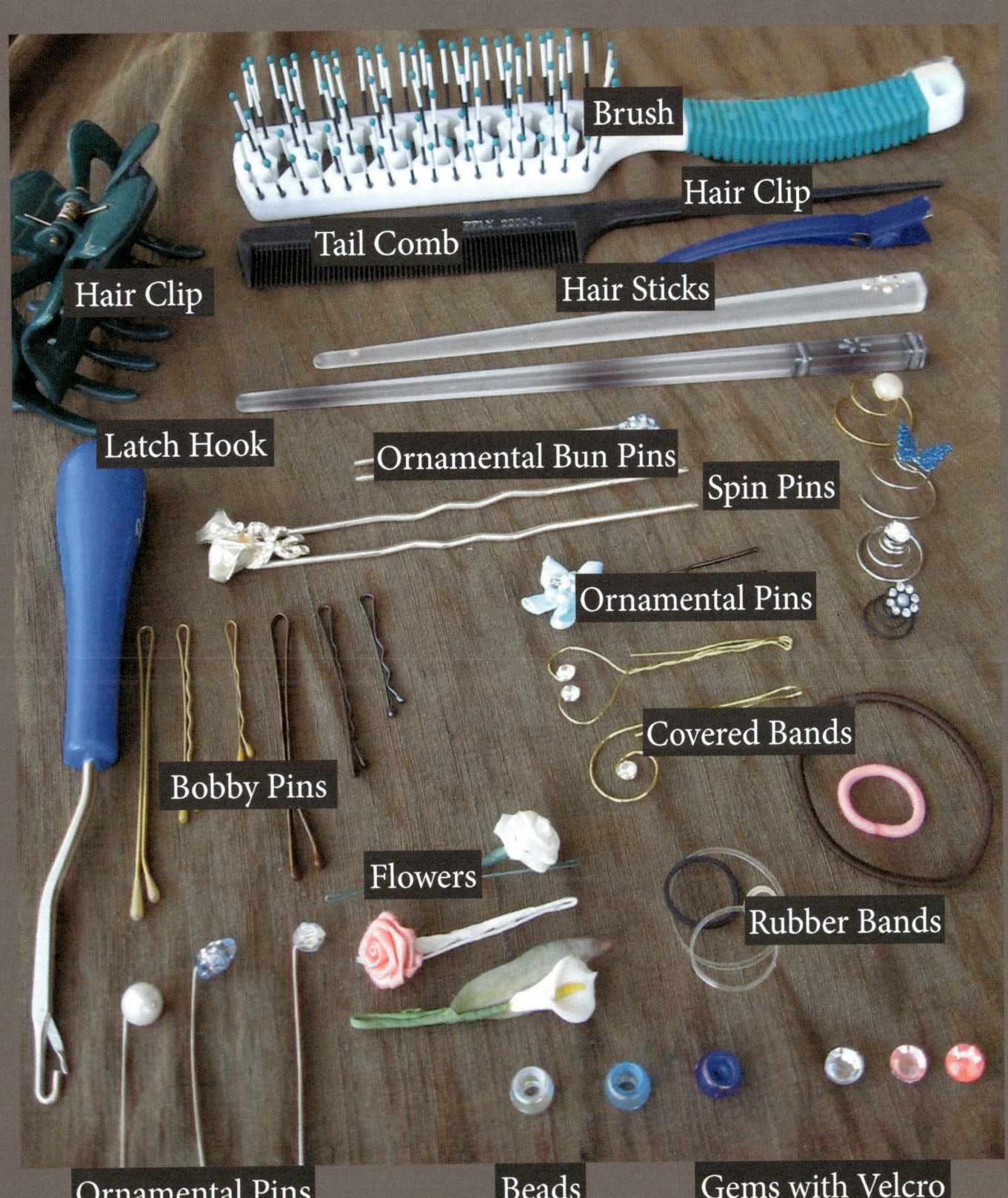

Learning

If you are not learning as quickly as you had hoped, try using a different part of your brain. I recommend borrowing a child for a few hours and teaching the child. As you teach, you will be surprised how differently you see the project.

The human brain fascinates me. While writing this book I spent time in the library reading about the human brain and the learning process. I also spent days googling the learning process. This is what I came across.

When we are young, our heads are filled with axons, neurons, and synaptic connections. We loose these, as we age. The only way to counter-act this loss is to fill our heads with new knowledge. The more we use a specific knowledge, the stronger the synaptic connections become. When a specific knowledge is not used, those pathways become weak and disintegrate.

Learning new stuff = hard. It has been proven that the more you emotionally care about something, the easier it is to learn.

The brain is made up of three parts. You cannot learn with only one part of your brain. They are all interconnected. One part is for basic sensory motor functions. Another is for emotions, memory, and biorhythms. The last is for reasoning, language, and the higher intelligence.

By approaching a subject from different angles you get different perspectives on it, thus making it easier to learn. So, as you are learning, be sure to see it, feel it, and hear it. And when you use hair products while you learn to braid you can also smell it and taste it:)

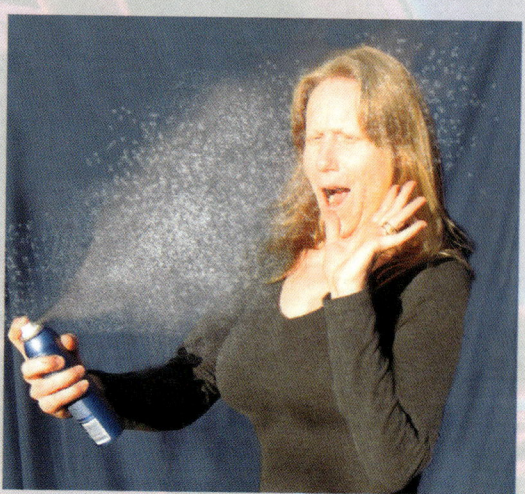

Finally, I would like to push you to seek out how-to videos. There are so many for sale and even more free ones online. Try the popular Youtube website and find hundreds of them.

Those who attain any excellence, commonly spend their life in pursuit of it, for excellence is not often gained on easier terms.
– Samuel Johnson

Tips

- This section will make more sense later. Please refer back here as you gain more experience.

- The braid goes where you go. This is the first thing I learned about braiding. Pretend the braid is attached to your belly button and stand where you want the braid to come. Be willing to tilt the head, gaining access to the part you need. Often this requires your subject be seated on a short stool. If you have trouble finding a subject that will sit still, a doll head from a beauty supply store works great.

- Extra long hair tangles less when you gather, separate and detangle with the tail of a tail comb. When I braid, I look like Captain Hook with a comb.

- Use a comb to distribute hair product evenly through the hair.

- Keep your knuckles on the head; it is the easiest way to braid tightly. If your subject tells you that you are hurting them, please relax. Keep a grip on their hair but relax your shoulders, then relax your hands, take a deep breath, loosening your death grip on their head. Ask if it still hurts. If it still does, repeat relaxation technique. Hair does not have to be pulled out, to be braided. Keeping your knuckles close to, or on the person's head should create a tight braid without pain.

- Extensions can be used in any hairstyle. The color does not need to tbe identical to their own hair. Most people have natural highlights. Extentions made with human hair look the most natural - if you are going for a natural look. Synthetic extensions are a lot of fun to work with and can spice up hairsyles with a more dramatic efffect.

- I would like to give my opinion on clean hair versus dirty hair. Practice makes perfet. Will you practice on diry or clean hair? I personally learned on clean hair. Looking back on my years of braiding , I am glad that I took the extra time.

- The morning before a braiding session, ask the subject to have their hair down and loose. Clips and rubber bands leave demarcations that have to be worked with.

- If your subject has a strong cowlick, work with it. Pushing it in the opposite dirction will only make it painful for them the next day.

- There is more than one way to part hair; try a zigzag, a diagonal, a square or curvy part.

- Cover up mistakes with decorations like push-in flowers or sparkle pins.

- If the person you are braiding is going to change into an evening gown or wedding dress, ask them to wear a button-up-the-front shirt.

No mans knowledge can go beyond his experience. – John Locke

List of Terms

Accent
Accents are created using hair left out of a braid. Accents add creativity to a hairstyle. Please do not limit yourself to the accents in this book.

Braid
A braid is the of folding or weaving of hair, straw or ribbon into a pattern. A braid with more than three strands is also known as a plait.

Cascade
The hair left out of a braid to showcase the length of your hair or to keep your neck warm.

Durable
A braid that will stay in over night is considered durable.

Dutch
Dutch braids gather hair into both sides and are not flush, they pop up.

Form
The shape a braid takes as it traverses your head.

Fragile
A braid that may not last overnight is considered fragile.

French
French braids gather hair into both sides. They lie flush, gathers fold in towards the head.

Gather
Extra hair added into a braid as you braid.

Inexpensive products
These are cheap products that can be purchased practically anywhere. They work if you are in a bind and need something at night when the salons are closed; otherwise I recommend salon quality products.

Hair product
Hair product is added to hair to maintain a tidy hairstyle, create shine and add hold to the hairstyle. (Gel, hairspray, palmade, paste, wax.)

Lace
Lace braids gather hair into only one side of a braid.

Long hair
Long hair is below the fastener of the bra. (If your a guy, you still know where that is.)

Medium length hair
Medium hair is between the shoulders and the fastener of the bra.

List of Terms

Merging
Connecting two separate braids into a single braid. The junction, teardrop, and heart all blend two braids into a single braid.

Pass
A pass, folds a single strand into place or completes a weave of several strands from one side. Several passes create a braid or plait.

Plait
A plait is a manner of folding or weaving multiple strands (hair, straw, ribbon) into a flat pattern. A braid with more than three strands is also known as a plait.

Practice
Repeat a lesson until improvement is seen. This requires the lesson to be repeated several times over several days until improvement is seen.

Salon quality products
More expensive, higher quality products **tend** to be gentler on your hands and hair.

Satin pillow case
Wrap your head in a satin wrap, and sleep on a satin pillowcase, creating a non-friction surface (preventing wisps).

Short hair
Short hair brushes the shoulders or layers above the shoulders.

Stitch
A stitch braid gathers hair into both sides. A stitch braid includes feather loose, dutch french, and taper braids.

Stretching
Something people rarely do even though it is essential to releave muscle tension. Stretch your hands, arms and shoulders after engaging in a new activity like braiding.

Tail braid
Tail braids do not gather hair; instead the braid pops out from the head or hangs loose.

Tapered
Taper braids gather hair into both sides. They are french on one side dutch on the other. Taper braids are created with four, six, and eight-strands.

Way
How many number of strands will you use when you braid?

Knowledge without wisdom is a load of books on an ass's back.
– Japanese Saying

Chapter One

If you are not an accomplished braider you will find your hands cramping as you practice the different ways to braid. Hand stretches help battle fatigue and cramping. Squeezing and playing with a small squishy ball strengthens hands and releases muscle tension. Do not be surprised if you develop soreness in your forearms and shoulders.

Mentally, try to stay relaxed while you are braiding, this will help lessen these pains. A simple and effective way to stretch your shoulders is to lock your fingers behind your head and stretch.

Learning each option, of each way, shown; will give you a good overveiw of the nature of braiding and you will be able to execute those options with ways of braiding not shown. This book breaks down braiding in an organized manner applicable elsewhere. There are other options for each way of braiding that I choose not to show here. Seek them out and add them to your repetuior.

The four-strand plait section could easily be doubled due to the amount of information available on that particular way of braiding, but I selected the most pertinent for this book. There are four weaving patterns that I know of for executing the four-strand round dutch stitch. I chose one for this book, while also choosing to ignore the french stitch.

This book contains a quarter of the amount of braiding information that I possess. That leaves you with plenty more to learn after you devour this book.

Chapter One ~ Ways

When you choose a way, you are choosing two different components:

1. How many numbers will you be braiding with?

2. How will you gather into that number?

In other words, the way you braid is a two part process involving a number of strands and a gathering option.

There are three options for gathering a one-strand braid, a nine-strand braid and every number in between.

1. Braid = no gathers

2. Stitch = gathers on both sides

3. Lace = gathers on one side

Is it that easy? - No.

Lace braids start out small on one side and incrementally grow larger as you braid across to the other side. This effect is magnified when working with thick hair. I use two tricks to decrease this effect while I braid. One is to start out with a large section of hair and decrease the size of each gather as you braid. Two is to cascade the hair as you go so that only small portions are being gathered into the braid. Chapter two teaches cascading.

Don't worry, it gets more complicated. Creating a braid with even-numbered stands is more difficult than odd-numbered because each hand carries out a different set of instructions. In even numbered braids the weaving instructions for each hand is different. However, in odd numbered braids the weaving pattern for each hand is the same.

This is a lot of information. Just ignore it! Find the number you wanted to learn and dive in.

Nature...has ordained that difficulty should precede every work of excellence.
-Quintillian

Introducing the fourteen ways we will be braiding with

Braid = no gathers.

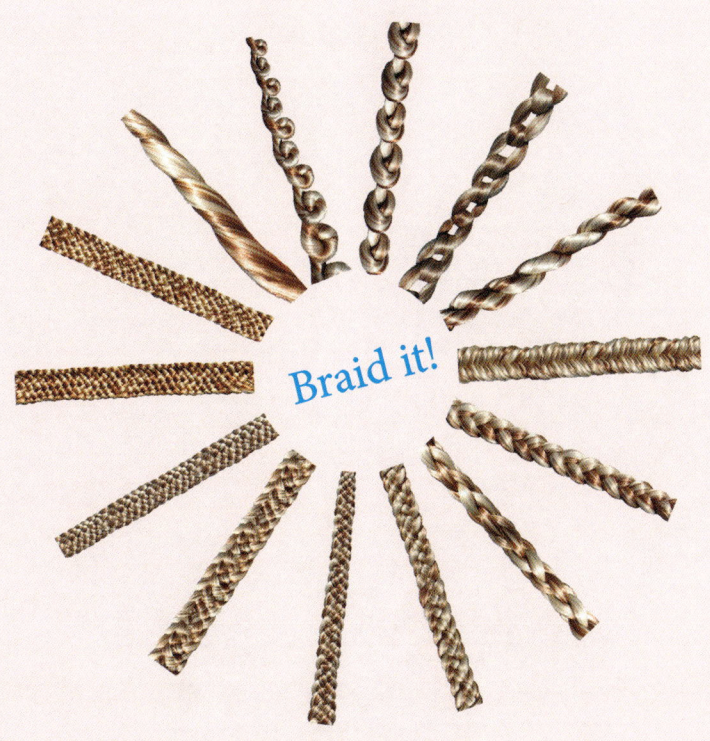

Braid it!

Stitch = gathers on both sides.

Lace = gathers on one side.

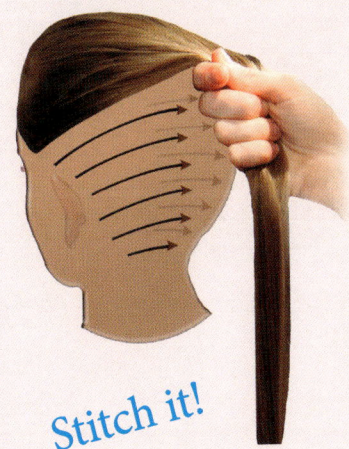

Stitch it!

Pick a number to braid and these icons will let you know which option we are on. Find them and maneuveur through the book with ease.

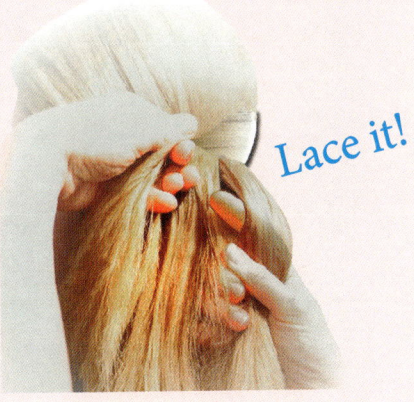

Lace it!

Pick a number of strands...then
braid it, stitch it, lace it!

One-Strand Twist

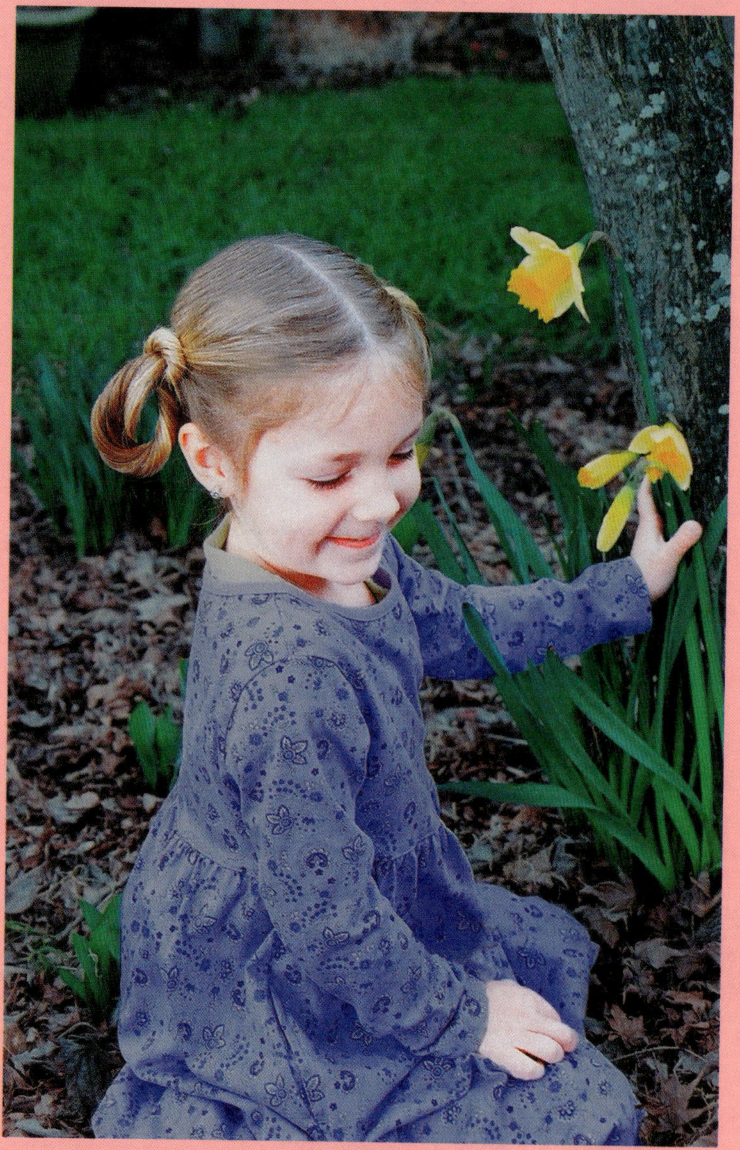

This is a beautiful and delicate braid that requires gel and hairspray to keep it in place. A good braid for one day if you are gentle with it during the day.

One-Strand Twist

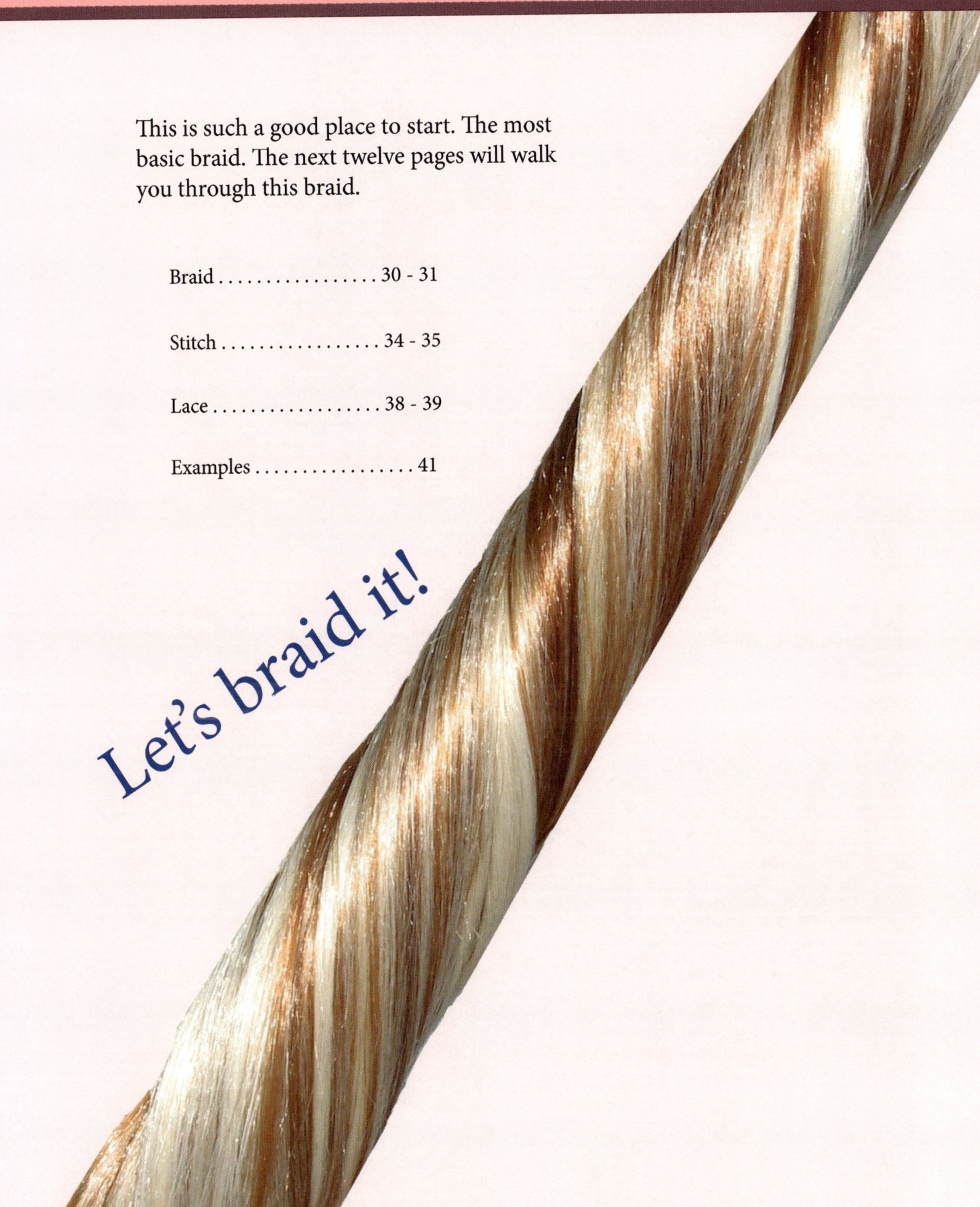

This is such a good place to start. The most basic braid. The next twelve pages will walk you through this braid.

Braid . . . . 30 - 31

Stitch . . . . 34 - 35

Lace . . . . 38 - 39

Examples 41

Let's braid it!

1 One-Strand Twist Braid

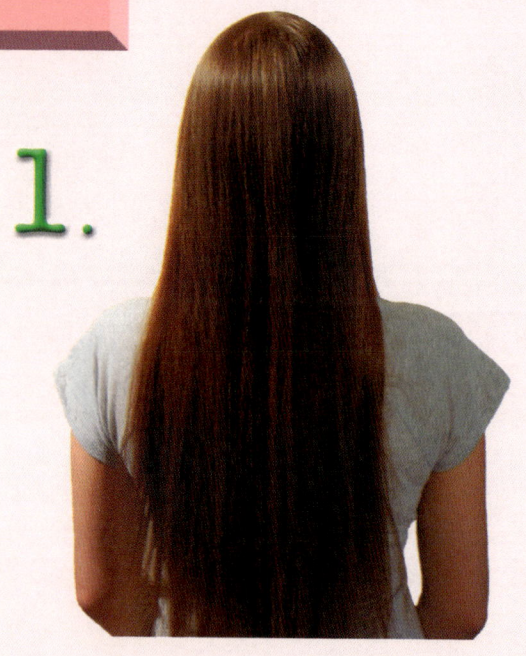

1. Begin with clean, brushed hair.

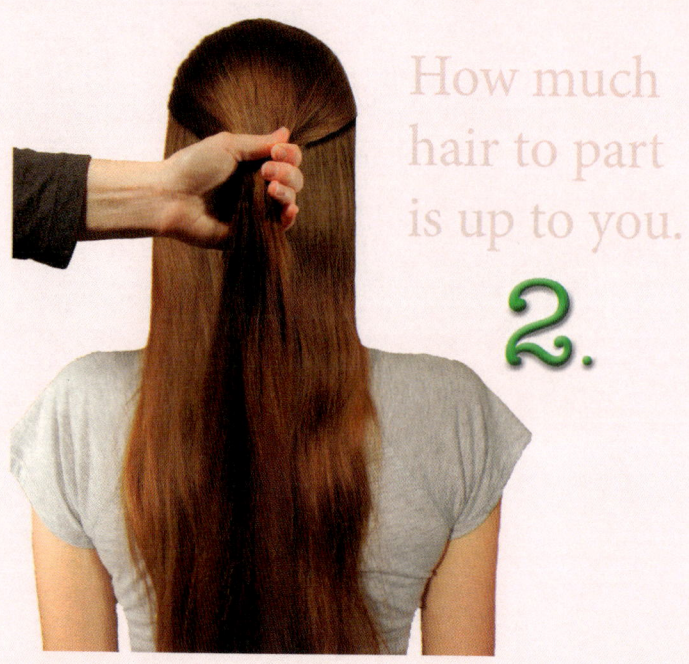

2. Take a section of hair.

How much hair to part is up to you.

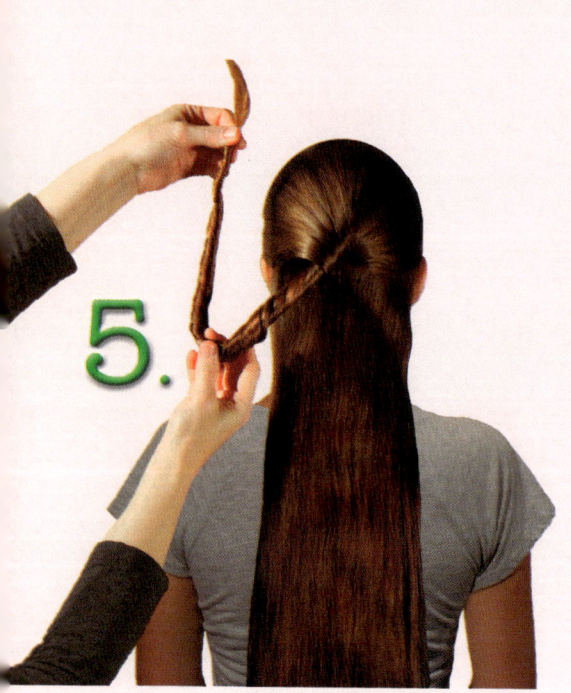

5. Let the strand coil as desired and twist more, if needed to keep it coiled.

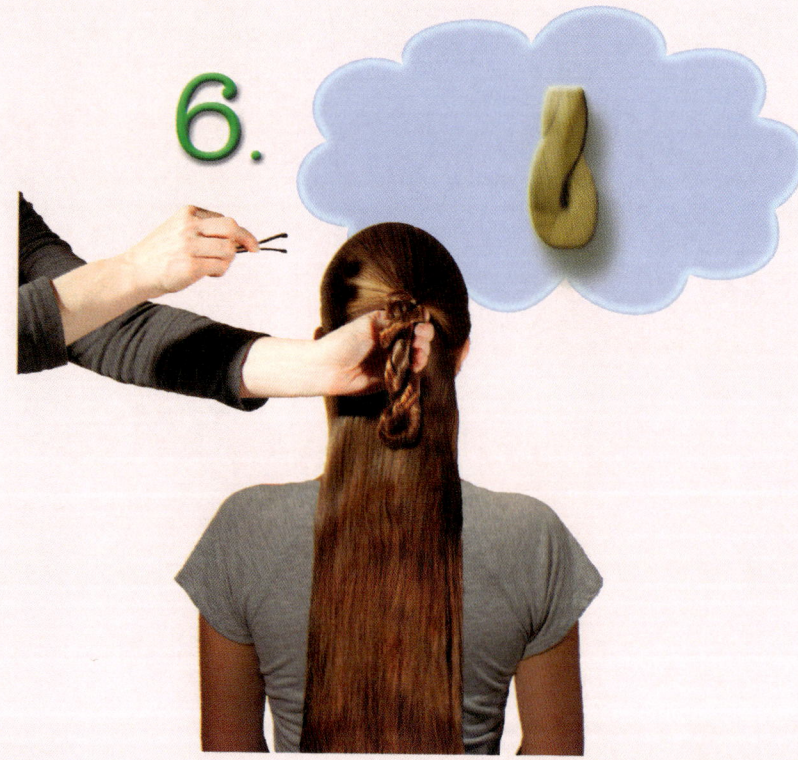

6. Fix the end of the braid with bobby pins to hold the braid in place.

30   www.findingbraids.com

One-Strand Twist Braid

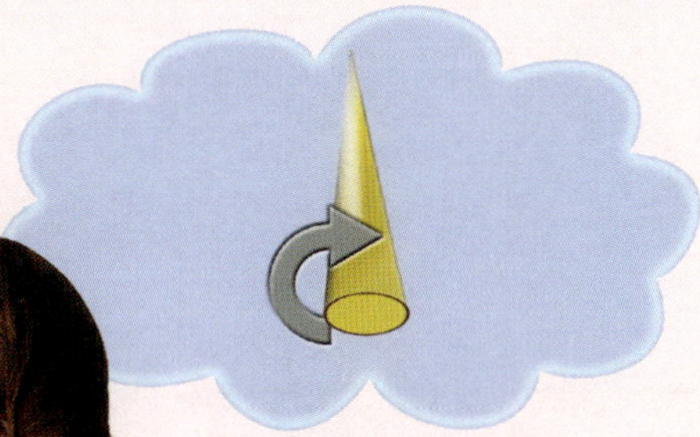

3. 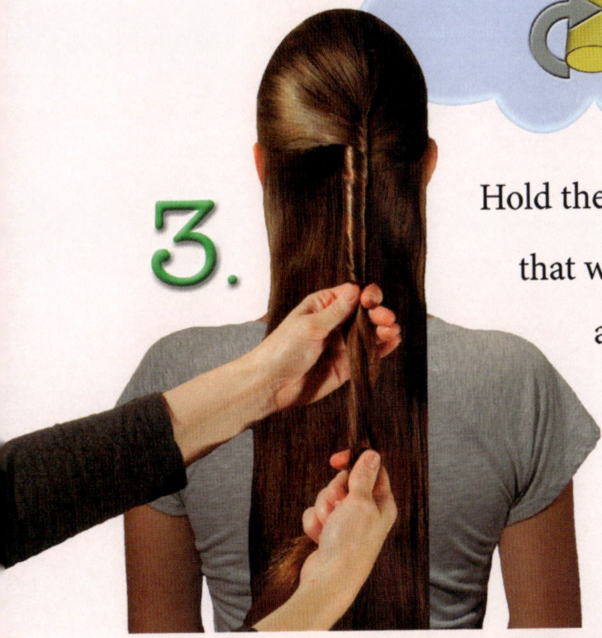 Hold the strand that will be braided and twist.

4. Secure with a rubber band.

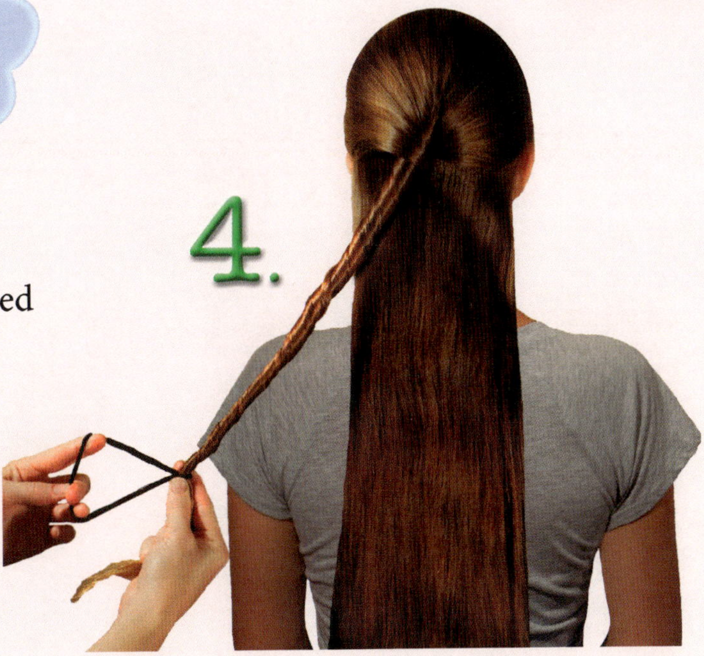

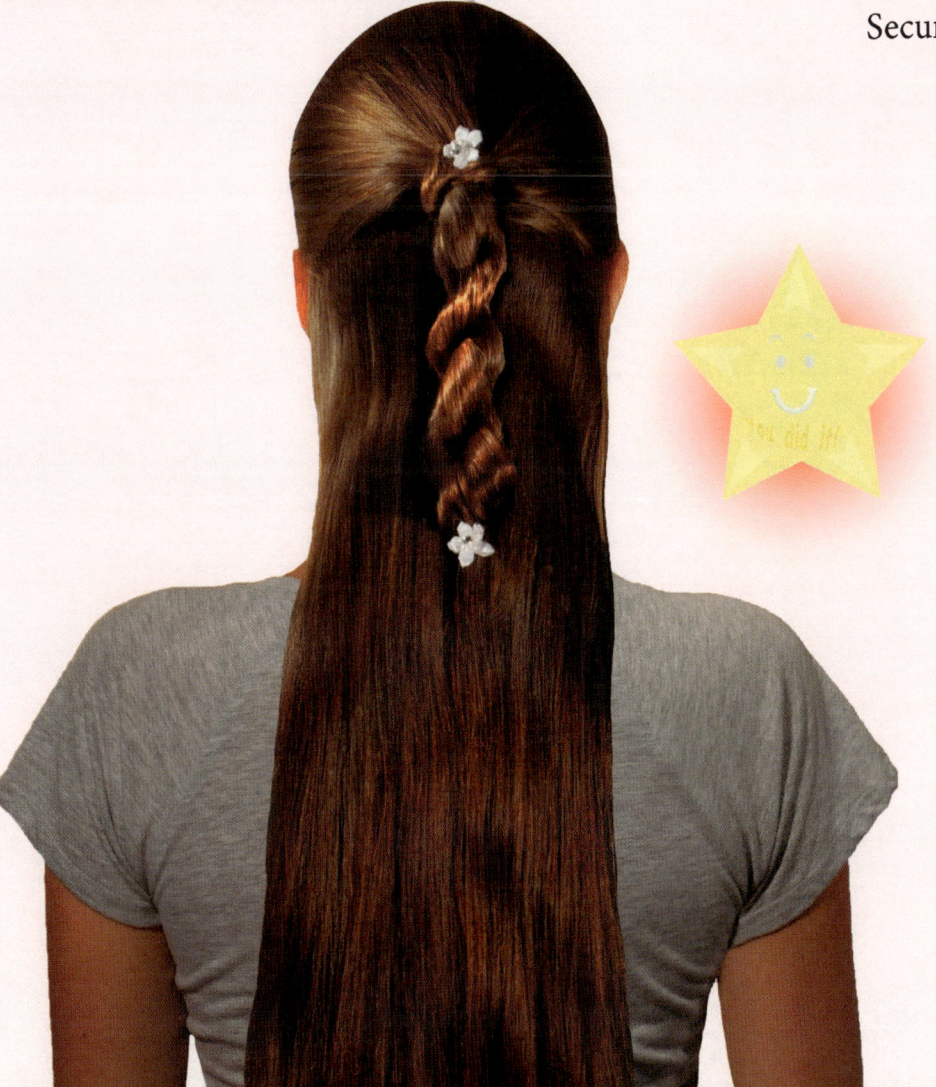

Why do I ask you to secure the end of a twist with a rubber band? It does seem silly. A band adds immense holding power when used with bobby pins. The pins grab the band and lock the braid in place. It is very much an anchor worth using.

One-Strand Twist

Notes

_____

_____

_____

_____

_____

_____

_____

This braid gathers differently on each side depending on which direction you twist the strand. When twisting to the right, the gather from the right is added to the strand by going under the strand first and wrapping around it back to the right while twisting it in with the braid. The left side gather is added from above and wrapping down with the twist of the braid. (shh...that makes it a taper braid)

One-Strand Twist

Gather from both sides

Let's stitch it!

Let's stitch it!

Let's stitch it!

Ways

1   One-Strand Twist Stitch

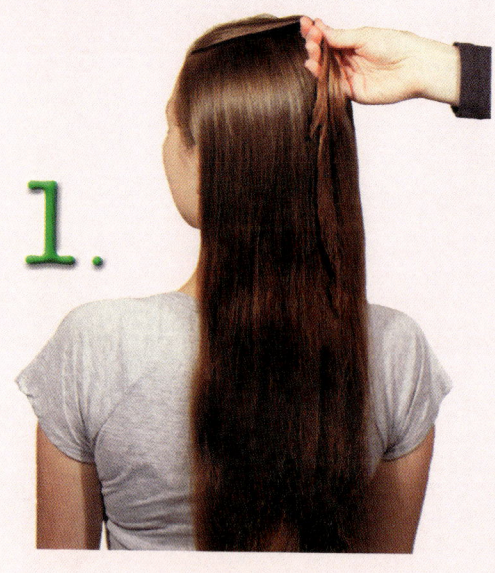

1. Take a section of hair as illustrated.

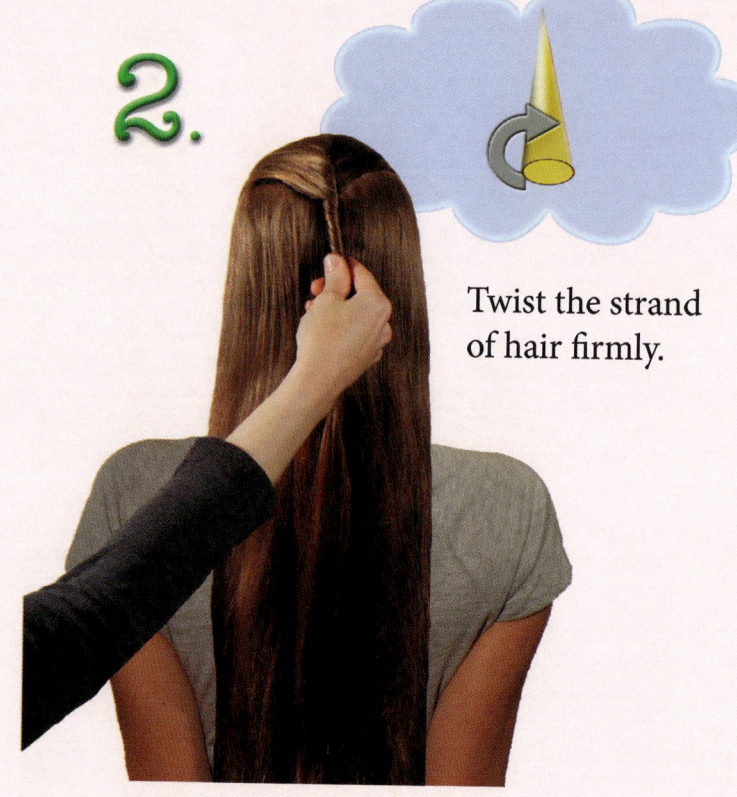

2. Twist the strand of hair firmly.

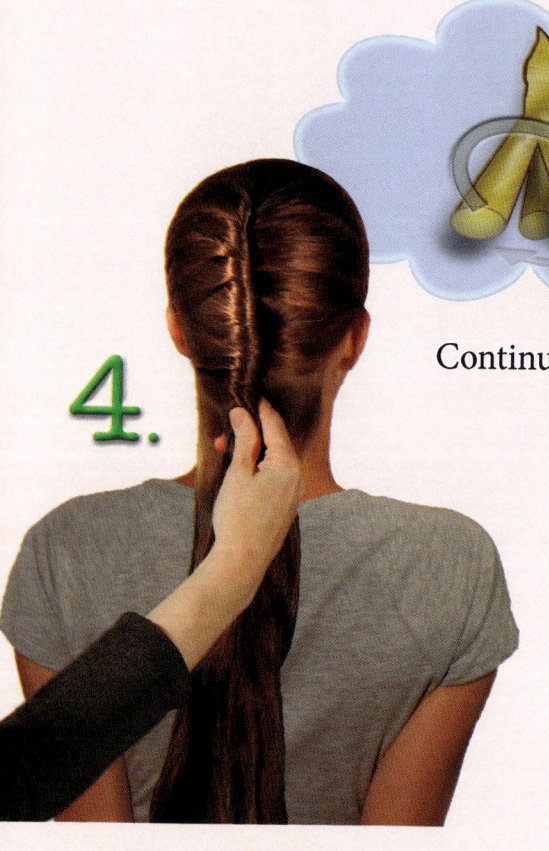

4. Continue gathering and twisting until you reach the end of the hair.

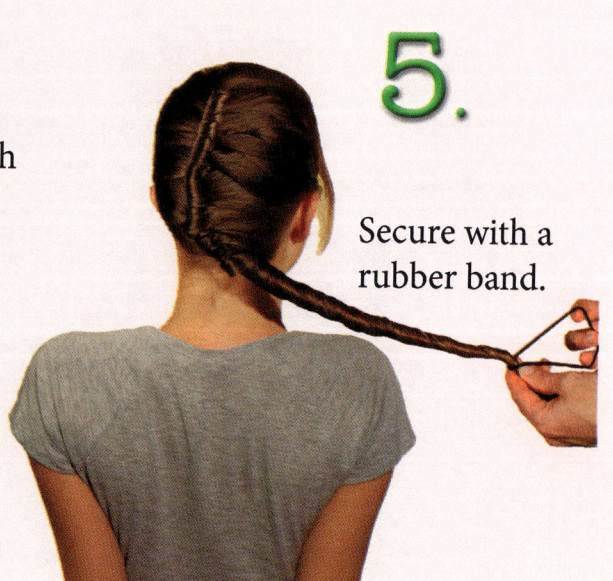

5. Secure with a rubber band.

One-Strand Twist Stitch

1

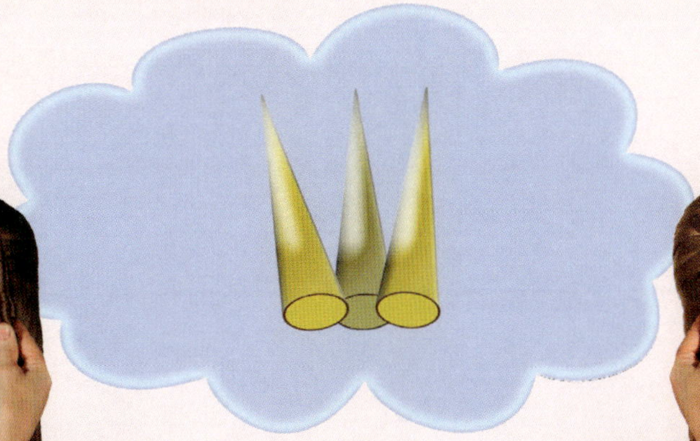

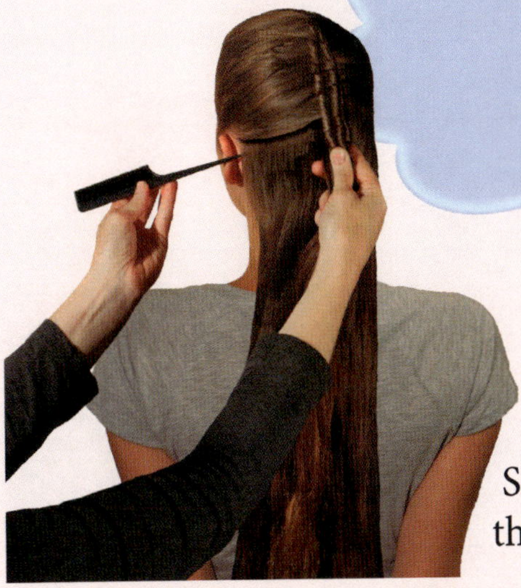

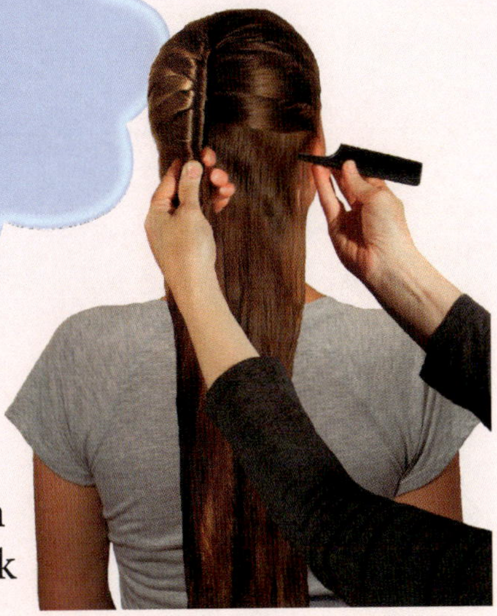

3.

Sliver off a gather from the face all the way back to the braid.

Gather into the braid from both sides. Twist the gathers with the strand.

6.

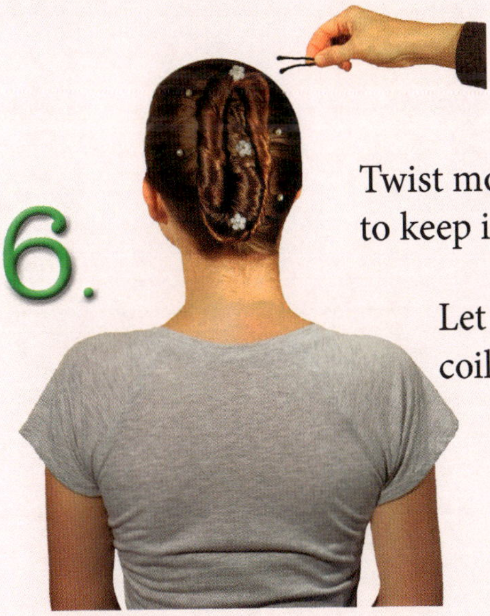

Twist more, if needed, to keep it braided.

Let the strand coil as desired.

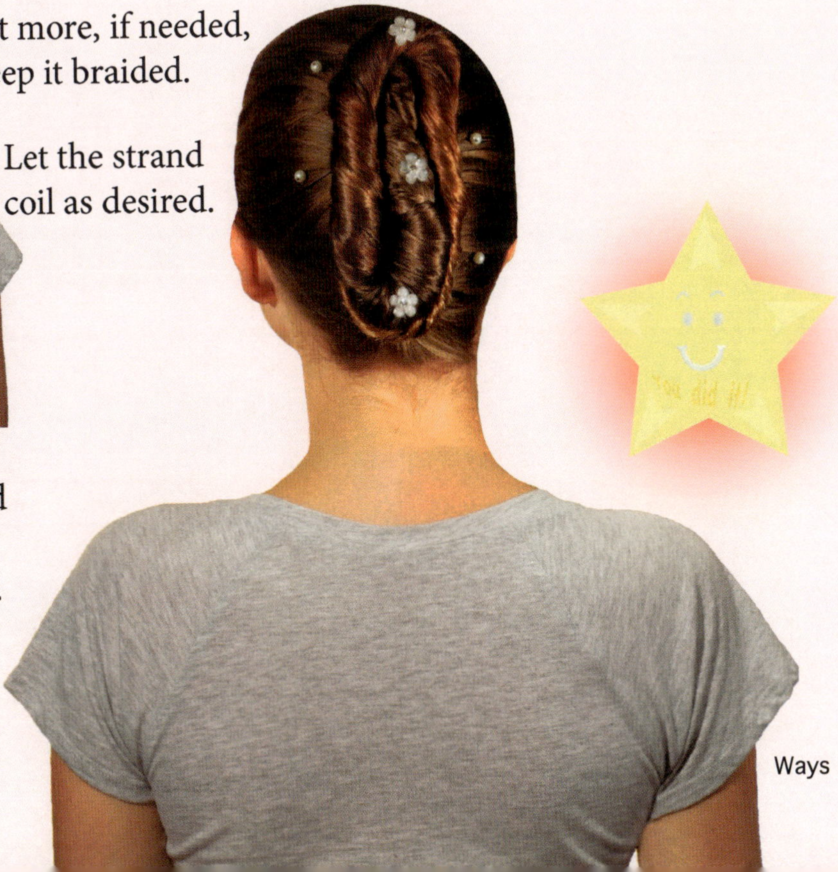

Fix the end of the braid with bobby pins to hold the braid in place.

Ways 35

One-Strand Twist

Notes

_____

_____

_____

_____

_____

_____

_____

_____

I like requests to do twist braids because twists are usually associated with updo hairstyles. Use this braid just like any other braid and create your own unique styles.

One-Strand Twist

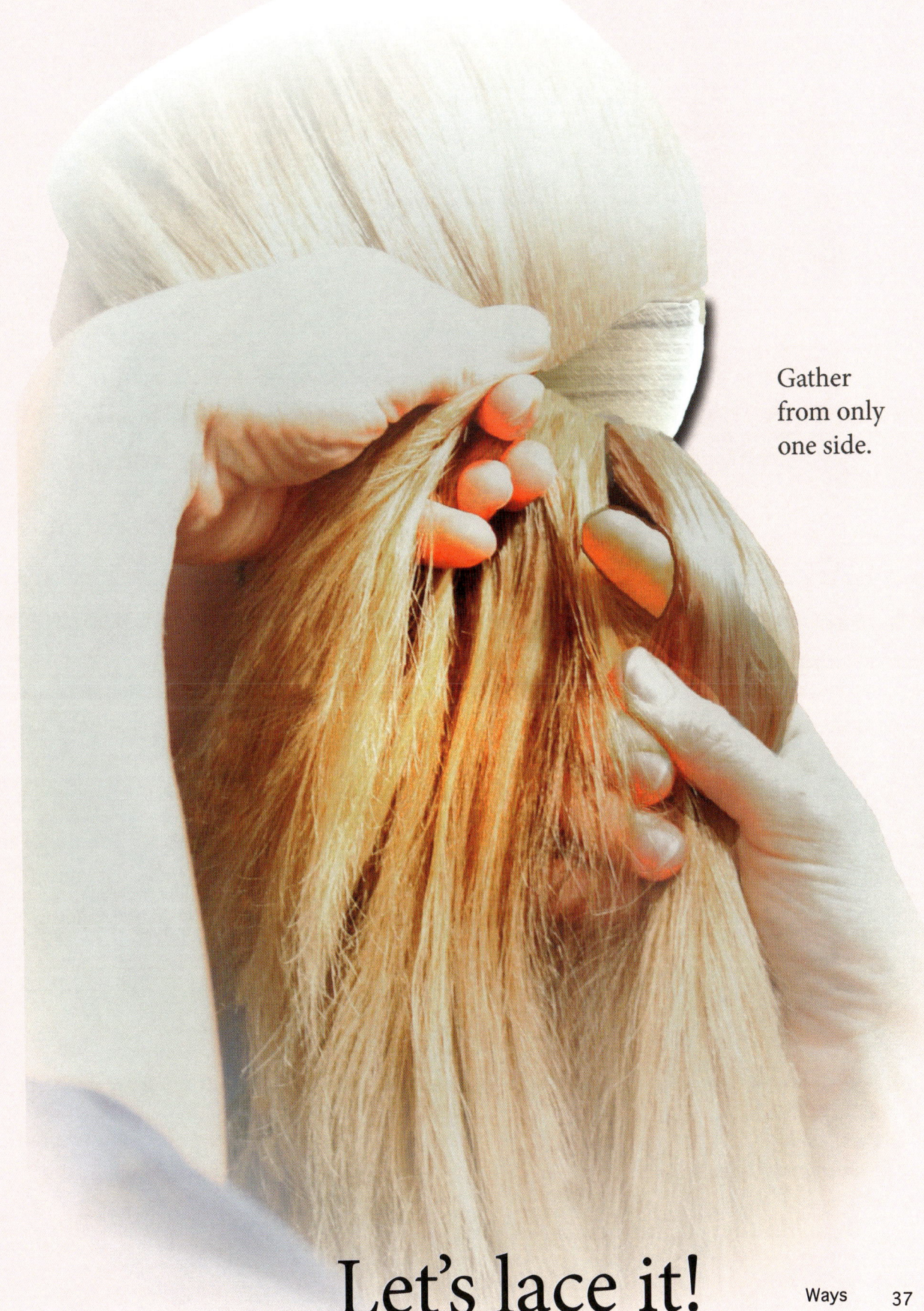

Gather from only one side.

Let's lace it!

One-Strand Twist Lace

1

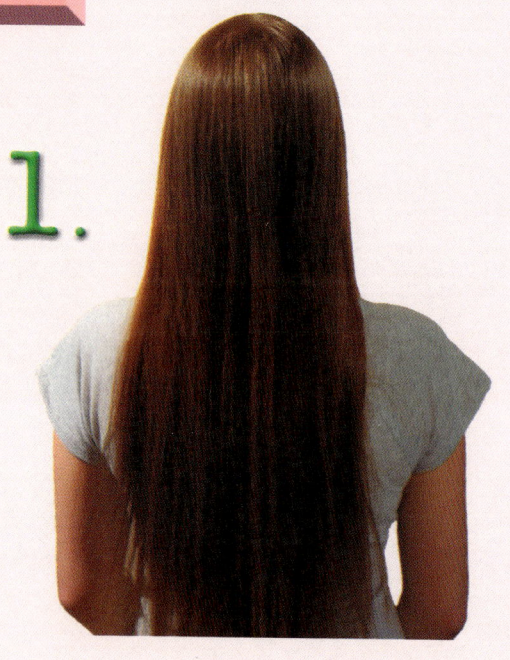

1. Begin with clean, brushed hair.

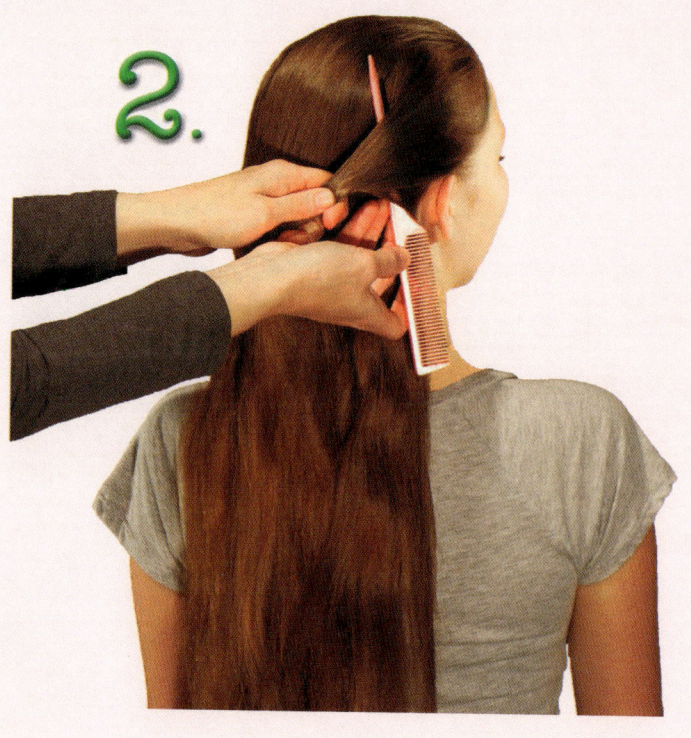

2. Take a section of hair as illustrated.

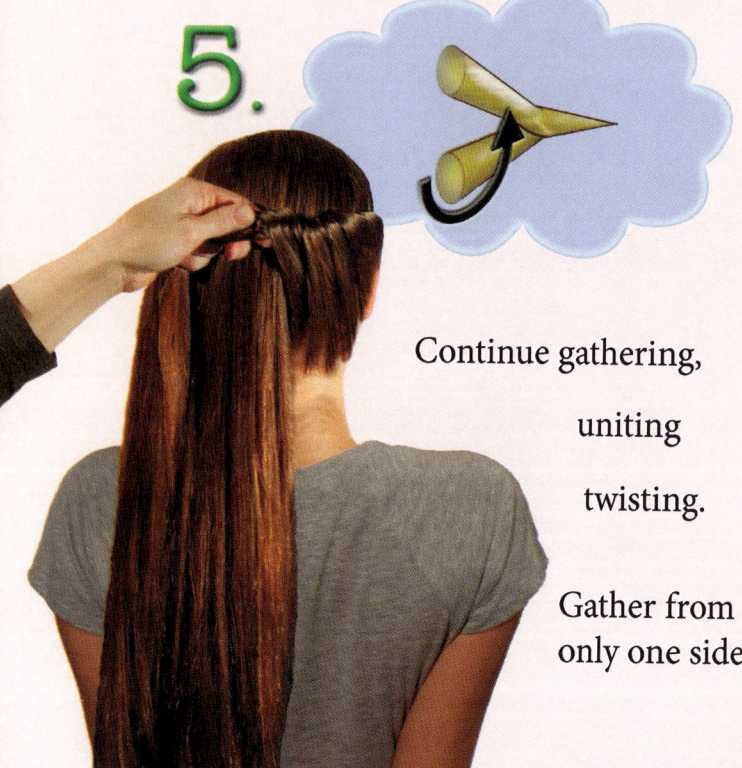

5. Continue gathering, uniting twisting.

Gather from only one side.

Twist until you reach the end of the hair.

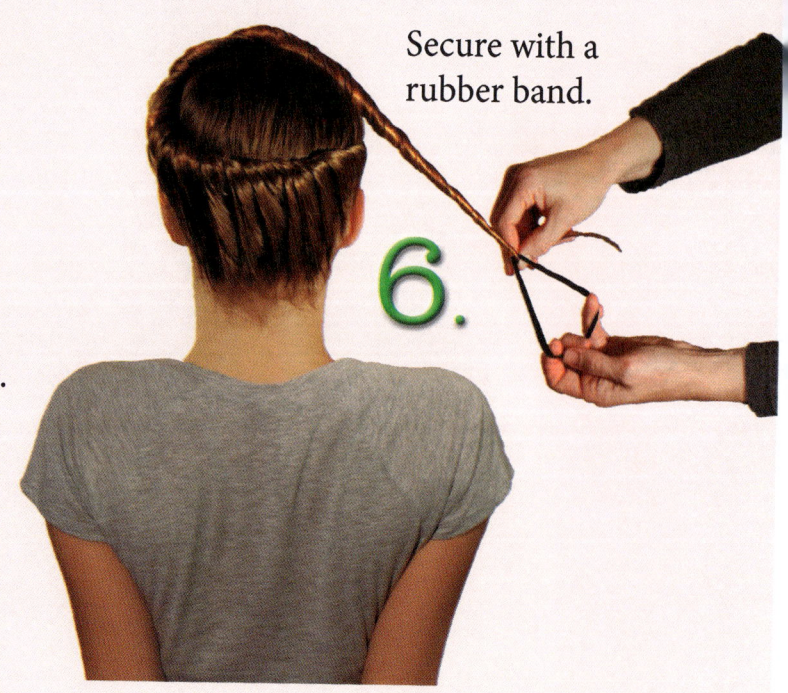

6. Secure with a rubber band.

38 www.findingbraids.com

One-Strand Twist Lace

1

3.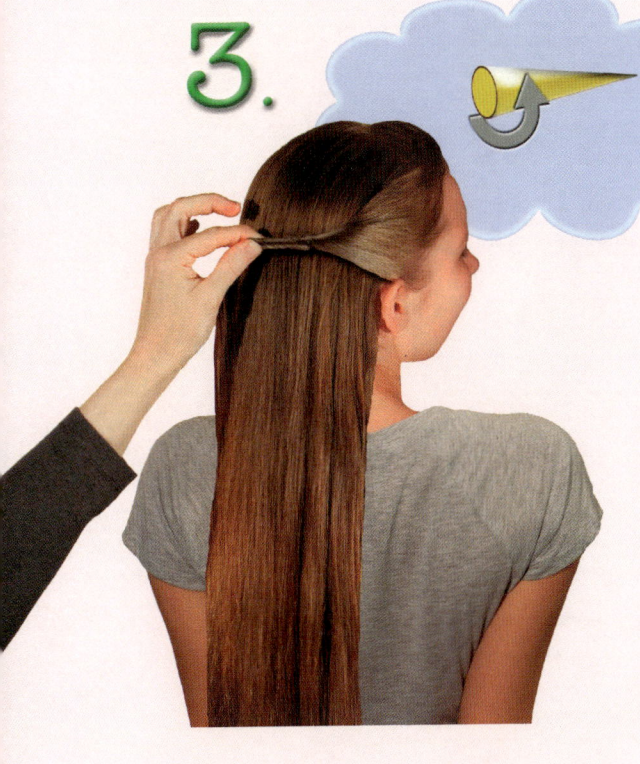

Twist the strand of hair firmly.

4.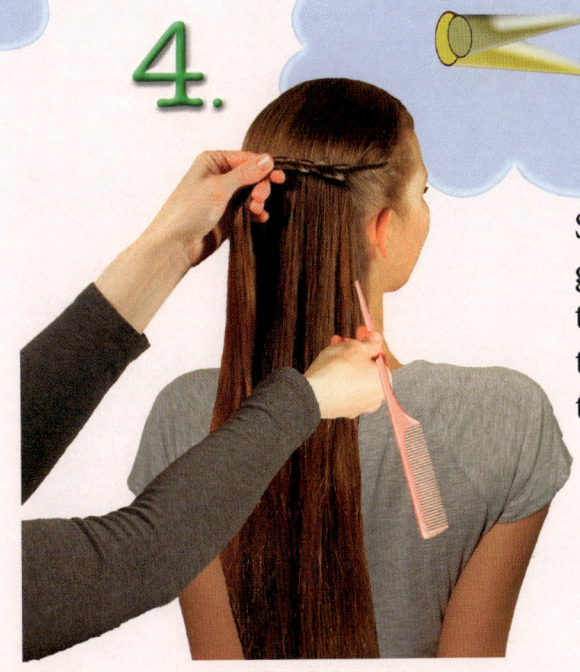

Sliver off a gather from the face all the way back to the braid.

Gather into the twist from only one side and unite the strands by twisting them together.

7. Fix the end of the braid with bobby pins to hold the braid in place.

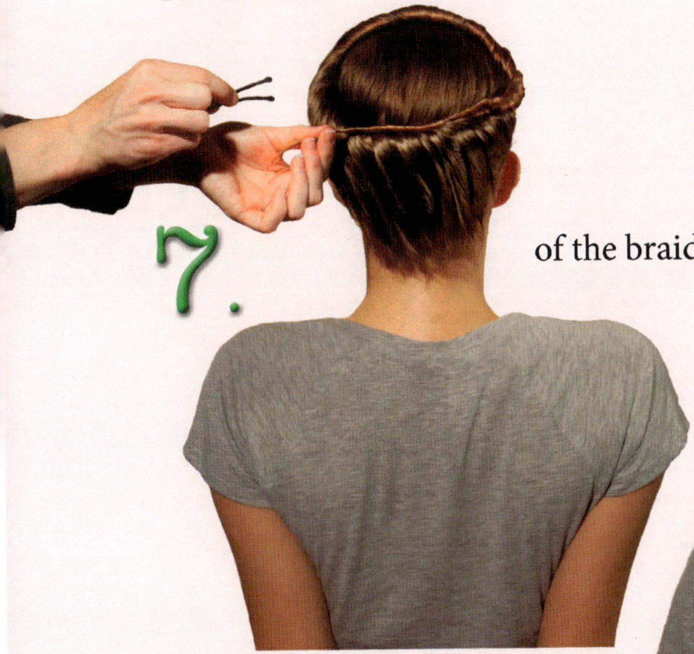

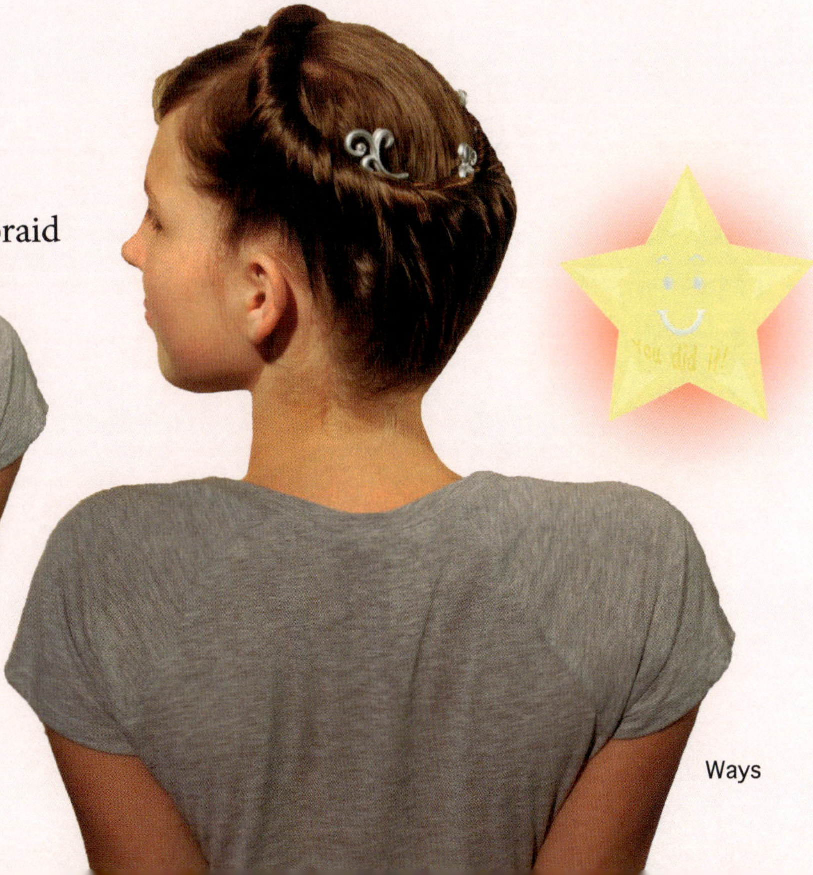

One-Strand Twist

Notes

_____

_____

_____

_____

_____

_____

_____

Give the examples a try now!

Examples of One-Strand Twist

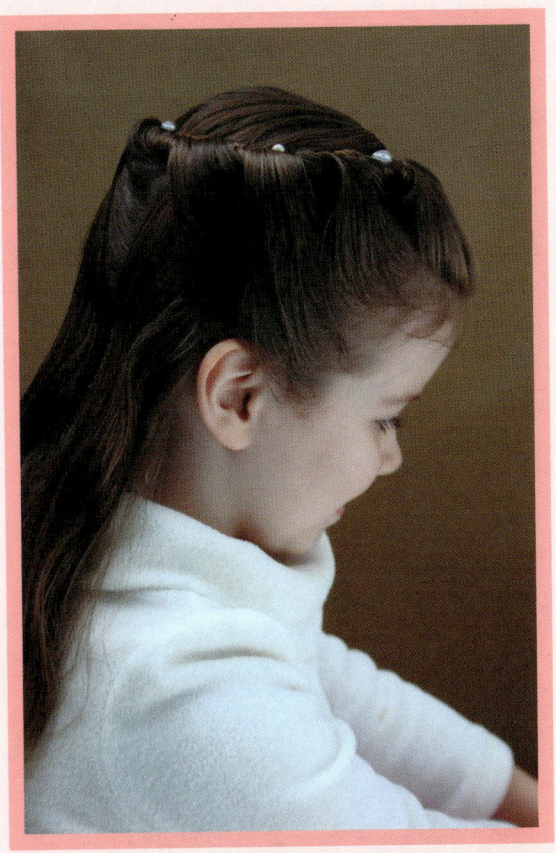
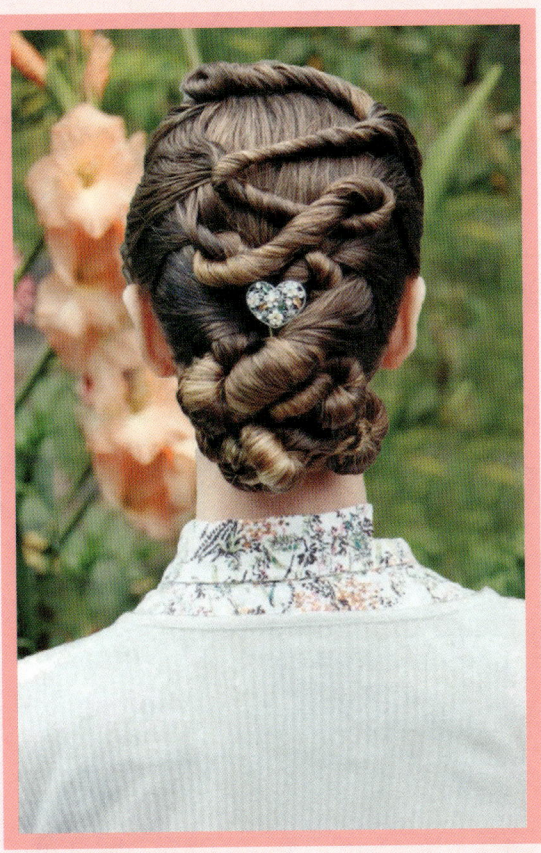
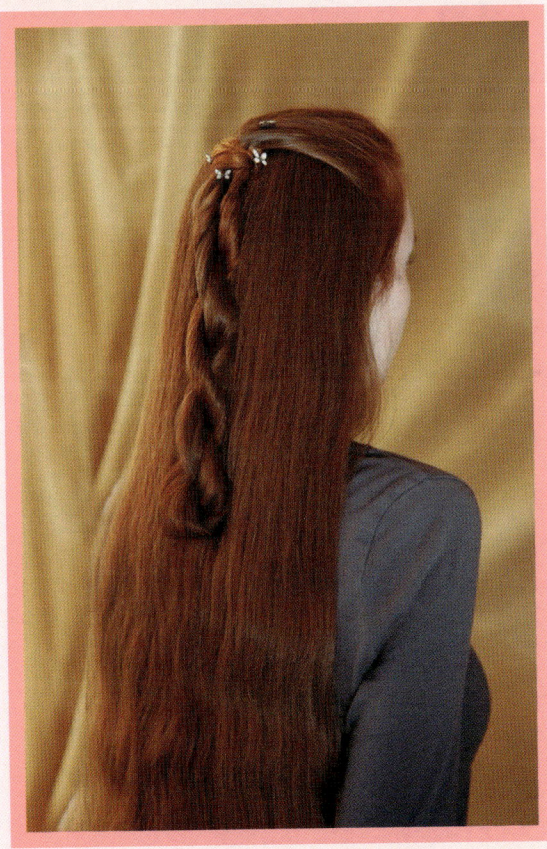
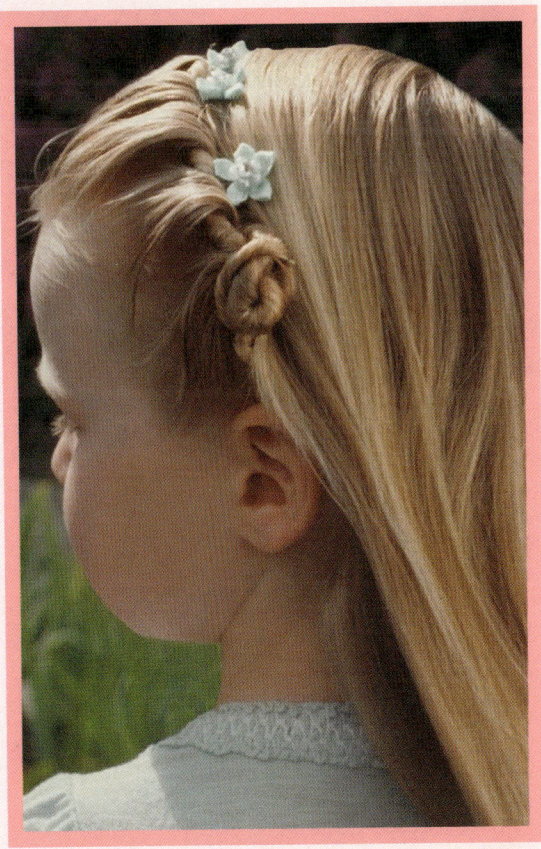

Visit my website to see more examples of the One-Strand Twist

One-Strand Rosette

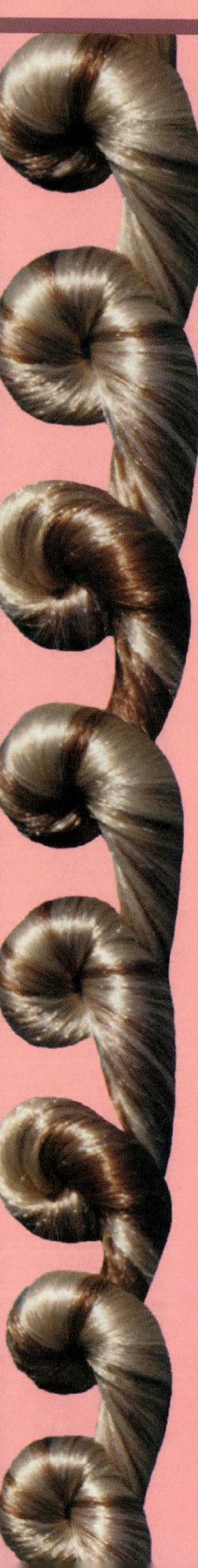

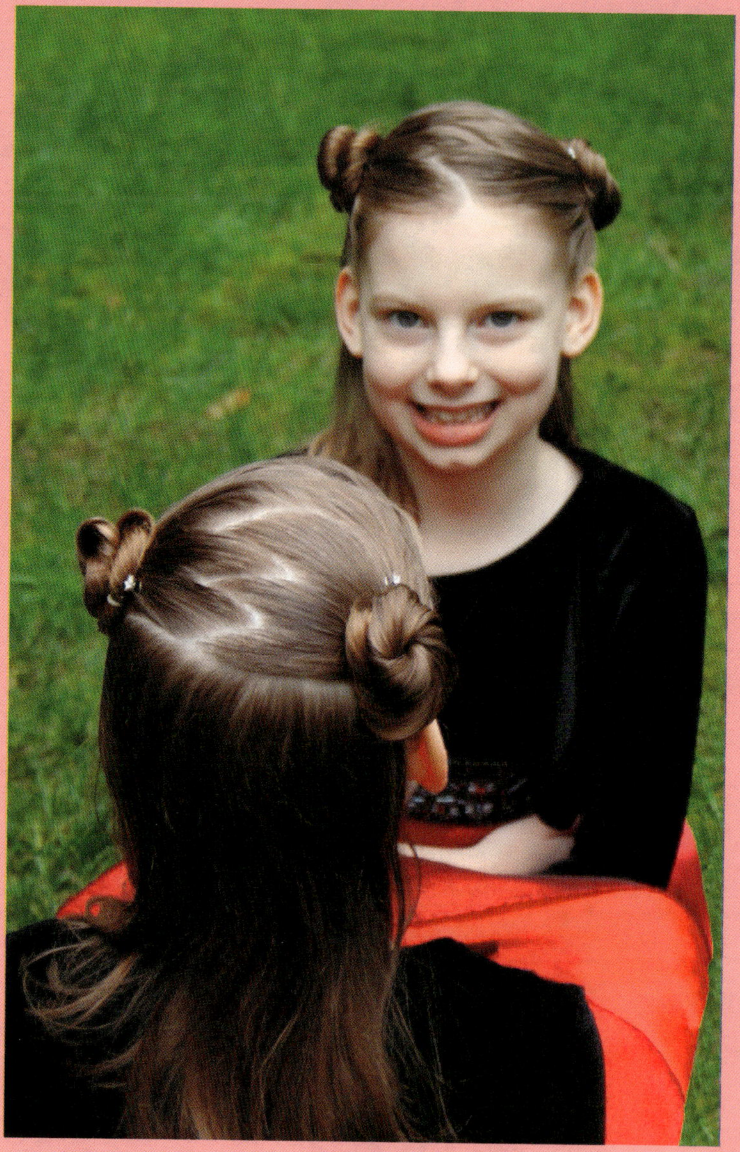

This is a braid that requires a gentle but steady hand. If the hair is twisted too tight it can cause damage. If it is twisted too loose, it will not stay.

One-Strand Rosette

Looking for something new and eye catching? The next fourteen pages will walk you through this braid.

Braid . . . . 44 - 45

Stitch . . . . 48 - 51

Lace . . . . 54 - 56

Examples 57

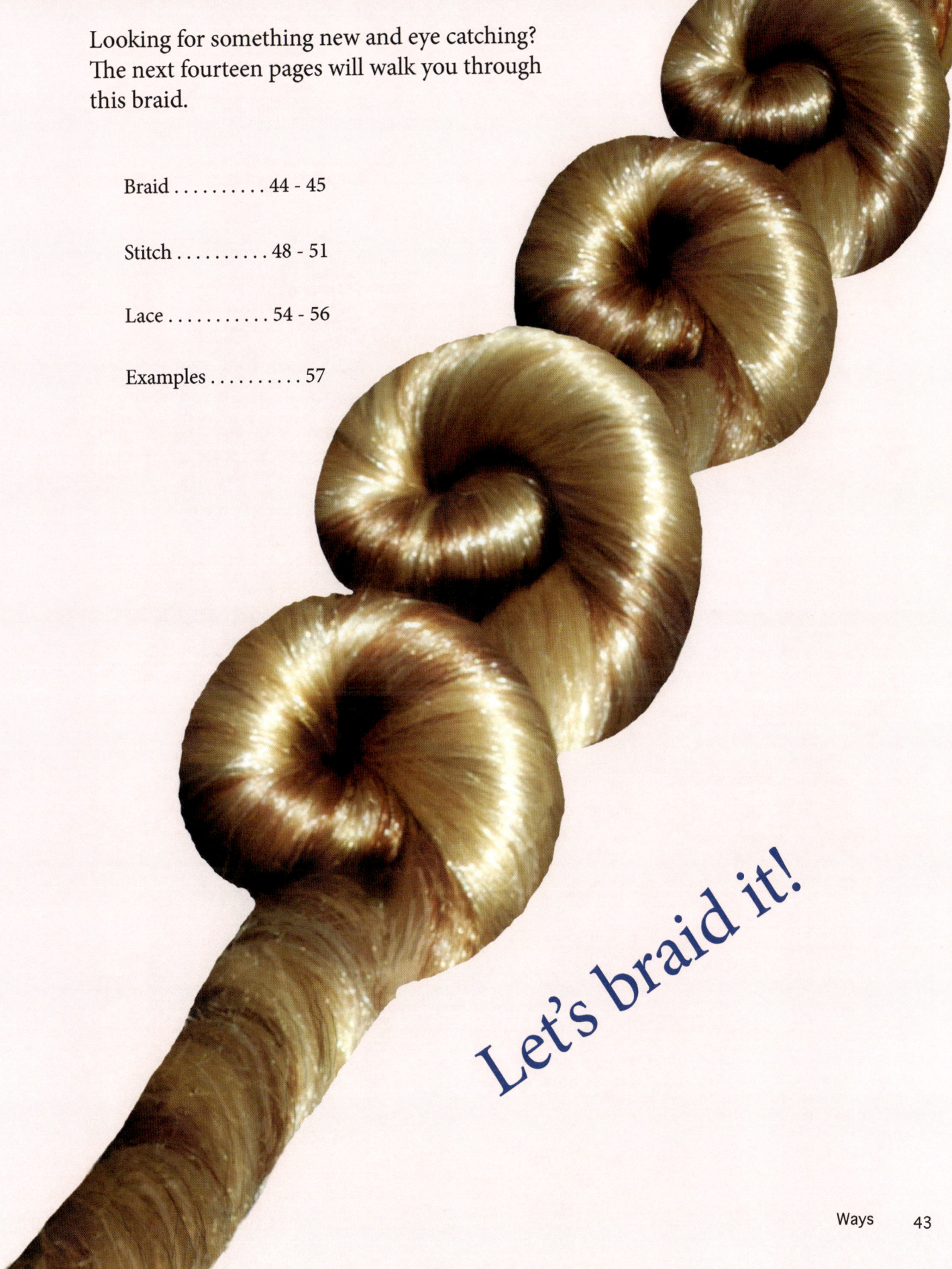

Let's braid it!

One-Strand Rosette Braid

1

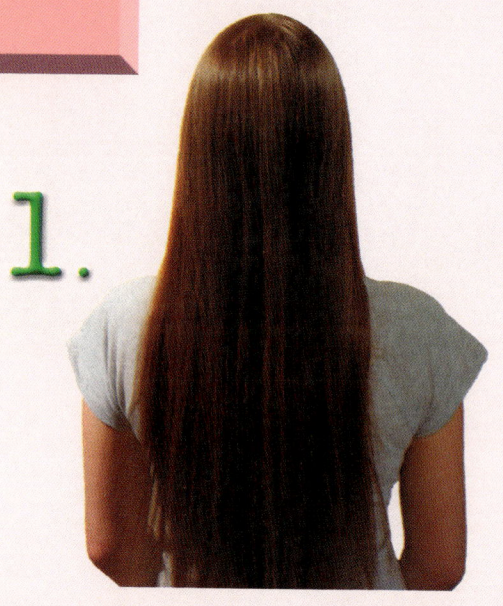

1. Begin with clean, brushed hair.

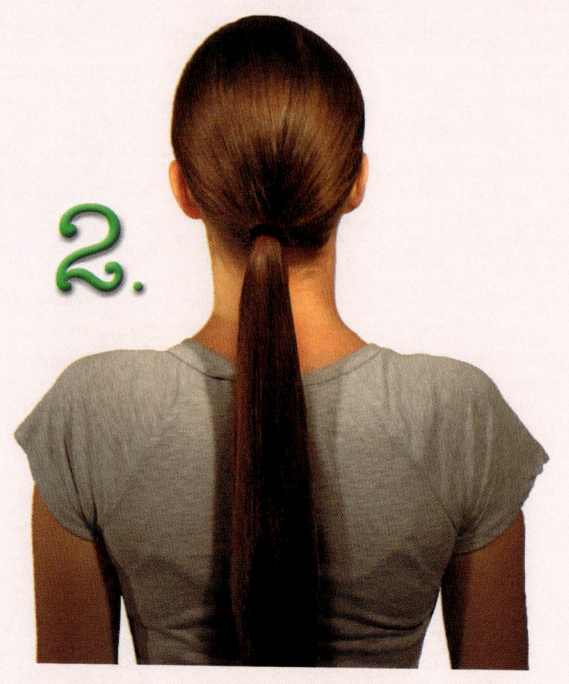

2. Take a section of hair.

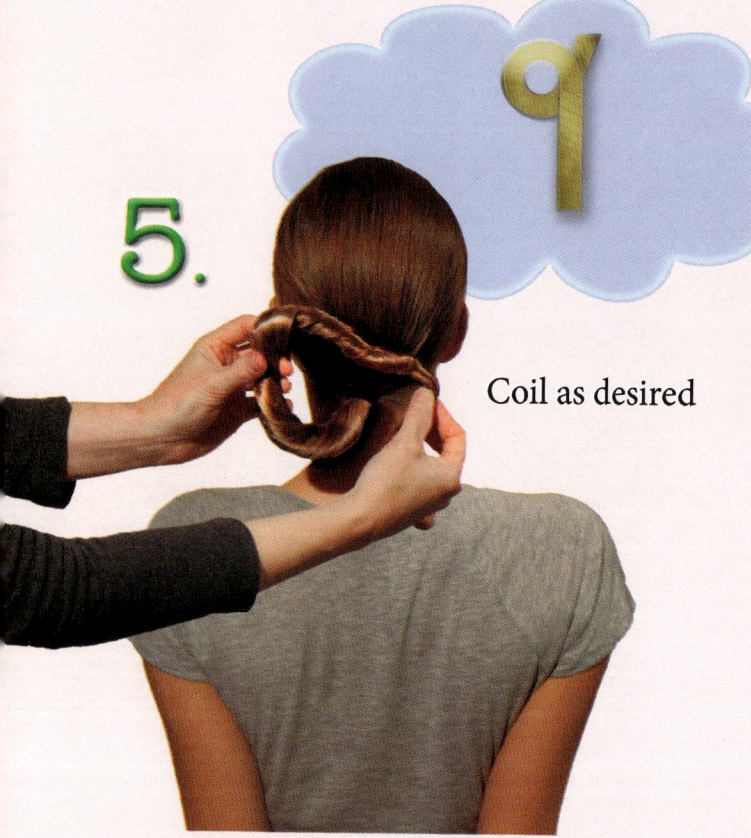

9

Coil as desired

5. and twist more if needed to keep it braided.

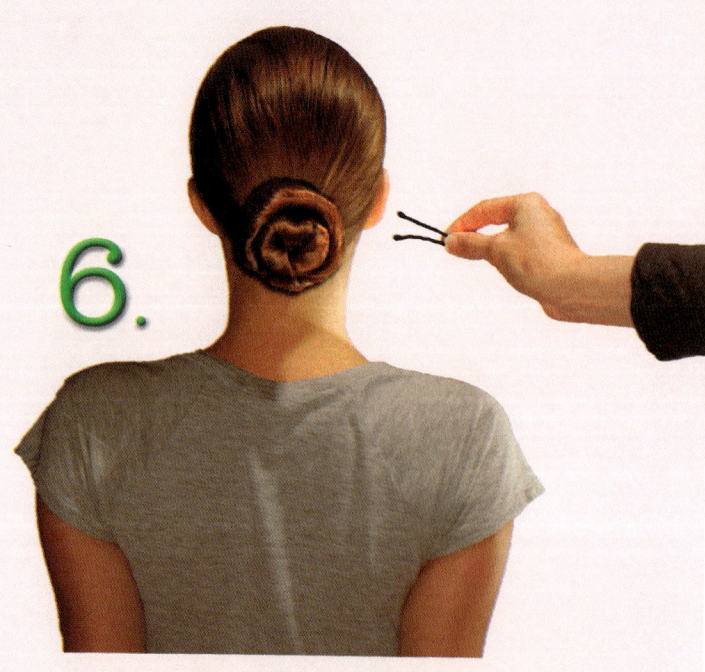

6. Fix the end of the braid with bobby pins to hold the braid in place.

One-Strand Rosette Braid

1

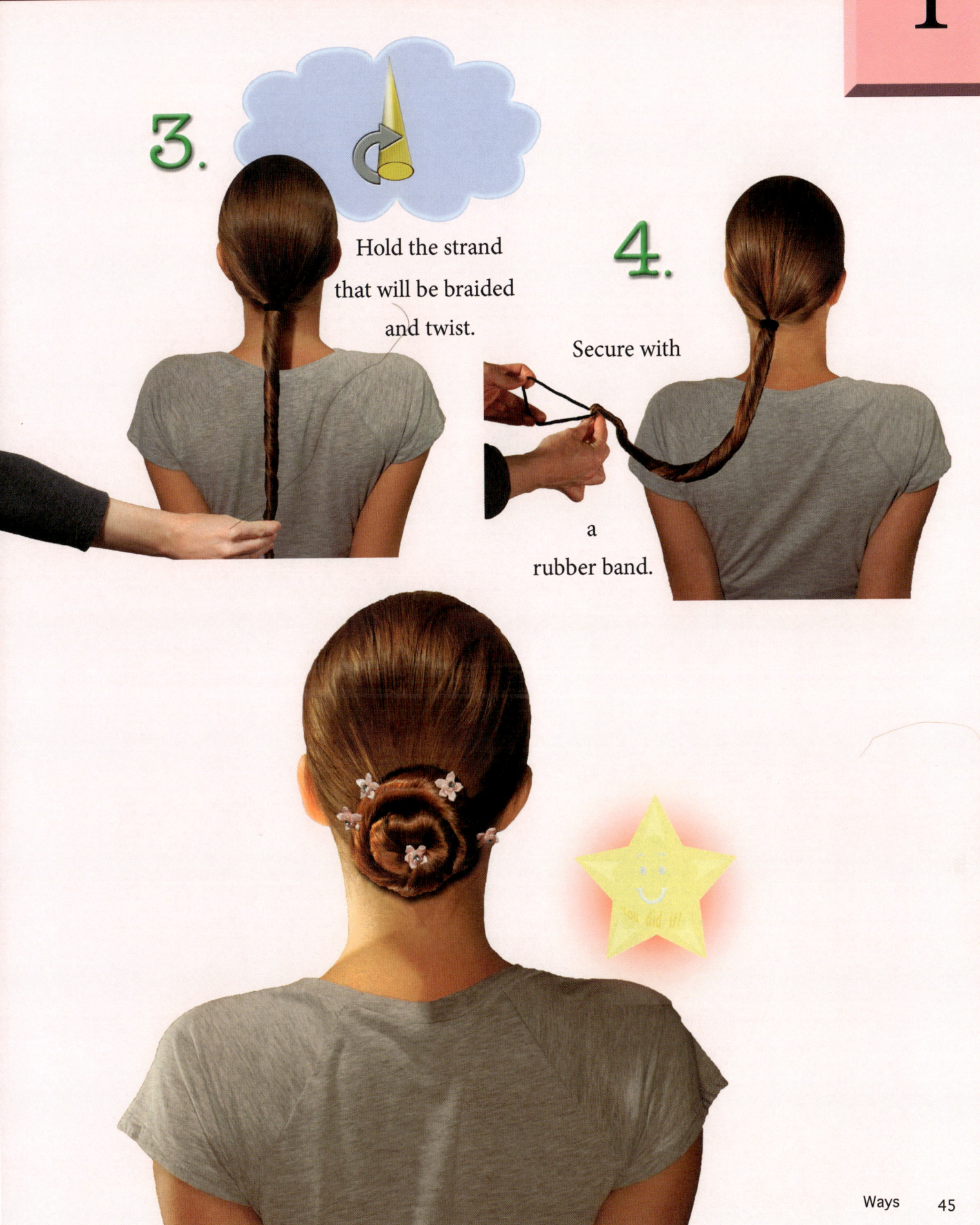

3. Hold the strand that will be braided and twist.

4. Secure with a rubber band.

Ways

One-Strand Rosette

Notes

_____

_____

_____

_____

_____

_____

The first time I came across this way of braiding, it was as if my brain had been slapped. How wonderful and strange this is as a braid. Its flowery pattern is unique. Many bobby pins are necessary to make this captivating braid sturdy. Be patient when learning this technique.

One-Strand Rosette

Gather from both sides

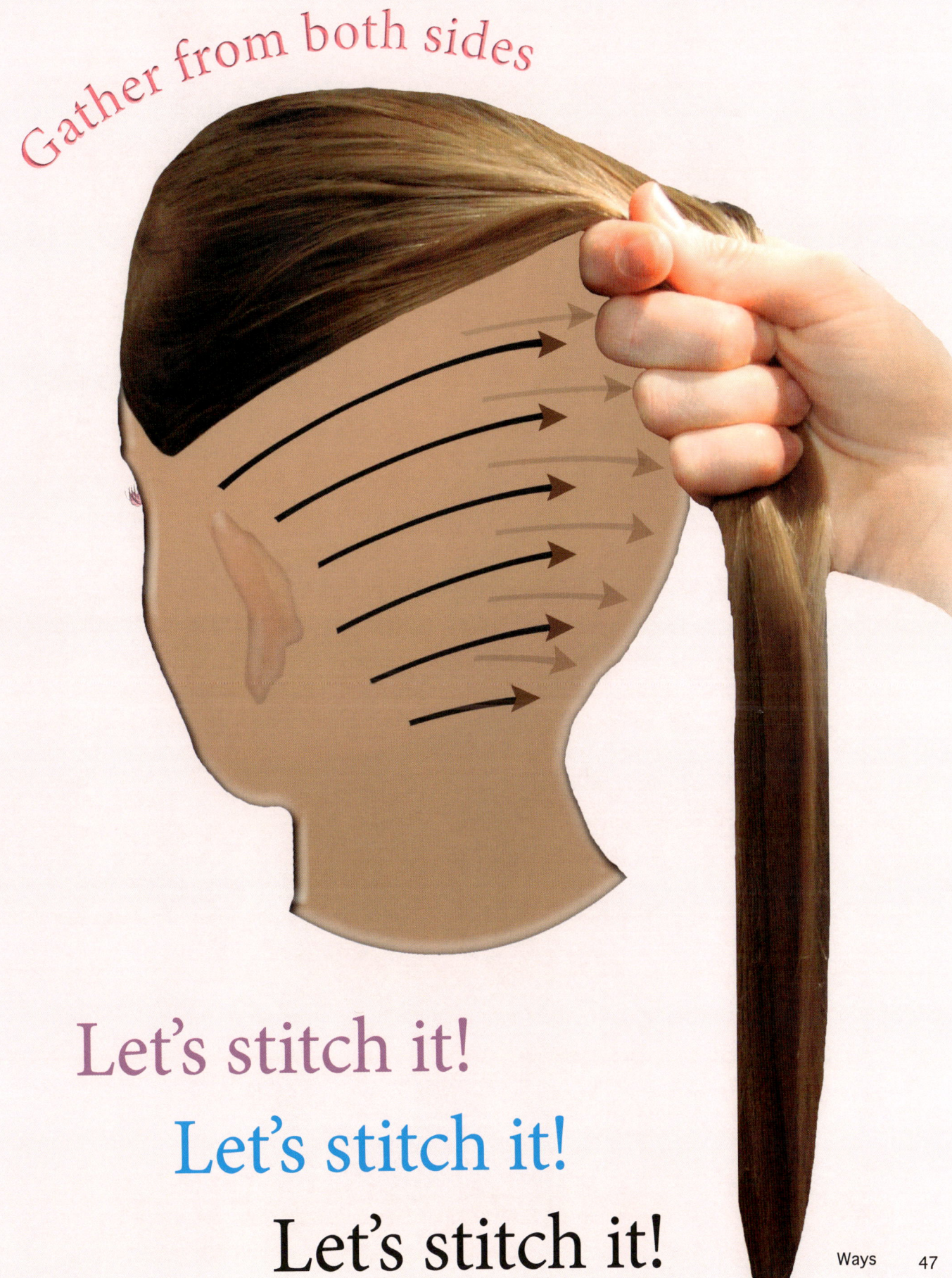

Let's stitch it!
Let's stitch it!
Let's stitch it!

One-Strand Rosette Stitch

1

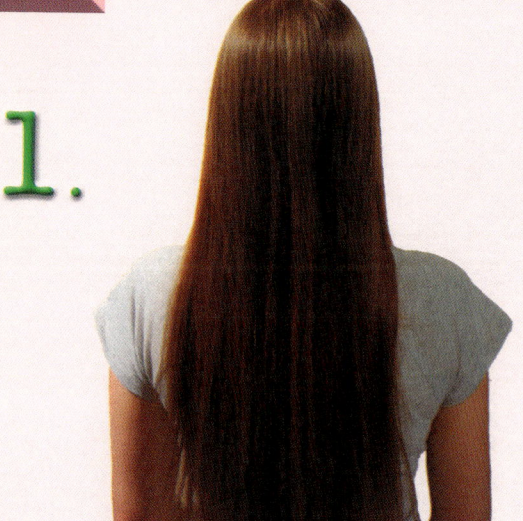

1.

Begin with clean, brushed hair.

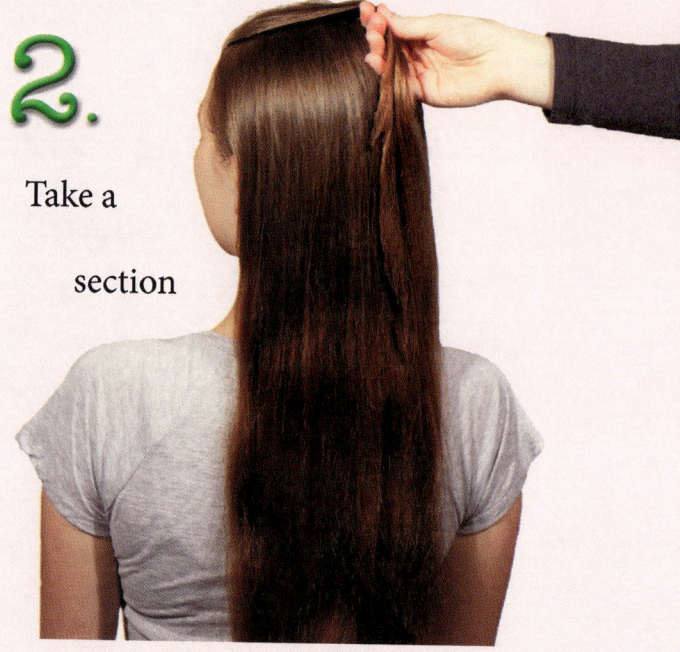

2.

Take a section of hair as illustrated.

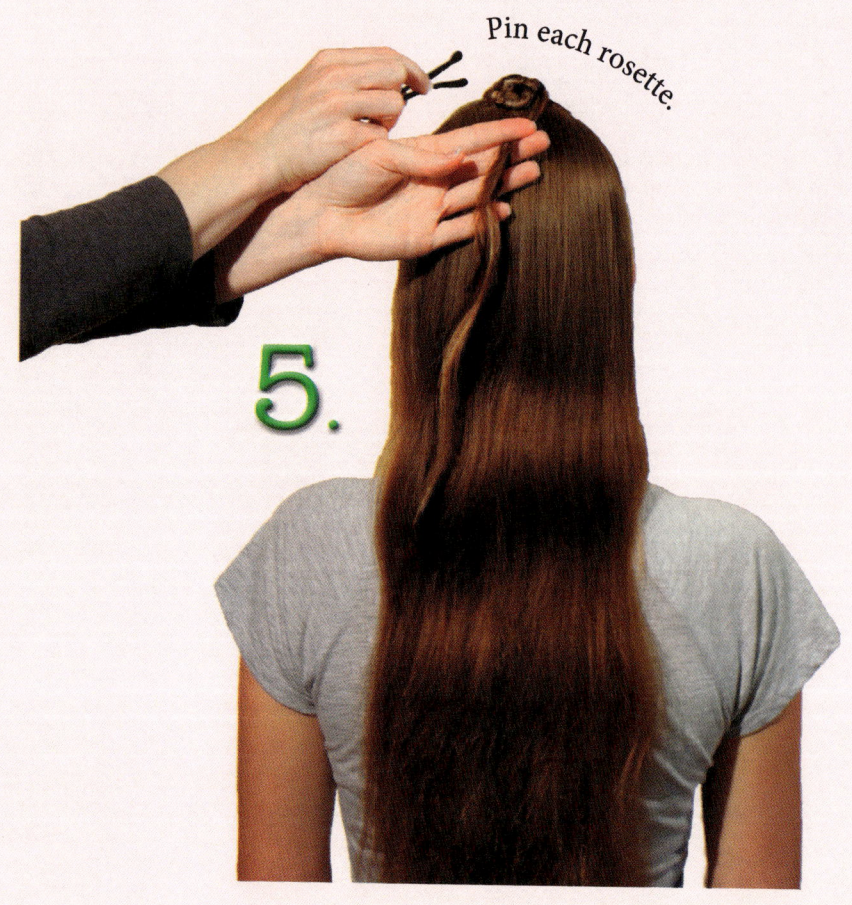

Pin each rosette.

5.

One-Strand Rosette Stitch

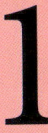

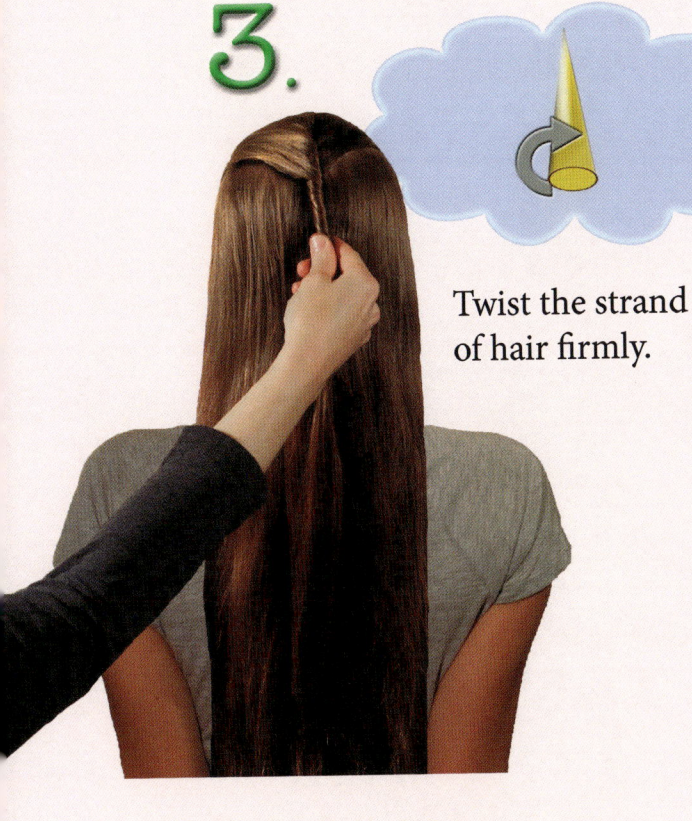

3. Twist the strand of hair firmly.

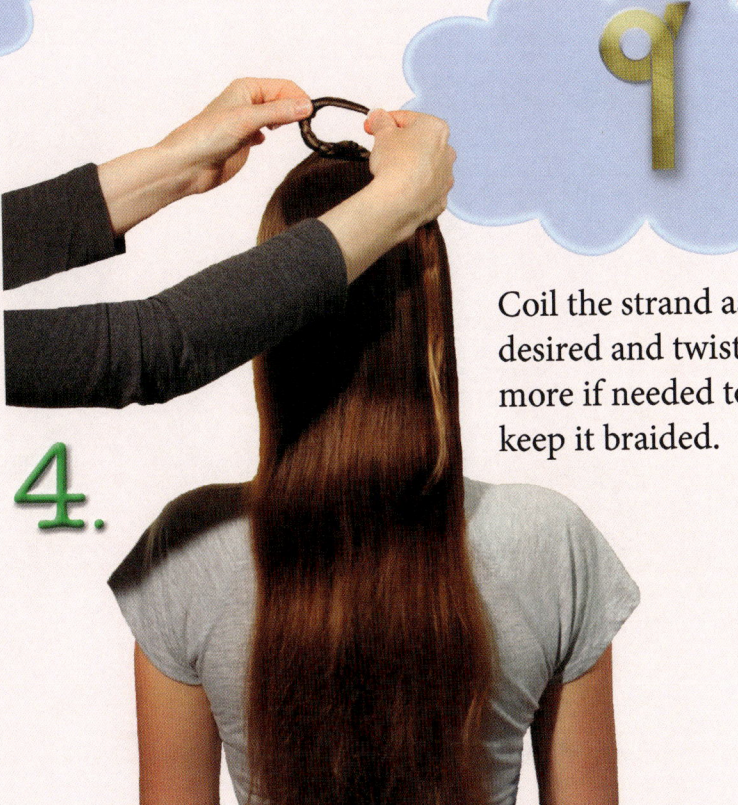

4. Coil the strand as desired and twist more if needed to keep it braided.

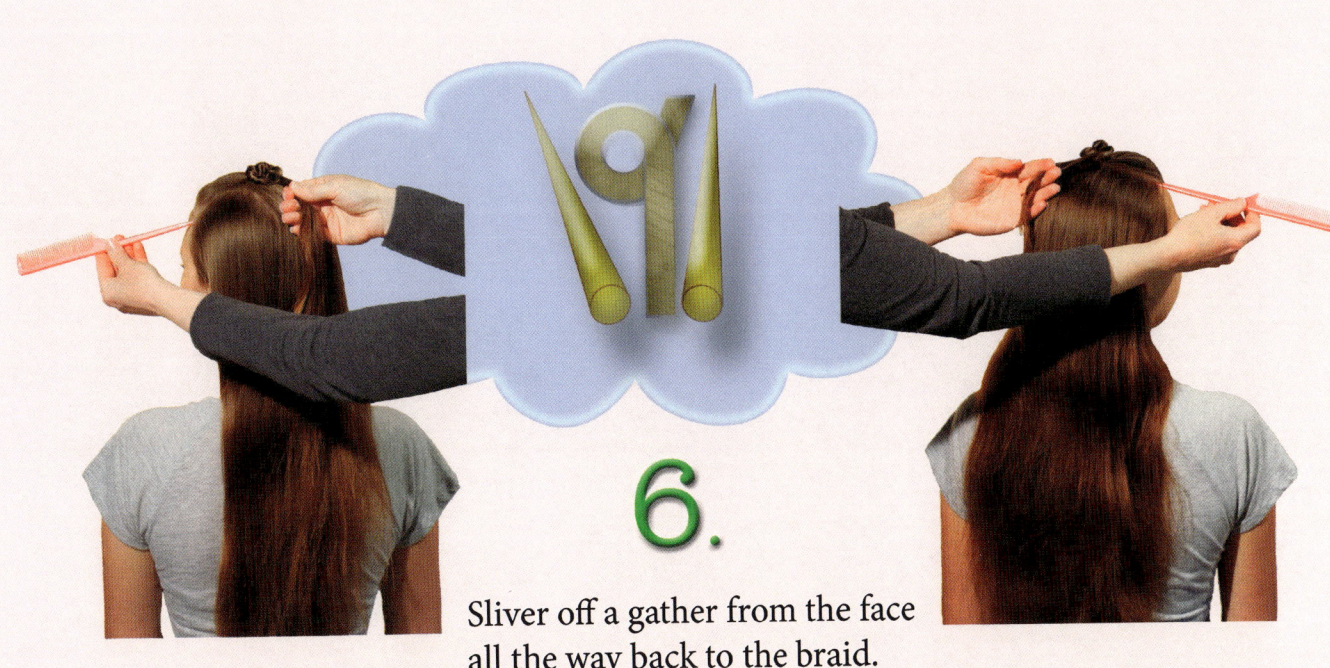

6. Sliver off a gather from the face all the way back to the braid. Gather into the braid from both sides.

Ways

1 Continuing

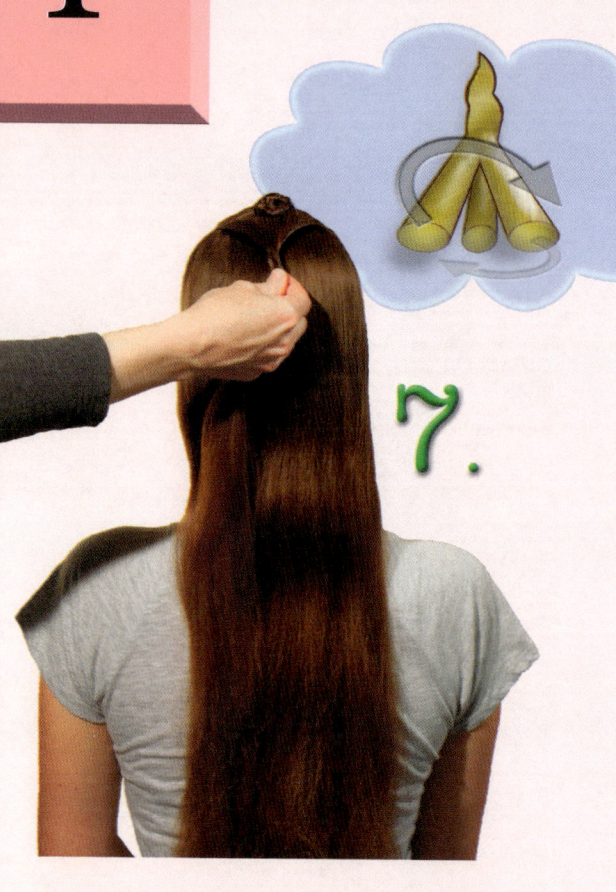

Twist the gathers into the strand.

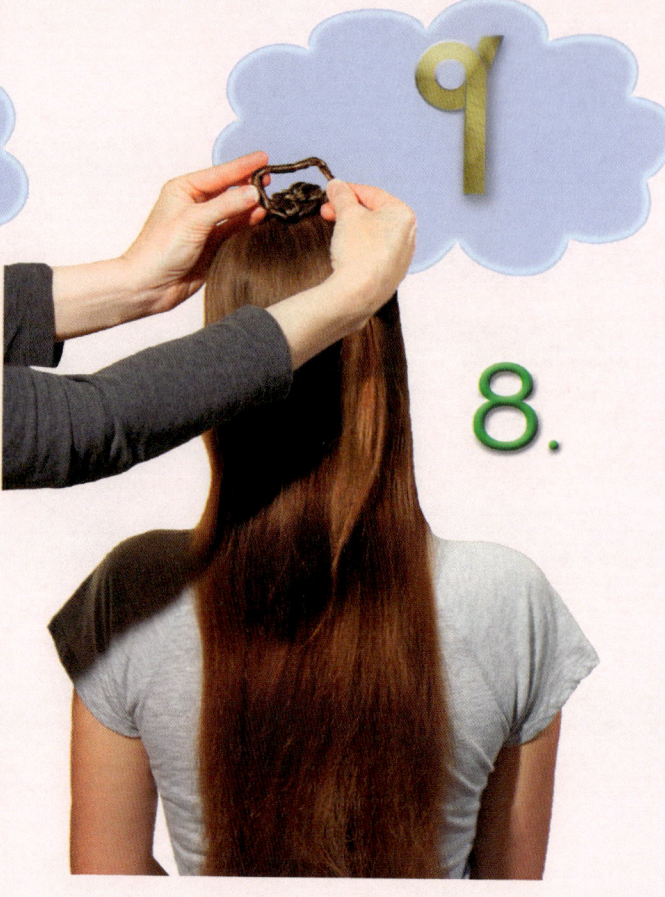

Coil as desired. Twist more if needed to keep it braided.

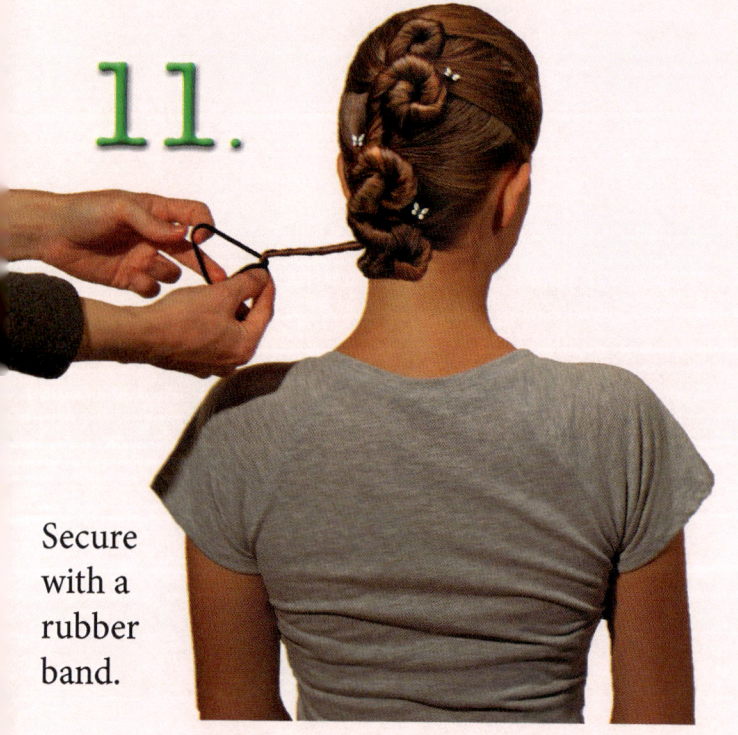

Secure with a rubber band.

Fix the end of the braid with bobby pins to hold the braid in place.

part 2. One-Strand Rosette Stitch

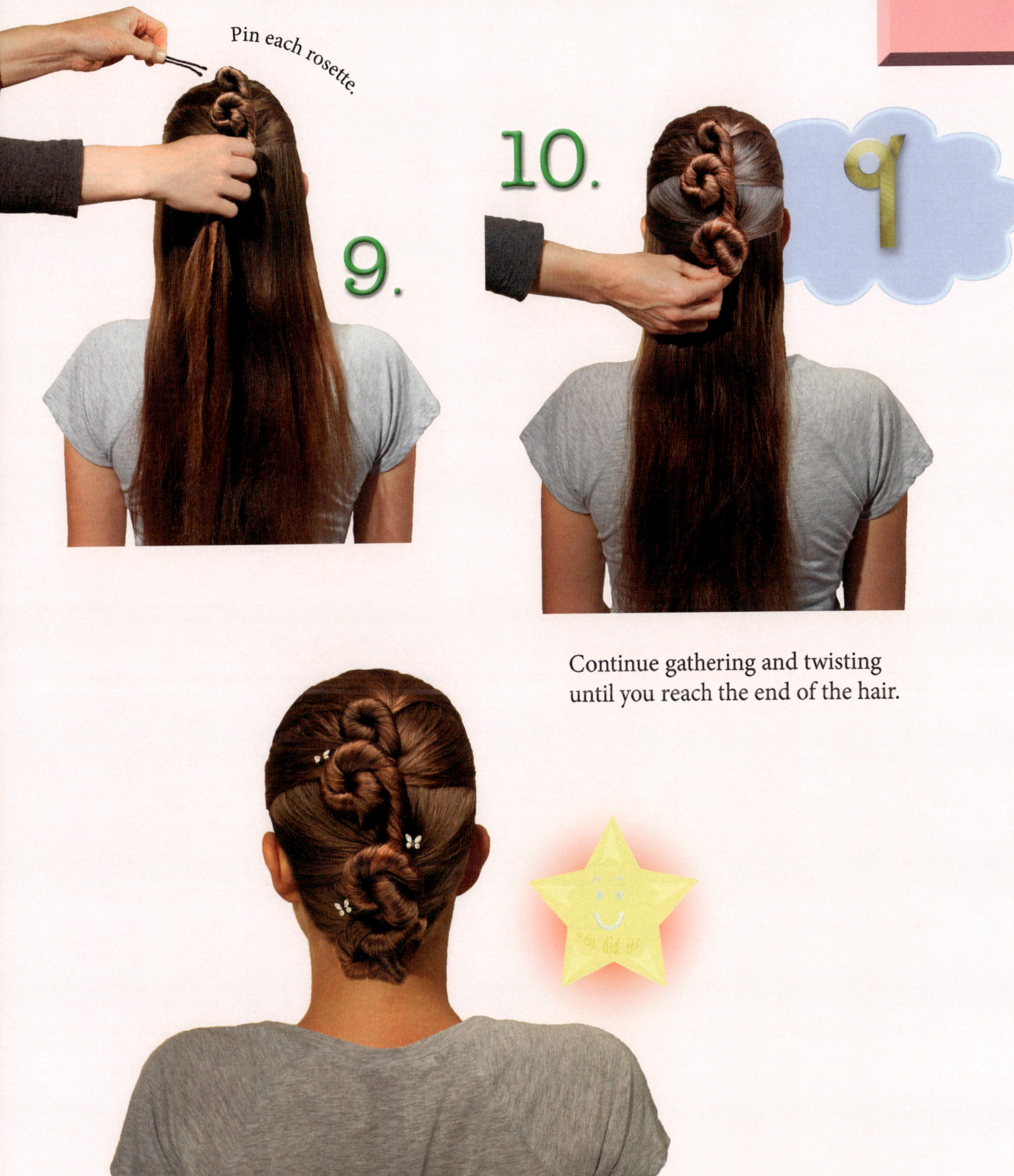

Pin each rosette.

9.

10.

Continue gathering and twisting until you reach the end of the hair.

One-Strand Rosette

Notes

One-Strand Rosette

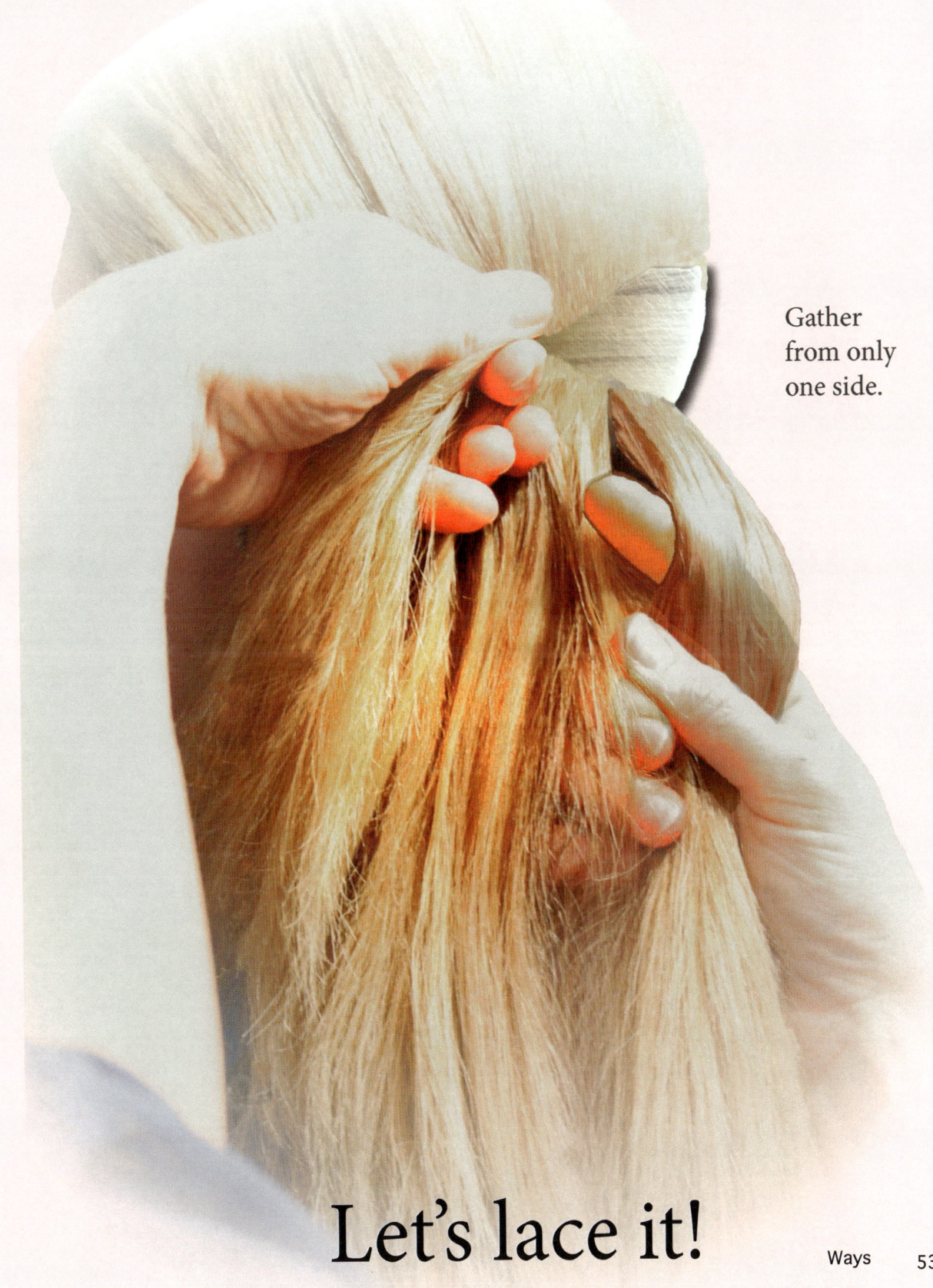

Gather from only one side.

Let's lace it!

One-Strand Rosette Lace

1.

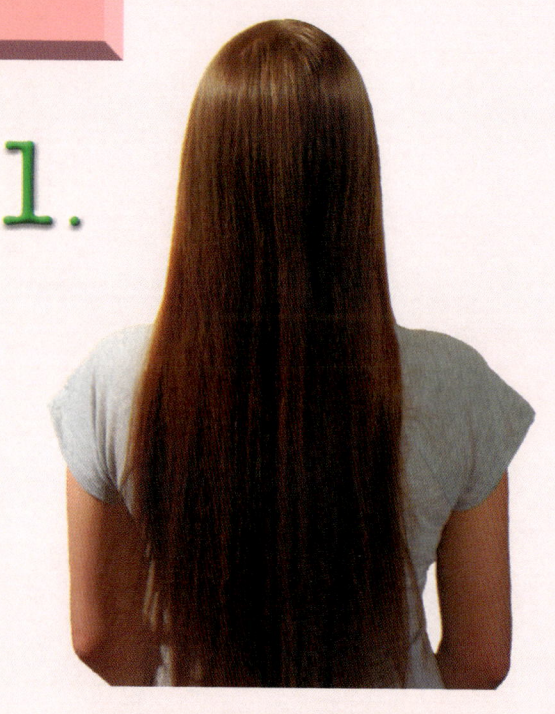

Begin with clean, brushed hair.

2.

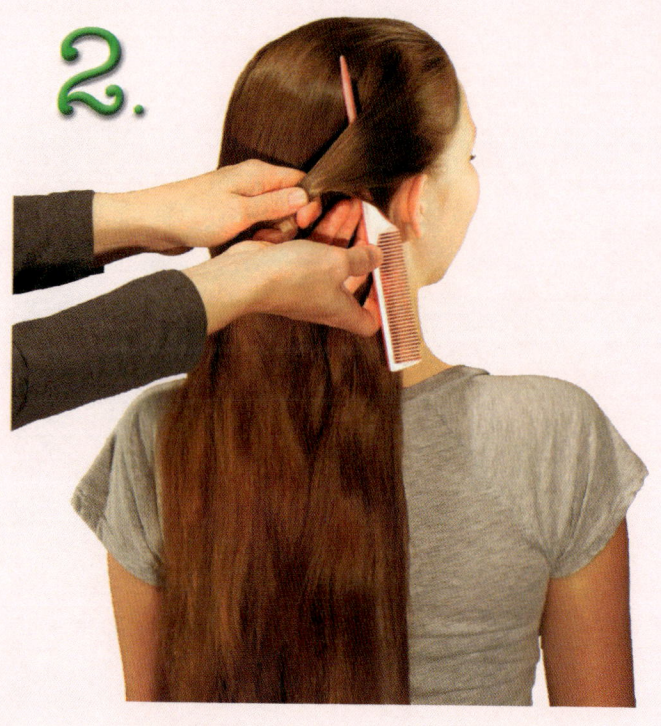

Take a section of hair illustrated.

Pin each rosette.

5.

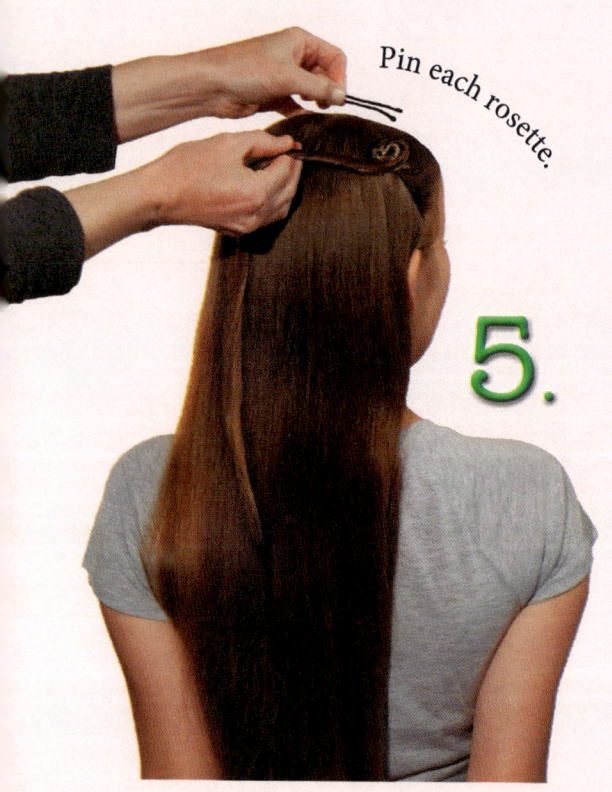

6.

Gather from only one side.

Sliver off a gather from the face all the way back to the braid.

One-Strand Rosette Lace

3.
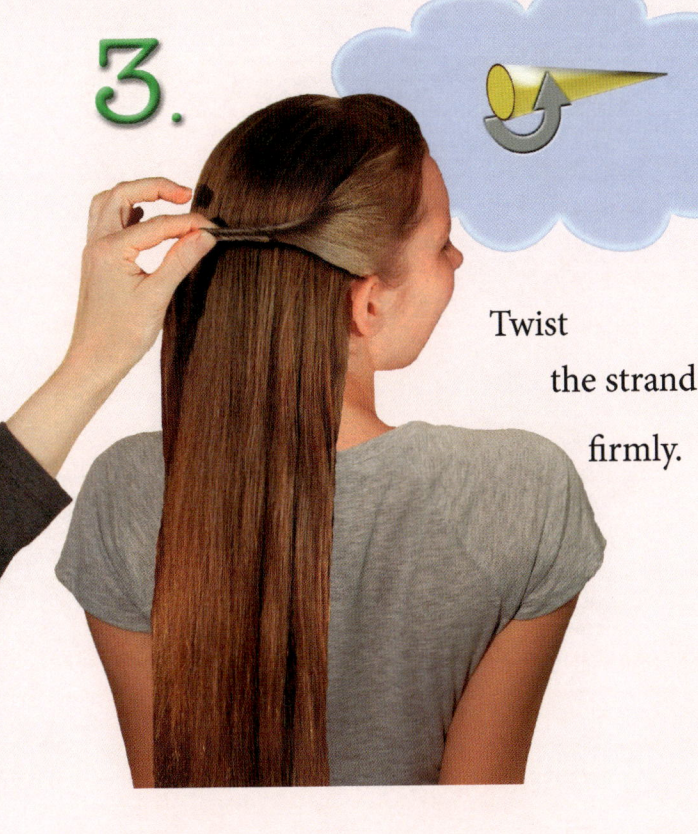
Twist the strand firmly.

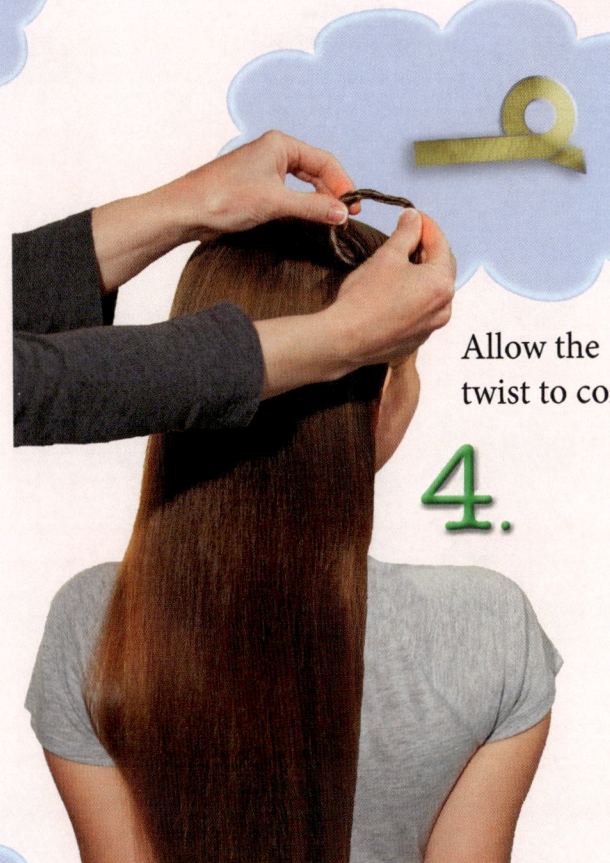
Allow the twist to coil.

4.

7.
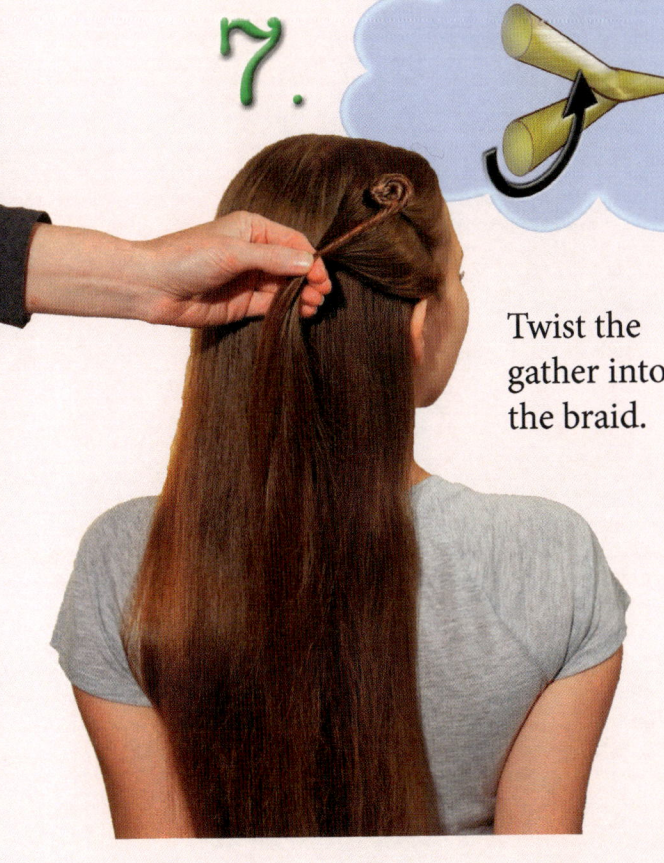
Twist the gather into the braid.

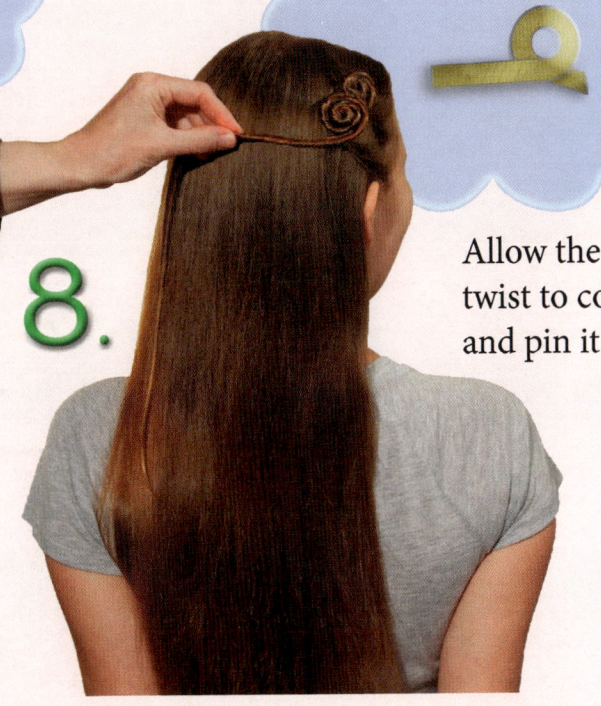
8.
Allow the twist to coil and pin it.

Ways 55

1 part 2. One-Strand Rosette Lace

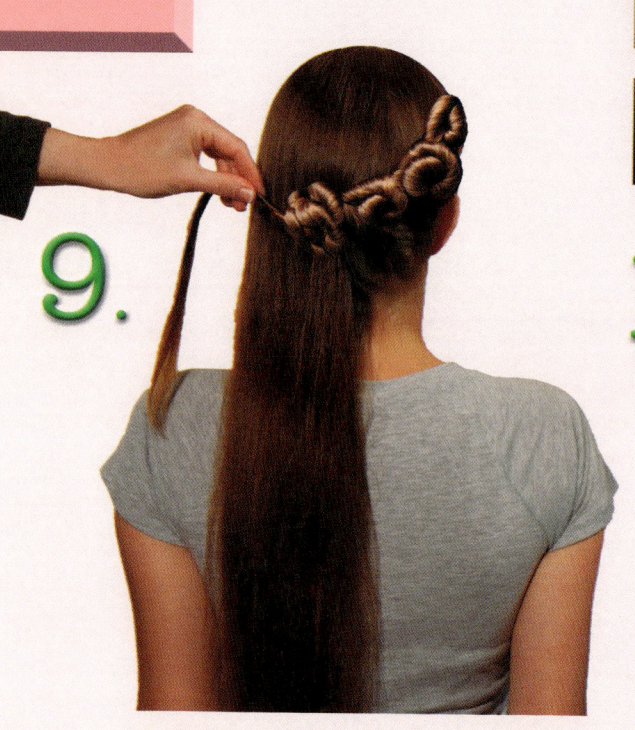

9.

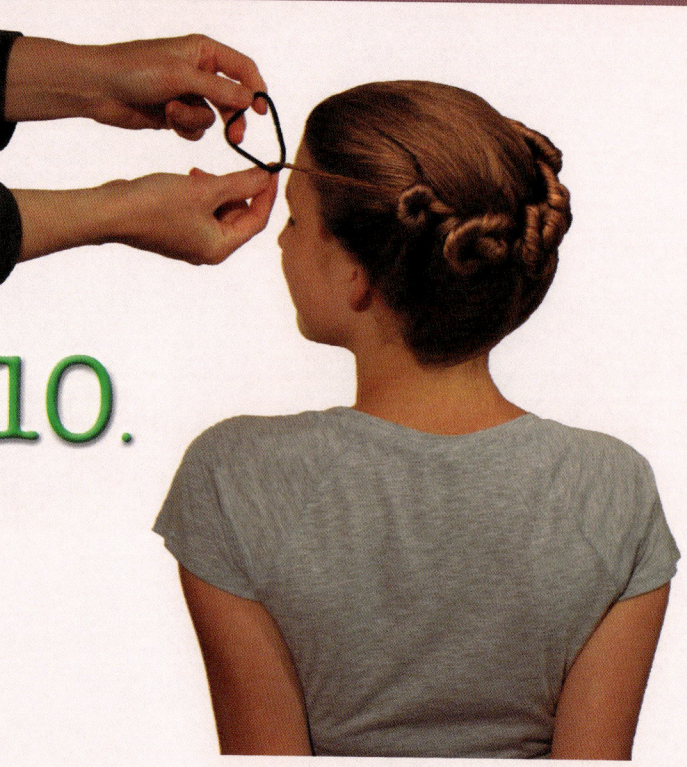

10.

Secure with a rubber band.

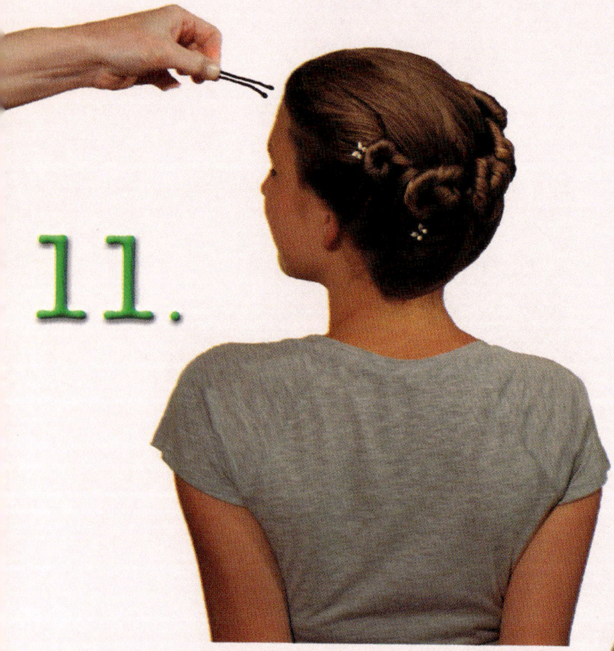

Continue gathering and twisting until you reach the end of the hair.

11.

Fix the end of the braid with bobby pins to hold the braid in place.

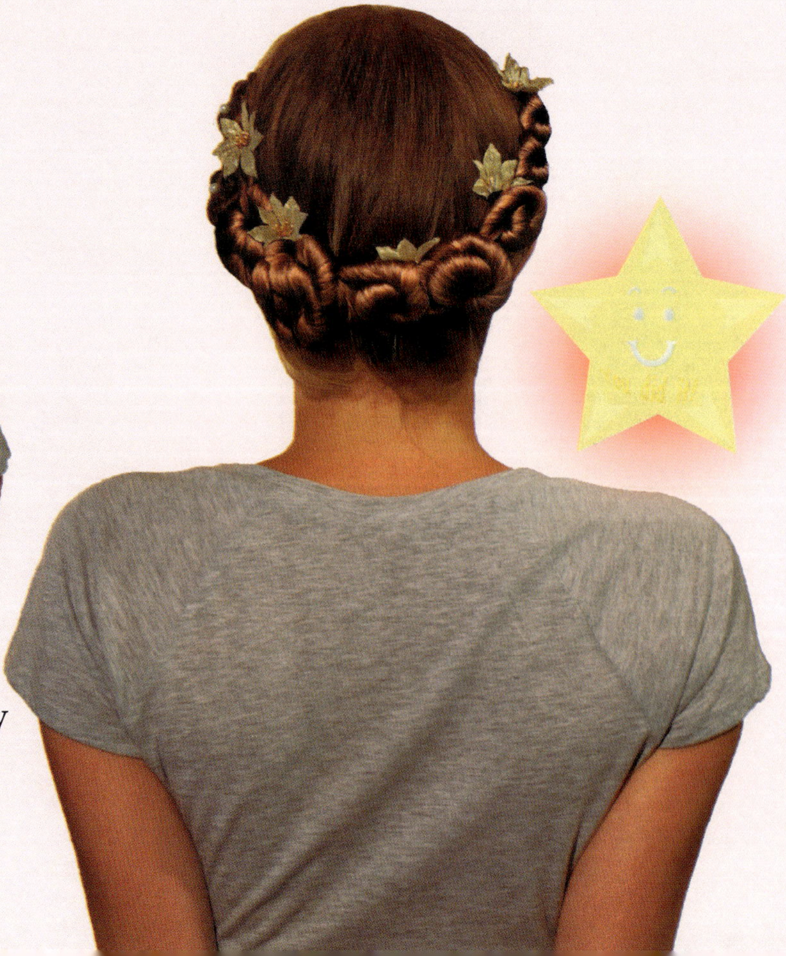

Examples of One-Strand Rosette

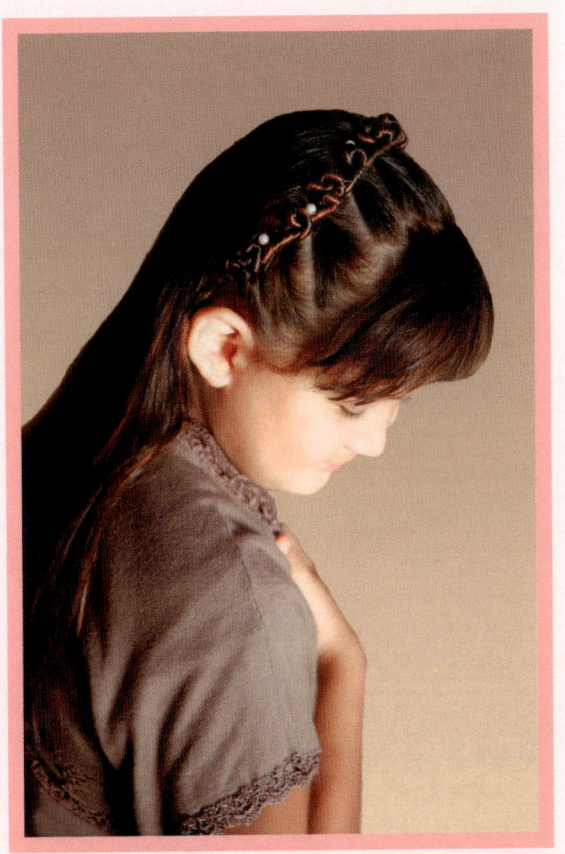
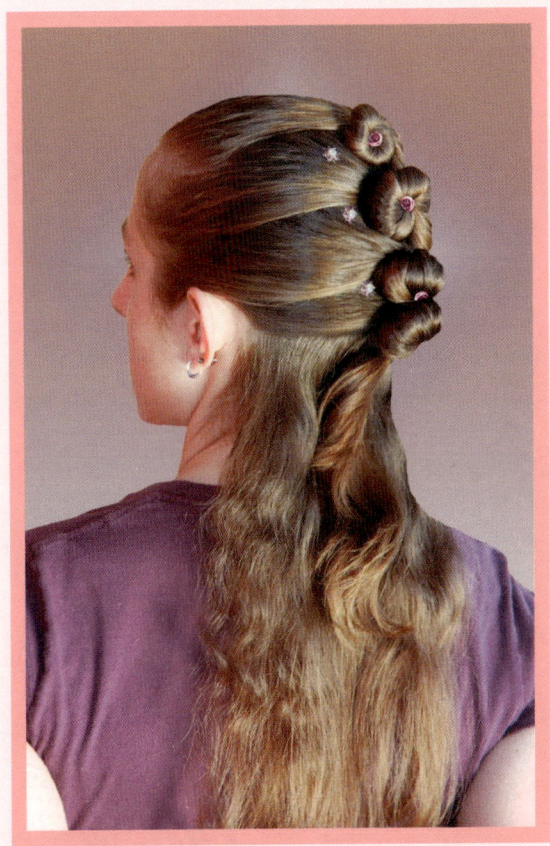
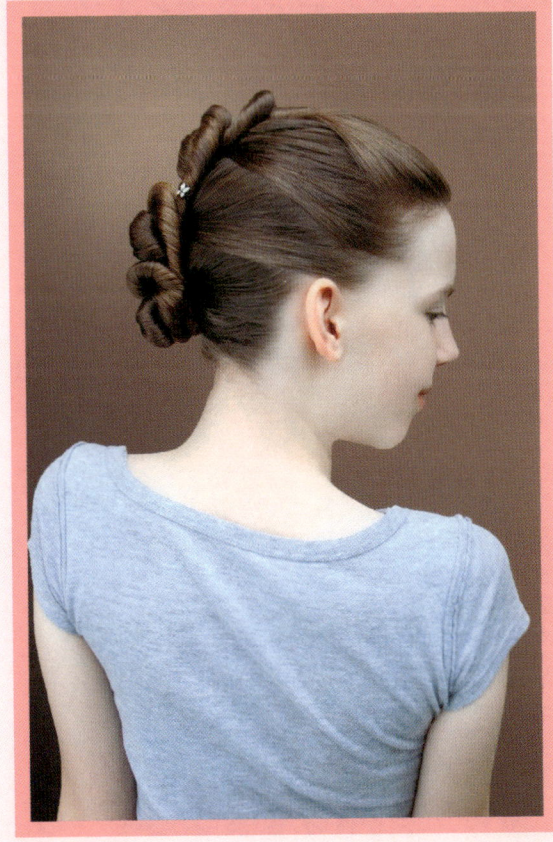
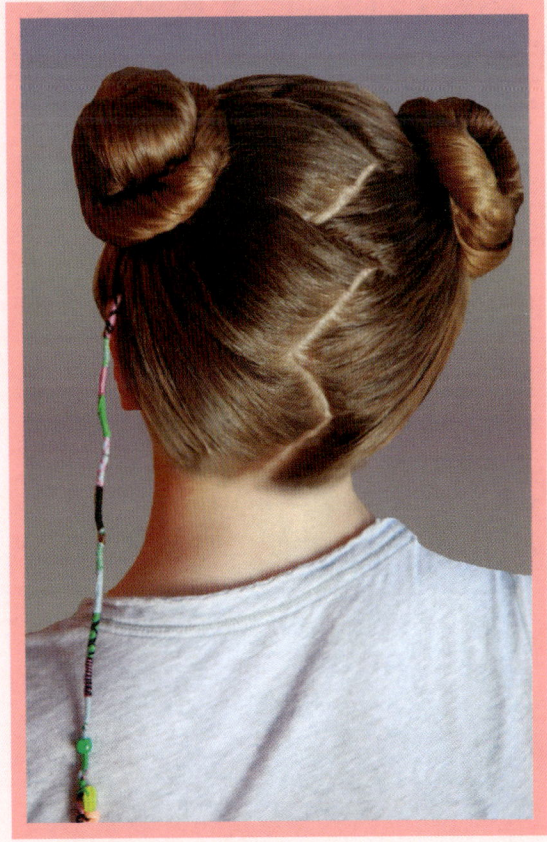

Visit my website to see more examples of the One-Strand Rosette

One-Strand Pretzel

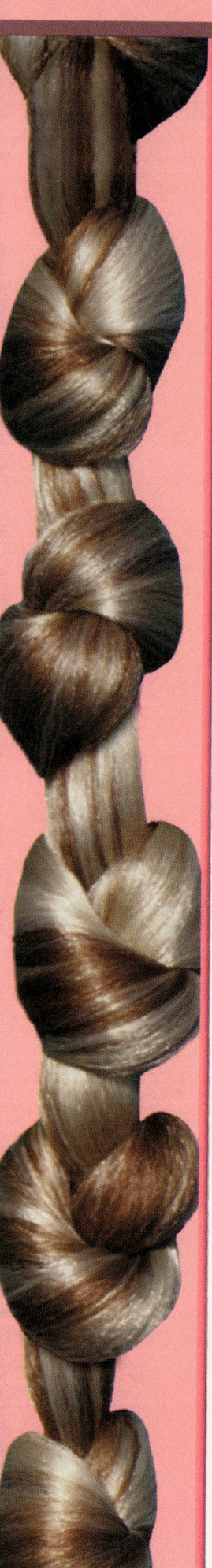

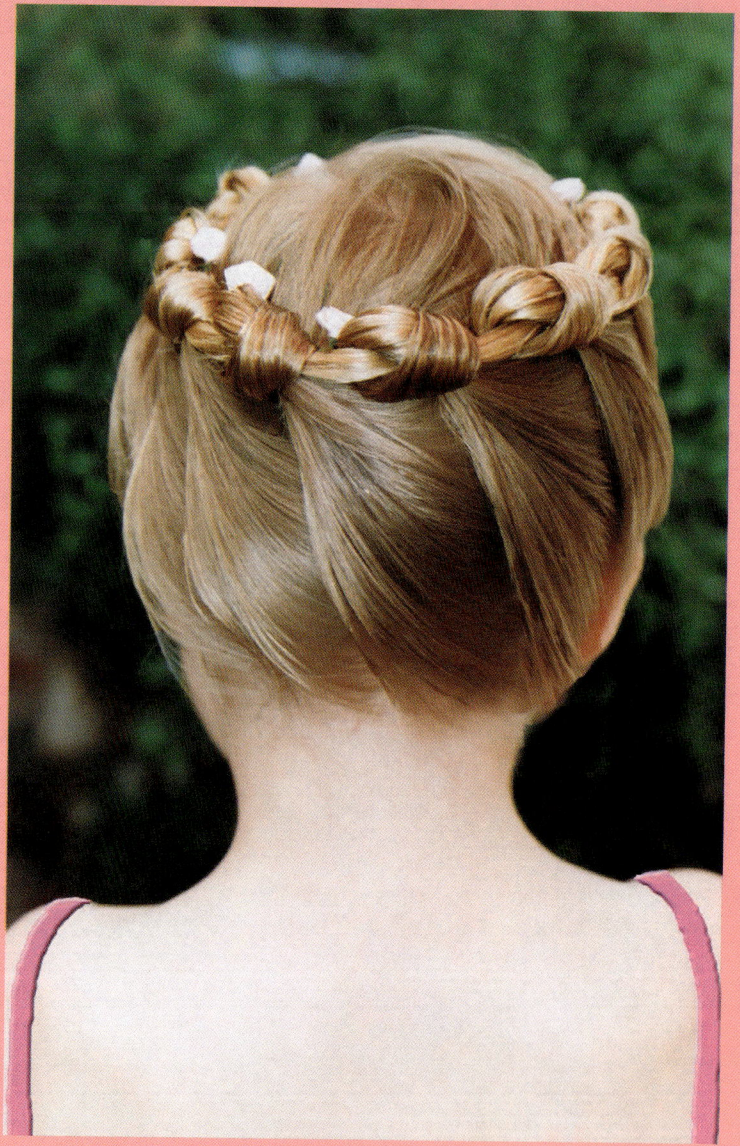

This braid takes practice. It adds a graceful touch to common styles. It can look like a garland. Add it to the flower girls hairstyle or the brides updo.

One-Strand Pretzel

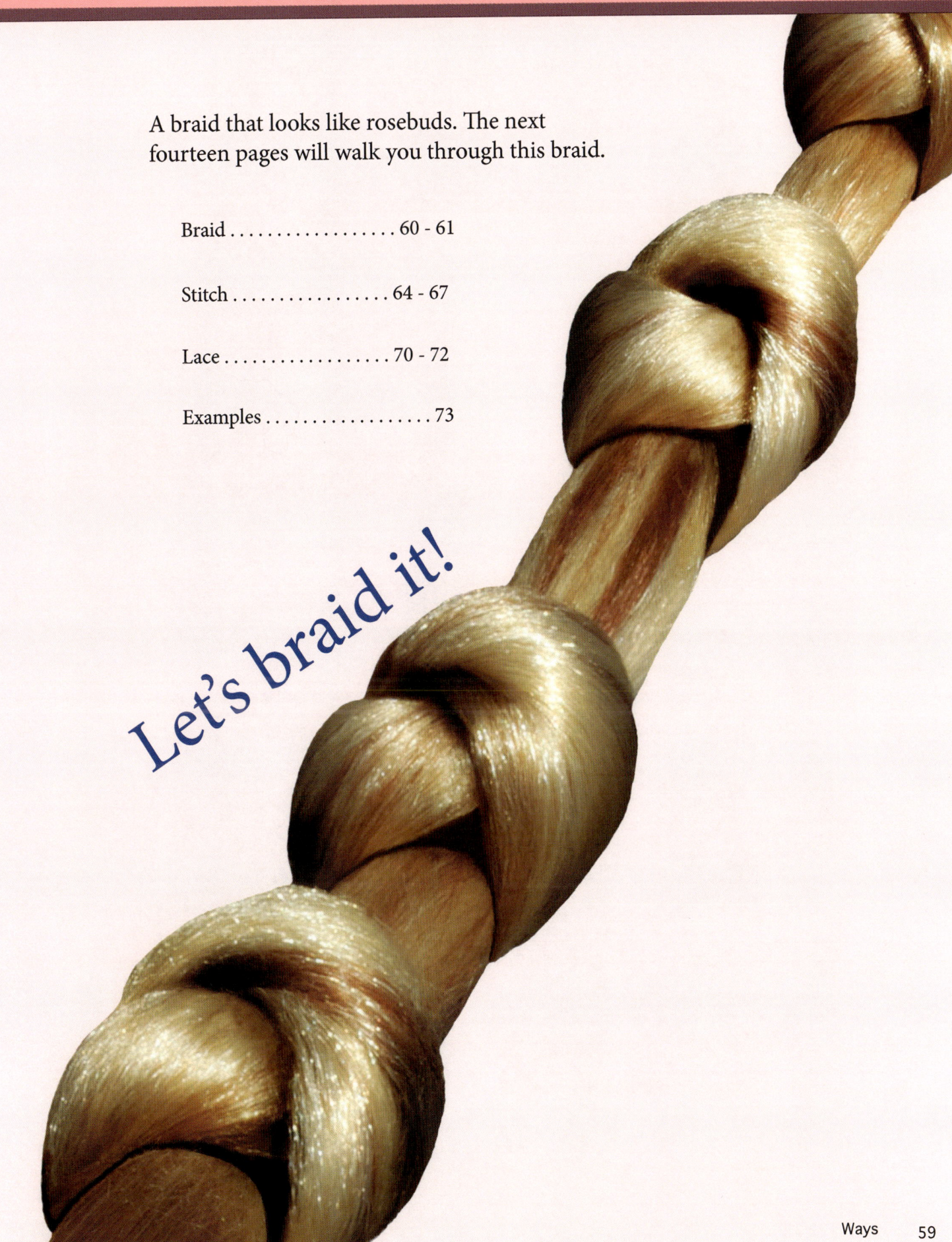

A braid that looks like rosebuds. The next fourteen pages will walk you through this braid.

Braid . . . . 60 - 61

Stitch . . . . 64 - 67

Lace . . . . 70 - 72

Examples 73

Let's braid it!

1 One-Strand Pretzel Braid

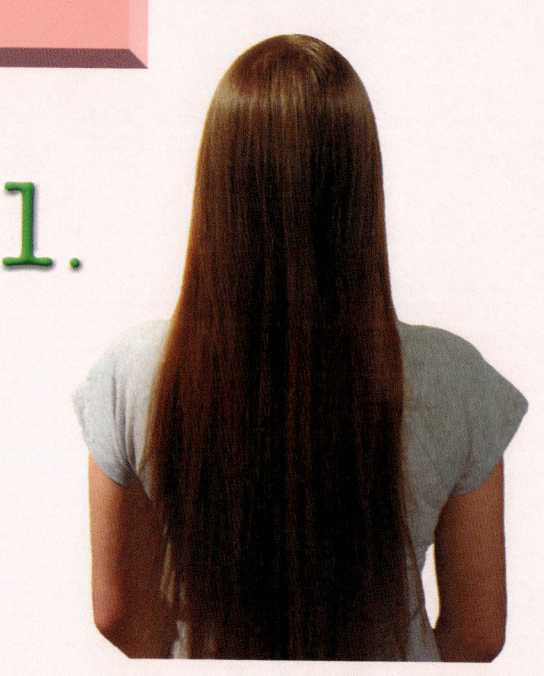

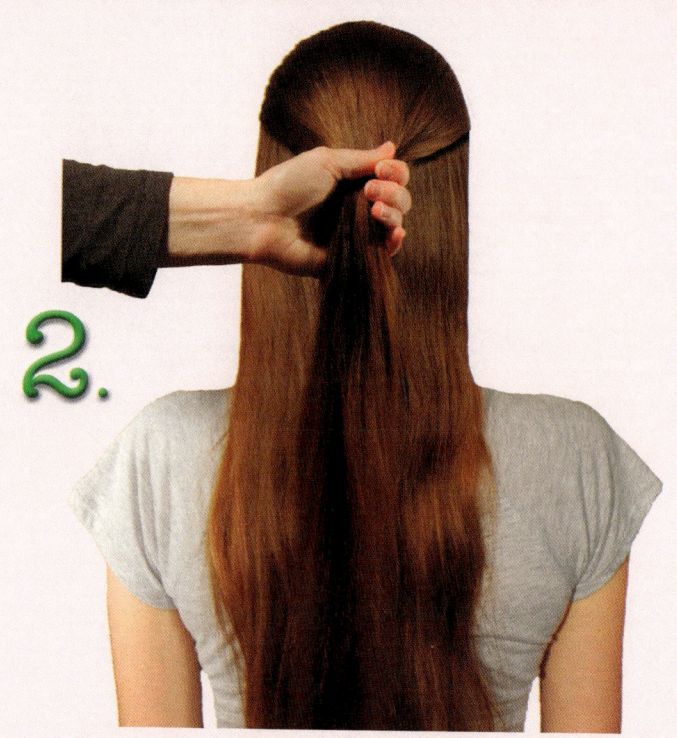

1. Begin with clean, brushed hair.

2. Take a section of hair.

Tuck the end of the braid under the bun to create a tidy, finished look.

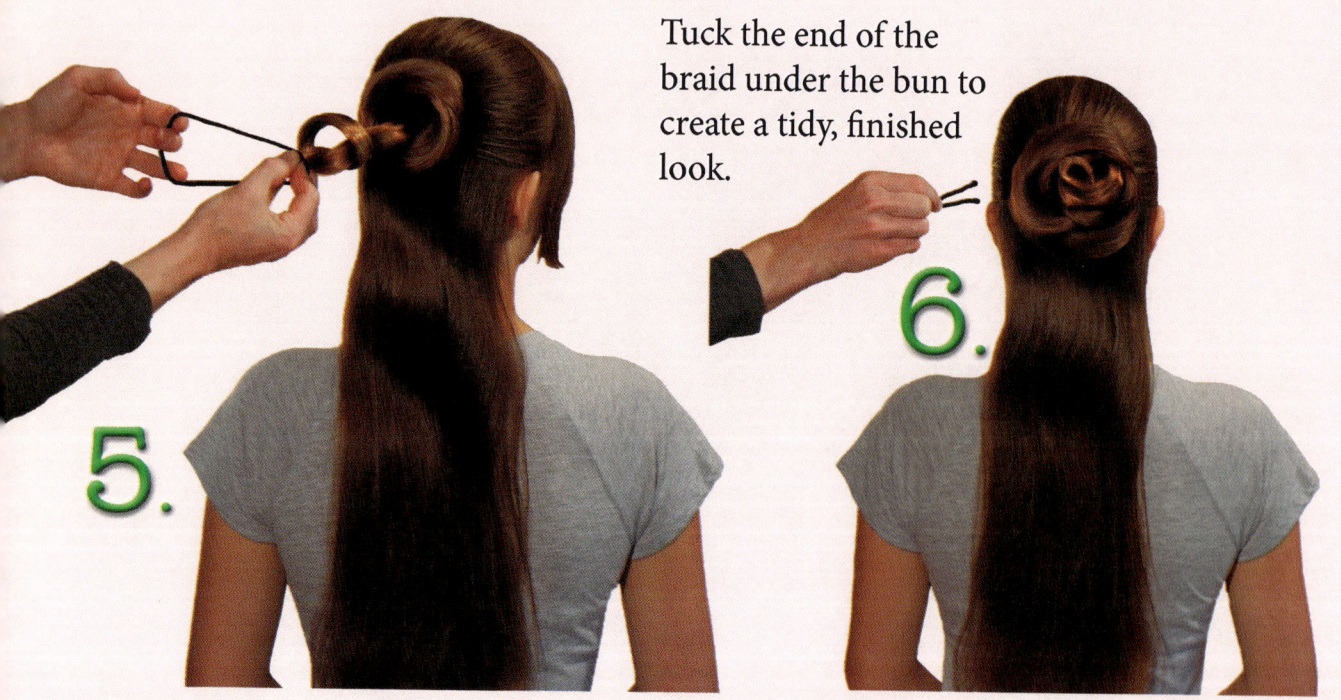

5. Secure with a rubber band.

6. Fix the end of the braid with bobby pins to hold the braid in place.

One-Strand Pretzel Braid

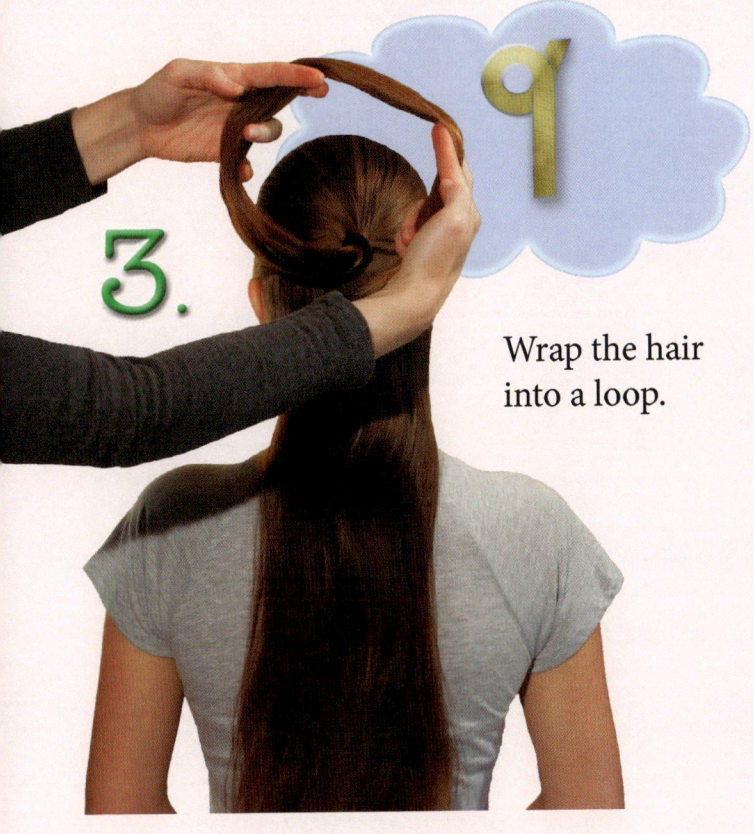

3.

Wrap the hair into a loop.

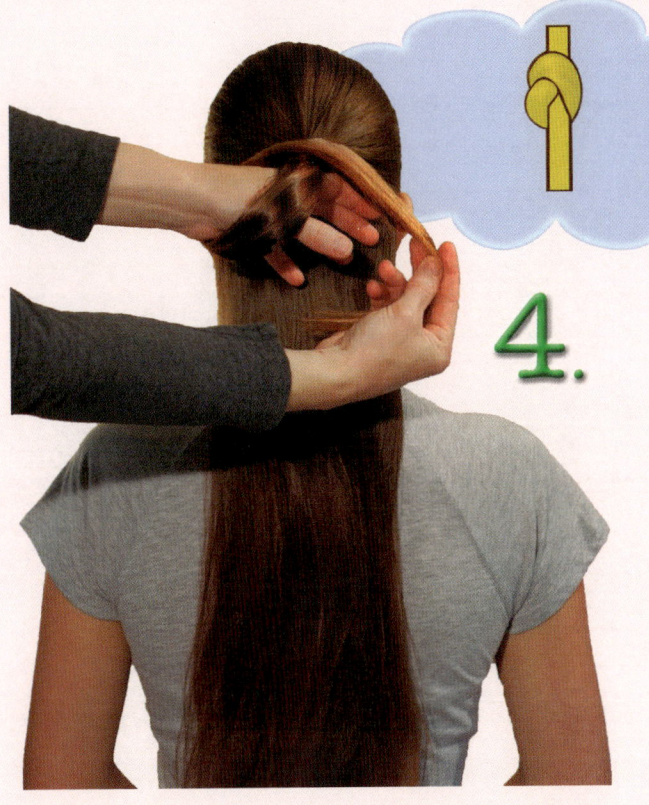

4.

Pull the end of the strand through the loop. Continue creating pretzel knots until you reach the end of the hair.

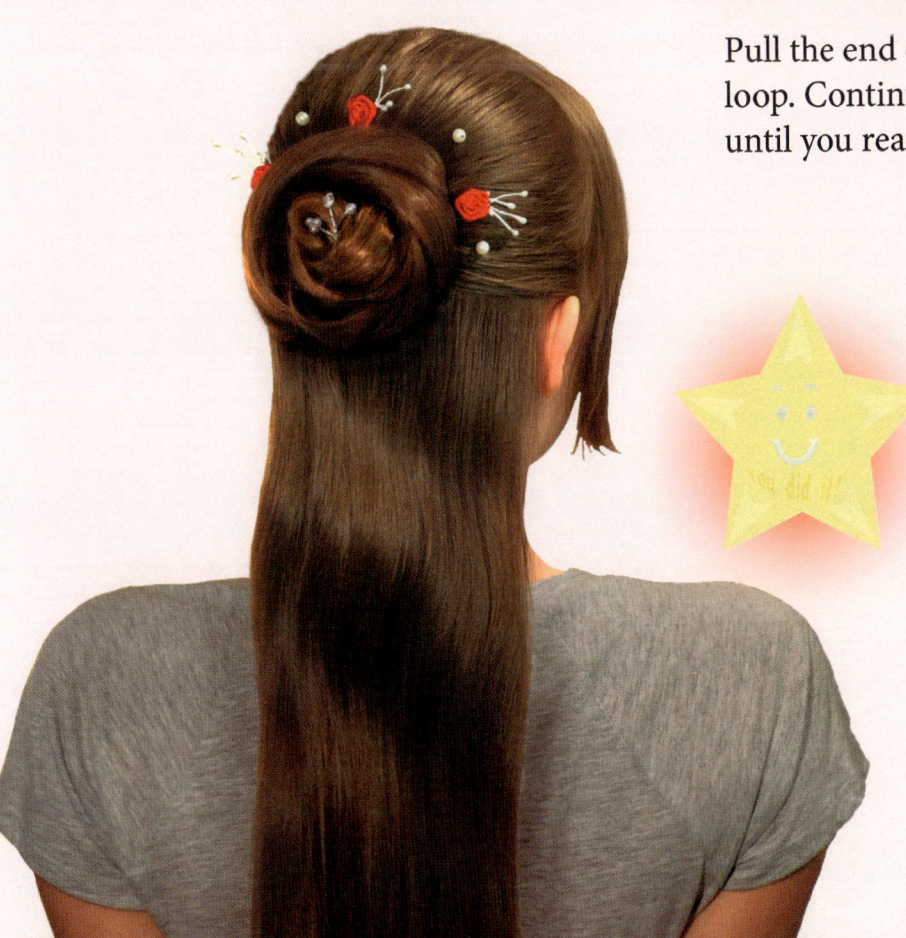

One-Strand Pretzel

Notes

I have seen this technique used in updos and quasi-braiding, but never as a full on braiding technique. I have used it in several photo shoots and clients love it. Many bobby pins are necessary to make this captivating braid sturdy.

One-Strand Pretzel

Gather from both sides

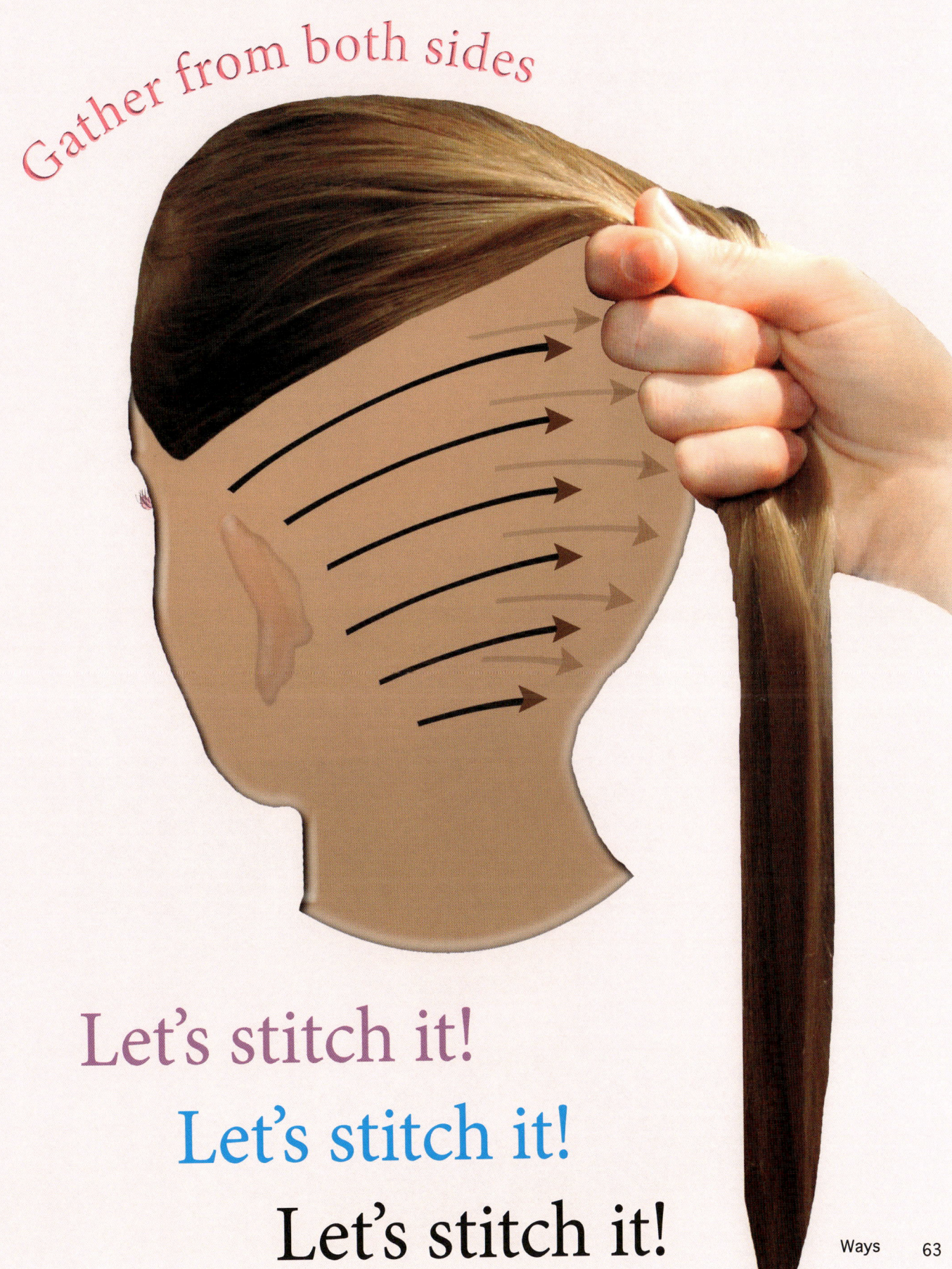

Let's stitch it!

Let's stitch it!

Let's stitch it!

One-Strand Pretzel Stitch

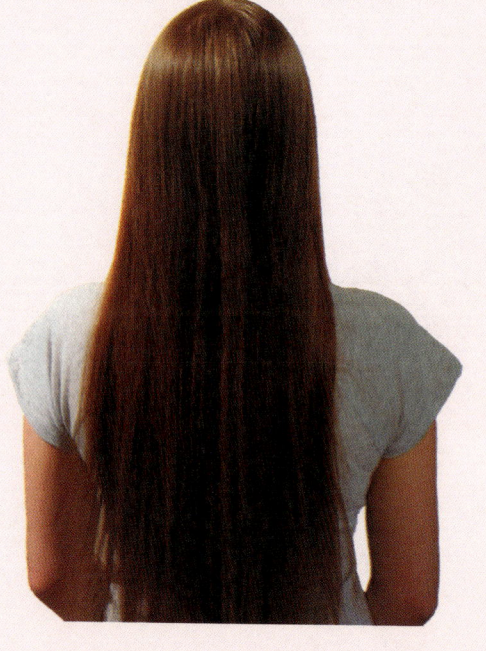

1. Begin with clean, brushed hair.

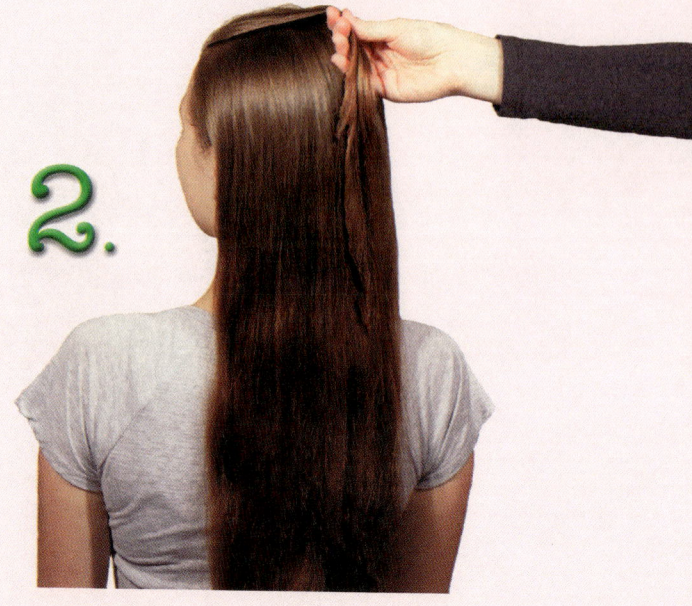

2. Take a section of hair as illustrated.

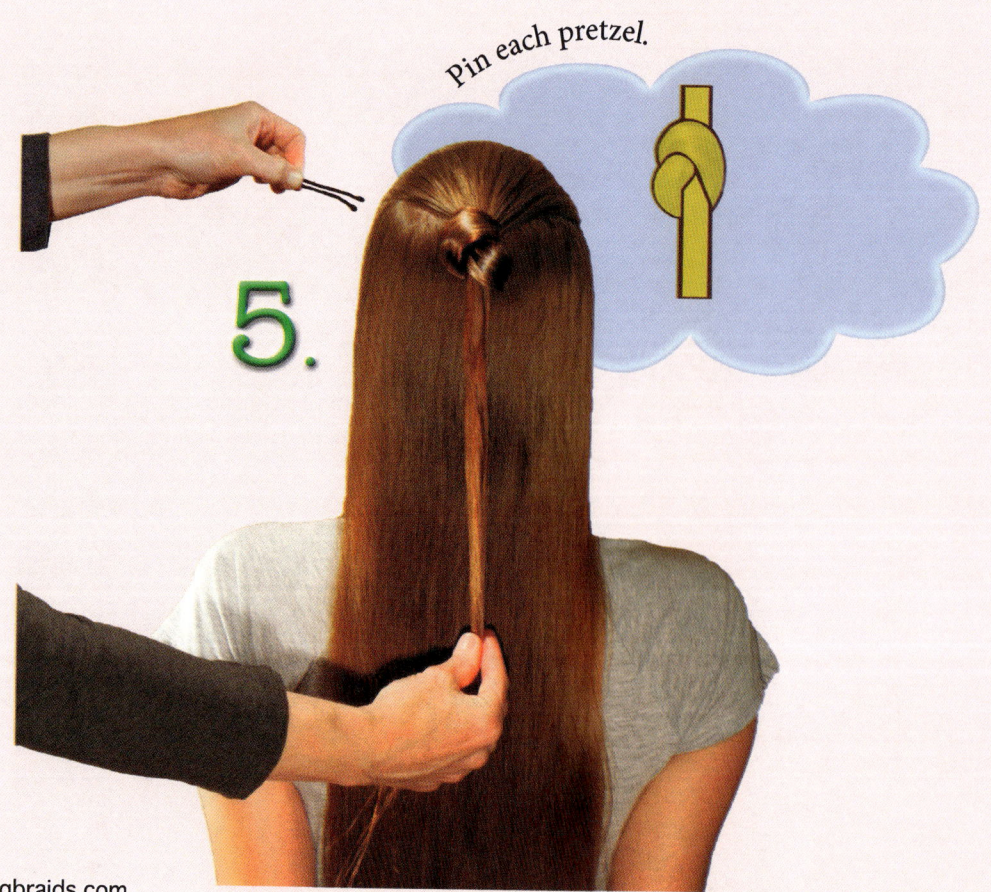

Pin each pretzel.

5.

One-Strand Pretzel Stitch

1

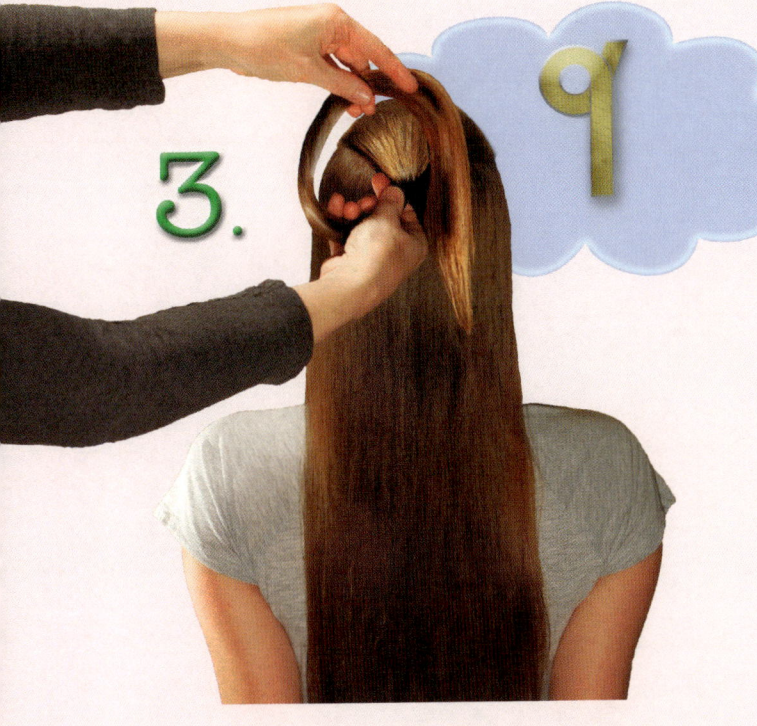

Wrap the hair into a loop.

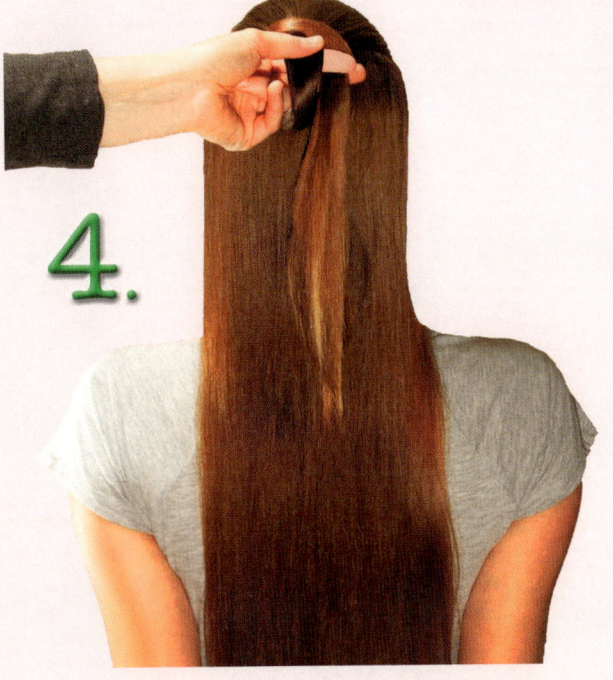

Pull the end through the loop.

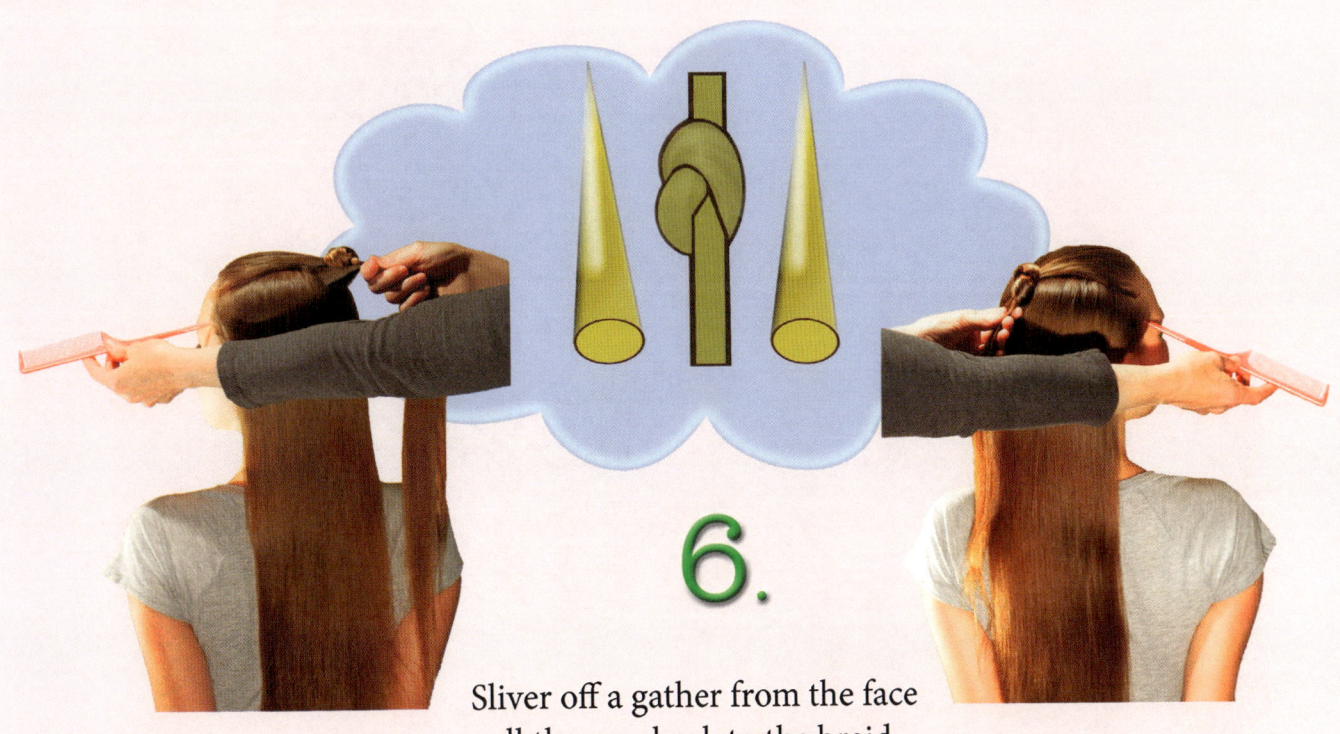

Sliver off a gather from the face
all the way back to the braid.
Gather into the braid from both sides.

1 Continuing

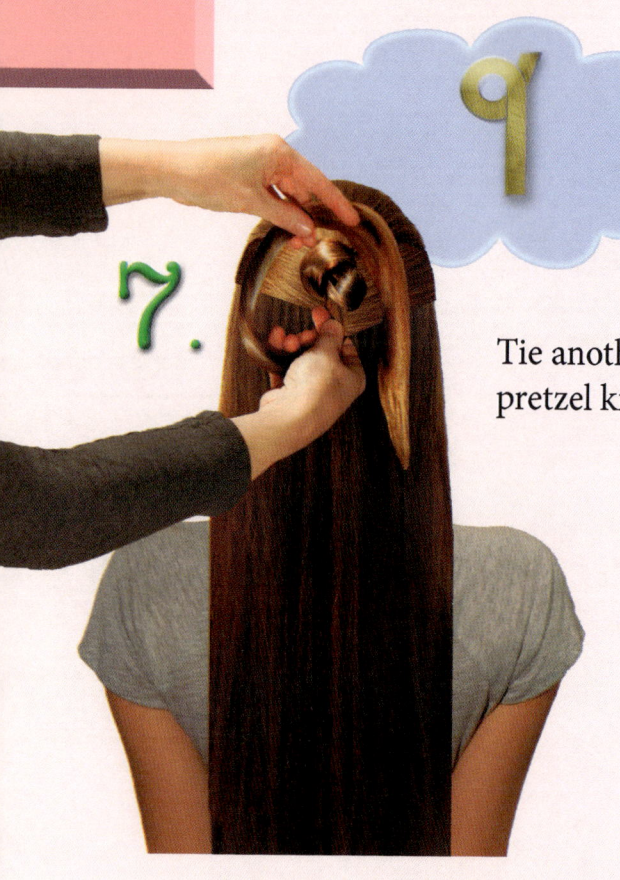

7.

9.

Tie another pretzel knot.

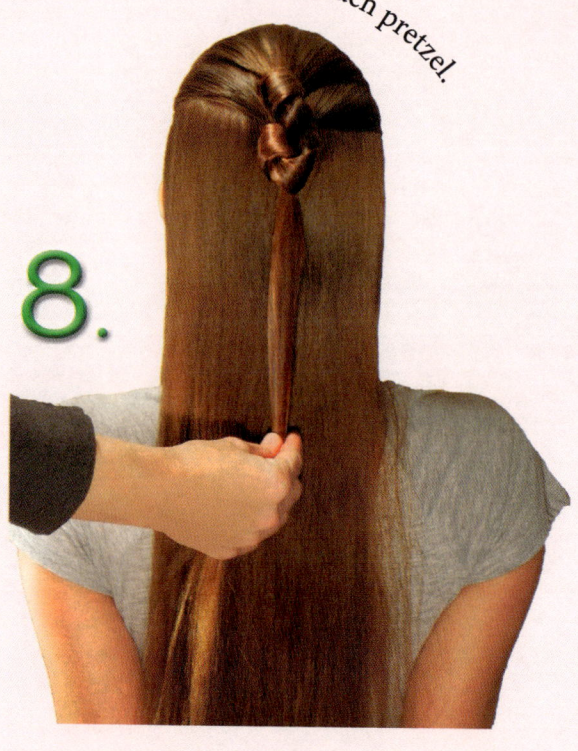

8.

Pin each pretzel.

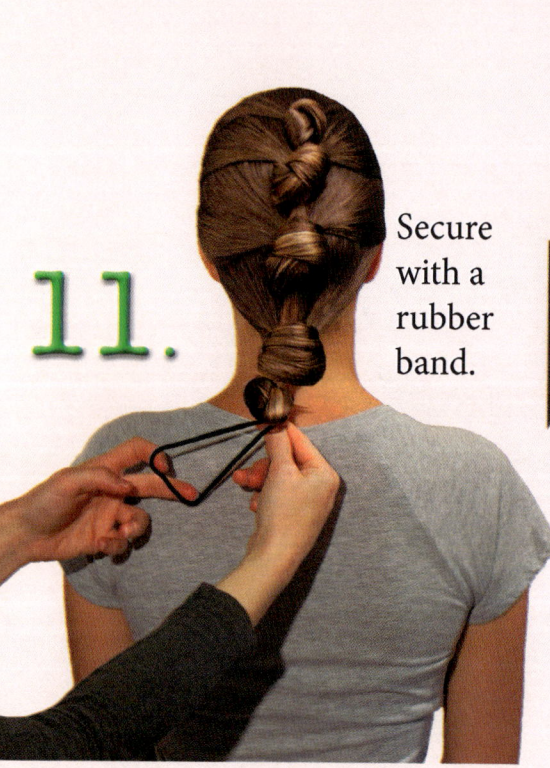

11.

Secure with a rubber band.

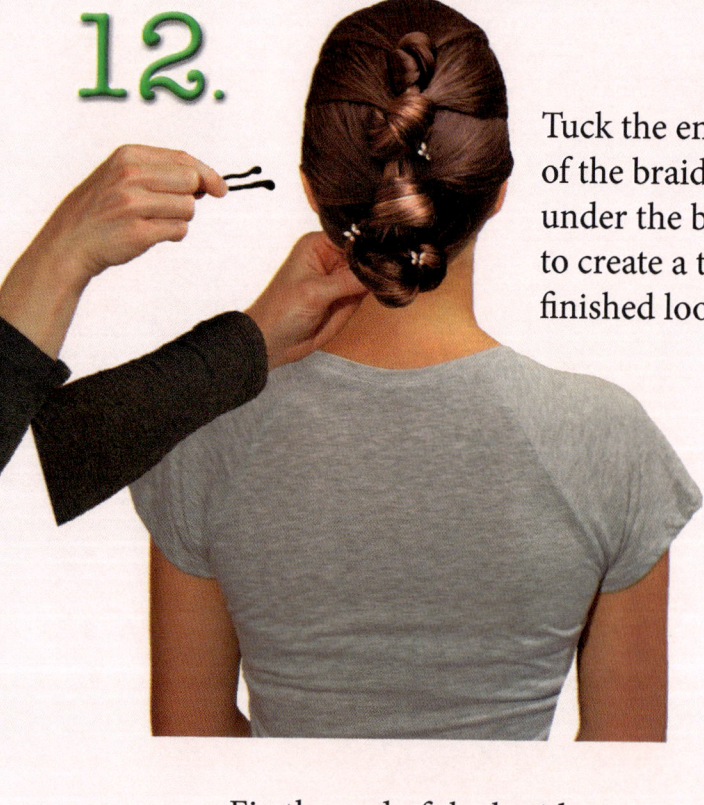

12.

Tuck the end of the braid under the bun to create a tidy finished look.

Fix the end of the braid with bobby pins to hold the braid in place.

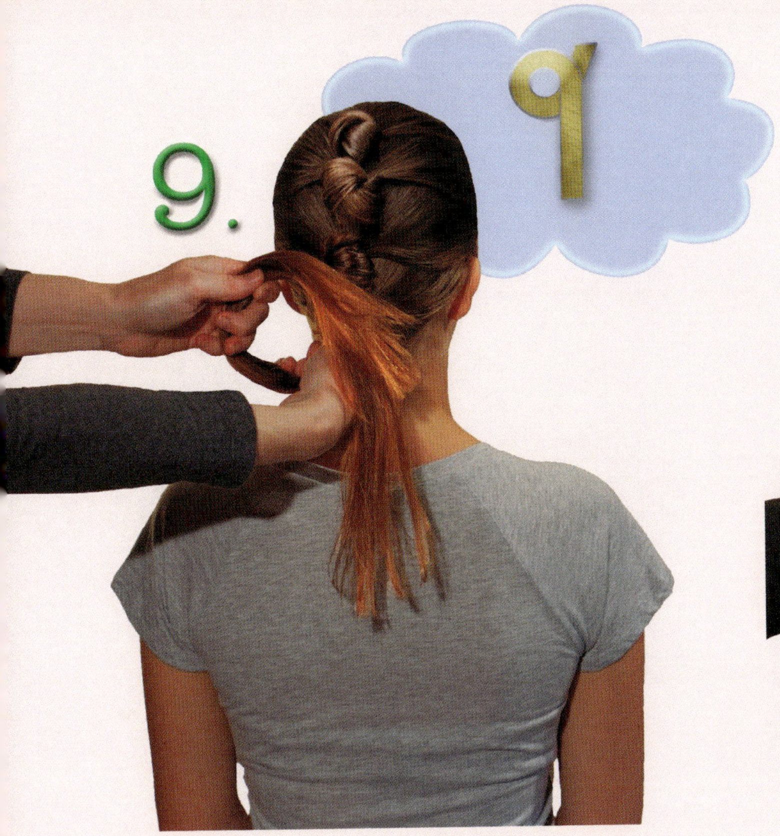

part 2. One-Strand Pretzel Stitch

9.

10.

Continue gathering and looping 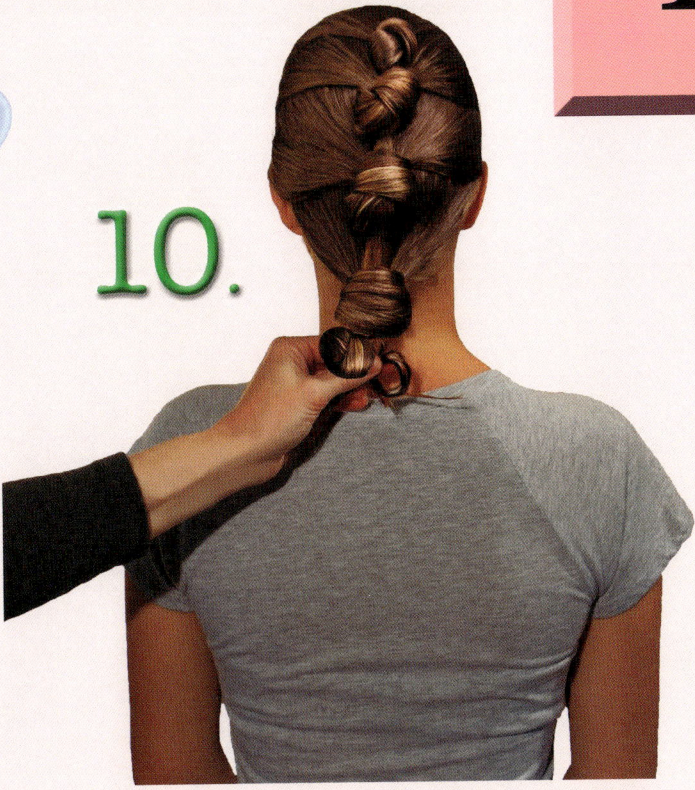 until you reach the end of the hair.

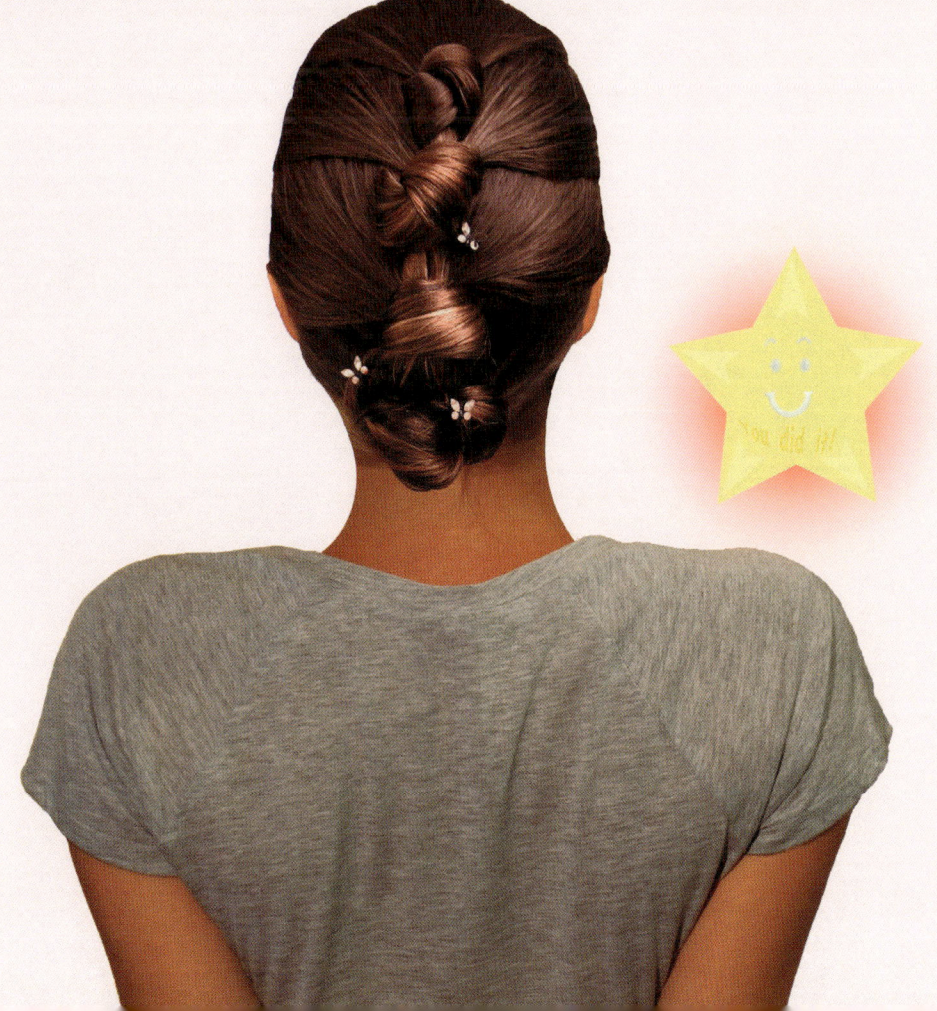

Ways 67

One-Strand Pretzel

Notes

One-Strand Pretzel

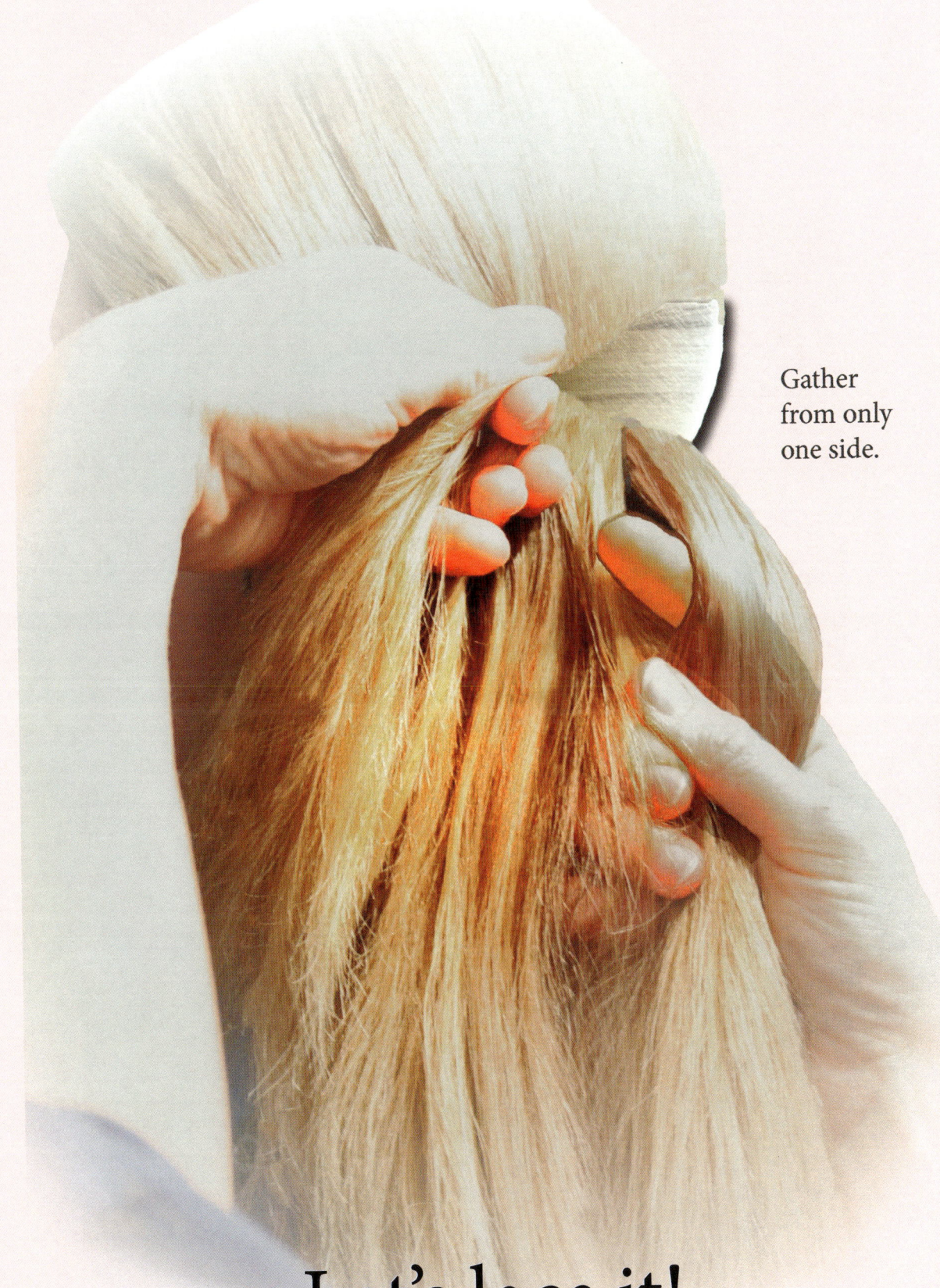

Gather from only one side.

Let's lace it!

1 — One-Strand Pretzel Lace

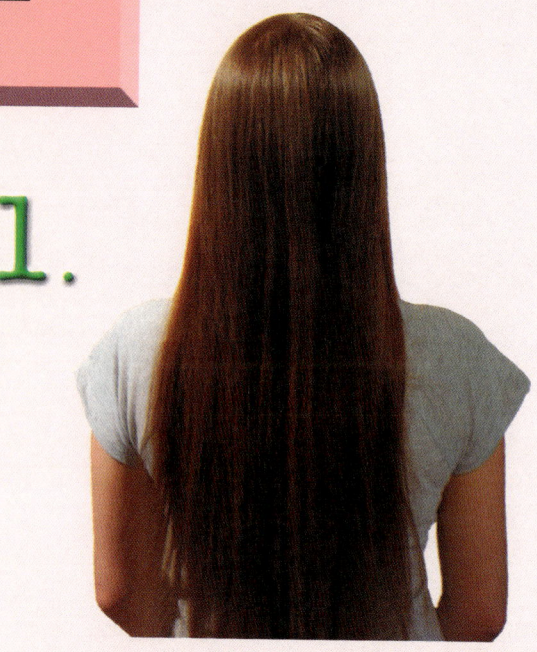

1. Begin with clean, brushed hair.

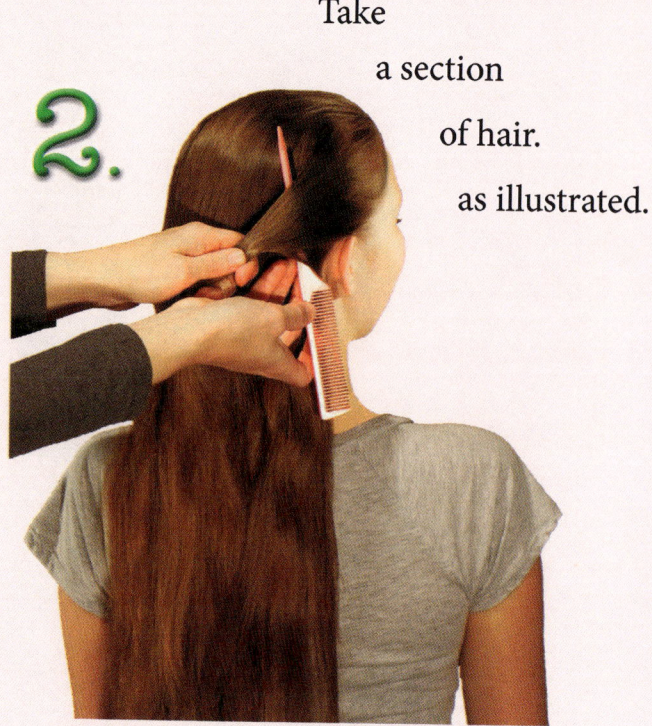

2. Take a section of hair. as illustrated.

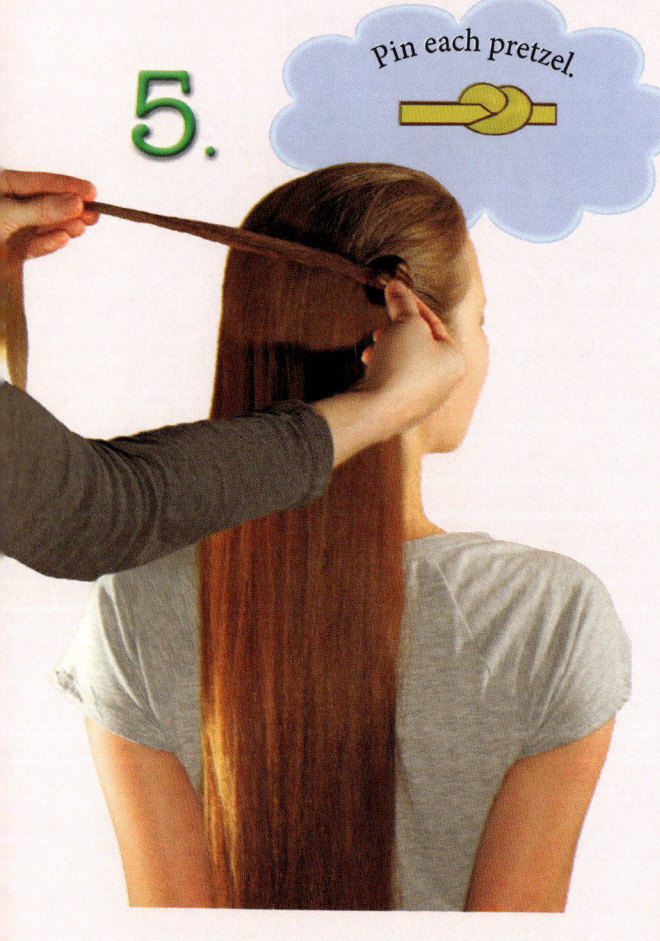

5. Pin each pretzel.

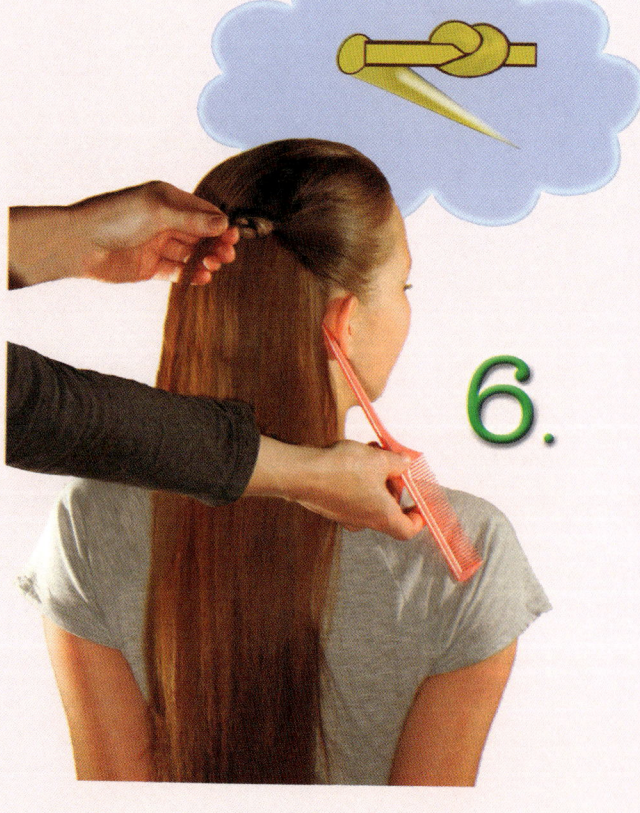

6. Sliver off a gather from the face all the way back to the braid.

One-Strand Pretzel Lace

1

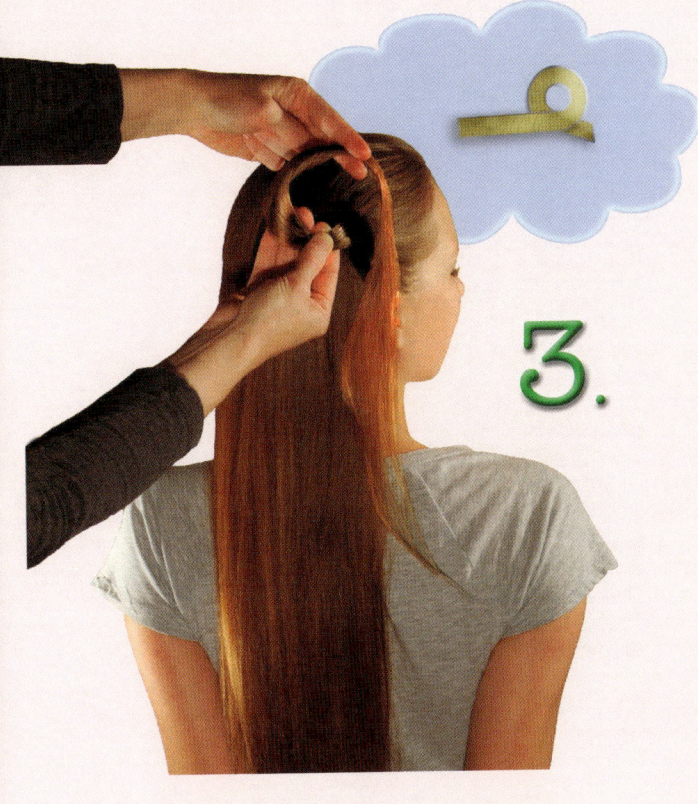

3.

Wrap the hair into a loop.

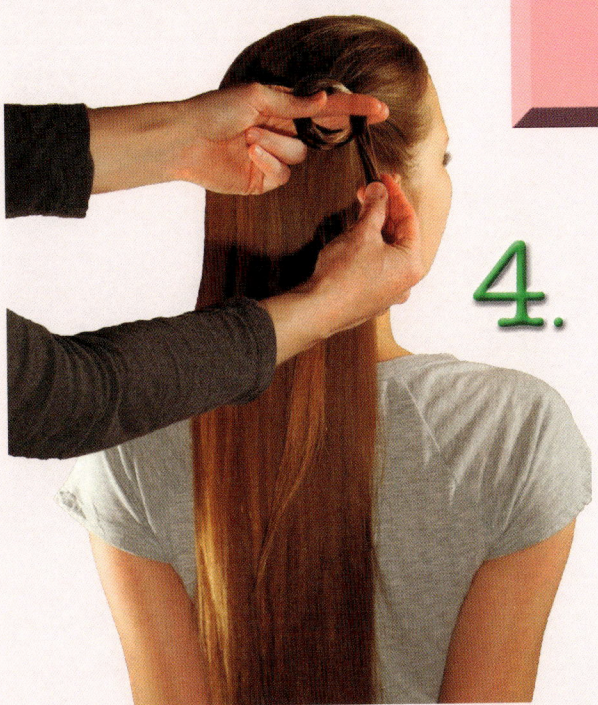

4.

Pull the end through the loop.

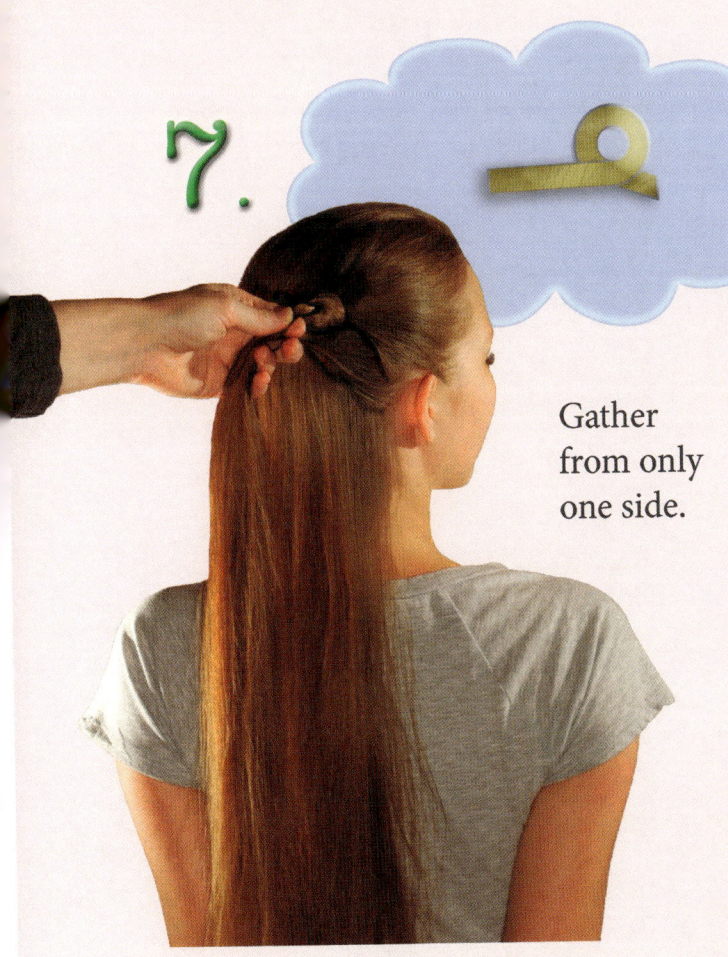

7.

Gather from only one side.

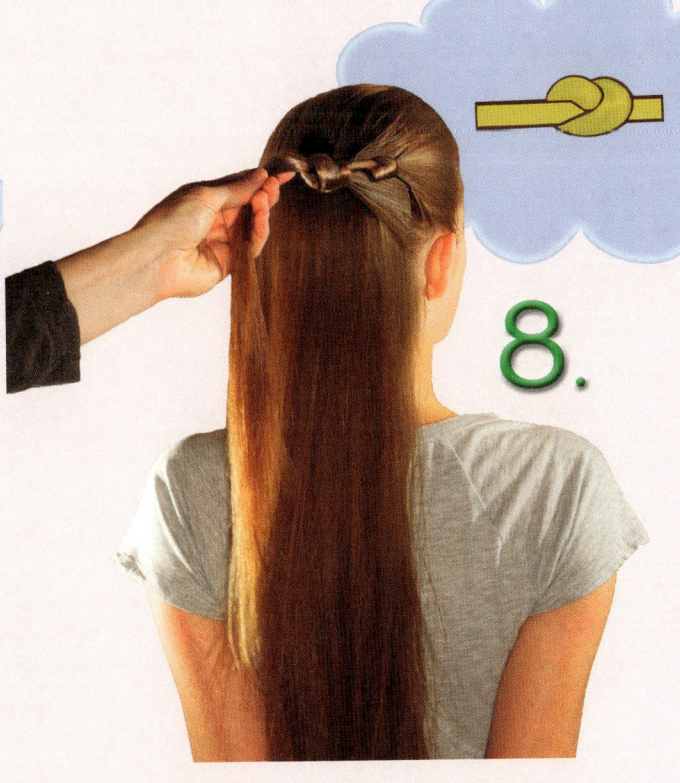

8.

Create the next pretzel knot with both the strand and the gather.

1 part 2. One-Strand Pretzel Lace

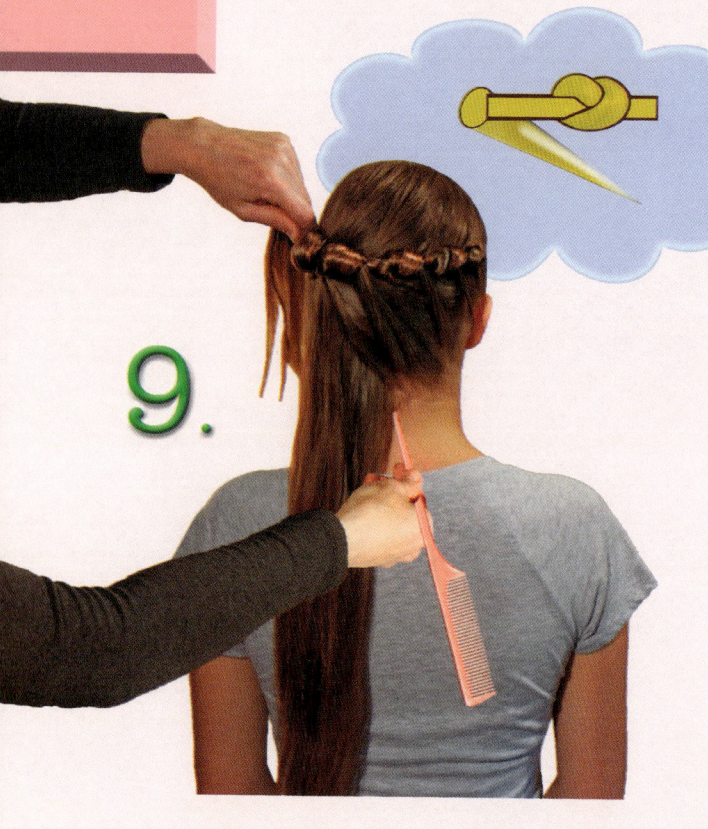

9. Continue gathering and tying until you reach the end of the hair.

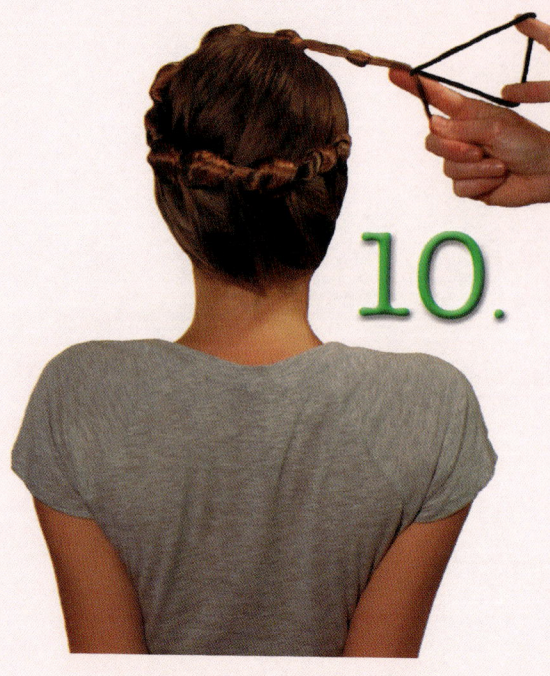

10. Secure with a rubber band.

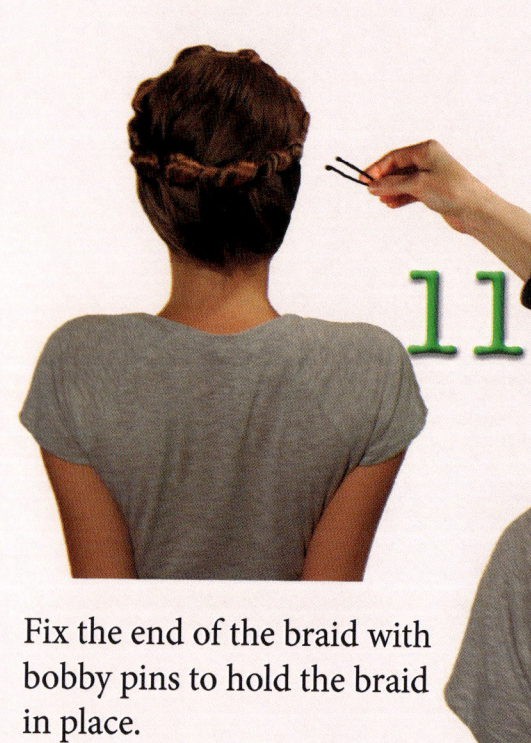

11. Fix the end of the braid with bobby pins to hold the braid in place.

Examples of One-Strand Pretzel

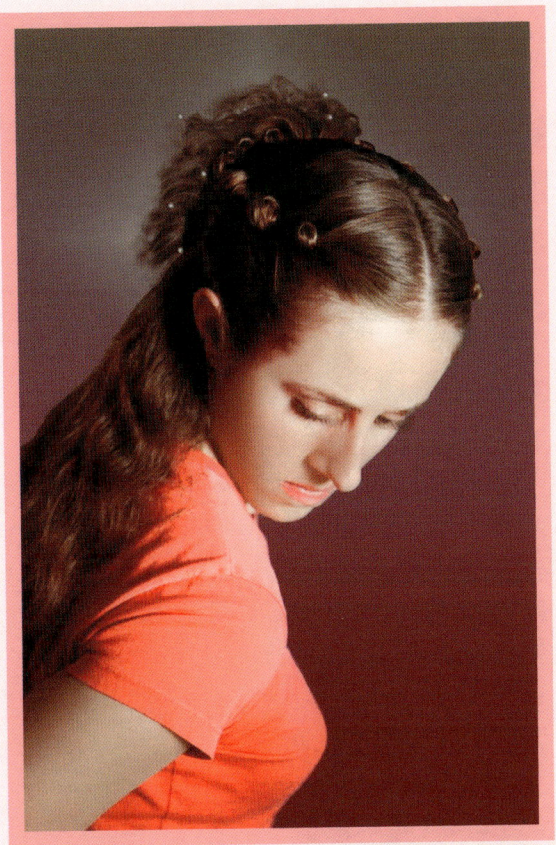
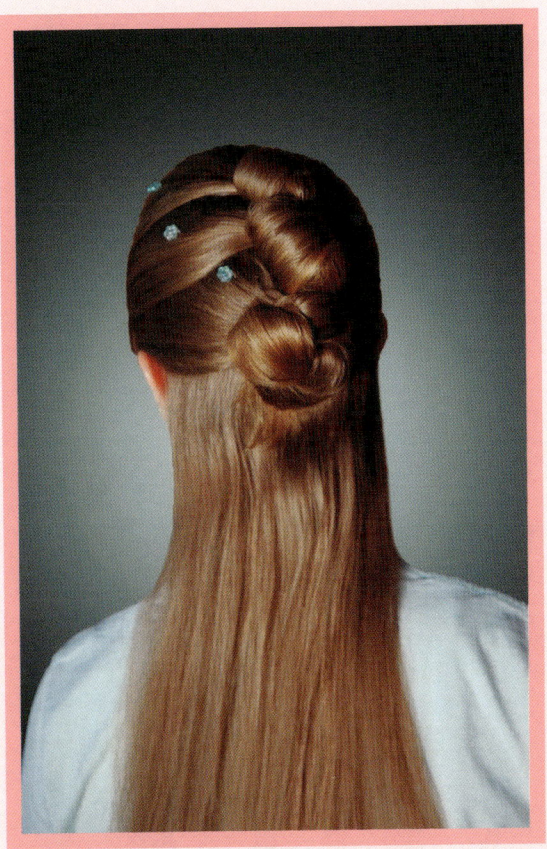
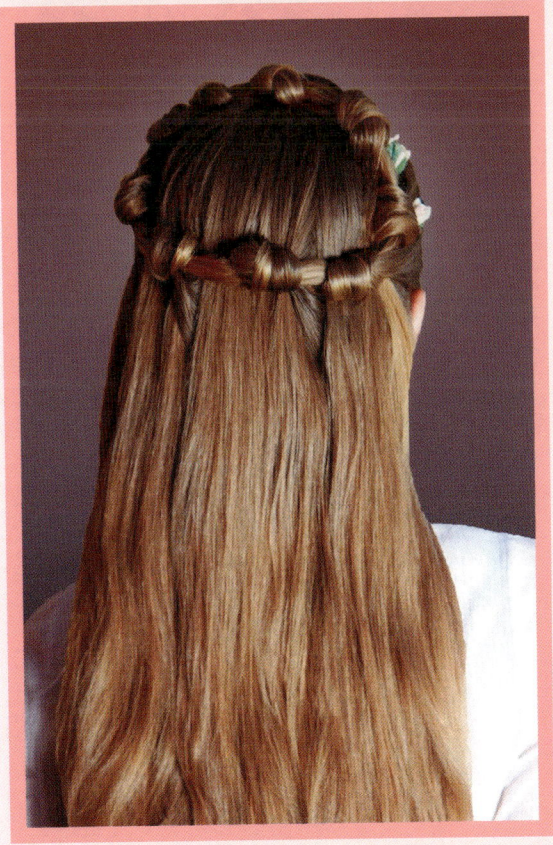
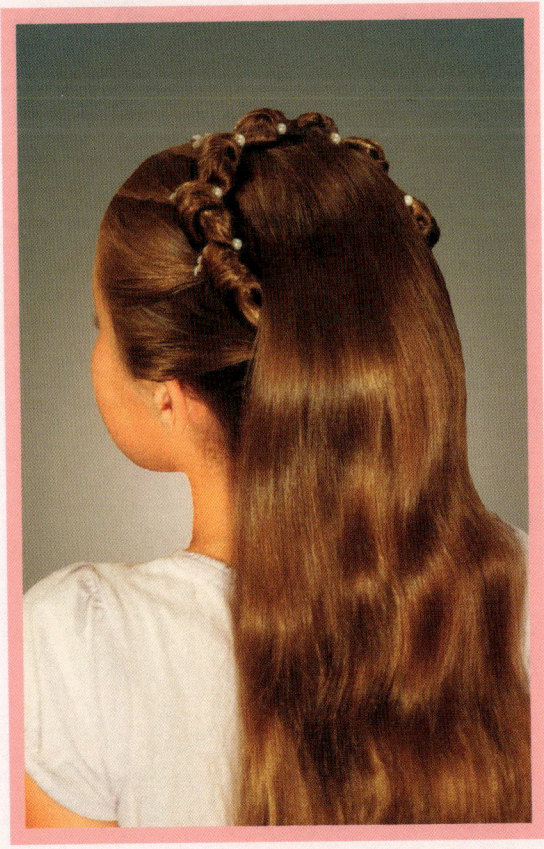

Visit my website to see more examples of the One-Strand Pretzel

Two-Strand Knot

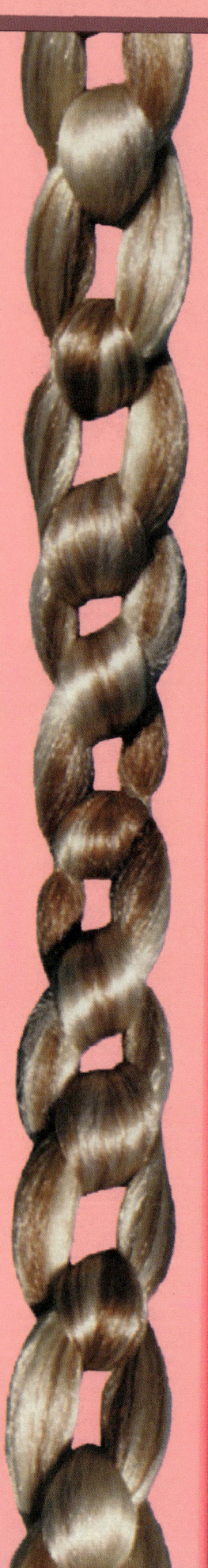

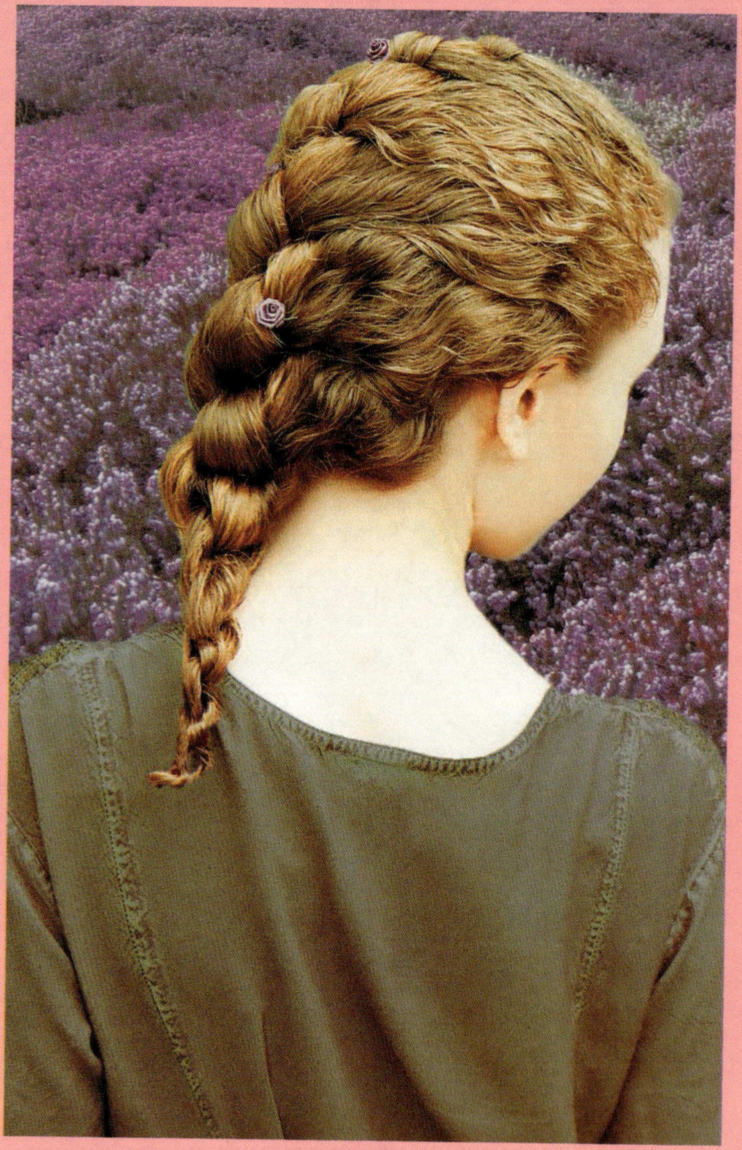

A fun and unique way to braid that seems to have become more popular with the internet. Gel and hairspray retain this way of braiding for the day.

Two-Strand Knot

A braid that looks like a chain. The next fourteen pages will walk you through this braid.

Braid . . . . 76 - 77

Stitch . . . . 80 - 82

Lace . . . . 84 - 87

Examples 89

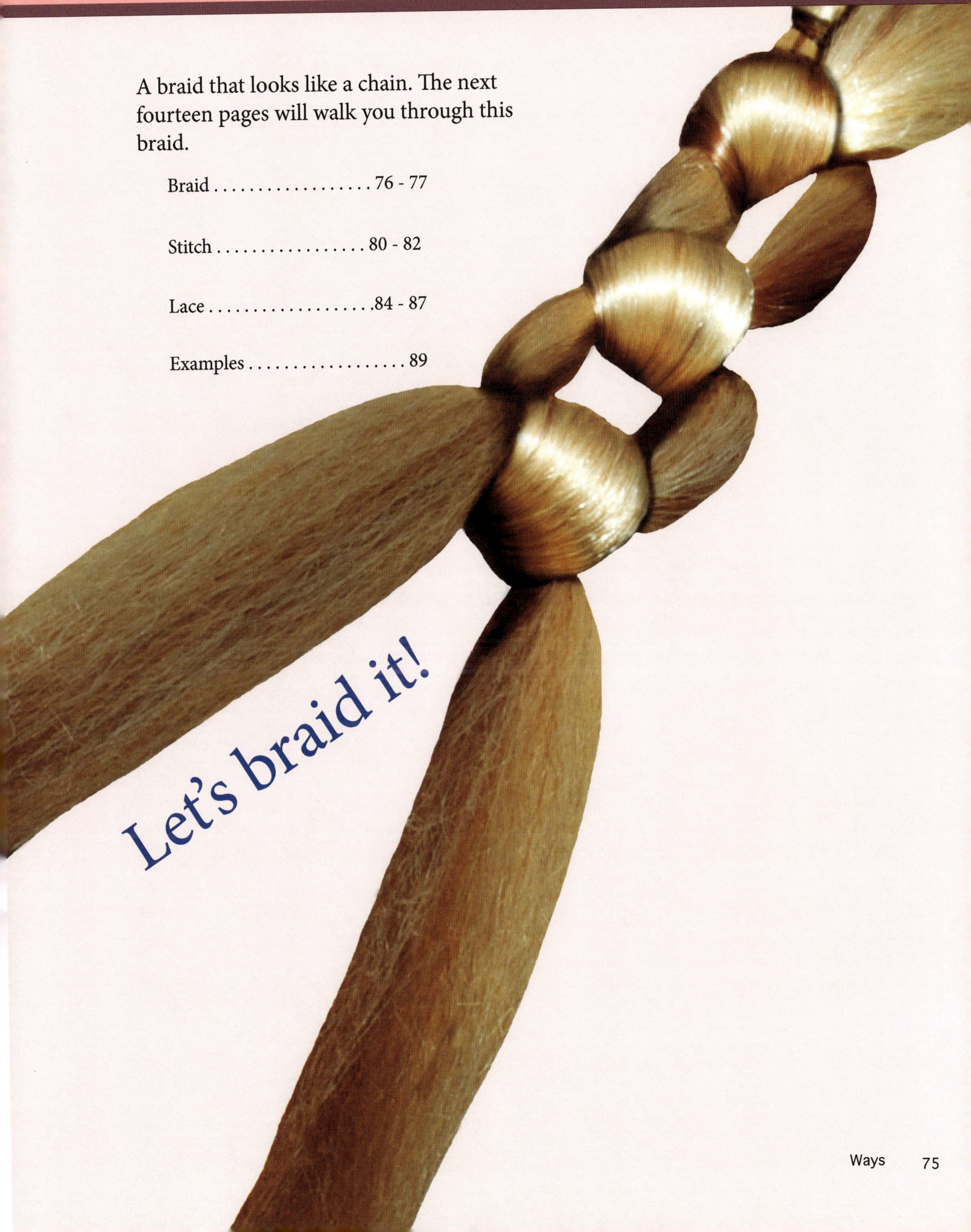

Let's braid it!

Two-Strand Knot Braid

1.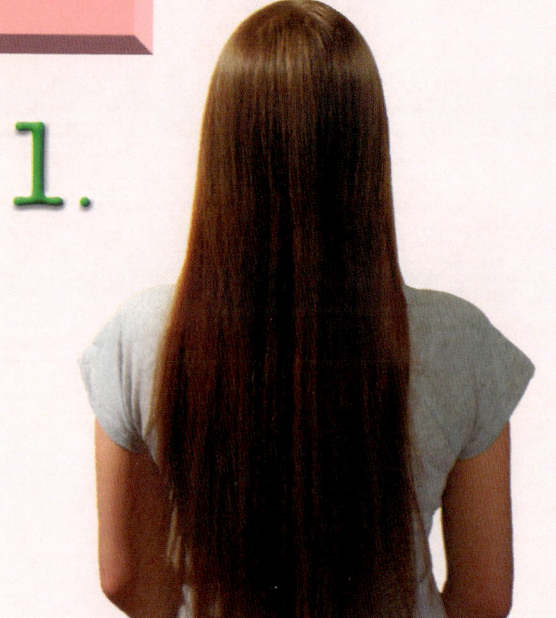

Begin with clean, brushed hair.

2.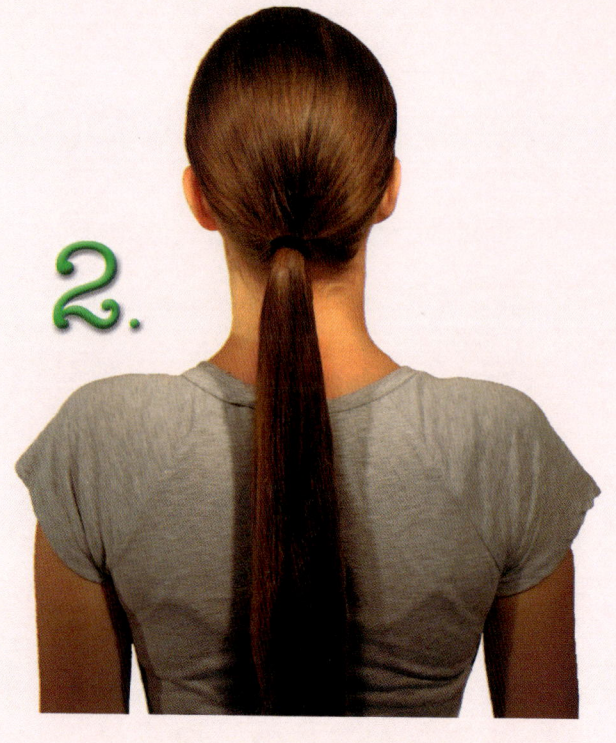

Take a section of hair.

5. Secure with a rubber band.

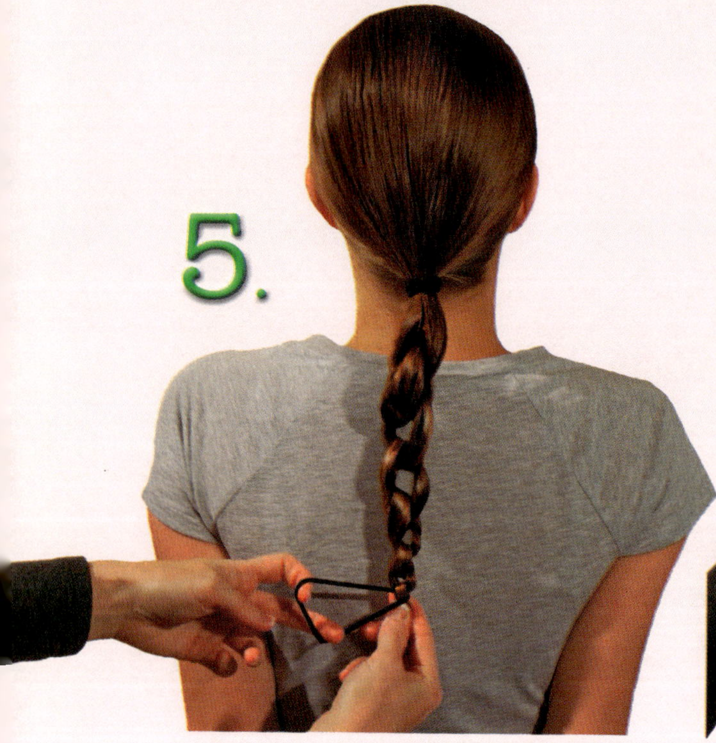

6. Coil the braid and tuck the end under, to finish the look.

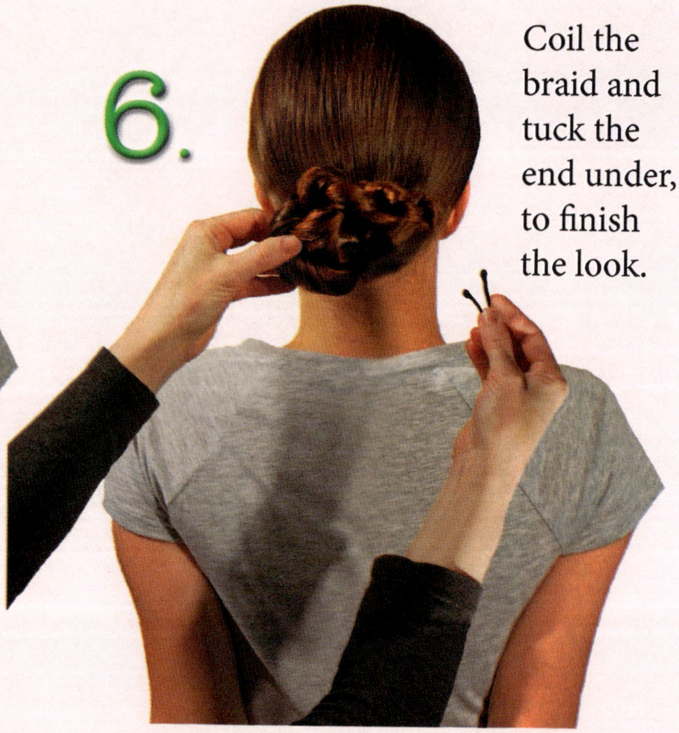

Fix the end of the braid with bobby pins to hold the braid in place.

Two-Strand Knot Braid

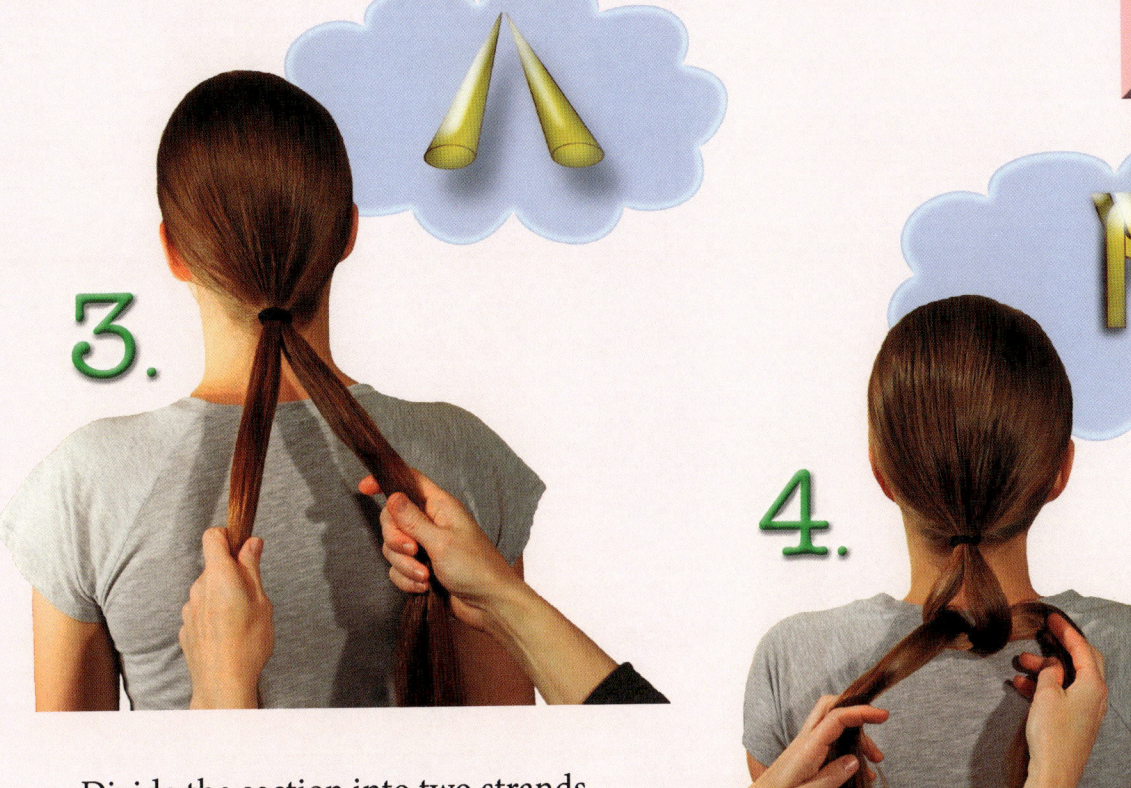

3. Divide the section into two strands.

4. Tie one strand around the other.

Two-Strand Knot

Notes

I learned this braid technique in Canada during a work day at the Renaissance Festival. When I look back on that day, I realize he wasn't crazy, however, at the time, I was pretty sure he was. This little old man was watching me braid and asked to show me his way of doing it. I gritted my teeth, flashed him the best smile I could muster, and said, "sure". The whole time he worked I could only think, "yeah, my clients will love this...can I tie knots in your hair?" For three months it pestered and plagued me till I finally tried it. It is now my favorite and most requested number of strands to work with.

Two-Strand Knot

Gather from both sides

Let's stitch it!

Let's stitch it!

Let's stitch it!

Two-Strand Knot Stitch

2

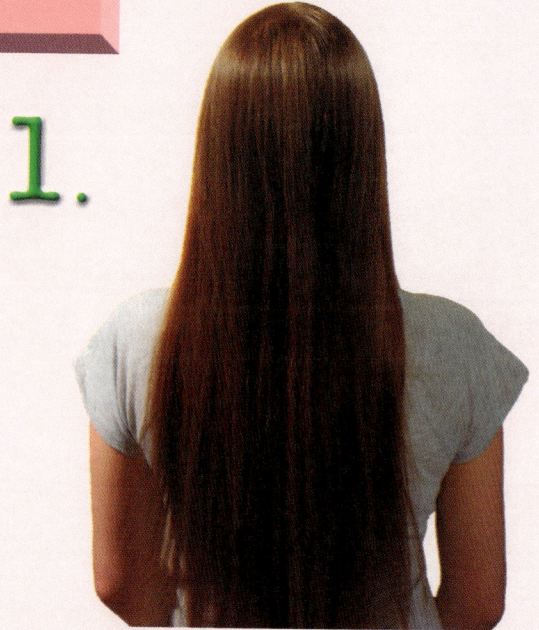

1. Begin with clean, brushed hair.

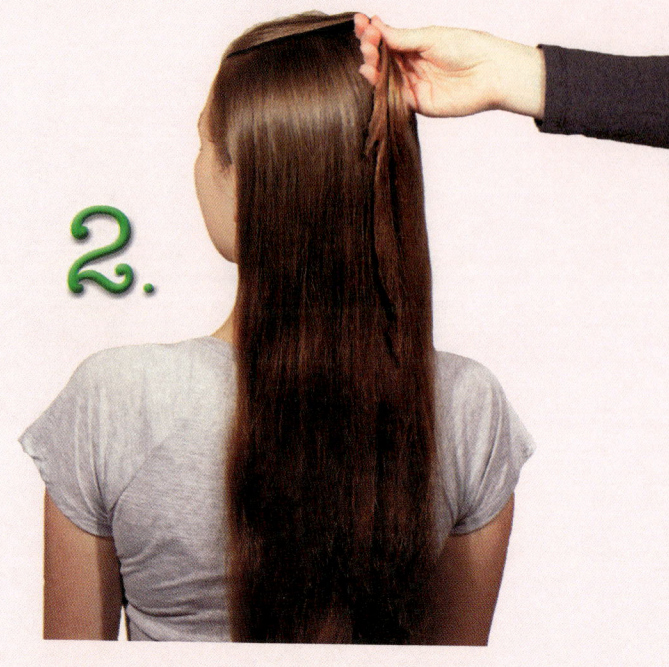

2. Take a section of hair as illustrated.

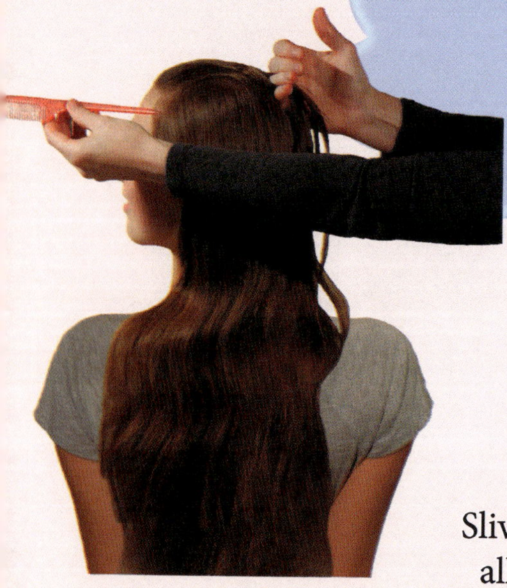

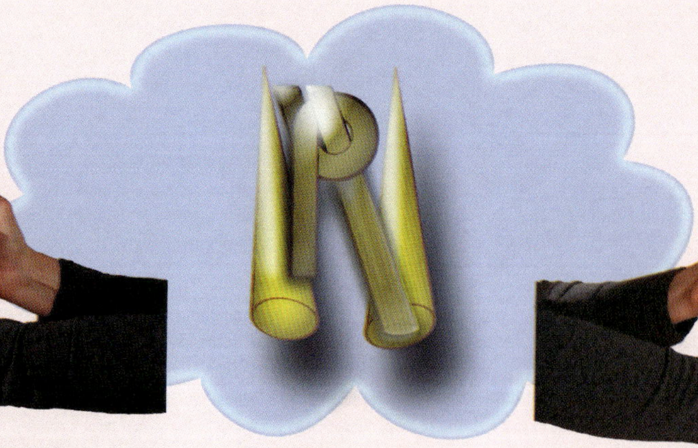

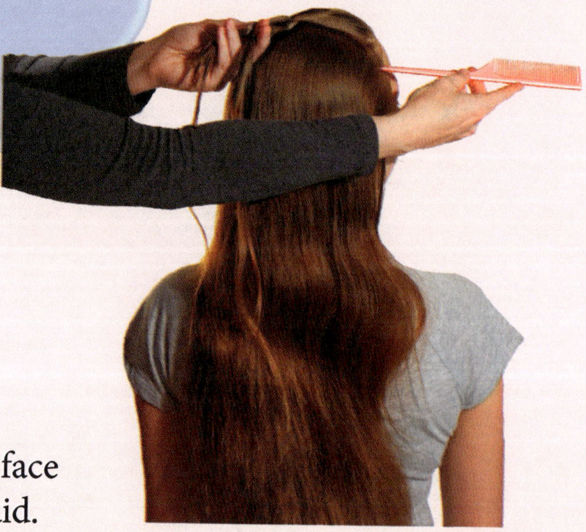

5. Sliver off a gather from the face all the way back to the braid. Gather into the braid from both sides. The right gather into the right strand.

Two-Strand Knot Stitch

2

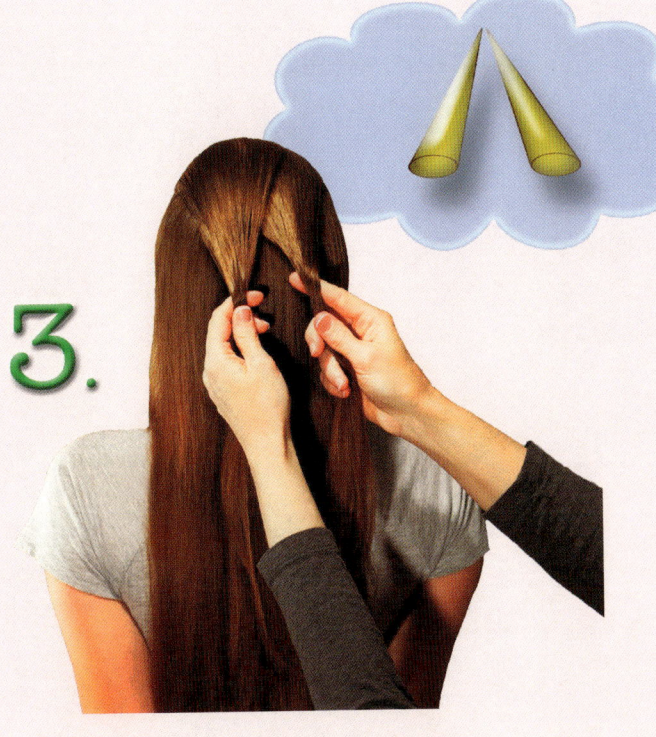

3.

Divide the section into two strands.

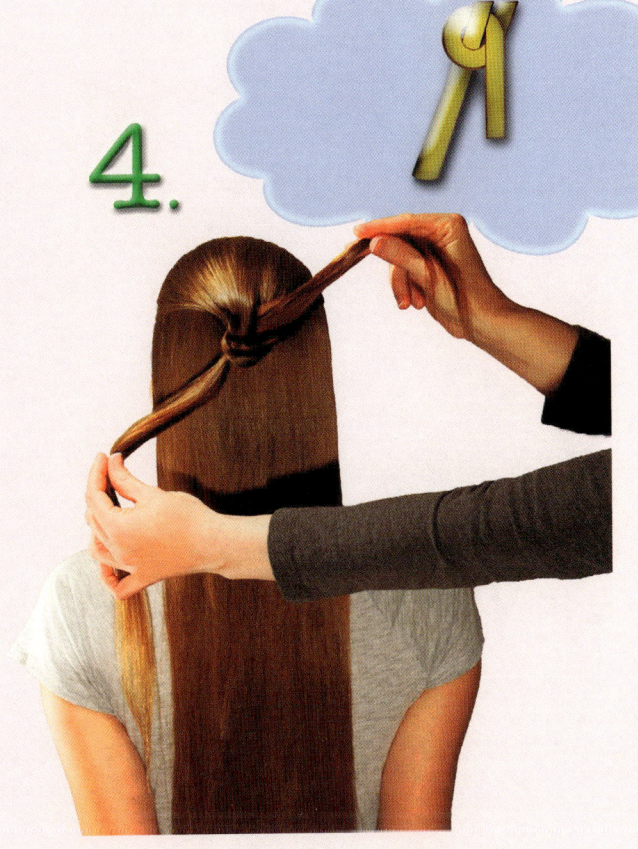

4.

Tie one strand around the other.

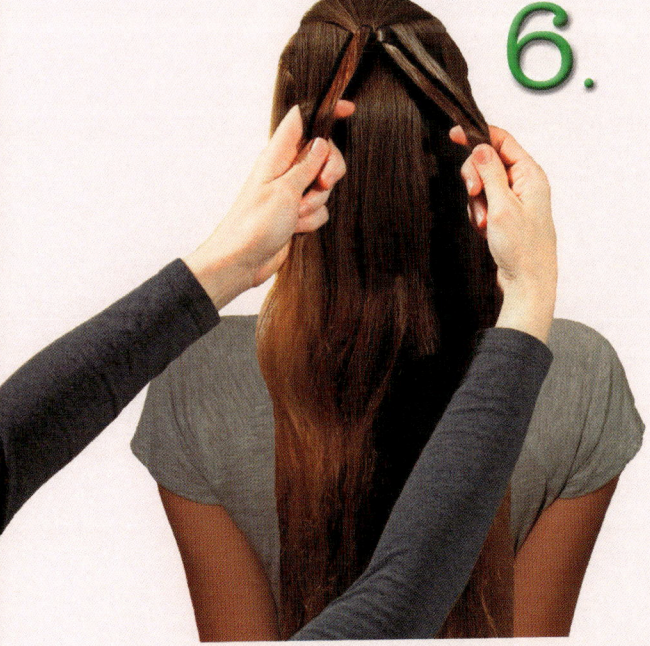

6.

The left gather into the left strand.

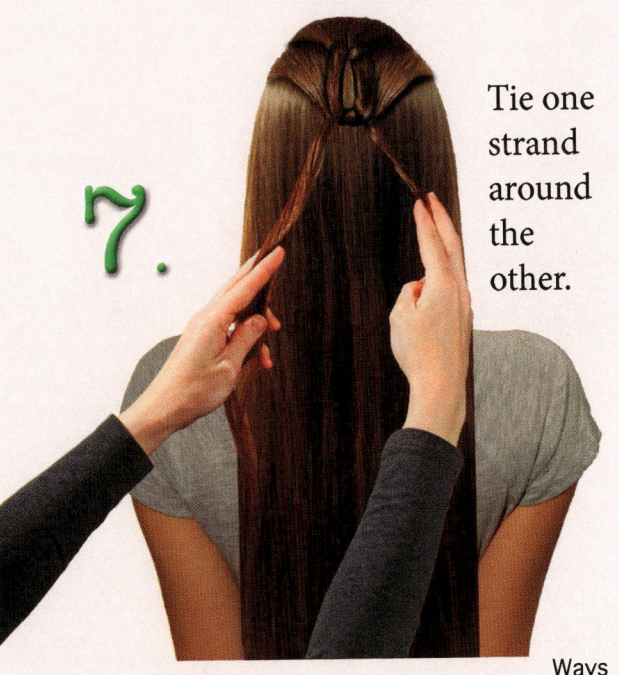

7.

Tie one strand around the other.

Ways

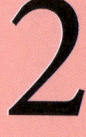

part 2. Two-Strand Knot Stitch

This braid looks very different when you always tie with the same strand versus alternating the strands you tie with. Try both and see what it looks like.

8.
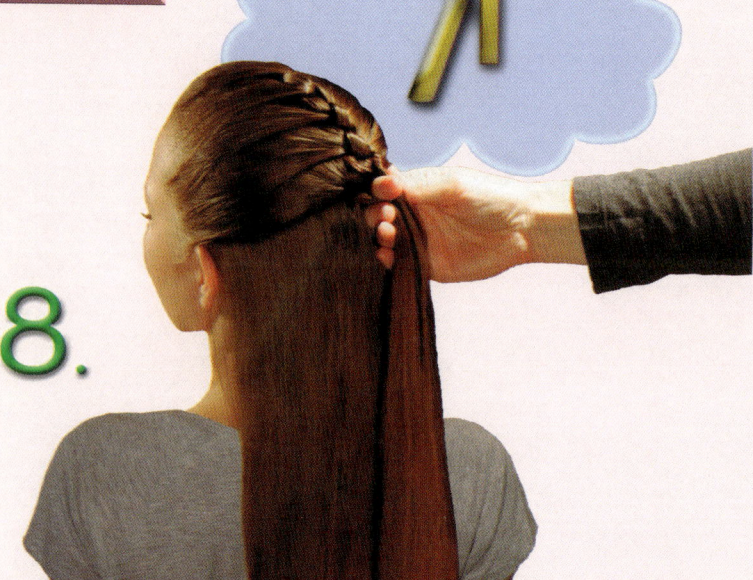

Continue gathering and tying until you reach the end of the hair.

9.
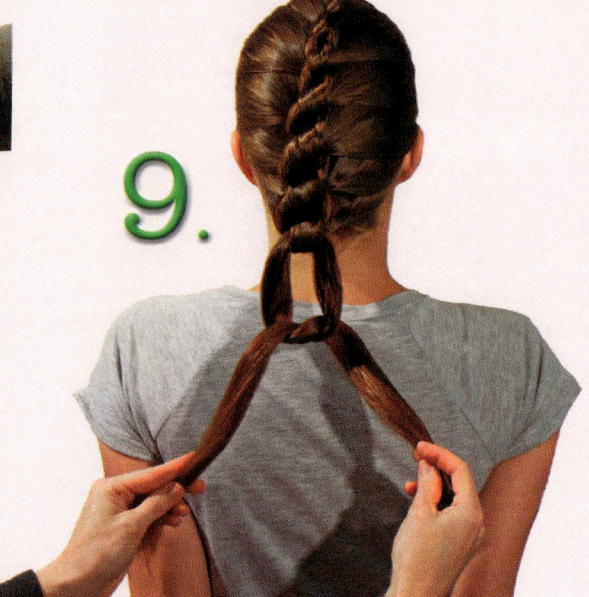

10.
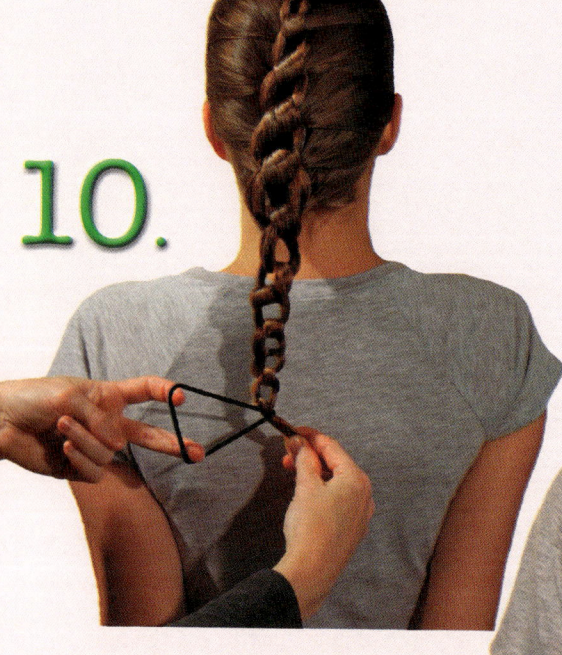

Secure with a rubber band.

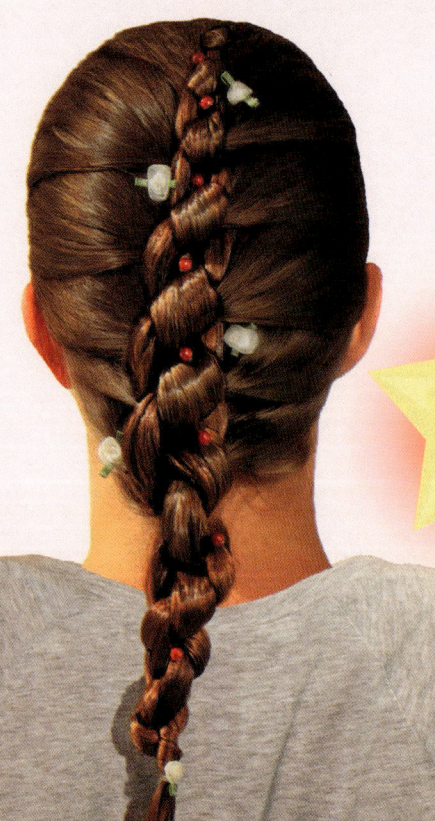

www.findingbraids.com

Two-Strand Knot

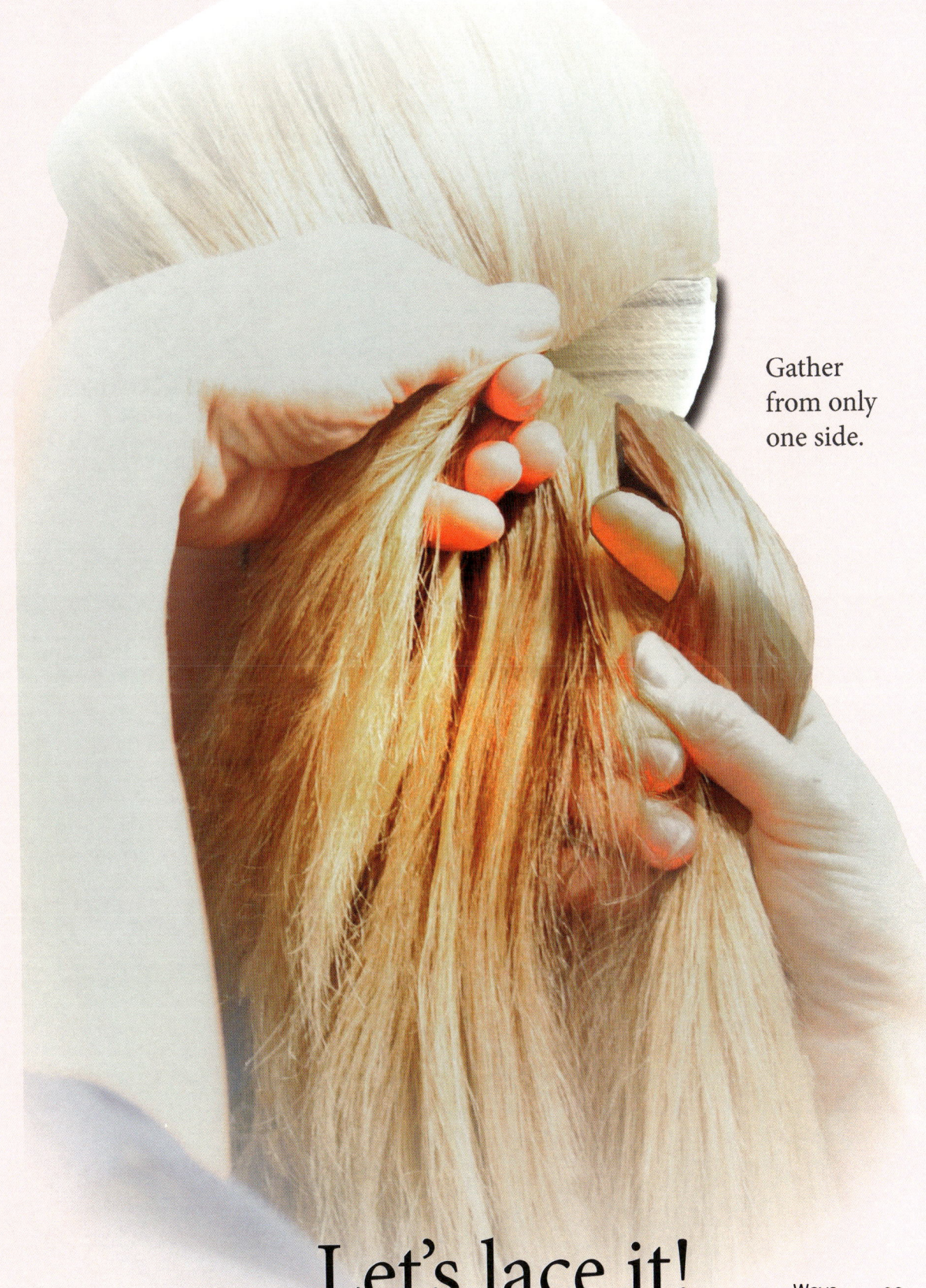

Gather from only one side.

Let's lace it!

Two-Strand Knot Lace

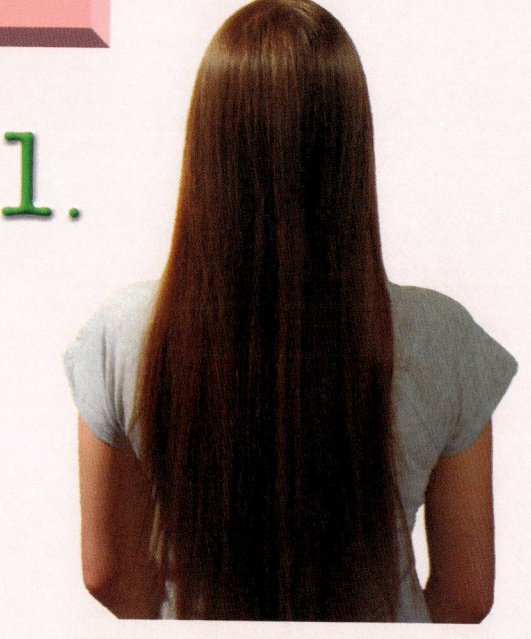

1. Begin with clean, brushed hair.

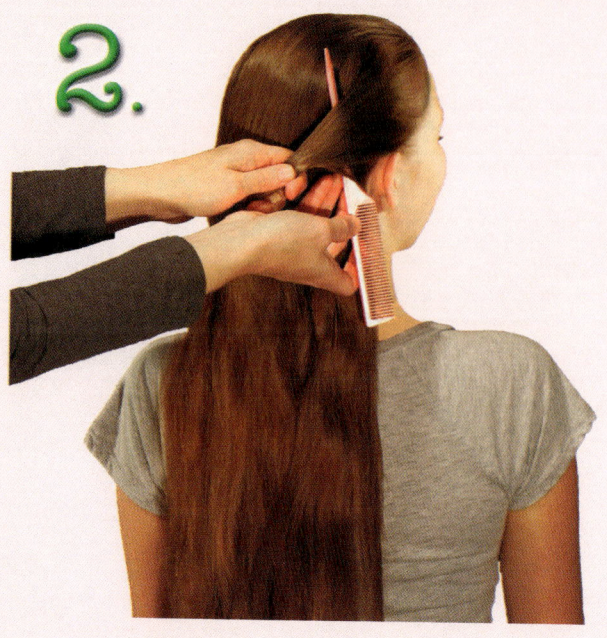

2. Take a section of hair as illustrated.

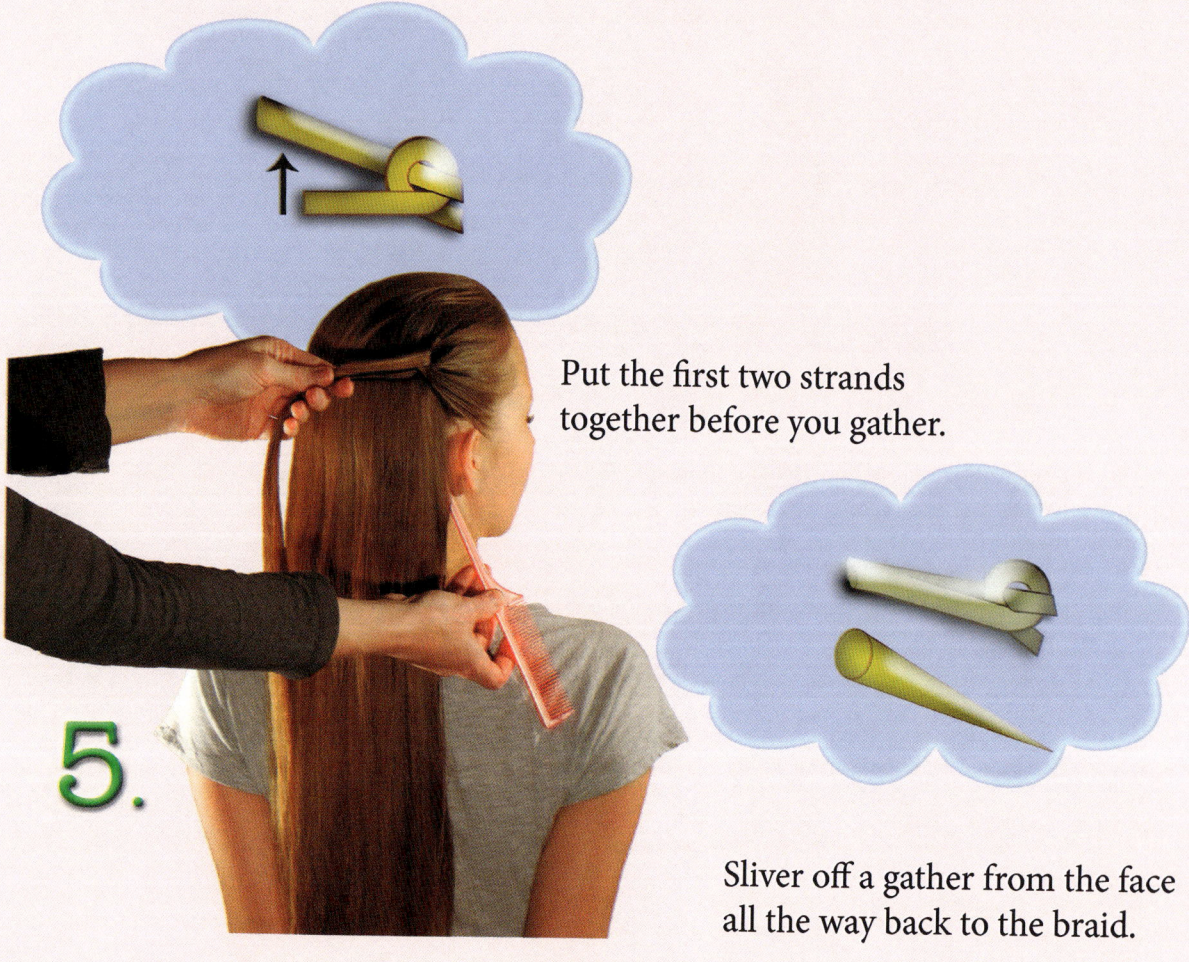

Put the first two strands together before you gather.

5. Sliver off a gather from the face all the way back to the braid.

84   www.findingbraids.com

Two-Strand Knot Lace

2

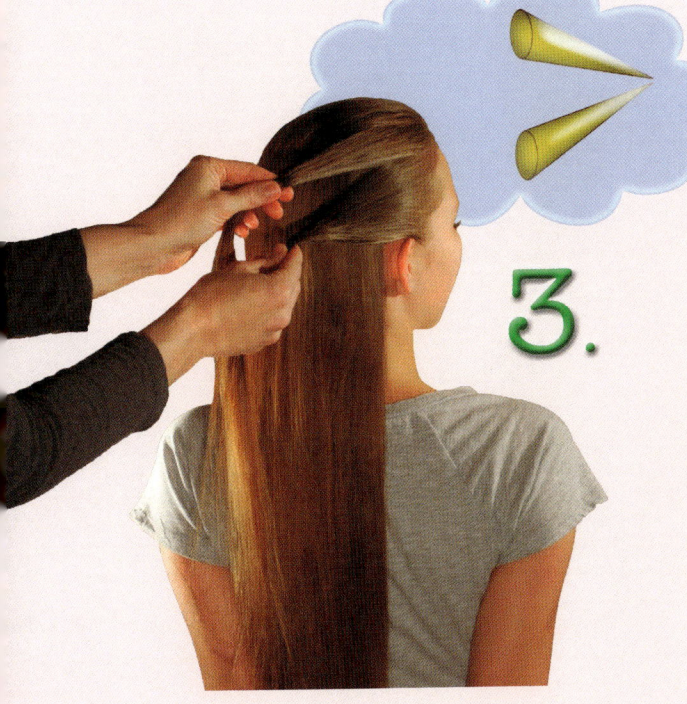

Divide the section into two strands.

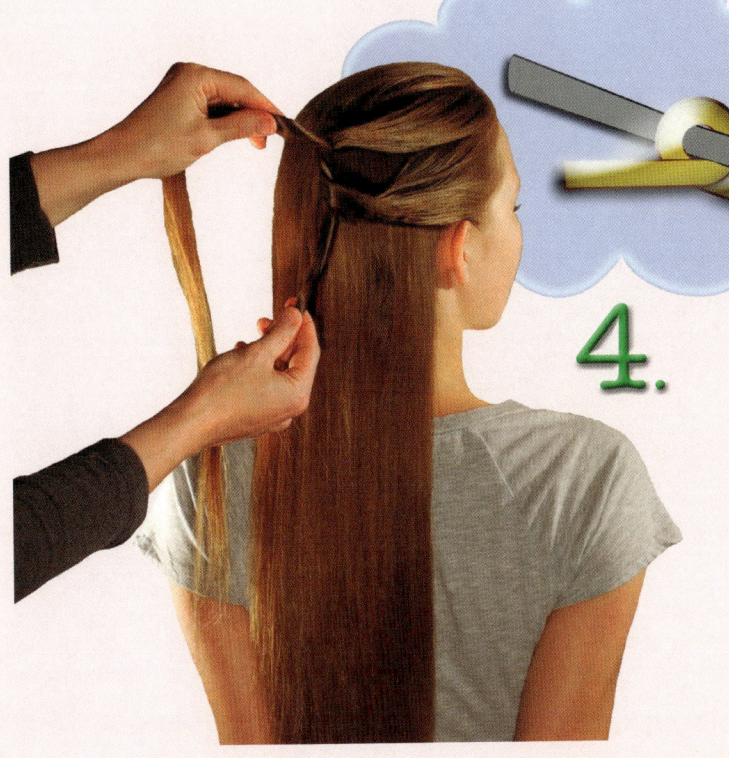

Tie one strand around the other.

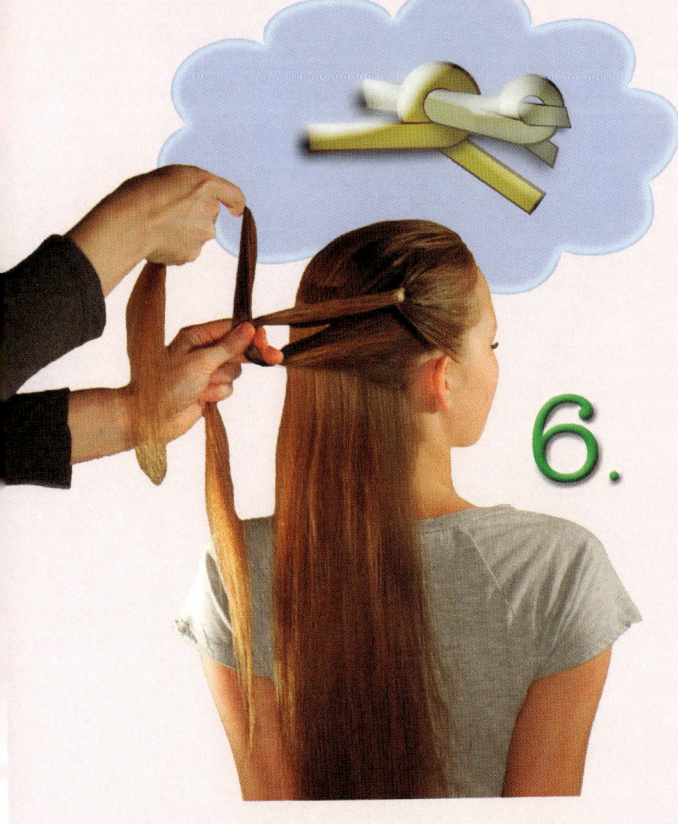

Tie the gather around the previous strands.

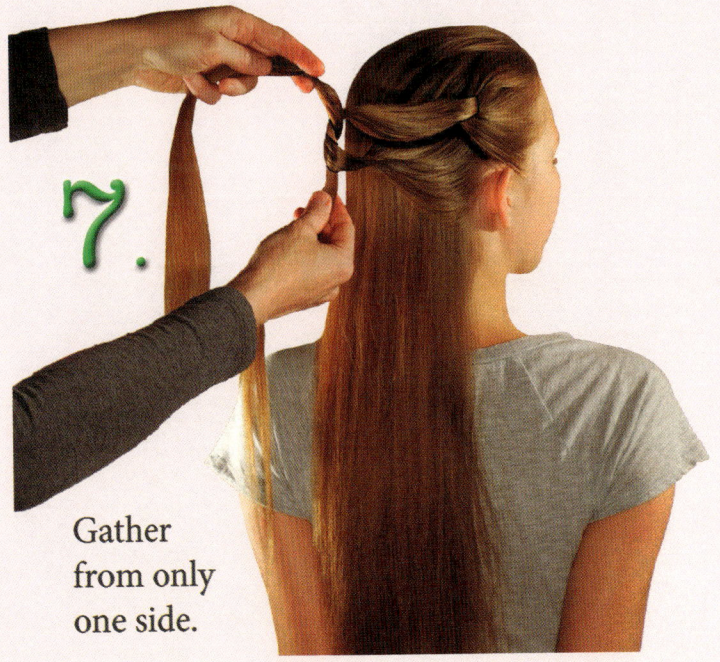

Gather from only one side.

2 Continuing

Put the two strands together before you gather.

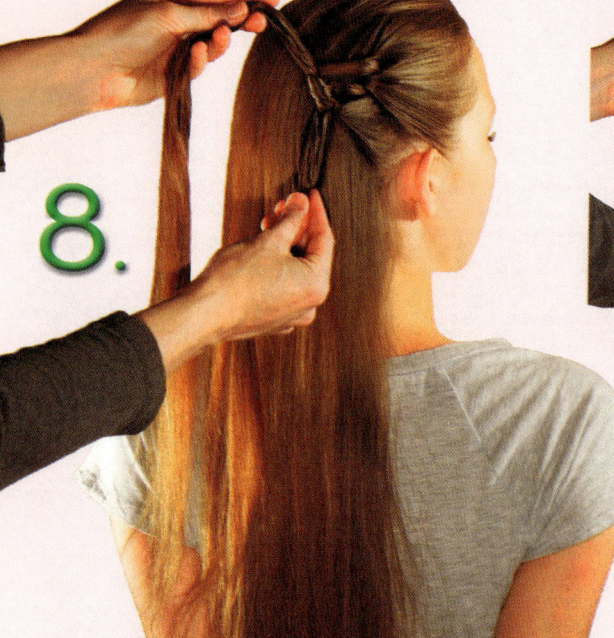

8.

9.

Sliver off a gather from the face all the way back to the braid.

The knot should be snug against the scalp.

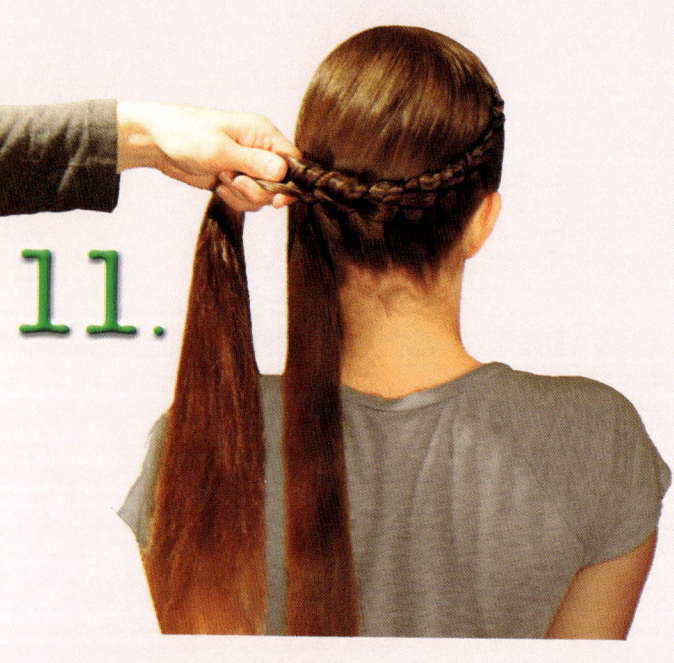

11.

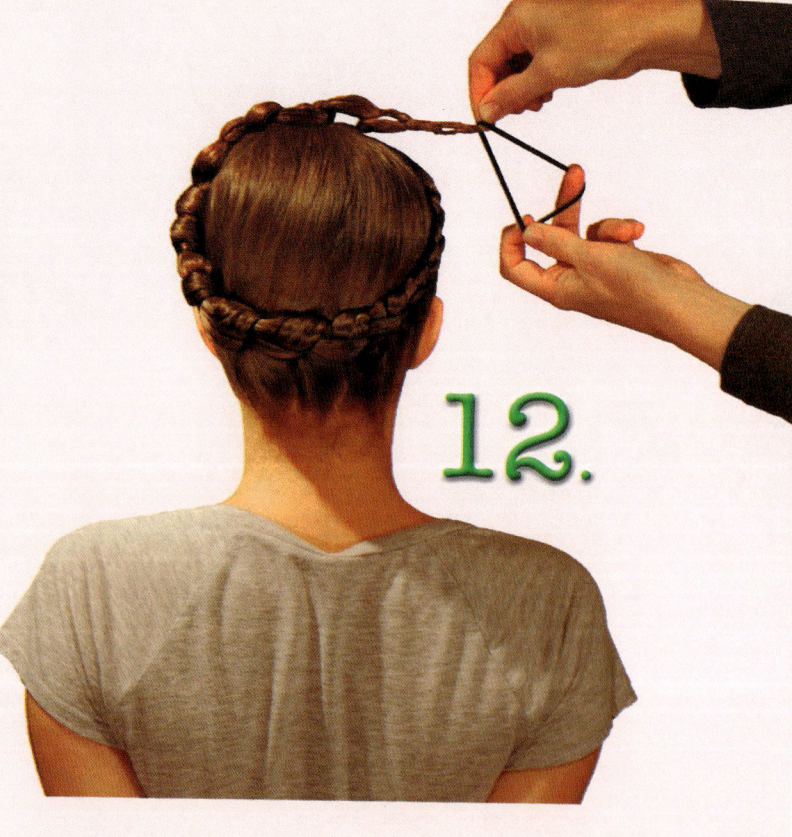

12.

Continue gathering and tying until you reach the end of the hair.

Secure with a rubber band.

part 2. Two-Strand Knot Lace

2

Tie the gather around the previous strands.

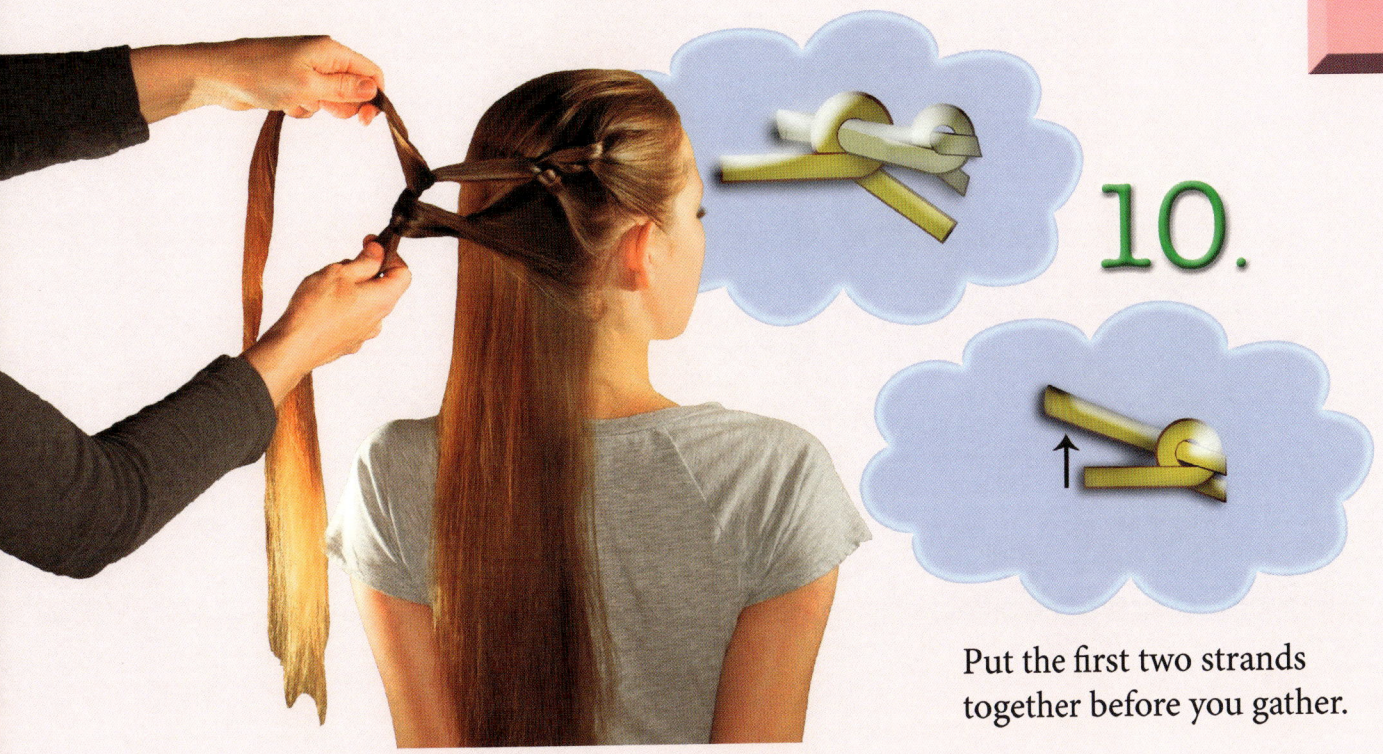

10.

Put the first two strands together before you gather.

13.

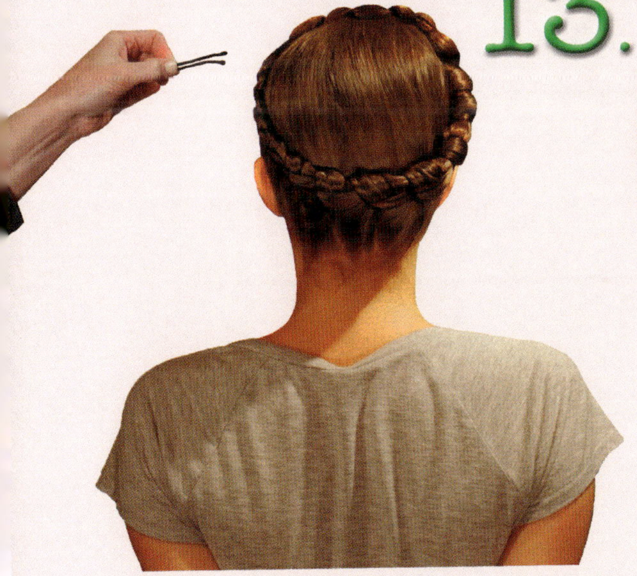

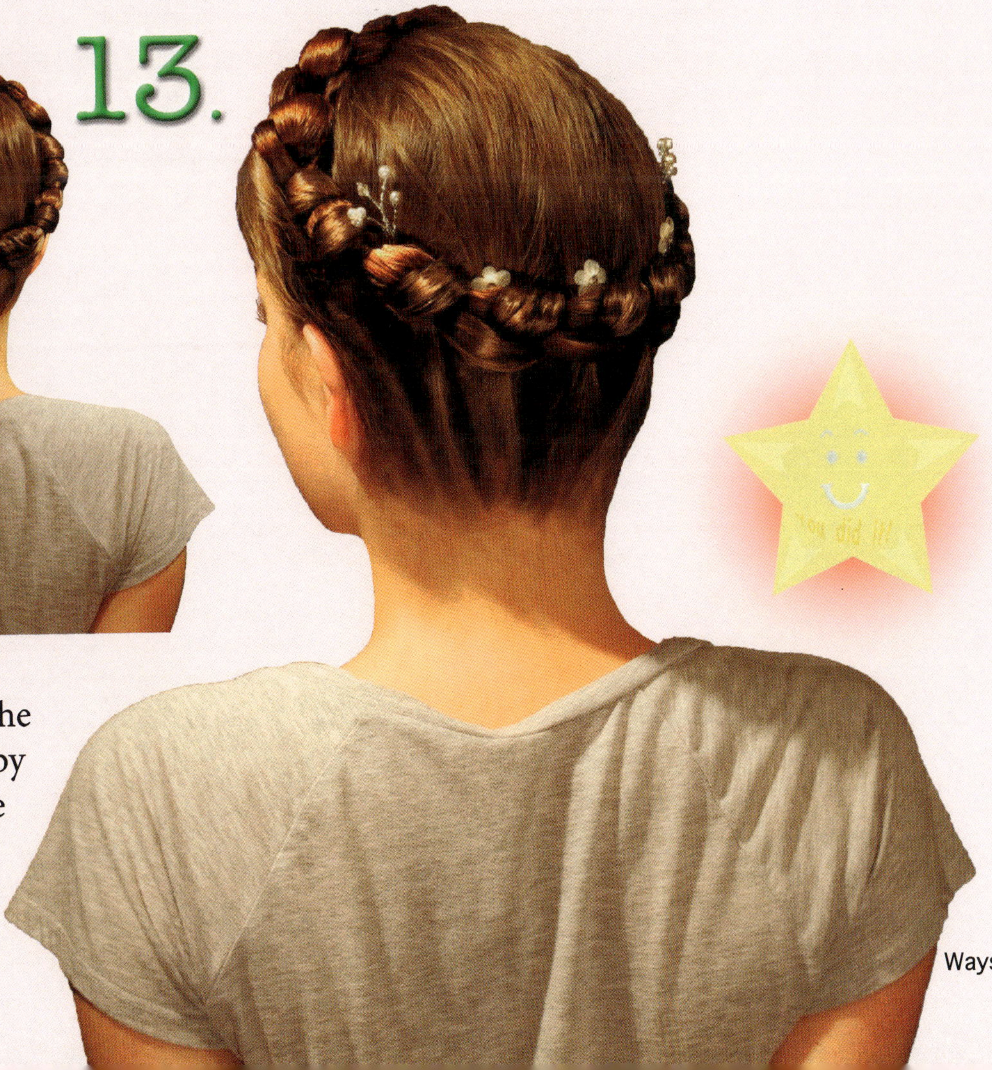

Fix the end of the braid with bobby pins to hold the braid in place.

Two-Strand Knot

Notes

Try out the examples with your new skills!

Examples of Two-Strand Knot

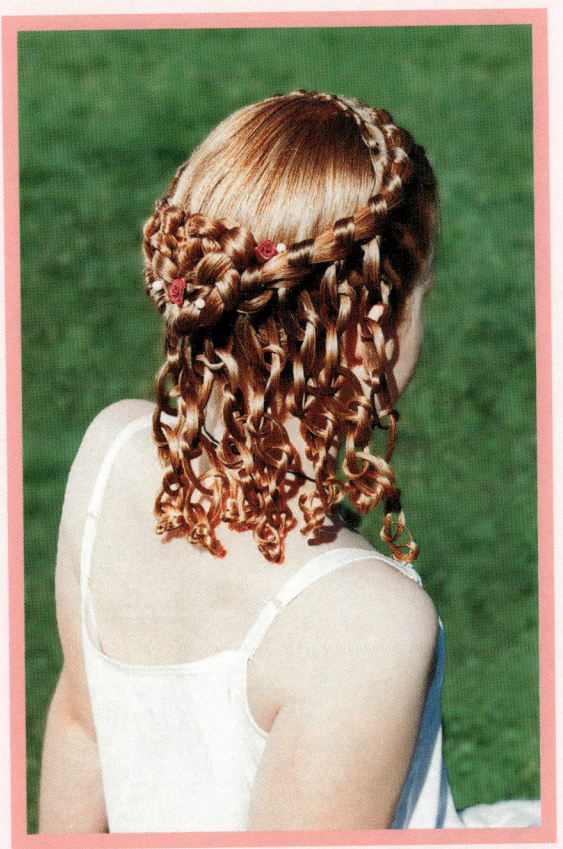
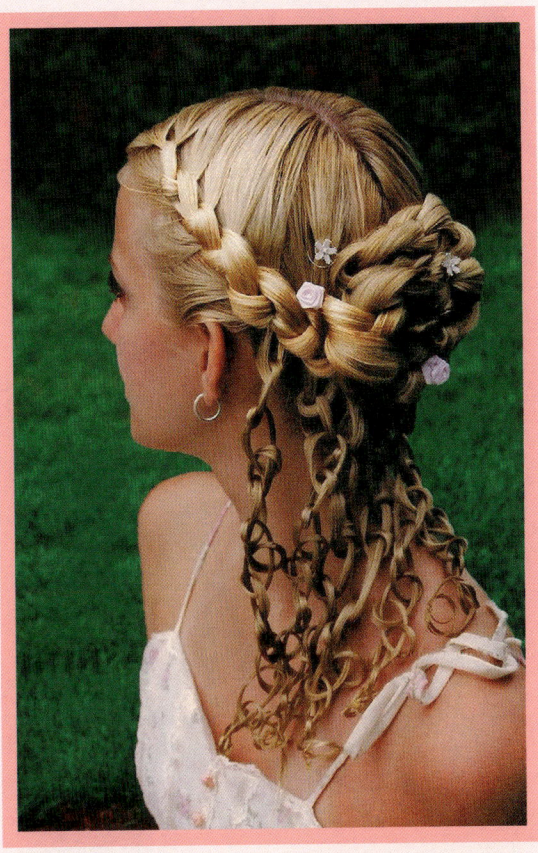
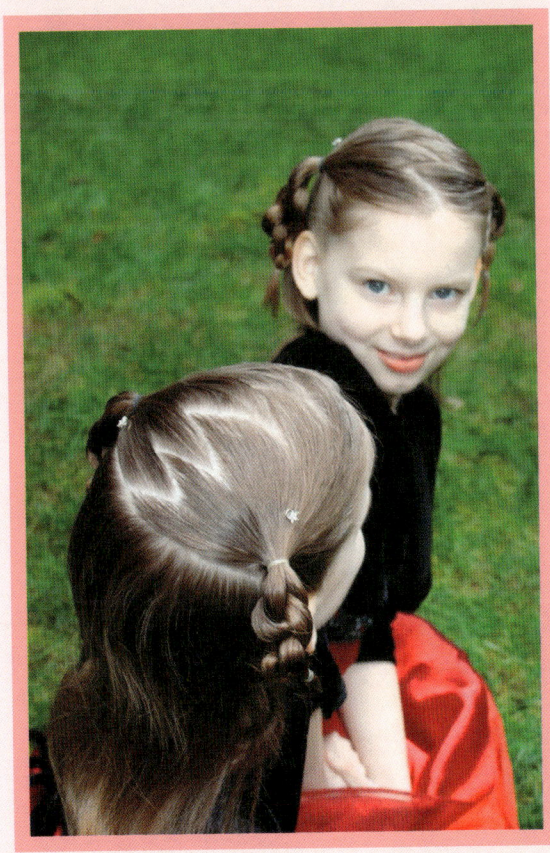
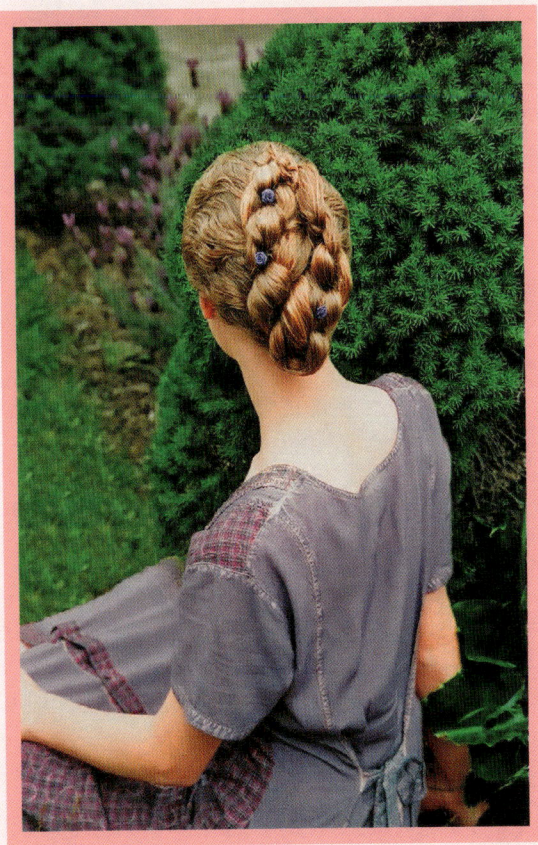

Visit my website to see more examples of the Two-Strand Knot

Two-Strand Rope

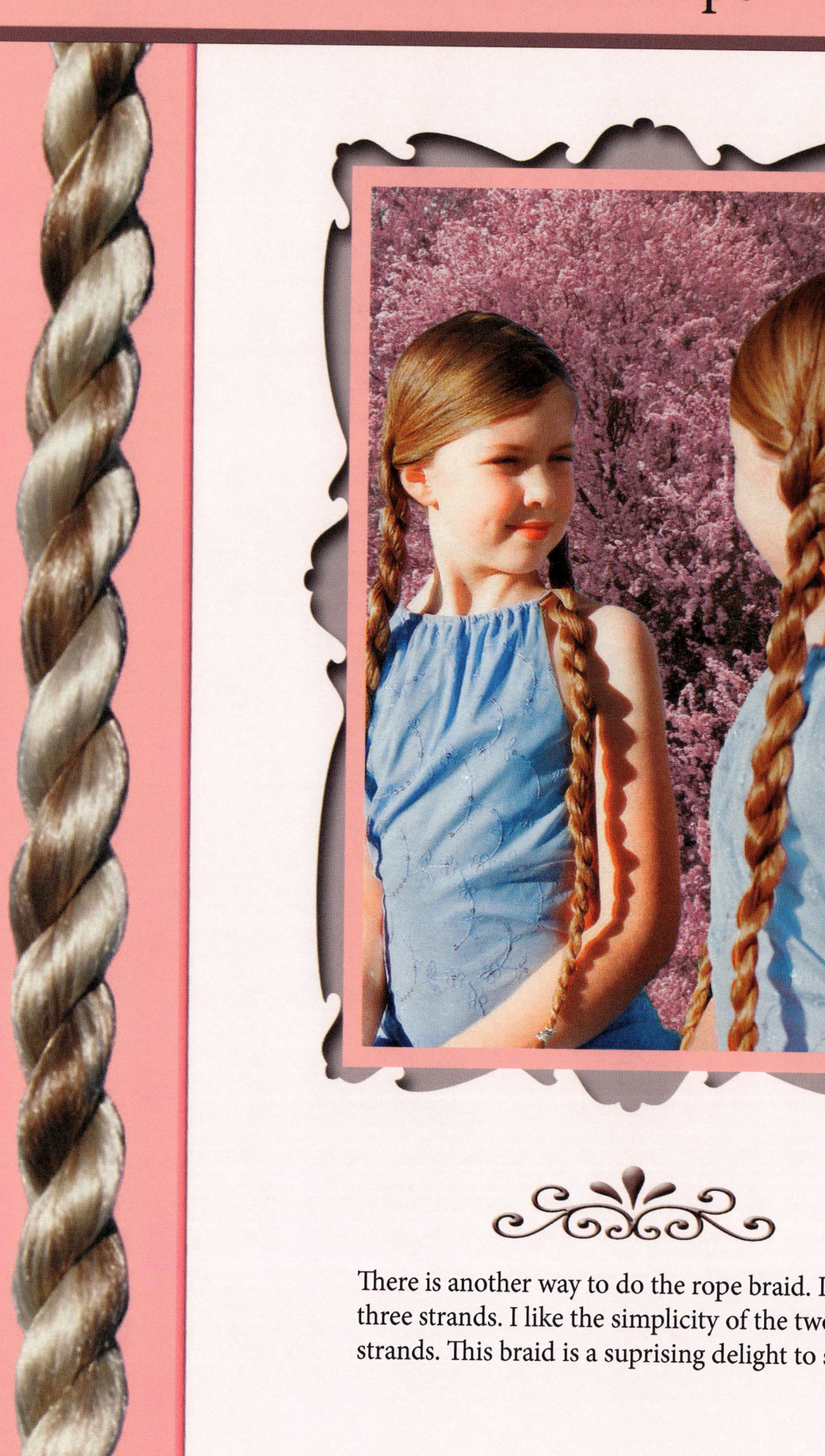

There is another way to do the rope braid. It uses three strands. I like the simplicity of the two strands. This braid is a suprising delight to see.

Two-Strand Rope

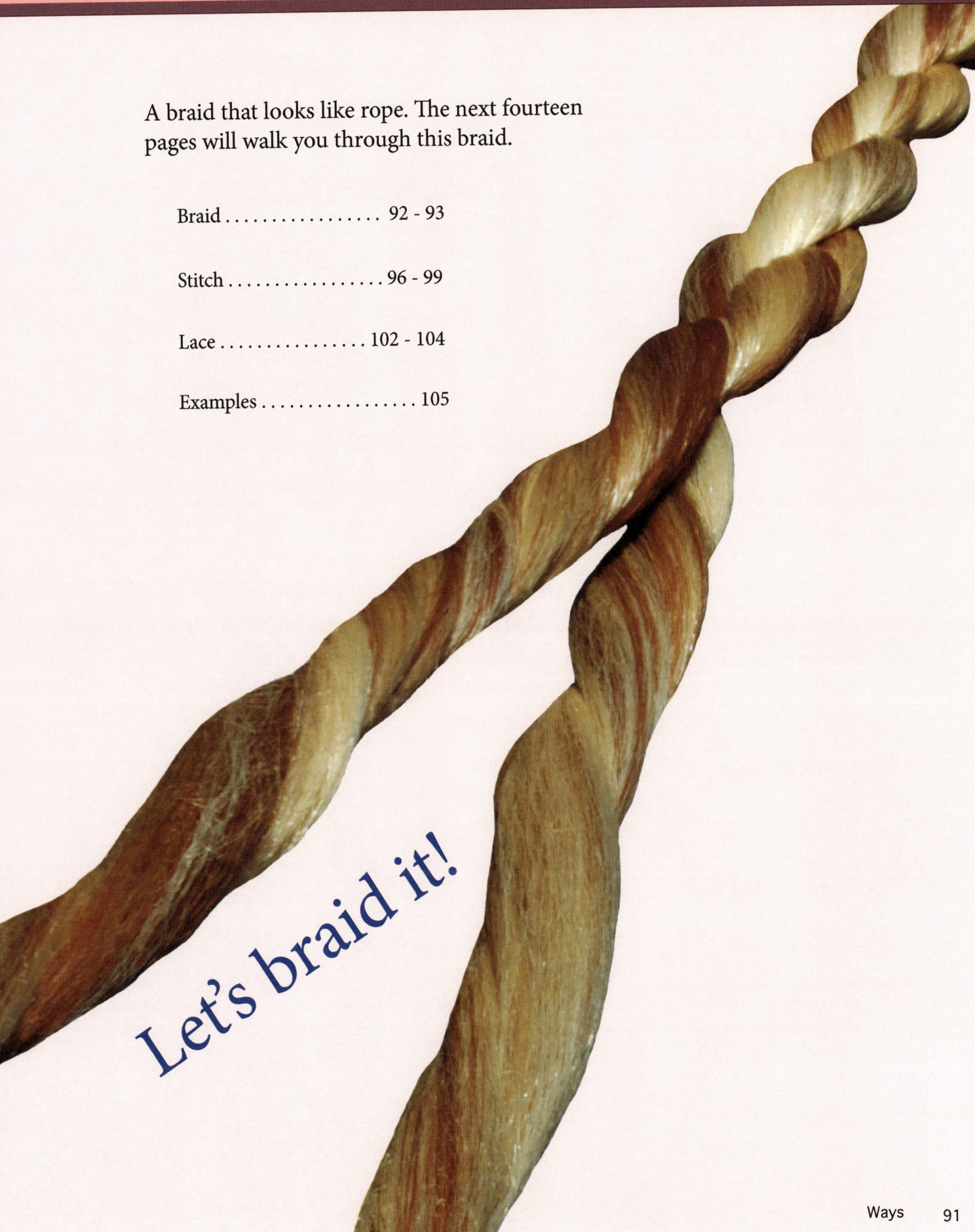

A braid that looks like rope. The next fourteen pages will walk you through this braid.

Braid . . . . 92 - 93

Stitch . . . . 96 - 99

Lace . . . . 102 - 104

Examples 105

Let's braid it!

Ways

Two-Strand Rope Braid

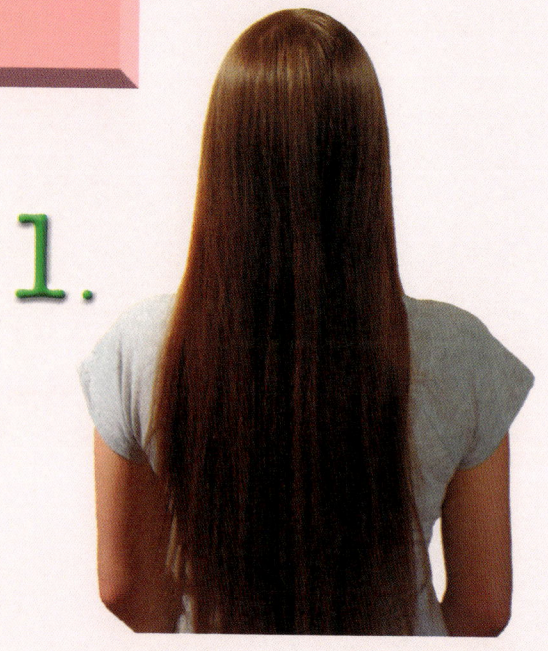

1. Begin with clean, brushed hair.

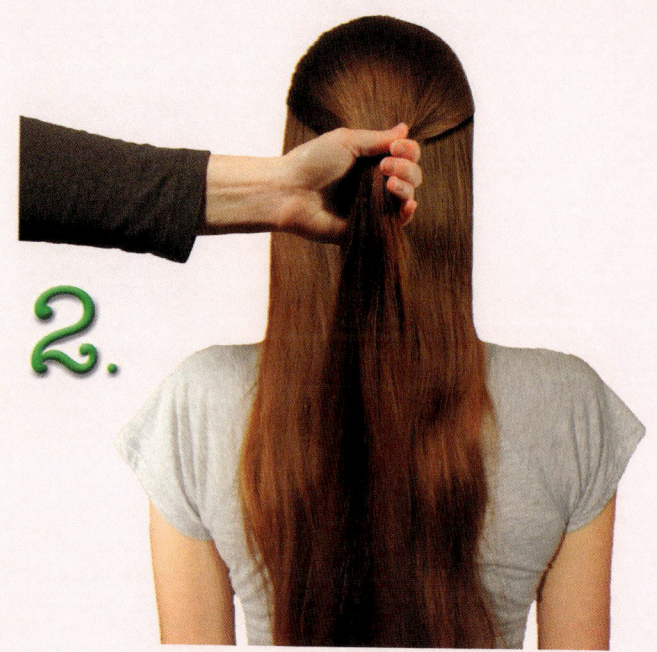

2. Take a section of hair.

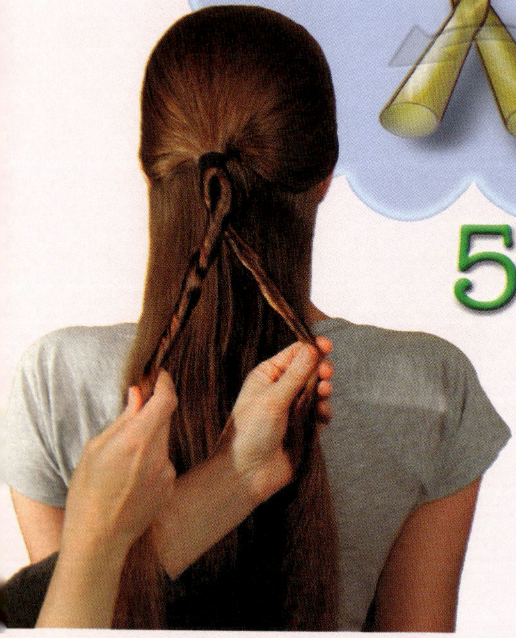

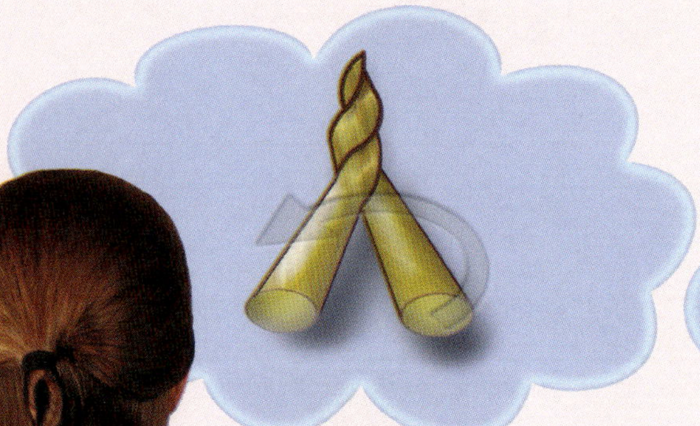

5. Wrap the strands around each other in the opposite direction.

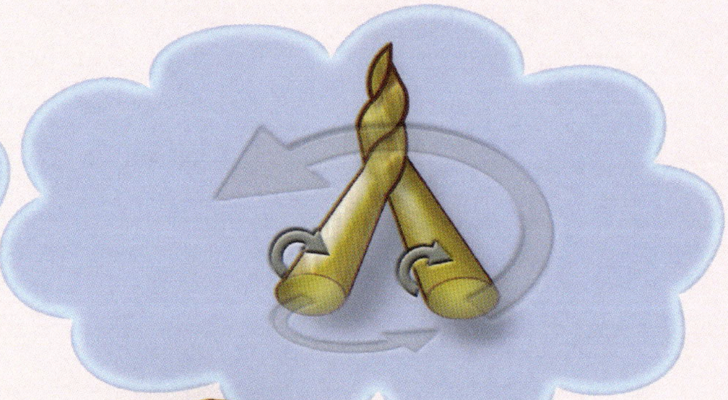

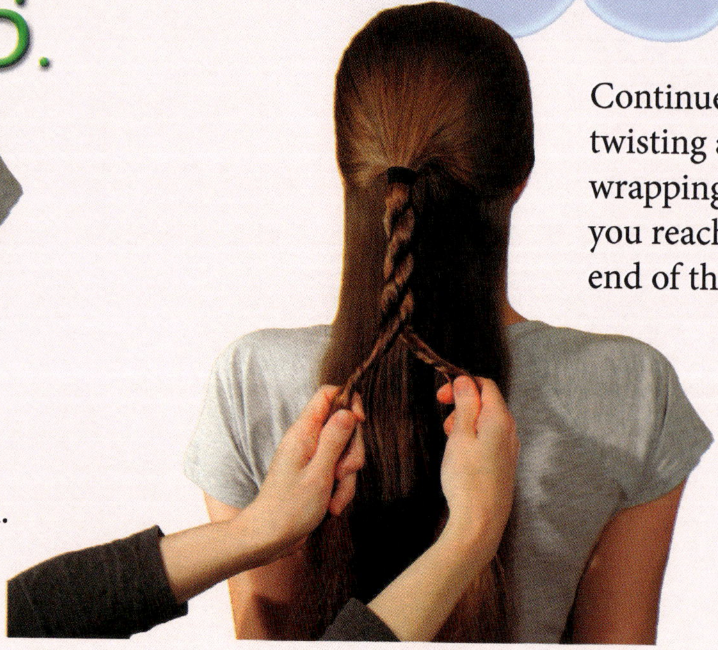

6. Continue twisting and wrapping until you reach the end of the hair.

92 www.findingbraids.com

Two-Strand Rope Braid

2

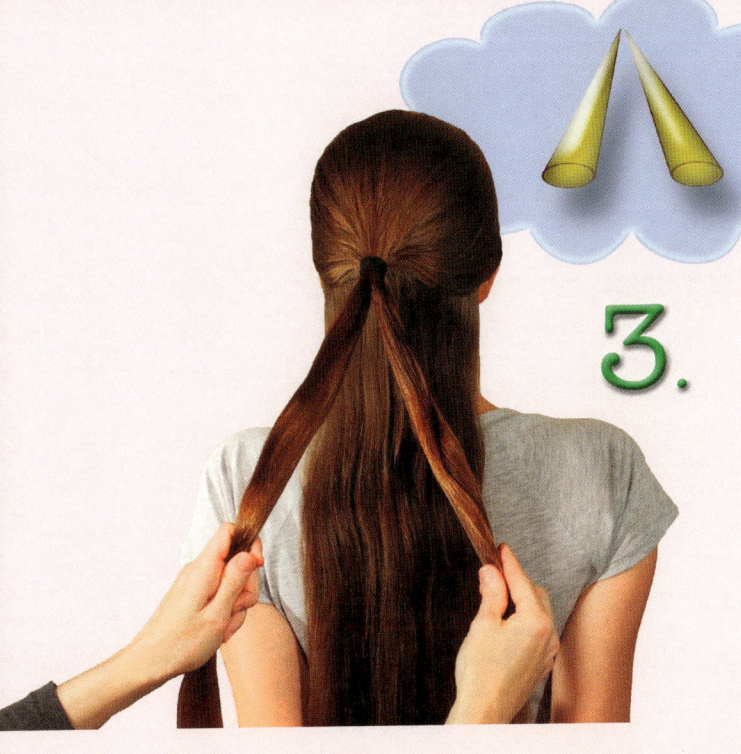

3.

Divide the section into two strands.

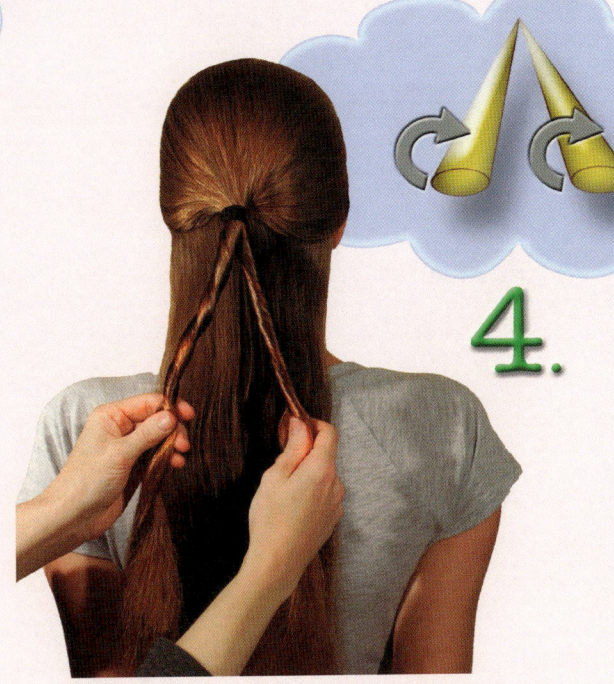

4.

Twist each strand individually in the same direction.

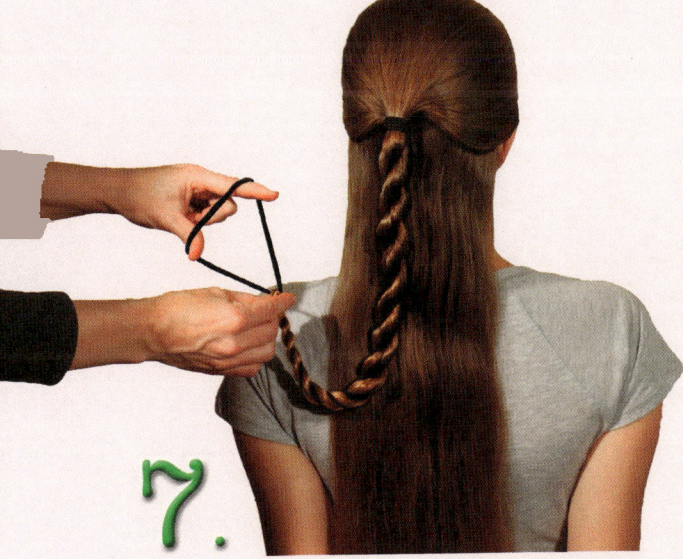

7.

Secure with a rubber band.

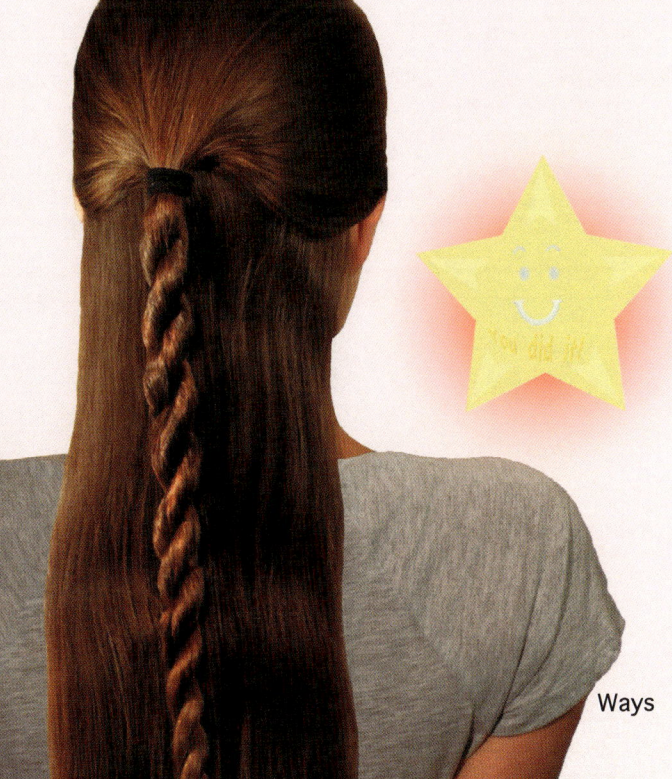

Ways 93

Two-Strand Rope

Notes

While the rope braid is very pretty, it requires a bit of coordination. I keep my knuckles as close to the clients scalp as possible when I braid. Keeping things snug and close makes it more likely for the hair to remain where you put it. You are also more likely to get a tight braid that way.

Two-Strand Rope

Gather from both sides

Let's stitch it!

Let's stitch it!

Let's stitch it!

Two-Strand Rope Stitch

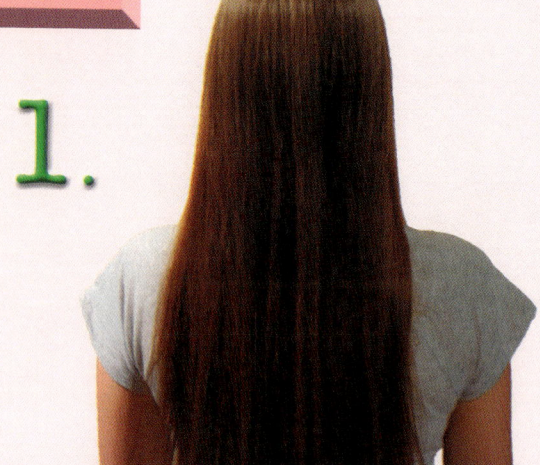

1. Begin with clean, brushed hair.

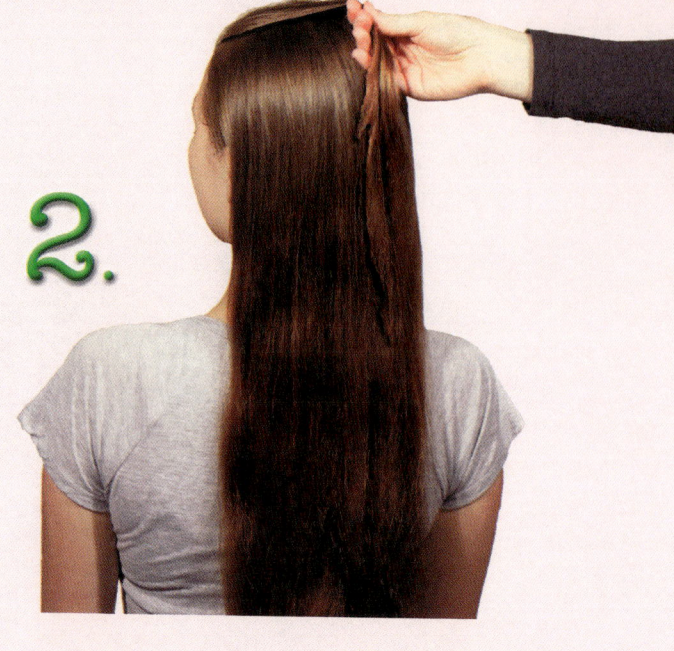

2. Take a section of hair as illustrated.

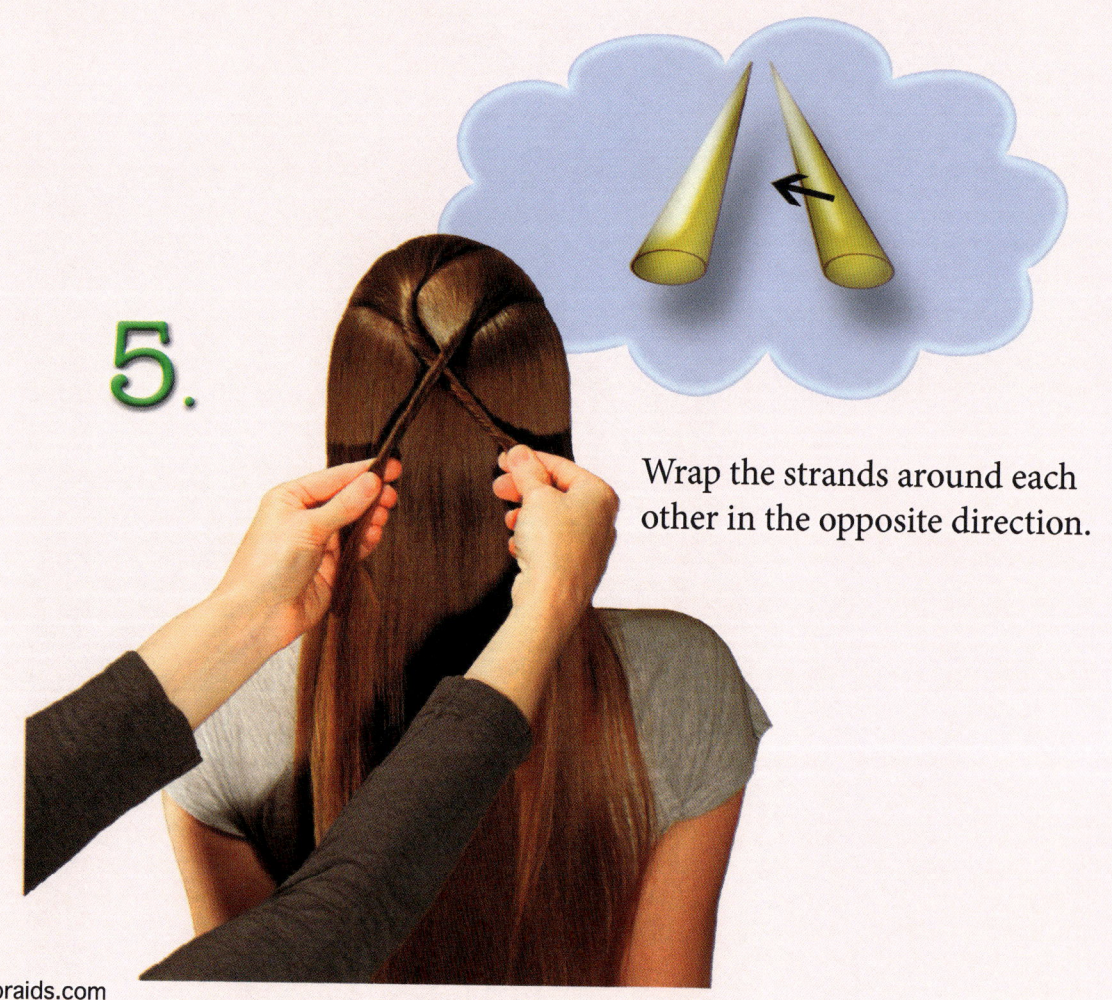

5. Wrap the strands around each other in the opposite direction.

Two-Strand Rope Stitch

2

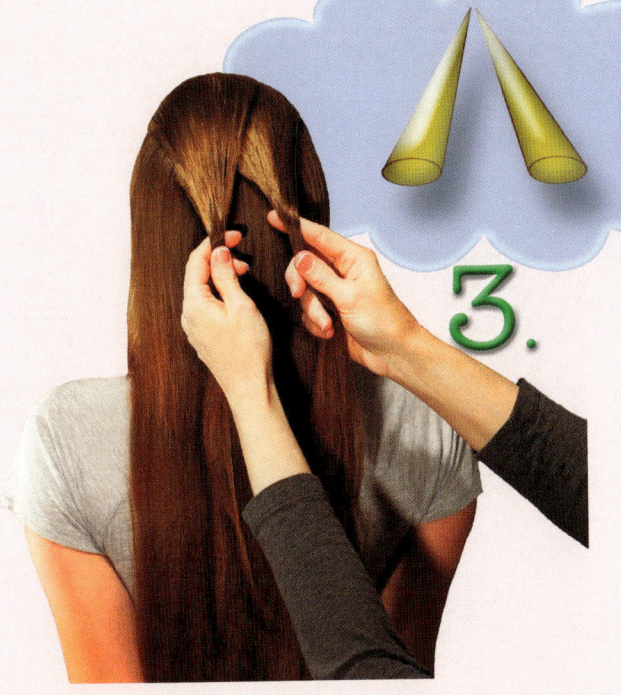

3.

Divide the section into two strands.

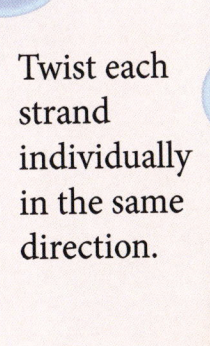

Twist each strand individually in the same direction.

4.

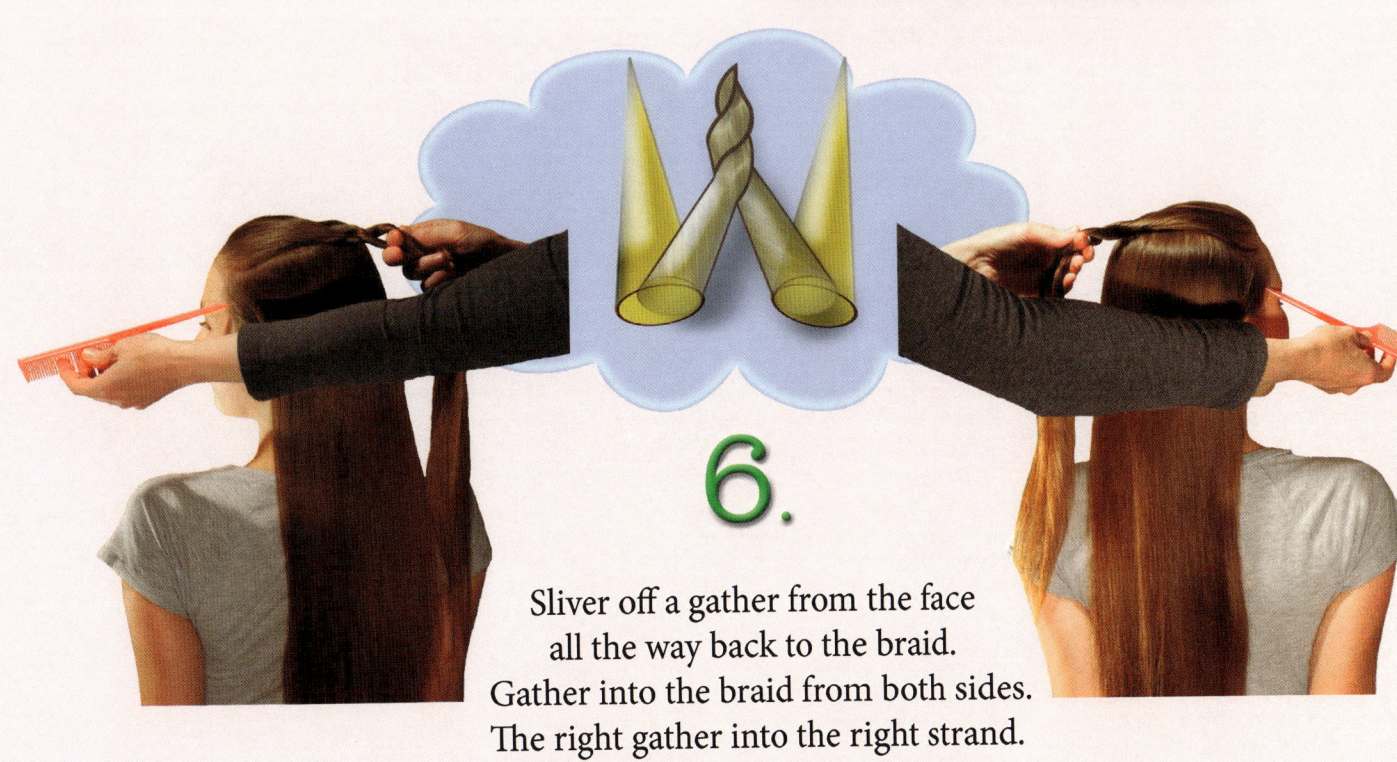

6.

Sliver off a gather from the face all the way back to the braid. Gather into the braid from both sides. The right gather into the right strand. The left gather into the left strand.

Ways 97

2 Continuing

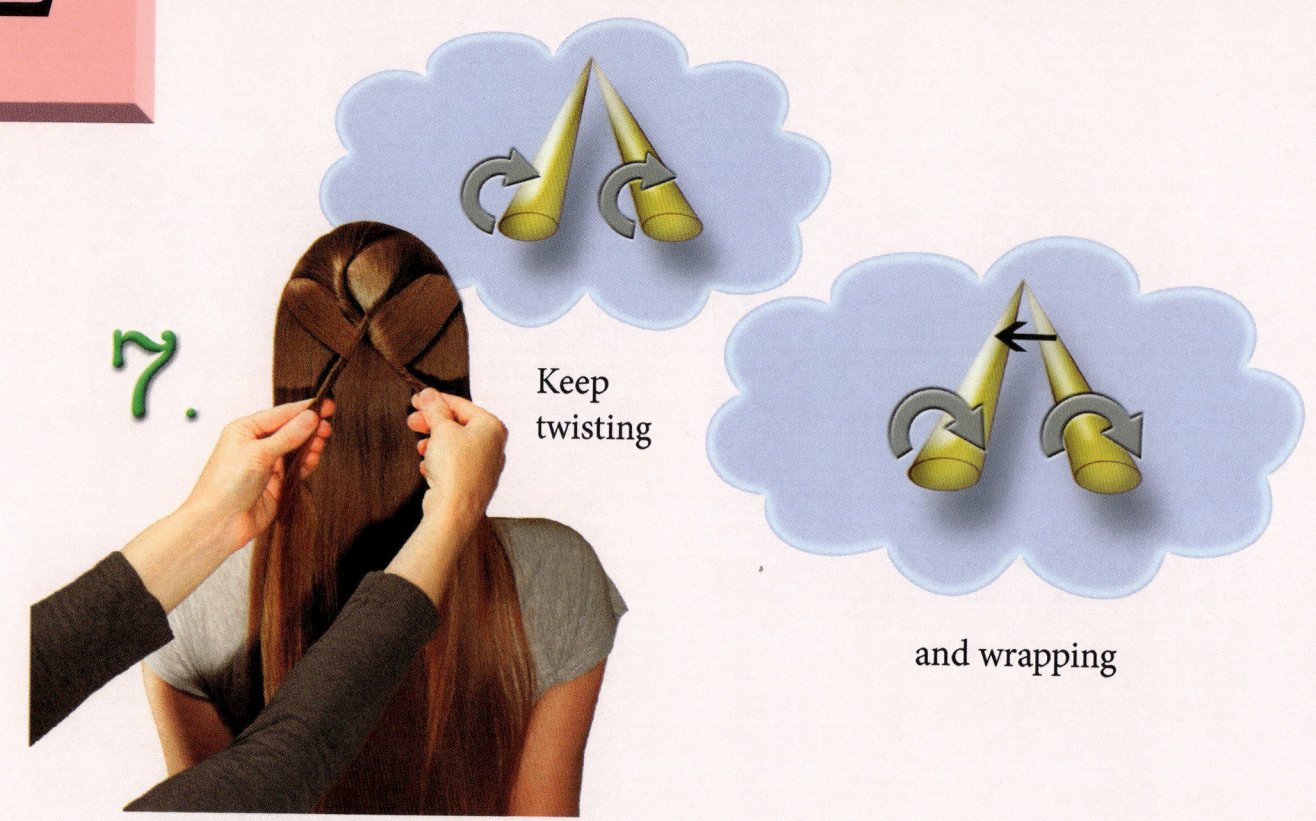

7. Keep twisting and wrapping

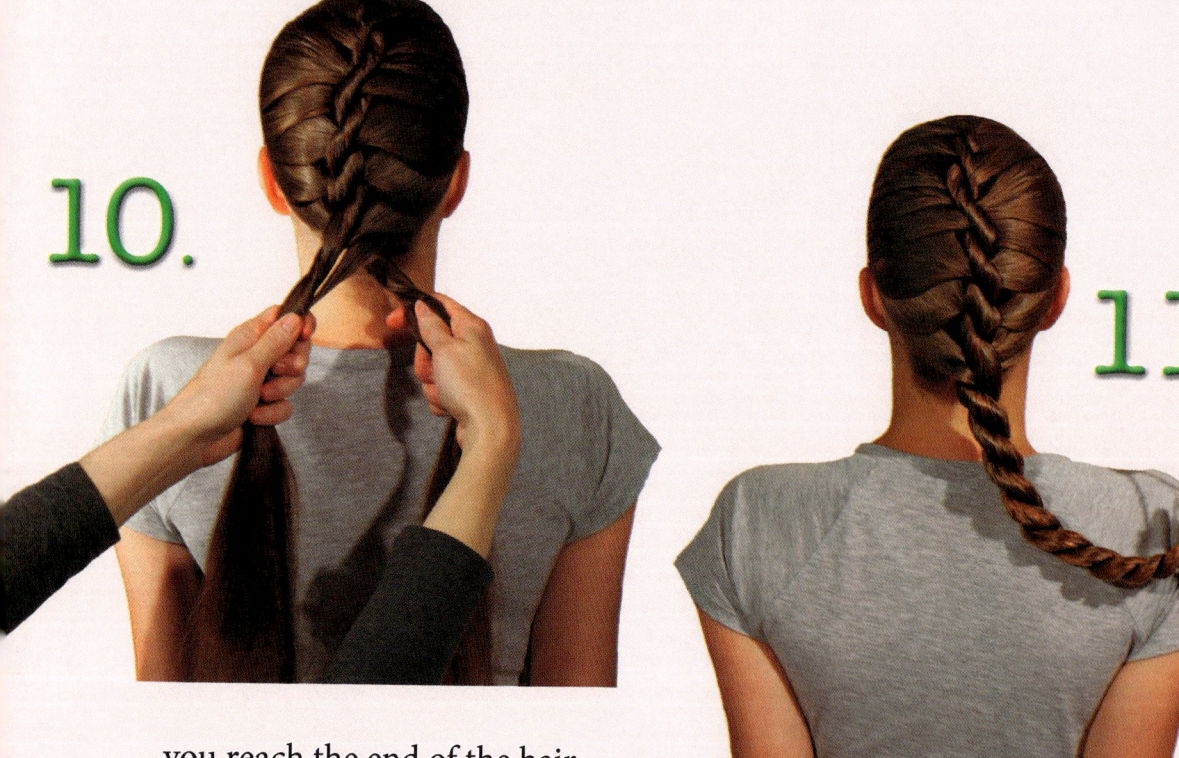

10. you reach the end of the hair.

11. Secure with a rubber band.

part 2. Two-Strand Rope Stitch

8. 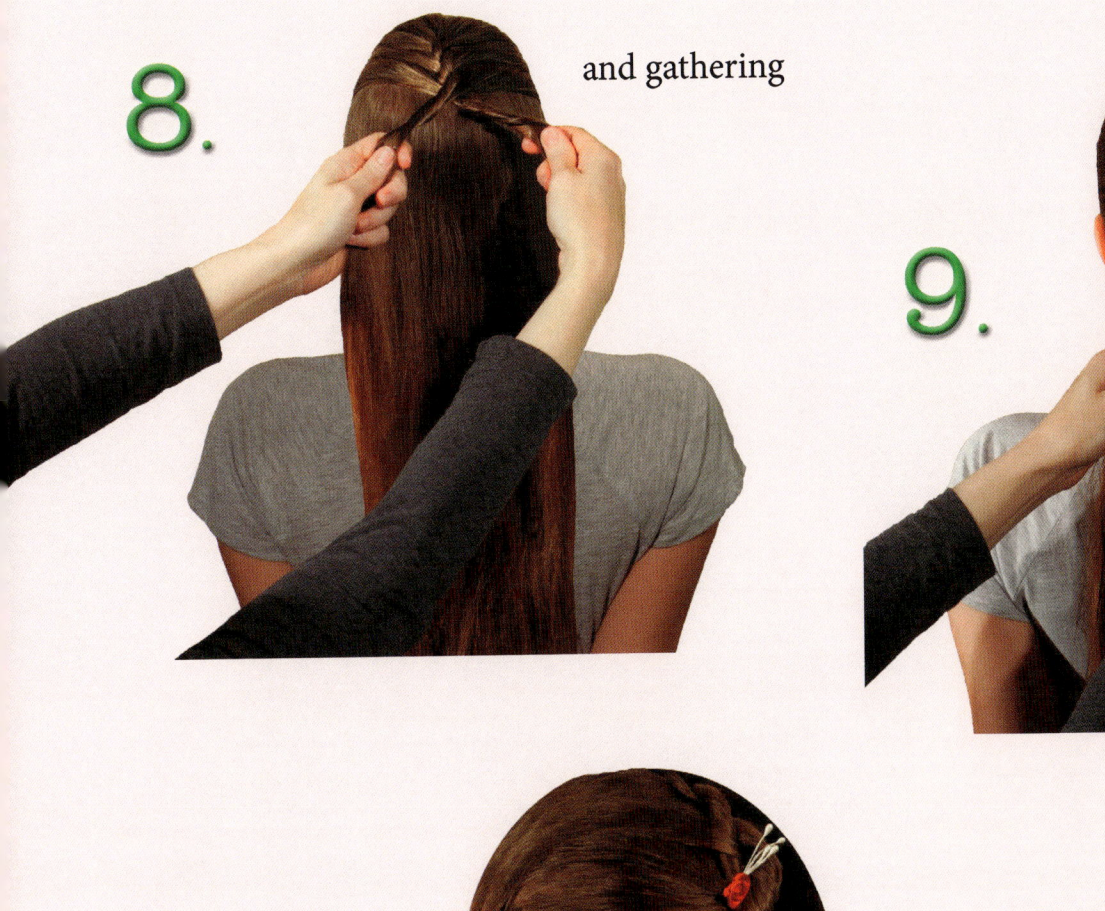 and gathering

9. 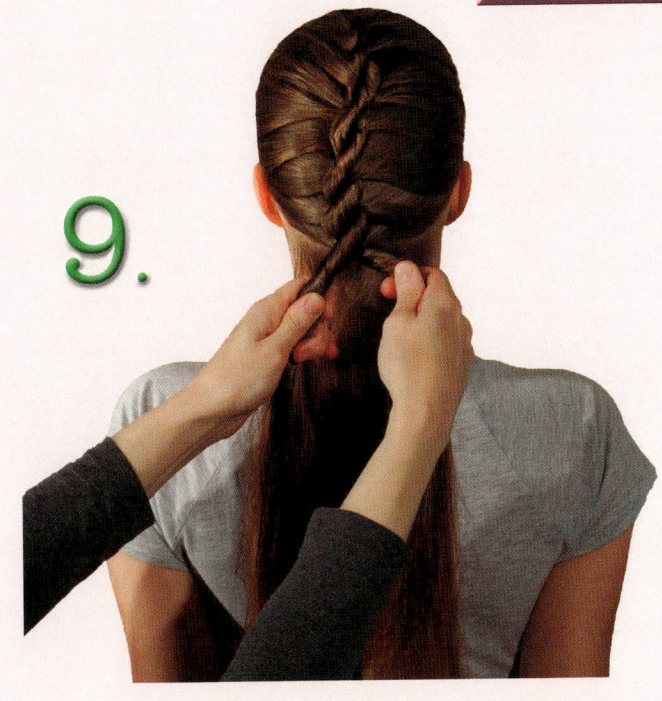 until

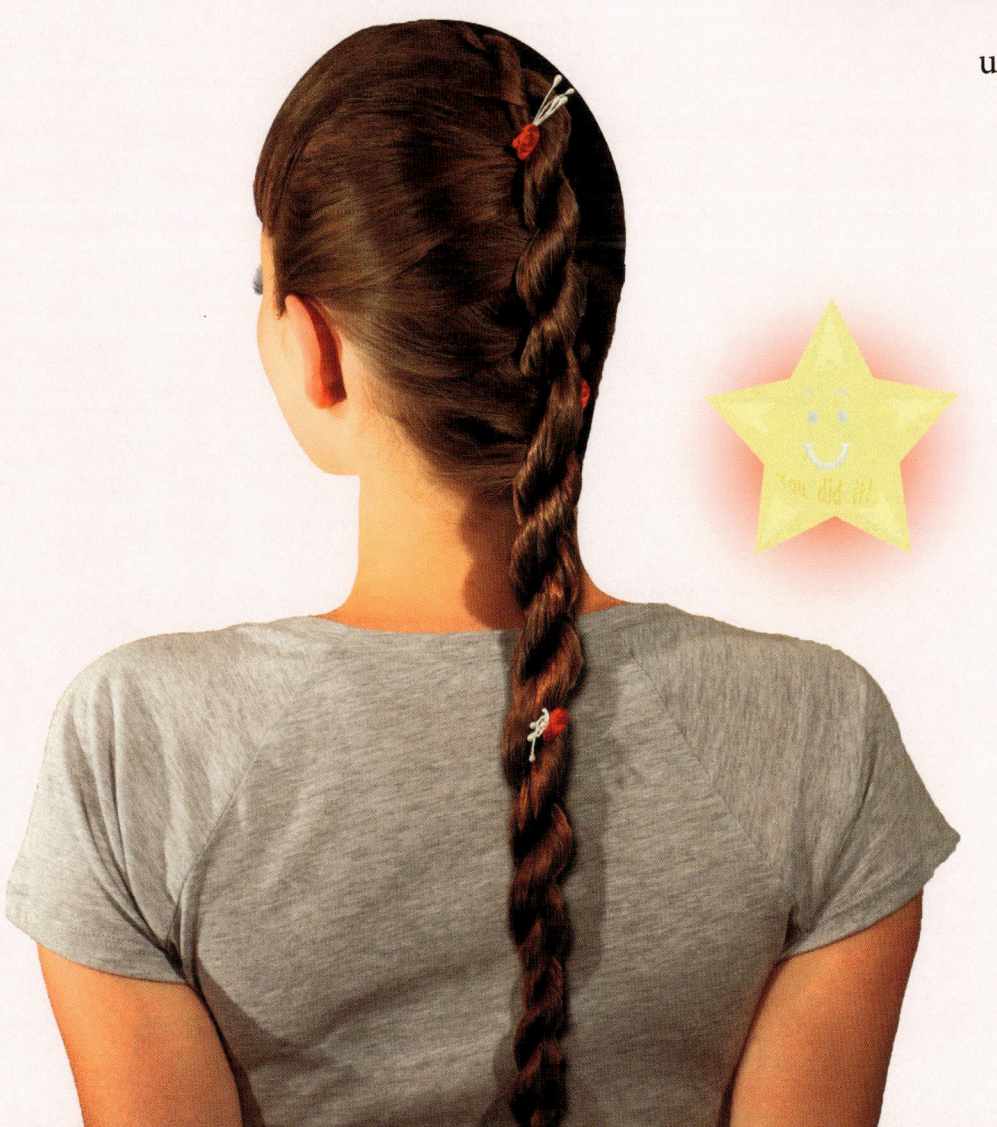

Ways 99

Two-Strand Rope

Notes

Two-Strand Rope

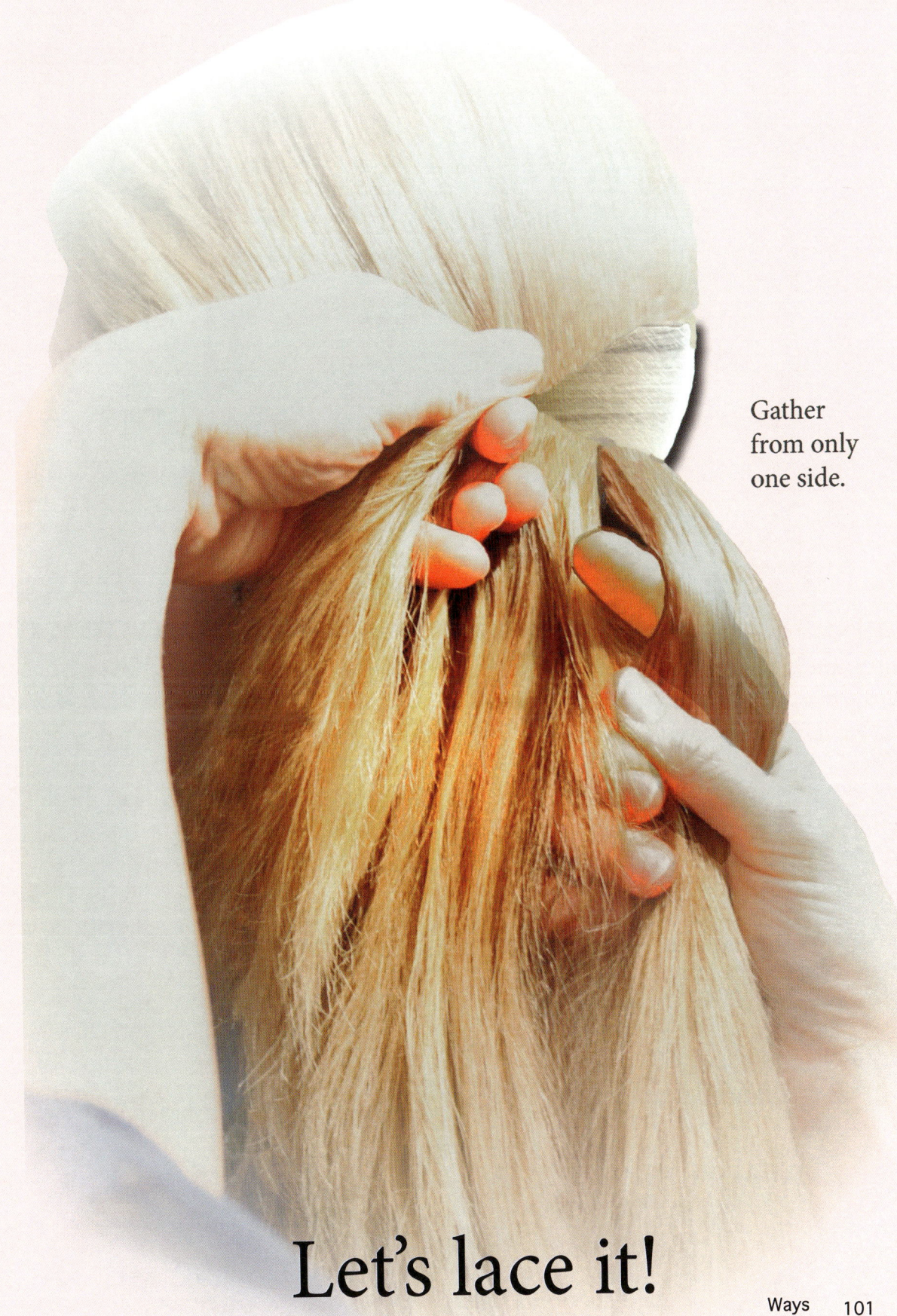

Gather from only one side.

Let's lace it!

2 Two-Strand Rope Lace

1. Begin with clean, brushed hair.

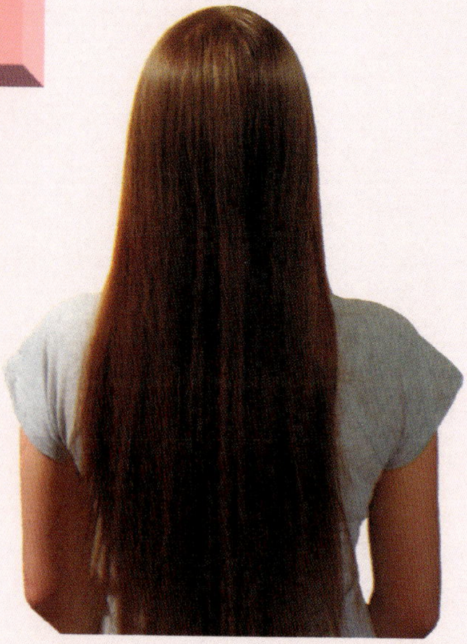

2. Take a section of hair as illustrated.

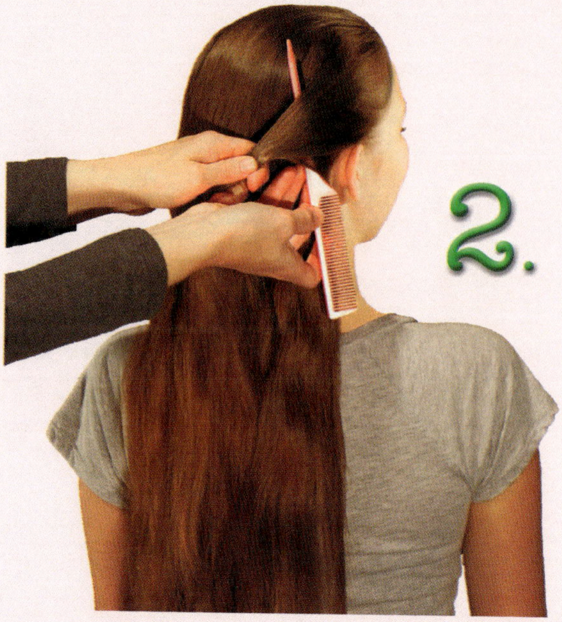

5. Wrap the strands around each other in the opposite direction.

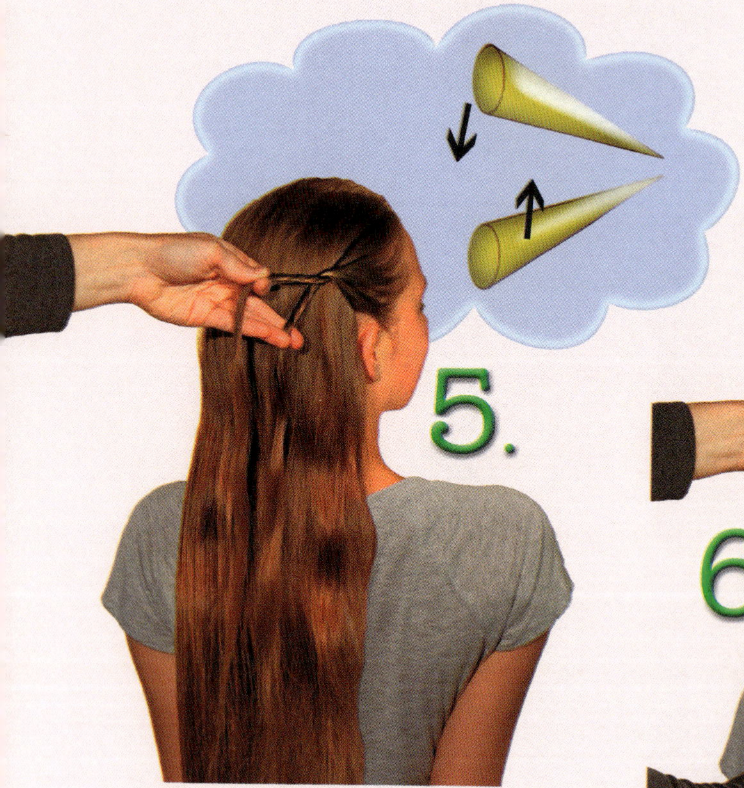

6. Sliver off a gather from the face all the way back to the braid. Gather from only one side, add the gather into the lower strand.

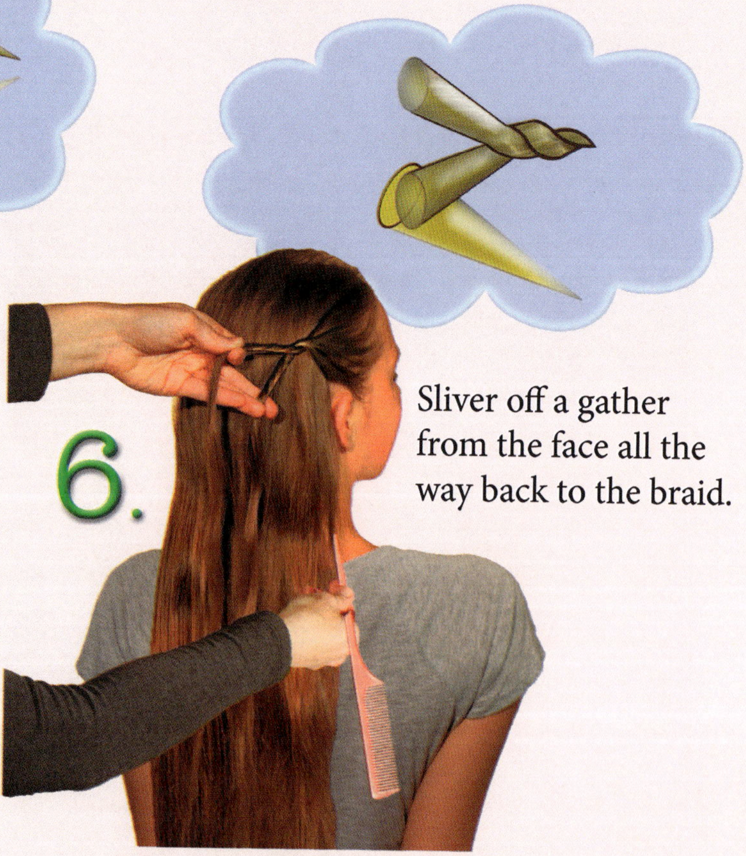

Two-Strand Rope Lace

2

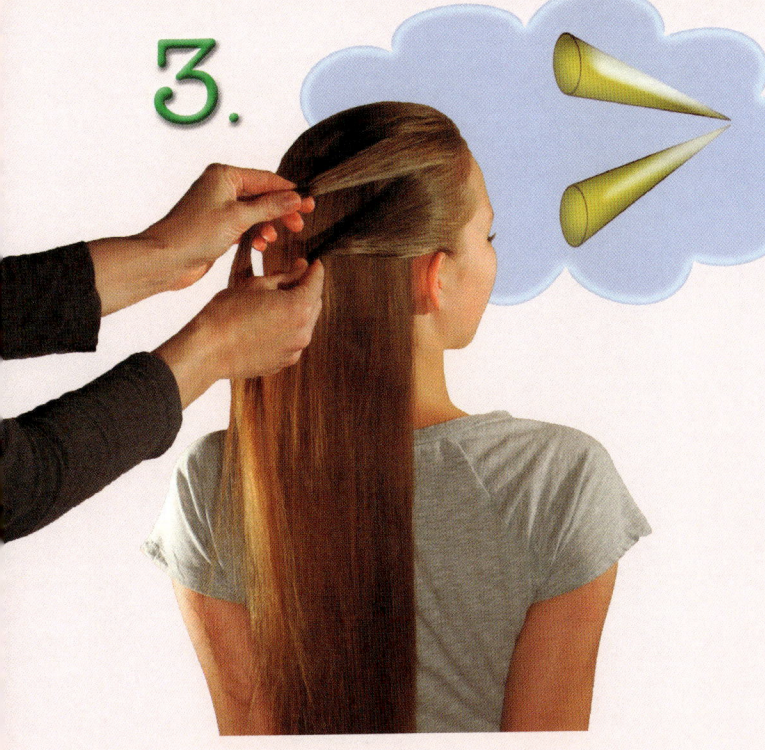

Divide the section into two strands.

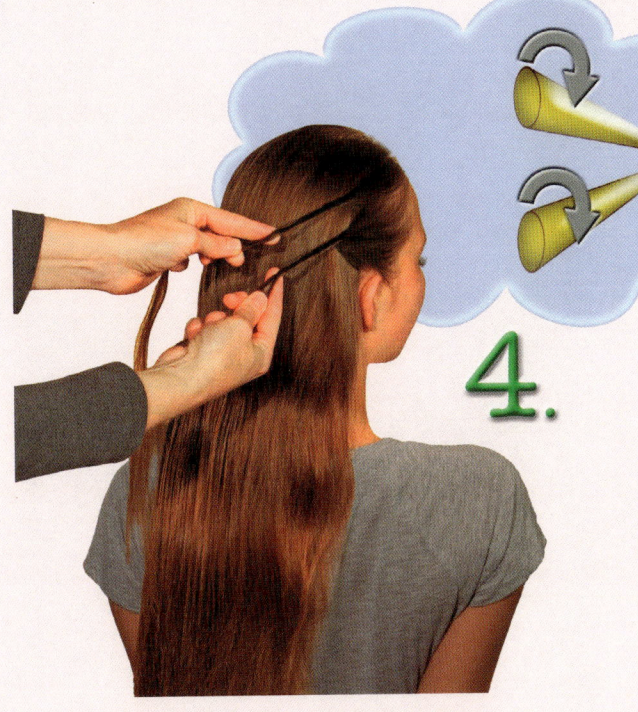

Twist each strand individually in the same direction.

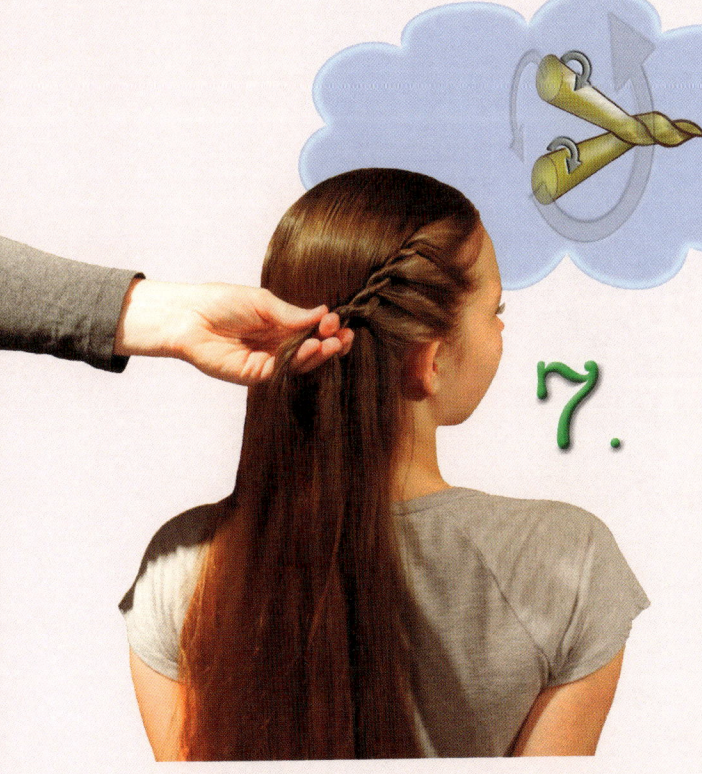

Twist the gather with the lower strand of the braid and cross them over the top strand.

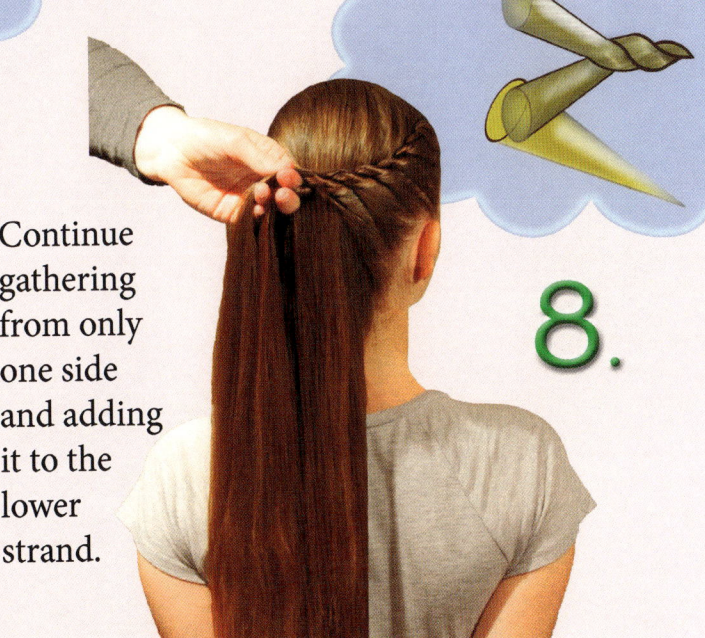

Continue gathering from only one side and adding it to the lower strand.

2 part 2. Two-Strand Rope Lace

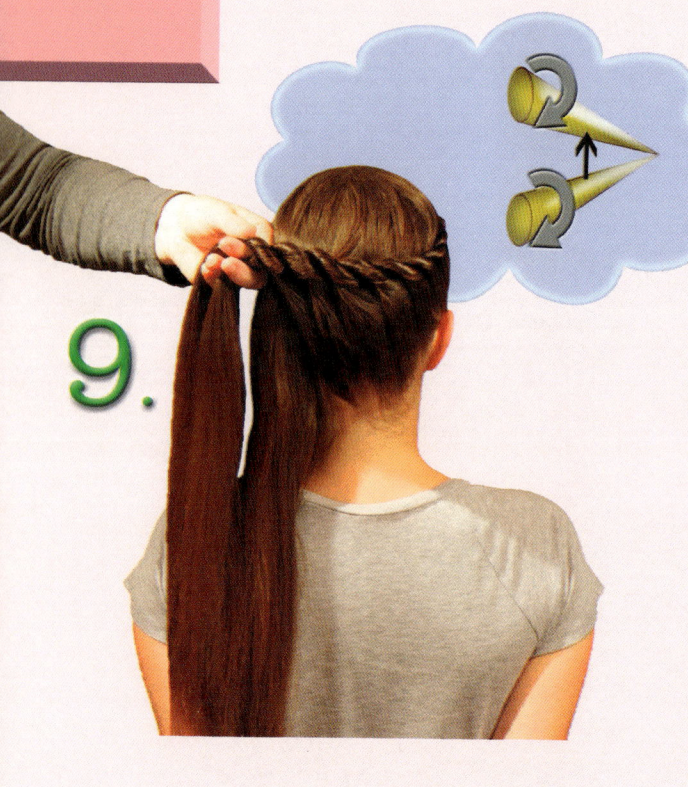

9.

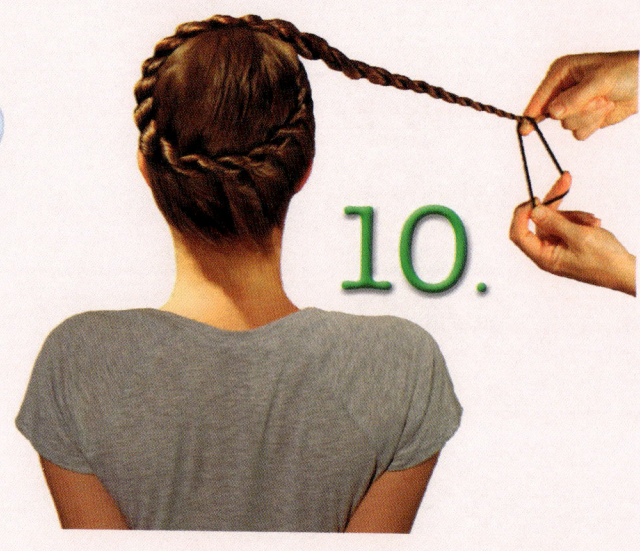

10.

Secure with a rubber band.

Continue gathering, twisting, and wrapping until you reach the end of the hair.

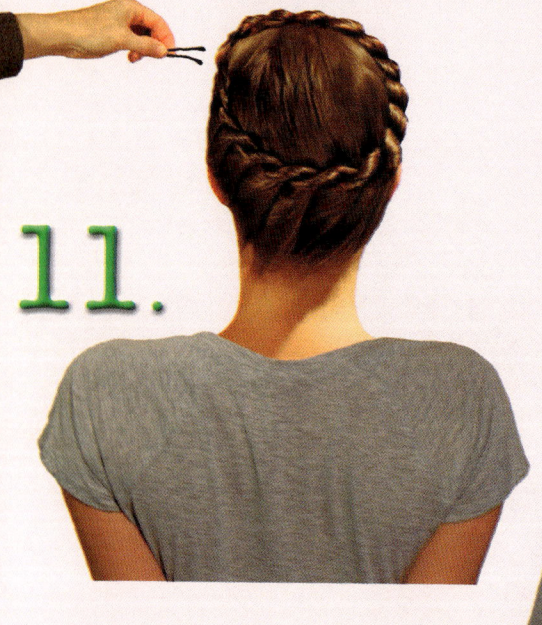

11.

Fix the end of the braid with bobby pins to hold the braid in place.

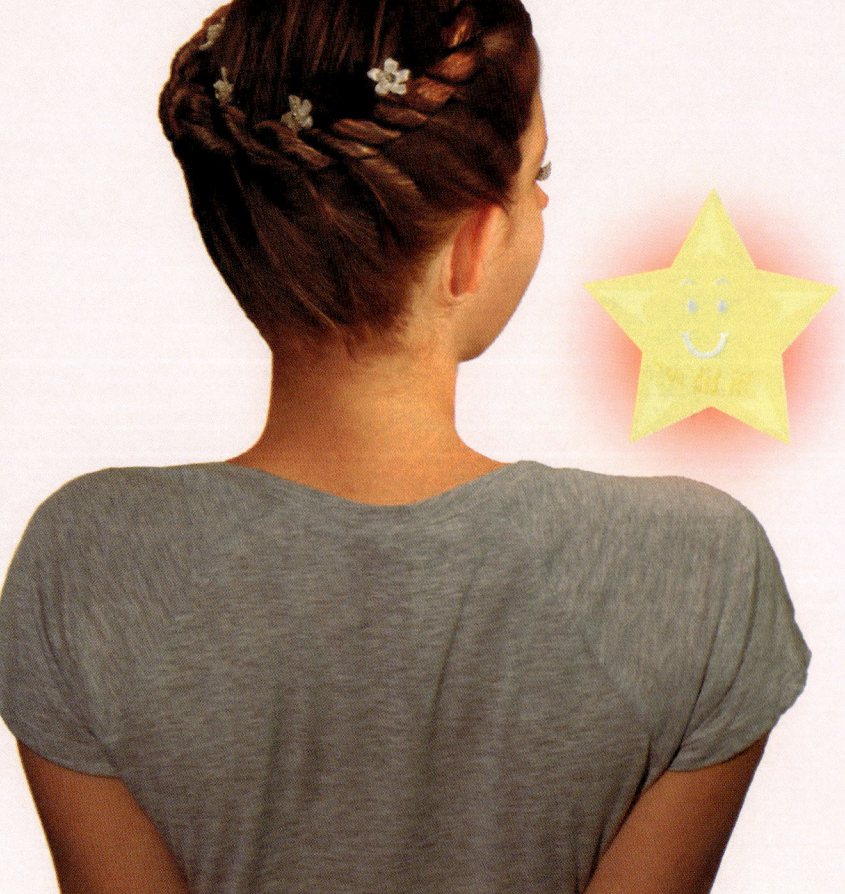

Examples of Two-Strand Rope

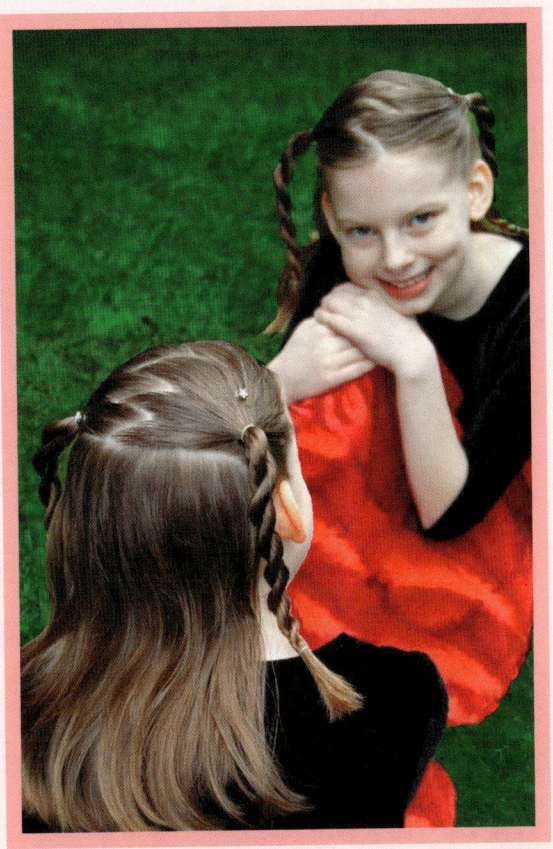
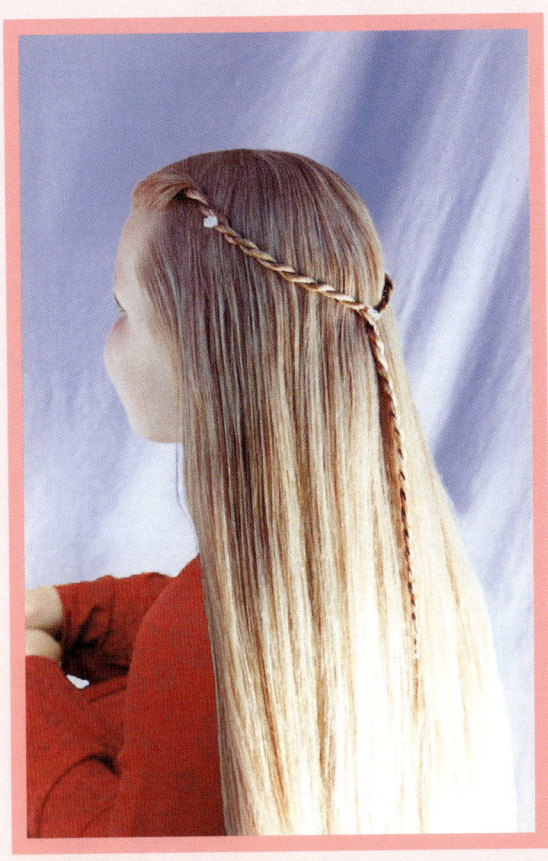
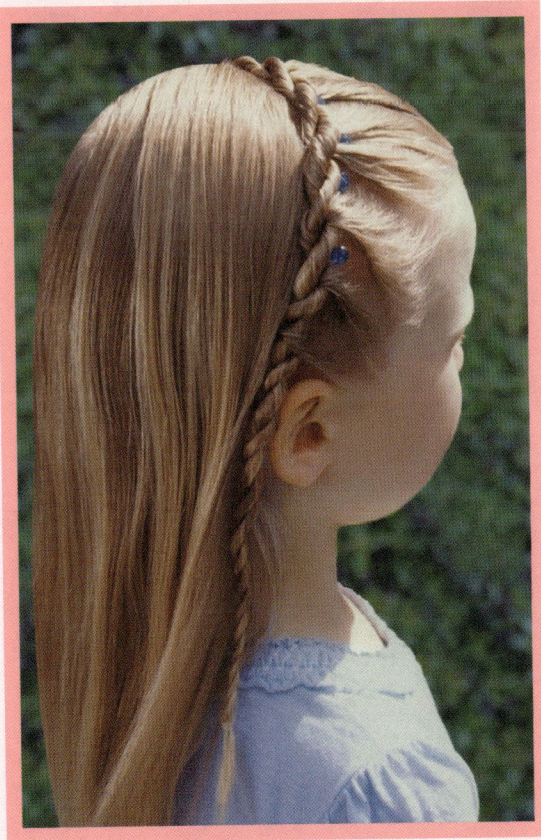
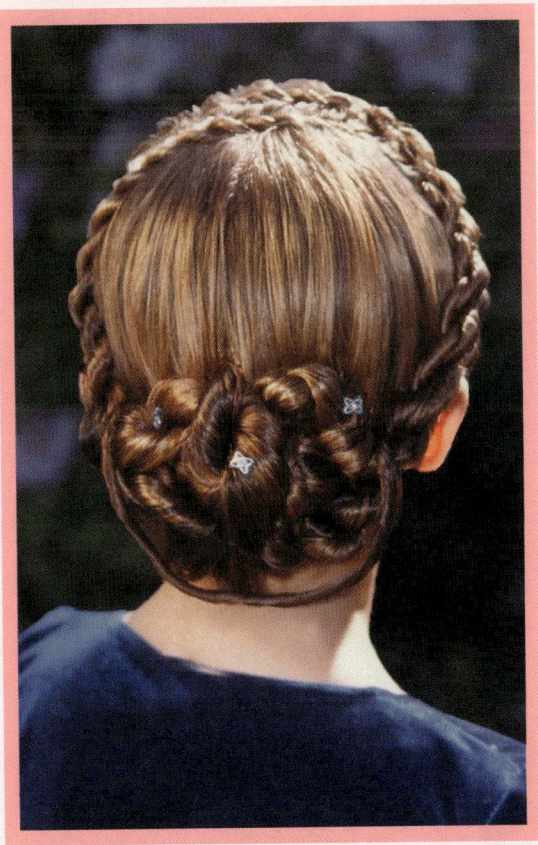

Visit my website to see more examples of the Two-Strand Rope

Two-Strand Herringbone

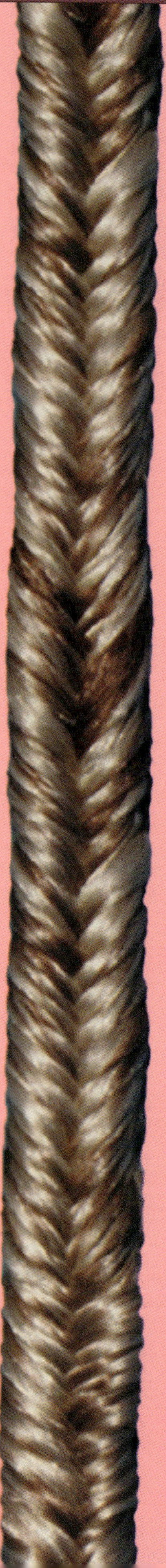

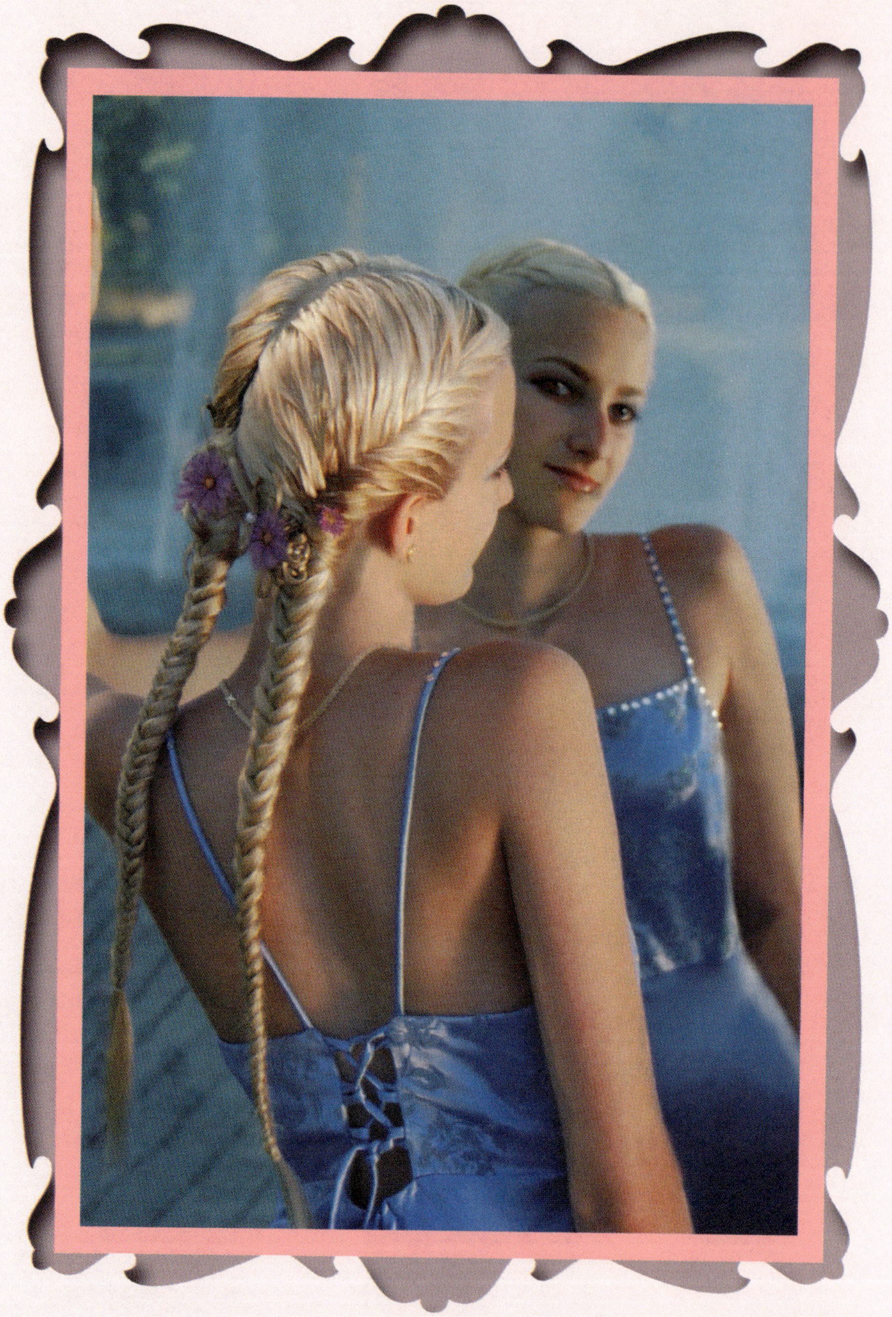

The intricacy of this braid draws the young and old. Also refered to as a fishbone because of the pattern it creates, it is a popular and pretty braid.

Two-Strand Herringbone

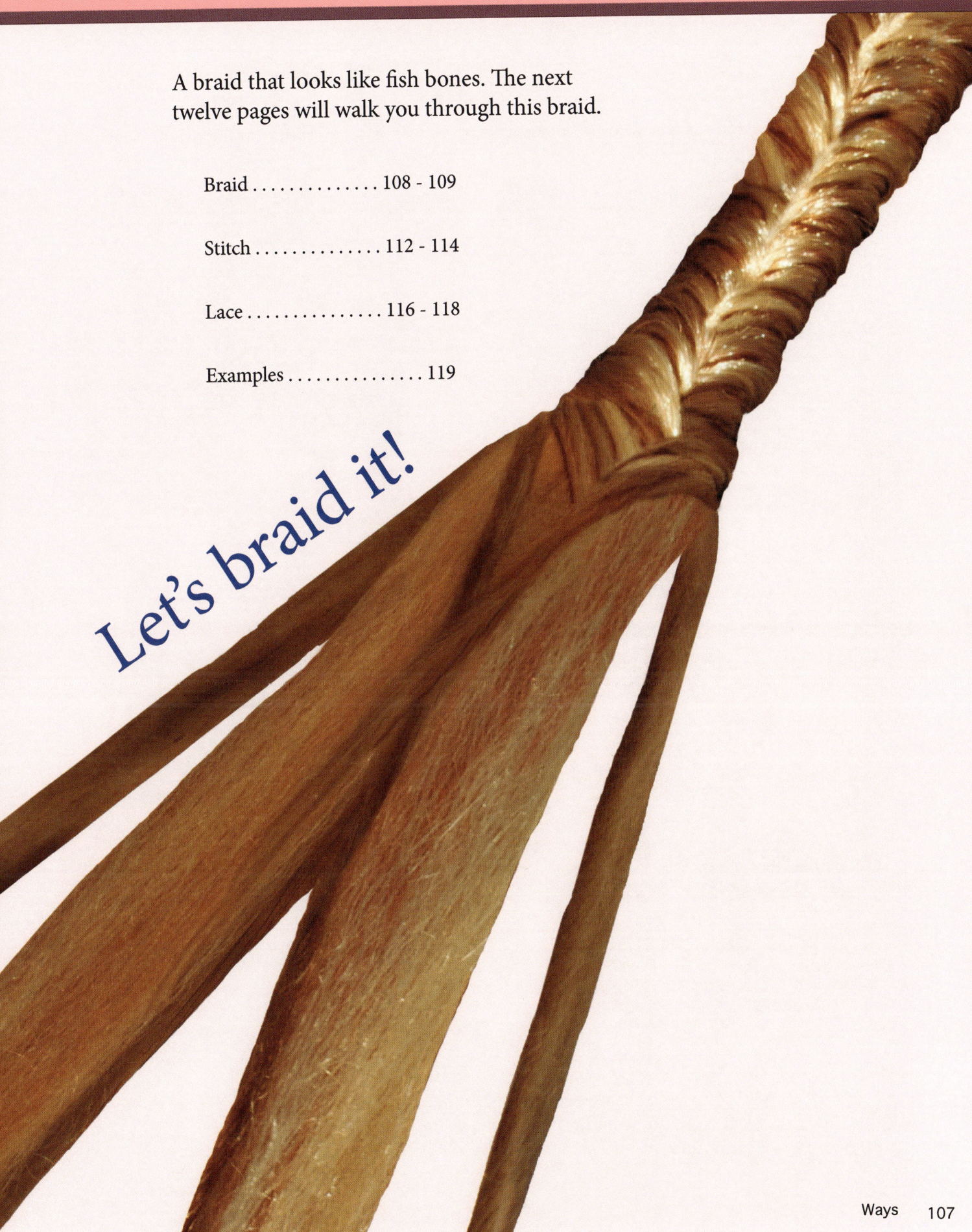

A braid that looks like fish bones. The next twelve pages will walk you through this braid.

Braid . . . . 108 - 109

Stitch . . . . 112 - 114

Lace . . . . 116 - 118

Examples 119

Let's braid it!

Ways

2 Two-Strand Herringbone Braid

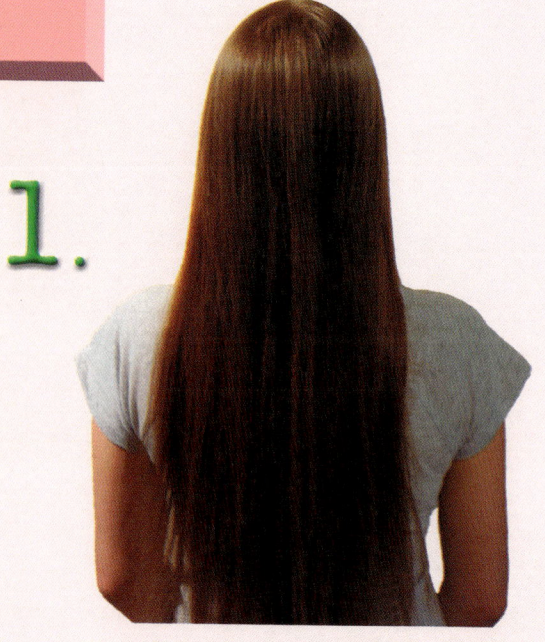

1. Begin with clean, brushed hair.

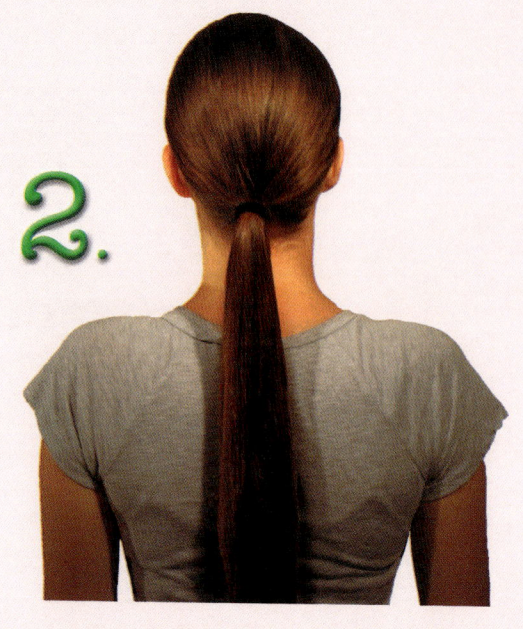

2. Take a section of hair.

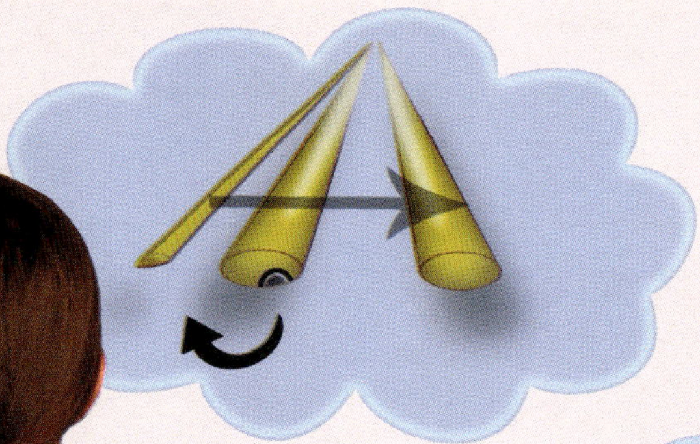

5. 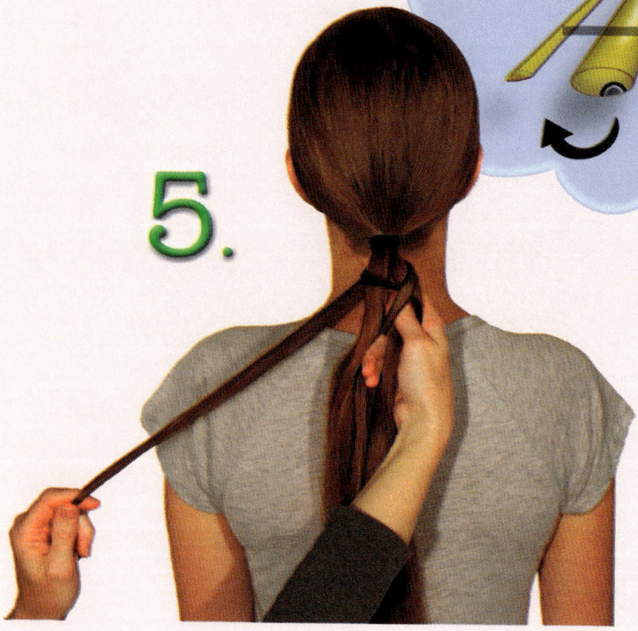 Using the same technique create an 'x' by slivering off a tiny bit from the underside of the other strand. Bring it over the top and combine it with the first strand.

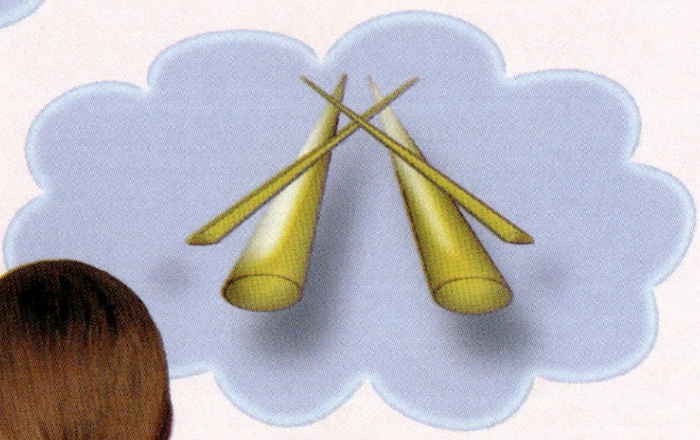

6. 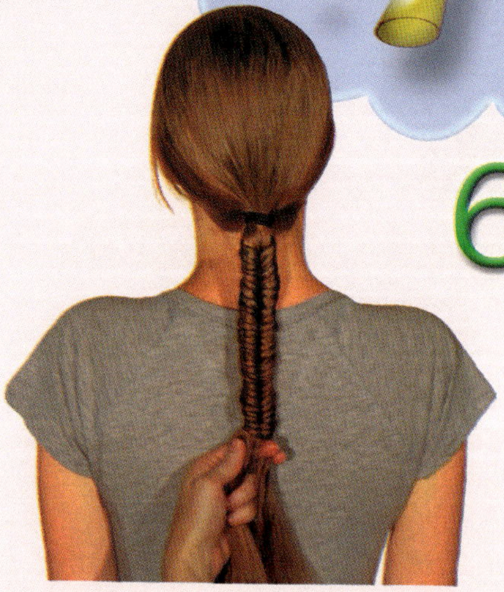 Continue making tiny 'x's by taking slivers from each side and alternating them over top.

108   www.findingbraids.com

Two-Strand Herringbone Braid

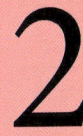

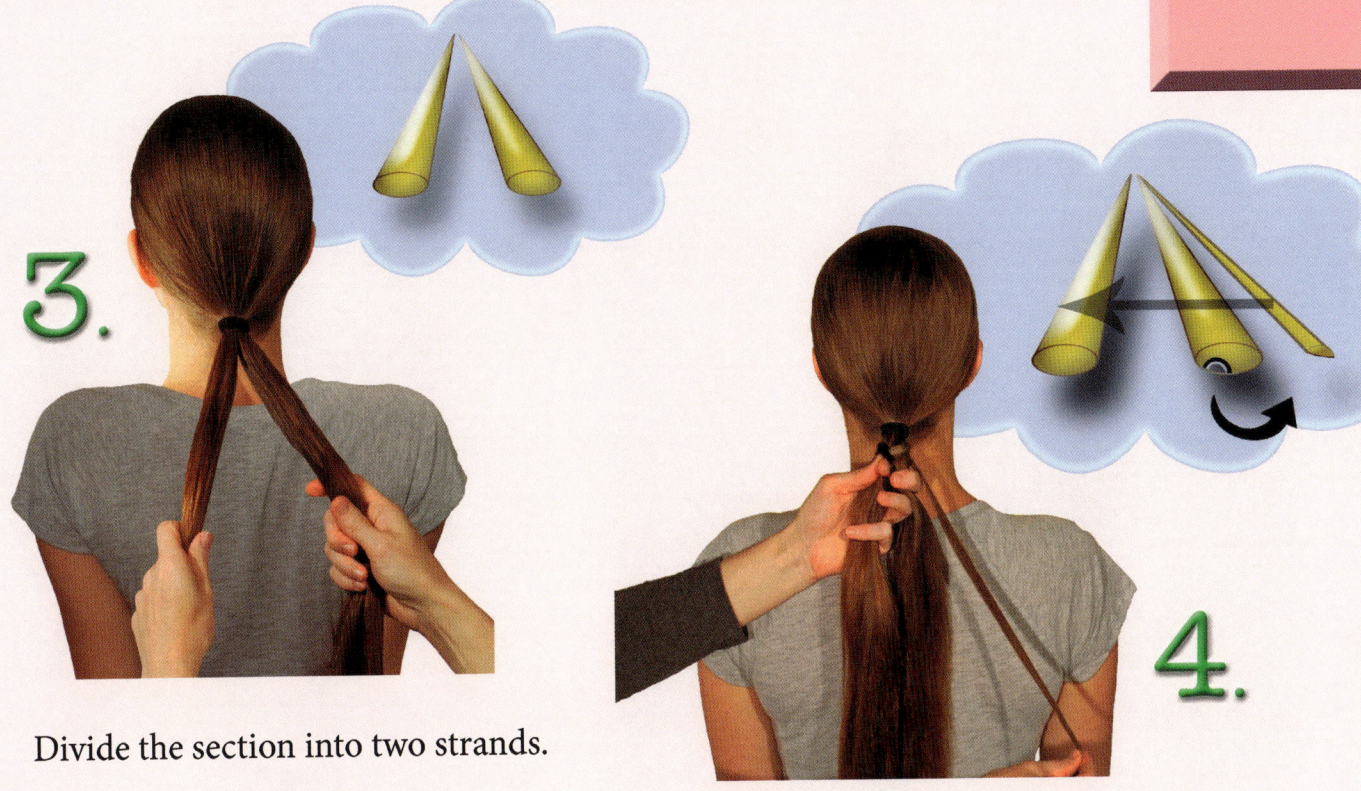

3. Divide the section into two strands.

4. Sliver off a tiny bit from the underside of one strand. Bring it over the top and combine it with the opposite strand.

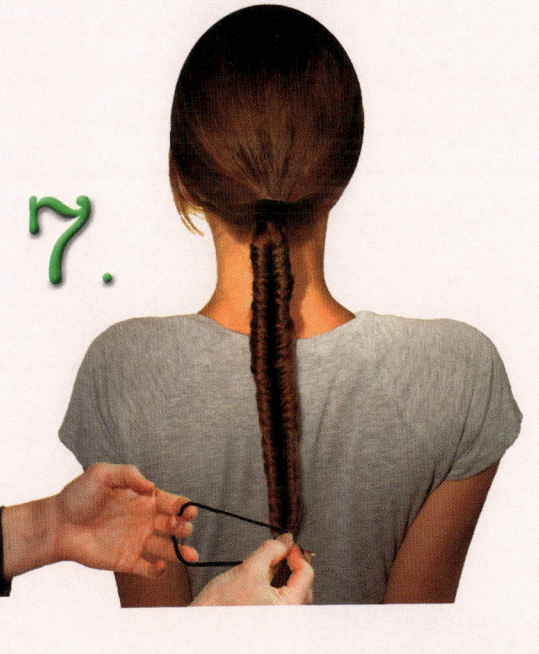

7. Secure with a rubber band.

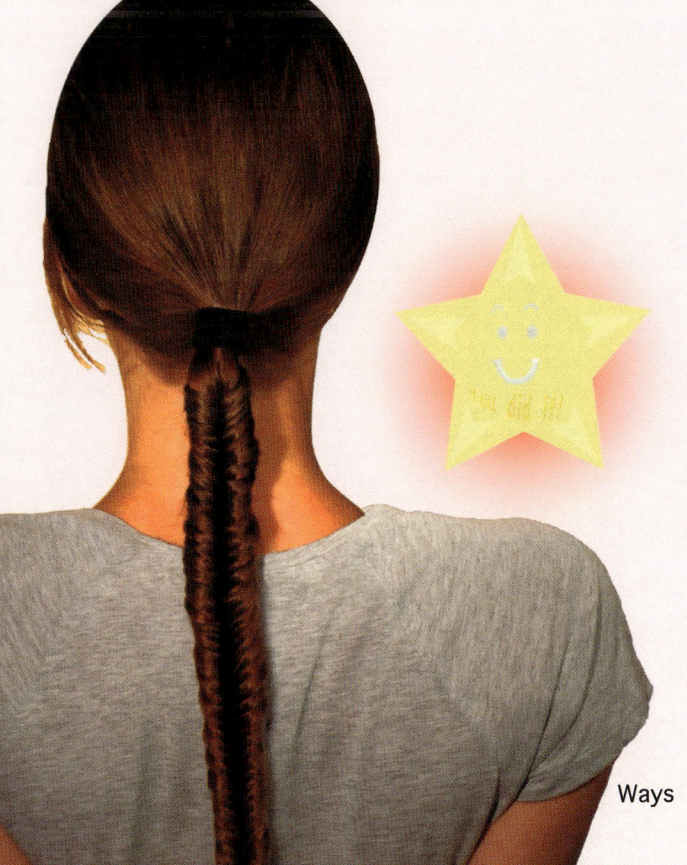

Two-Strand Herringbone

Notes

_____

_____

_____

_____

_____

_____

If patience ever was a virtue, it most certainly was here. It is entirely possible the only time I willingly did the herringbone braid was for this book. It is a mind numbingly tedious braid requiring time and slivers of hair moving back and forth.

Two-Strand Herringbone

Gather from both sides

Let's stitch it!

Let's stitch it!

Let's stitch it!

Ways 111

2 Two-Strand Herringbone Stitch

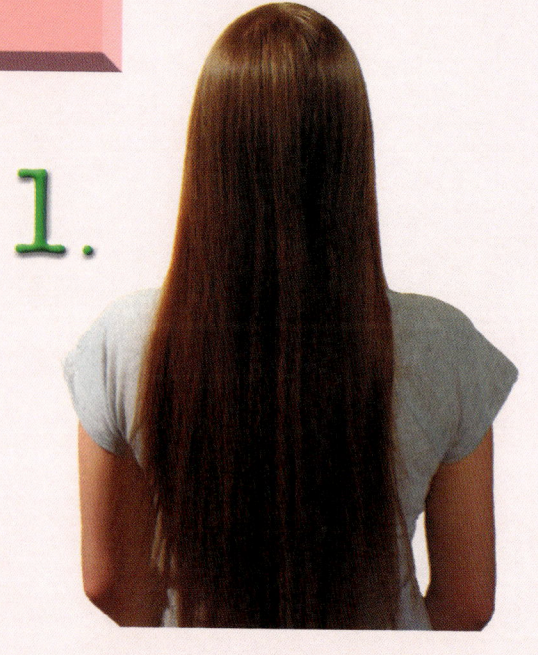

1. Begin with clean, brushed hair.

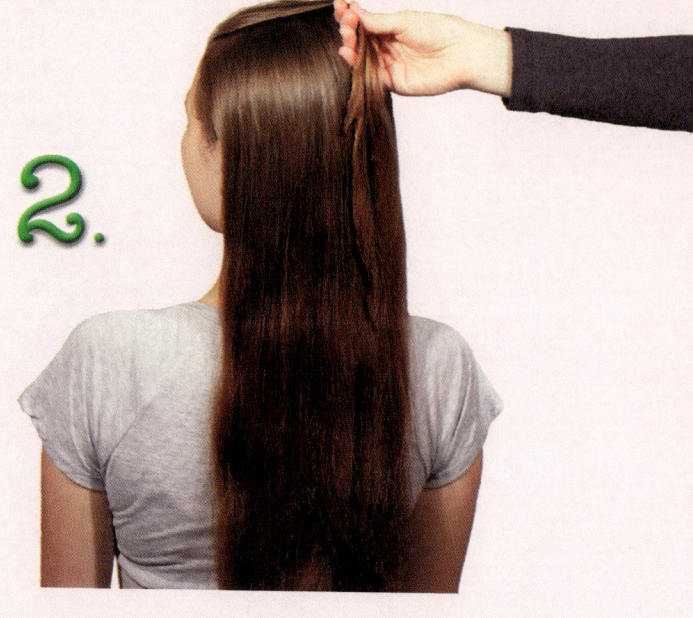

2. Take a section of hair as illustrated.

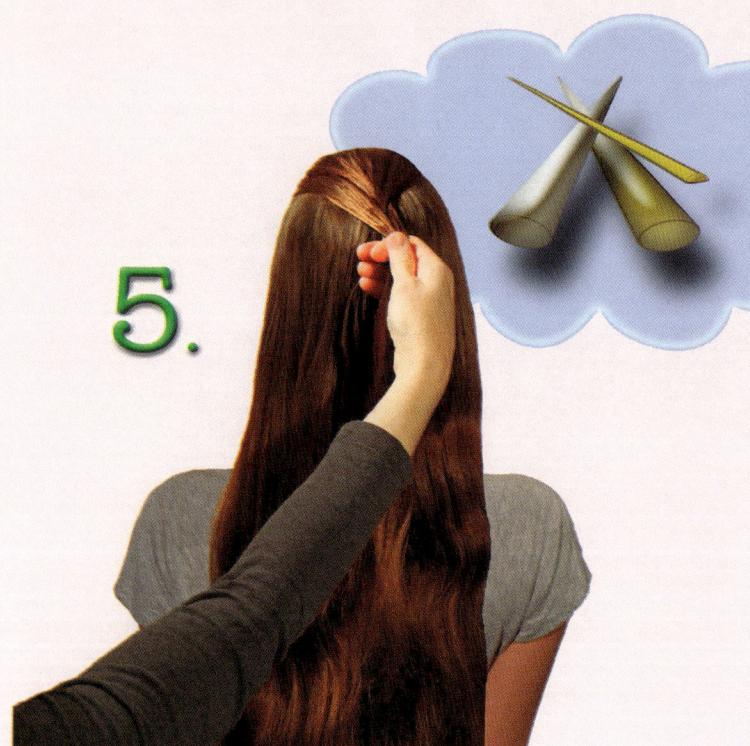

5. Cross the gather over the top and combine it with the opposite strand.

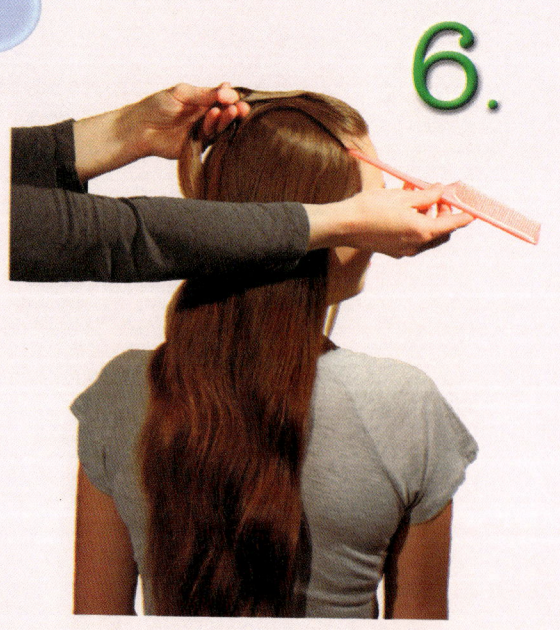

6. Sliver off a gather from the other side of the face all the way back to the braid.

Two-Strand Herringbone Stitch

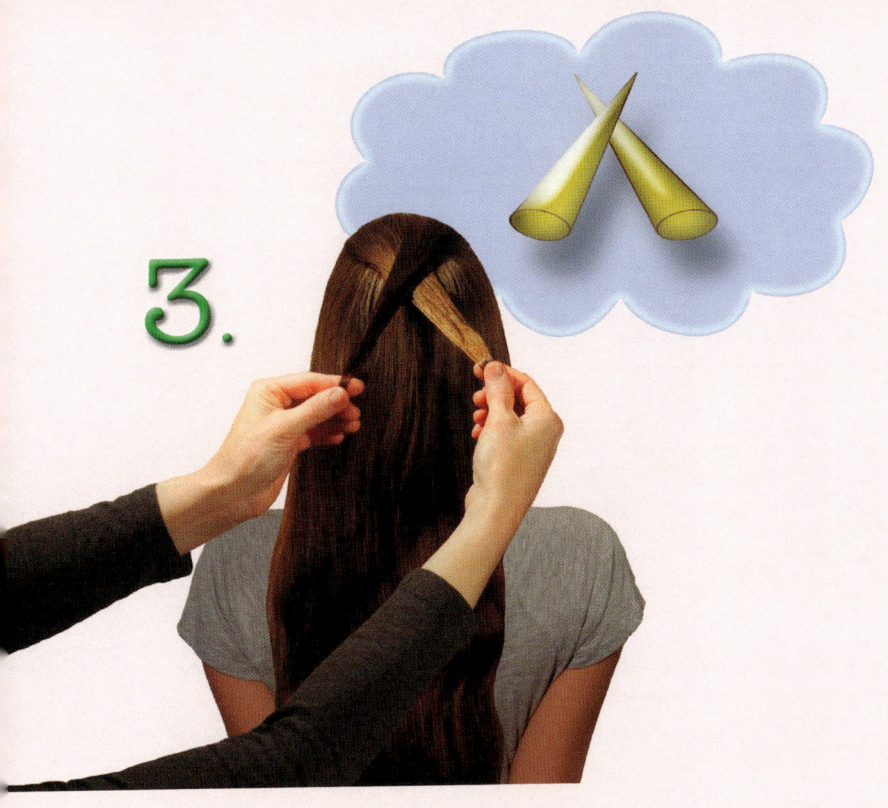

3. Divide the section into two strands. Cross the two strands to make an 'x'.

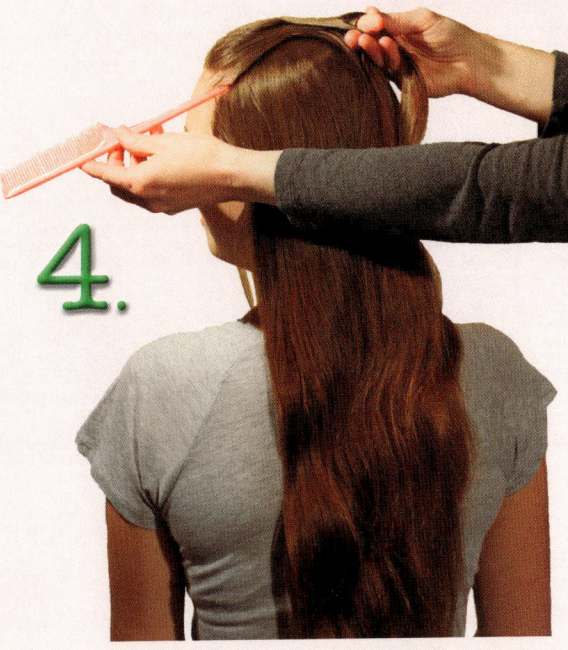

4. Sliver off a gather from the face all the way back to the braid.

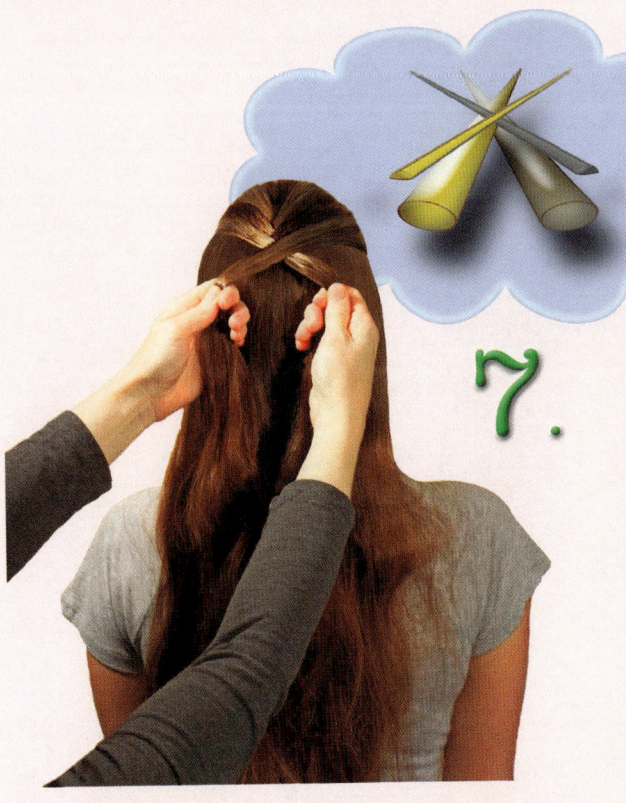

7. Cross the gather over the top and combine it with the opposite strand.

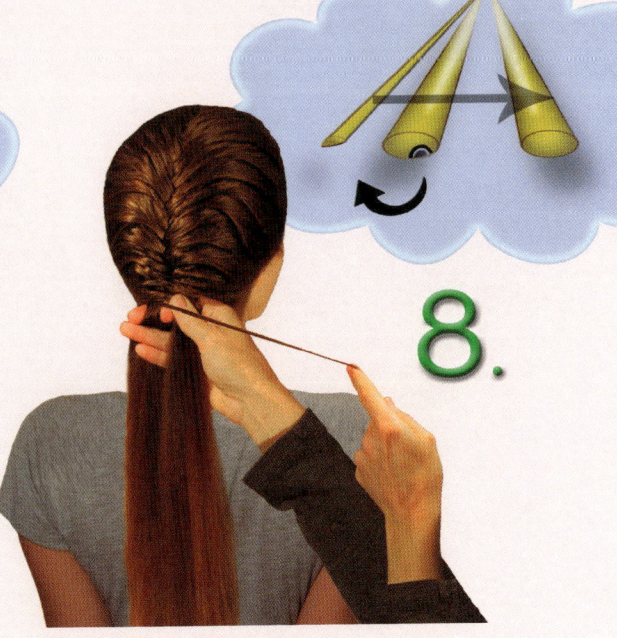

8. Once you run out hair to gather, continue making tiny 'x"s by taking slivers from underneath each strand and alternating them over top.

part 2. Herringbone Stitch

2

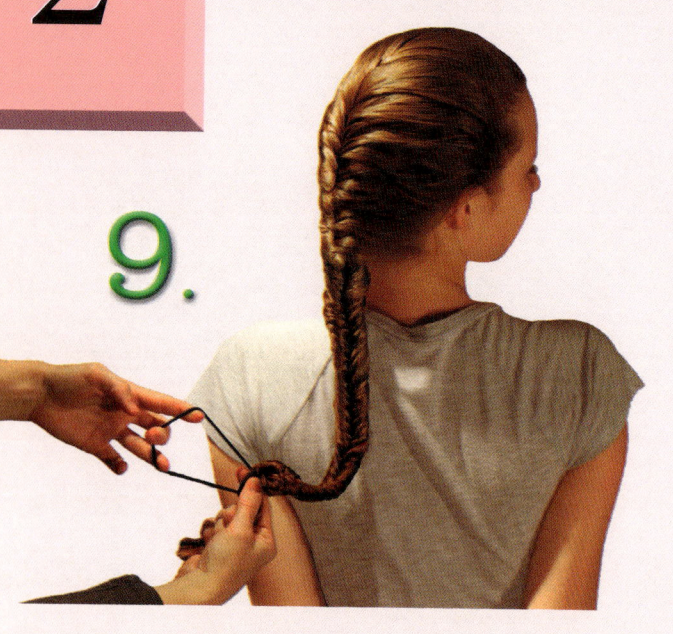

9.

Secure with a rubber band.

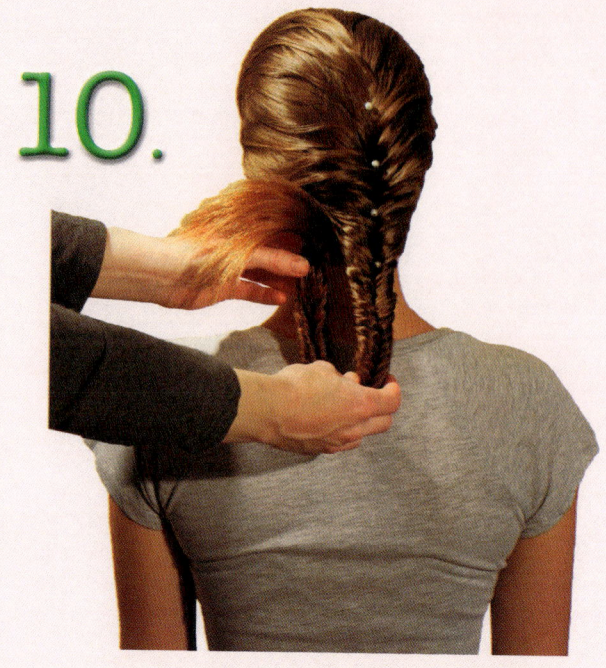

10.

This braid looks good tucked up and under.

11.

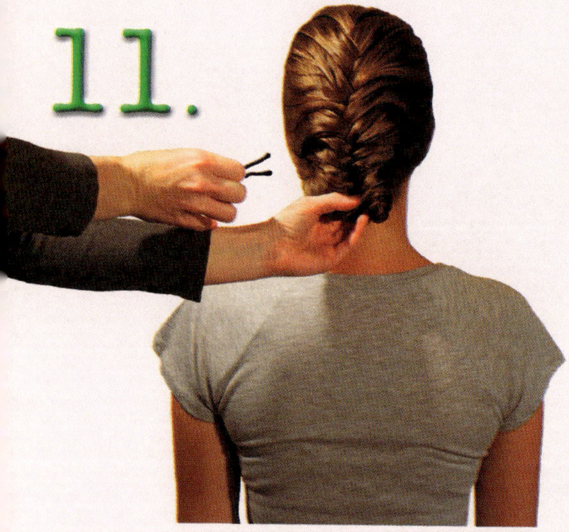

Fix the end of the braid with bobby pins to hold the braid in place.

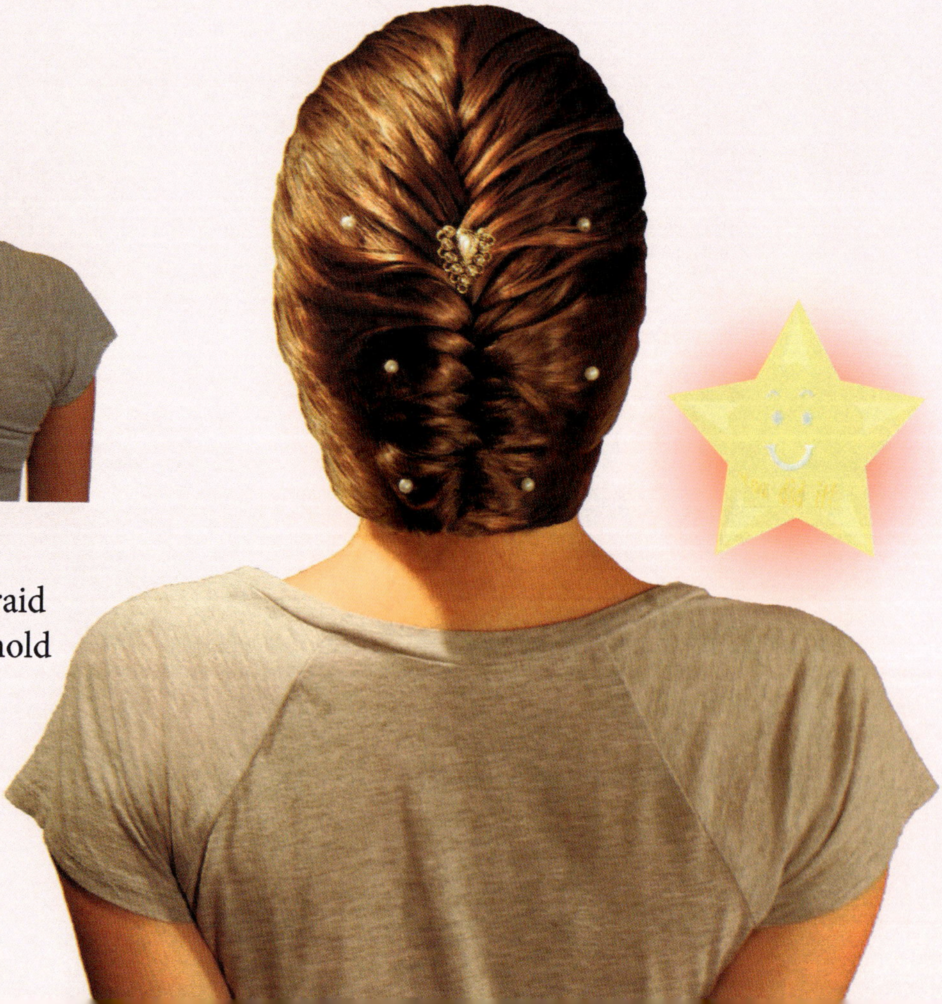

Two-Strand Herringbone

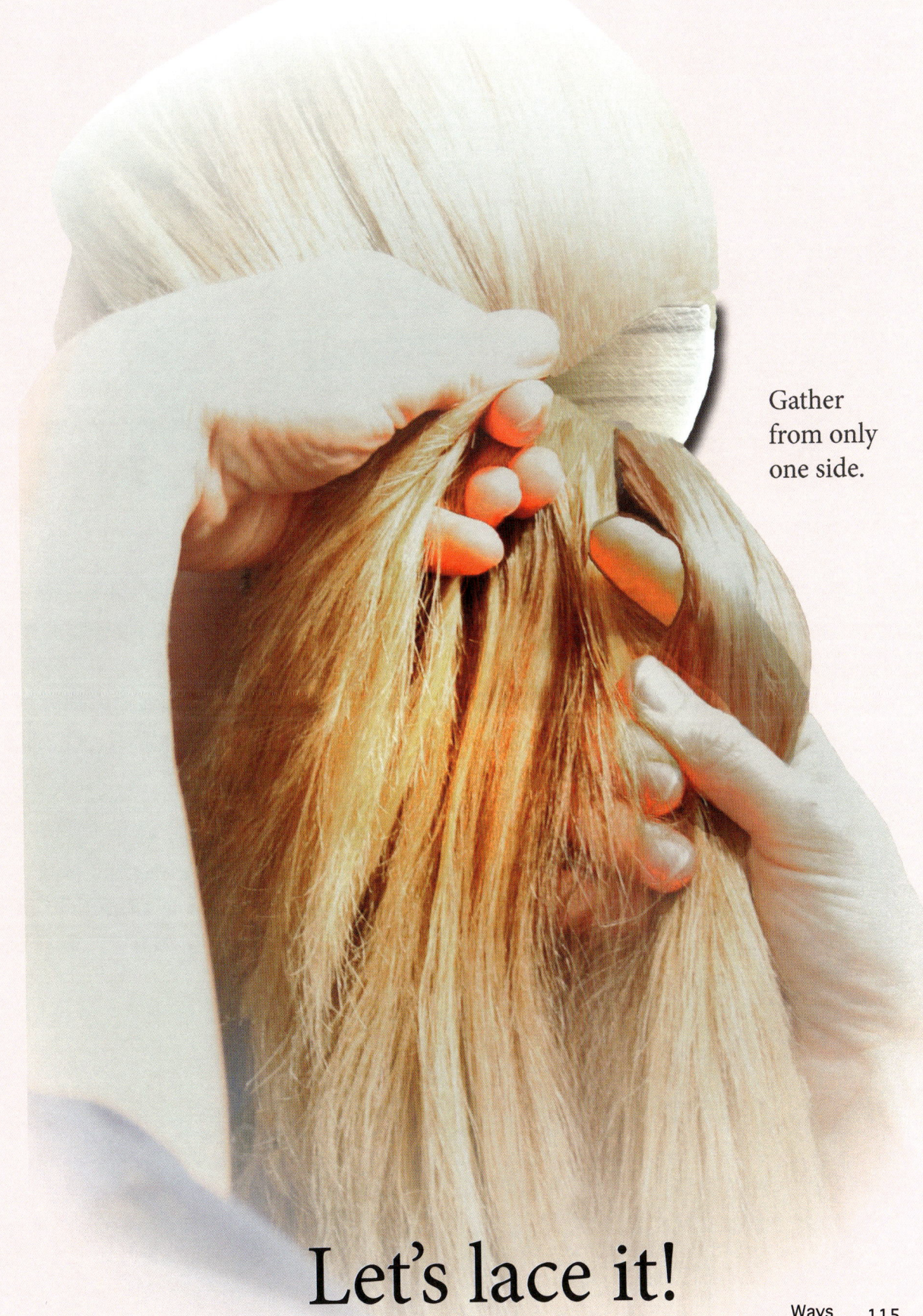

Gather from only one side.

Let's lace it!

2 Two-Strand Herringbone Lace

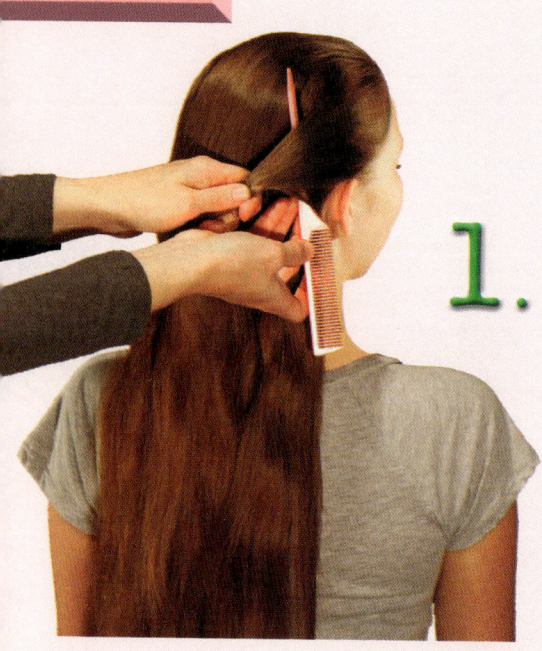

Take a section of hair as illustrated.

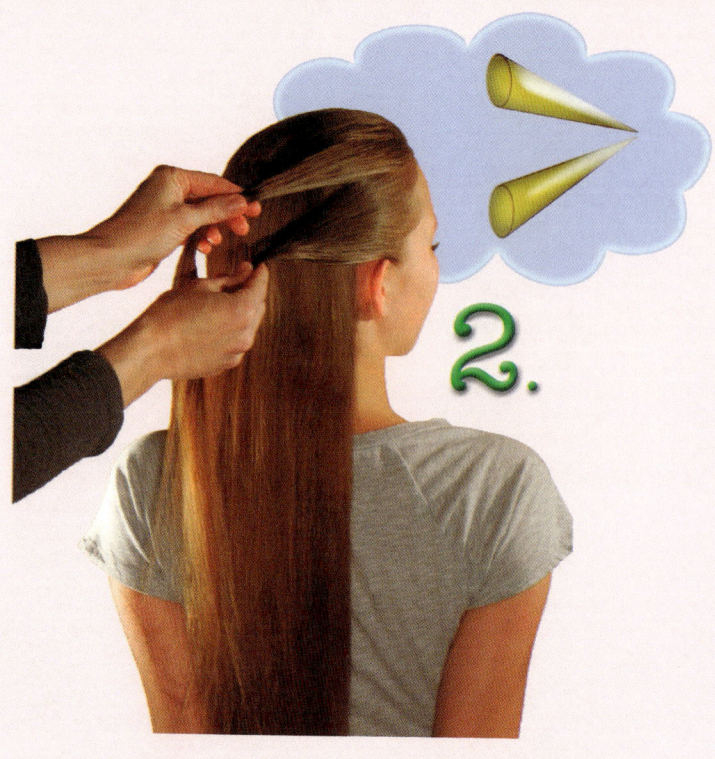

Divide the section into two strands.

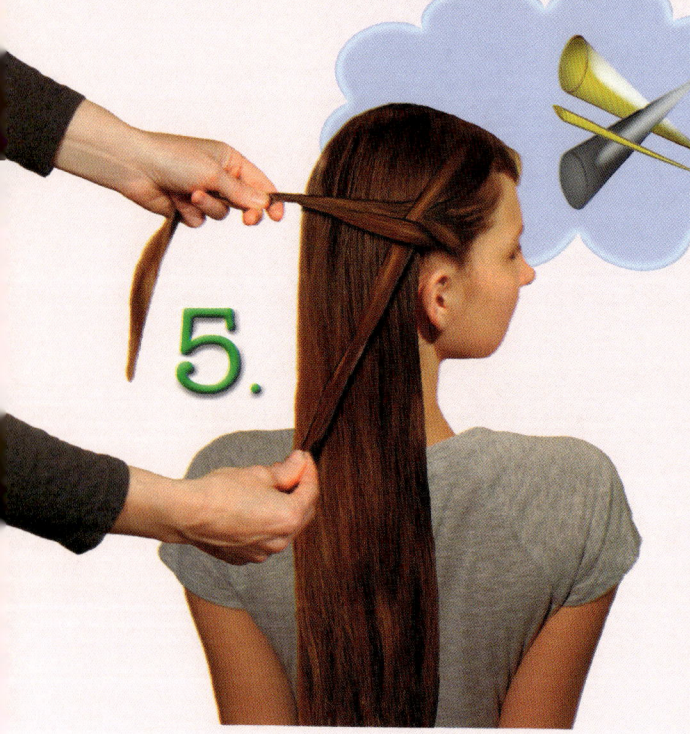

Cross the gather over the top and combine it with the opposite strand.

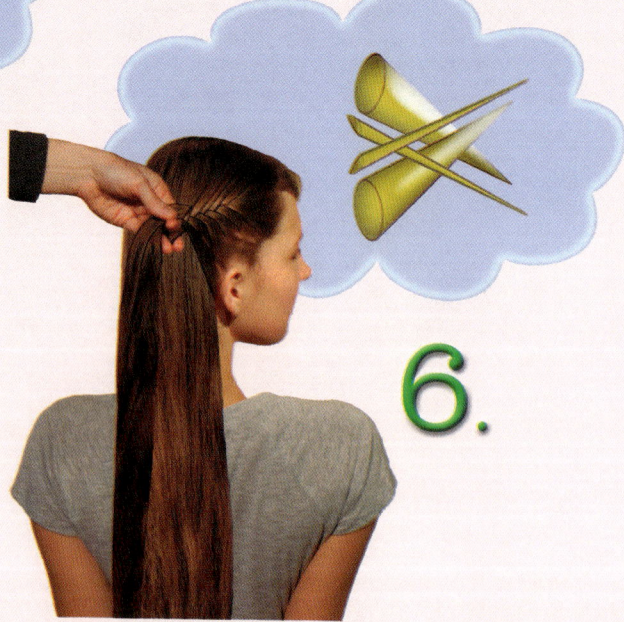

Gather from both sides for a few passes as illustrated. This anchors the braid to the head so you can lace across the back.

Two-Strand Herringbone lace

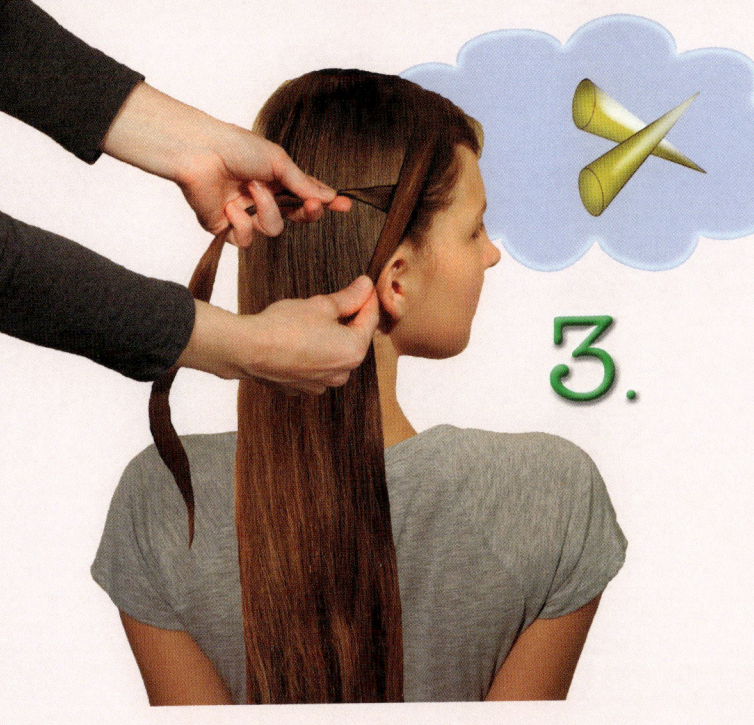

3.

Cross the two strands to make an 'x'.

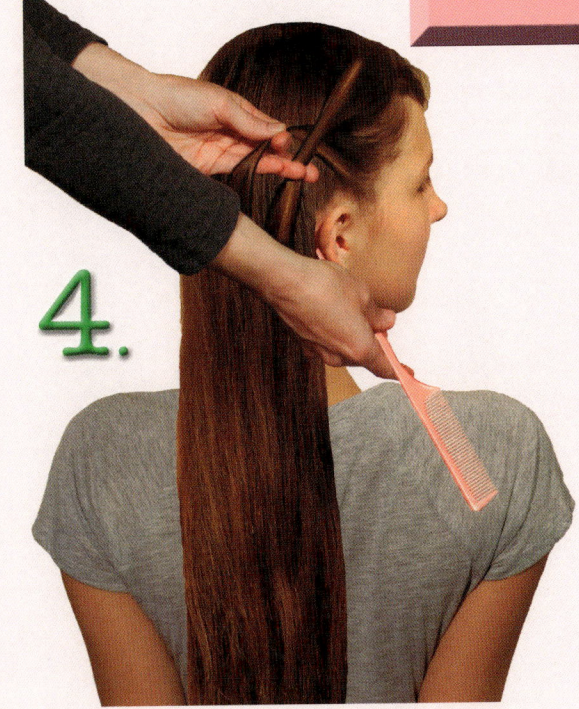

4.

Sliver off a gather from the face all the way back to the braid.

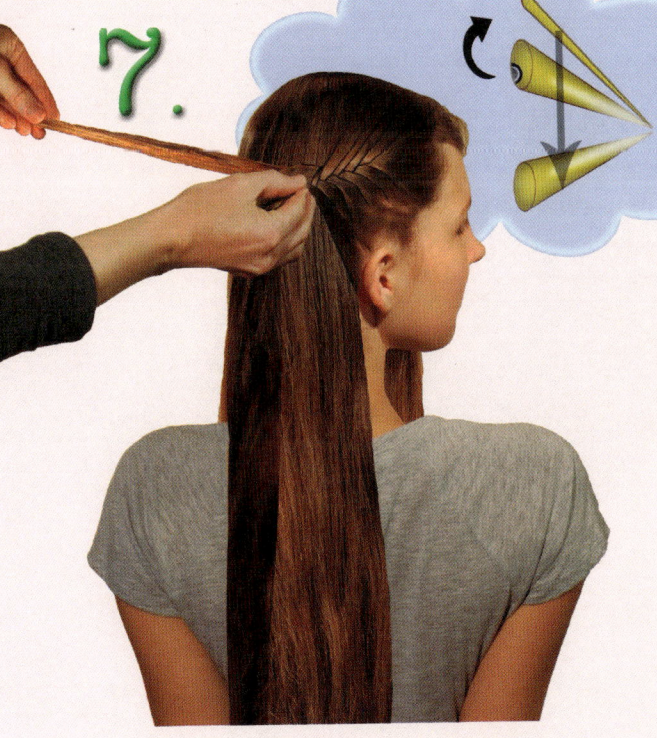

7.

To lace across the back, sliver off a tiny bit of hair from the top strands from now on and cross it over to the bottom strand, instead of gathering from the top.

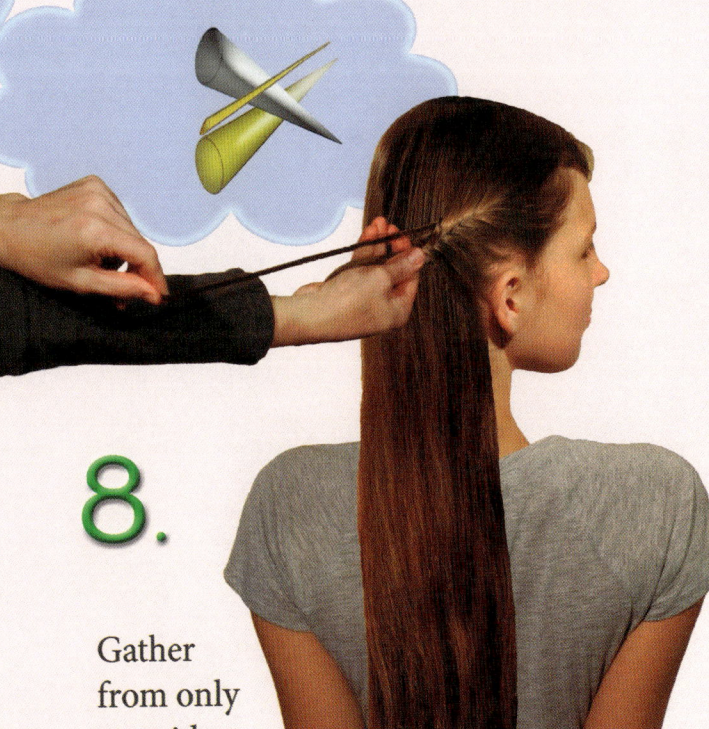

8.

Gather from only one side.

Ways

2   part 2. Herringbone Lace

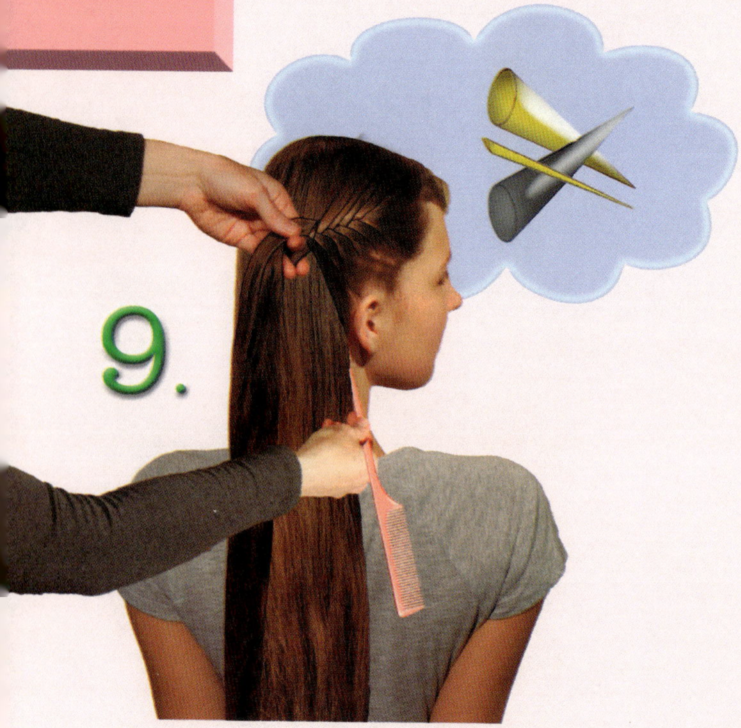

9.

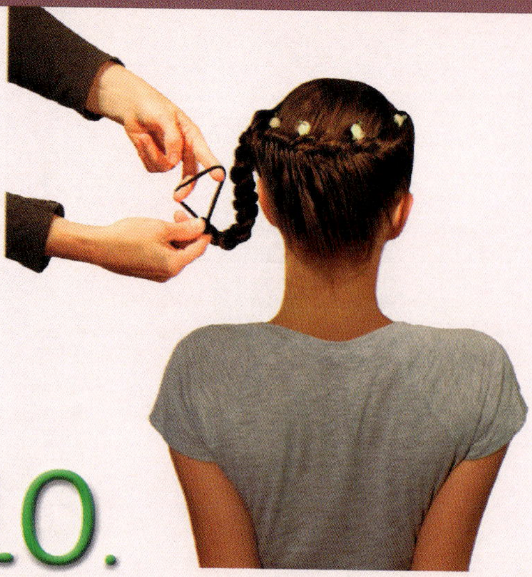

10. Secure with a rubber band.

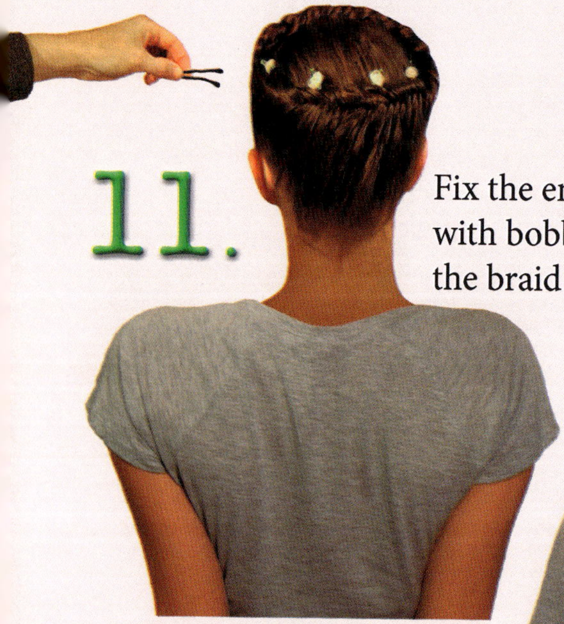

Continue gathering and making "x"'s until you reach the end of the hair.

11. Fix the end of the braid with bobby pins to hold the braid in place.

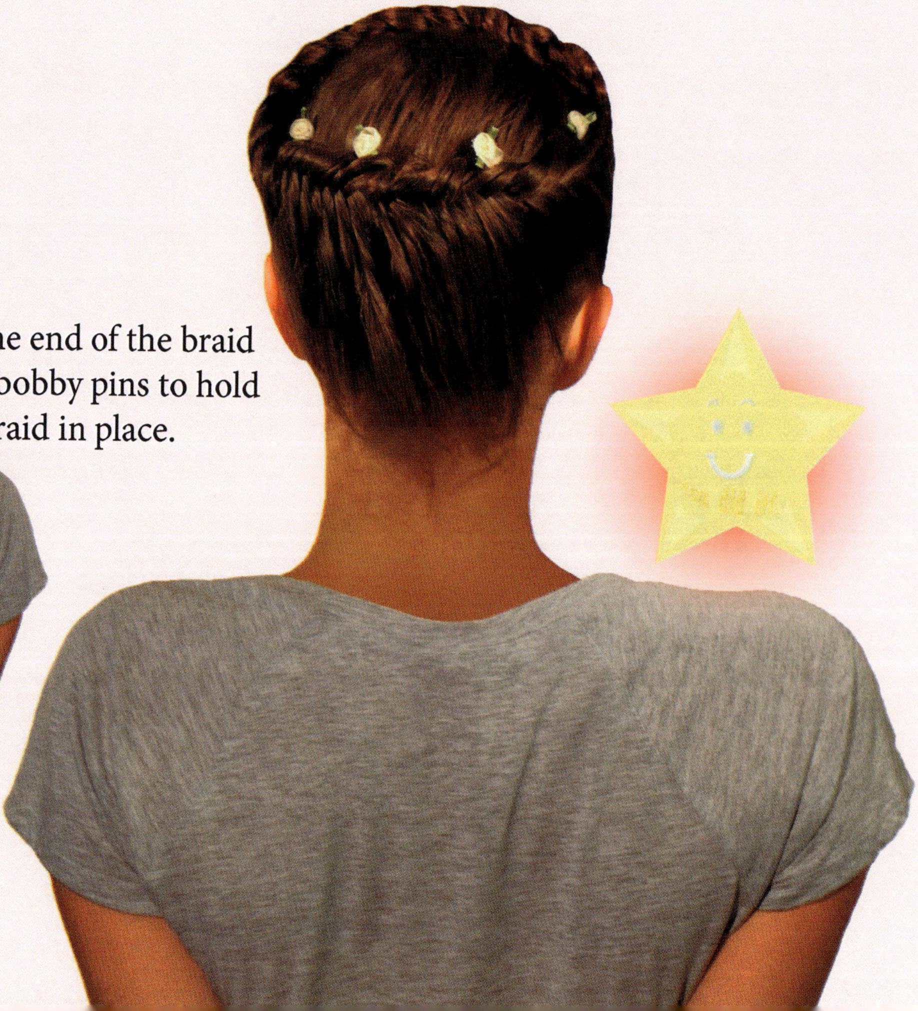

Examples of Two-Strand Herringbone

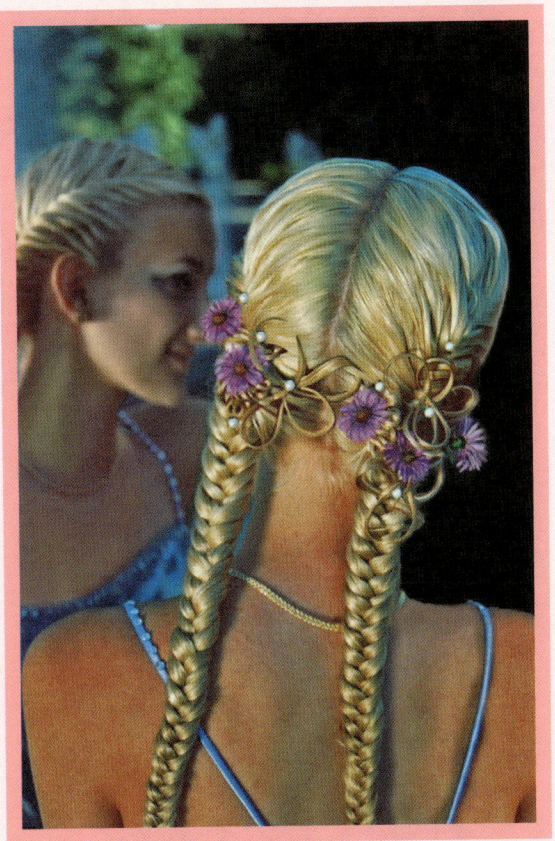
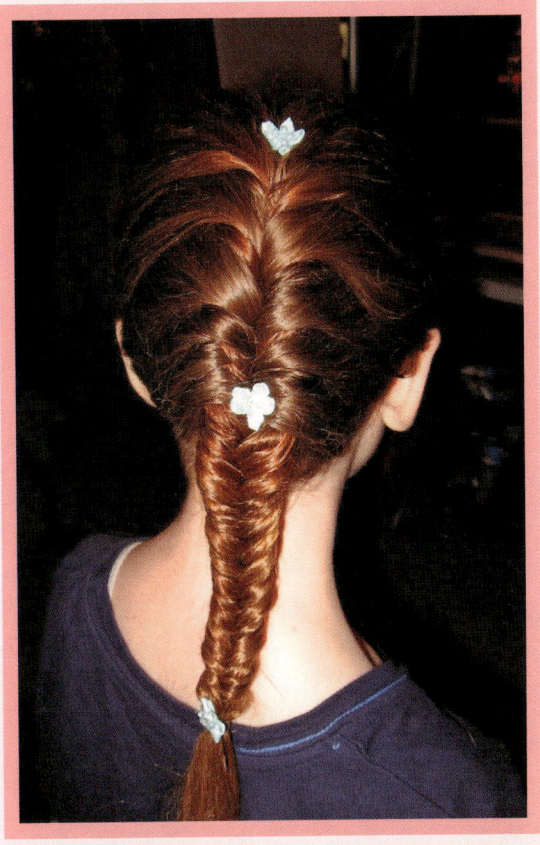
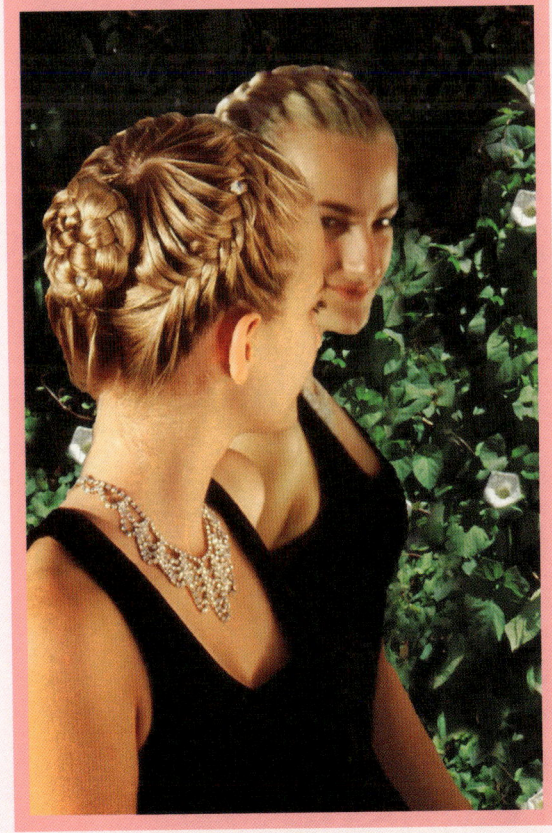
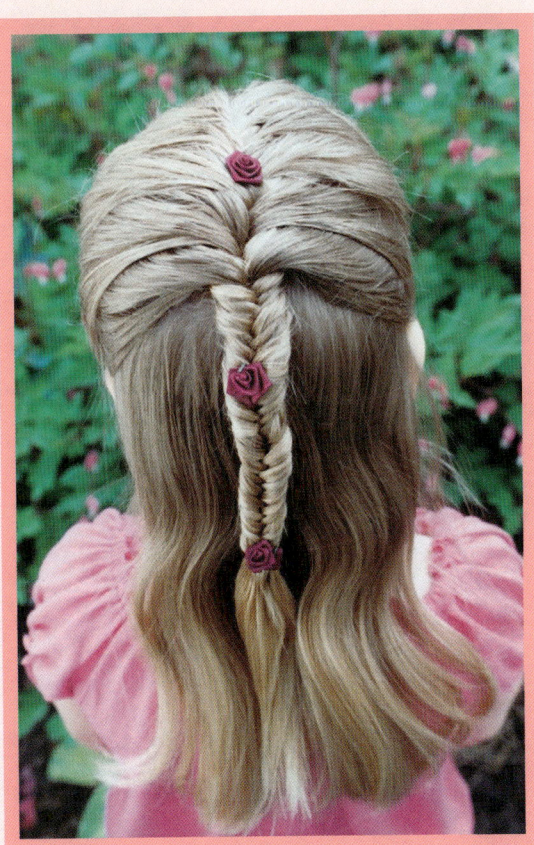

Visit my website to see more examples of the Two-Strand Herringbone

Three-Strand

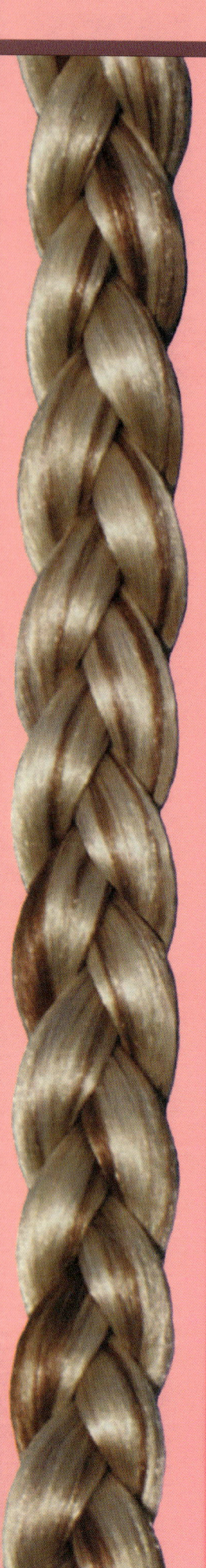

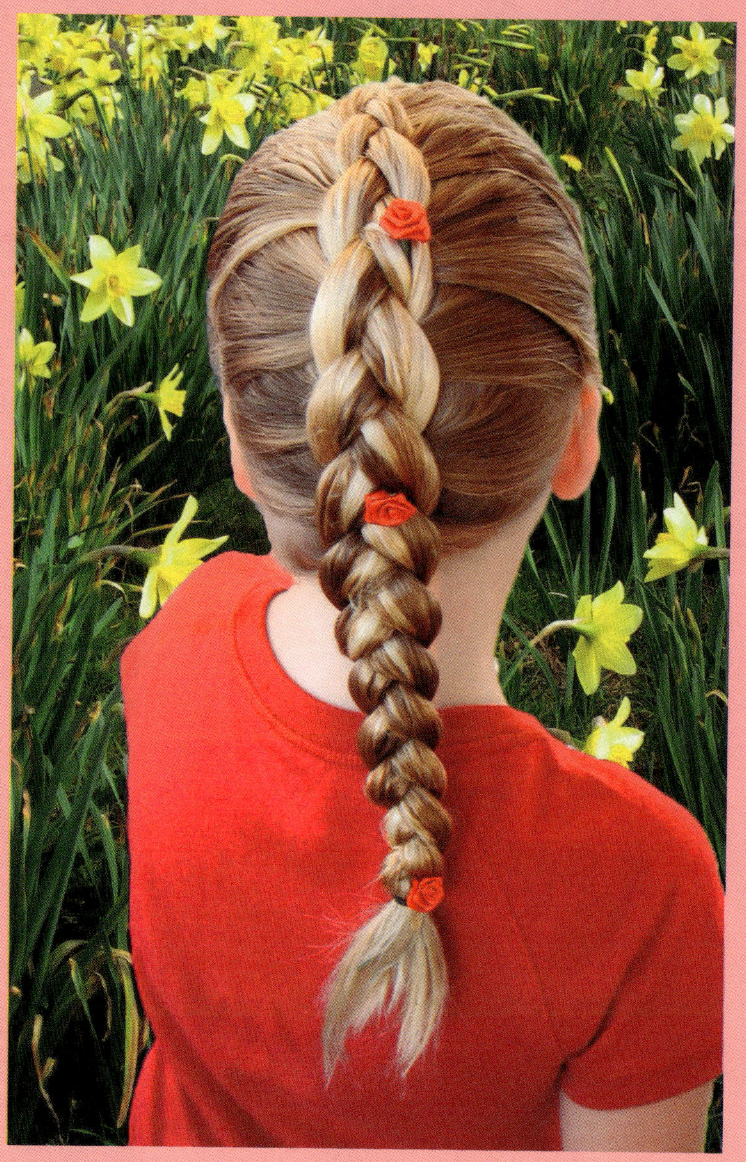

The most recognized braid around the world, the three strand is passed down from generation to generation. Done dutch it is a giant cornrow.

Three-Strand

The most known braid out there. The next thirty-two pages will walk you through this braid.

Braid . . . . 122 - 123

Stitch French . . . . .126 - 129

Feather Loose . . . . 132 - 135

French Lace . . . . 138 - 140

Stitch Dutch . . . . 142 - 148

Dutch Lace . . . . 150 - 152

Examples 153

Let's braid it!

Three-Strand Braid

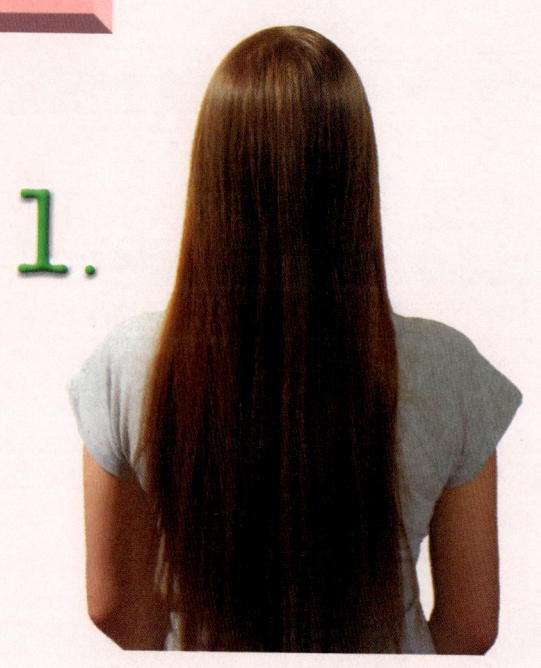

1. Begin with clean, brushed hair.

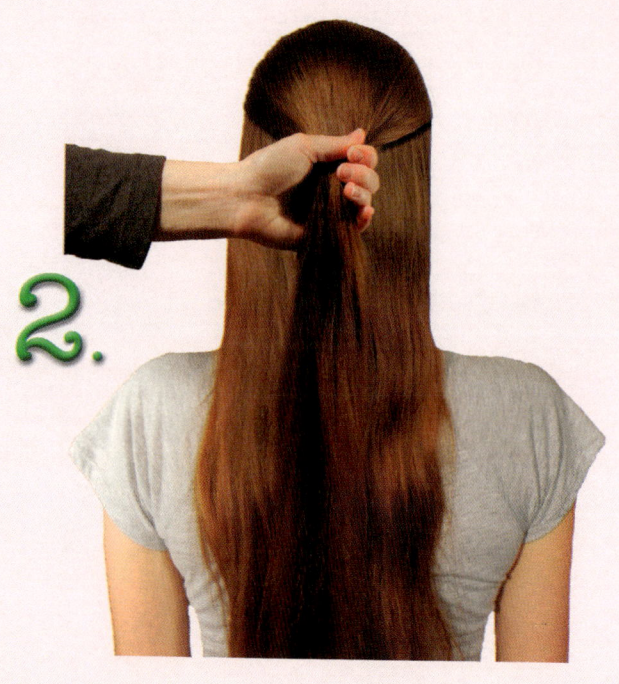

2. Take a section of hair.

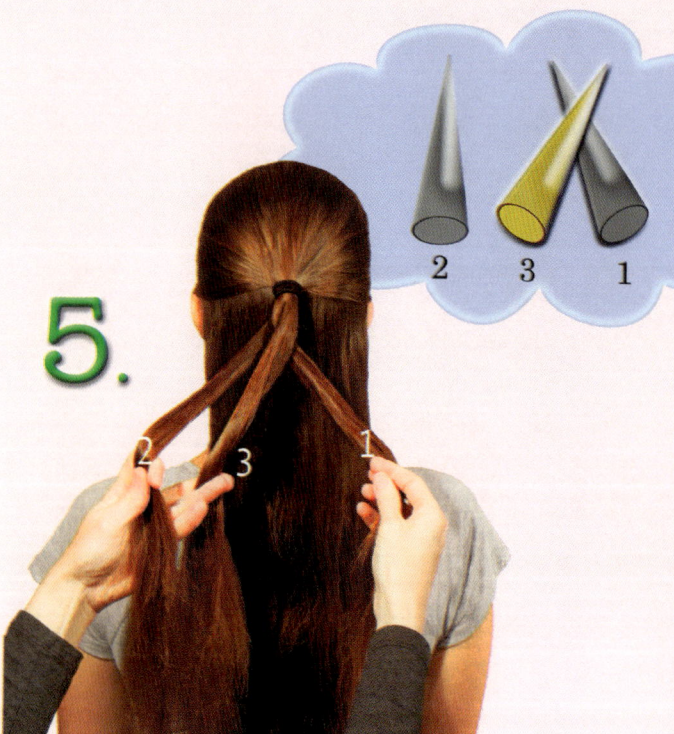

5. Strand 3 crosses over strand 1 to become the new center strand.

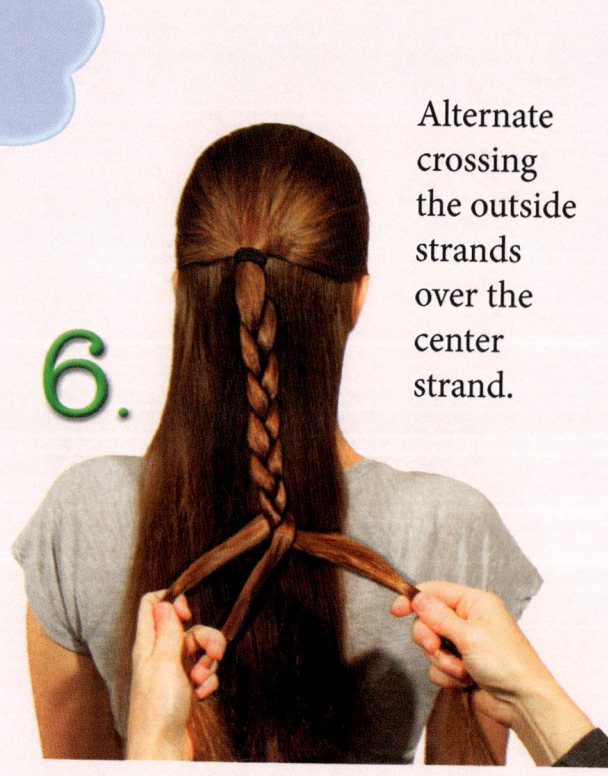

6. Alternate crossing the outside strands over the center strand.

Three-Strand Braid

3

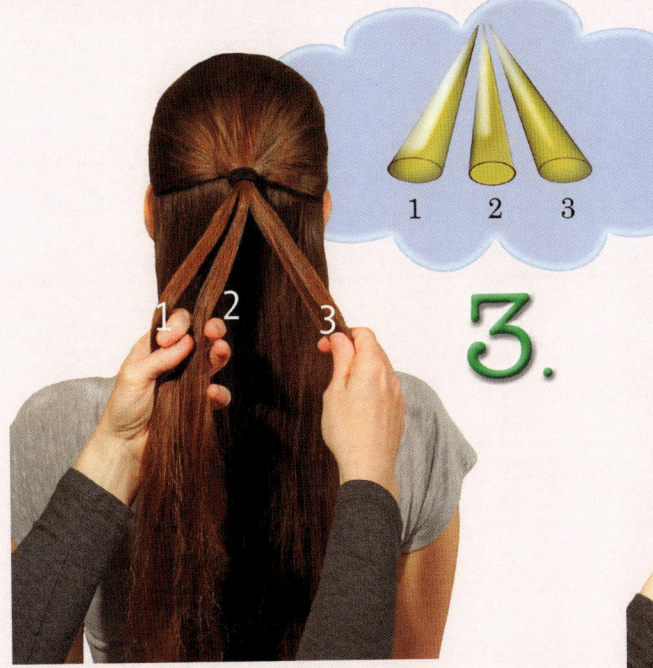

3.

Divide the section into three equal strands.

Maybe you noticed how strand 2 went from my middle finger to my pointer finger? As you braid with any number of strands you will need to shift the strands around your fingers to make the weaving process easier.

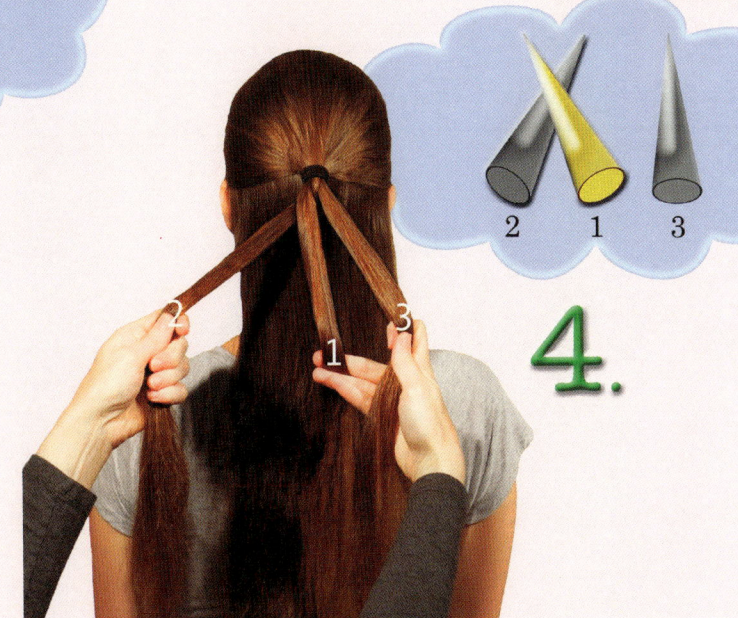

4.

Strand 1 crosses over strand 2 to become the new center strand.

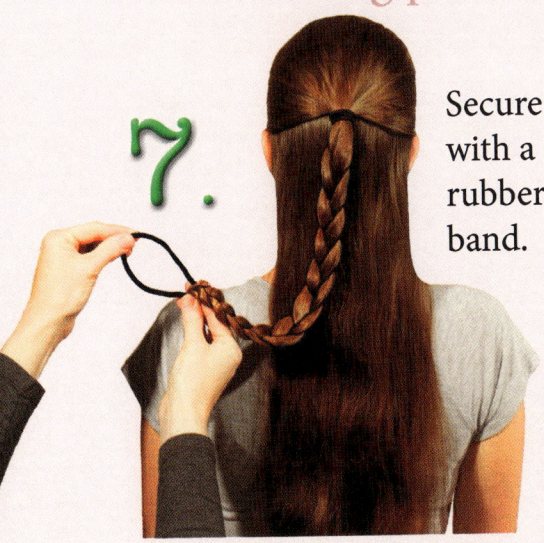

7.

Secure with a rubber band.

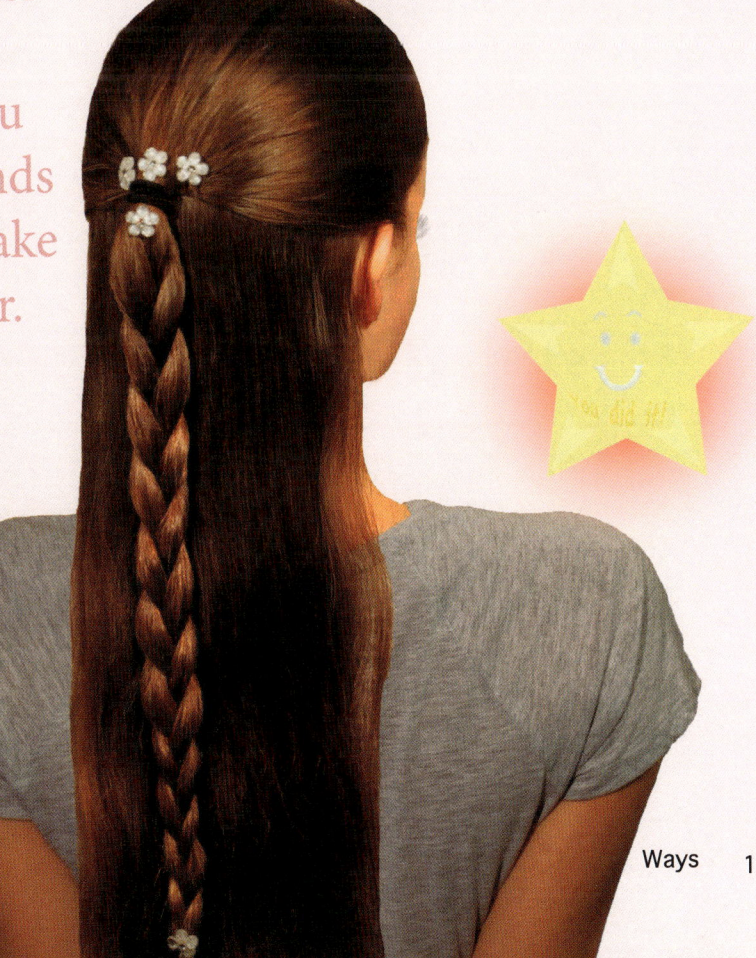

Three-Strand

Notes

Until you reach page 212 there is flexability in which fingers you choose to use. You probably have five fingers on each hand. When there is less than five strands...you don't really have to take the first strand with your pinky. I give explisite directions here because it is a book. Logic is in the background whispering that it doesn't matter which finger you use as long as the strands are weaving the proper pattern.

Three-Strand

Gather from both sides

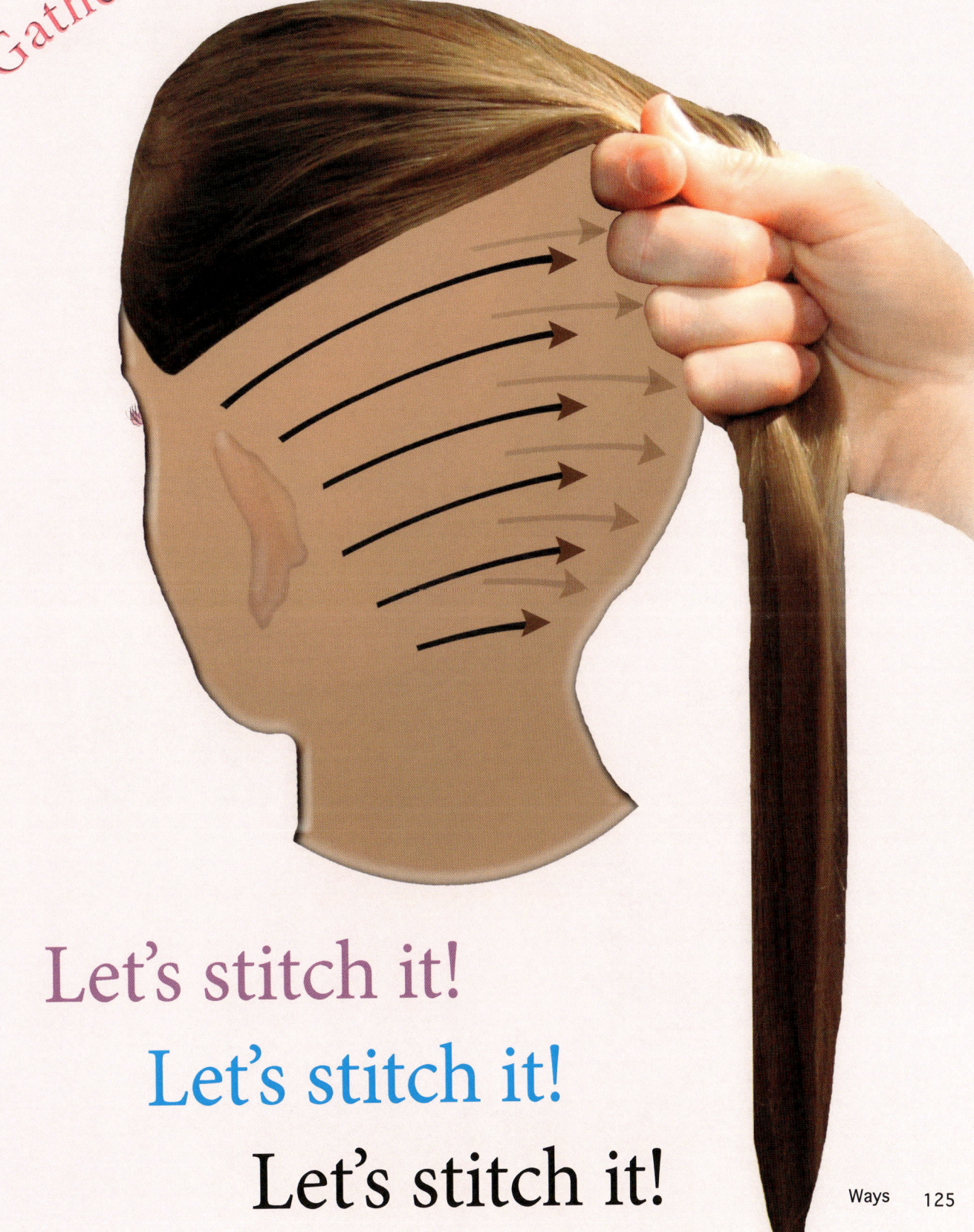

Let's stitch it!

Let's stitch it!

Let's stitch it!

Three-Strand French Stitch

1. Begin with clean, brushed hair.

2. Take a section of hair as illustrated.

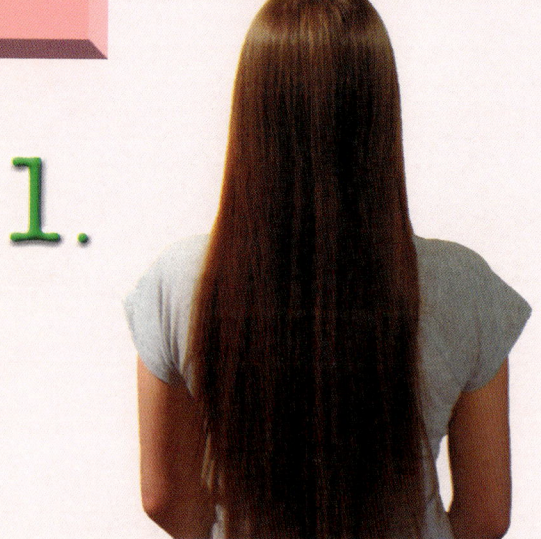

5. Strand 3 crosses over strand 1 to become the new center strand.

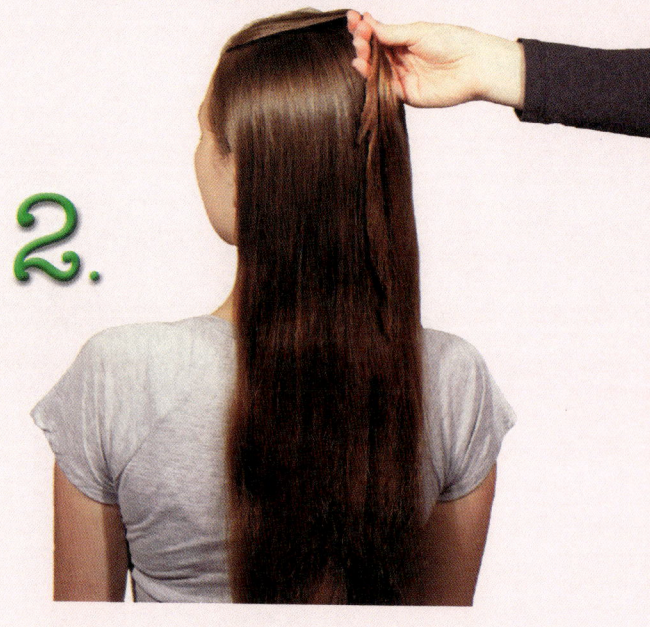

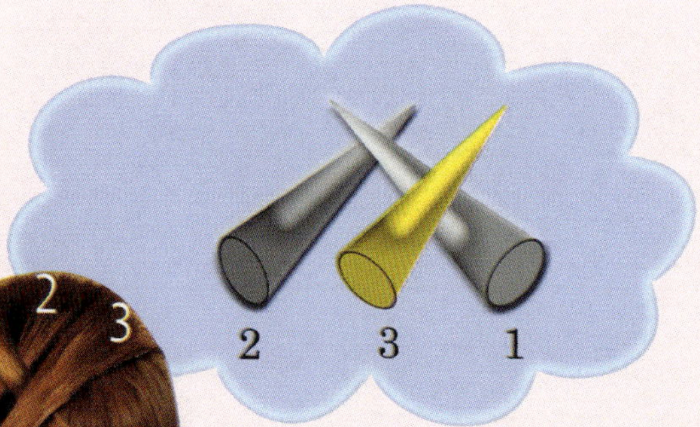

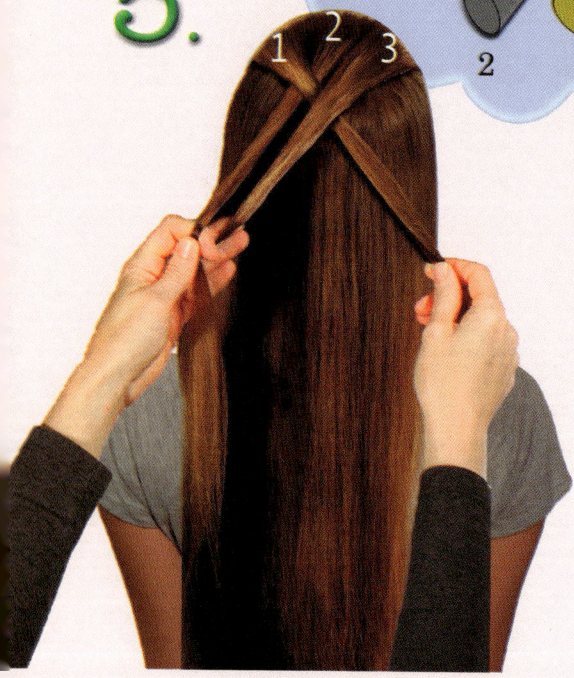

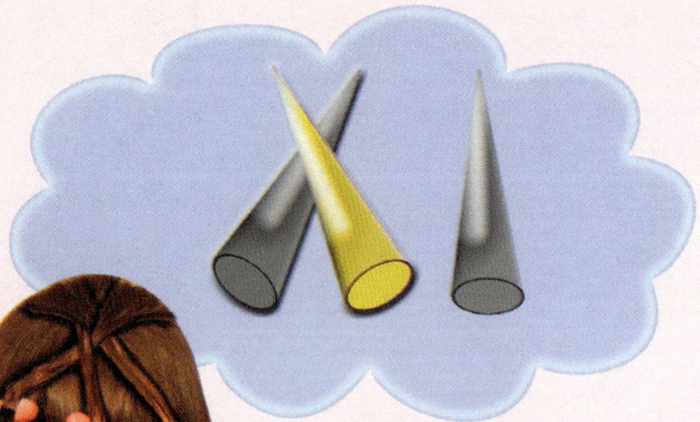

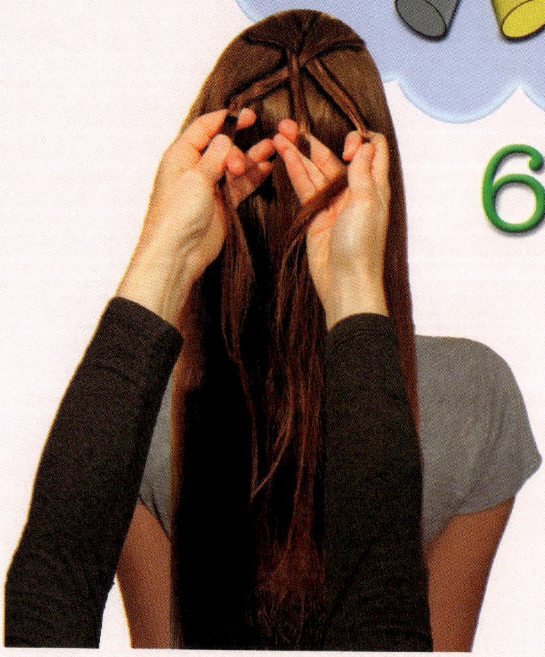

6. Maybe you have noticed that the outside strands are taking turns jumping up and into the middle?

Three-Strand French Stitch

3

3.

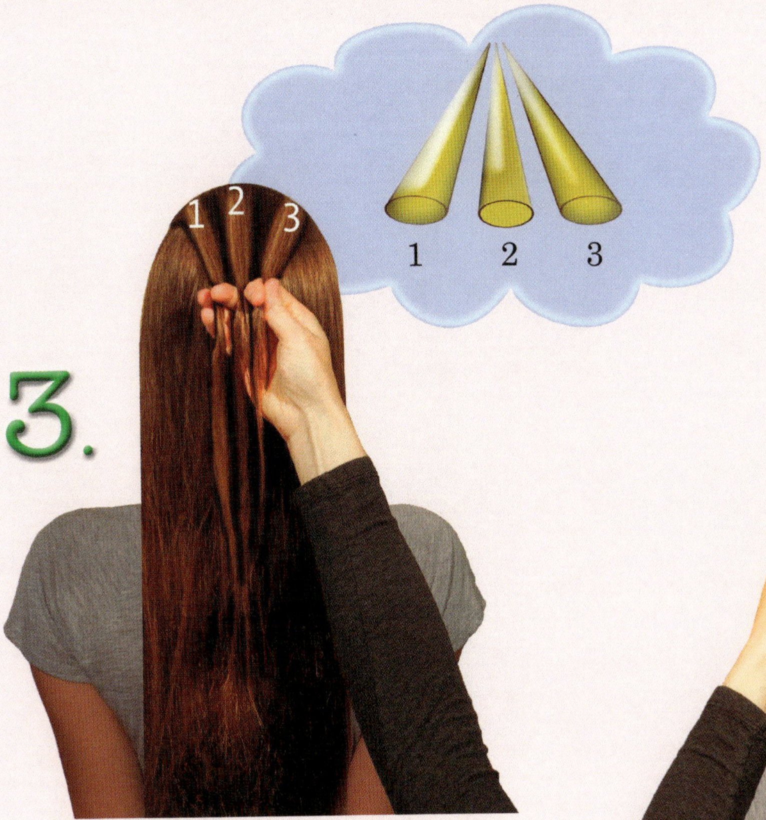

Divide the section into three equal strands.

4.

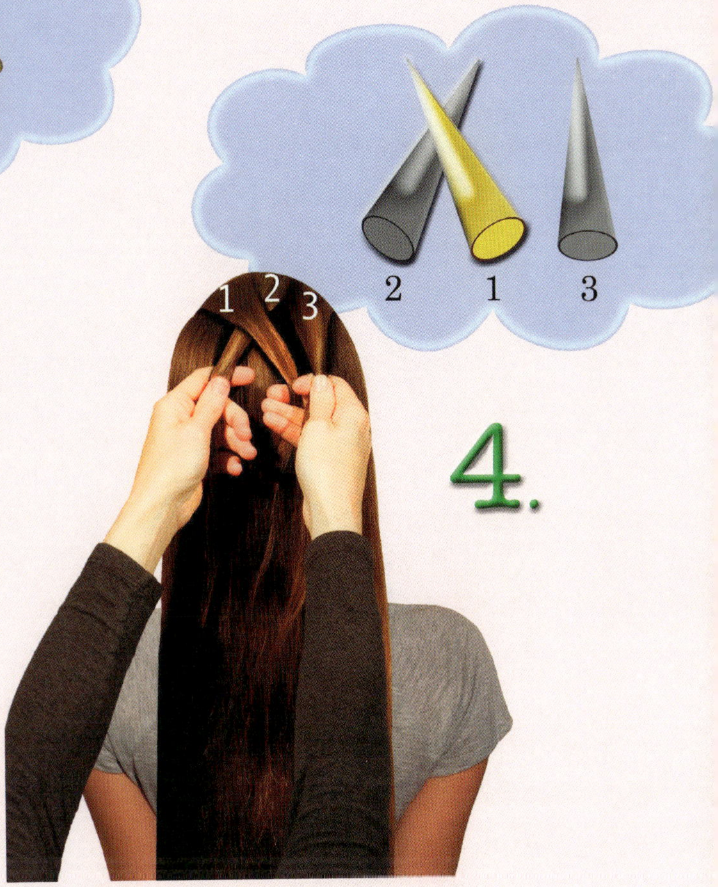

Strand 1 crosses over strand 2 to become the new center strand.

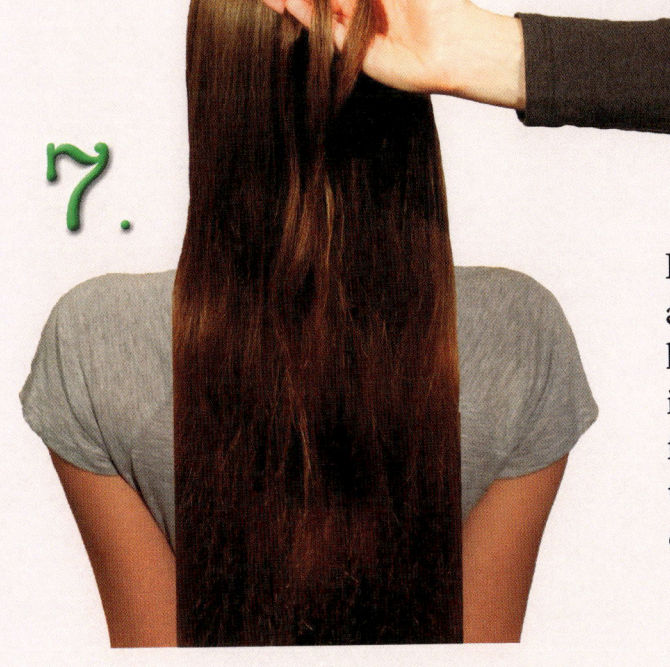

7.

In order to gather hair to make a french braid you need a free hand, so place all three strands into one hand. You will have a free hand to turn the page and then pick up the comb to part off a bit of hair for your gather.

Ways 127

3 Continuing

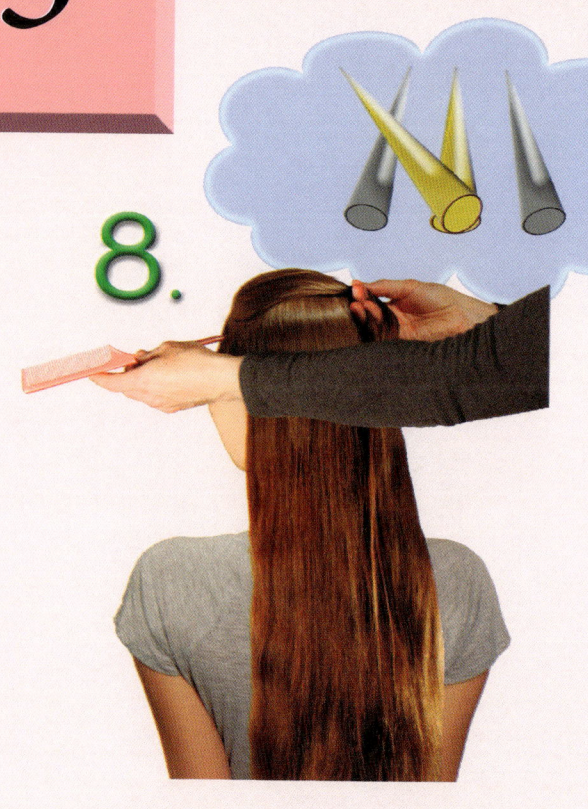

8. Sliver off a gather from the face all the way back to the braid, and then add the gather into the center strand.

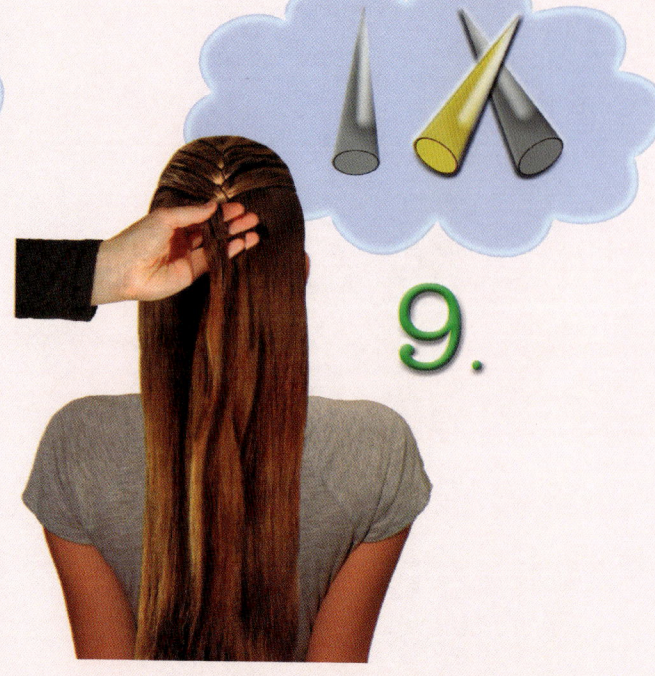

9. Cross the right outside strand over into the center. You now need your right hand free to gather, so place all three strands into the left hand to free your right hand.

How big are my gathers supposed to be? For a large chunky braid, take large uneven gathers. For a graceful look, take slivers.

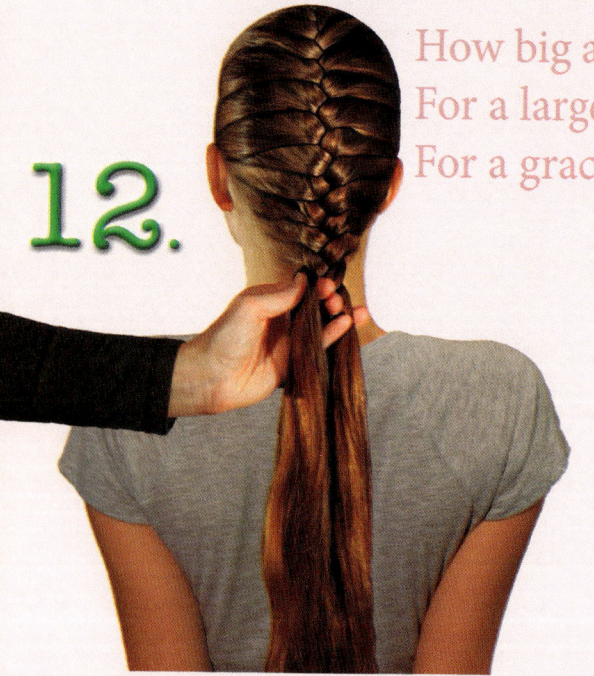

12. Braid until you reach the end of the hair.

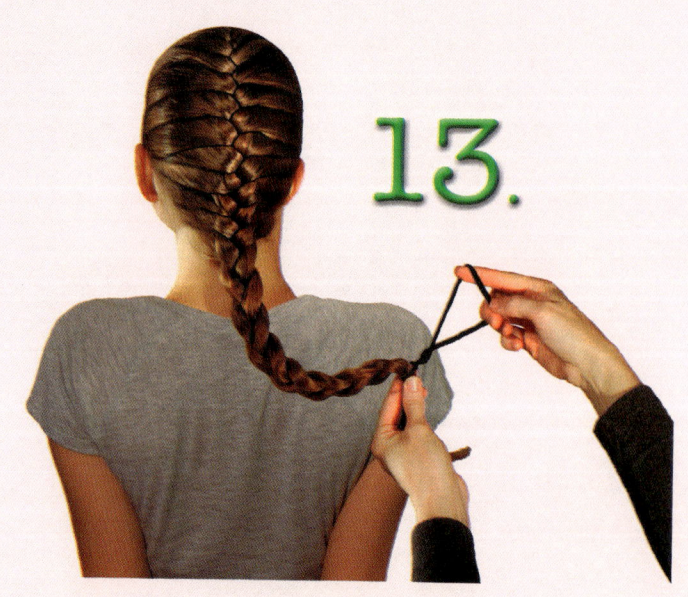

13. Secure with a rubber band.

128   www.findingbraids.com

part 2. Three-Strand French Stitch

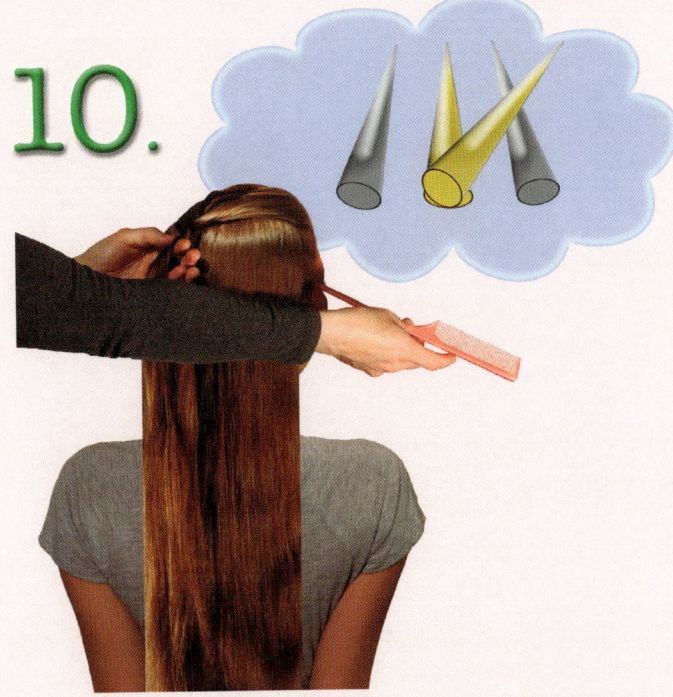

10. Sliver off a gather from the face all the way back to the braid, and then add the gather into the center strand.

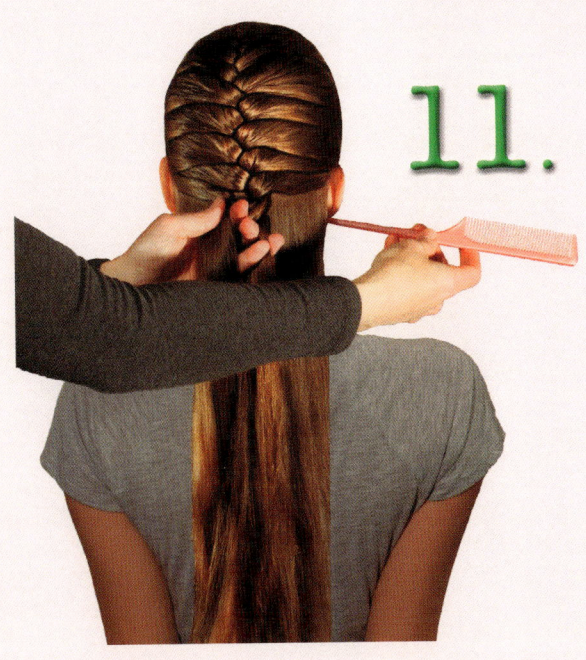

11. Continue alternating outside strands into the center and gathering into them.

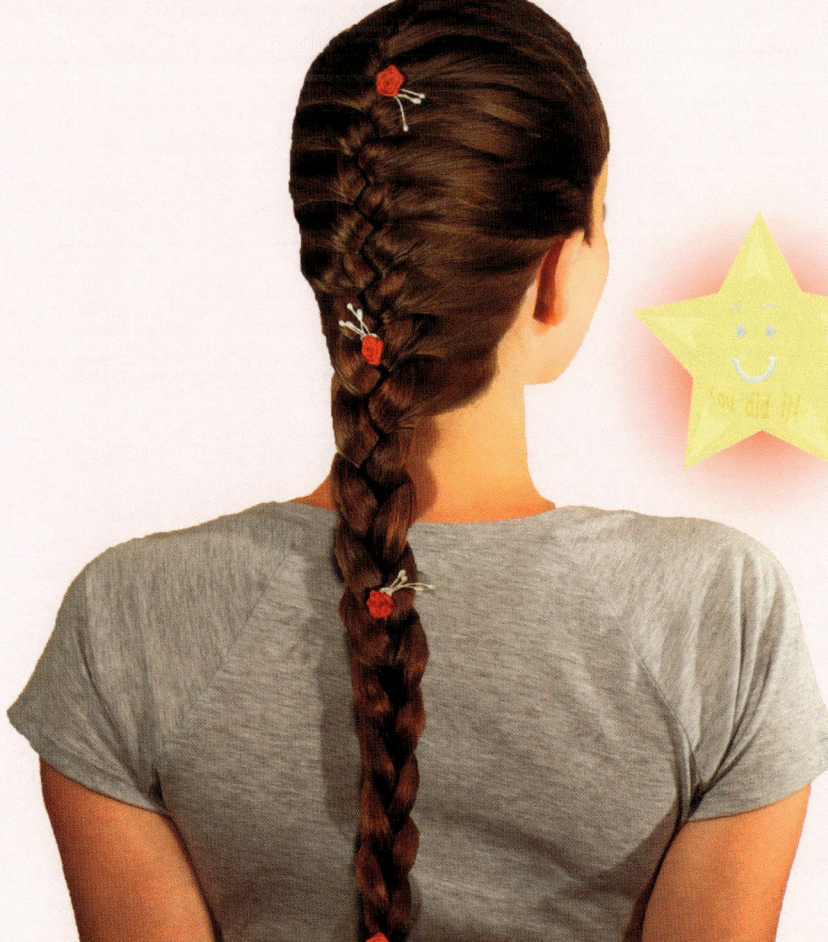

Do you have a system in place to keep the strands seperate while you gather?

Consider the fact that there are only three strands and five fingers. I suggest using your fingers to keep the strands seperate. You won't need to have two strands in a single finger until we reach the six-strand braids.

Three-Strand

Notes

Three-Strand

Gather from both sides

Let's stitch it!

Let's stitch it!

Let's stitch it!

3 Three-Strand Feather Loose

1. Take a section of hair as illustrated.

2. Divide the section into three equal strands.

5. Sliver off a gather from the face all the way back to the braid.

Add the gather into the new center strand.

132 www.findingbraids.com

Three-Strand Feather Loose

3

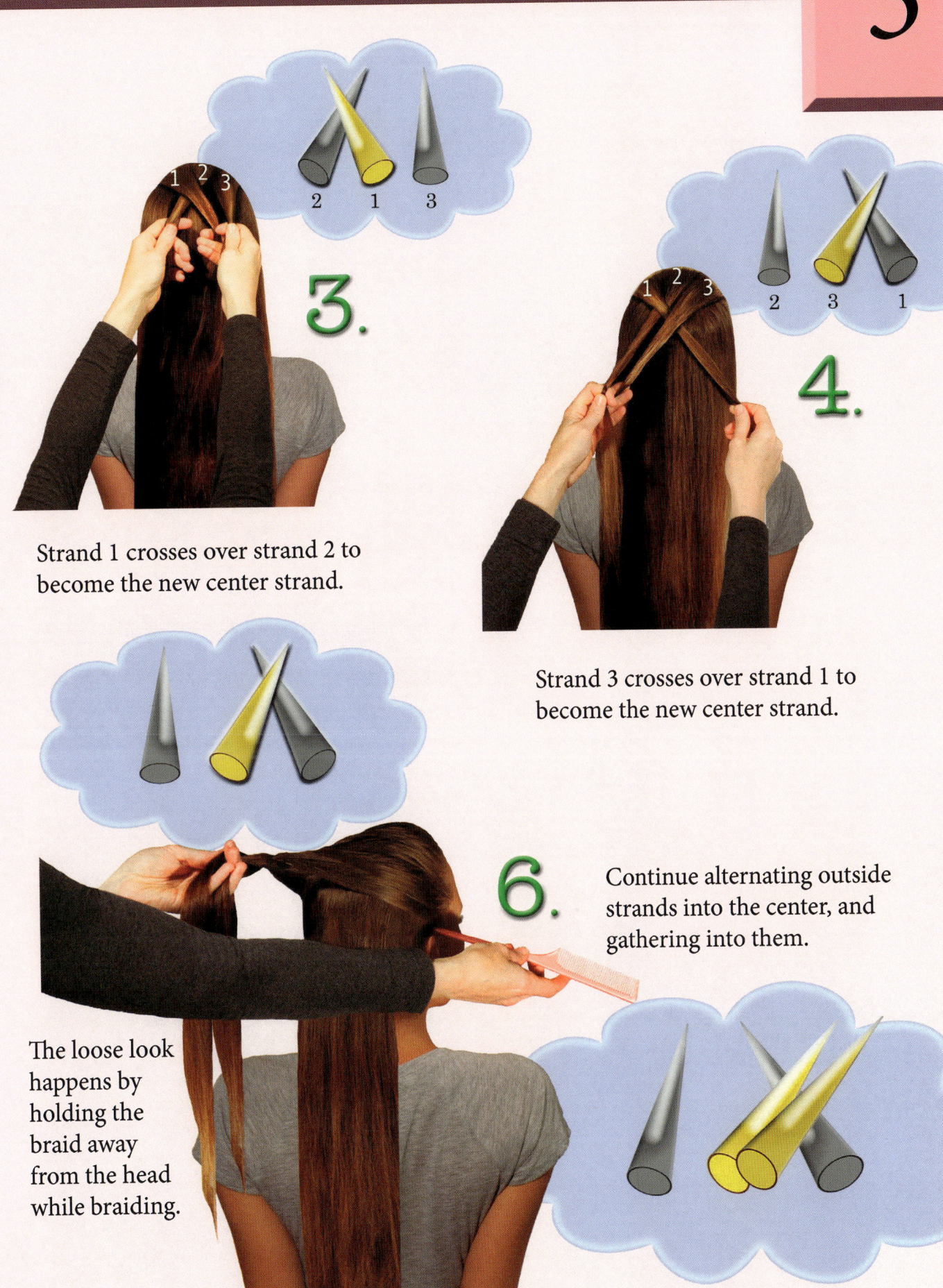

3.

Strand 1 crosses over strand 2 to become the new center strand.

4.

Strand 3 crosses over strand 1 to become the new center strand.

6.

Continue alternating outside strands into the center, and gathering into them.

The loose look happens by holding the braid away from the head while braiding.

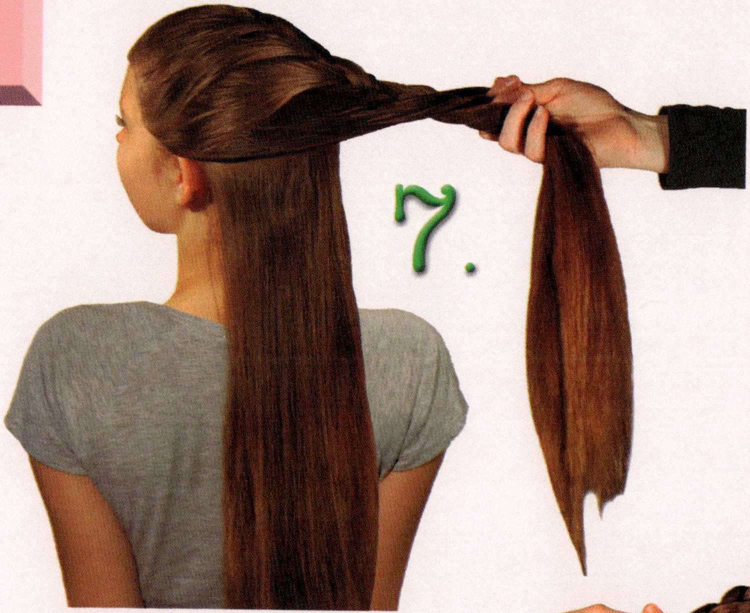

3 Continuing

7. Braid until you reach the end of the hair.

8. Keep the braid held away from the head.

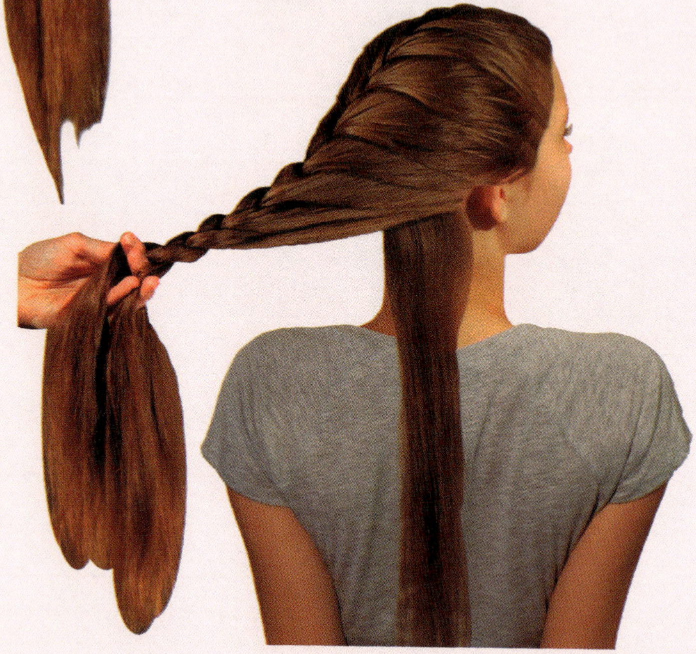

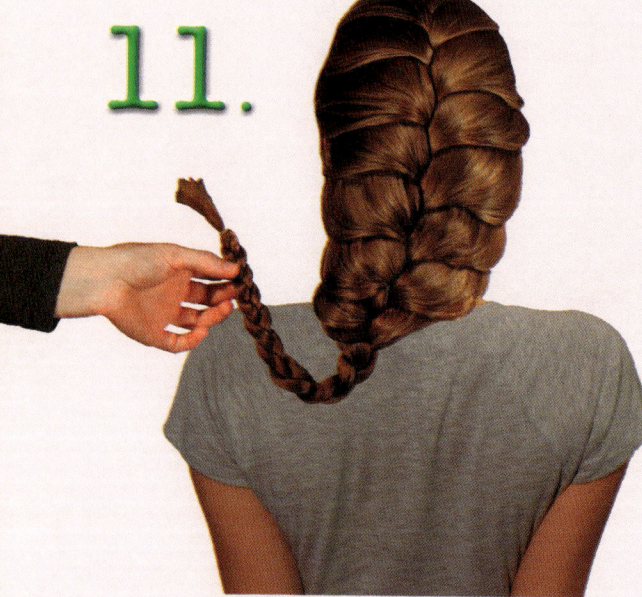

11. This braid looks good tucked up and under.

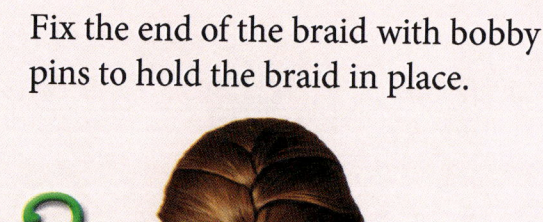

Fix the end of the braid with bobby pins to hold the braid in place.

12.

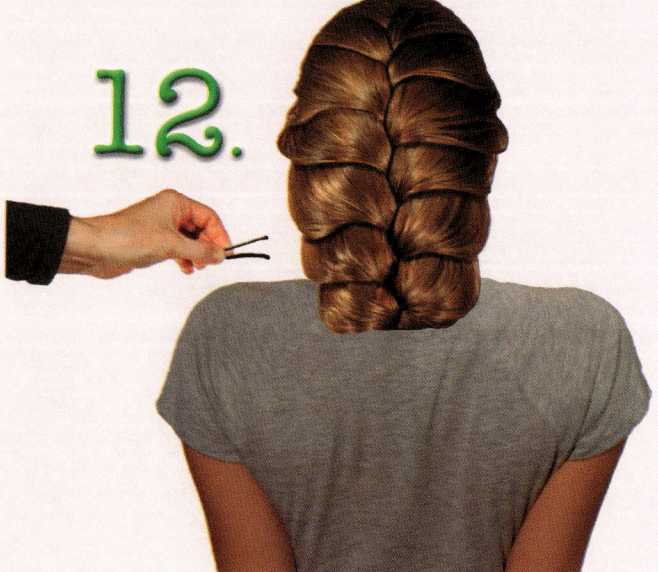

www.findingbraids.com

part 2. Three-Strand Feather Loose 3

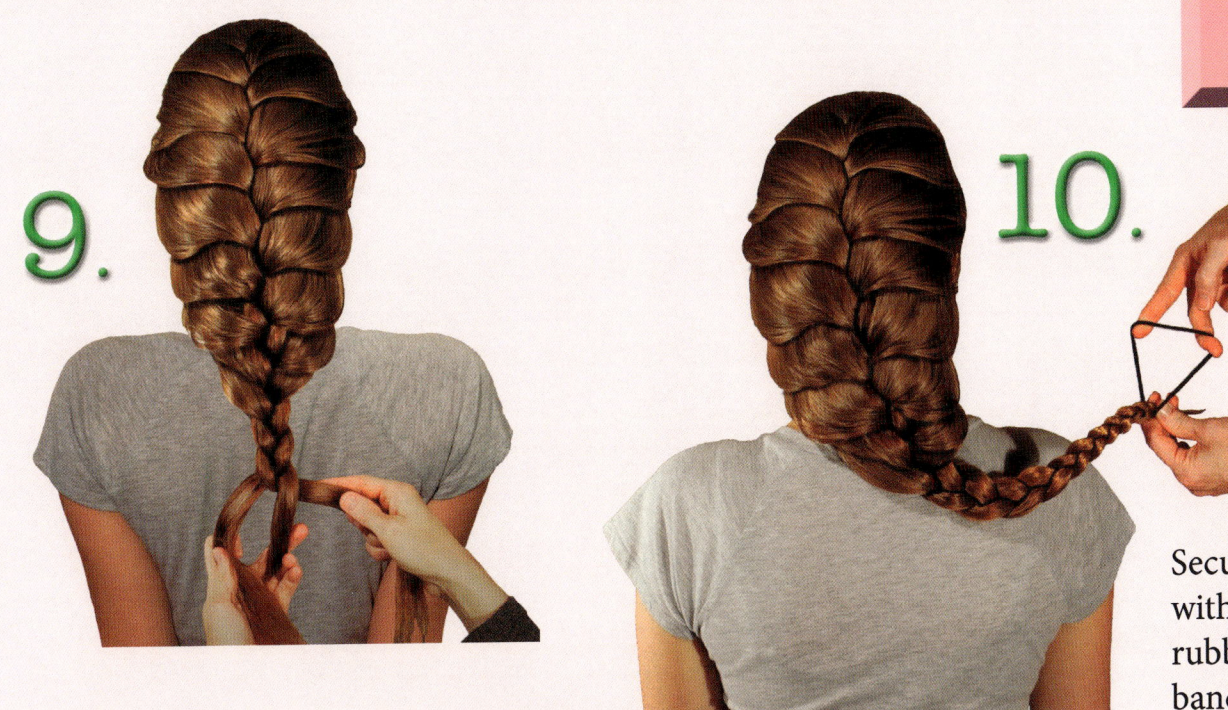

9.

10. Secure with a rubber band.

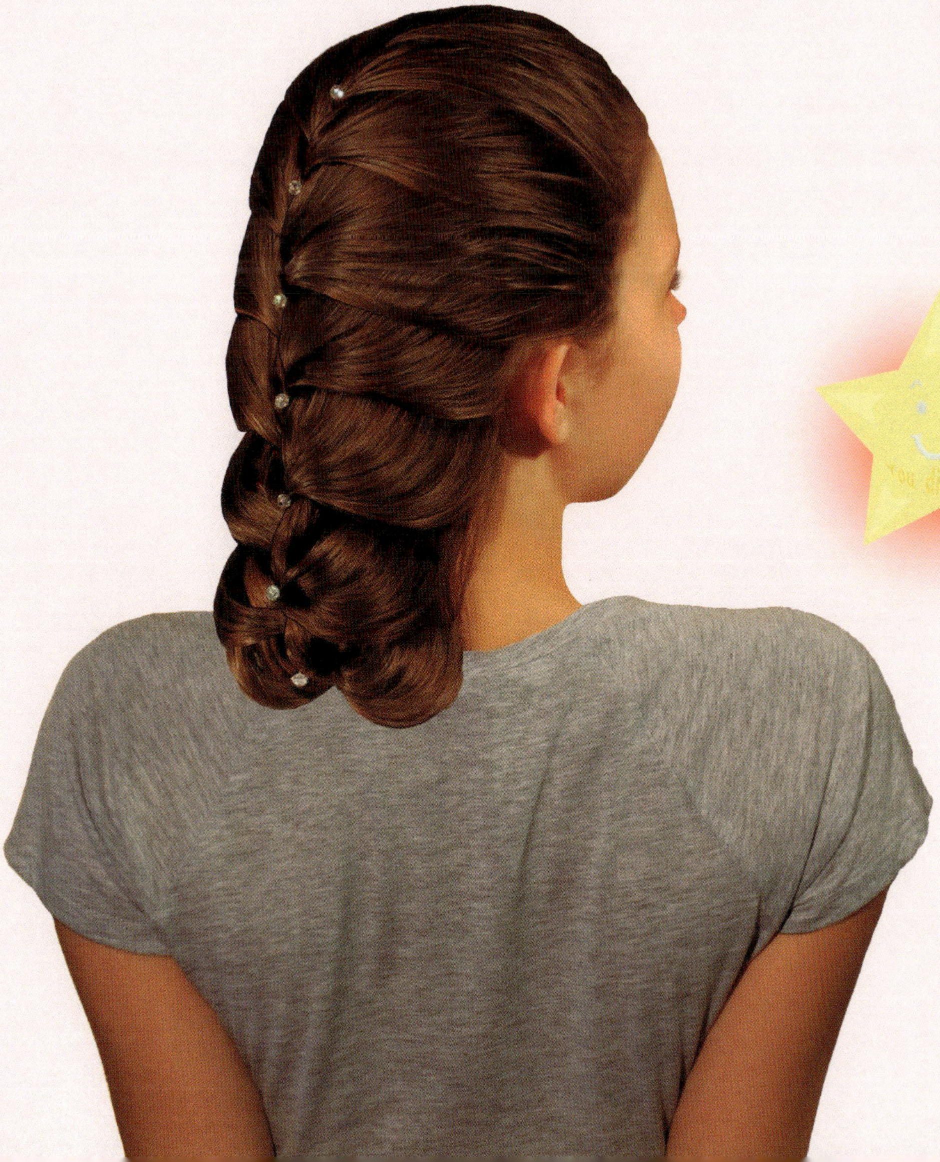

Ways 135

Three-Strand Notes

Three-Strand

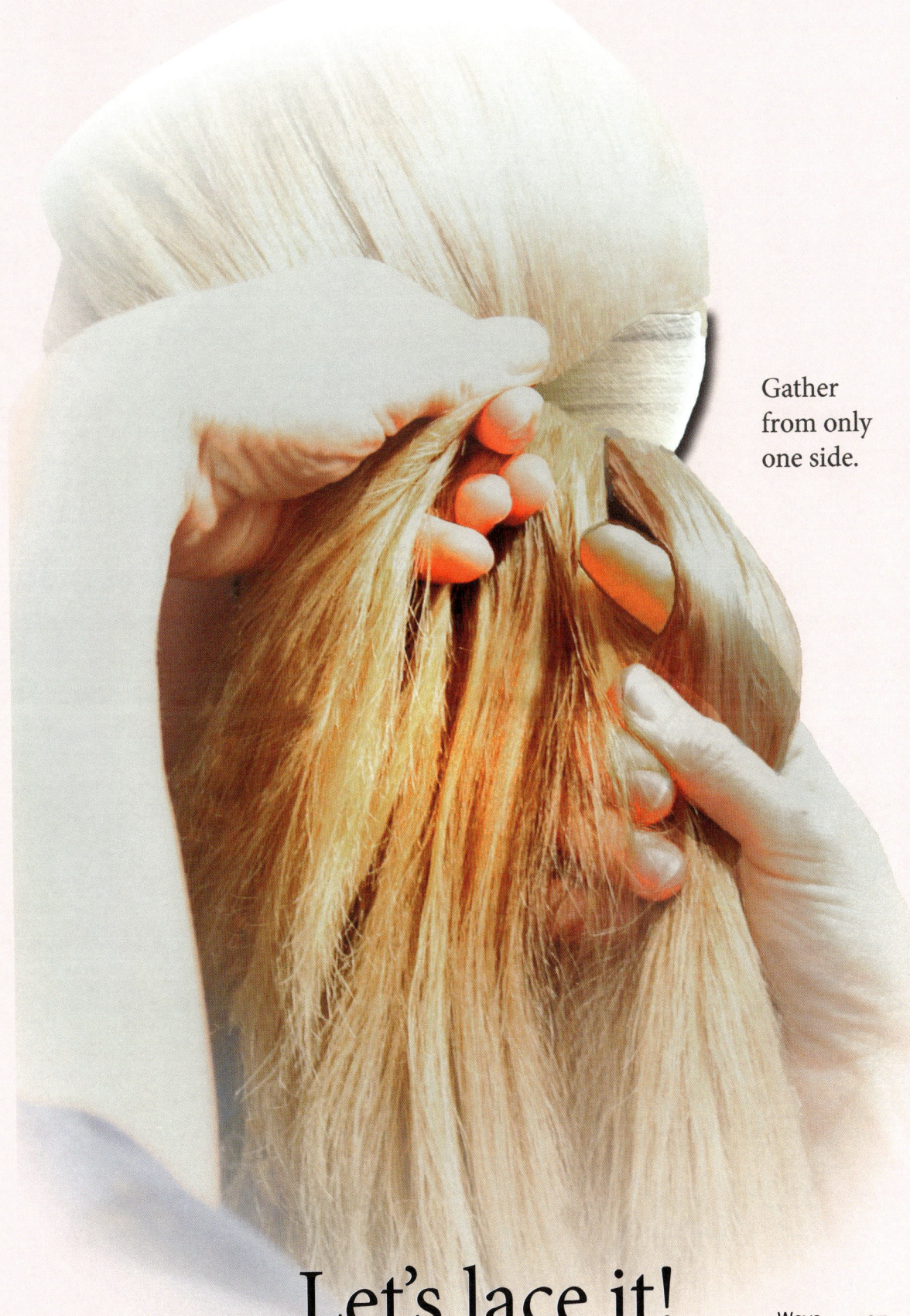

Gather from only one side.

Let's lace it!

3 Three-Strand French Lace

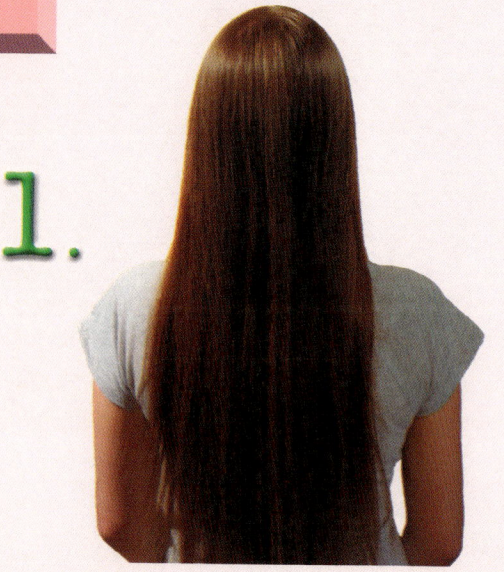

1. Begin with clean, brushed hair.

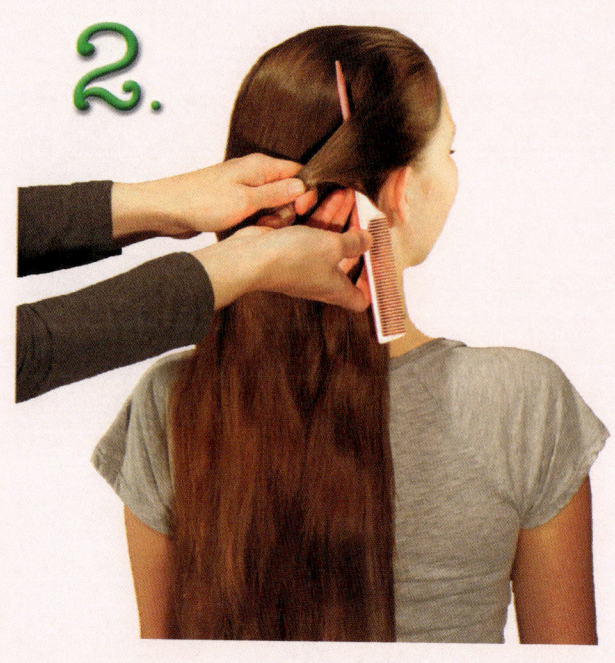

2. Take a section of hair as illustrated.

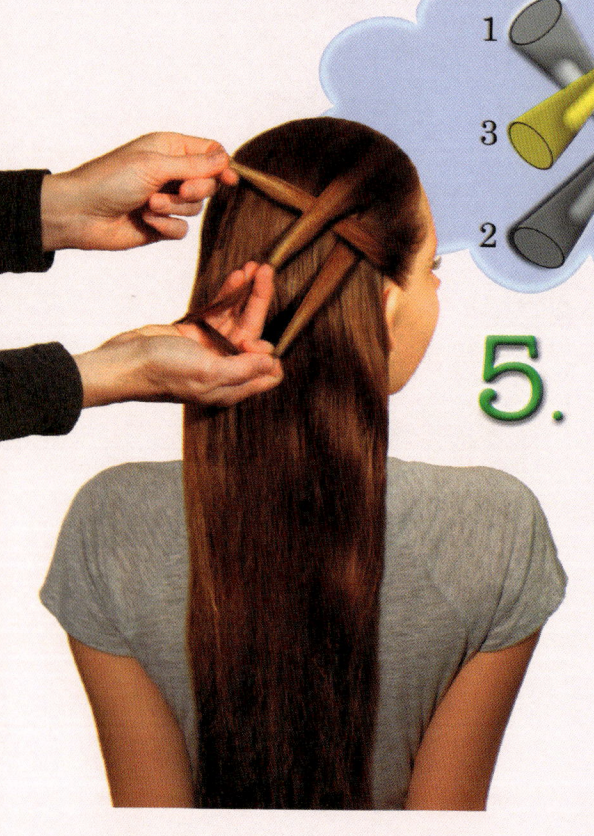

5. Strand 3 crosses over strand 1 to become the new center strand.

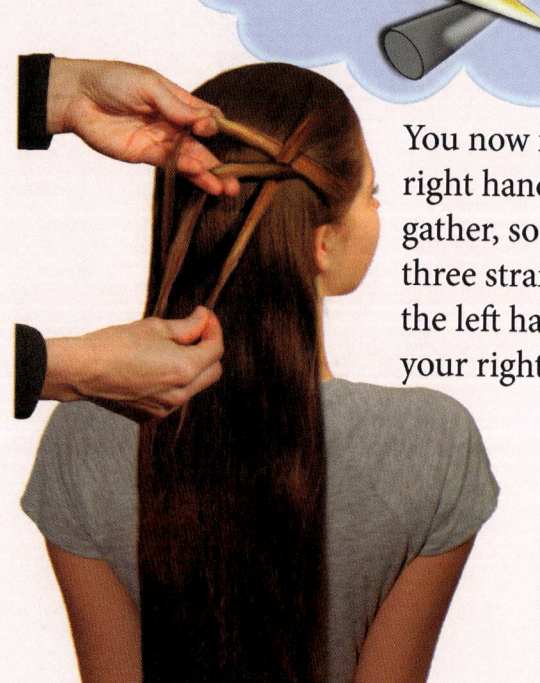

6. You now need your right hand free to gather, so place all three strands into the left hand to free your right hand.

www.findingbraids.com

Three-Strand French Lace

3

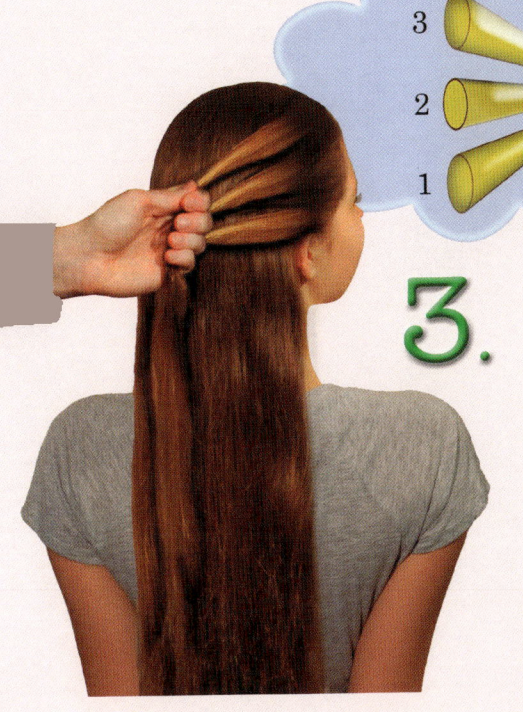

3.

Divide the section into three strands.

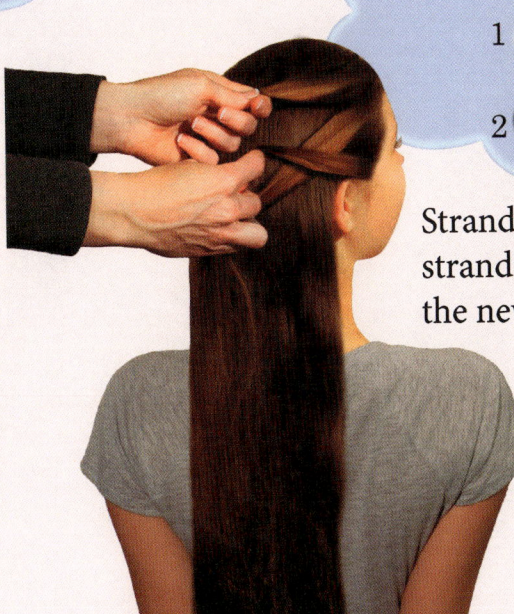

Strand 1 crosses over strand 2 to become the new center strand.

4.

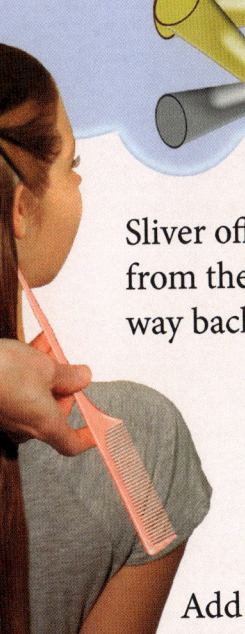

Sliver off a gather from the face all the way back to the braid.

7.

Add the gather into the center strand.

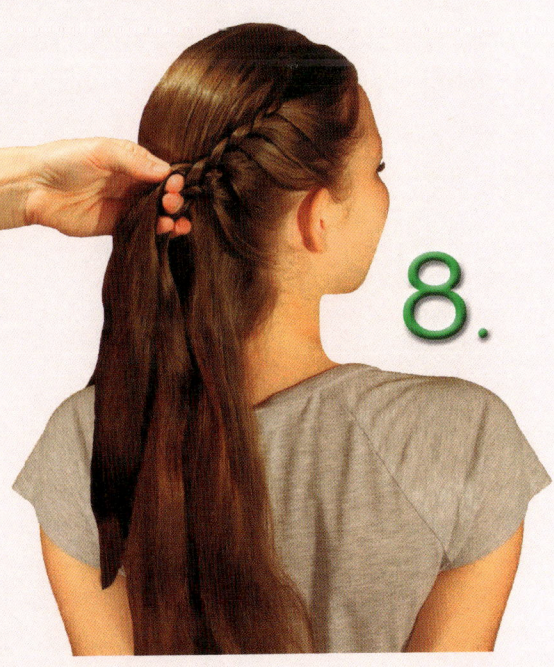

8.

Gather from only one side.

Ways

3 part 2. Three-Strand French Lace

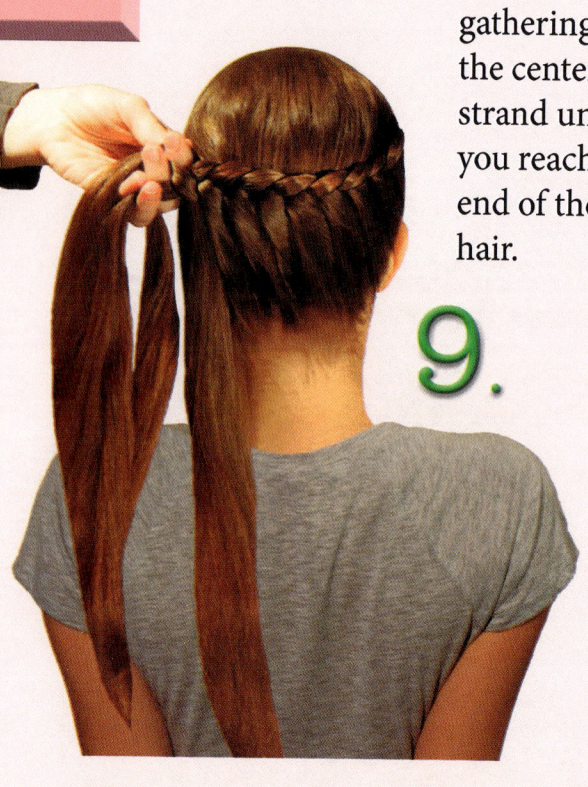

Continue gathering into the center strand until you reach the end of the hair.

9.

10.

Secure with a rubber band.

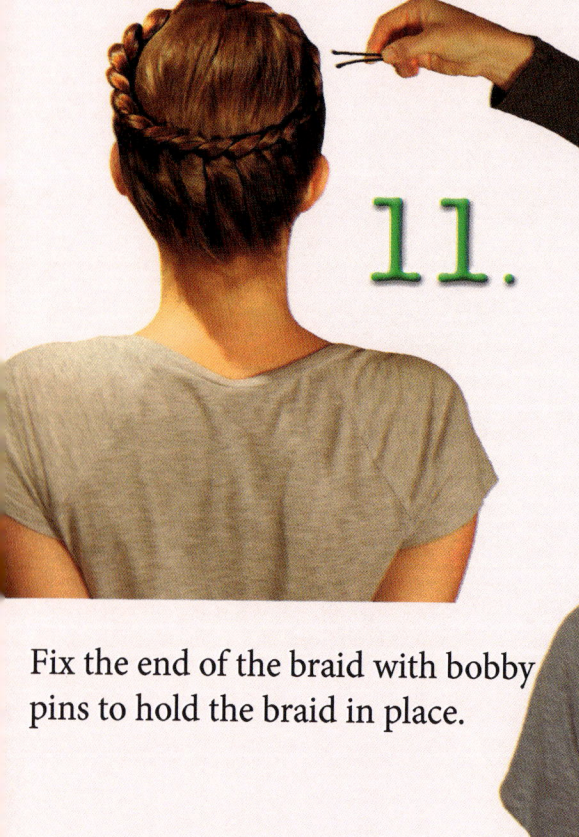

11.

Fix the end of the braid with bobby pins to hold the braid in place.

Three-Strand

Gather from both sides

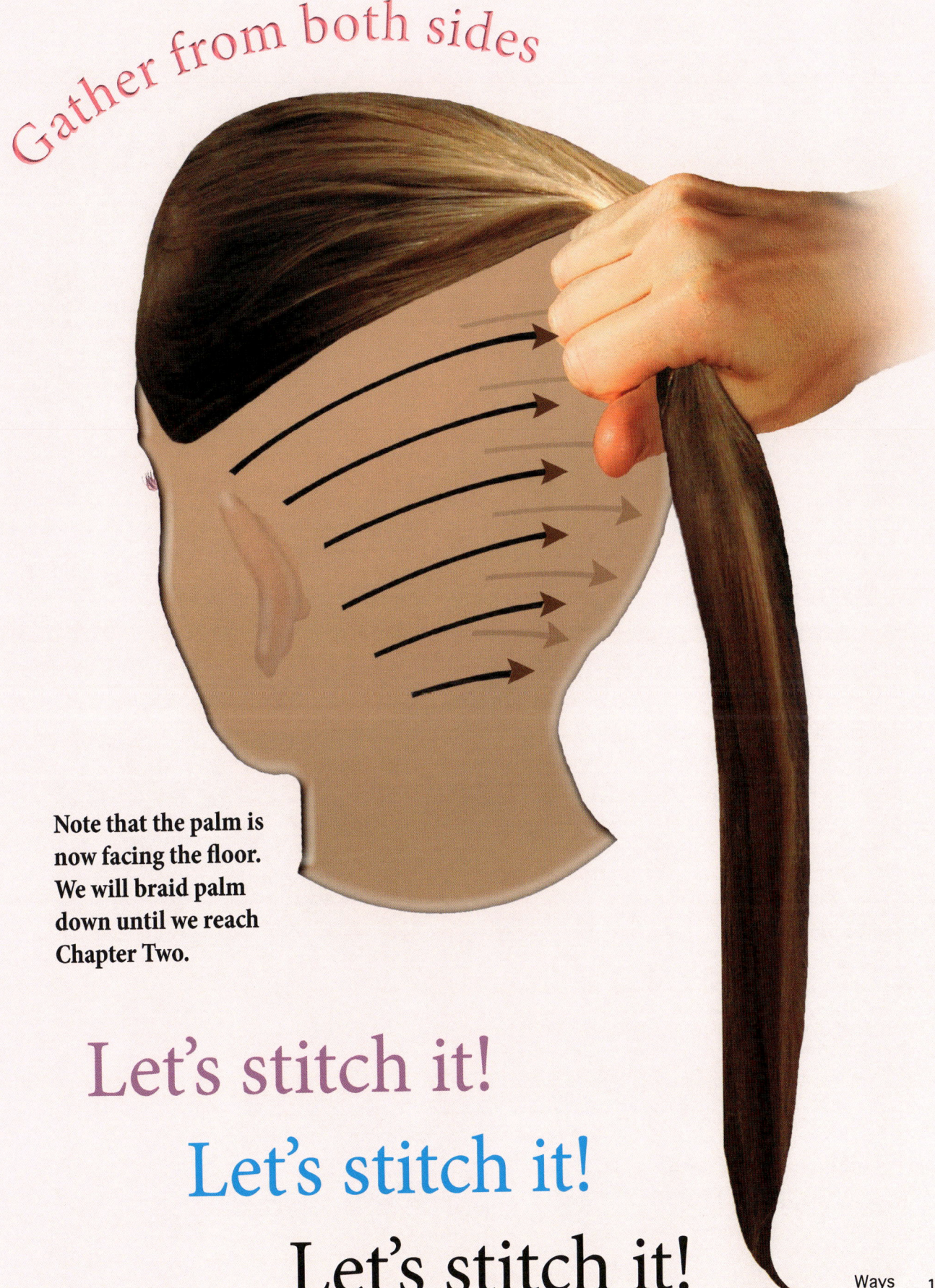

Note that the palm is now facing the floor. We will braid palm down until we reach Chapter Two.

Let's stitch it!
Let's stitch it!
Let's stitch it!

Ways

3 Three-Strand Dutch Stitch

1.

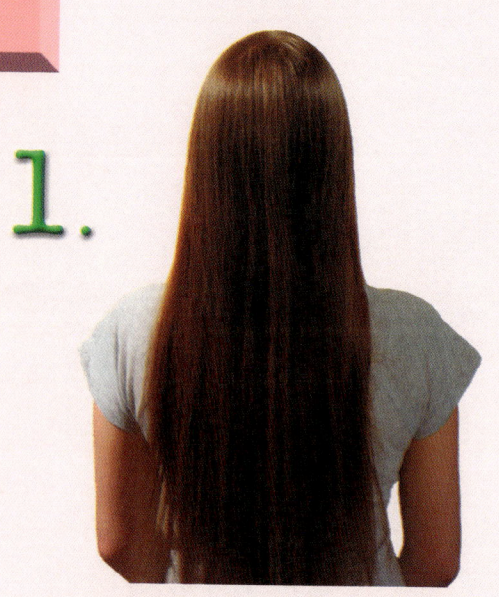

Begin with clean, brushed hair.

2.

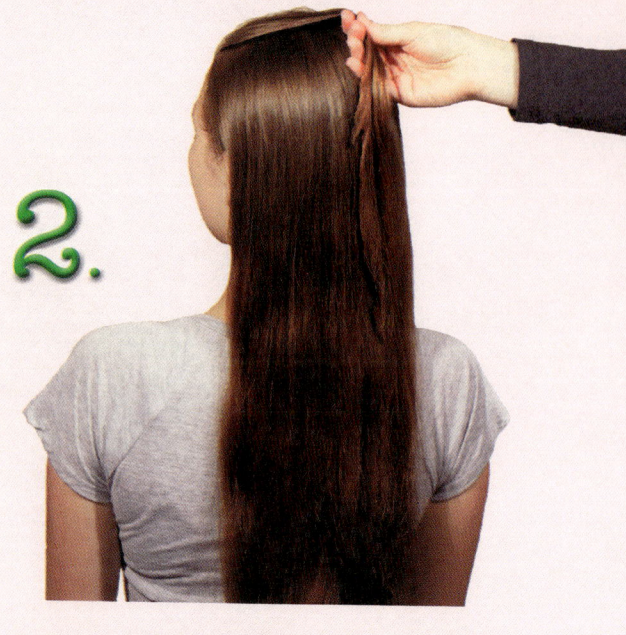

Take a section of hair as illustrated.

This specific handhold is required through much of the book, so practice it here.

5.

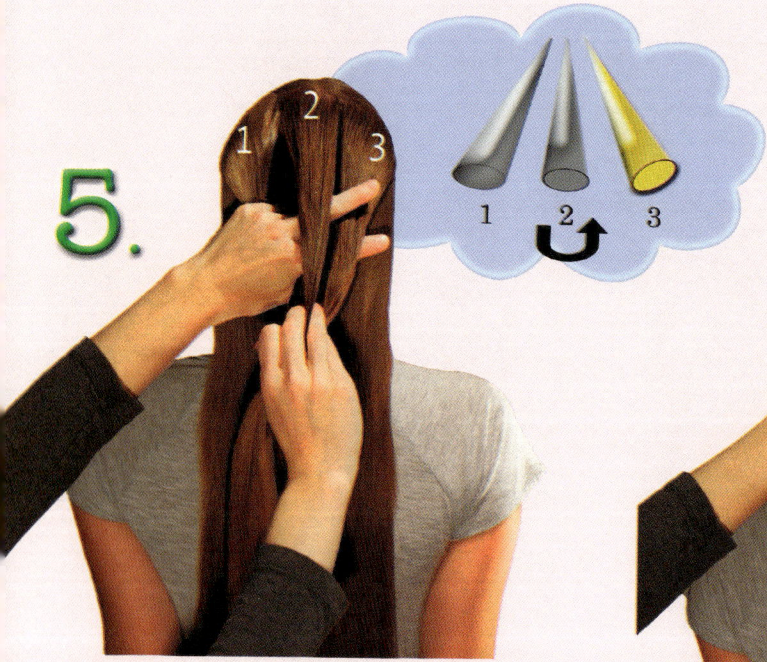

Reach under strand 2 and hook strand 3 with your middle finger.

6.

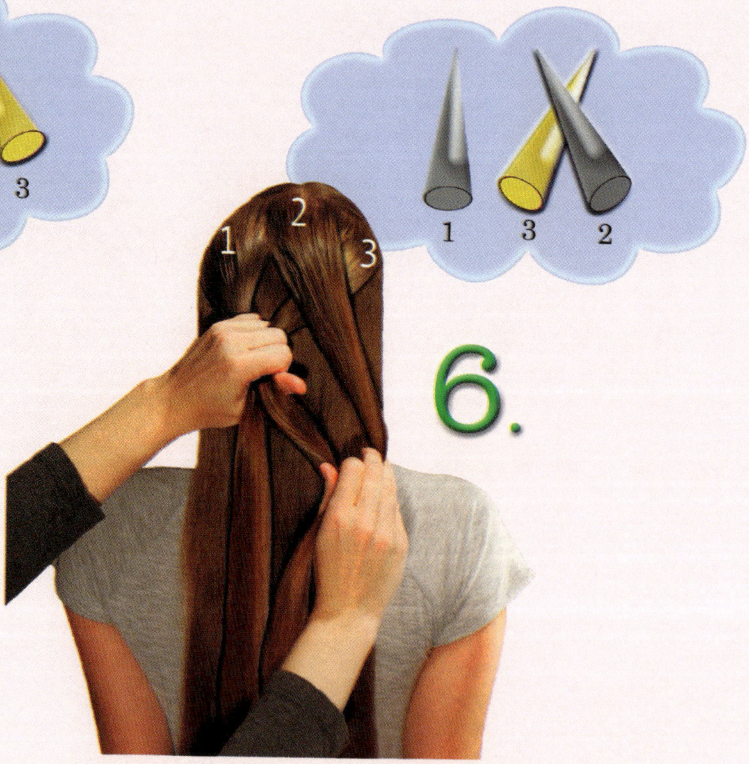

Bring it beneath strand 2 and make it the new center strand.

142   www.findingbraids.com

Three-Strand Dutch Stitch

3

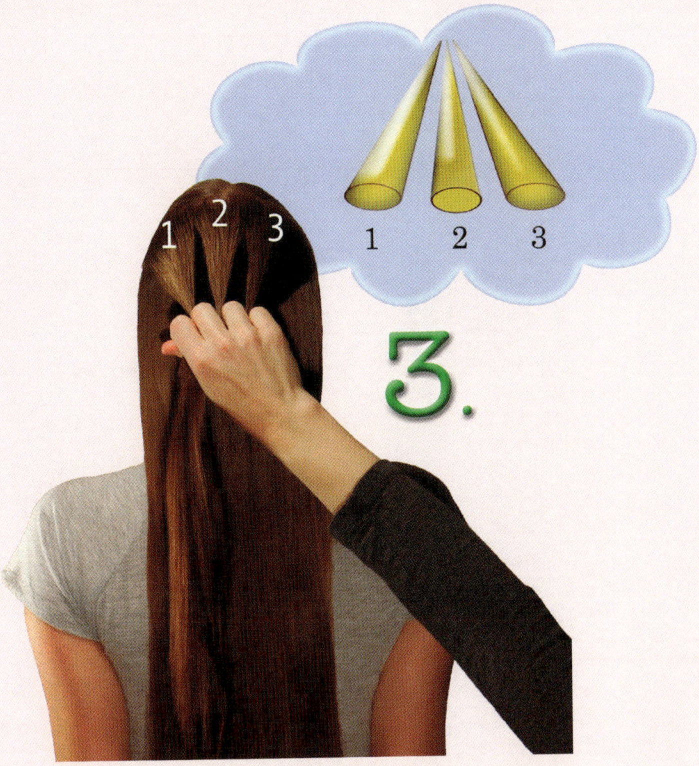

3. Divide the section into three strands.

4. Start braiding by grabbing strand 1 with your palm down and your thumb facing your belly button.

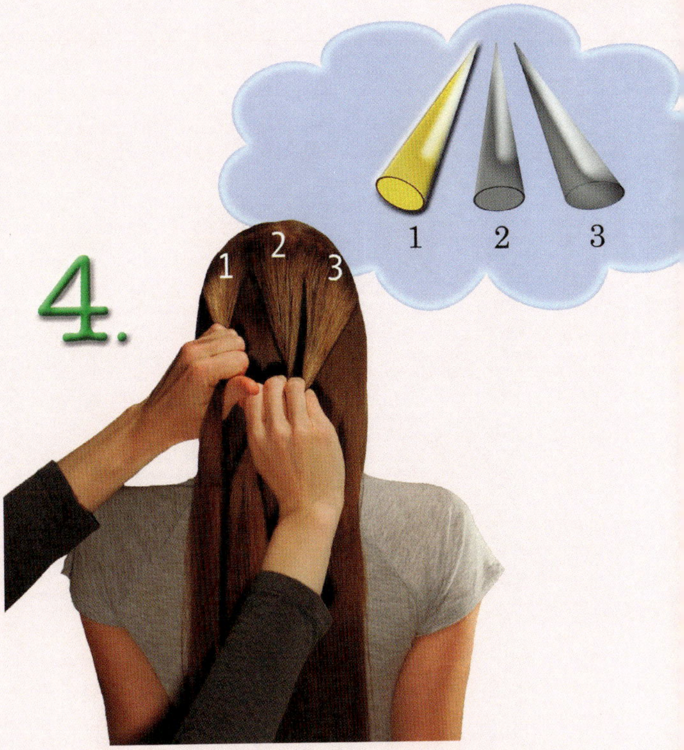

Close-up.

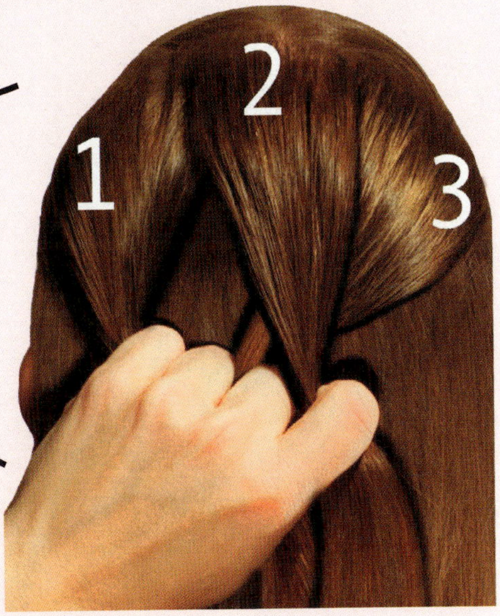

Now you have a free hand to braid the other direction.

7. Place strand 2 in your pointer finger.

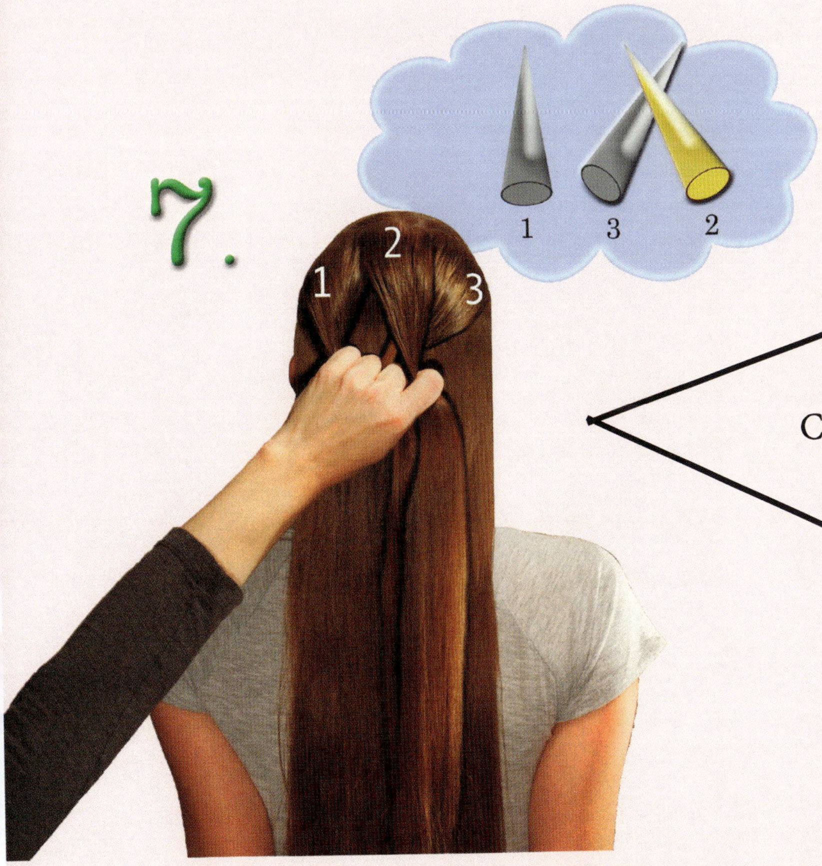

Ways 143

3 Continuing

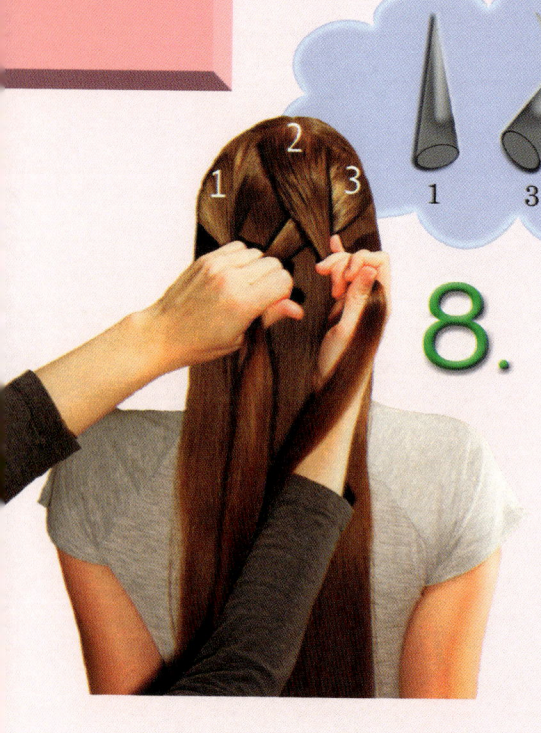

8. Continue braiding by grabbing strand 2 with your palm down and your thumb facing your belly button.

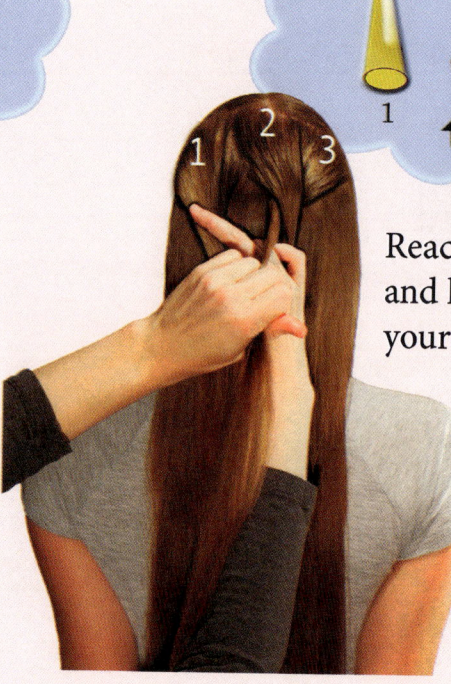

9. Reach under strand 3 and hook strand 1 with your middle finger.

12. Continue braiding by grabbing the outside strand.

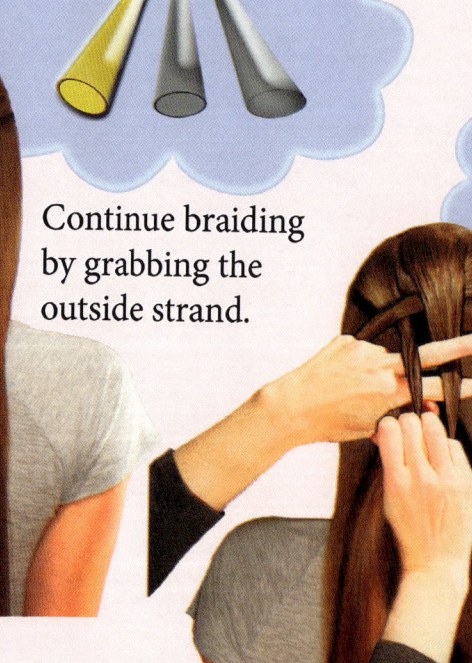

13. Reach under the middle strand and hook the outside strand with your middle finger. Bring it beneath the center strand and make it the new center strand.

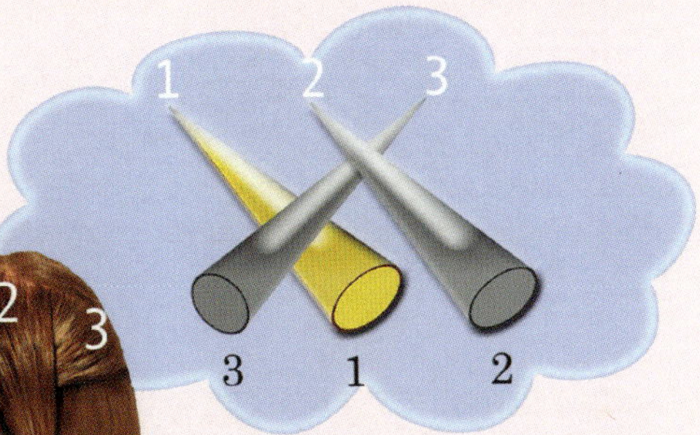

part 2. Three-Strand Dutch Stitch

10.

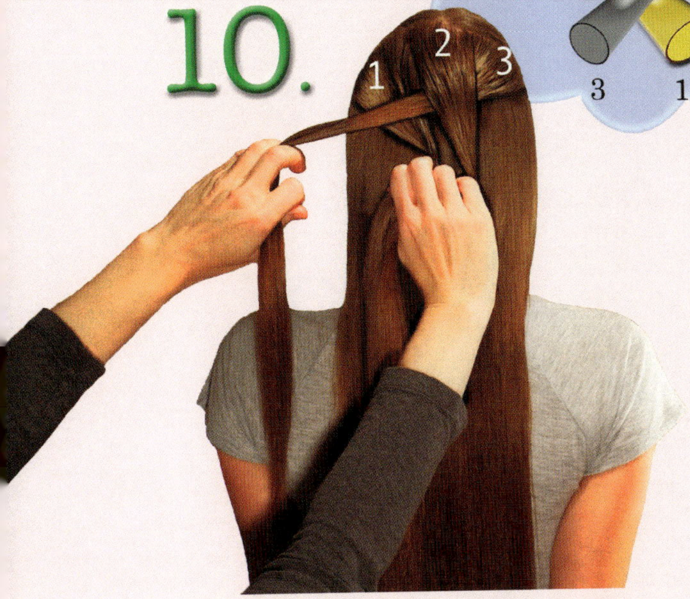

Bring it beneath strand 3 and make it the new center strand.

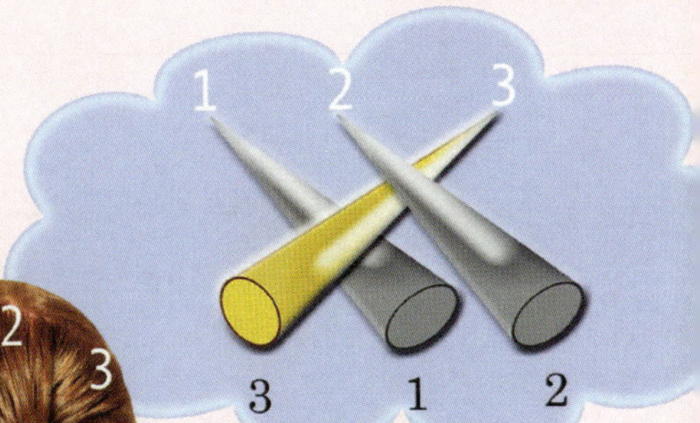

11.

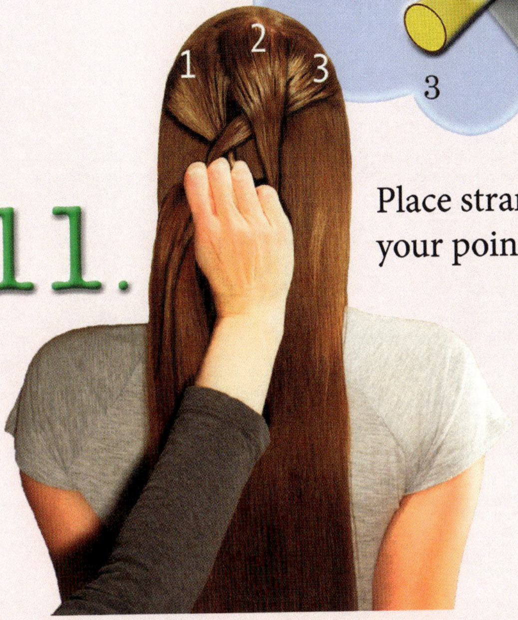

Place strand 3 in your pointer finger.

Now you have a free hand to braid the other direction.

Maybe you are noticing the pattern your hands are weaving. The outside strands alternate going down and into the center.

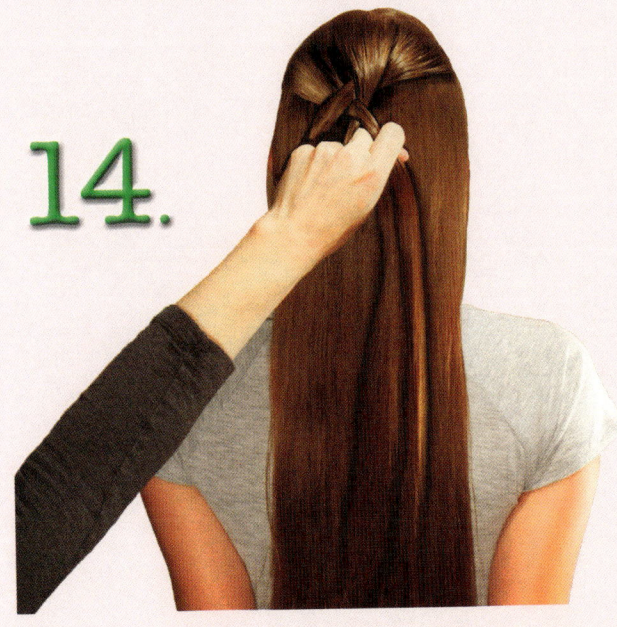

14.

Place the strand still remaining in your right hand into the pointer finger in your left hand. Now you have a free hand to braid the other direction.

Each strand is seperated by a finger. The ends of the hair should come out of the fist at the thumb.

Ways 145

Continuing

3

15. Sliver off a gather from the face all the way back to the braid.

16. From underneath add the gather into the center strand.

19. Reach under the middle strand and hook the furthest away outside strand with your middle finger.

20. Bring that outside strand under the center strand and make it the new center strand.

part 3. Three-Strand Dutch Stitch

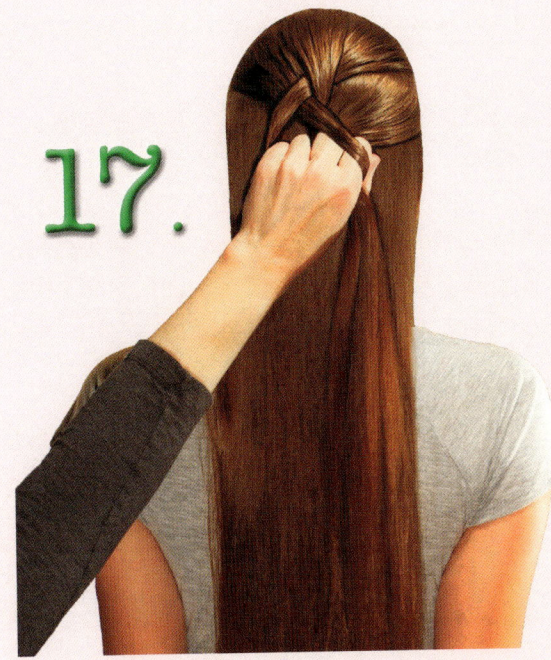

17.

Your right hand is free to braid the other direction.

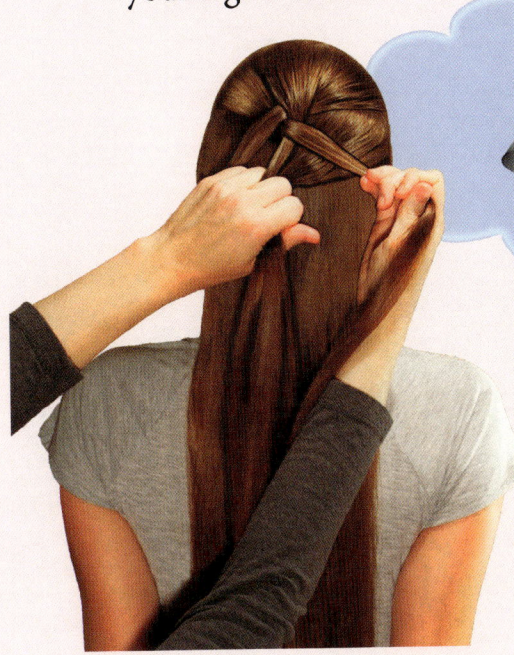

Grab the strand nearest your right hand.

18.

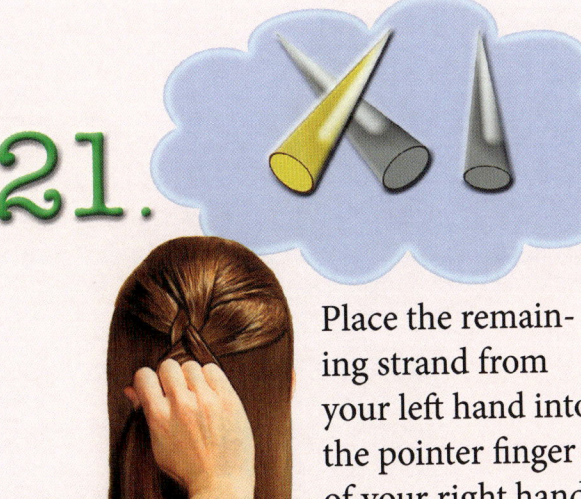

21.

Place the remaining strand from your left hand into the pointer finger of your right hand.

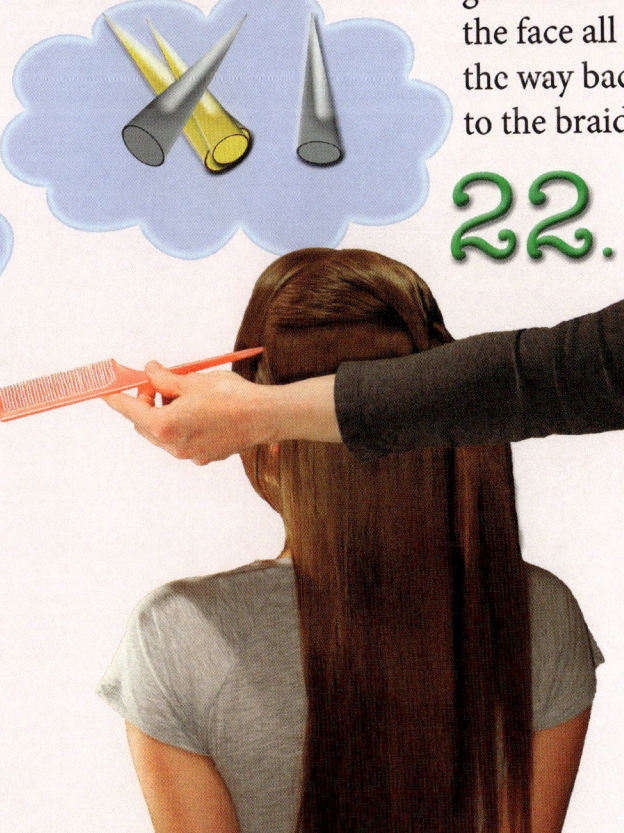

Sliver off a gather from the face all the way back to the braid.

22.

part 4. Three-Strand Dutch Stitch

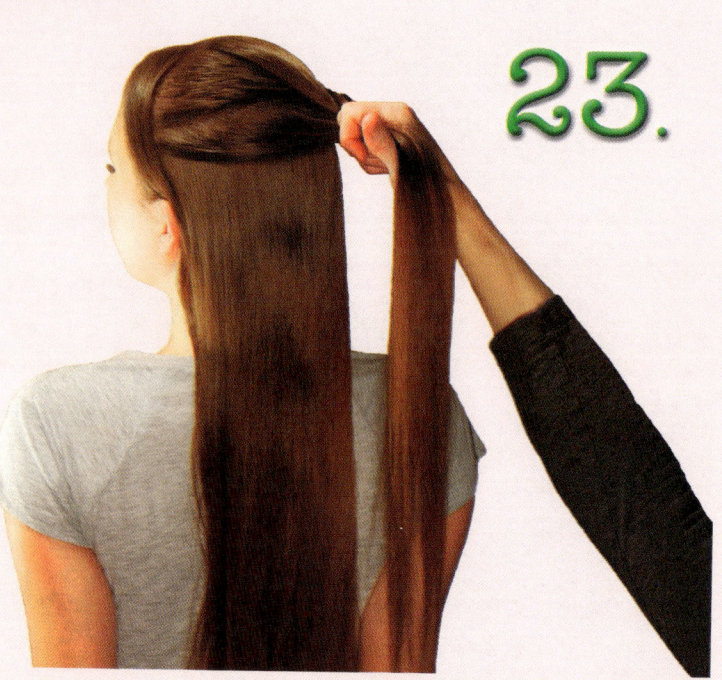

23.

From underneath add the gather into the center strand.

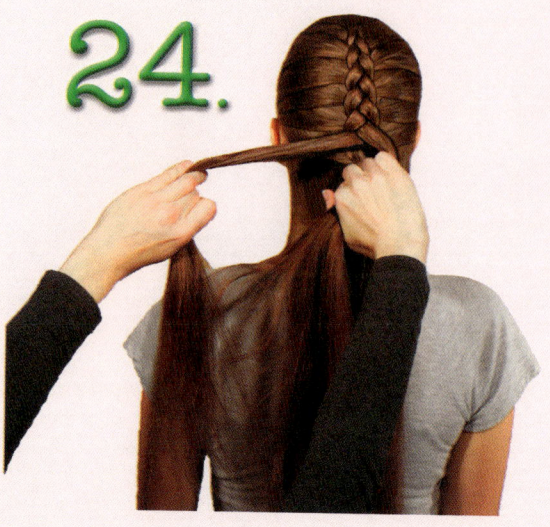

24.

Continue crossing alternate outside strands under and into the center while gathering into the new center strand until you reach the end of the hair.

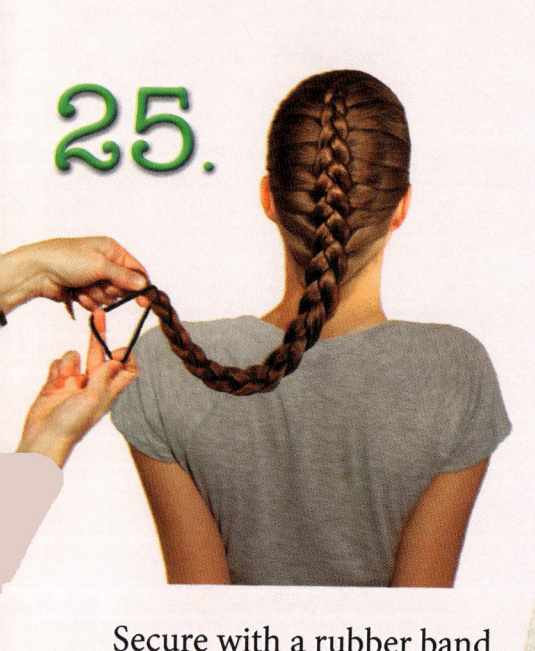

25.

Secure with a rubber band.

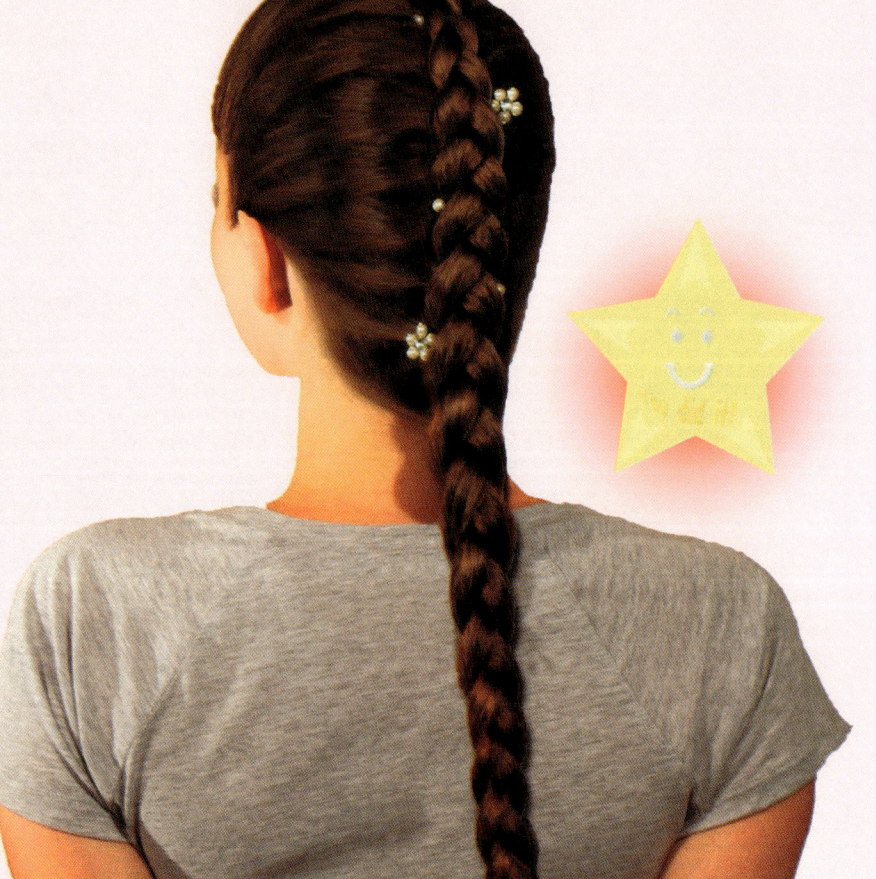

Three-Strand

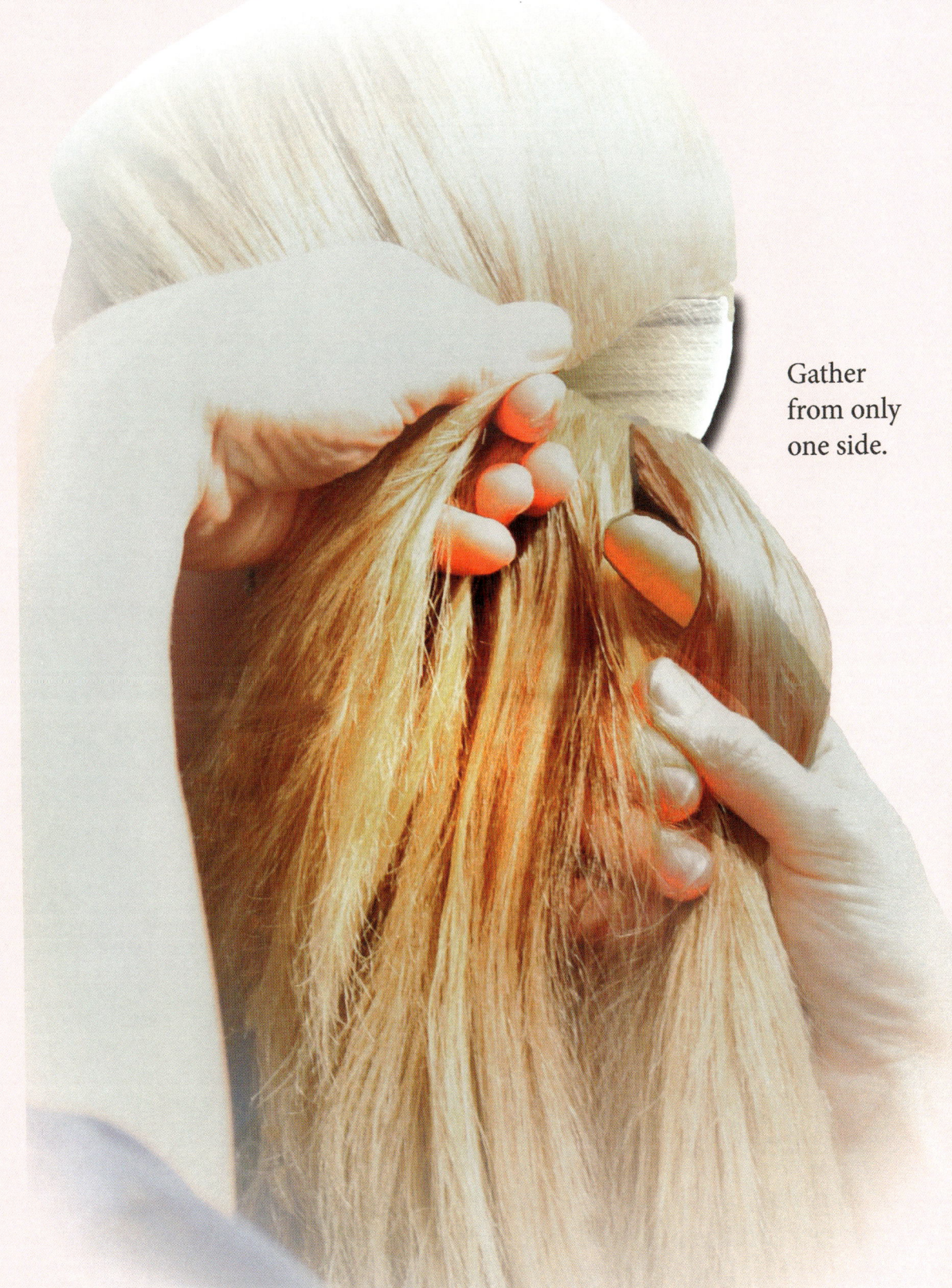

Gather from only one side.

Let's lace it!

3 Three-Strand Dutch Lace

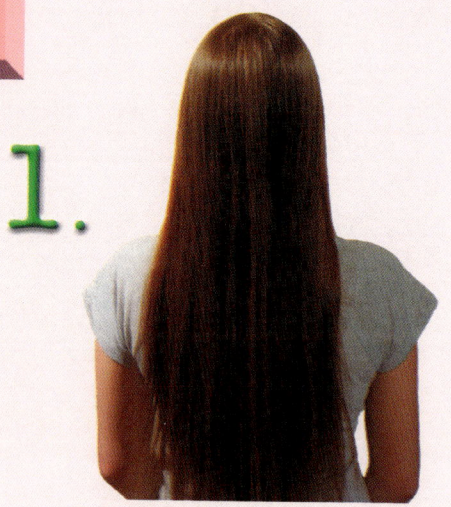

1.

Begin with clean, brushed hair.

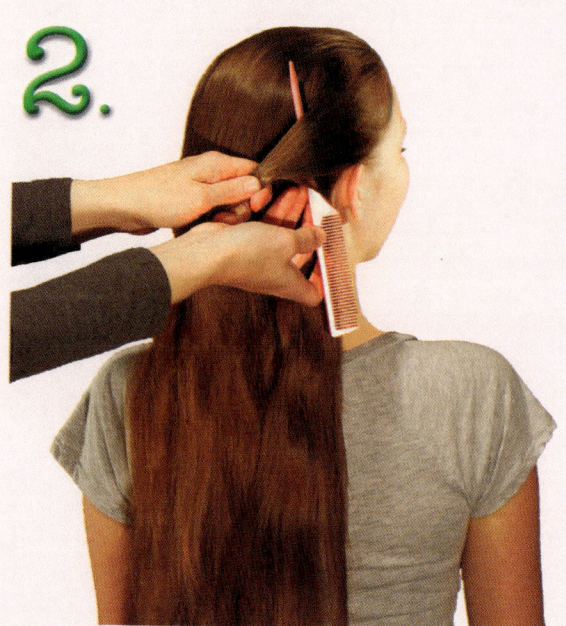

2.

Take a section of hair illustrated.

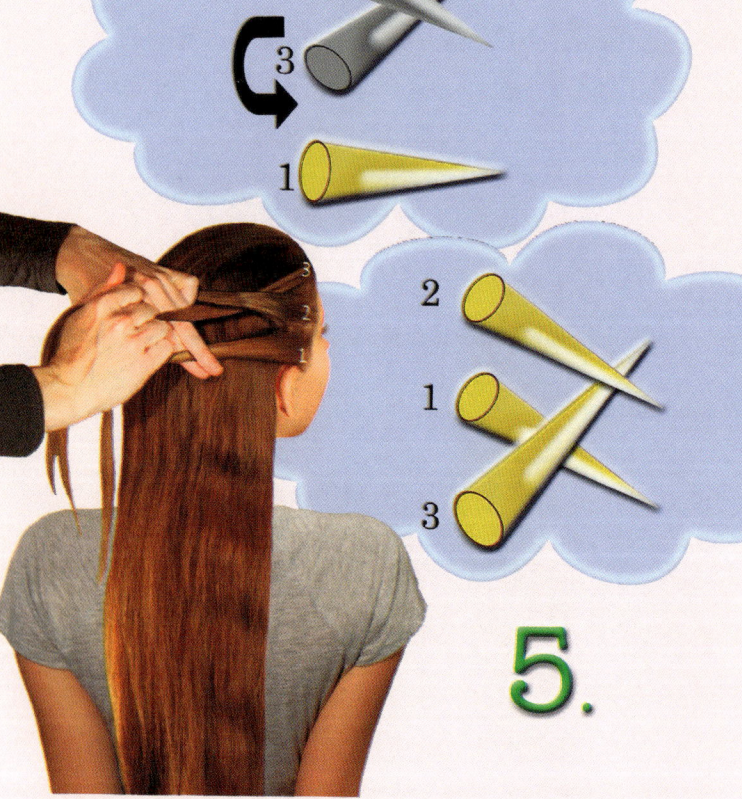

5.

After taking strand 2, reach under strand 3 and hook strand 1 with your middle finger. Place strand 3 in your pointer finger.

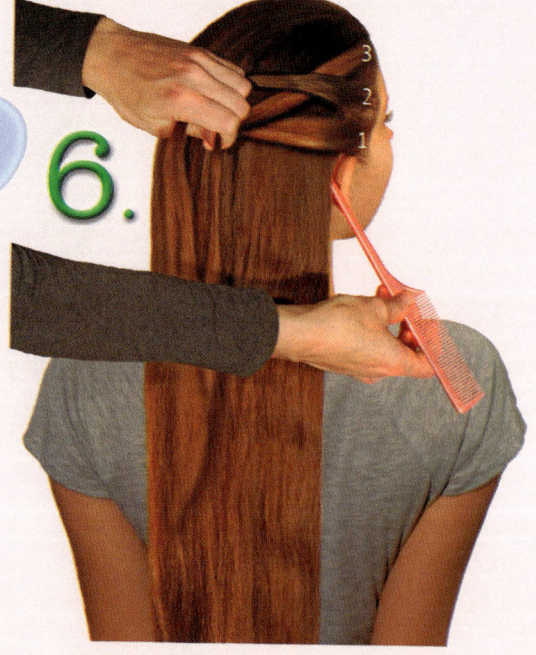

6.

Sliver off a gather from the face all the way back to the braid.

150   www.findingbraids.com

Three-Strand Dutch Lace

3

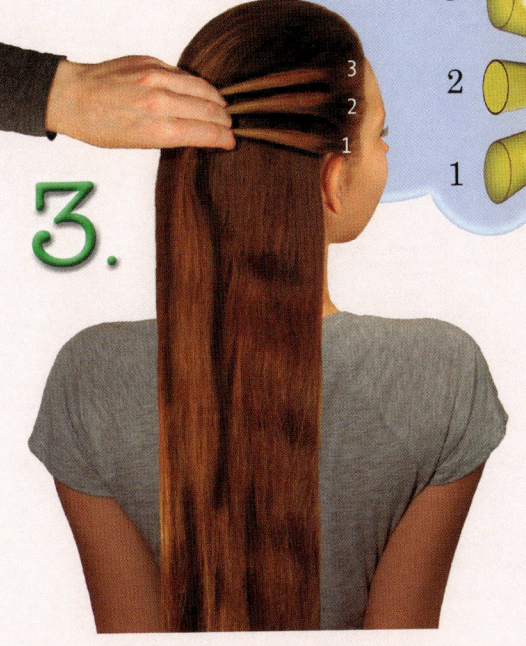

3.

Divide the section into three strands.

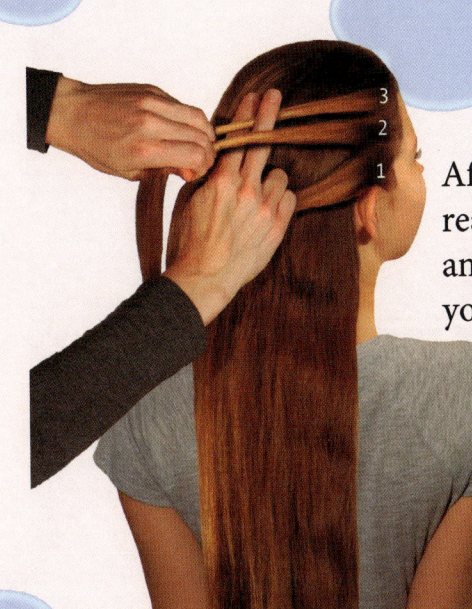

4.

After taking strand 1, reach under strand 2 and hook strand 3 with your middle finger.

Place strand 2 in your pointer finger.

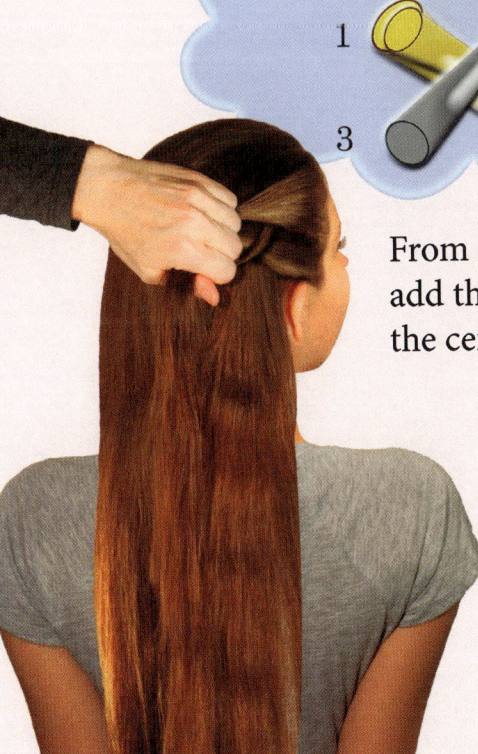

7.

From underneath add the gather into the center strand.

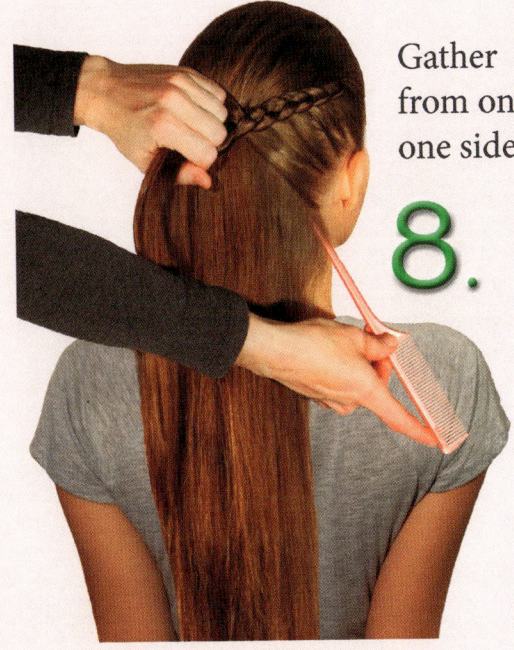

8.

Gather from only one side.

Ways 151

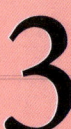

part 2. Three-Strand Dutch Lace

Continue gathering into the center strand from beneath until you reach the end of the hair.

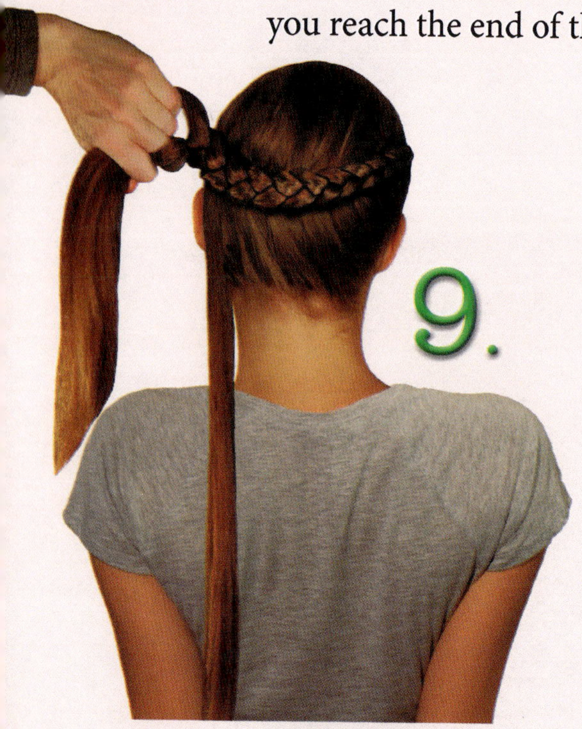

9.

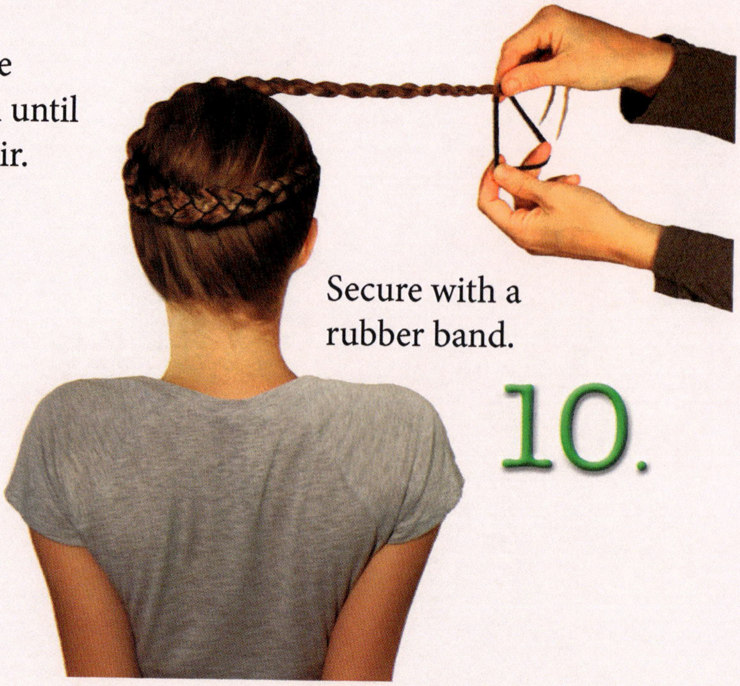

Secure with a rubber band.

10.

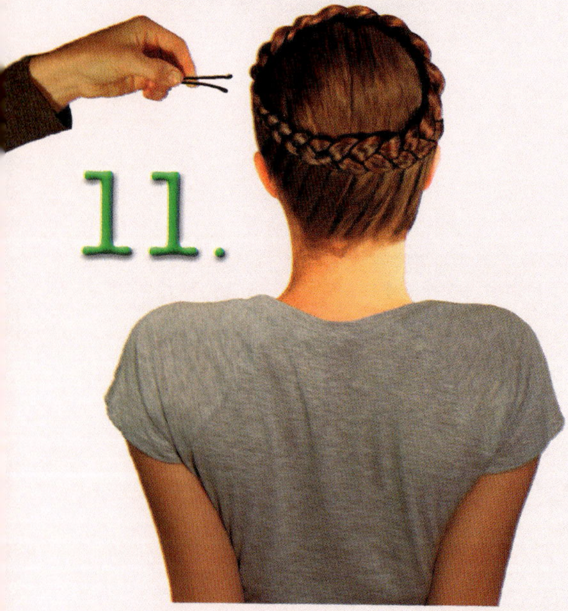

11.

Fix the end of the braid with bobby pins to hold the braid in place.

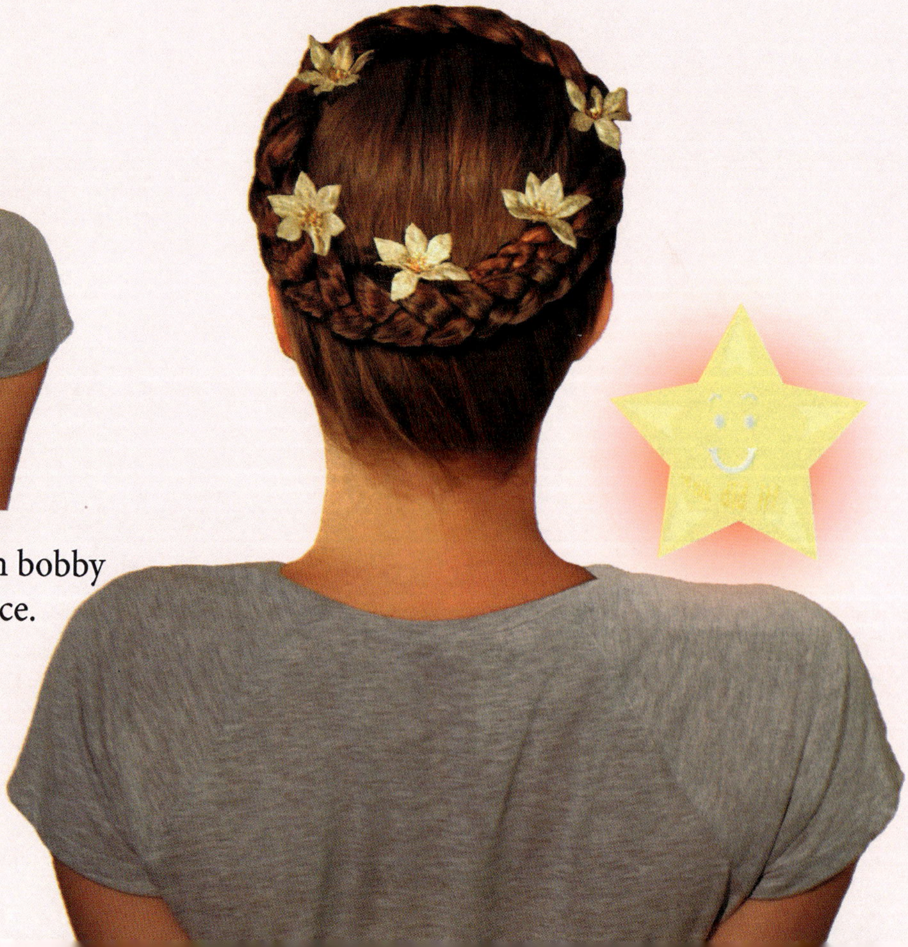

152   www.findingbraids.com

Examples of Three-Strand

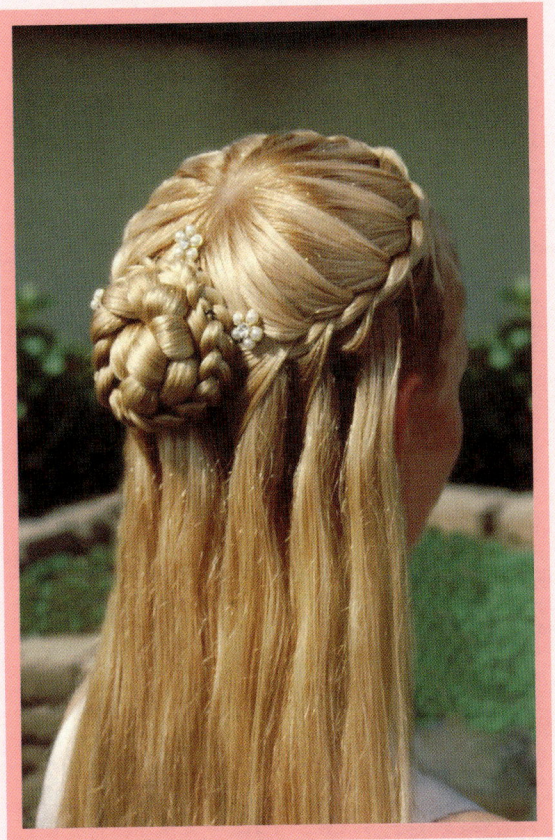
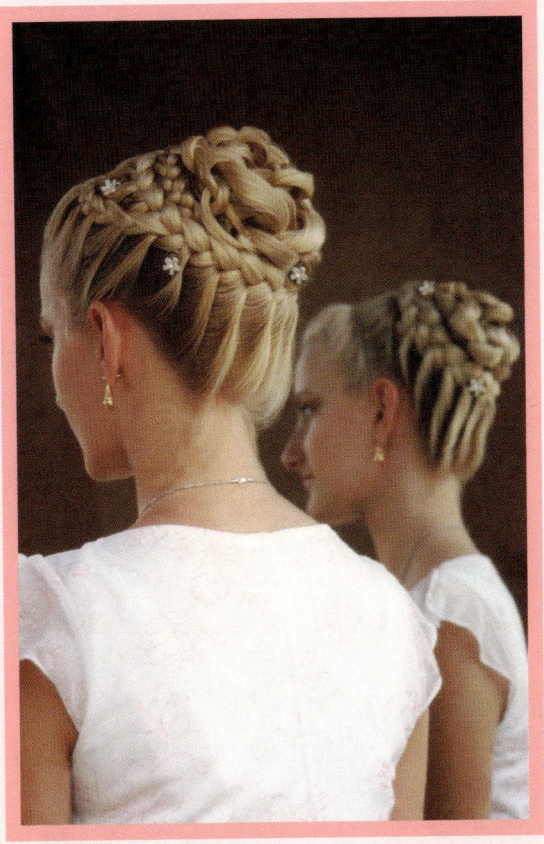
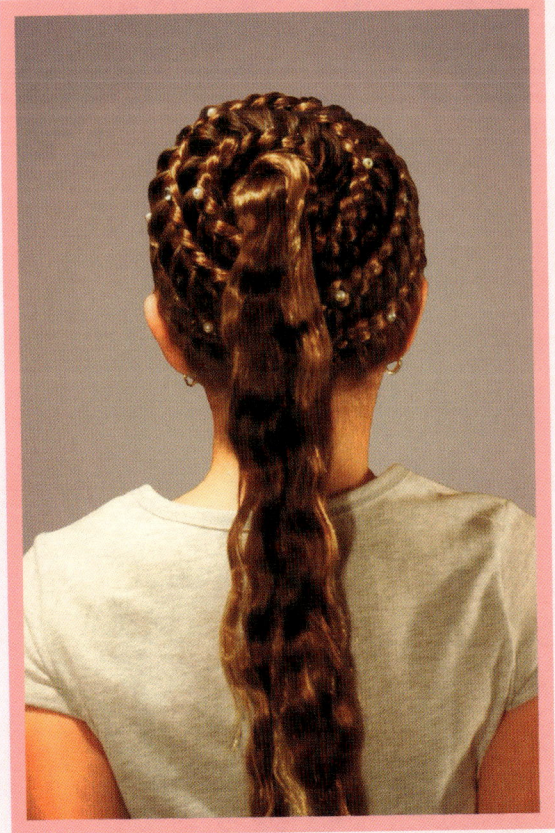
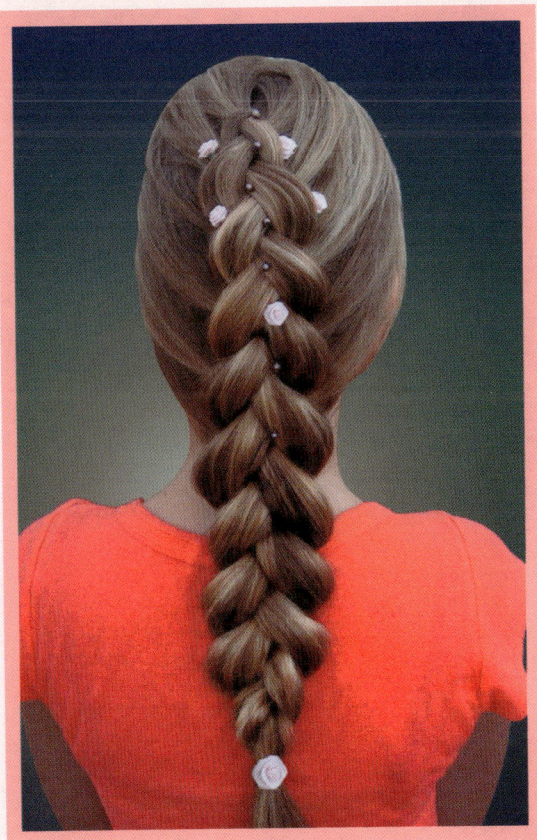

Visit my website to see more examples of the Three-Strand Ways

Four-Strand Round

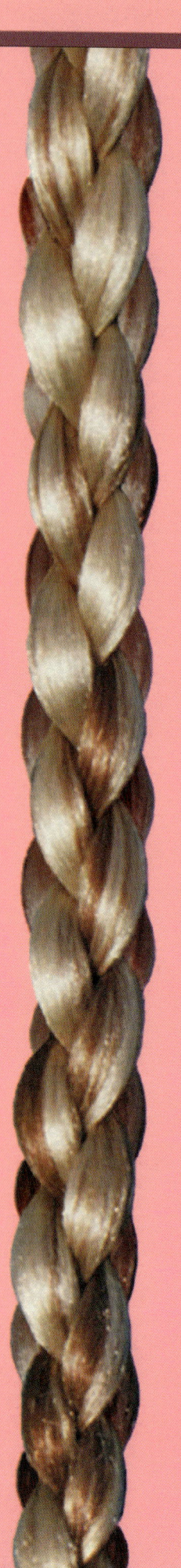

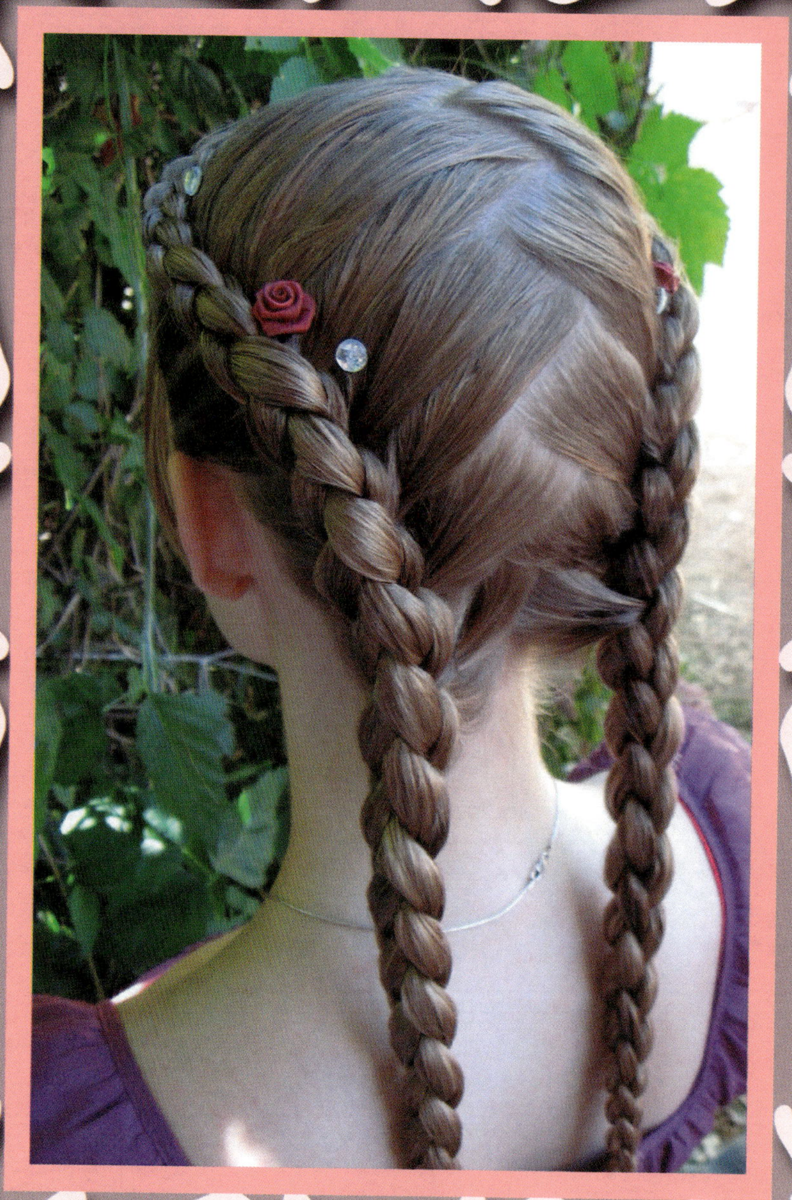

Tricky to master, fun to create, awesome to see, this braid is worth the challenge to learn. It is easy to loose track of the strands while you are braiding. Long hair without layers works best and impresses.

Four-Strand Round

A braid that looks like a friendship bracelette. The next nineteen pages will walk you through this braid.

Braid . . . . 156 - 158

Stitch . . . . 160 - 165

Lace . . . . 168 - 173

Examples 174

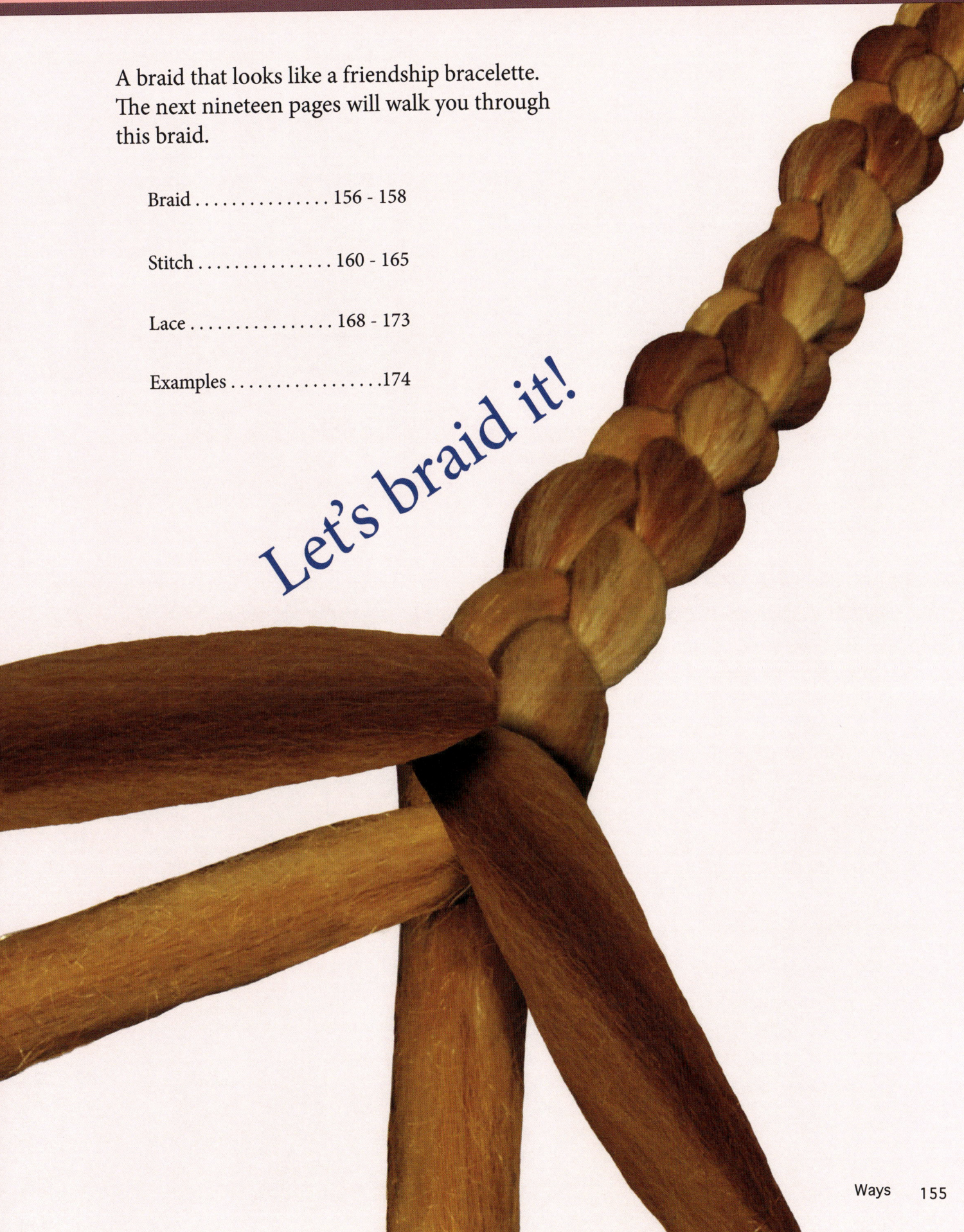

4 Four-Strand Round Braid

By making the effort we vastly improve the odds of achievement.
  - Dan Millman

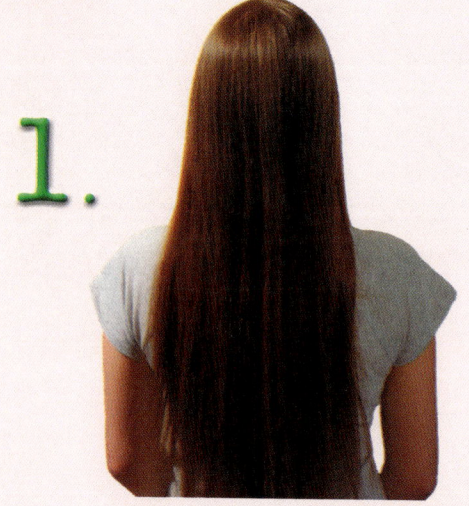

Begin with clean, brushed hair.

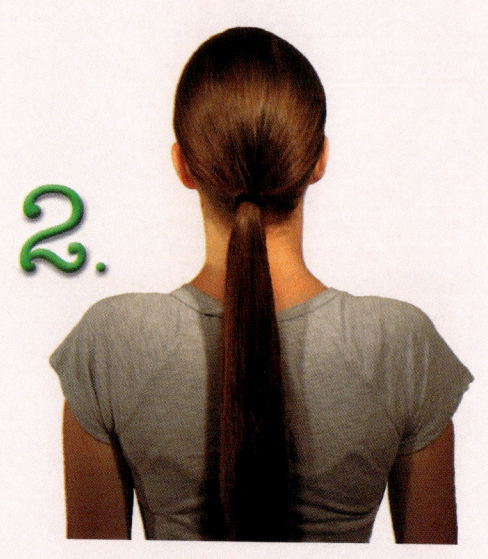

Take a section of hair.

Can you learn this braid?

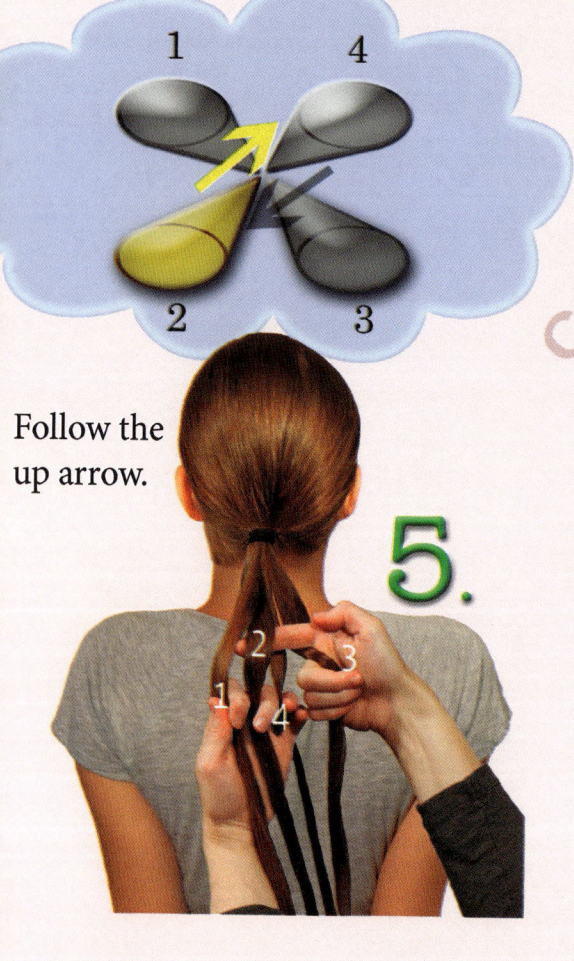

Follow the up arrow.

Before crossing strands 1 and 3, transfer strand 4 to the middle finger of the left hand.

Follow the down arrow.

Continue switching corners.

www.findingbraids.com

Four-Strand Round Braid

4

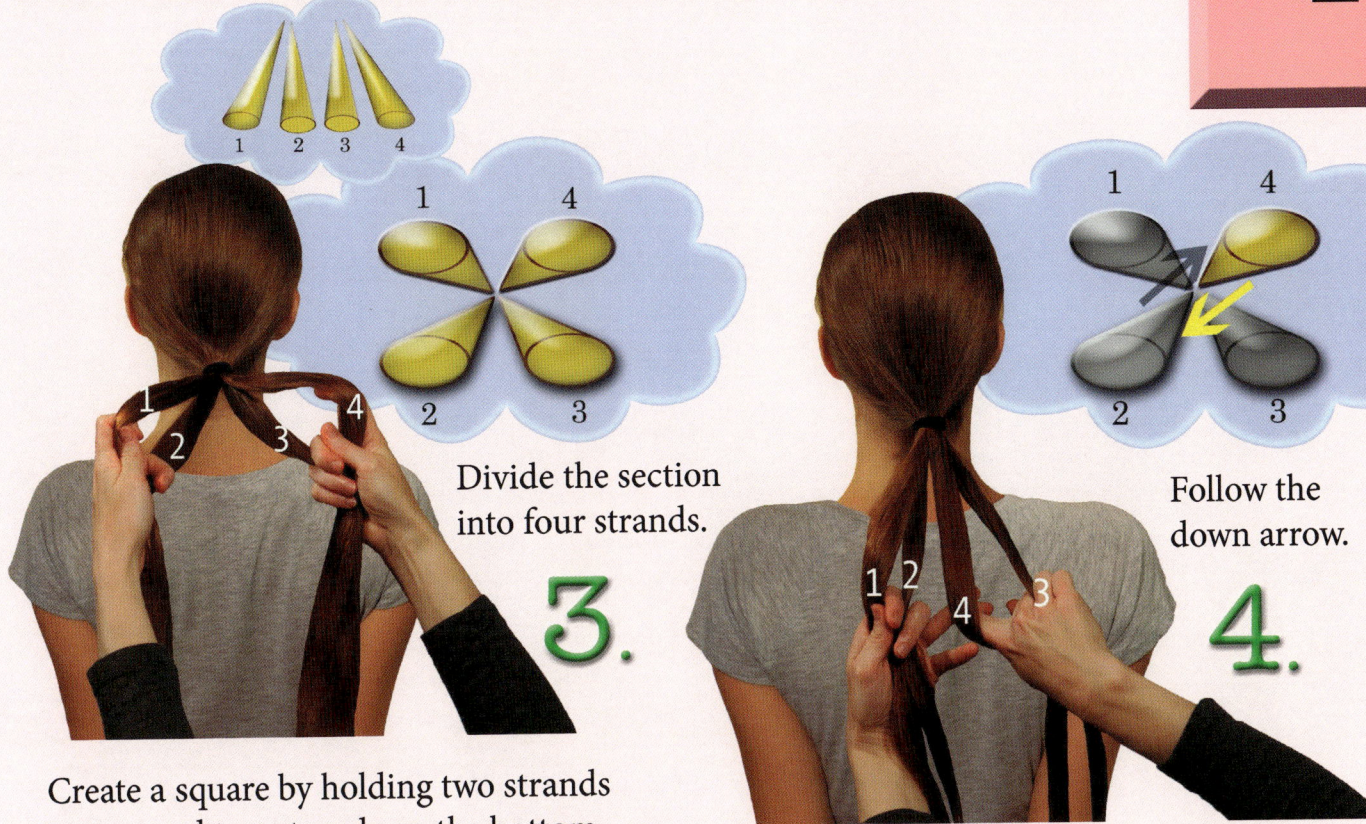

3. Divide the section into four strands.

Create a square by holding two strands on top and two strands on the bottom.

4. Follow the down arrow.

Opposite corners of the square cross to trade places.

It is tricky and complicated. See if you can.

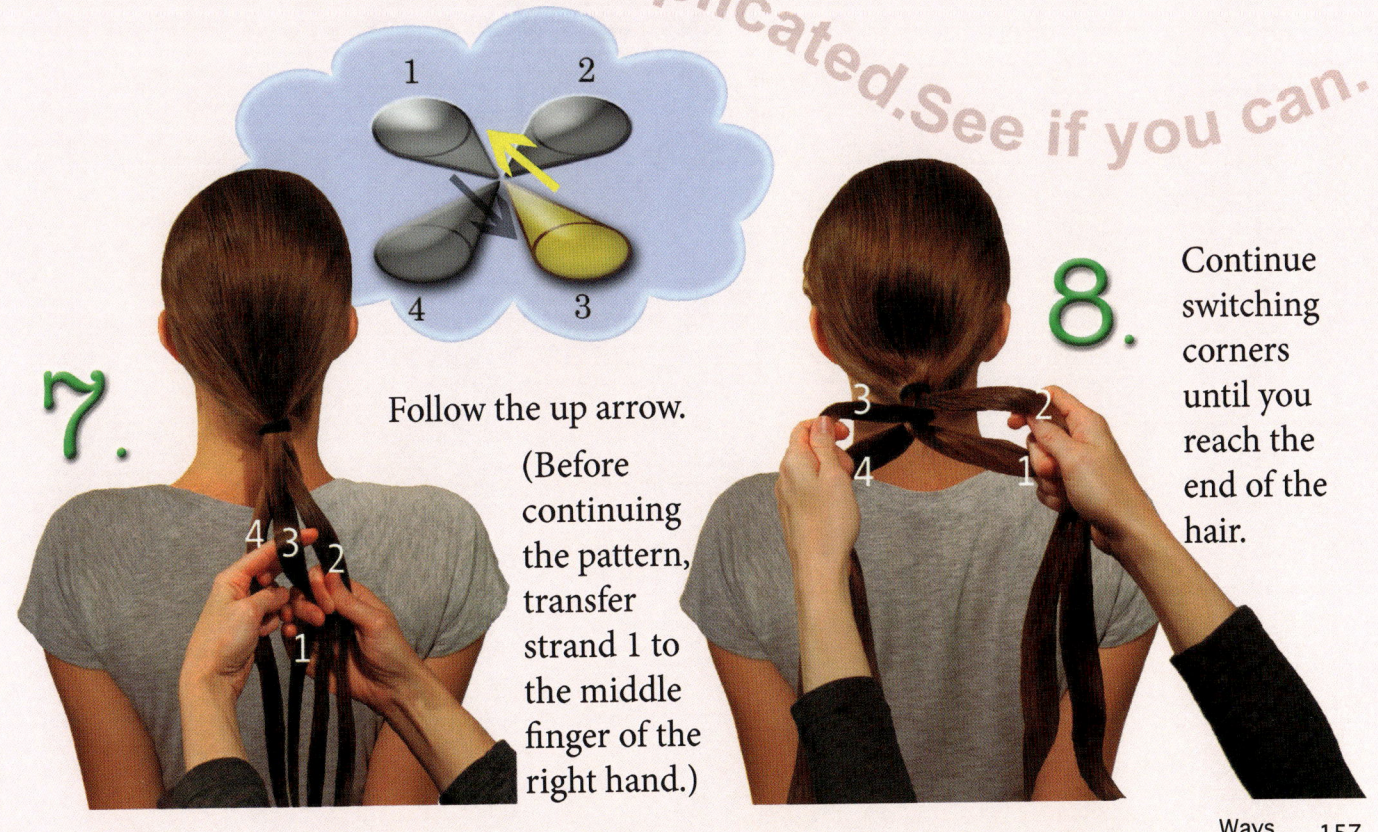

7. Follow the up arrow. (Before continuing the pattern, transfer strand 1 to the middle finger of the right hand.)

8. Continue switching corners until you reach the end of the hair.

Ways 157

part 2. Four-Strand Round Braid

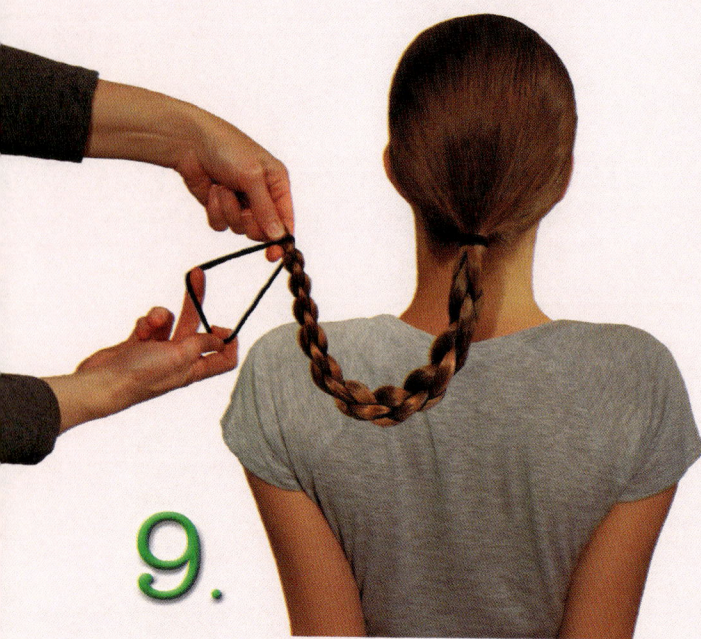

9.

Secure with a rubber band.

I invite you to find a happy zen place in your mind and emotions as you move forward in these lessons. As you have just seen, I am showing you complicated weaving patterns. They will be difficult to comprehend. Time and practice is needed to fully understand what is happening with the strands and your fingers.

Videos may help, as the weave patterns will be shown in motion. Give your brain a chance to make the neccessary pathways for this new information before deciding to give up. I recommend trying a lesson once a day for a week. The time in between practicing is important because that is when you will process what you have tried. Try each day.

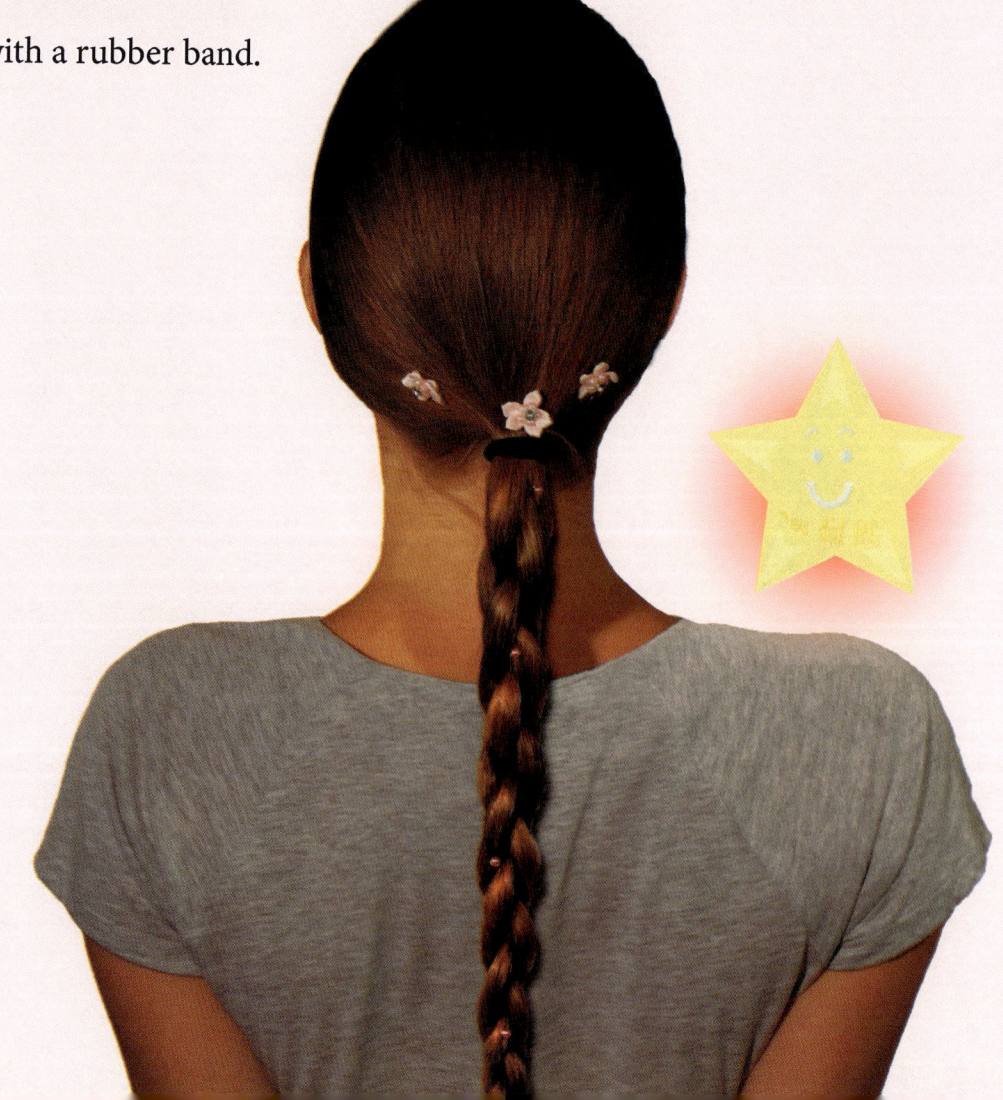

Four-Strand Round

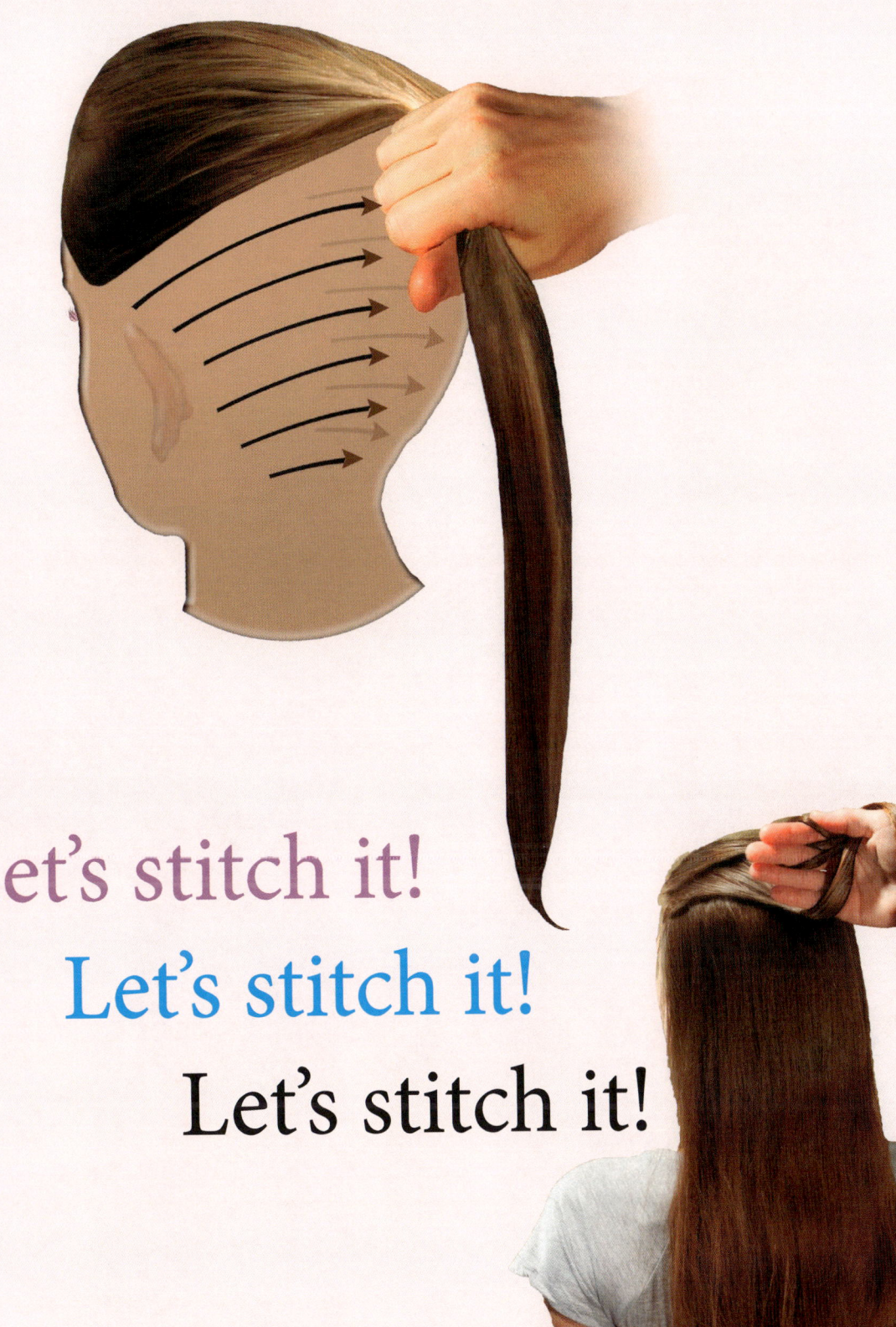

Let's stitch it!

Let's stitch it!

Let's stitch it!

As you braid, the strands of hair should be held through the palms of the hand like this.

Ways 159

4 Four-Strand Round Stitch

Patience, persistence, perseverance and practice.

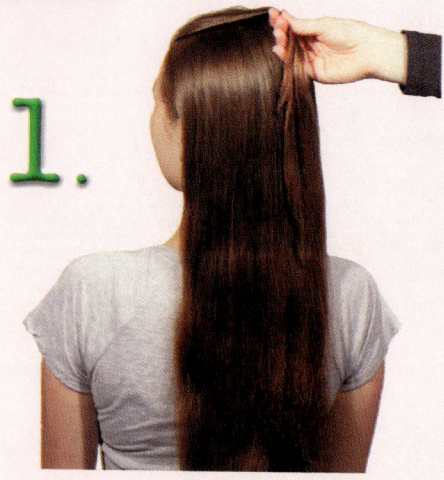

1. Take a section of hair as illustrated.

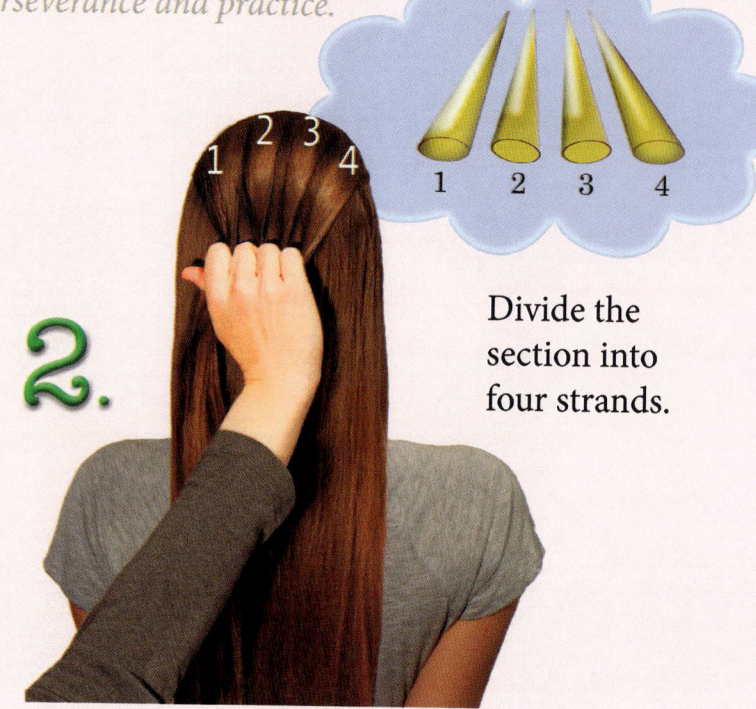

2. Divide the section into four strands.

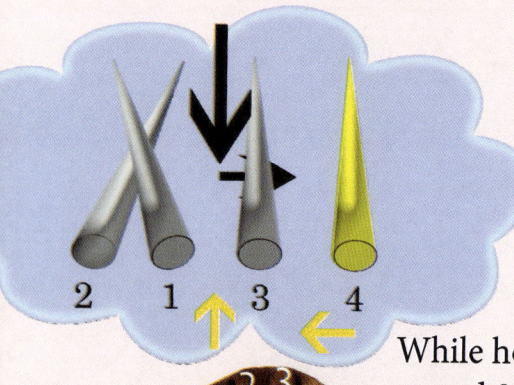

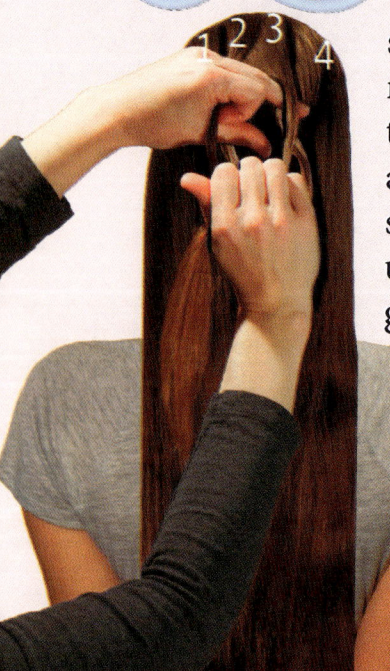

5. While holding strand 2 with the ring finger, weave the middle finger and thumb above strand 1 and under strand 3 to grab strand 4.

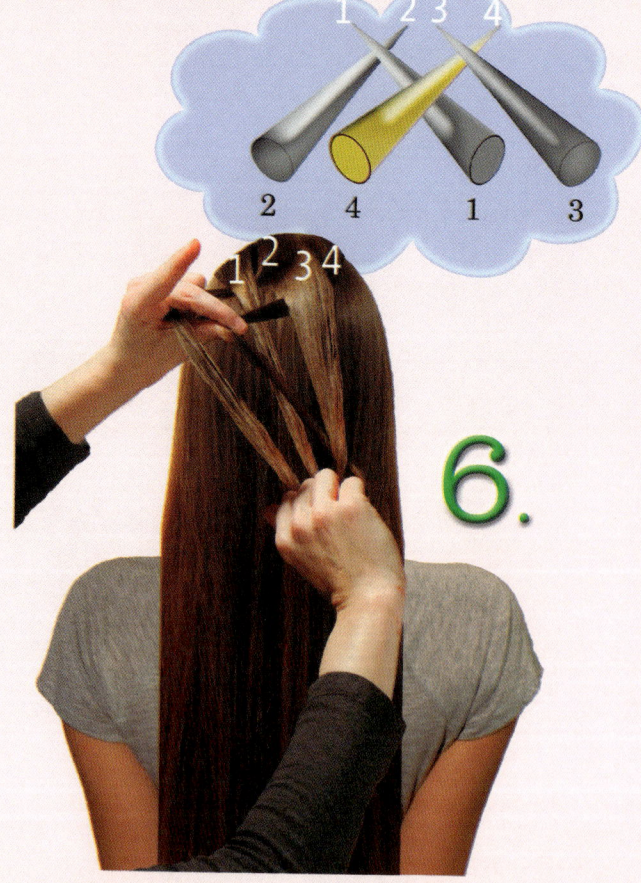

6. Bring strand 4 under strand 3 and above strand 1 with the middle finger. Keep strand 4 in the middle finger.

Four-Strand Round Stitch

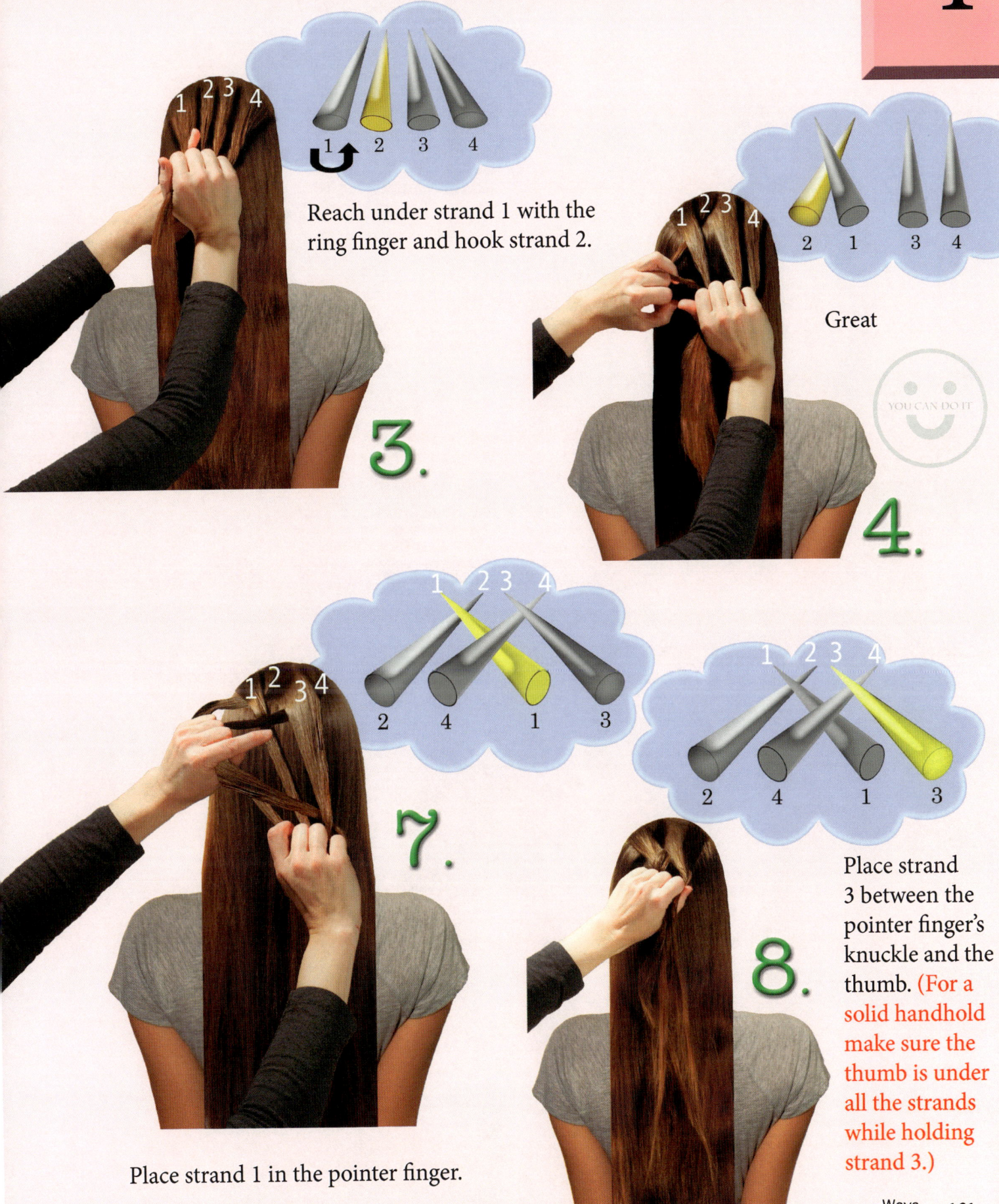

3. Reach under strand 1 with the ring finger and hook strand 2.

4. Great

7. Place strand 1 in the pointer finger.

8. Place strand 3 between the pointer finger's knuckle and the thumb. (For a solid handhold make sure the thumb is under all the strands while holding strand 3.)

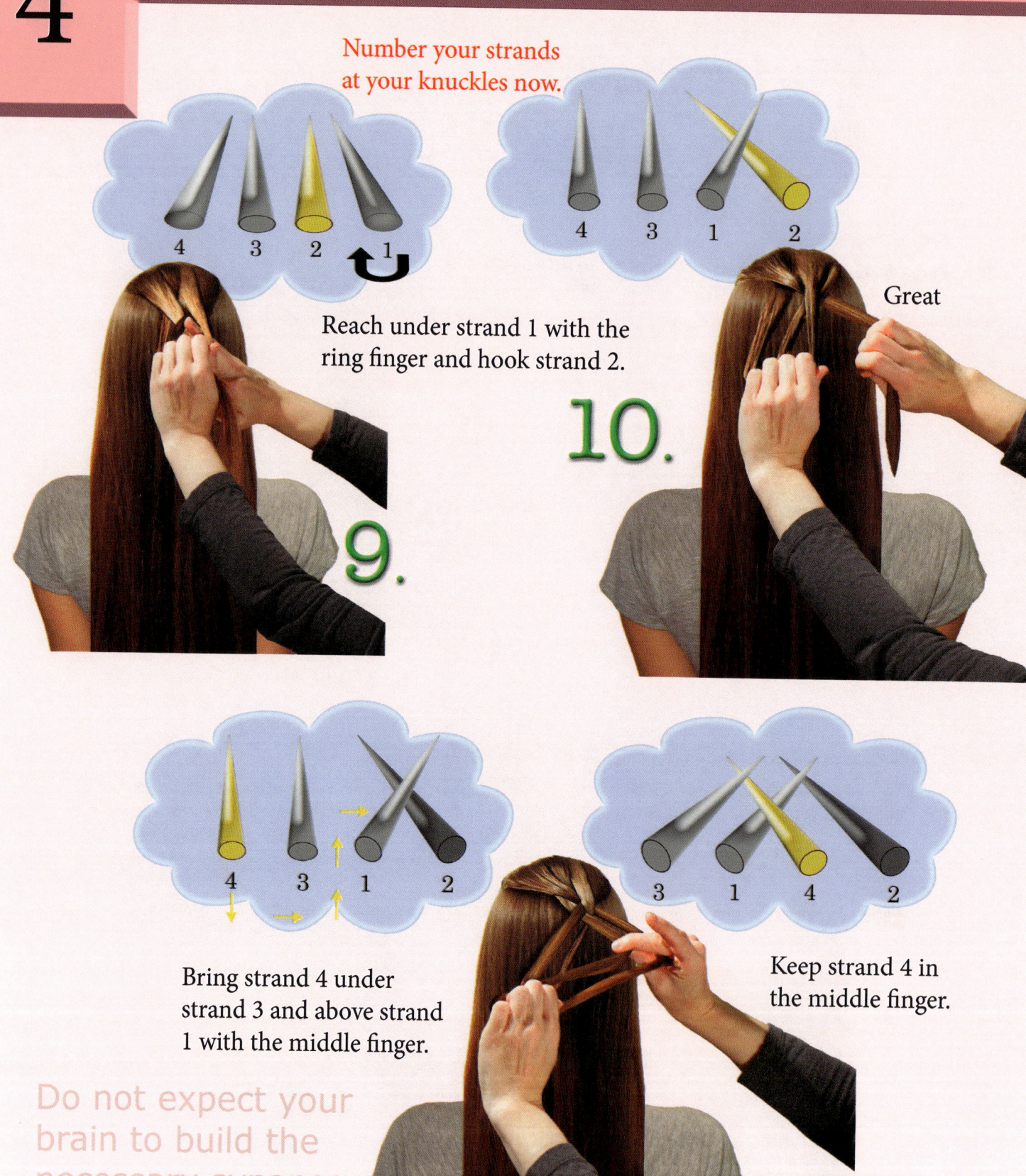

4 Continuing

Number your strands at your knuckles now.

9. Reach under strand 1 with the ring finger and hook strand 2.

10. Great

11. Bring strand 4 under strand 3 and above strand 1 with the middle finger.

12. Keep strand 4 in the middle finger.

Do not expect your brain to build the necessary synapse until you try this at least a dozen times.

162 www.findingbraids.com

part 2. Four-Strand Round Stitch

4

How many graphics does it take to show how to move a single strand of hair? Hopefully steps 11 and 12 get the point across.

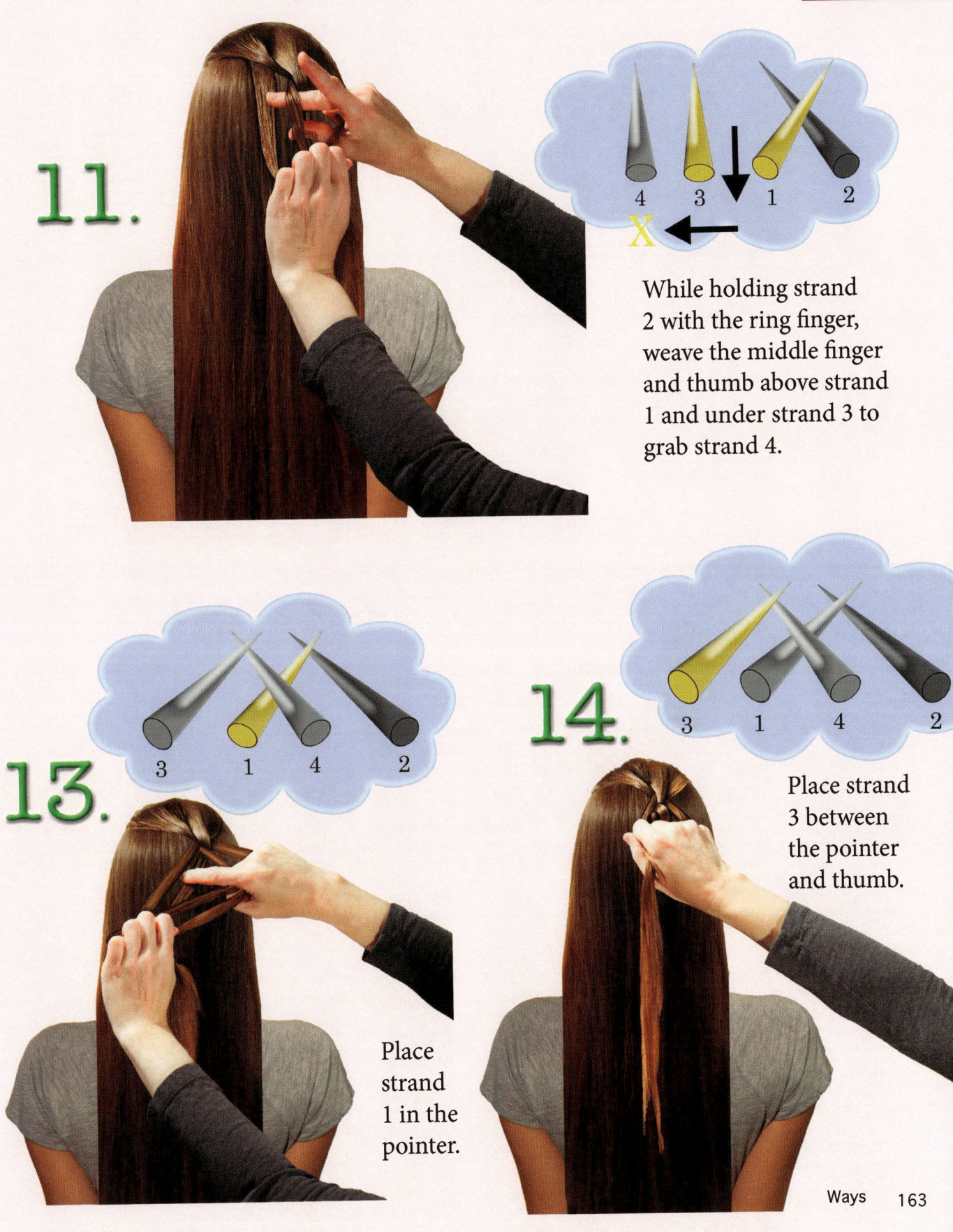

11.

While holding strand 2 with the ring finger, weave the middle finger and thumb above strand 1 and under strand 3 to grab strand 4.

13.

Place strand 1 in the pointer.

14.

Place strand 3 between the pointer and thumb.

Ways

4 Continuing

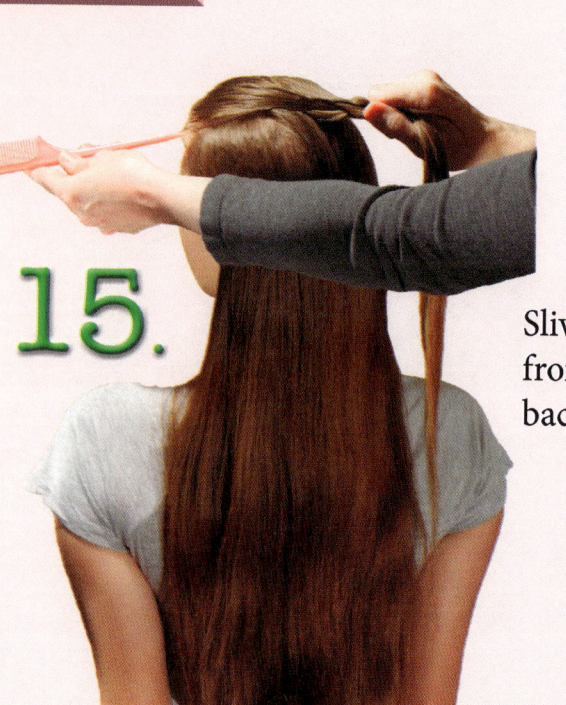

15.

Sliver off a gather of hair from the face all the way back to the braid.

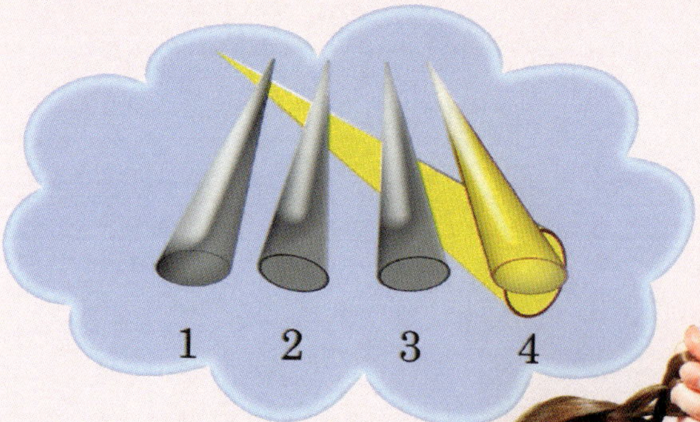

Combine that gather with strand 4 from underneath.

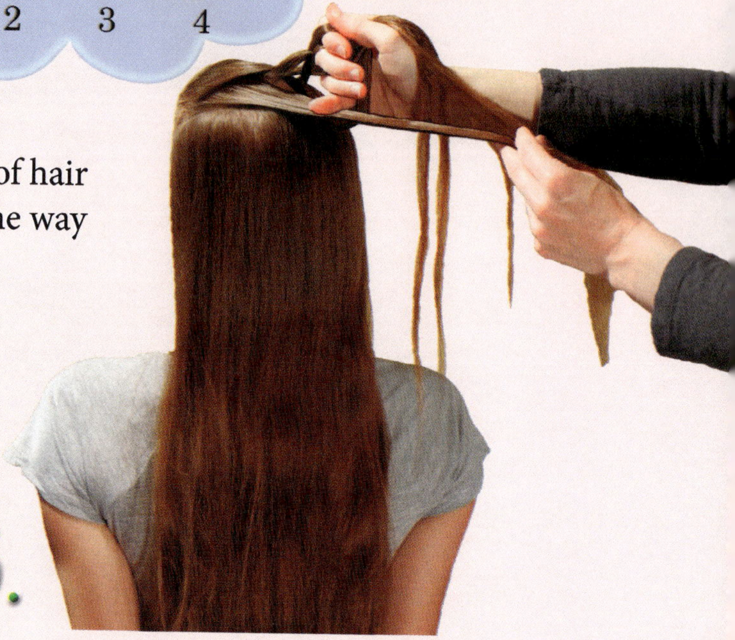

16.

19. Some of you may find it easier to switch to the four-strand round braid for the tail part of this braid.

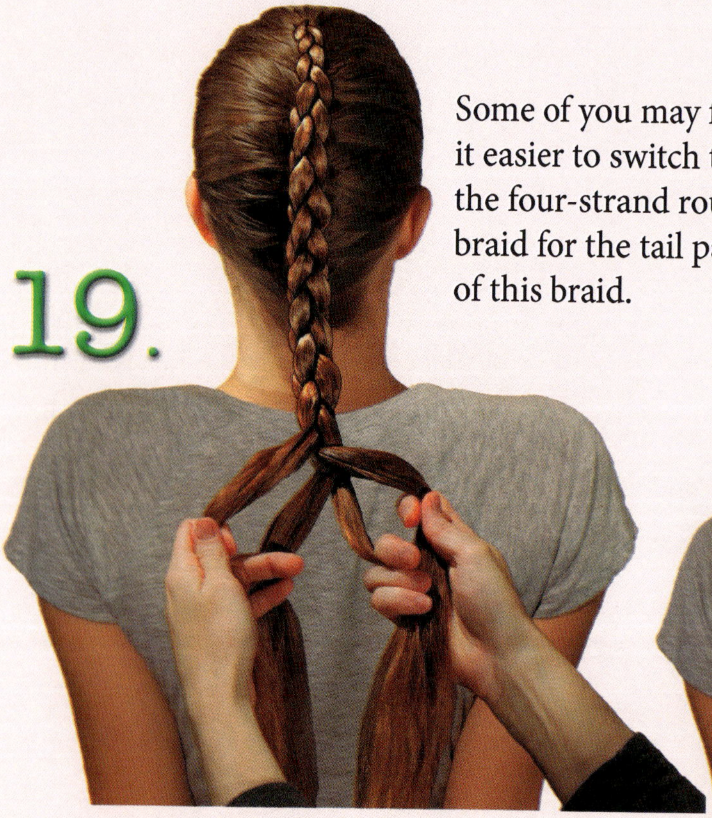

Secure with a rubber band.

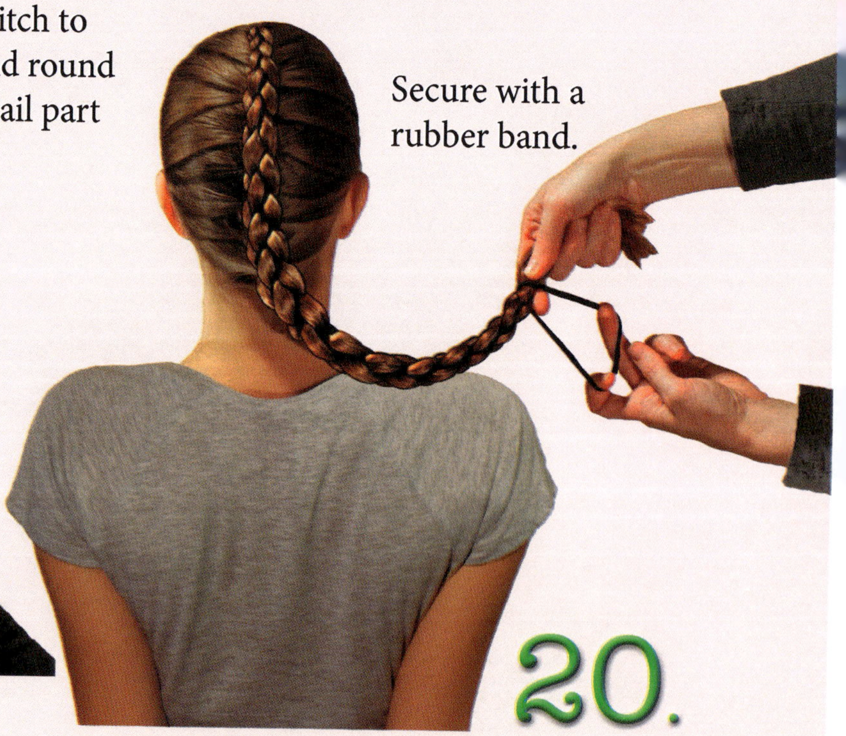

20.

164 www.findingbraids.com

part 3. Four-Strand Round Stitch

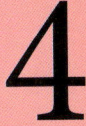

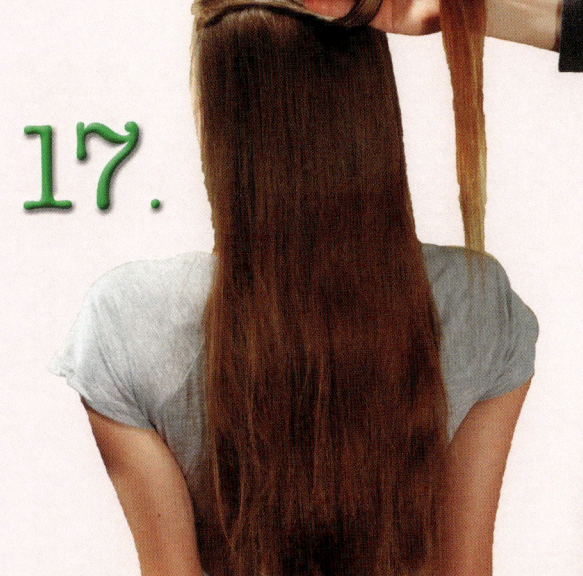

17.

Continue weaving and gathering until you reach the end of the hair.

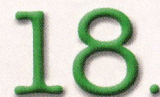

18.

Remember the hair is woven through the palm and out the fist with the other hair.

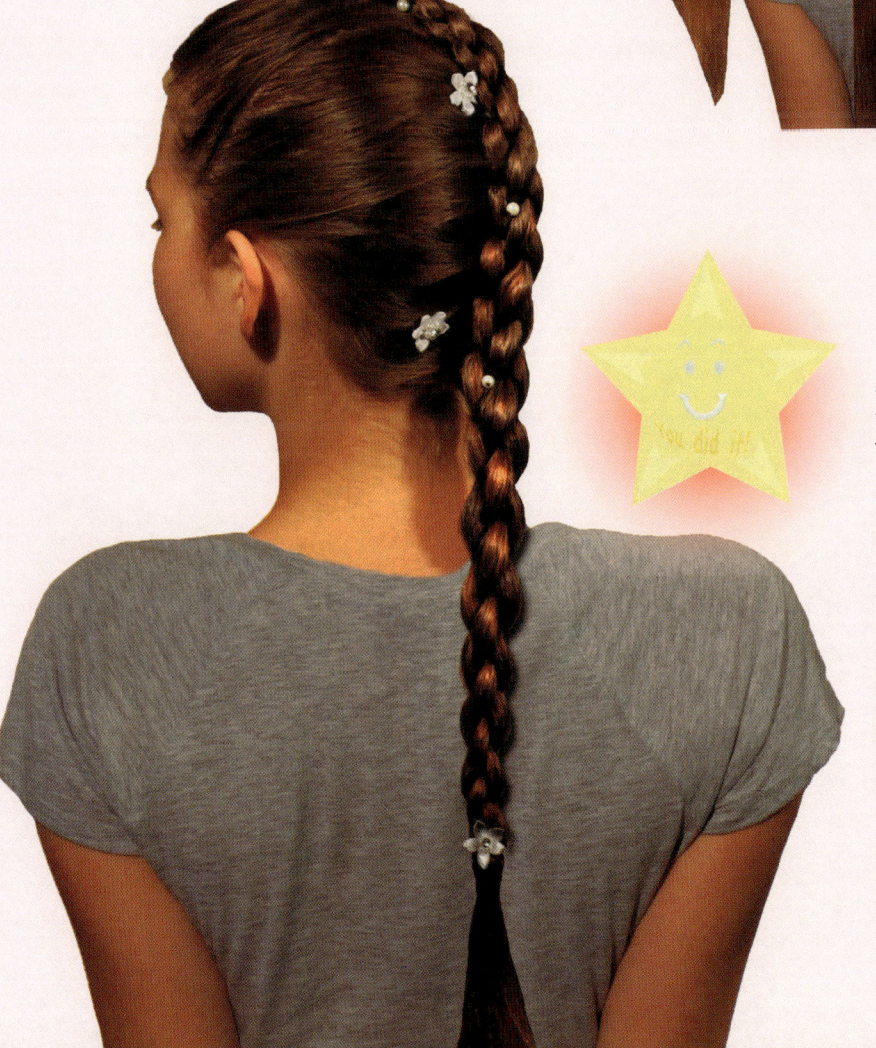

Learning how to "french" this was pure frustration. I call it stitch because french is folded inward and dutch is popping up. Technically this is dutch because it pops up quite a bit. I ended up creating my own gathering system that I have never seen before. It sure is complicated. But, it is also the only one I can remember when I braid.

Ways 165

Four-Strand Round

Notes

My braid mentor, Melaine, taught me this braid a few times and I never retained the information. When I started writing this book I wanted to include it and looked in many braid books. I found two books that taught this braid but I could not figure out how to do it. So, I looked online. That was in 2005, I found a tutorial and two videos. The information that worked the best for me ended up being a leather braiding tutorial.

Four-Strand Round

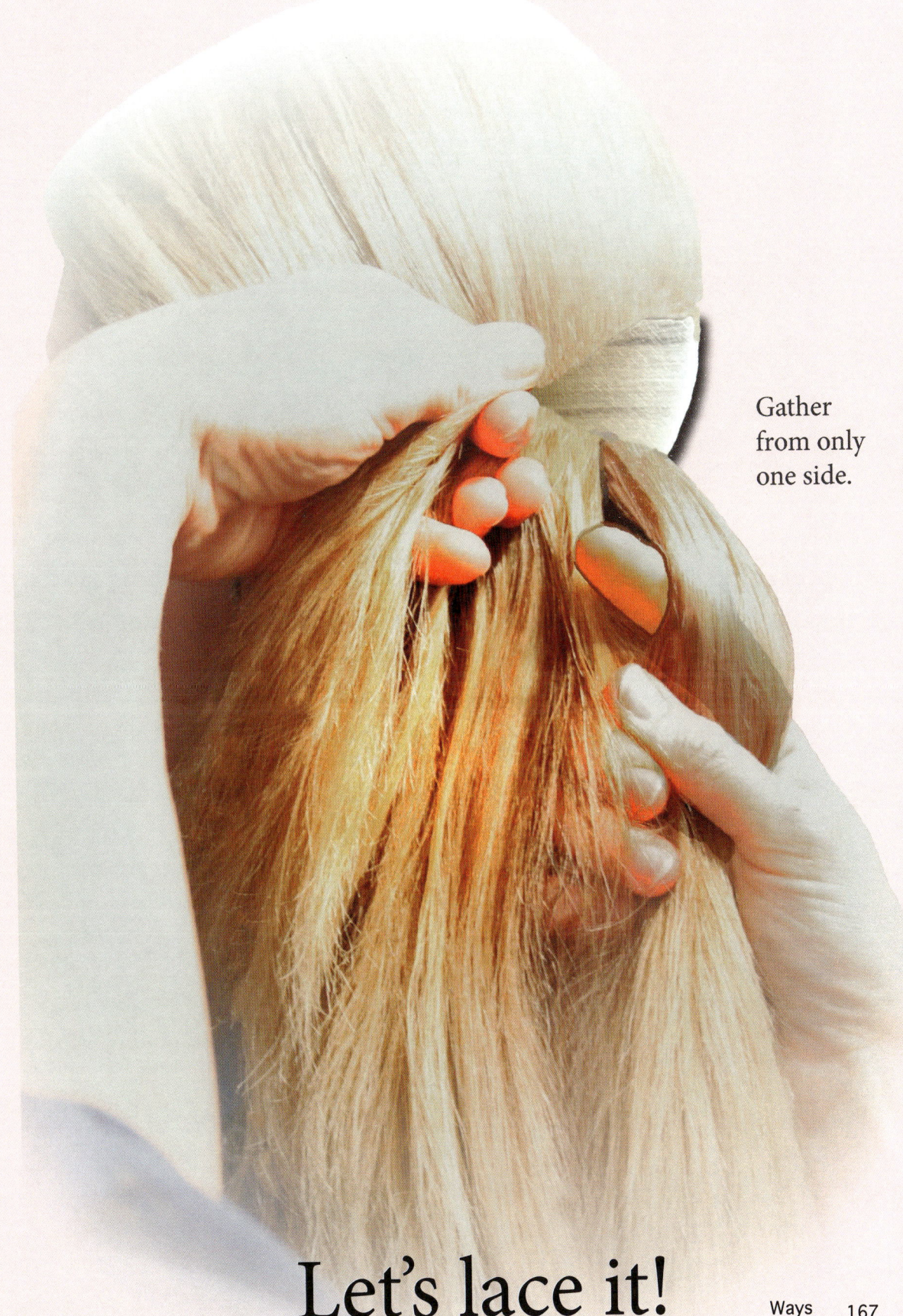

Gather from only one side.

Let's lace it!

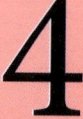

Four-Strand Round Lace

Determination: Ascertainment after investigation.

1. Take a section of hair as illustrated.

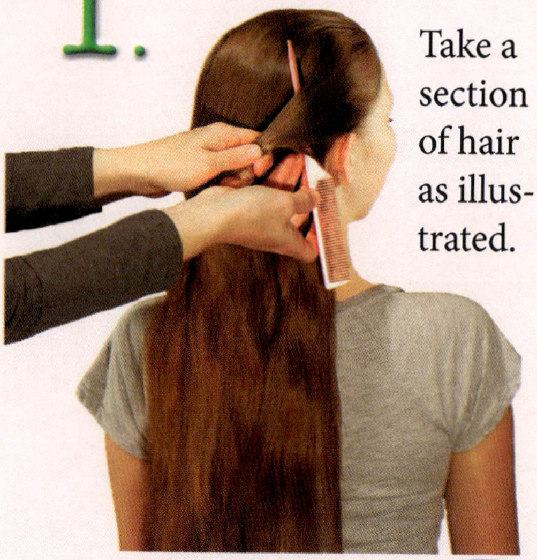

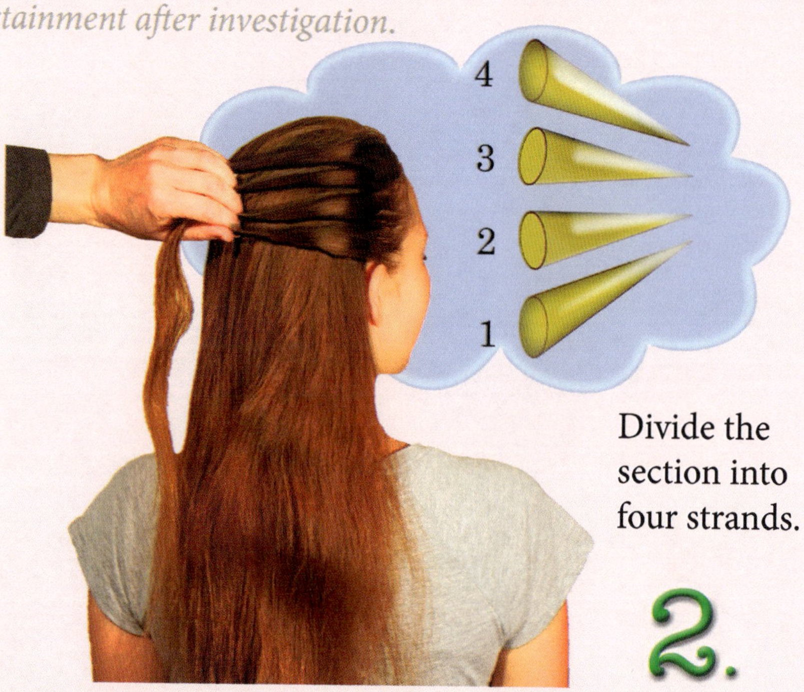

2. Divide the section into four strands.

5. While holding strand 2 with the ring finger, weave the middle finger and thumb above strand 1 and under strand 3 to grab strand 4.

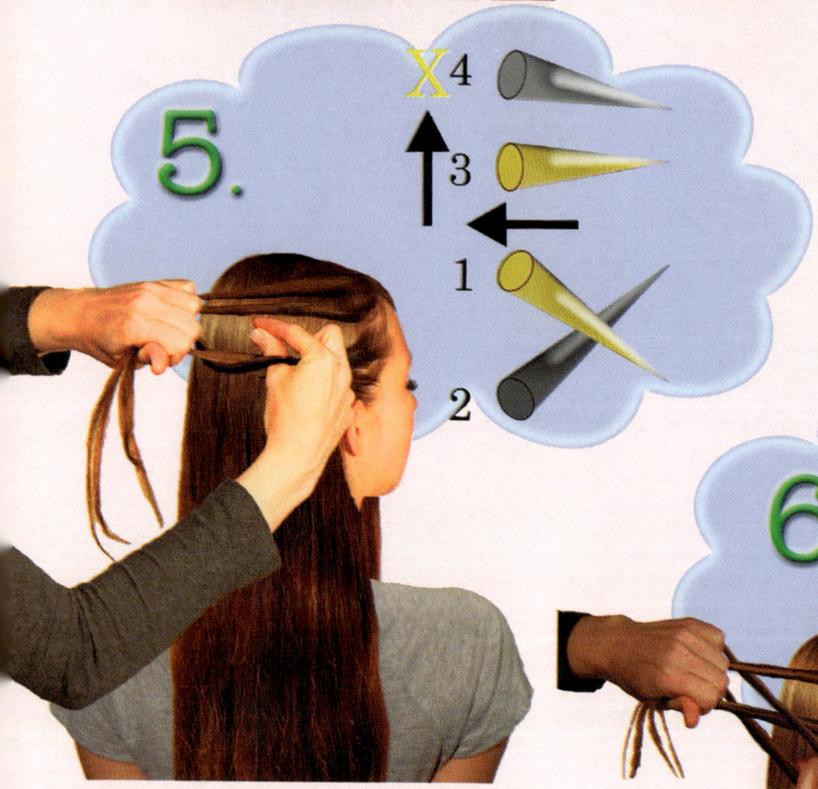

6. Bring strand 4 under strand 3 and above strand 1 with the middle finger.

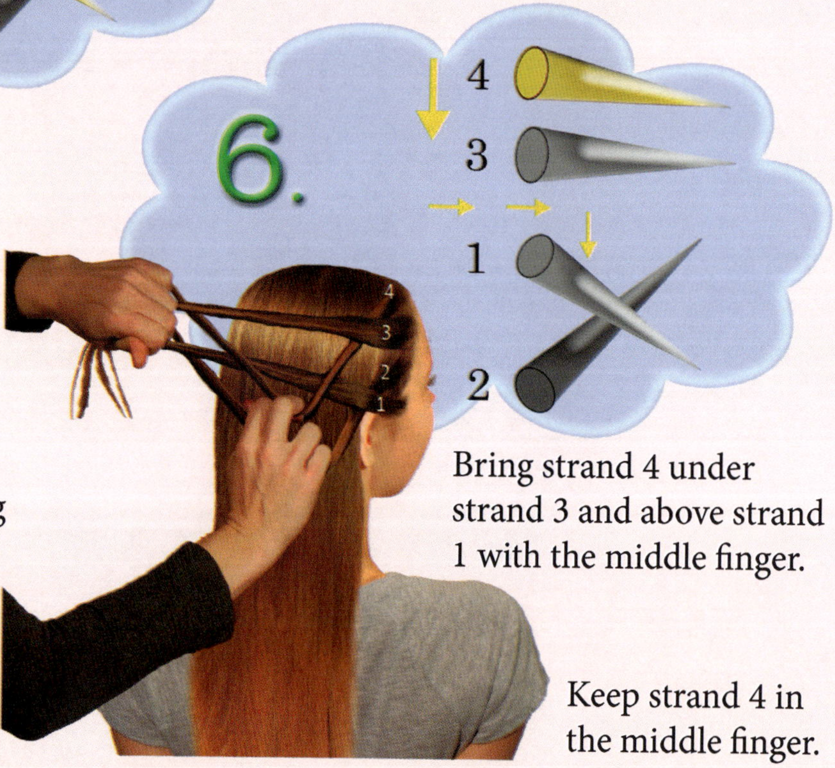

Keep strand 4 in the middle finger.

168 www.findingbraids.com

Four-Strand Round Lace

4

3.

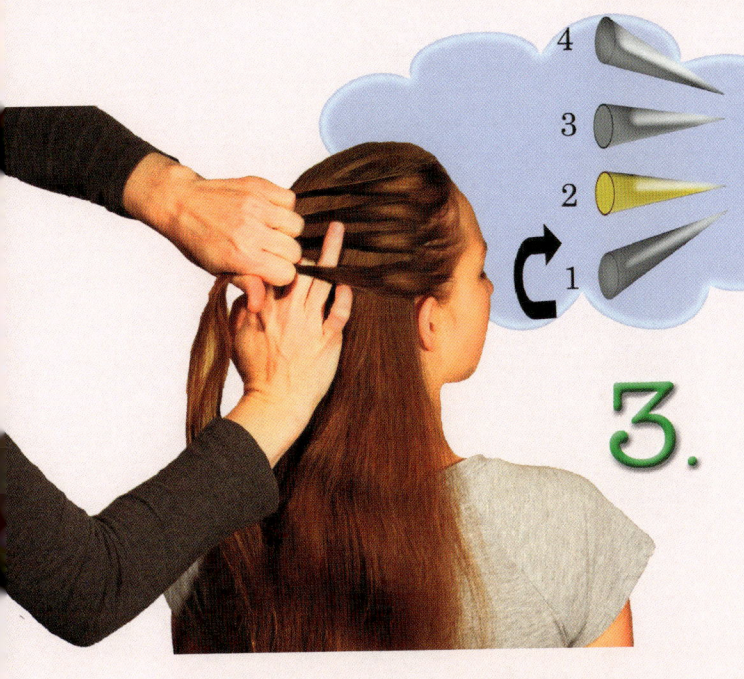

Reach under strand 1 with the ring finger and hook strand 2.

4.

Great

7.

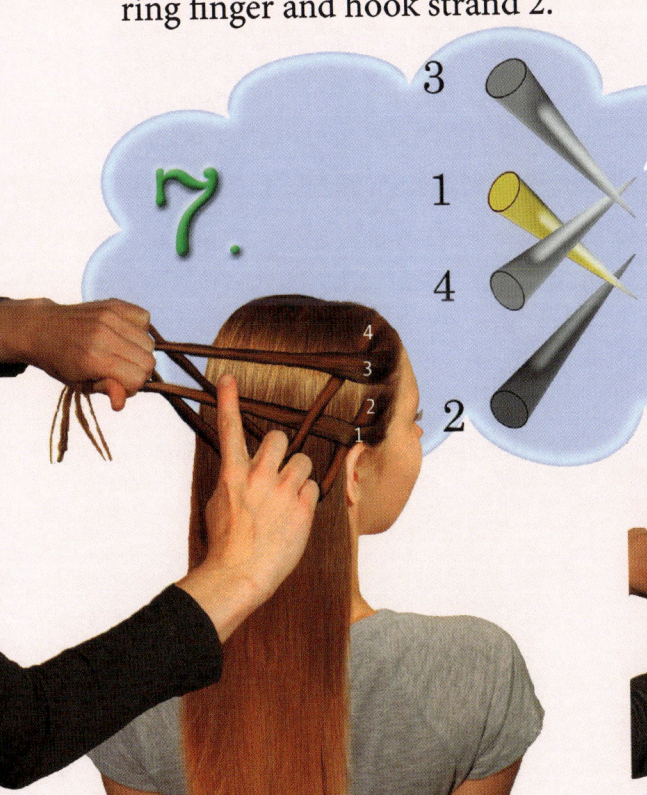

Place strand 1 in the pointer.

8.

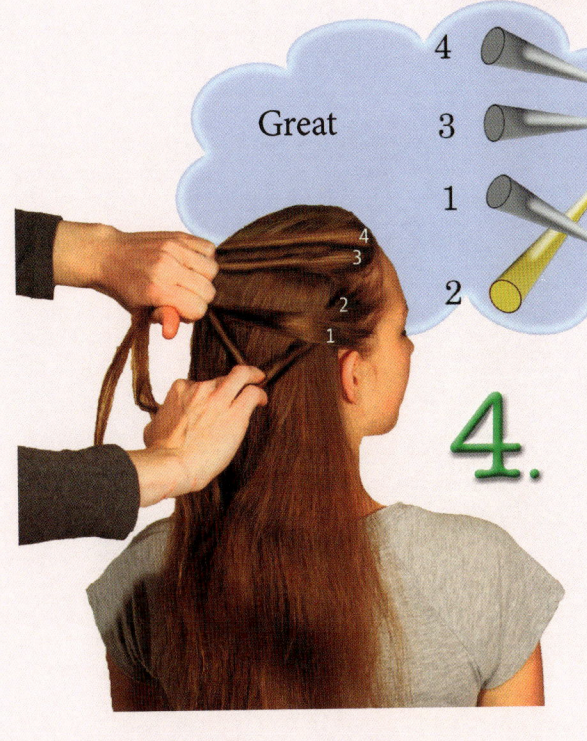

Place strand 3 between the pointer and thumb.

(For a solid handhold make sure the thumb is under all the strands holding strand 3.)

4 Continuing

9. Number your strands at your knuckles now.

10. Great!

13. Reach under strand 1 with the ring finger and hook strand 2. Place strand 1 in the pointer.

14. Place strand 3 between the pointer and thumb. For a solid handhold make sure the thumb is under all the strands holding strand 3.

part 2. Four-Strand Round Lace

4

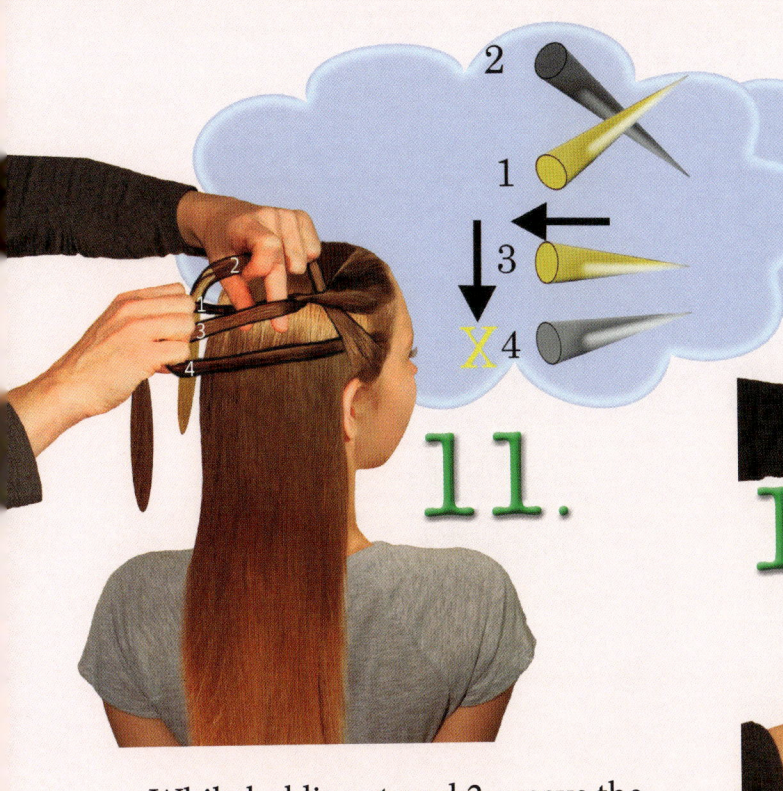

11. While holding strand 2, weave the middle finger and thumb over strand 1 and under strand 3 to grab strand 4.

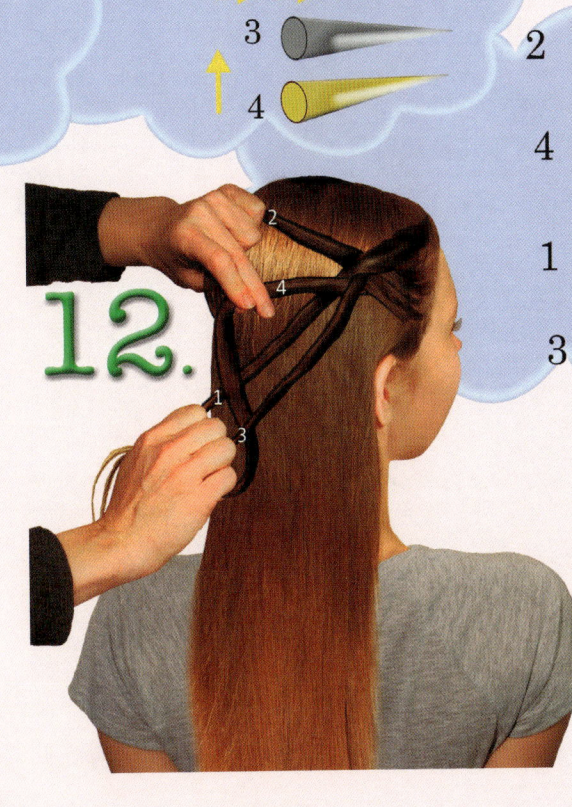

12. Bring strand 4 under strand 3 and above strand 1 with the middle finger.

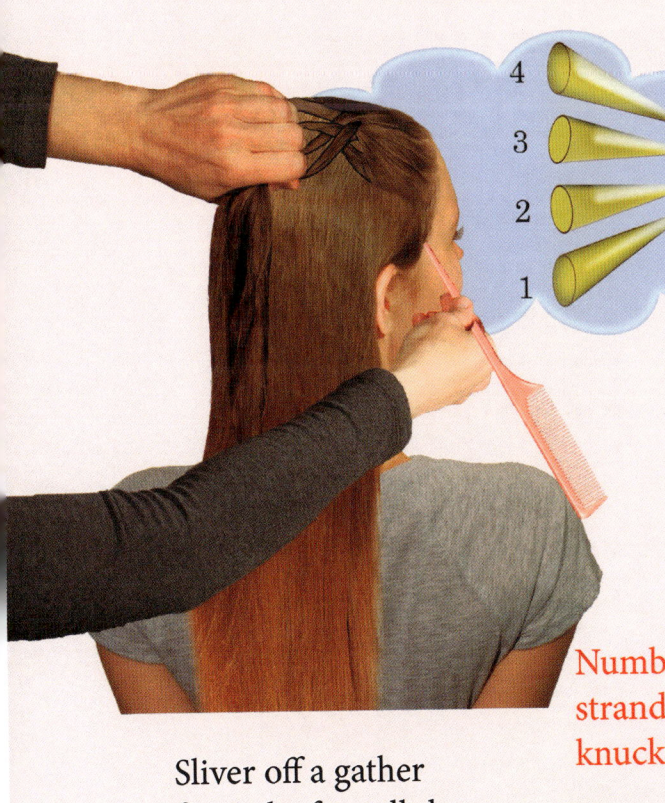

15. Sliver off a gather from the face all the way back to the braid.

Number your strands at your knuckles now.

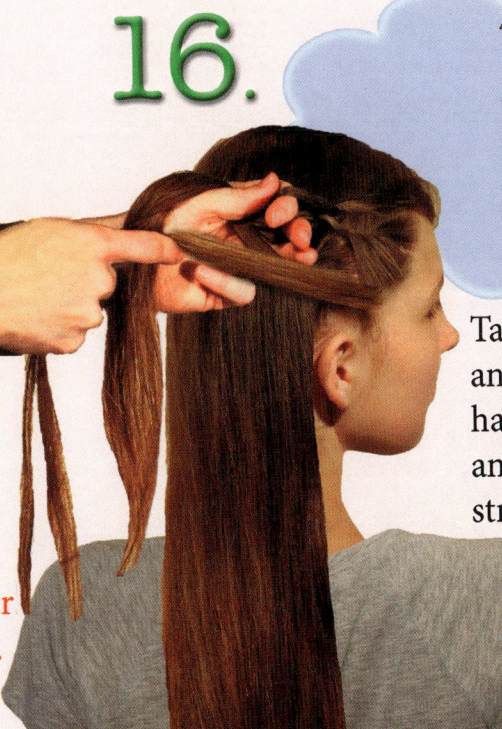

16. Take that gather and split it. Add half to strand 3 and the rest to strand 4.

Ways 171

4 Continuing

17.
Notice how the two gather halves are woven through the palm and out the fist with the other strands.

18.
You're ready to weave back the other direction.

21.
Secure with a rubber band.

22.
Fix the end of the braid with bobby pins to hold the braid in place.

part 3. Four-Strand Round Lace 4

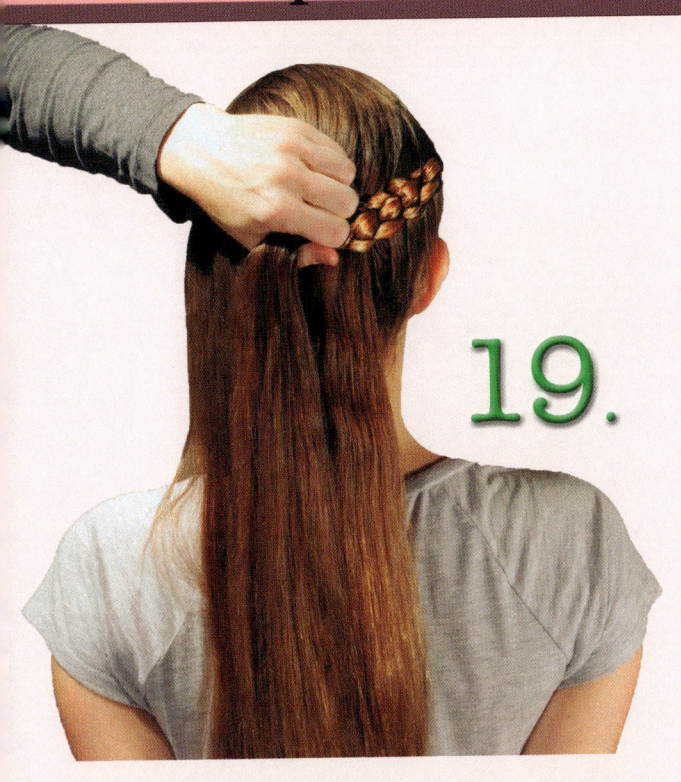

Continue weaving and gathering.

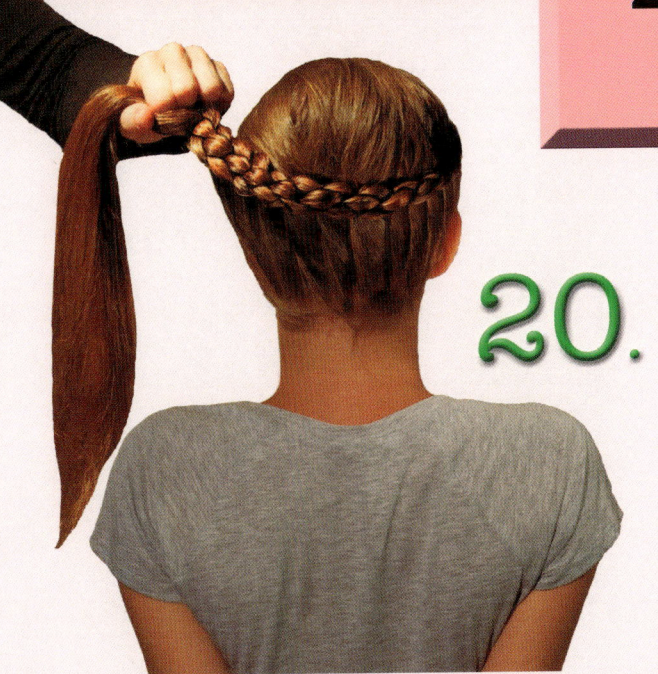

Gather from only one side.

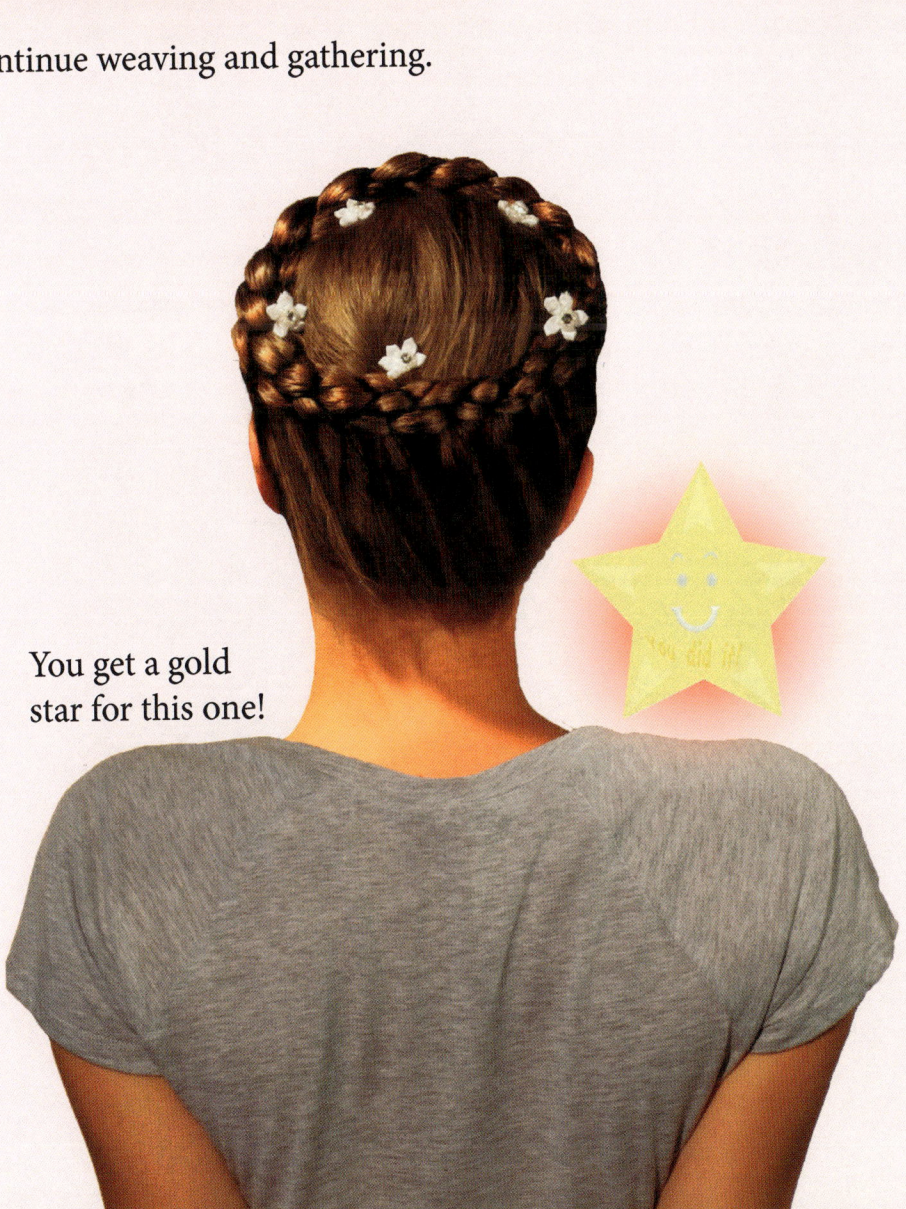

You get a gold star for this one!

Let's chat about the tail that is always tangling. In photograph #20 (just above) the hair of the tail is all smooth and pretty like. There are three things happening while I braid to make that happen. First, while I weave, I never try to get the tail ends seperated, I just weave with my fingers. Second, after I have woven with my fingers... I need to get the tail ends seperate. I use the hand that is letting go of the strands (in order to gather) and I swipe it down the length of the tail detangling and seperating those strands and tail ends. I never do it while I am weaving. If you are, I need you to stop. Third, I brush the tail ends when they are starting to get out of control when I have a free hand.

Ways 173

Examples of Four-Strand Round

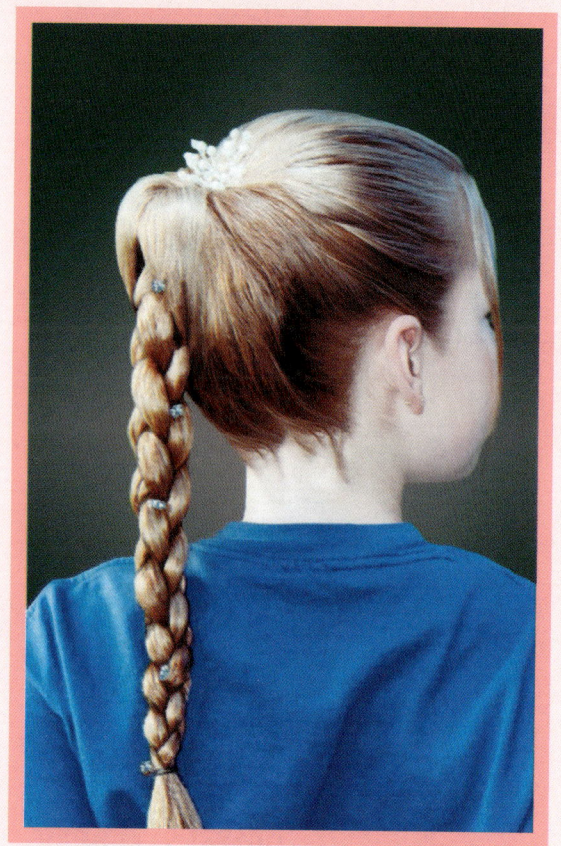
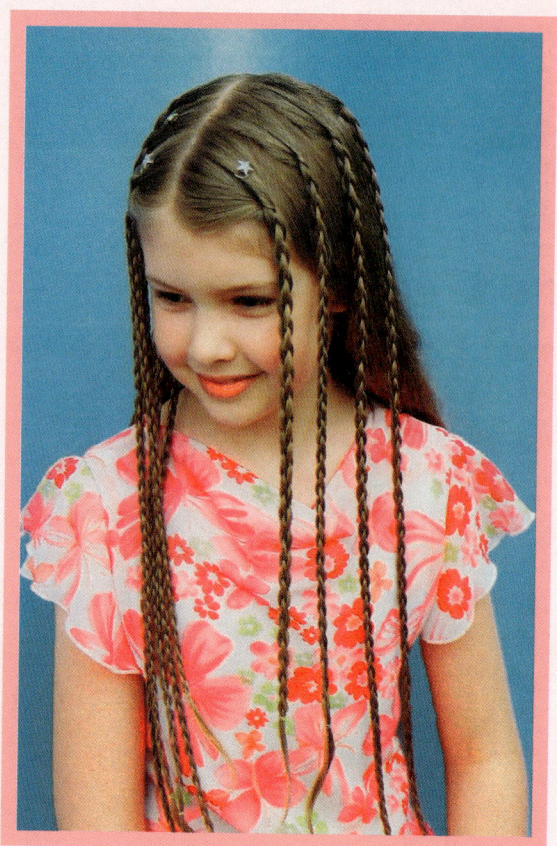
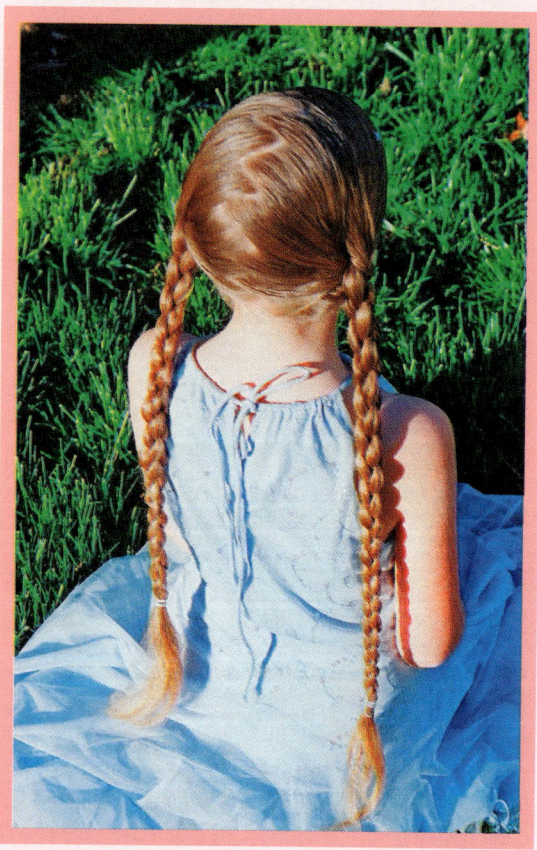
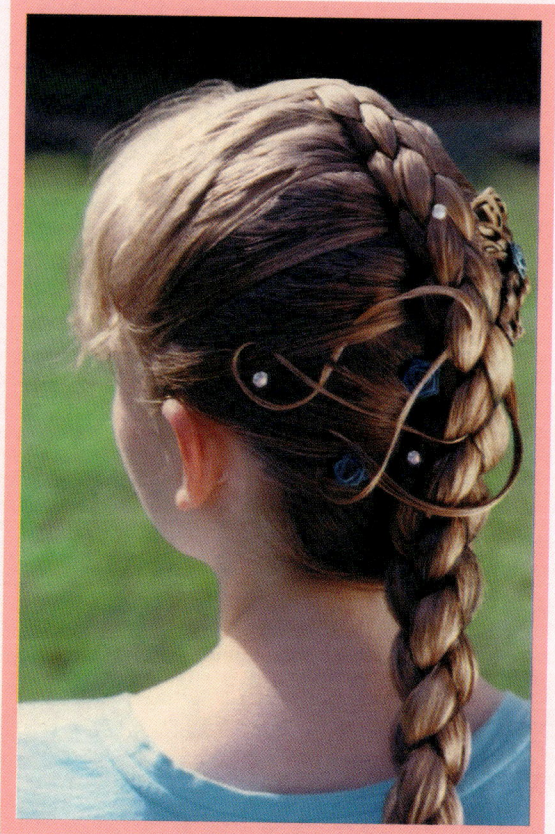

Four-Strand

After the first weave of a multiple stranded braid it gets very difficult to grab the correct strand because confusion and chaos try to take over.

Maybe paying close attention helps, maybe it doesn't. I believe that varies person to person. Practice is the only real remedy. I also suggest watching some how-to videos, probably online. When you are confused and ready to cry, take a deep breath and when you are calm; try again. The strands move if you twist your wrists. (as in - it is harder to tell which one is the first and second strand when you tilt your hands) So, keep your palms facing the floor as much as possible, especially when taking the first strand.

How easy is it to grab the wrong strand? Pretty easy. The strands cross so many times in the making of a braid there is only one honest place to look for the correct strand while braiding. The knuckles. Keep your eyes on the knuckles to know which strand to take. The closer to the knuckle you hook a strand the more likely you will be to take the correct strand.

This will be especially true on page 299 when you start learning the nine-strand braids.

As you get more proficient at braiding, the patterns you create will begin to make sense. You will recognize the over under patterns. Each strand takes turns going over and under its neighbors. In time you will realize when you grab the wrong strand because you will be able to follow that strand with your eye back to see if it is going under after going over.

I like to tell my students to just keep going if they make a mistake. Often a mistake is lost to the eye in such complicated patterns. Most people just see loveliness. Silk or live flowers are amazing at covering up mistakes and make braids that much more beautiful. Don't beat yourself up trying to get it perfect before you are ready. Focus on learning the pattern. Eventually you will get it correct all the way to the end of the braid.

Make up your own hairsyles with this way of braiding.

Four-Strand Plait

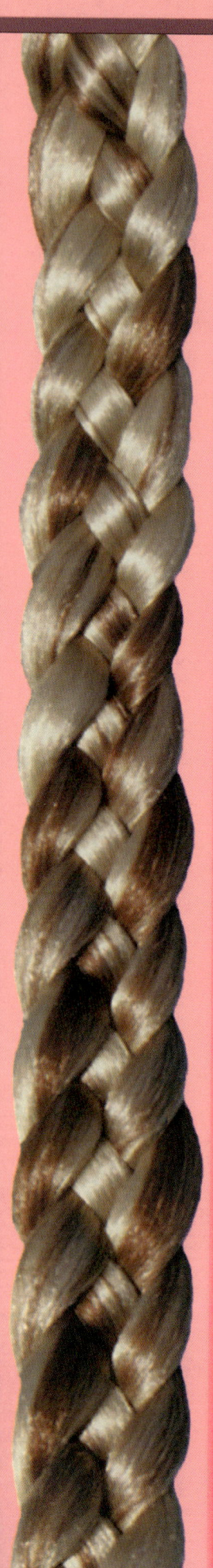

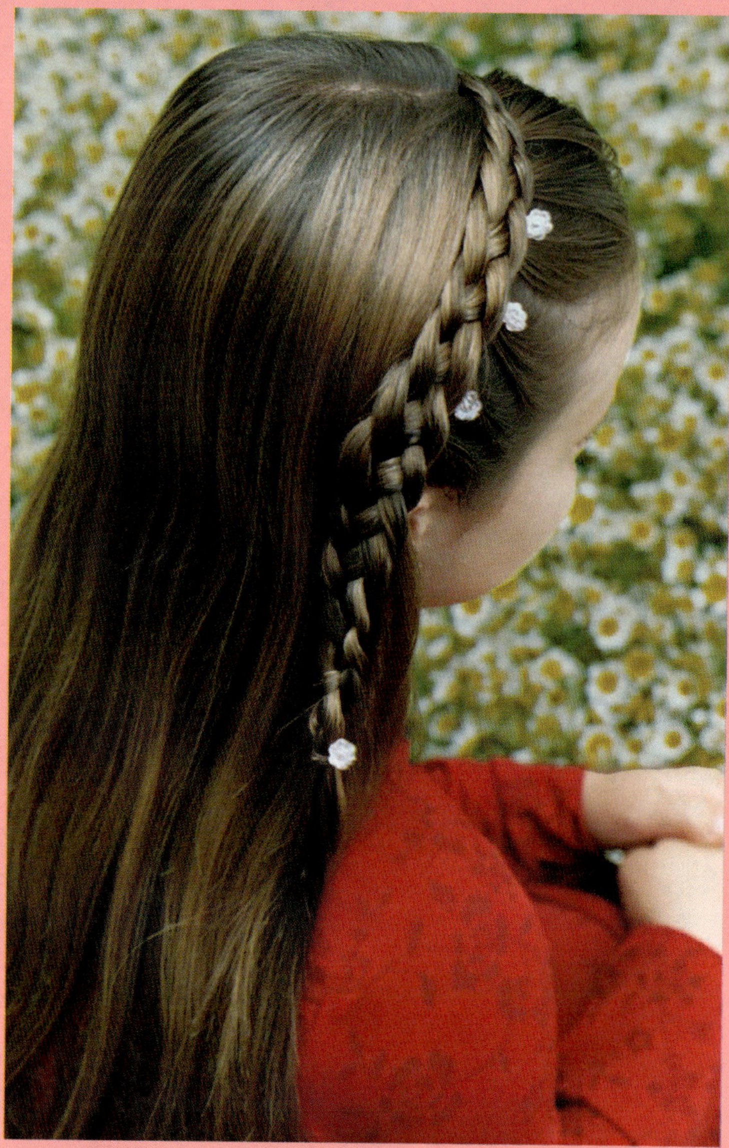

Ornate and intruiging, this is a puzzling braid to learn. The extra strand adds a sweet quality. A must have in any braiders box of tricks.

Four-Strand Plait

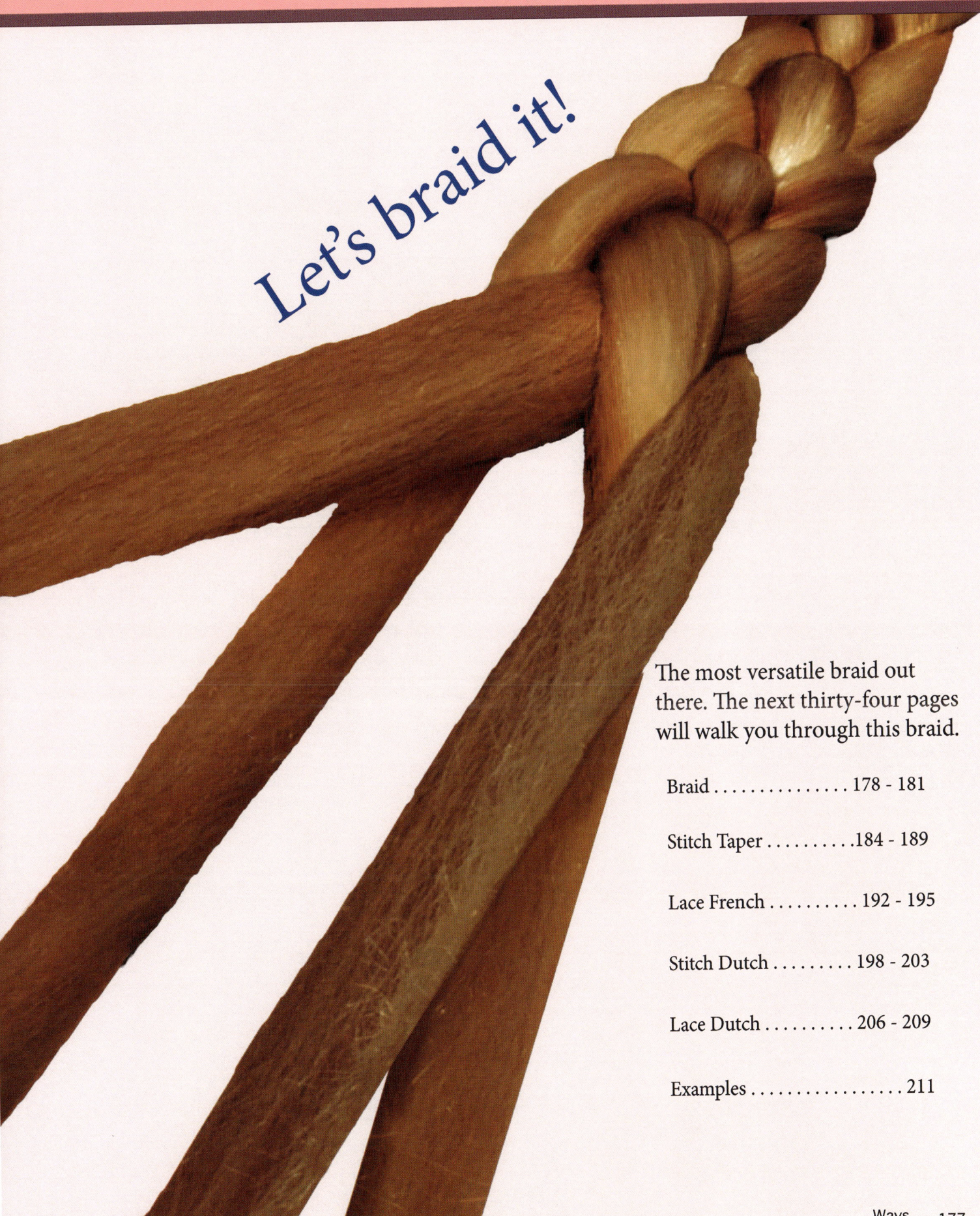

Let's braid it!

The most versatile braid out there. The next thirty-four pages will walk you through this braid.

Braid . . . . 178 - 181

Stitch Taper . . . . 184 - 189

Lace French . . . . 192 - 195

Stitch Dutch . . . . 198 - 203

Lace Dutch . . . . 206 - 209

Examples 211

Ways 177

Four-Strand Plait Braid

If people knew how hard I worked to gain my mastery, it wouldn't seem so wonderful. — Michelangelo

1.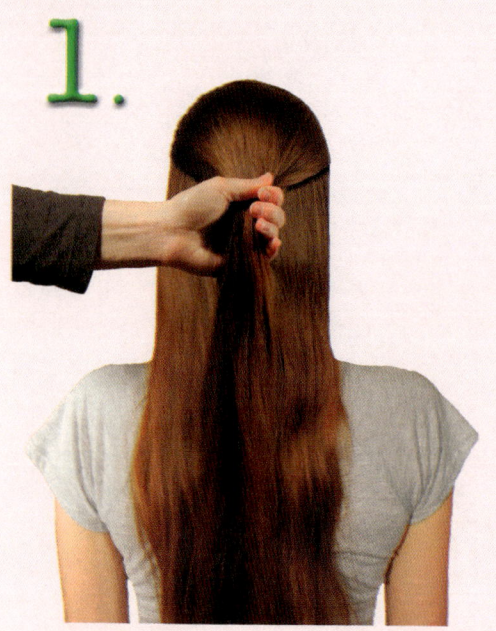

Take a section of hair.

2.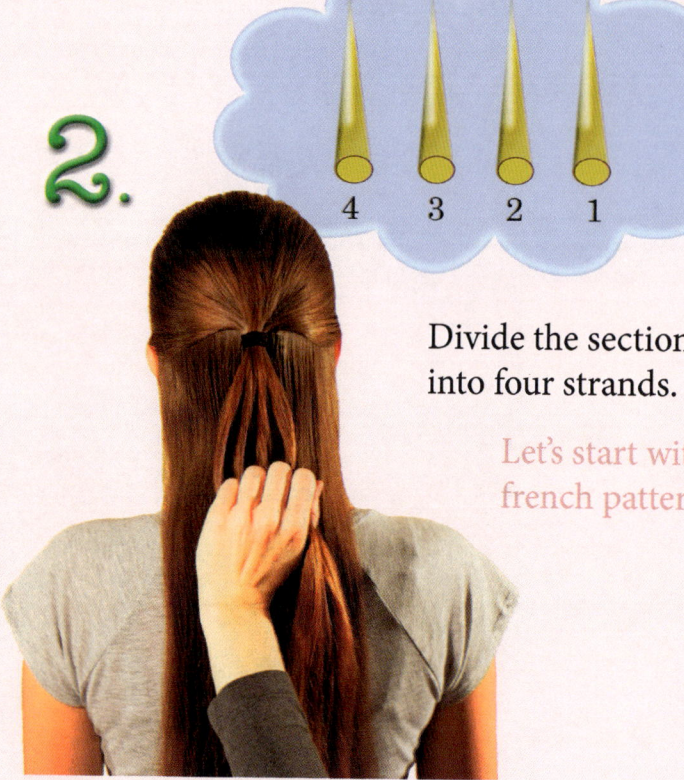

Divide the section into four strands.

Let's start with a french pattern.

5.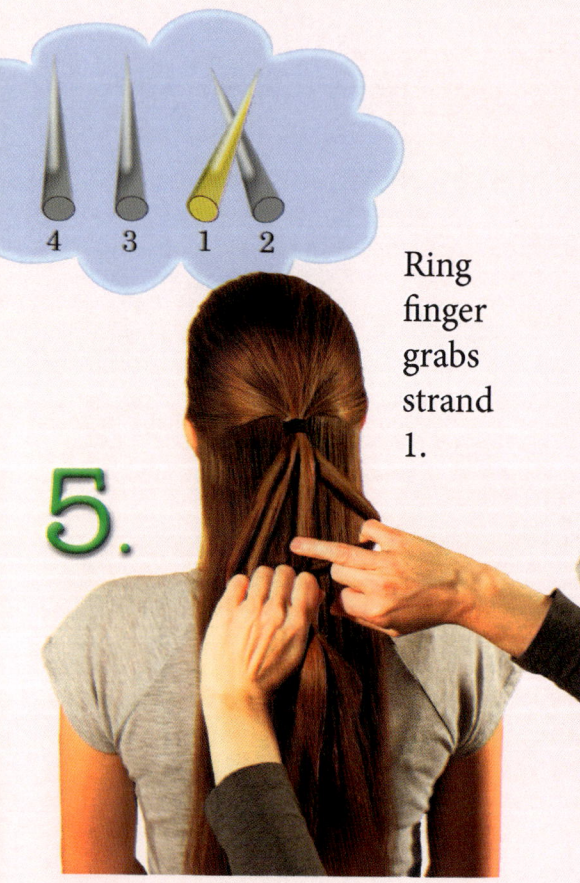

Ring finger grabs strand 1.

6. Reach under strand 3 with the middle finger and hook strand 4.

www.findingbraids.com

Four-Strand Plait Braid

4

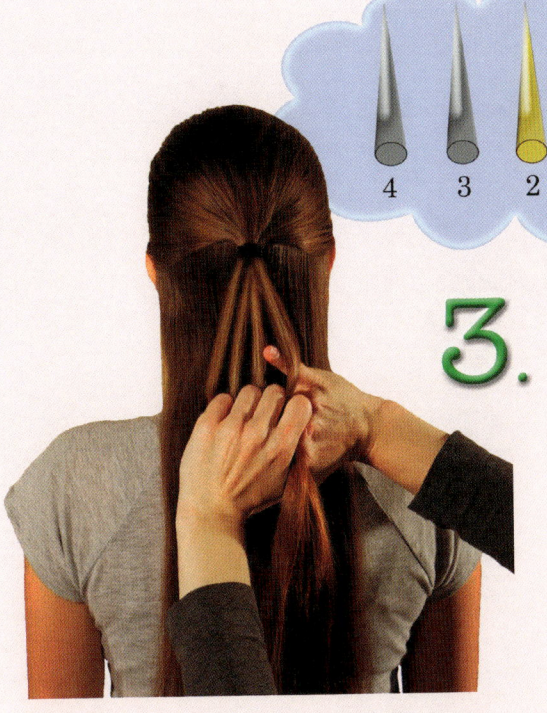

3.

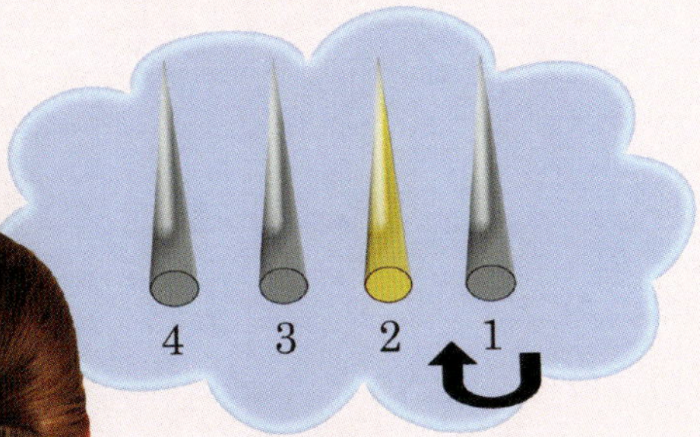

Reach under strand 1 with the pinky finger and hook strand 2.

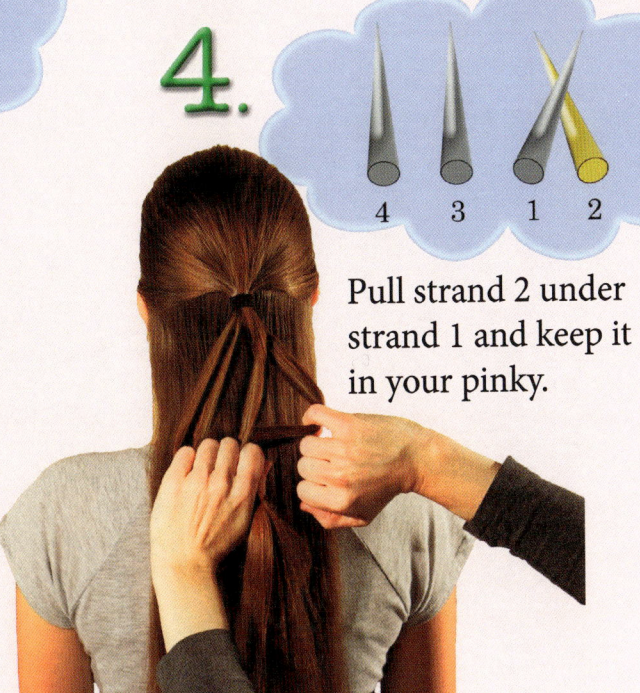

4.

Pull strand 2 under strand 1 and keep it in your pinky.

7.

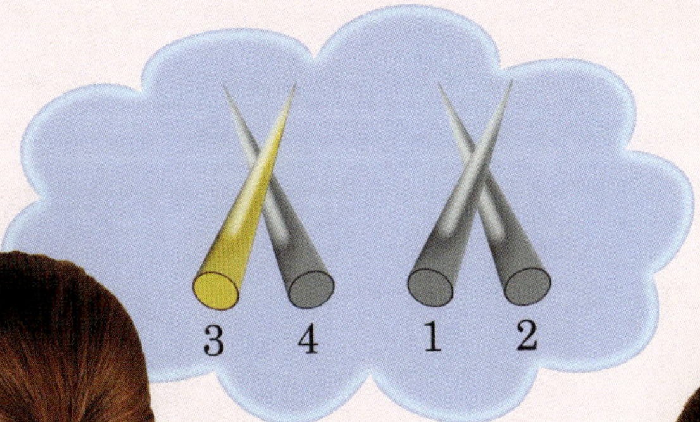

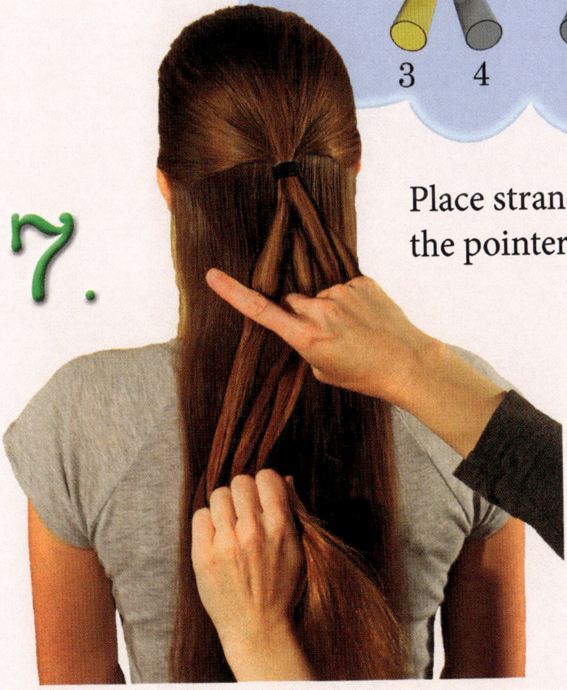

Place strand 3 in the pointer finger.

8.

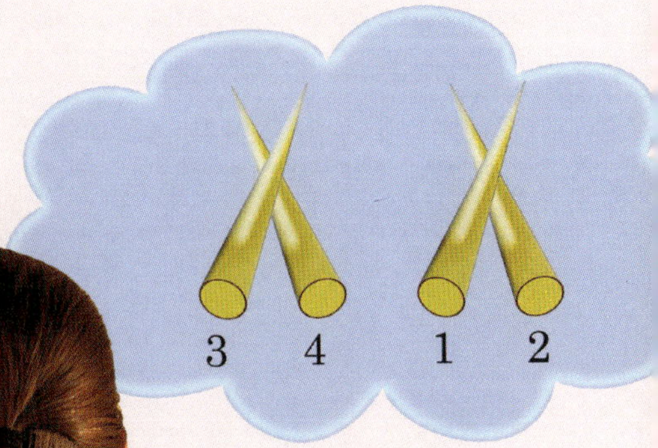

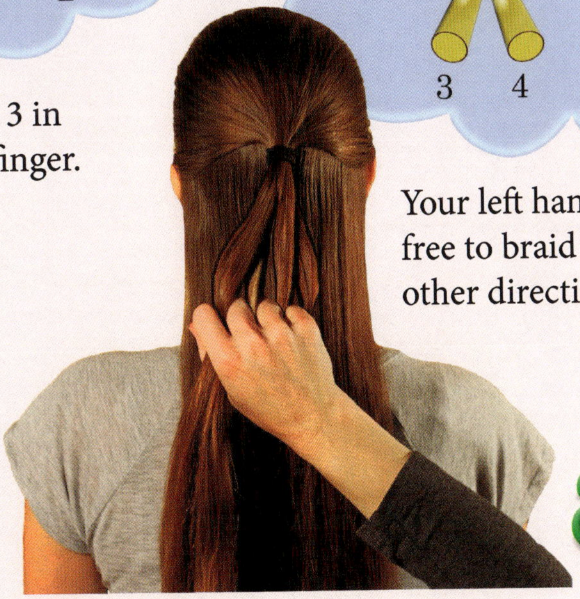

Your left hand is free to braid the other direction.

Ways 179

4 Continuing

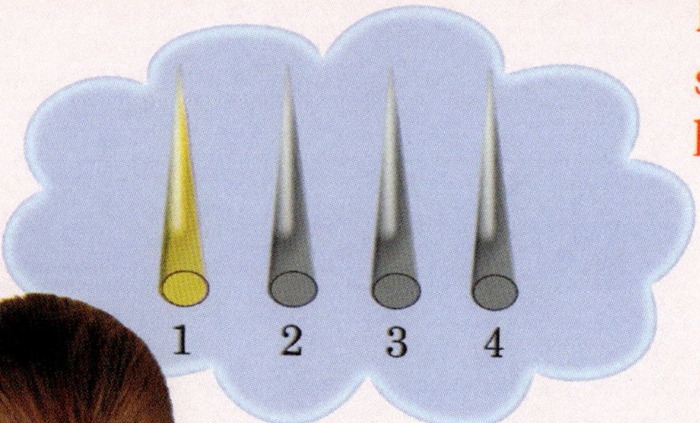

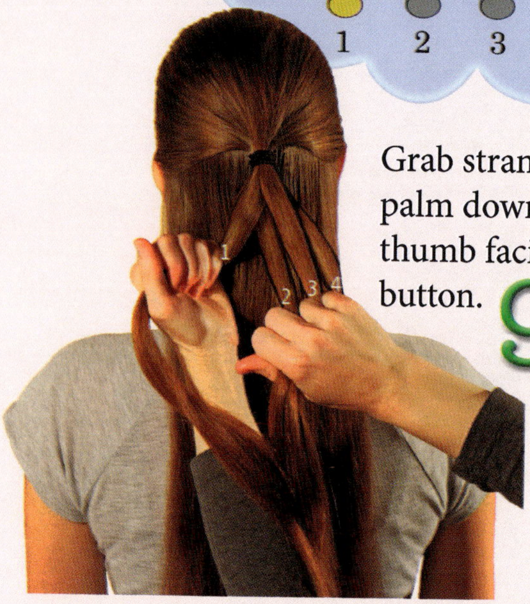

Number your strands at your knuckles now.

9. Grab strand 1 with your palm down and your thumb facing your belly button.

Time for the dutch pattern.

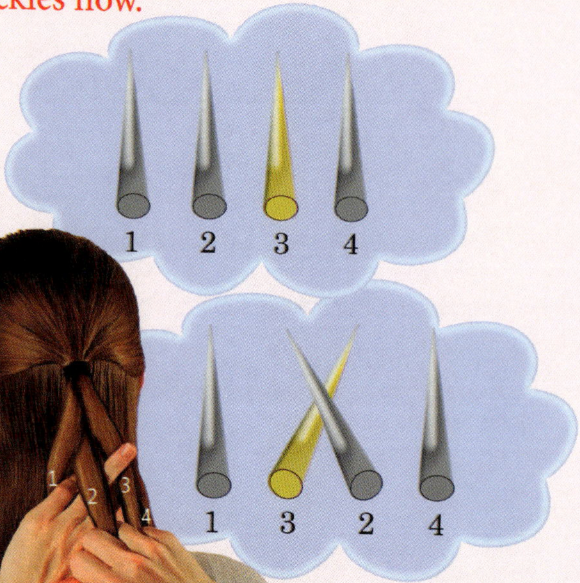

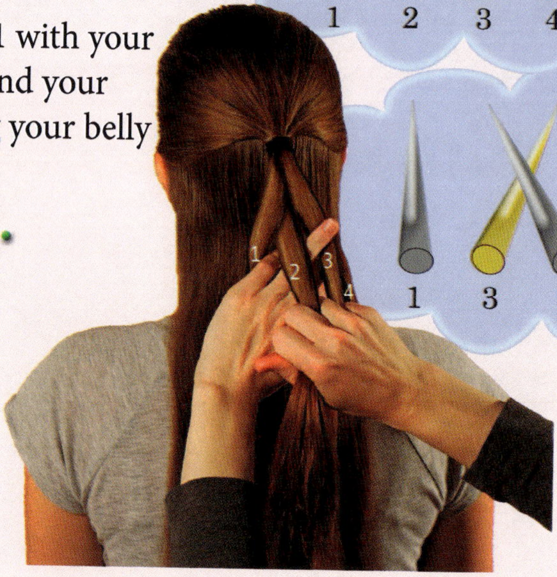

10. Reach under strand 2 and hook strand 3 with the ring finger.

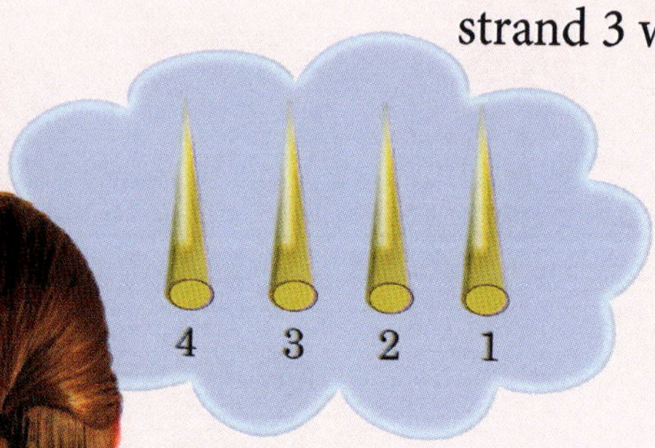

13. 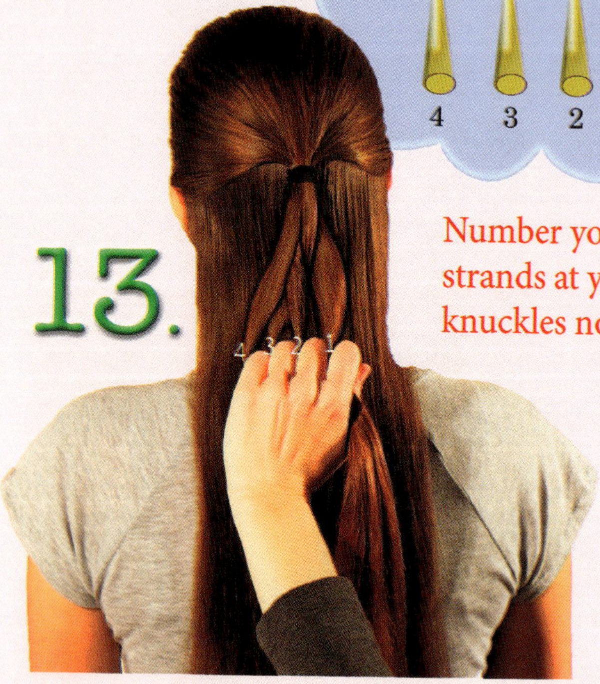 Number your strands at your knuckles now.

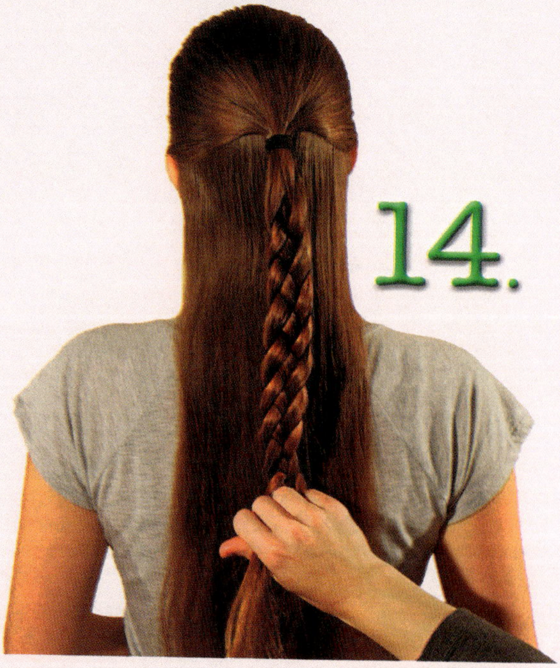

14. Continue alternating the french and dutch weaves until you reach the end of the hair.

part 2. Four-Strand Plait Braid

4

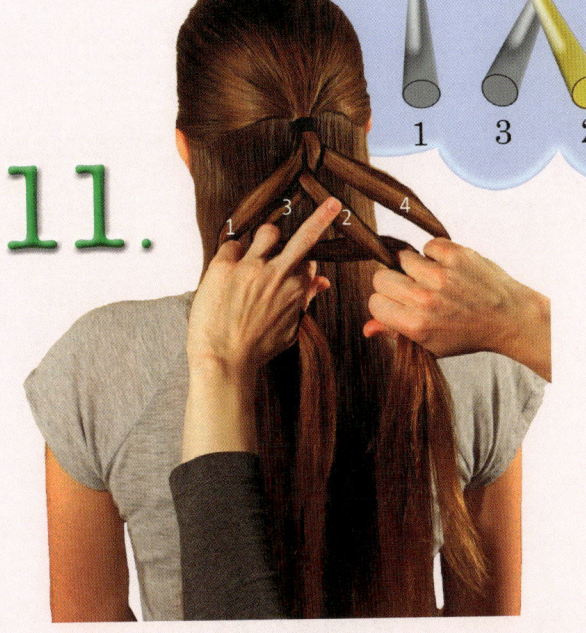

11.

Grab strand 2 with the middle finger.

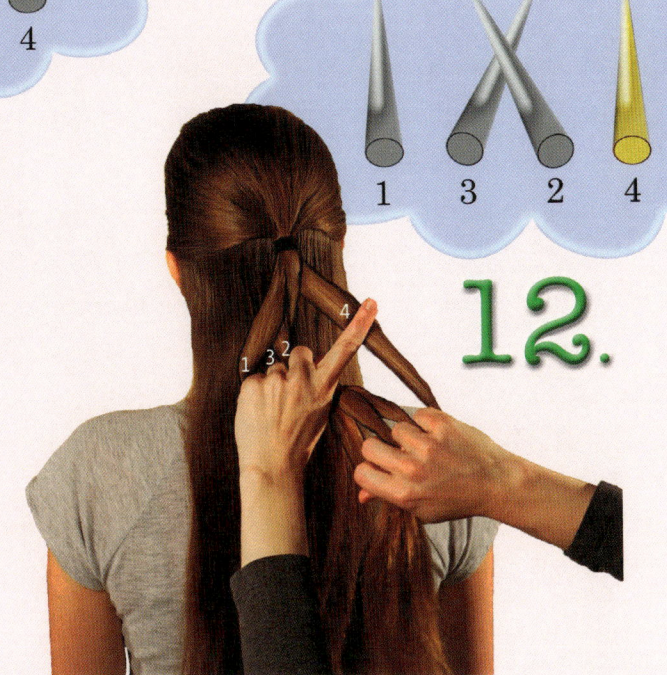

12.

Place strand 4 in the pointer finger.

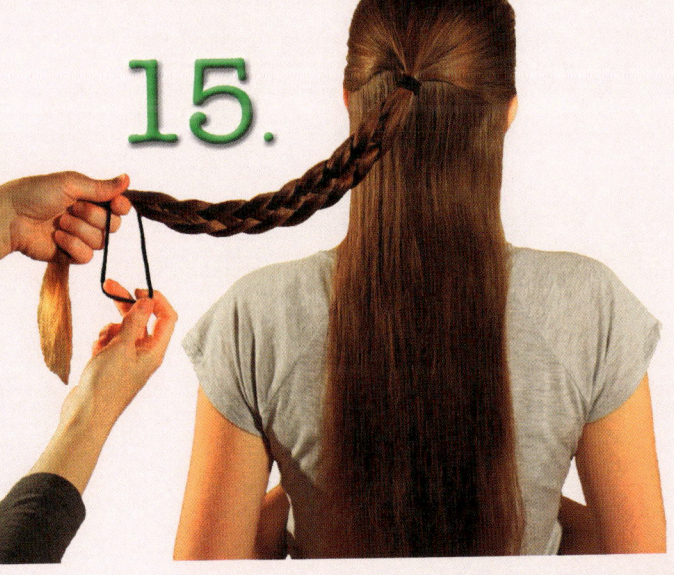

15.

Secure with a rubber band.

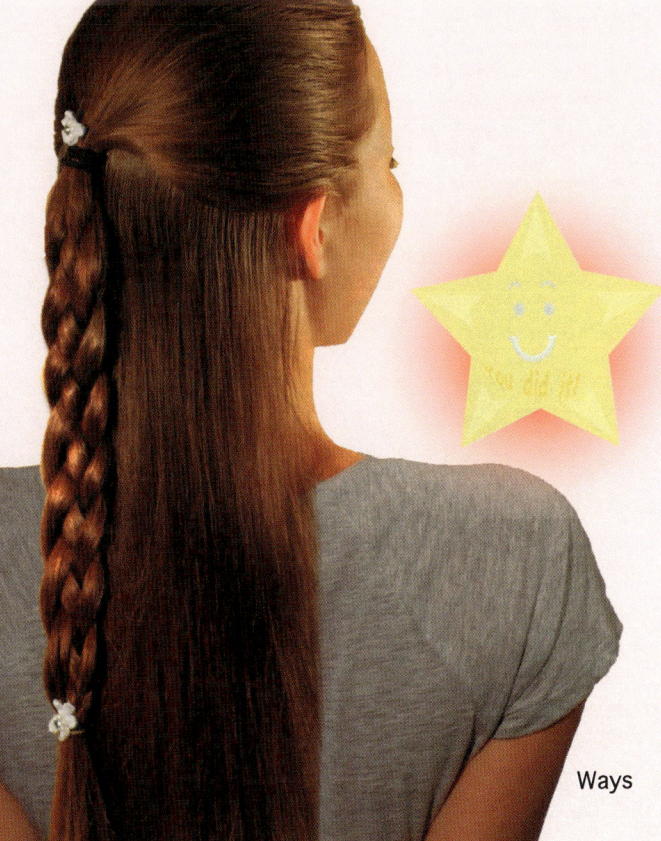

Ways 181

Four-Strand Plait

I would like to take some time to talk about braids that use an even number of strands. There are two weaving patterns with these braids. Even numbered braids are dutch braided with one hand and french braided with the other hand. It is difficult to remember who does what. If a hand accidently switches patterns you will find yourself unbraiding.

Decide which hand will do which pattern and then stick to it through the whole braid. When forms are involved while braiding, the patterns can effect the aesthetics of the style. The look of a halo braid changes depending on which side of the halo is dutched and which side is frenched.

An interesting effect of these braids is the twisting of the braid when done in a straight line. One side is popped up while the other is woven down. So when the braid transitions into a tail, it twists. There are some forms less likely to contort with this braid. Even numbered braids behave better when done in a form without tails or with buns.

To change the side that is frenched or dutched just flip the patterns. **When the gather is added into the first strand that side is french braided. When the gather is added into the second strand that side is dutch braided.** Interestingly, even numbered braids can be done solely dutch if gathered into the second strand on the dutch side and the third strand on the french side. (see page 198) But it is not possible to only french braid even numbered braids.

So, how do you make a french braid versus a dutch braid? If you study this manual you will find that french braids are created when outside strands cross over the second strand. Dutch braids are created when the outside strands cross under the second strand.

You can control which side is frenched or dutched. Learn the patterns and create the most amazing styles how you want them.

Please apply this knowledge to the six and eight strand braids in this book as I do not show the dutch only option. Nor do I show the mirror version of taper braids.

The unique appearance of even numbered weaves is worth the extra effort needed to learn it.

Four-Strand Plait

Gather from both sides

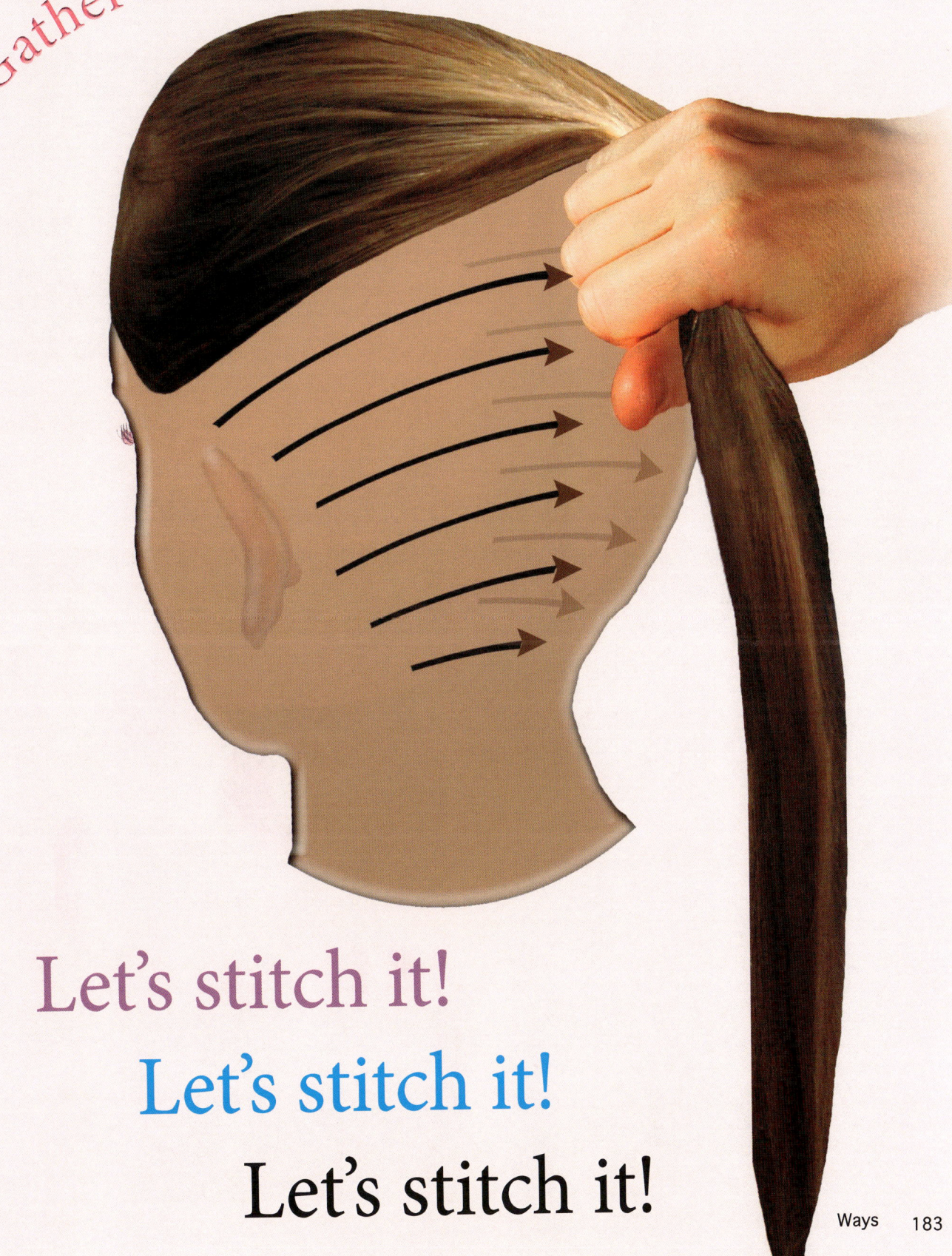

Let's stitch it!
Let's stitch it!
Let's stitch it!

Four-Strand Plait Stitch

He conquers who endures. - Persius

1. Begin with clean, brushed hair.

2. Take a section of hair as illustrated.

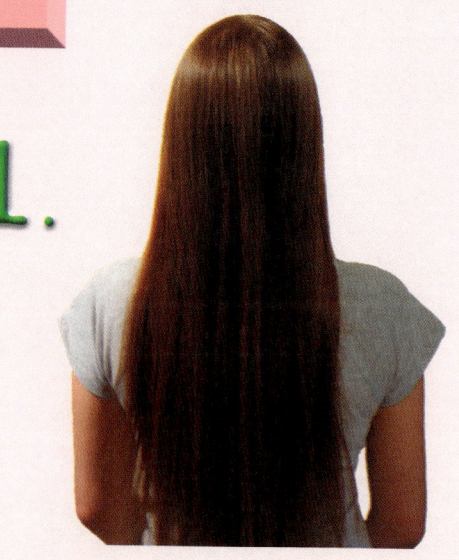

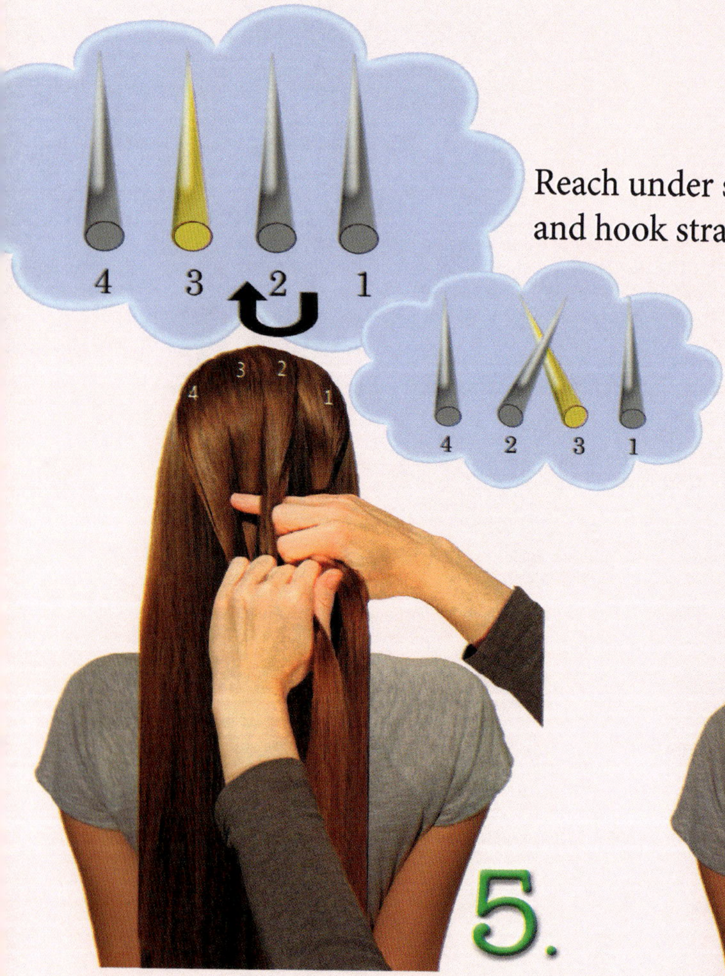

Reach under strand 2 and hook strand 3.

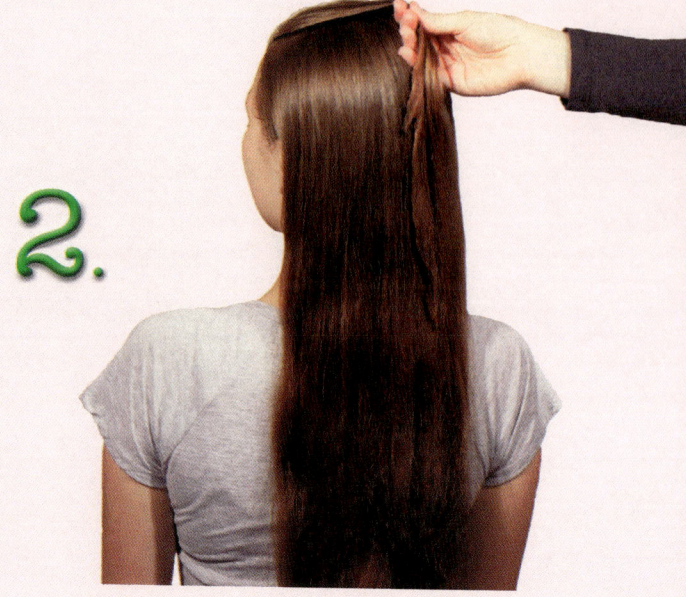

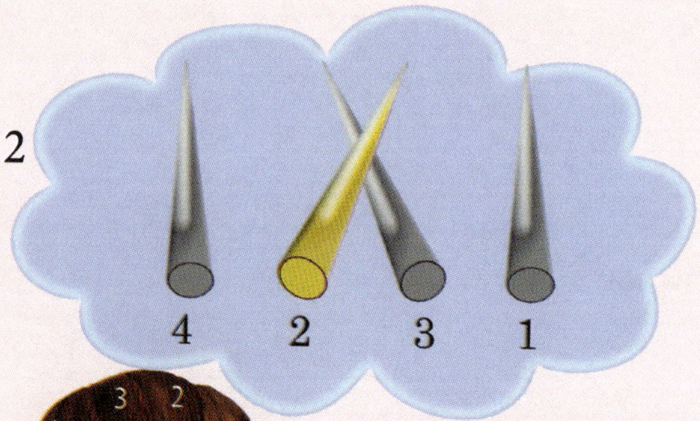

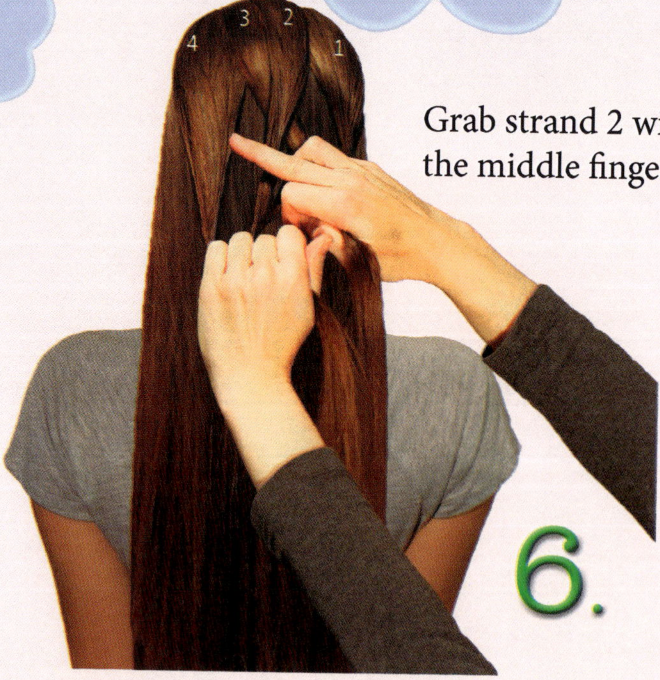

Grab strand 2 with the middle finger.

5.

6.

Four-Strand Plait Taper Stitch

4

3.

Divide the section into four strands.

Let's start with a dutch pattern.

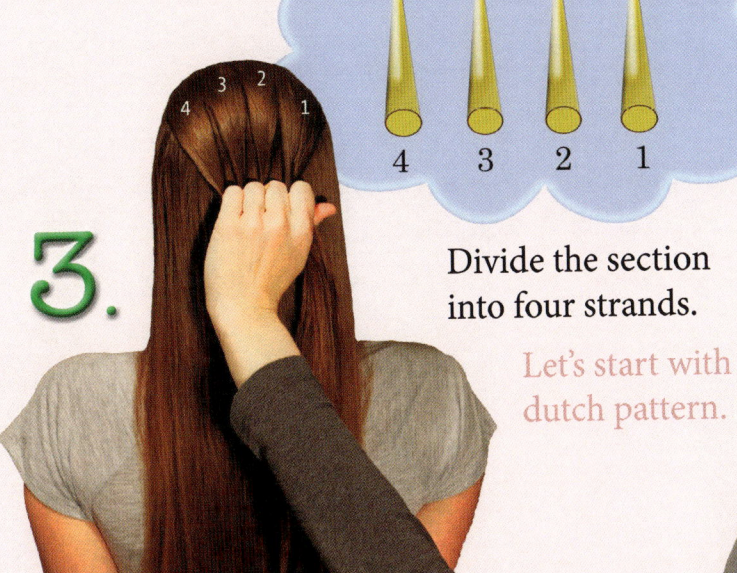

4.

Start braiding by grabbing strand 1 with your palm down and your thumb facing your belly button.

7.

Place strand 4 in the pointer finger.

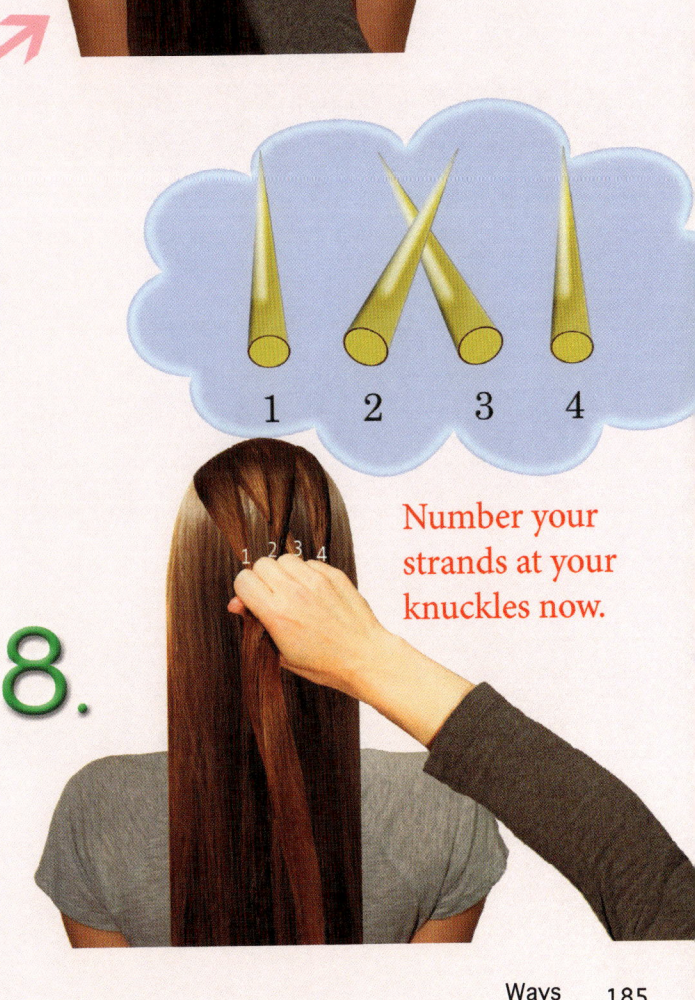

8.

Number your strands at your knuckles now.

Ways   185

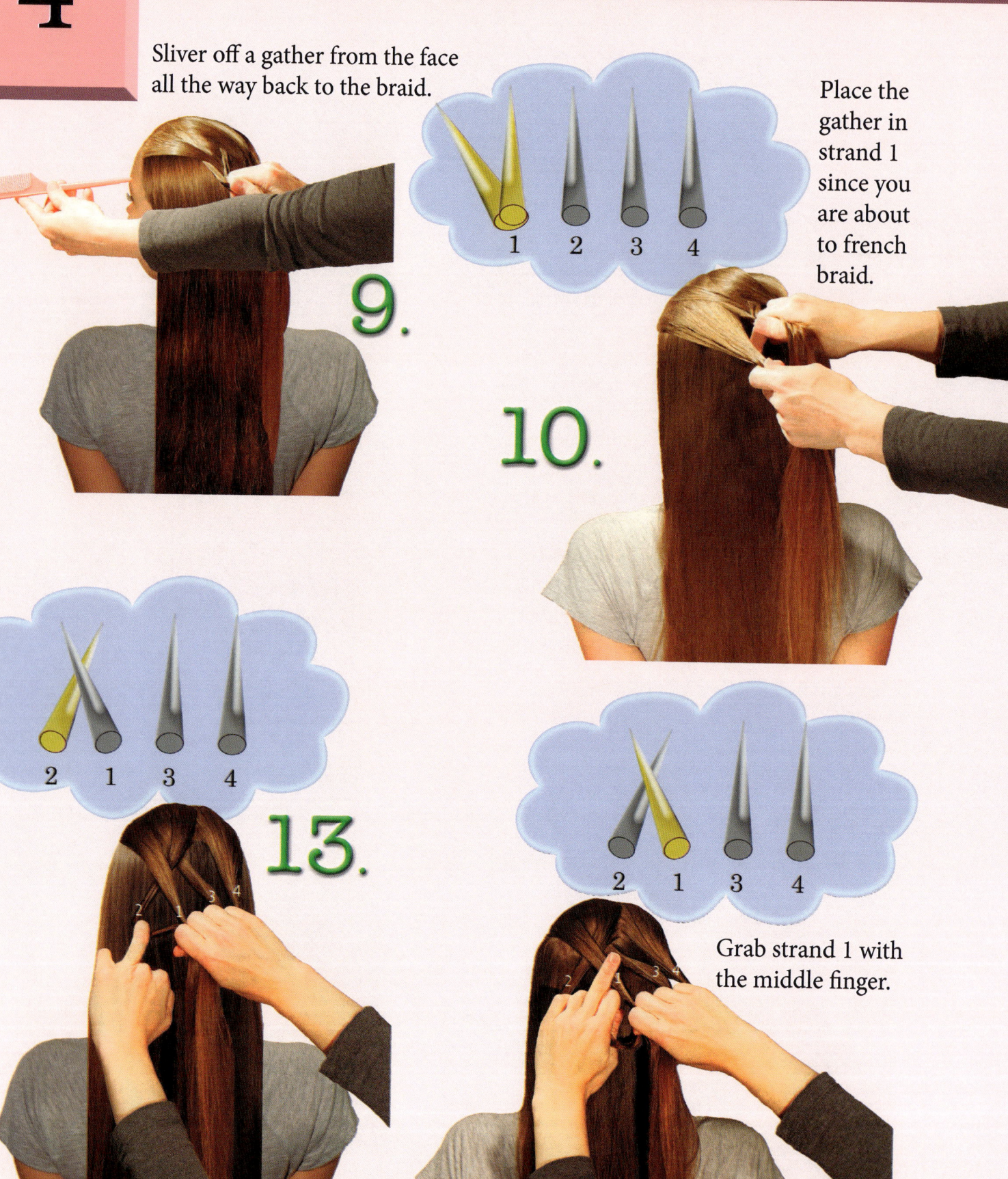

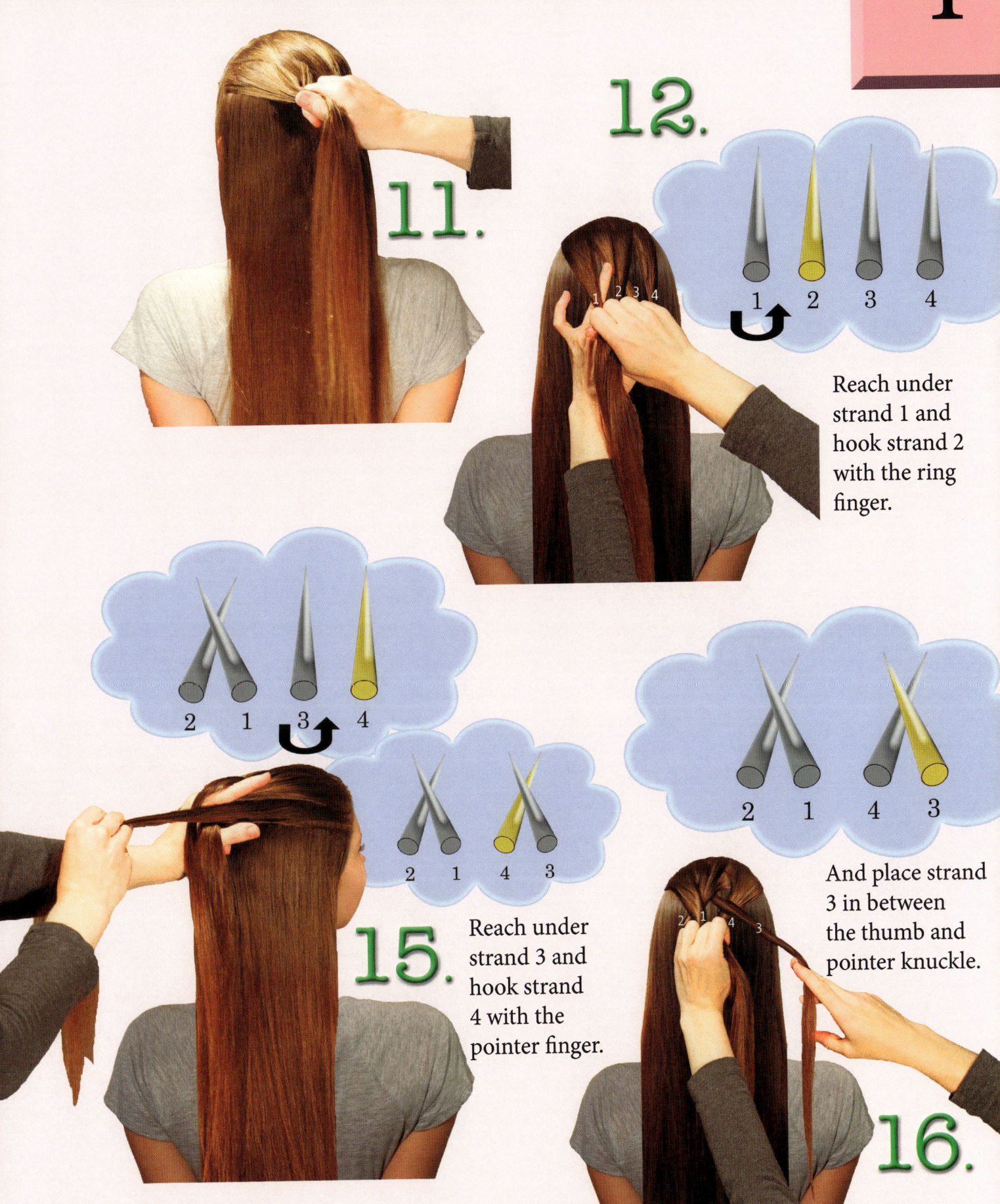

4 Continuing

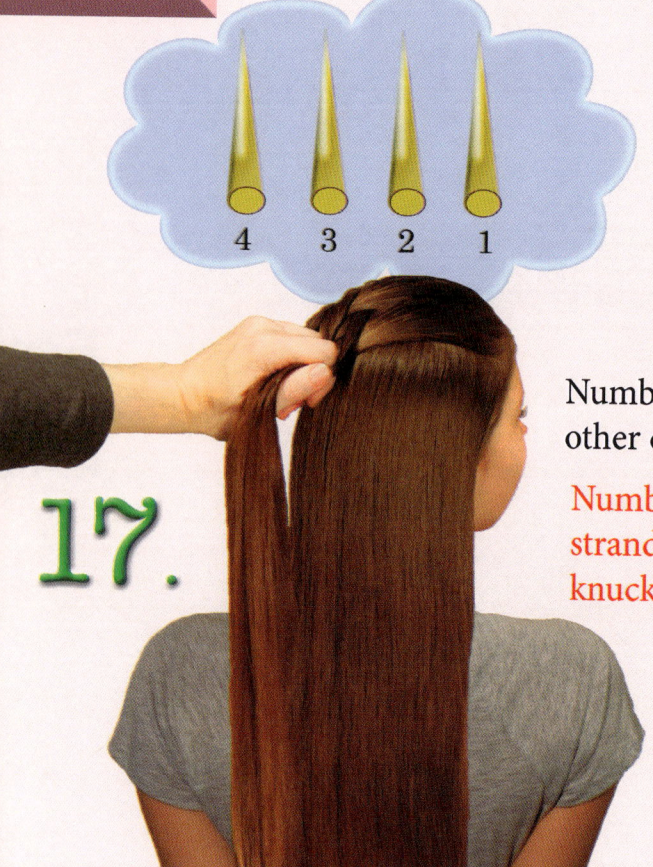

17.

Number back the other direction.

Number your strands at your knuckles now.

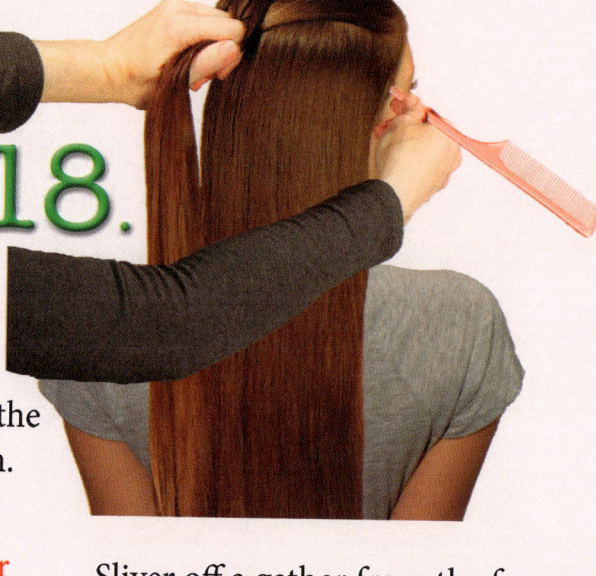

18.

Sliver off a gather from the face all the way back to the braid.

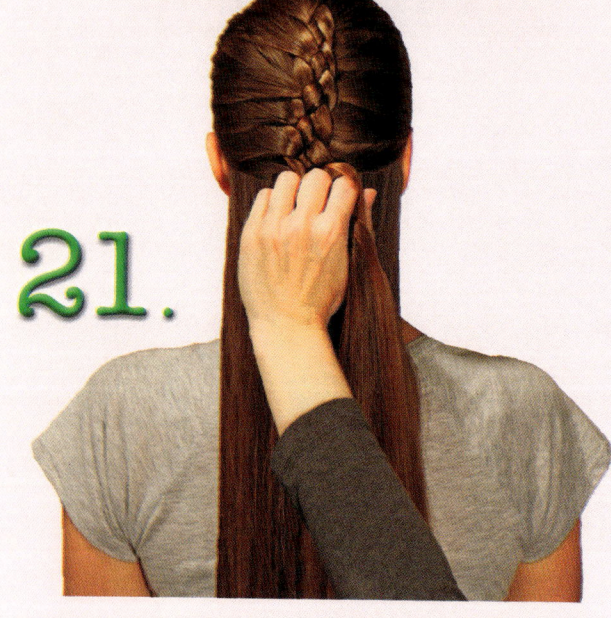

21.

Continue weaving and gathering the french and dutch patterns until you reach the end of the hair.

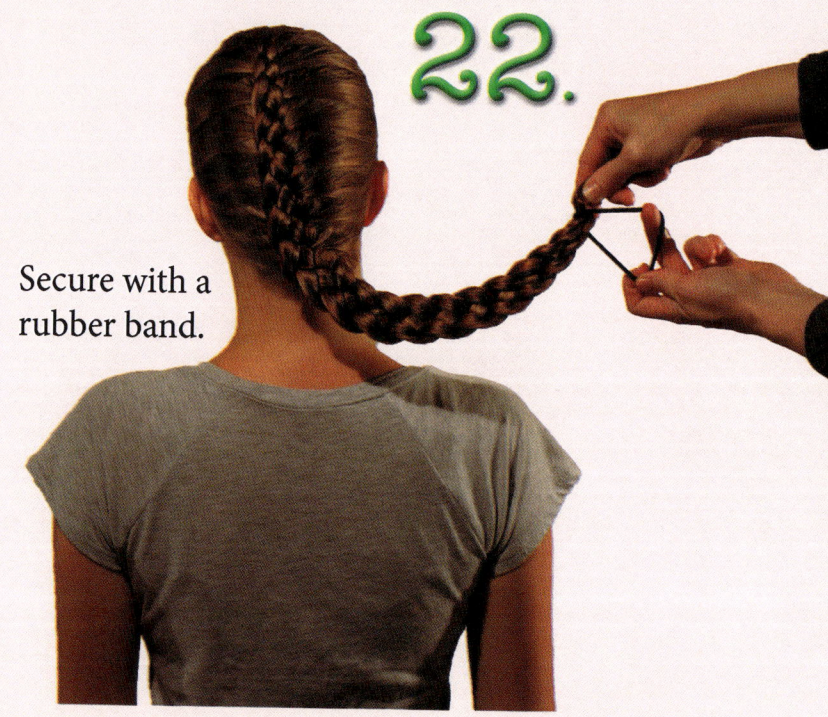

22.

Secure with a rubber band.

part 3. Four-Strand Plait Taper Stitch

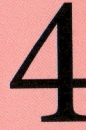

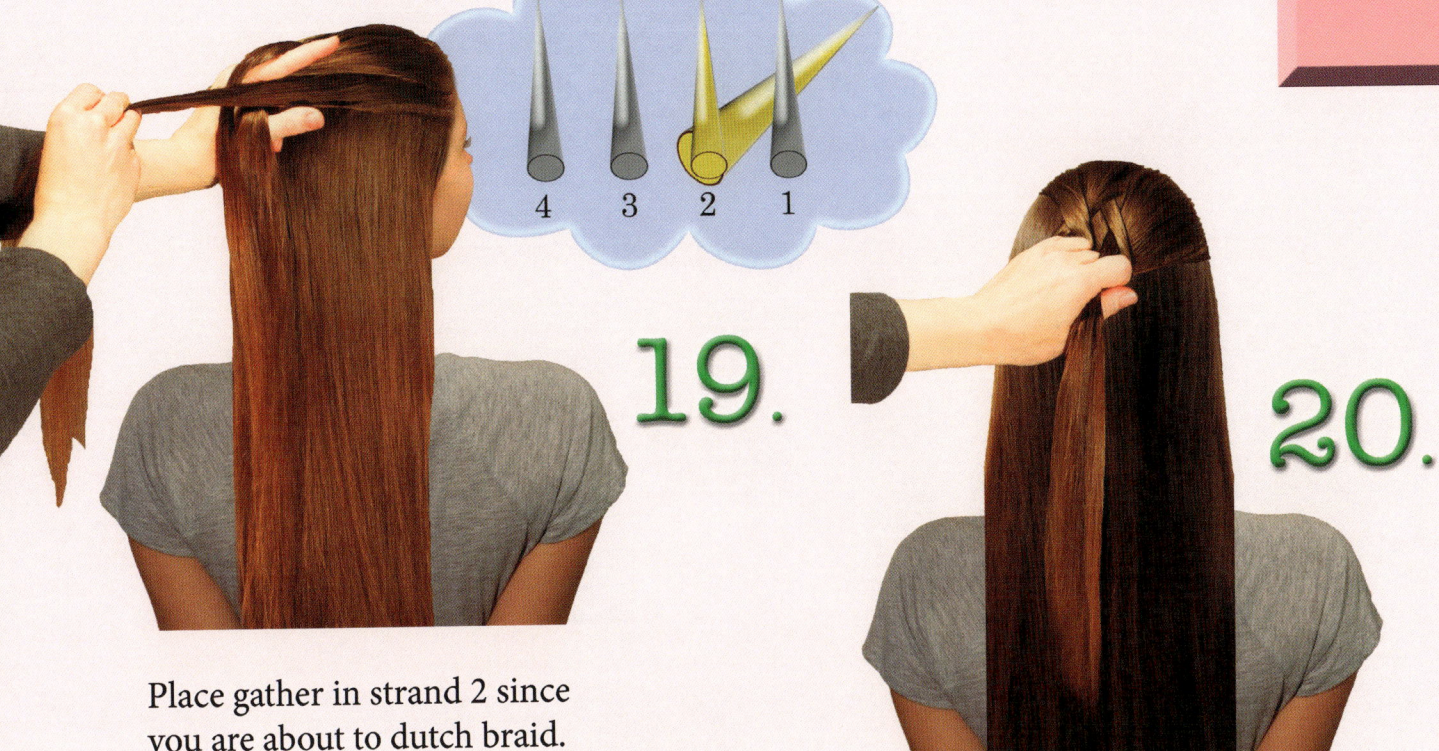

19.

Place gather in strand 2 since you are about to dutch braid.

20.

Notice how it is woven through the palm and out the fist with the other hair.

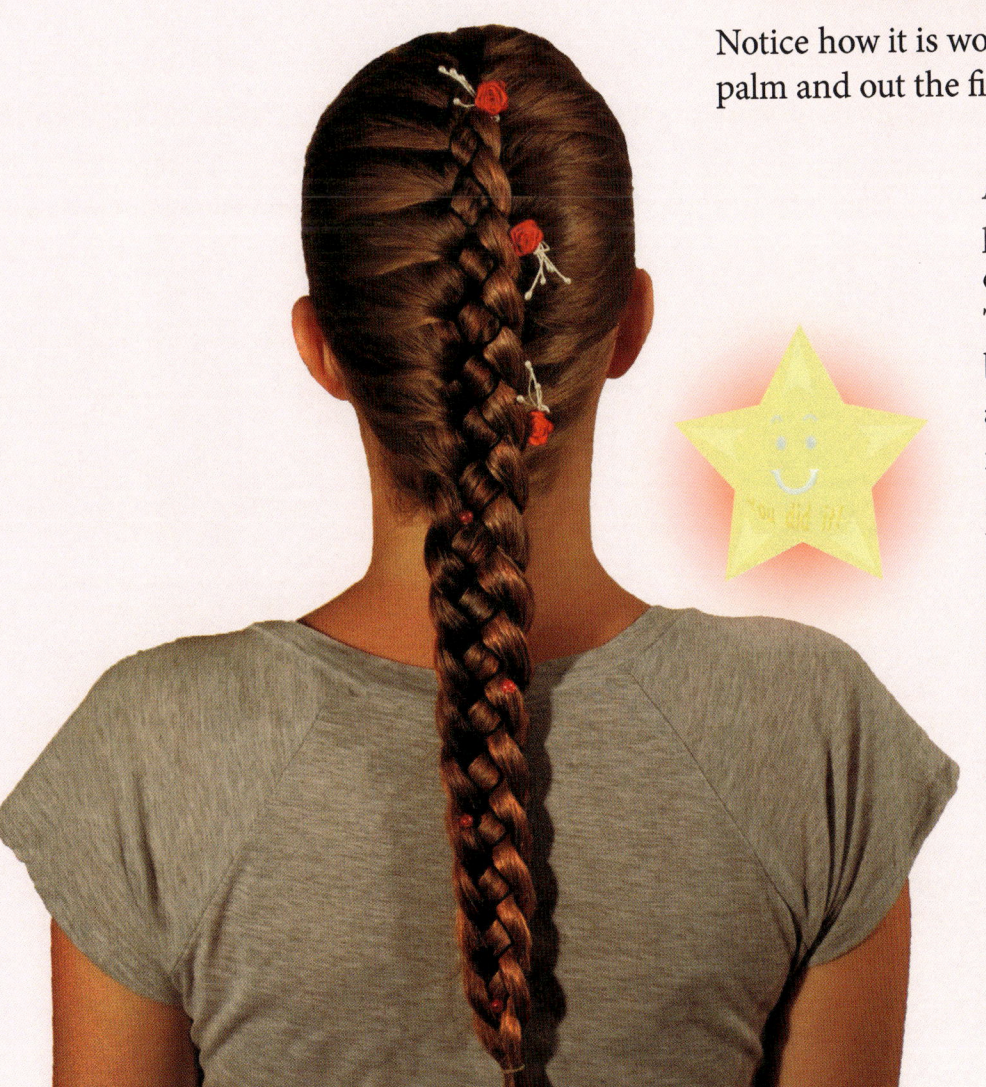

As you can see, the patterns you weave create certain braids. This braid has a french braid on the left and a dutch braid on the right. I did not feel right calling it a french braid or calling it a dutch braid. It is a plait. It is not round. I call it a taper braid because it tapers from dutch to french. I use the word stitch to indicate that there are gathers added into the braid on both sides.

Ways   189

Four-Strand Plait

Notes

_____

_____

_____

_____

_____

_____

_____

The knowledge in the next few pages can be applied later in the book to the six and eight strand braids. I do not show how to lace either of those yet it is entirely possible to lace both of them.

Four-Strand Plait

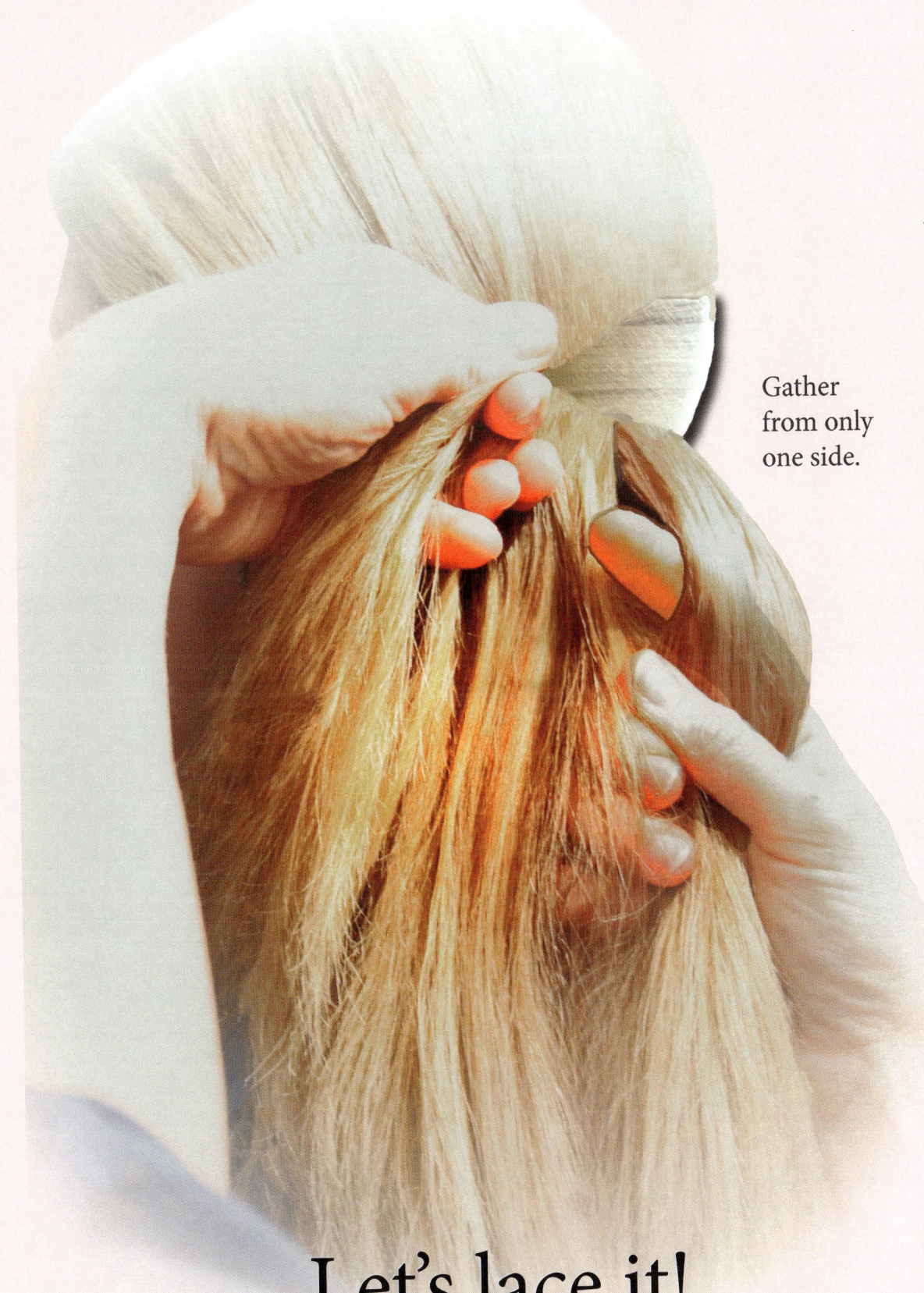

Gather from only one side.

Let's lace it!

4 Four-Strand Plait Lace: French option

Don't limit your challenges; challenge your limits.

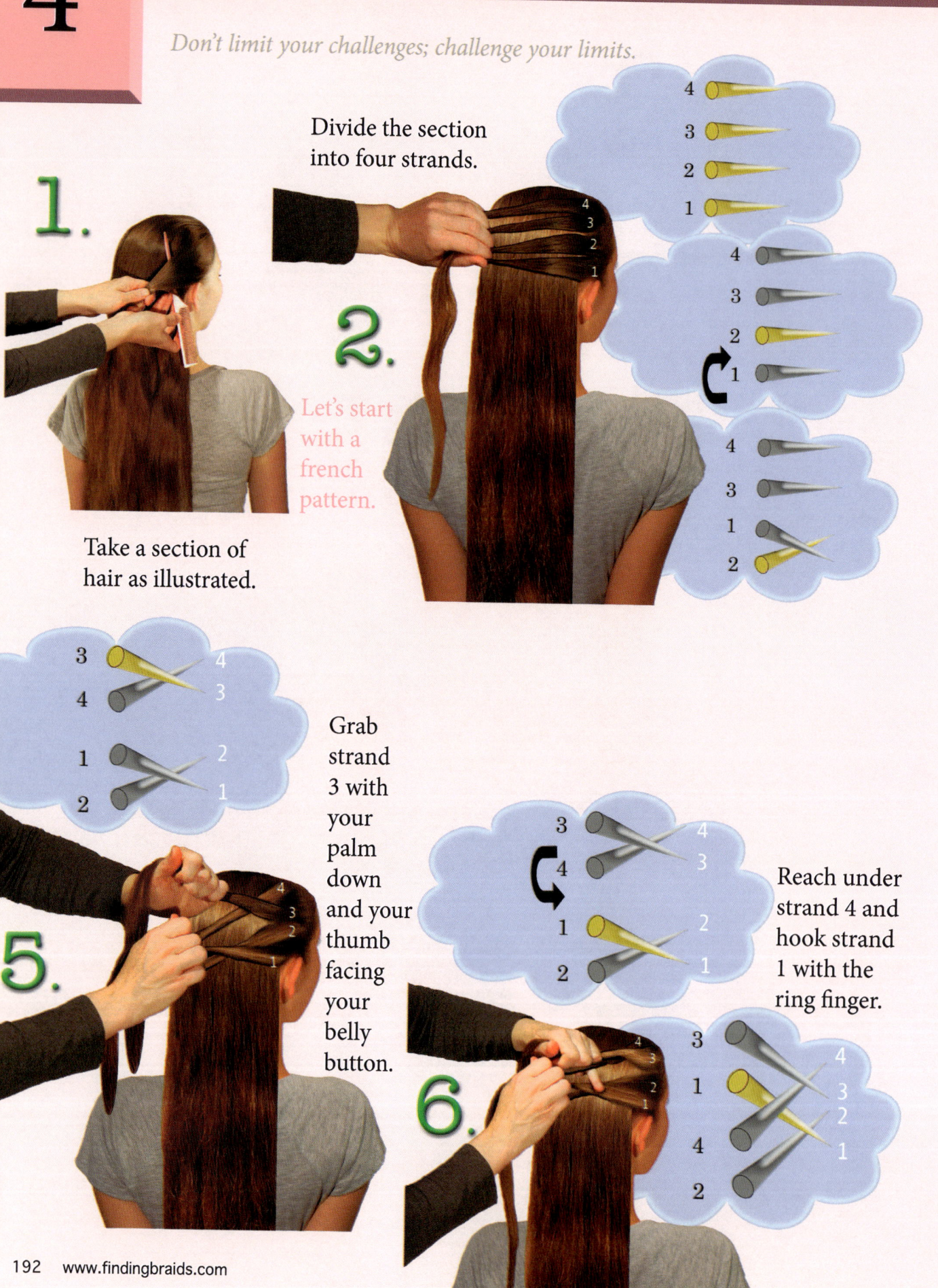

1. Take a section of hair as illustrated.

2. Divide the section into four strands.

   Let's start with a french pattern.

5. Grab strand 3 with your palm down and your thumb facing your belly button.

6. Reach under strand 4 and hook strand 1 with the ring finger.

Four-Strand Plait Lace: French option

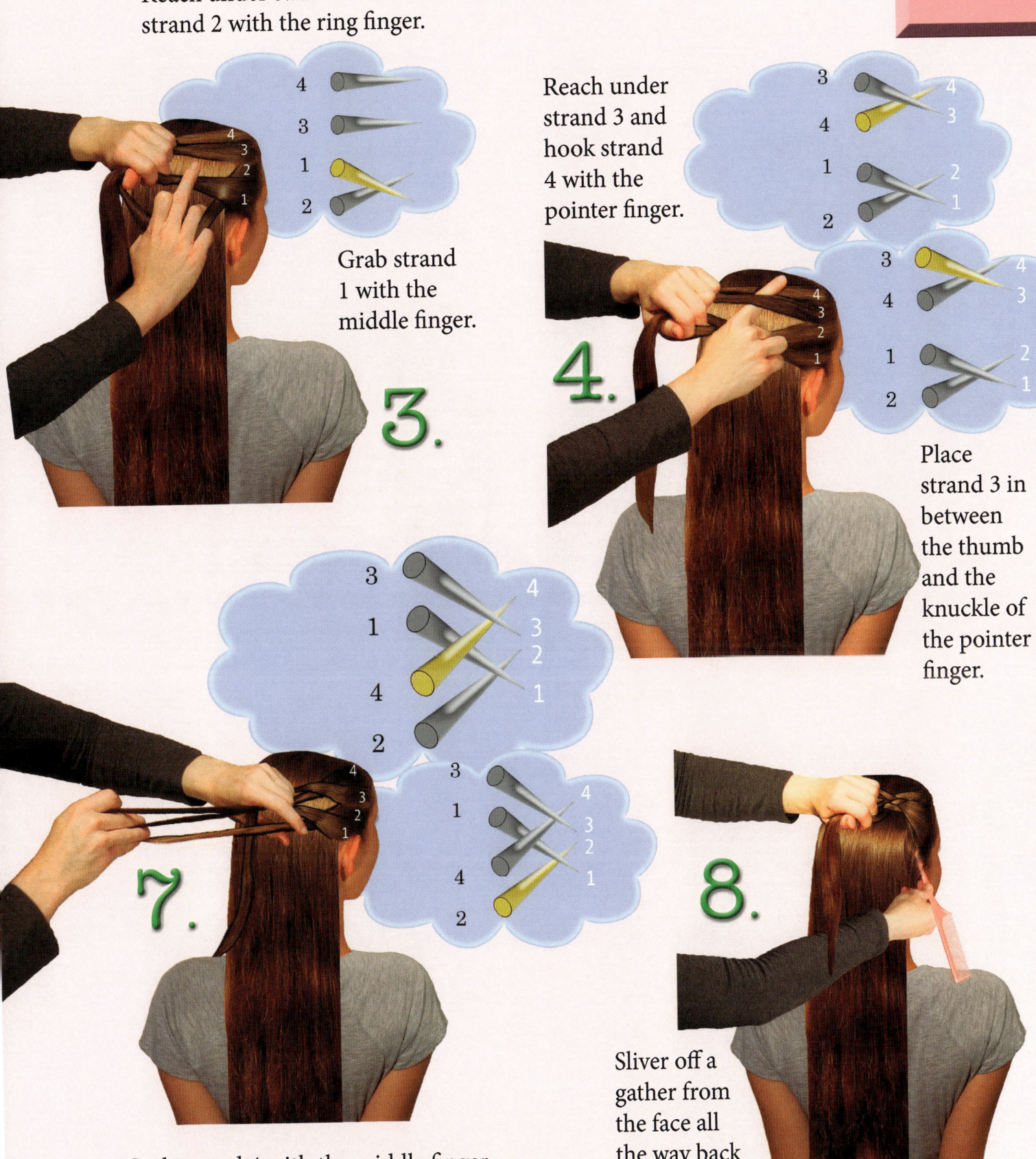

Reach under strand 1 and hook strand 2 with the ring finger.

Grab strand 1 with the middle finger.

3.

Reach under strand 3 and hook strand 4 with the pointer finger.

Place strand 3 in between the thumb and the knuckle of the pointer finger.

4.

7.

Grab strand 4 with the middle finger. Place strand 2 in the pointer finger.

8.

Sliver off a gather from the face all the way back to the braid.

4 Continuing

9.

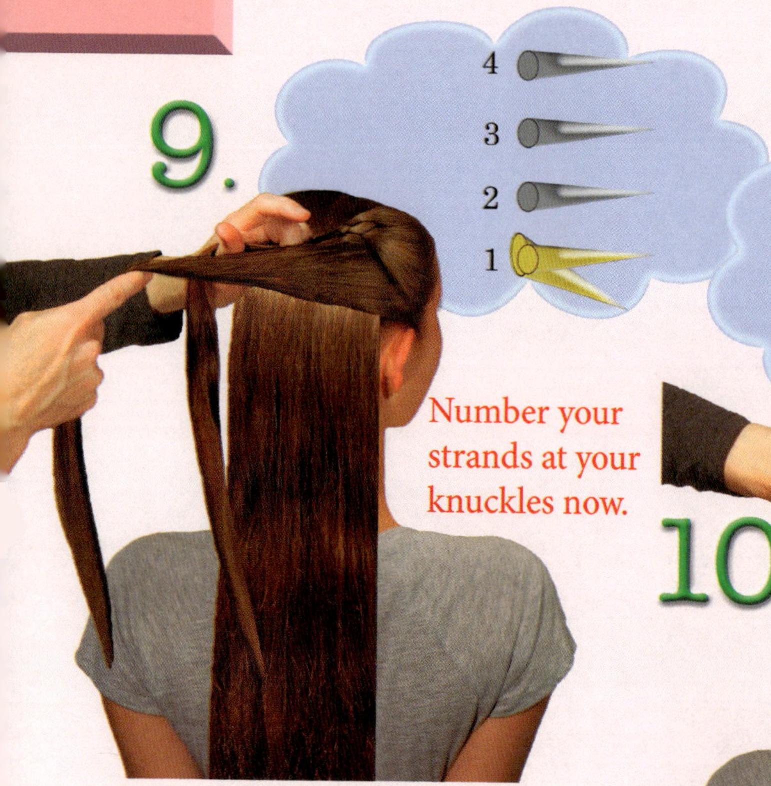

Number your strands at your knuckles now.

Place gather in strand 1 since you are about to french braid.

10.

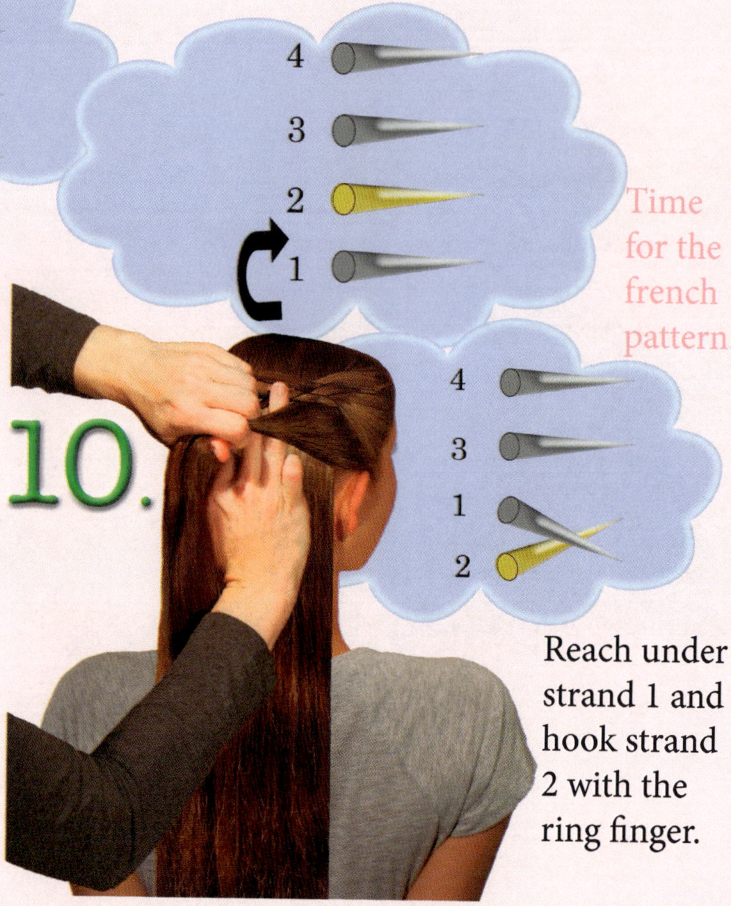

Time for the french pattern.

Reach under strand 1 and hook strand 2 with the ring finger.

13.

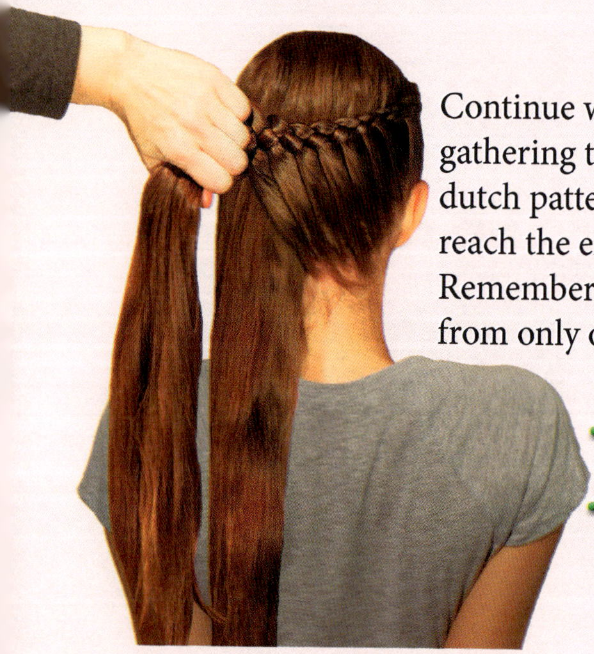

Continue weaving and gathering the french and dutch patterns until you reach the end of the hair. Remember to gather from only one side.

14.

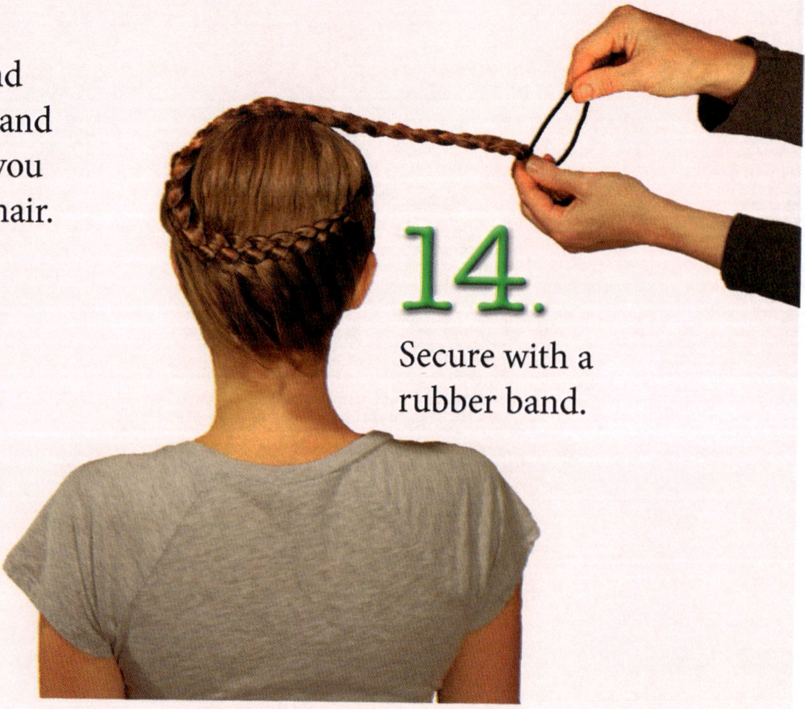

Secure with a rubber band.

www.findingbraids.com

part 2. Four-Strand Plait Lace: French 4

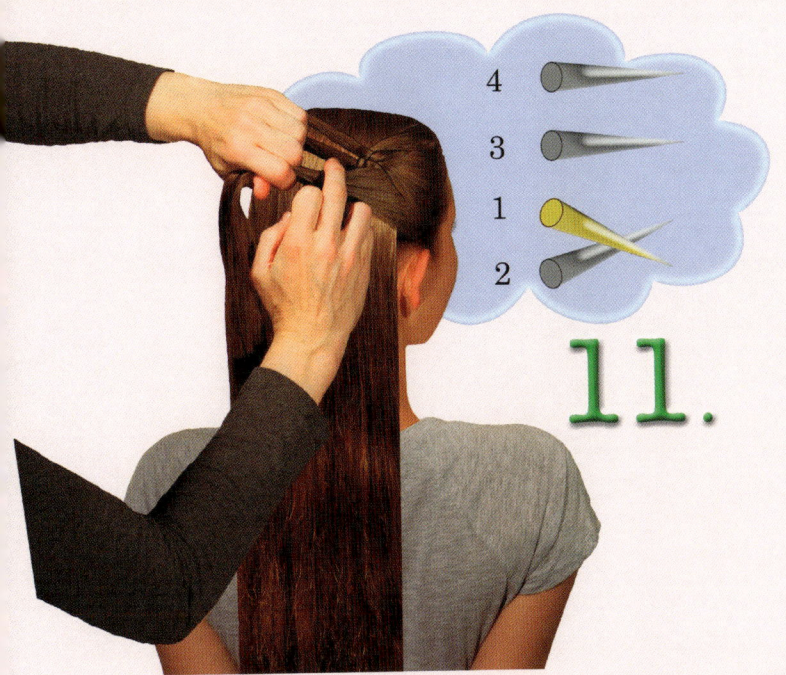

11.

Grab strand 1 with the middle finger.

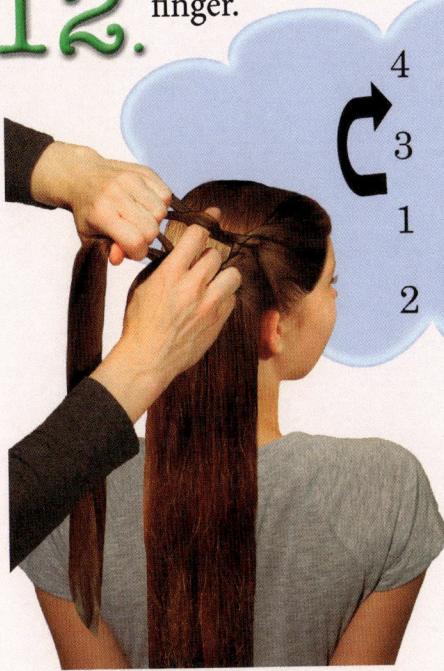

12.

Reach under strand 3 and hook strand 4 with the pointer finger.

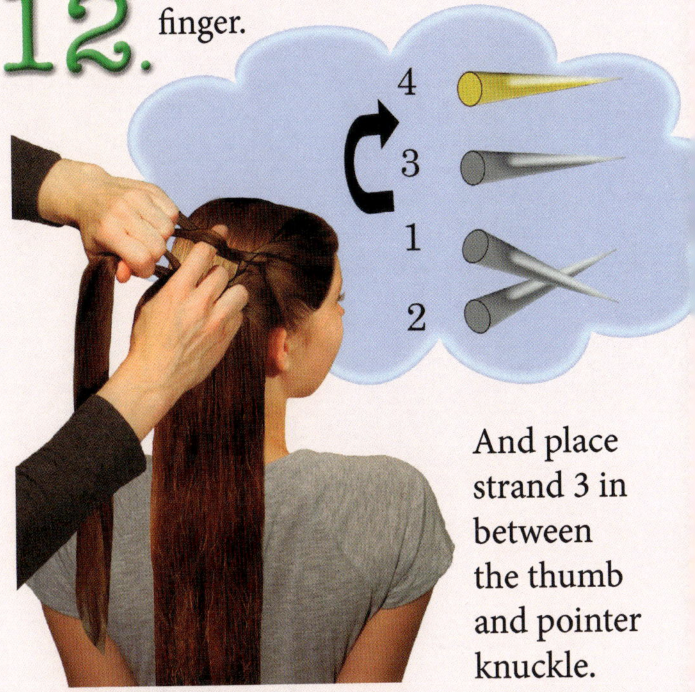

And place strand 3 in between the thumb and pointer knuckle.

15.

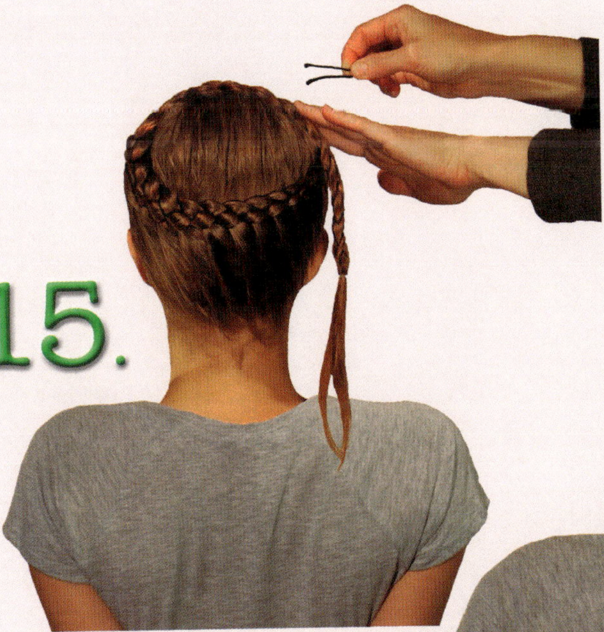

Fix the end of the tail with bobby pins to hold the braid in place.

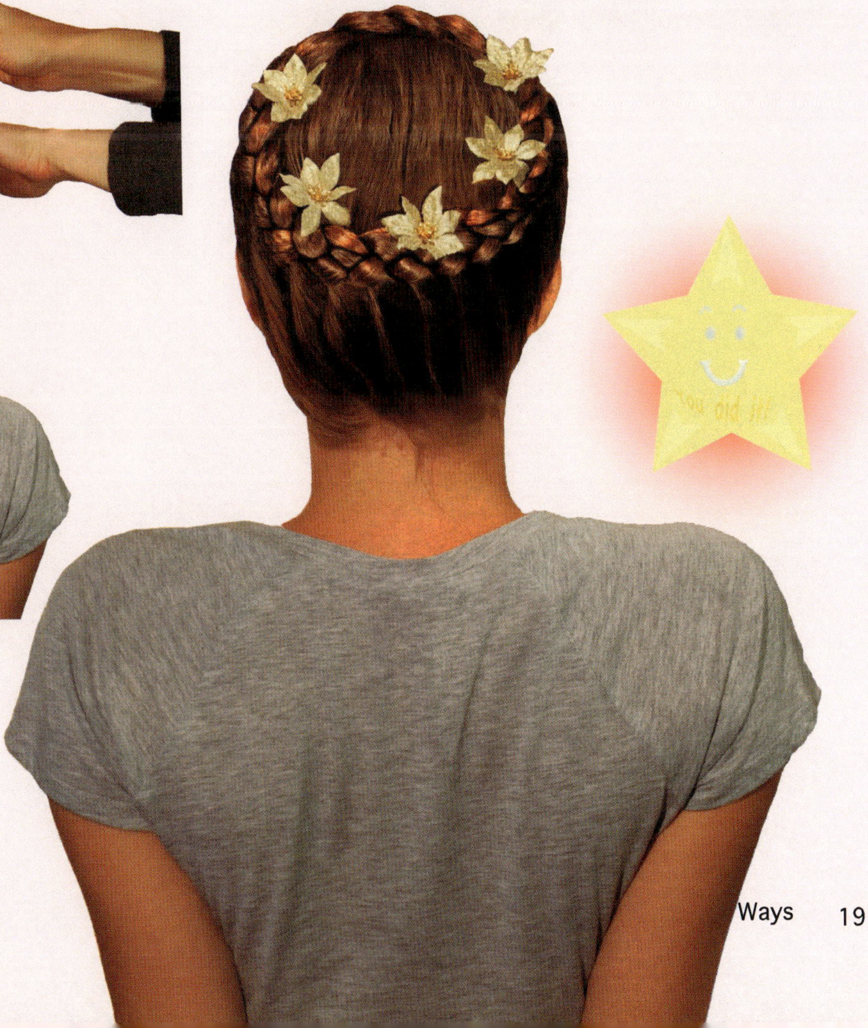

195

Four-Strand Plait

Notes

_____

_____

_____

_____

_____

_____

Let's talk about weaving and taking strands. When you hook a strand, you may want the entire length of that strand to be free of the other strands. It doesn't need to be. If it is seperated from the other strands with your fingers at the scalp, then it can be seperated later at the bottom when you finish weaving all the strands on that sides weave. There is a magic moment when you finish a weave on one side. You are about to let go with one hand in order to gather. Before you let go, slide that hand down the length of the tail to detangle the strands from each other. This is the best time to brush the tail as well.

Four-Strand Plait

Gather from both sides

Let's stitch it!

Let's stitch it!

Let's stitch it!

Four-Strand Plait Dutch Stitch

What we learn to do, we learn by doing. - Aristotle

1.

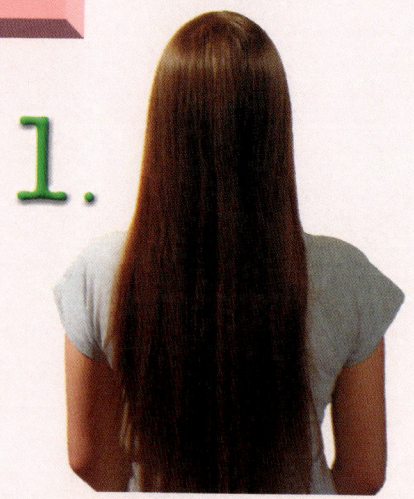

Begin with clean, brushed hair.

2.

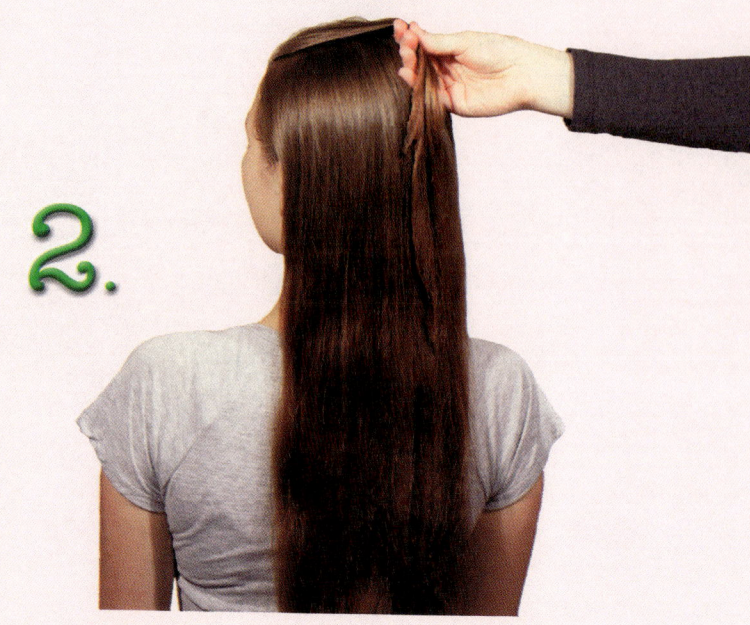

Take a section of hair as illustrated.

5.

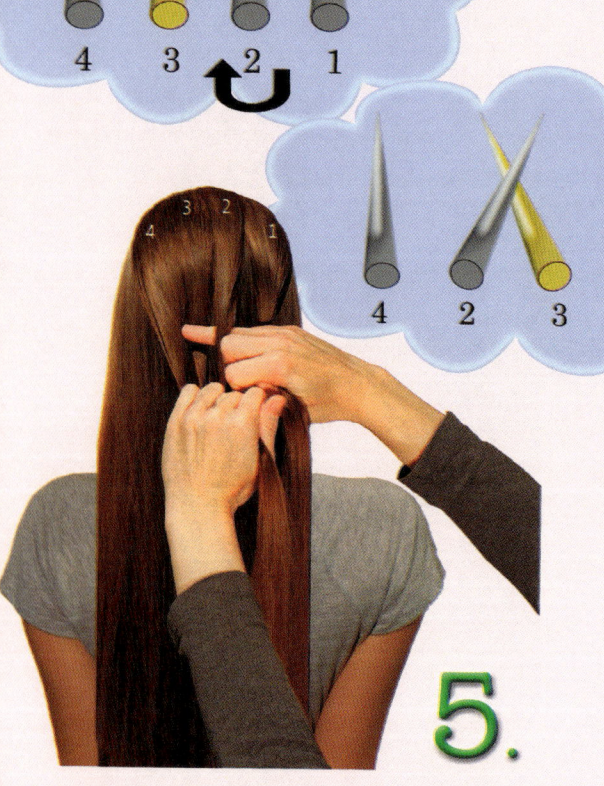

Reach under strand 2 and hook strand 3.

6.

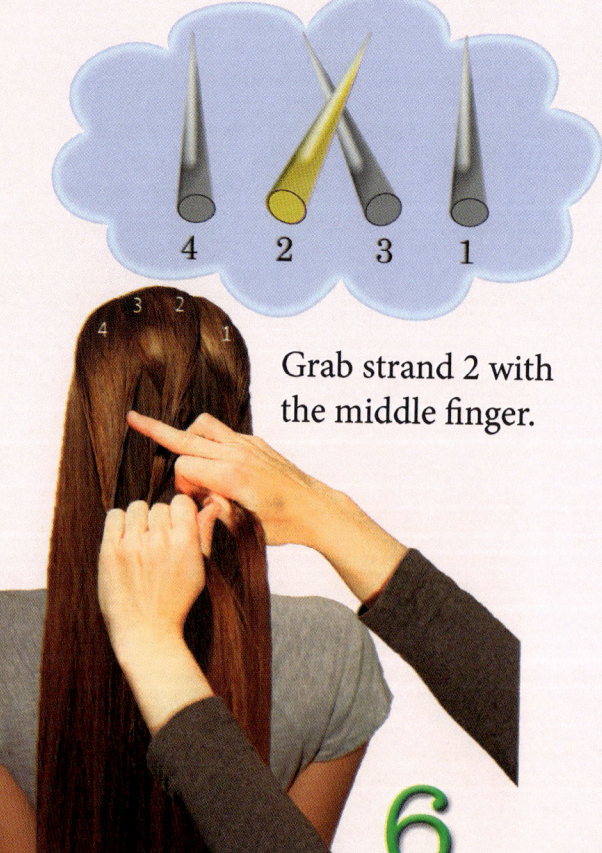

Grab strand 2 with the middle finger.

198   www.findingbraids.com

Four-Strand Plait Dutch Stitch

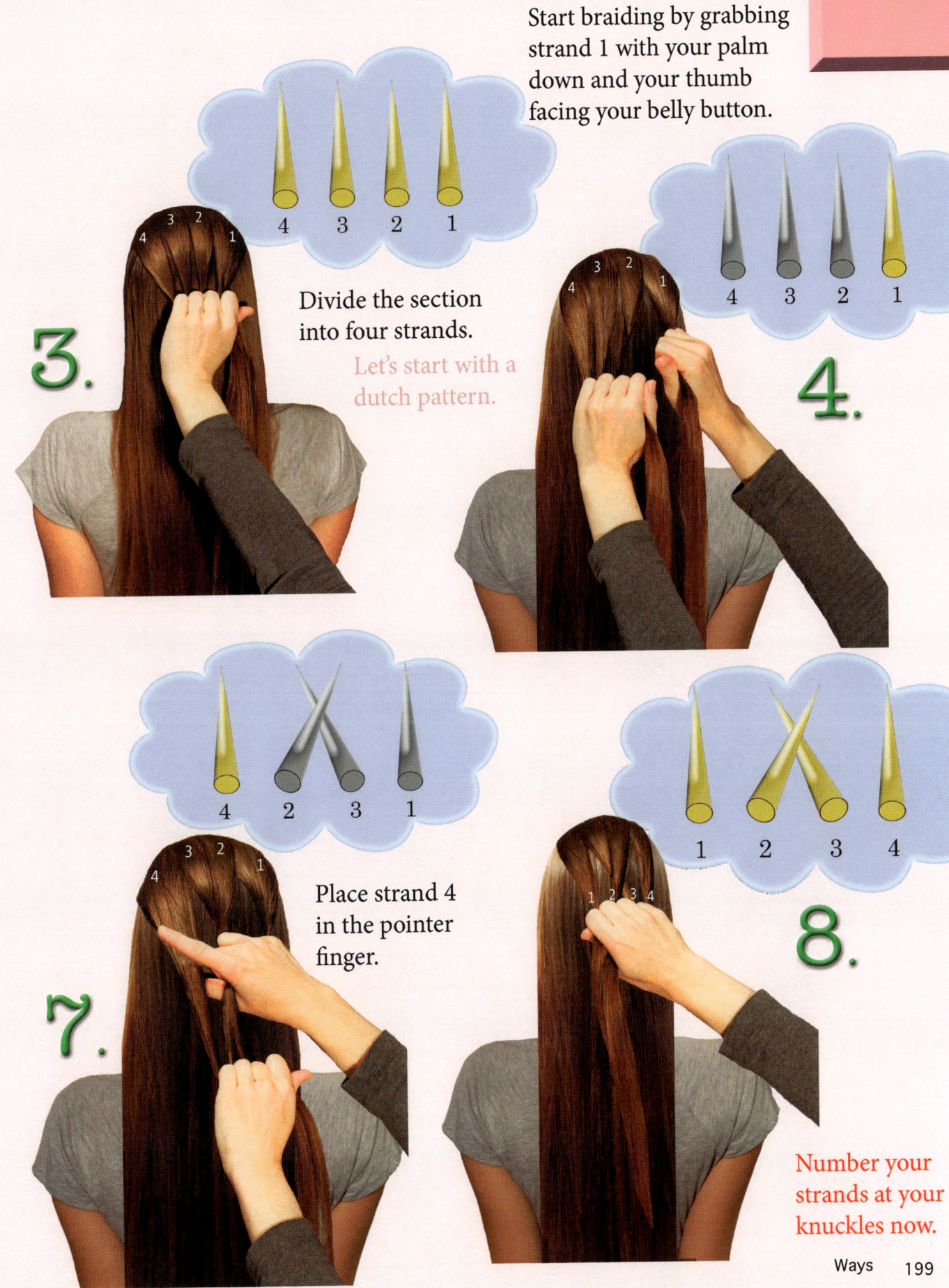

Start braiding by grabbing strand 1 with your palm down and your thumb facing your belly button.

Divide the section into four strands.

Let's start with a dutch pattern.

Place strand 4 in the pointer finger.

Number your strands at your knuckles now.

4 Continuing

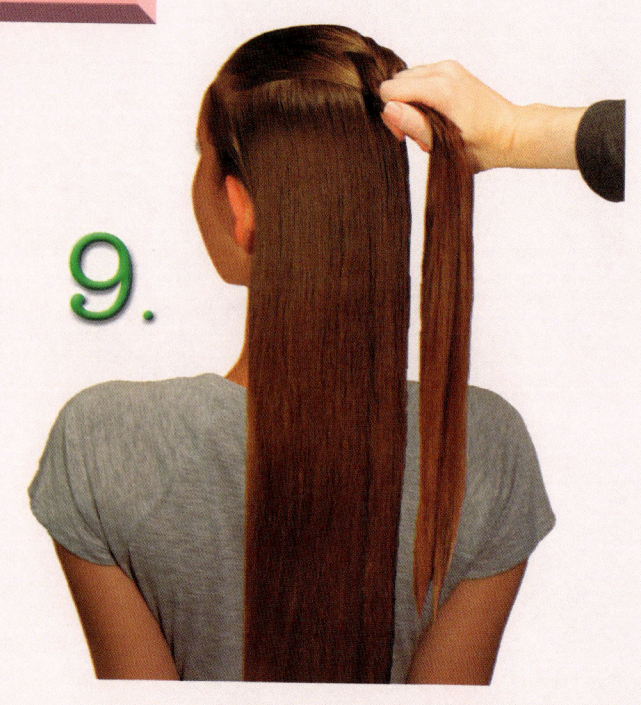

9.

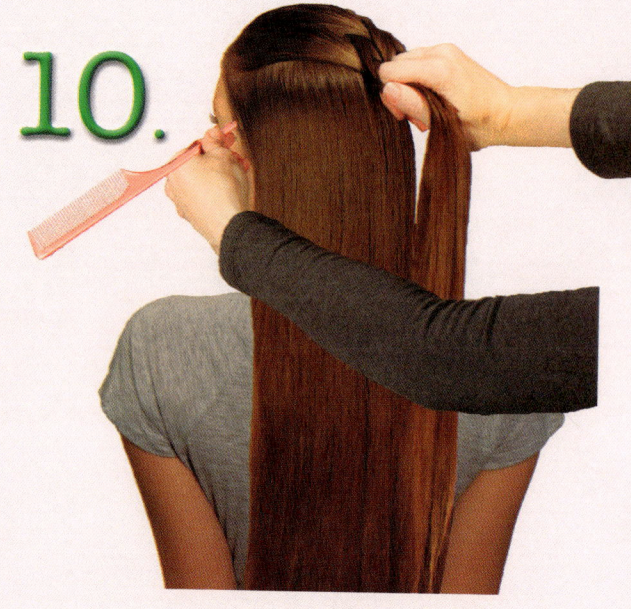

10.

Sliver off a gather from the face all the way back to the braid.

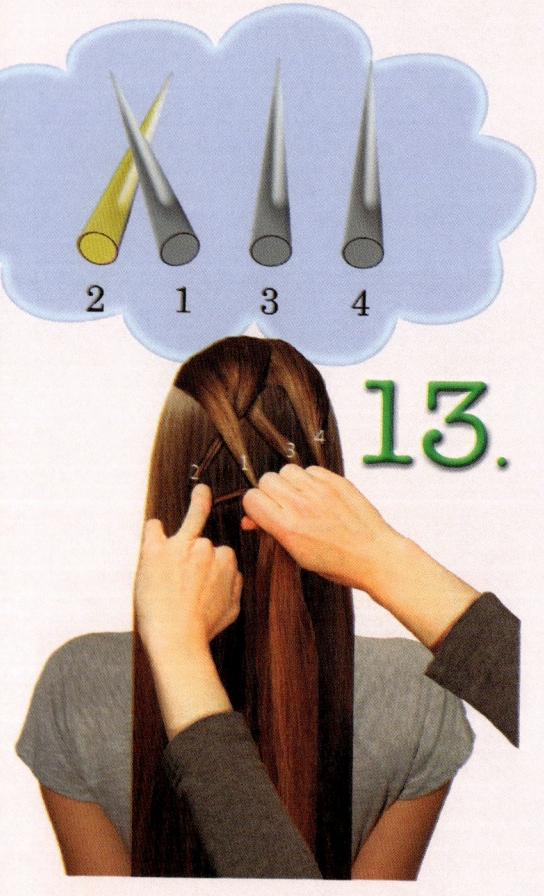

13.

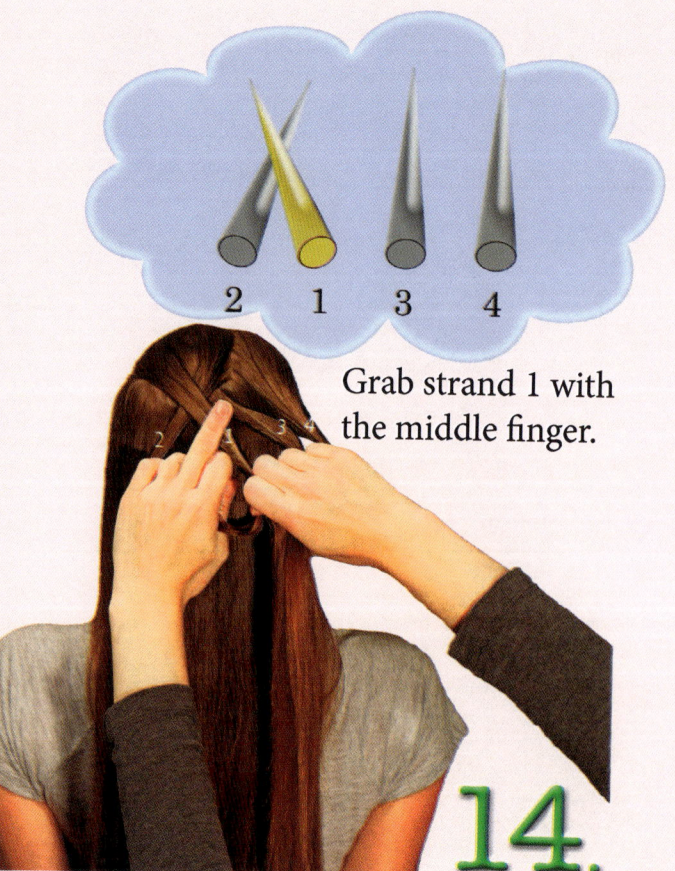

Grab strand 1 with the middle finger.

14.

part 2. Four-Strand Plait Dutch Stitch

4

Since this is the "french" side, gather into strand 3 to simulate a dutch braid.

Time for the "french" pattern.

11.

12. Reach under strand 1 and hook strand 2 with the ring finger.

15. Reach under strand 3 and hook strand 4 with the pointer finger.

16. And place strand 3 in between the thumb and pointer knuckle.

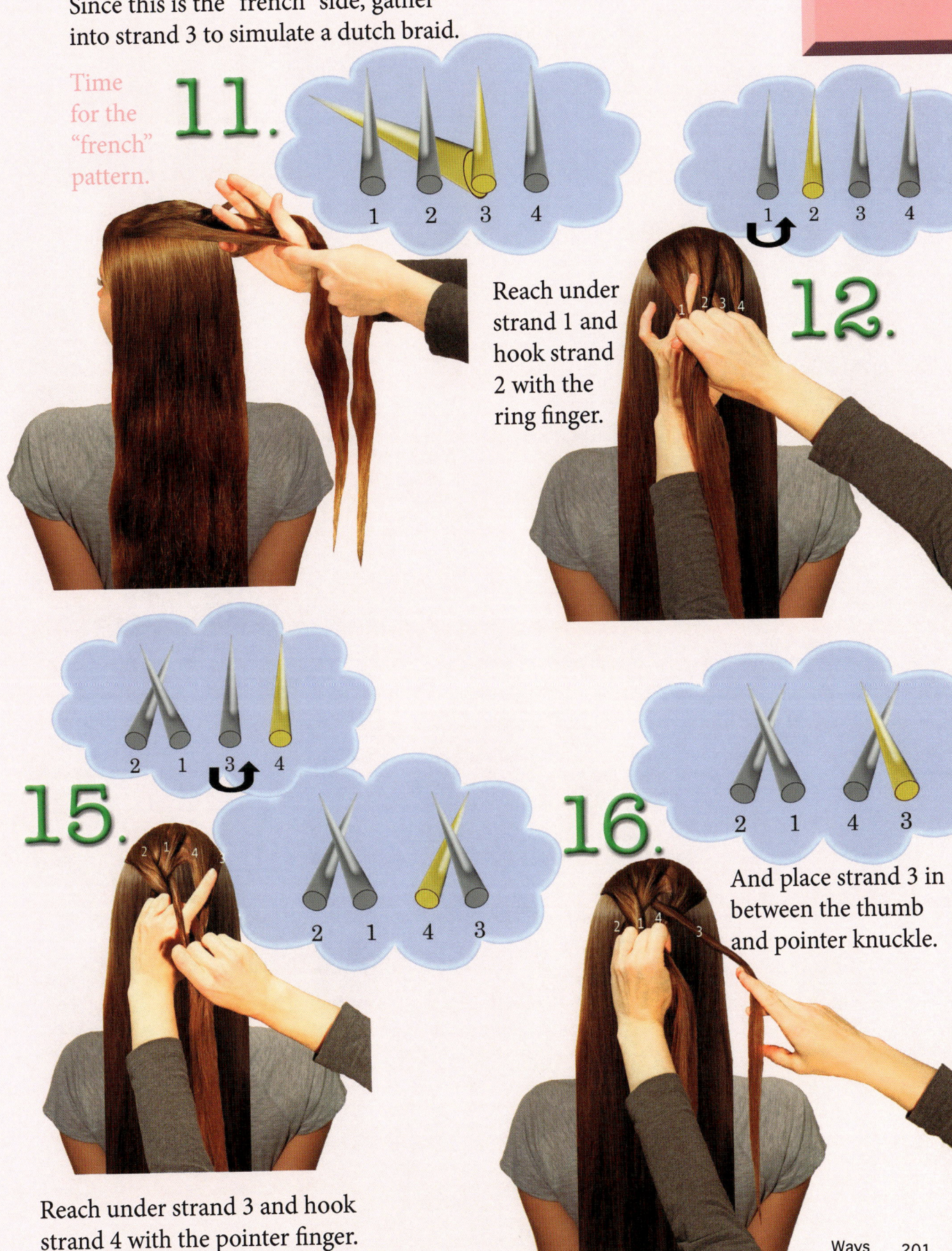

Ways 201

4   Continuing

17.

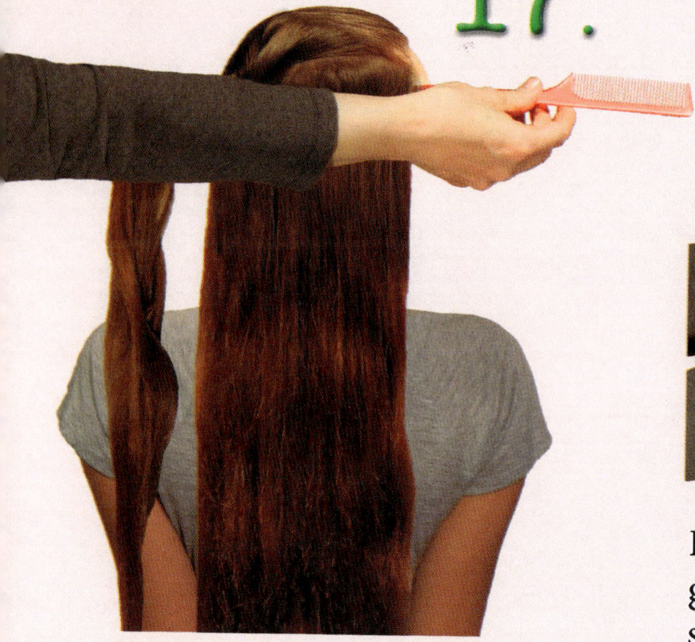

Sliver off a gather from the face all the way back to the braid.

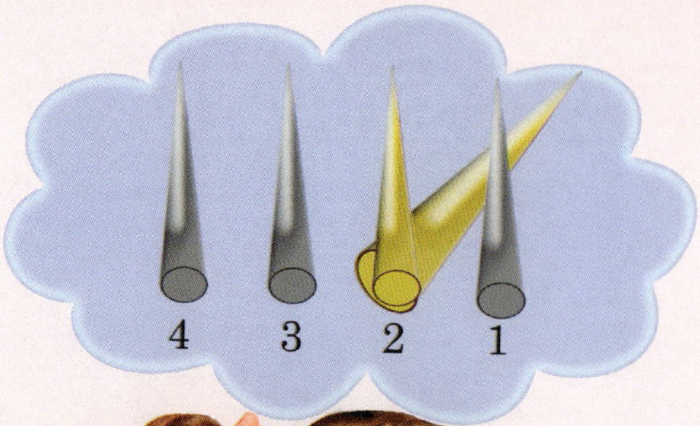

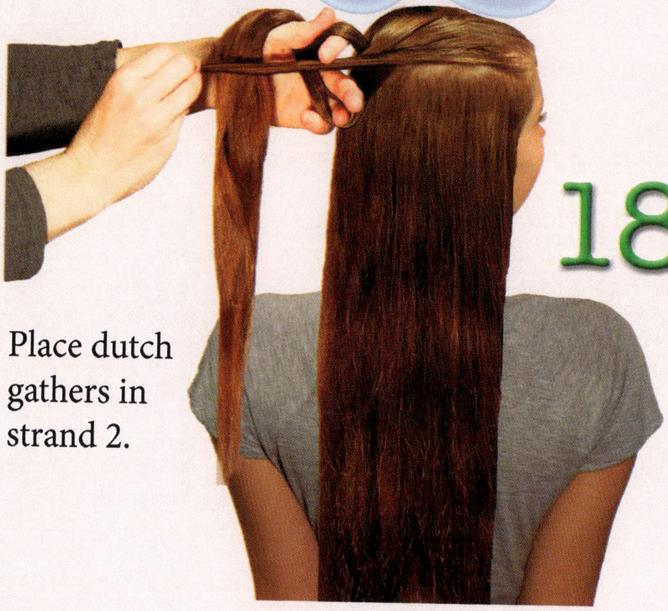

18. Place dutch gathers in strand 2.

21. Secure with a rubber band.

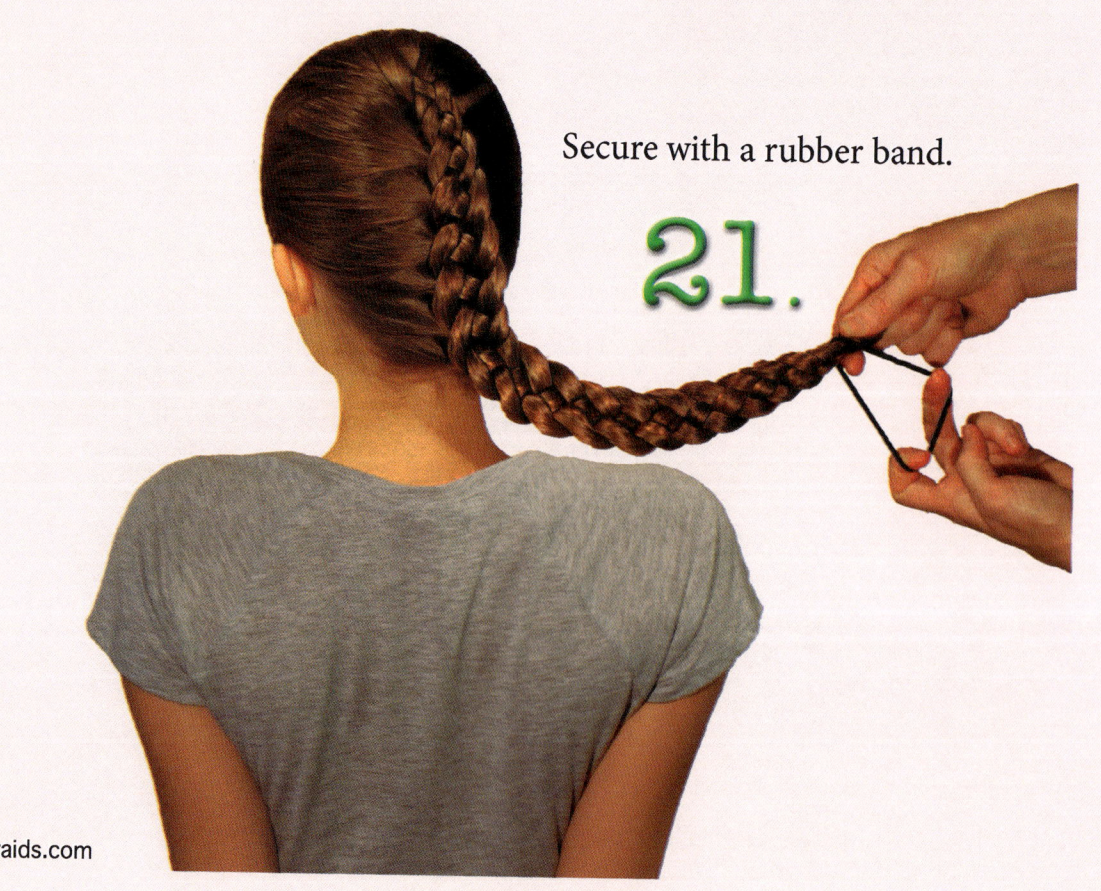

part 3. Four-Strand Plait Dutch Stitch

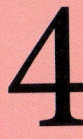

Notice how it is woven through the palm and out the fist with the other hair.

19.

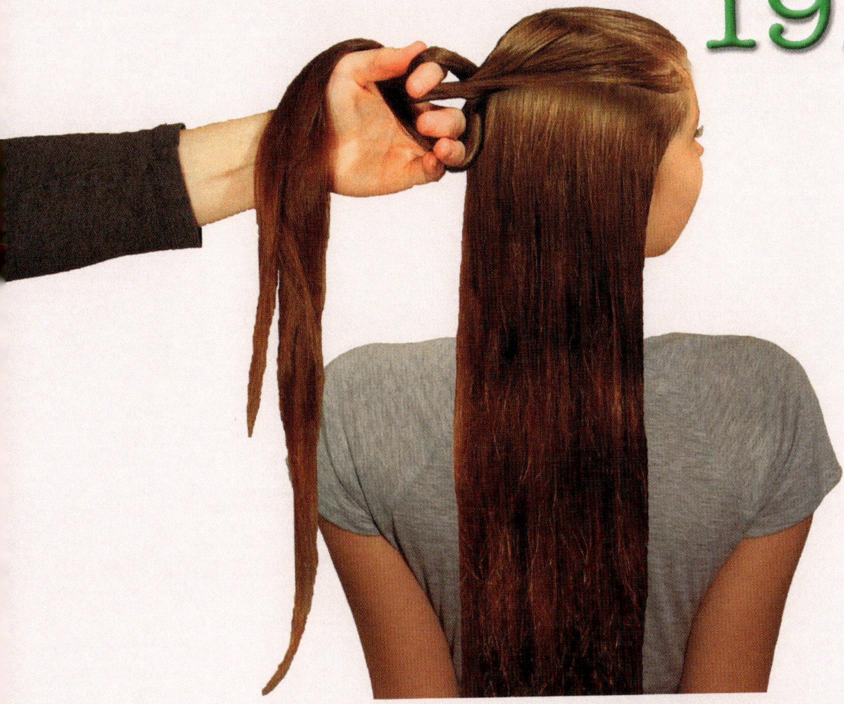

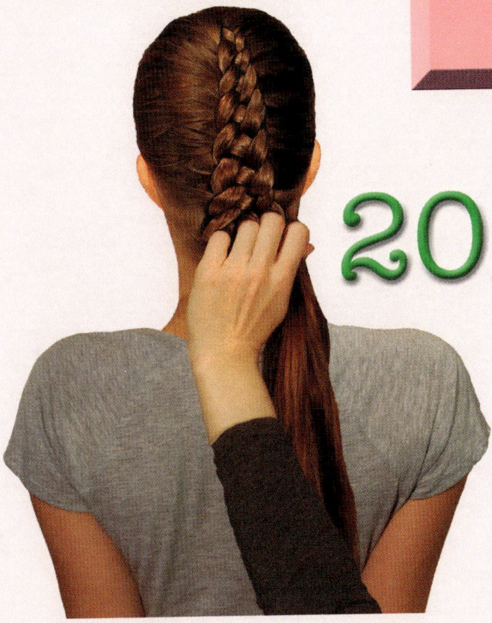

20.

Continue weaving the dutch and "french" patterns while placing the gathers in a dutch and dutch simulated fashion until you reach the end of the hair.

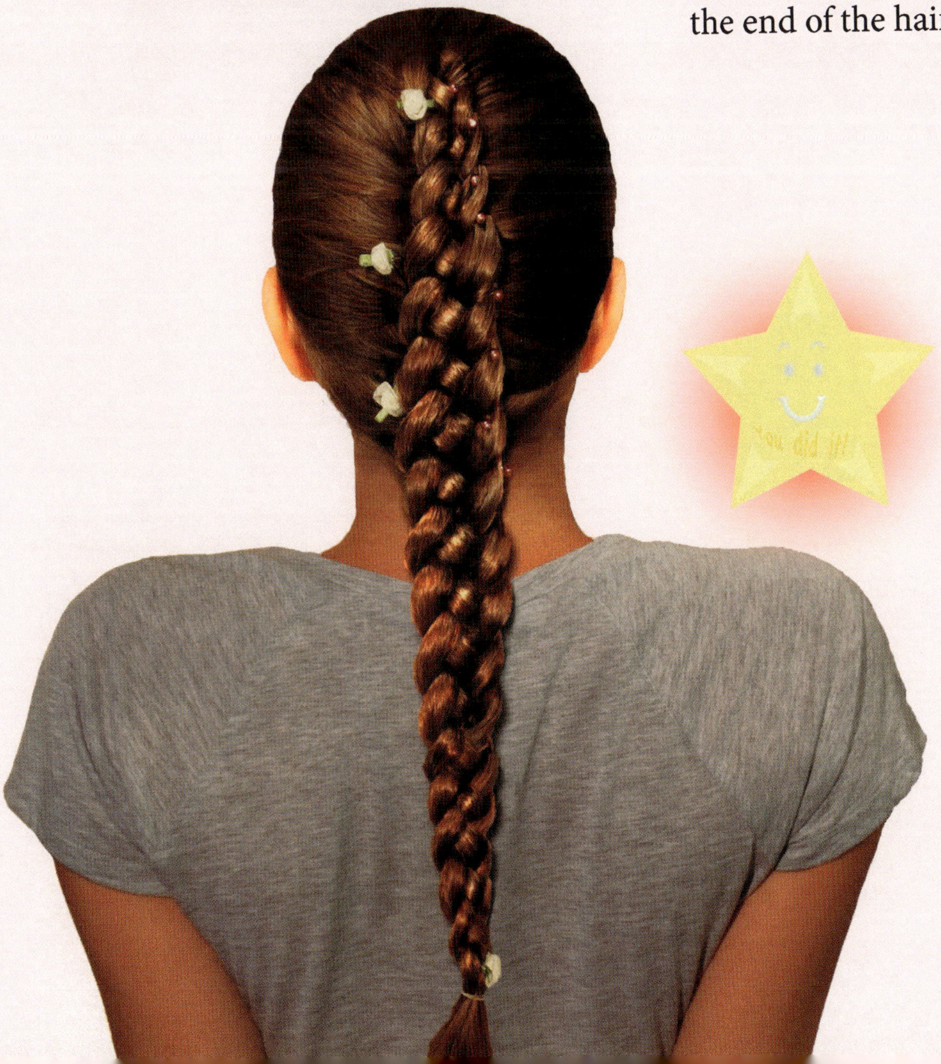

Four-Strand Plait

Notes

_____

_____

_____

_____

_____

_____

_____

The knowledge in the next few pages can be applied later in the book to the six and eight strand braids. I do not show how to lace either of those yet it is entirely possible to lace both of them.

Four-Strand Plait

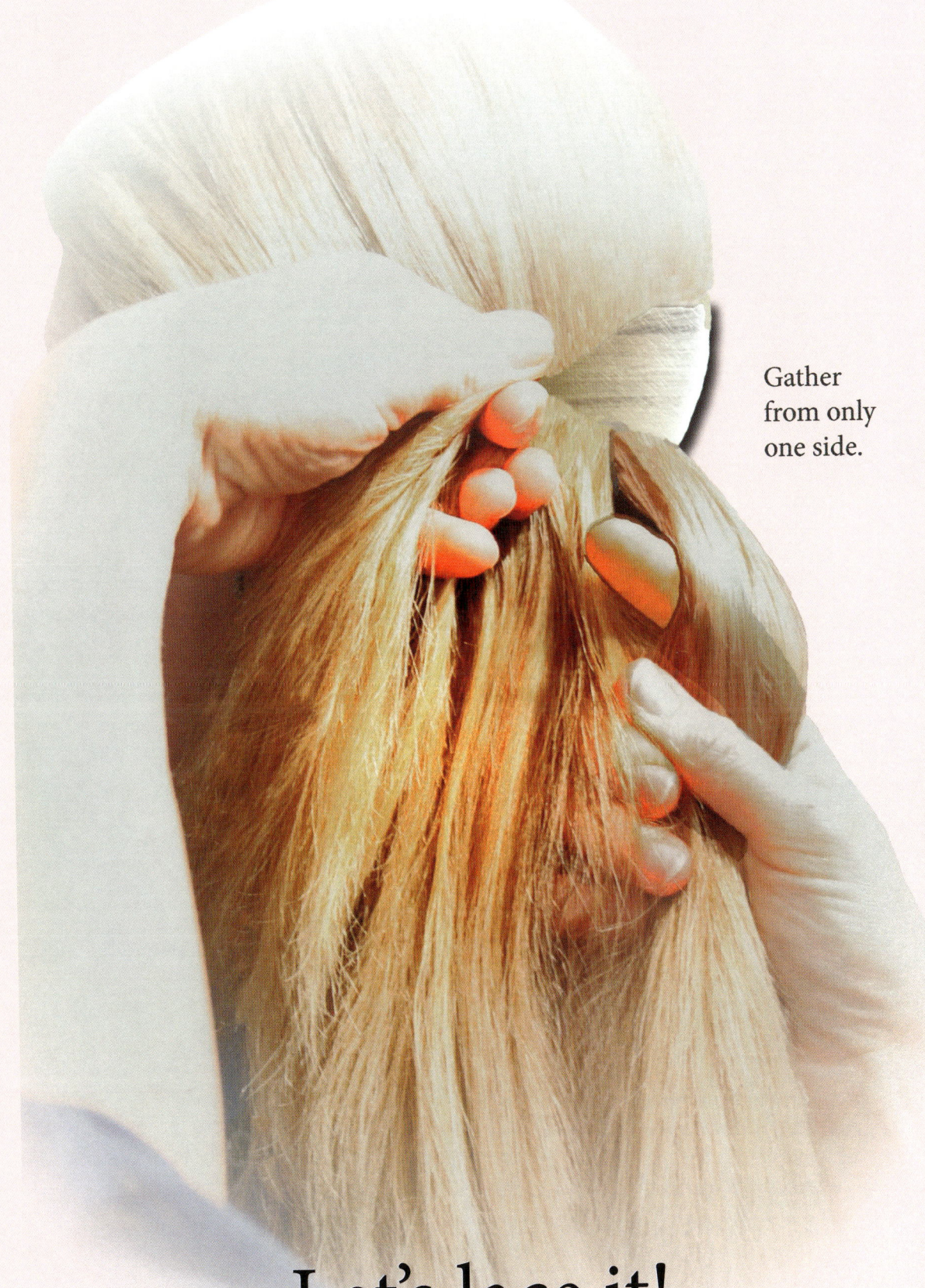

Gather from only one side.

Let's lace it!

4 Four-Strand Plait Lace: Dutch option

A person, who never made a mistake, never tried anything new.
- Albert Einstein

1. Take a section of hair as illustrated.

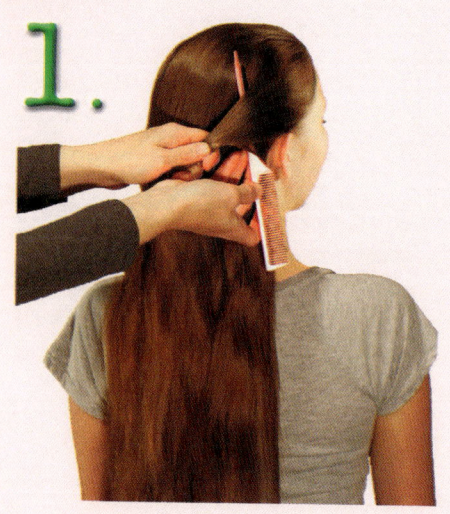

2. Divide the section into four strands.

Let's start with a french pattern.

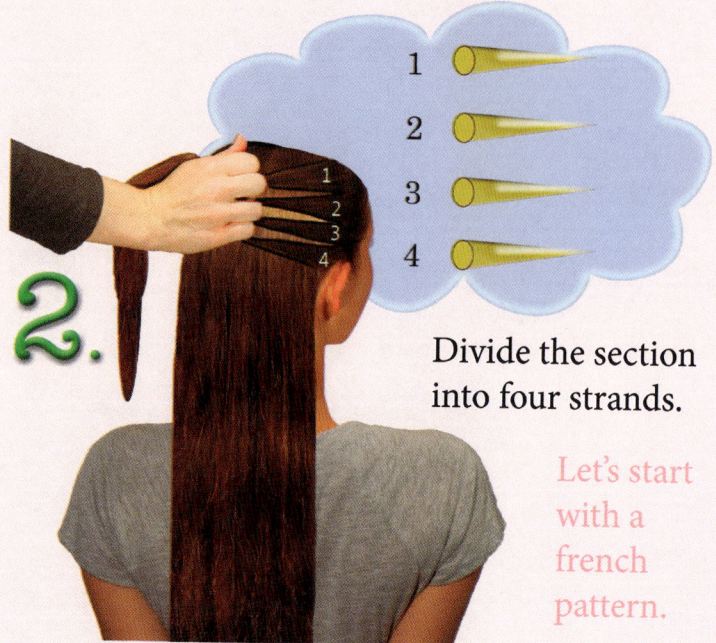

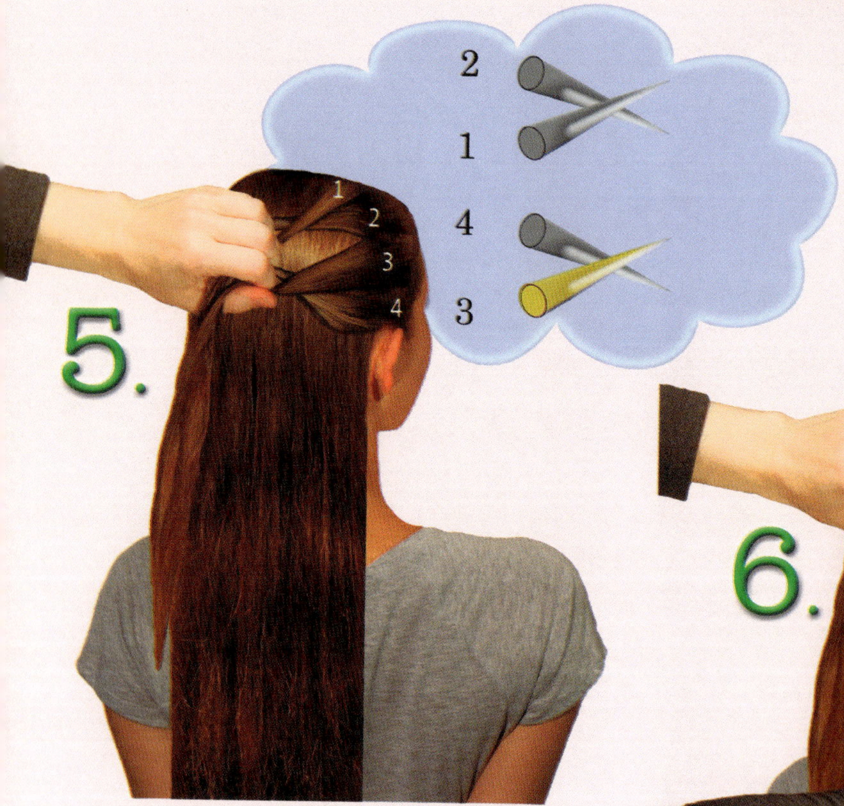

5. Place strand 3 between the thumb and the knuckle of the pointer finger.

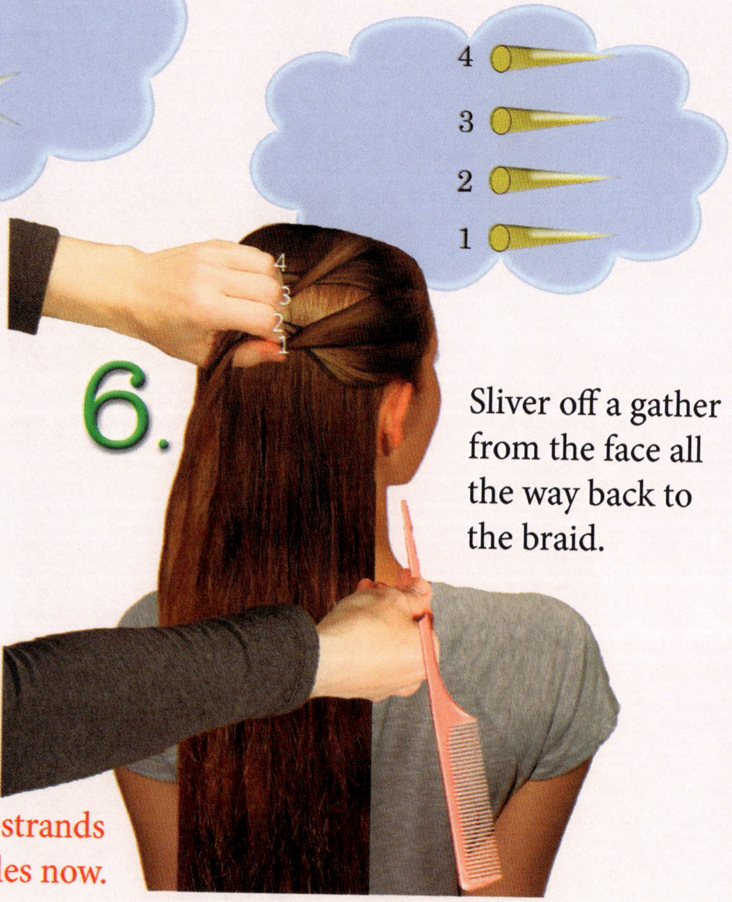

Number your strands at your knuckles now.

6. Sliver off a gather from the face all the way back to the braid.

206   www.findingbraids.com

Four-Strand Plait Lace: Dutch option

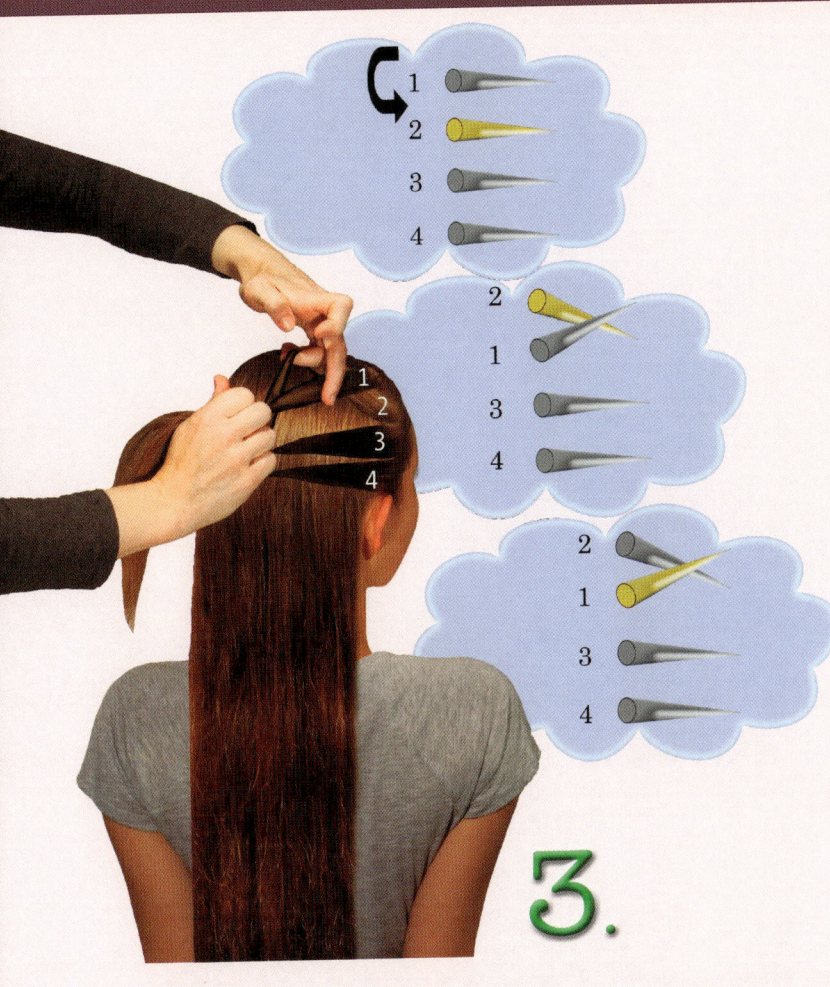

3.

Reach under strand 1 and hook strand 2 with the ring finger. Grab strand 1 with the middle finger.

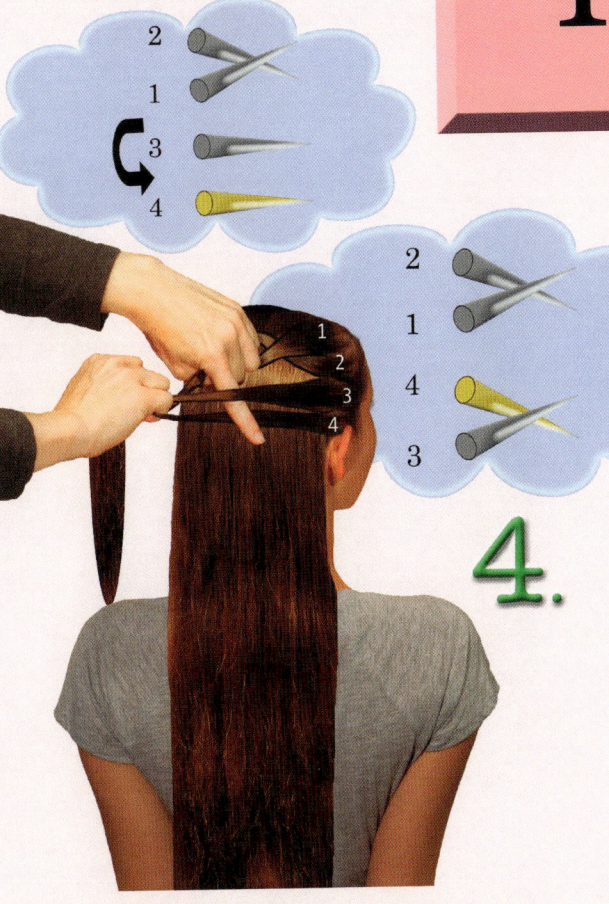

4.

Reach under strand 3 and hook strand 4 with the pointer finger.

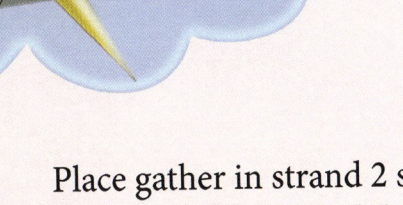

7.

Place gather in strand 2 since you are about to dutch braid.

Ways 207

4 Continuing

Time for the dutch pattern.

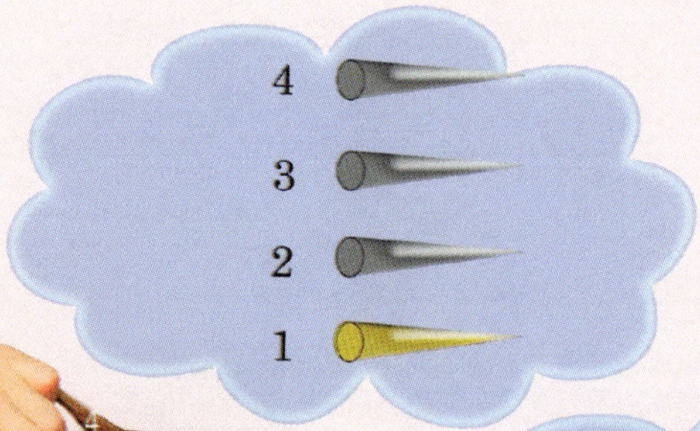

Grab strand 1 with the pinky finger.

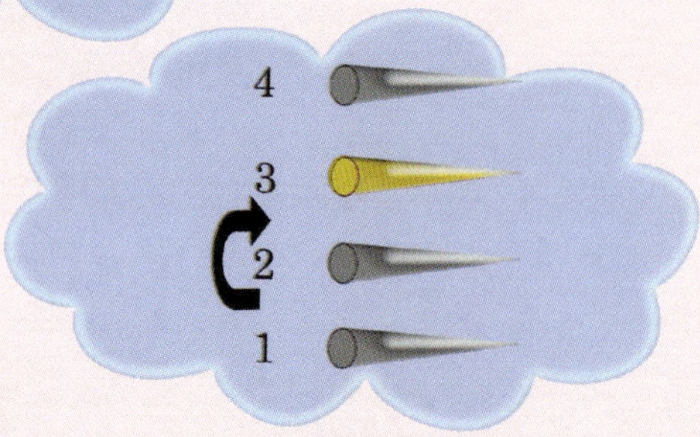

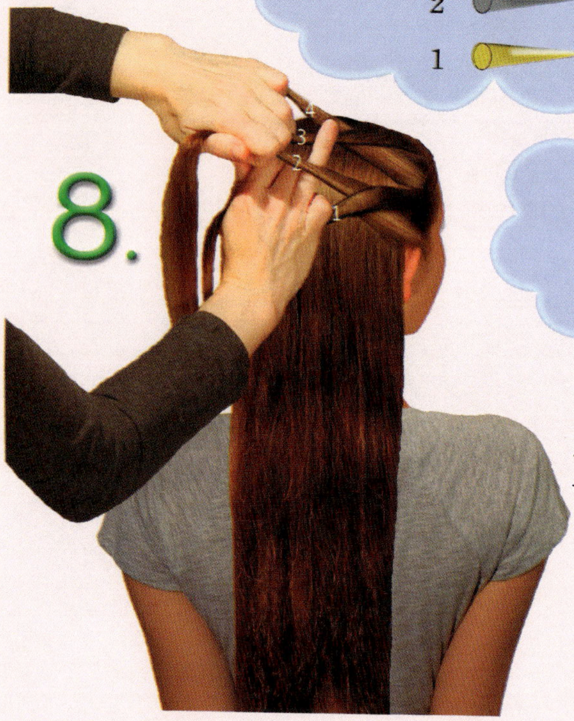

Reach under strand 2 and hook strand 3 with the ring finger.

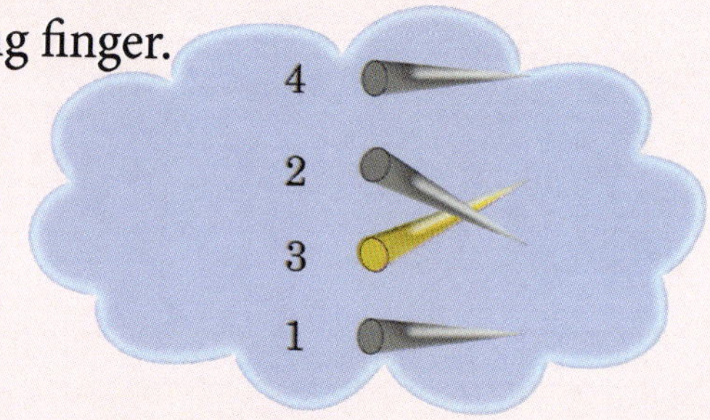

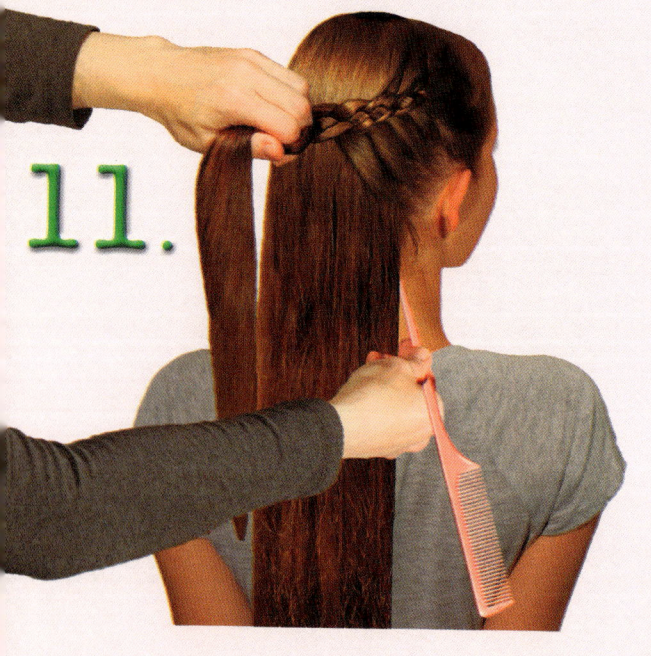

8.

11.

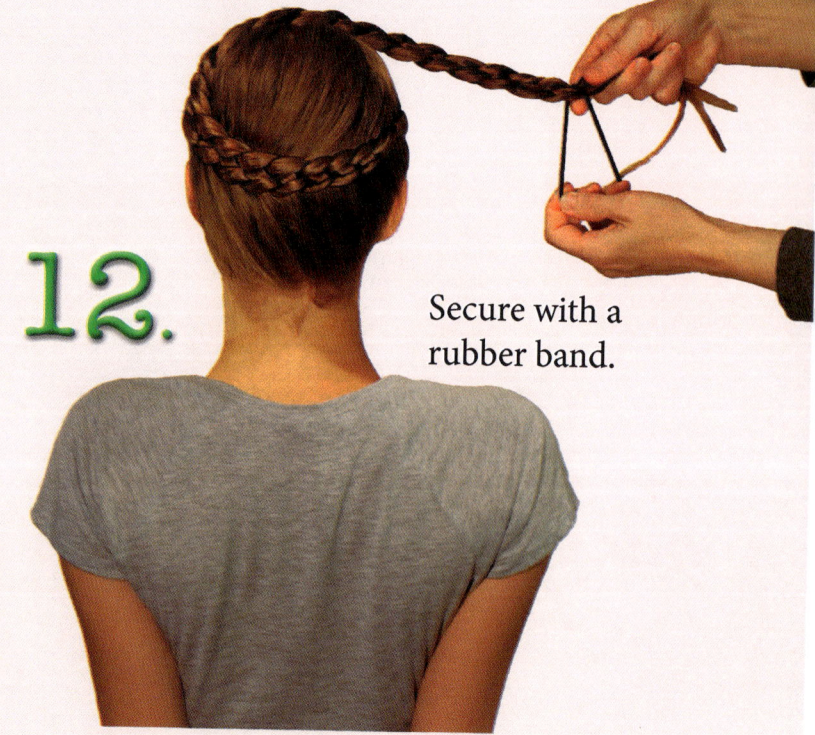

12.

Secure with a rubber band.

part 2. Four-Strand Lace: Dutch

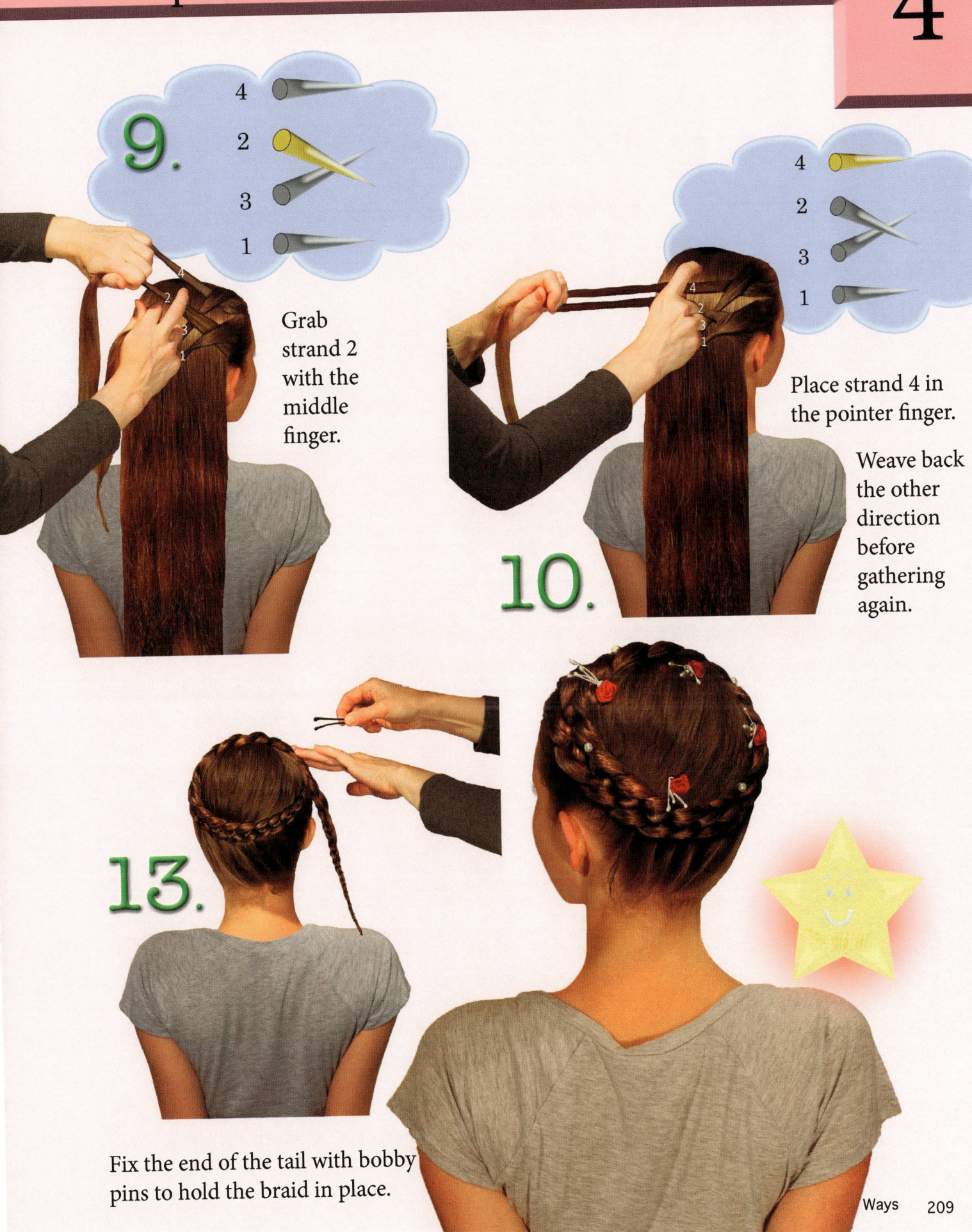

9. Grab strand 2 with the middle finger.

10. Place strand 4 in the pointer finger. Weave back the other direction before gathering again.

13. Fix the end of the tail with bobby pins to hold the braid in place.

Four-Strand Plait

Notes

After trying these examples, create your own!

Examples of Four-Strand Plait

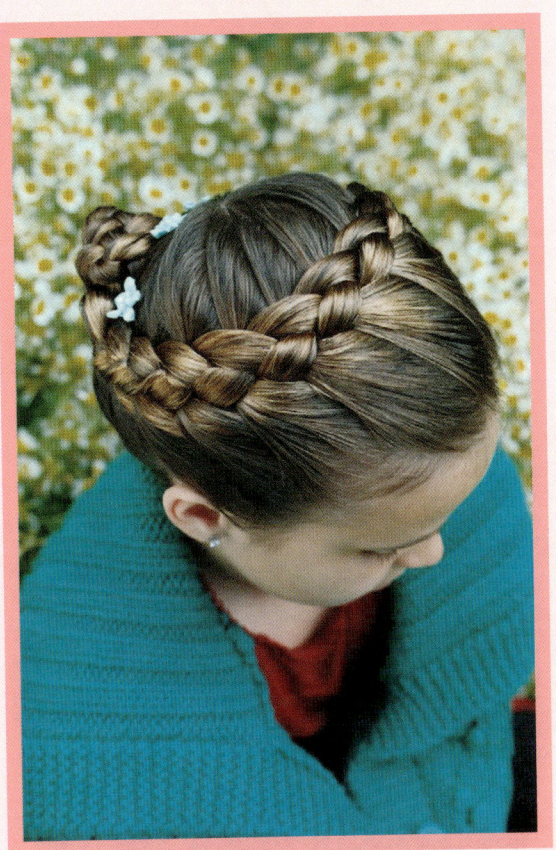
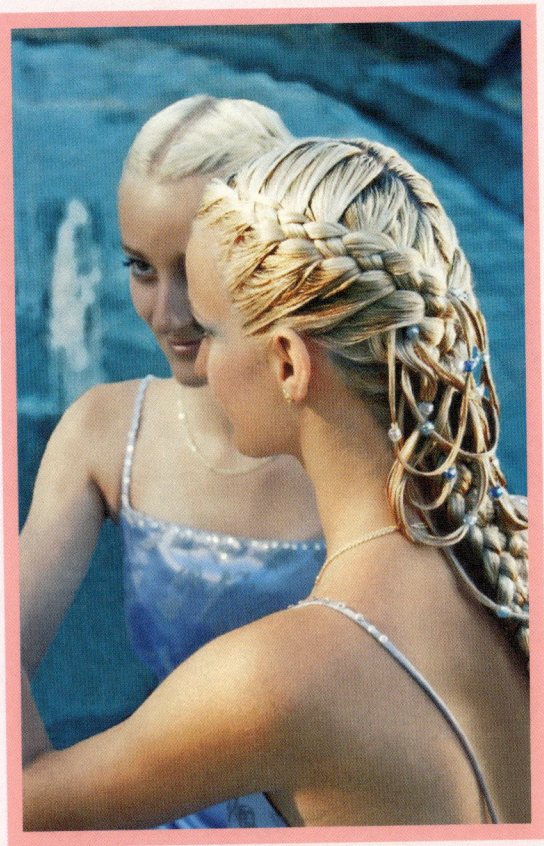
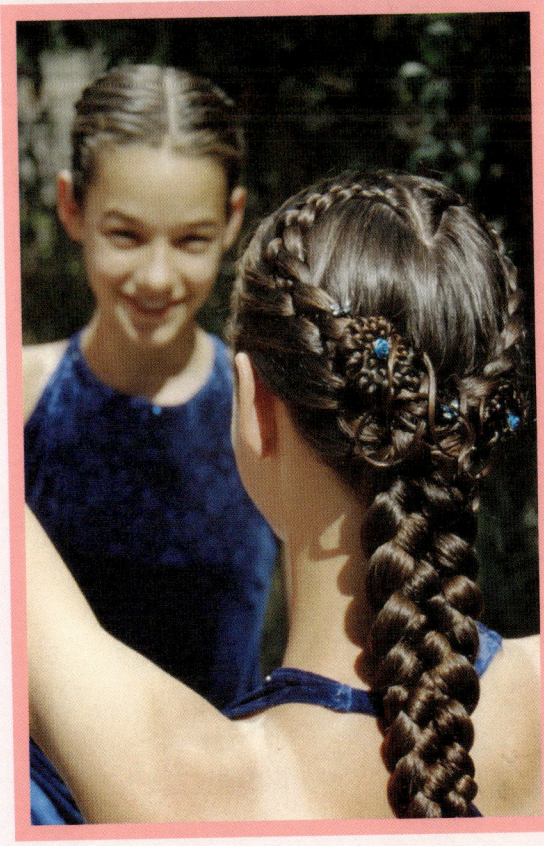
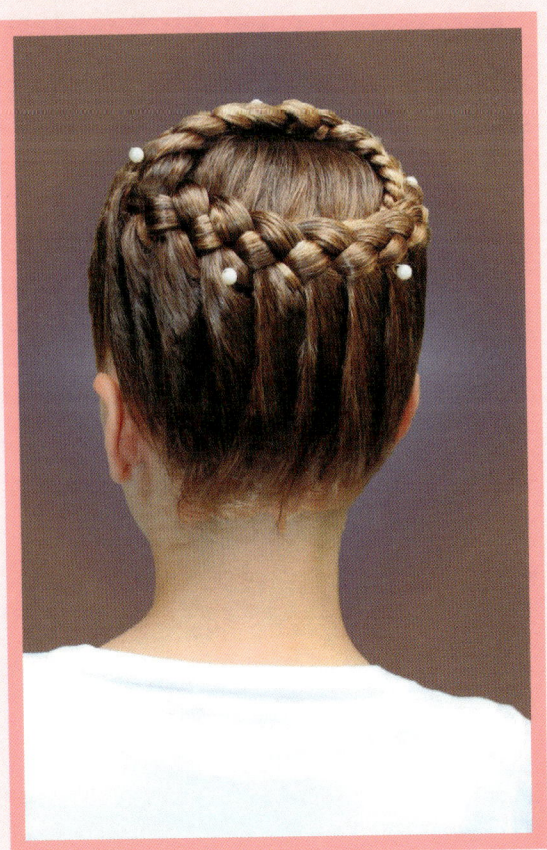

Visit my website to see more examples of the Four-Strand Plait

Five-Strand

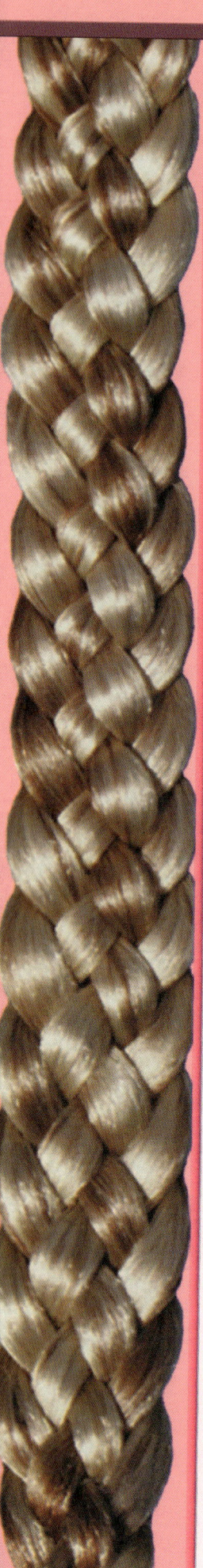

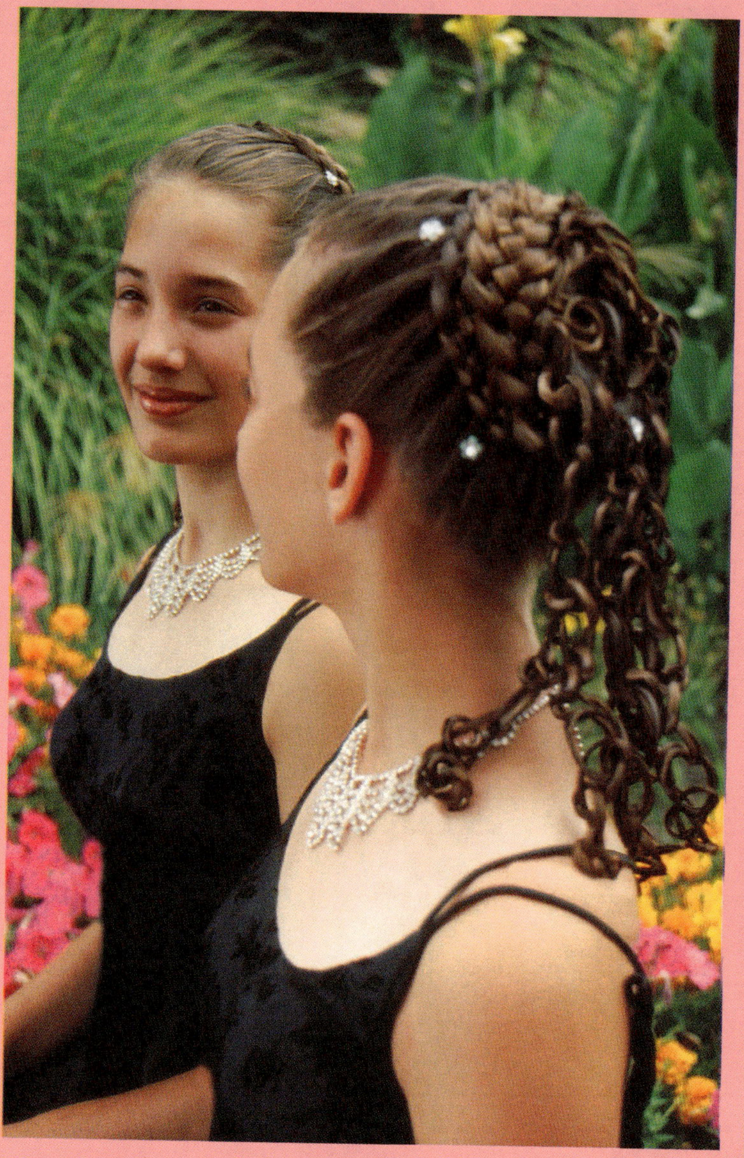

The good thing is you have five fingers, one for each strand. This braid is possible with a little perseverance. After you learn it you will enjoy it.

Five-Strand

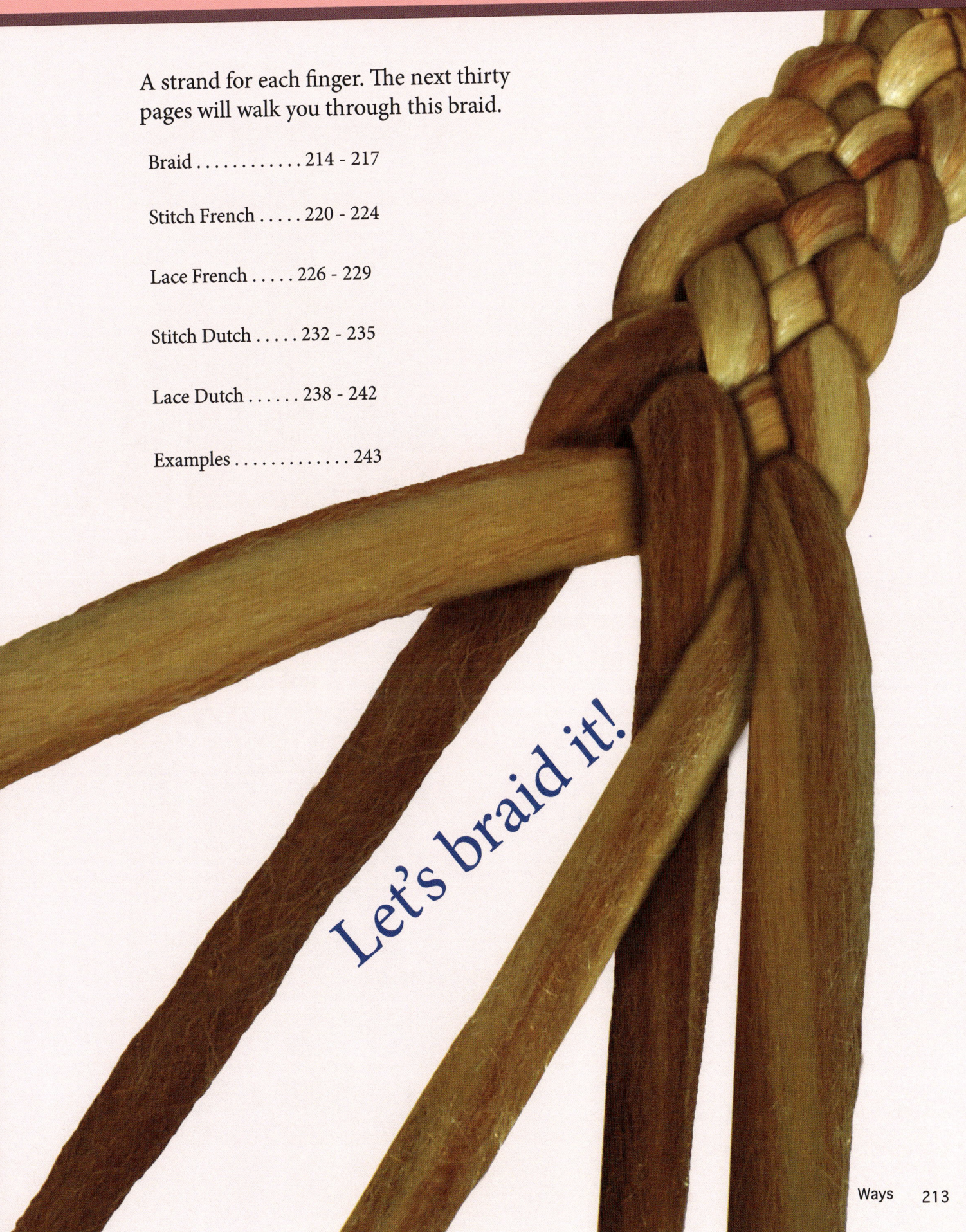

A strand for each finger. The next thirty pages will walk you through this braid.

Braid . . . . 214 - 217

Stitch French . . . . . 220 - 224

Lace French . . . . . 226 - 229

Stitch Dutch . . . . . 232 - 235

Lace Dutch . . . . . . 238 - 242

Examples 243

Let's braid it!

Five-Strand Braid

Attitude, not aptitude, determines altitude. - Jesse Jackson

1.

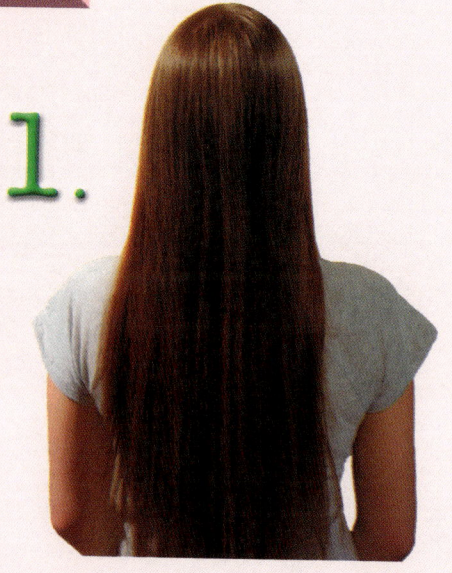

Begin with clean, brushed hair.

2.

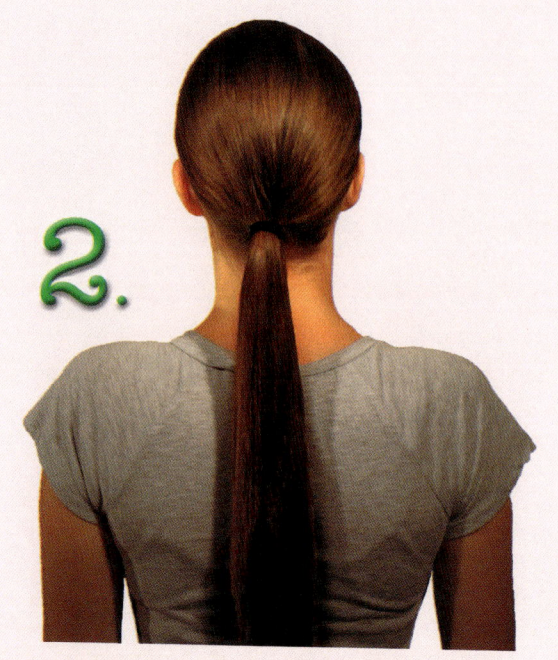

Take a section of hair.

5.

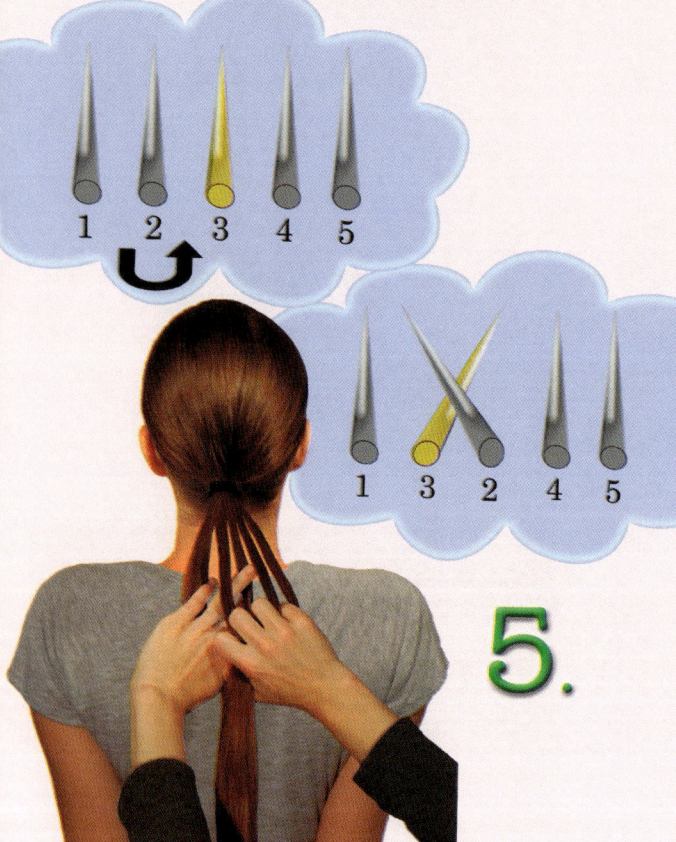

Reach under strand 2 and hook strand 3 with the ring finger.

6.

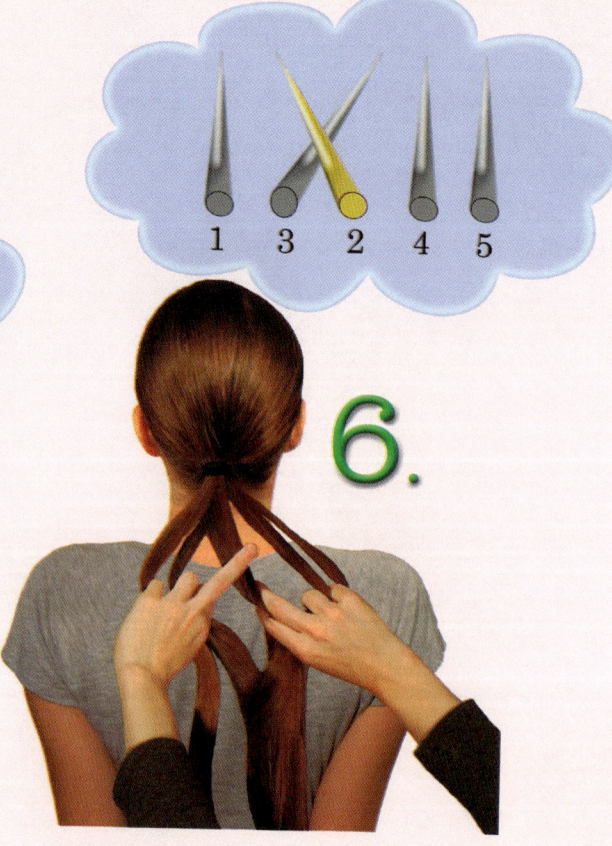

Grab strand 2 with the middle finger.

214   www.findingbraids.com

Five-Strand Braid

5

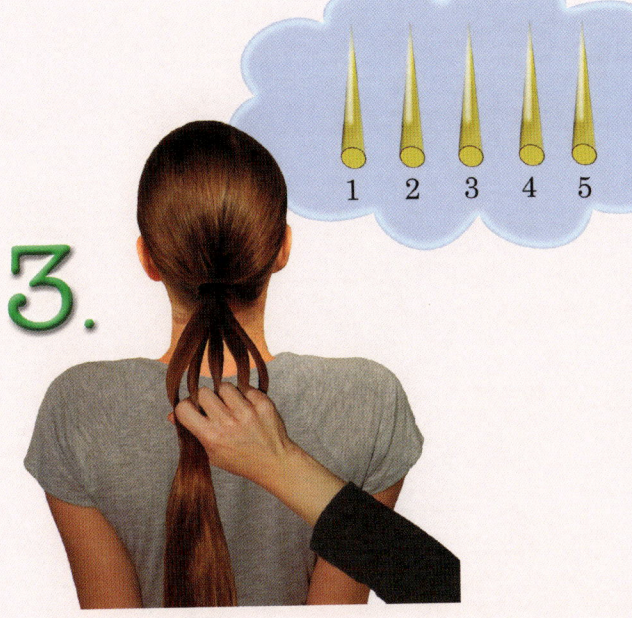

3.

Divide the section into five strands.

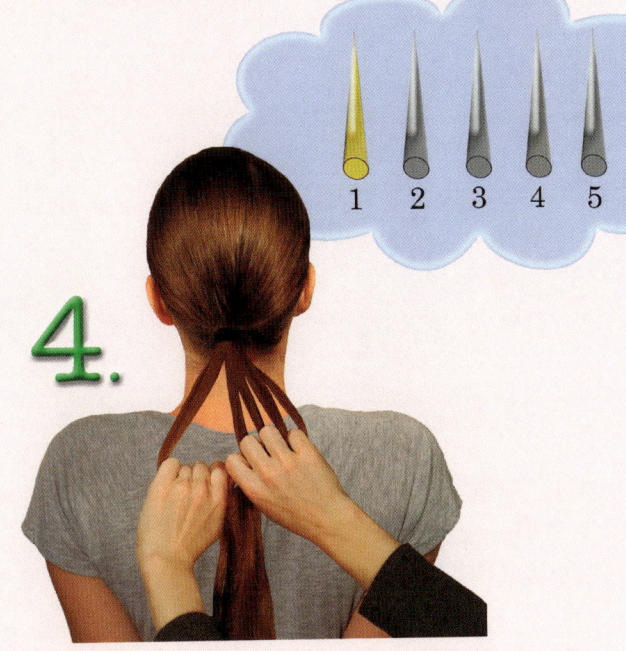

4.

Start braiding by grabbing strand 1 with your palm down and your thumb facing your belly button.

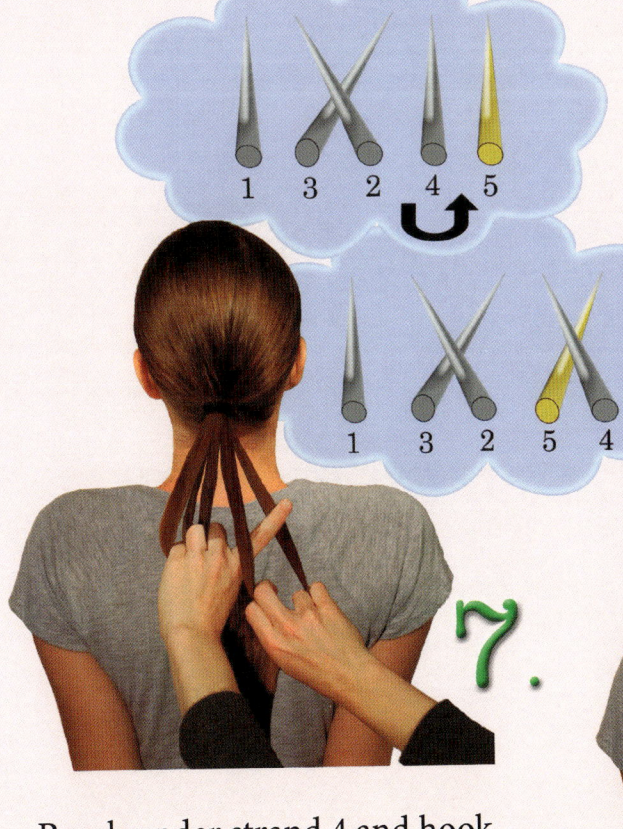

7.

Reach under strand 4 and hook strand 5 with the pointer finger.

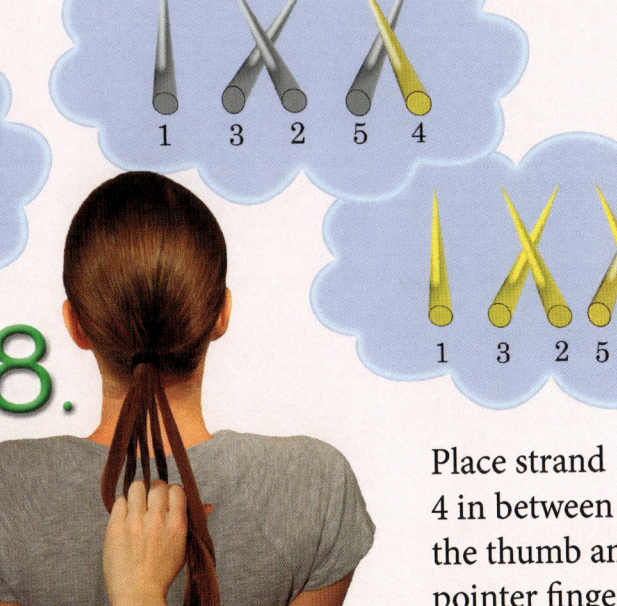

8.

Place strand 4 in between the thumb and pointer finger.

Continuing

5

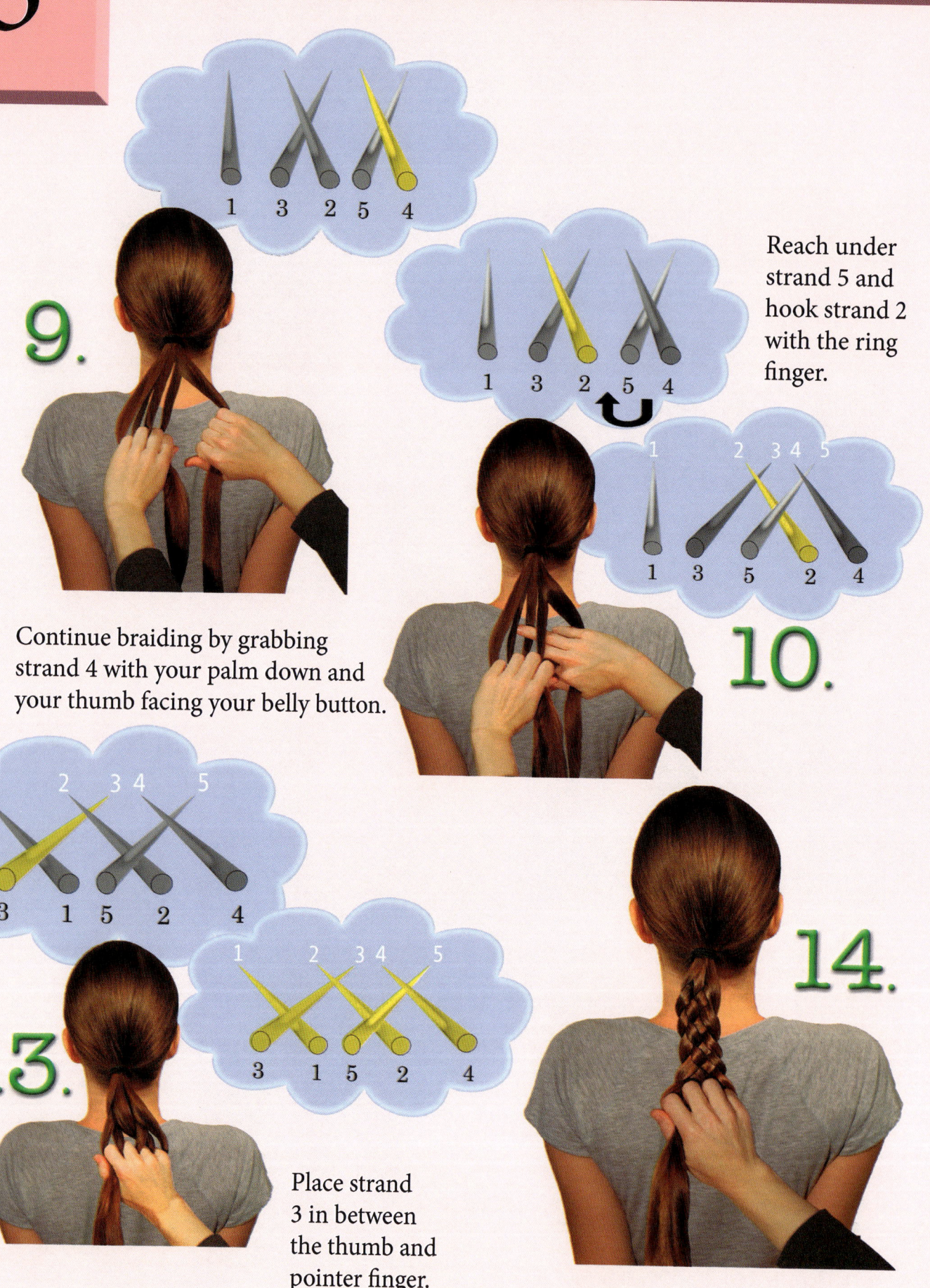

9. Continue braiding by grabbing strand 4 with your palm down and your thumb facing your belly button.

10. Reach under strand 5 and hook strand 2 with the ring finger.

13. Place strand 3 in between the thumb and pointer finger.

14. Continue weaving until the end of the hair.

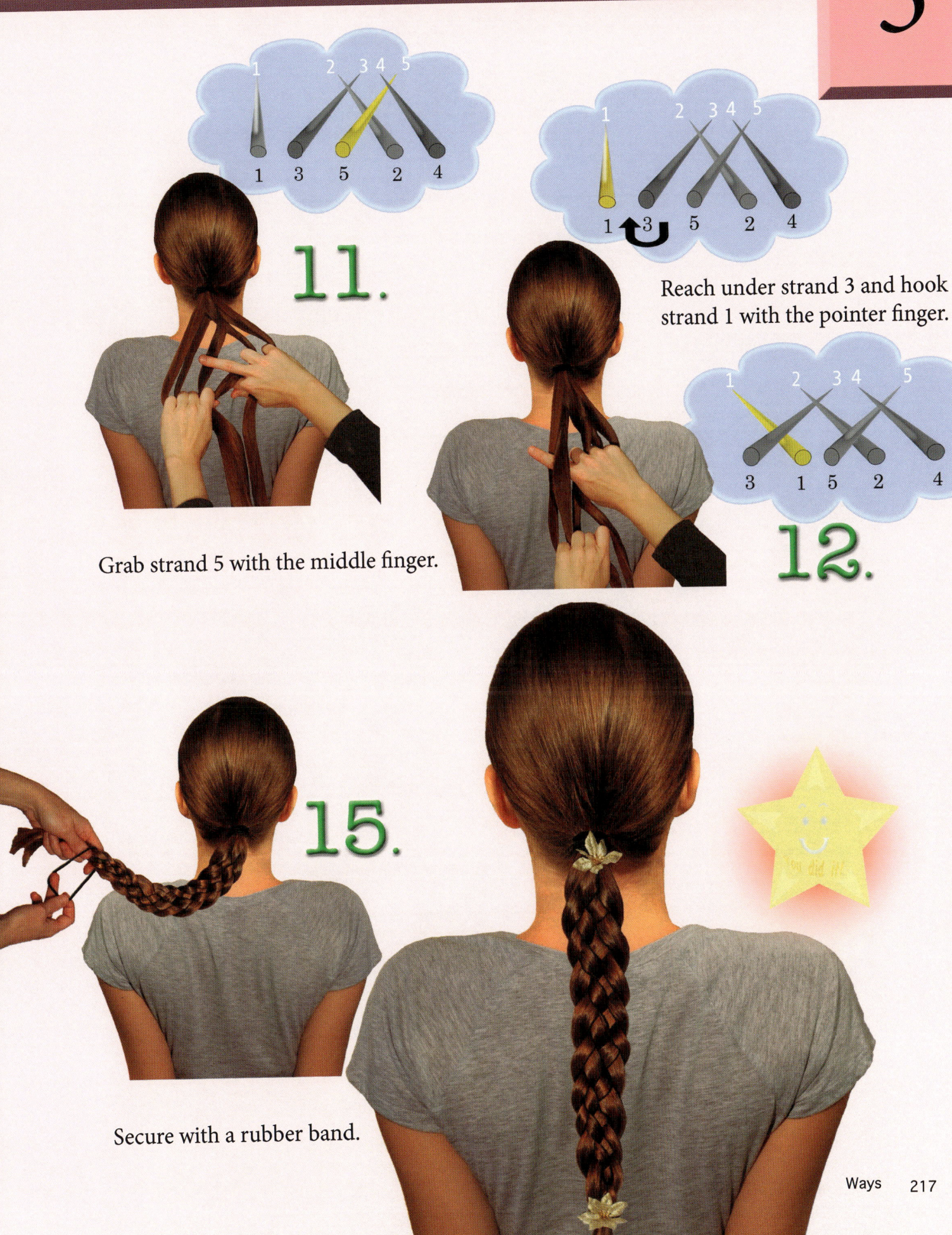

Five-Strand

Notes

Five-Strand

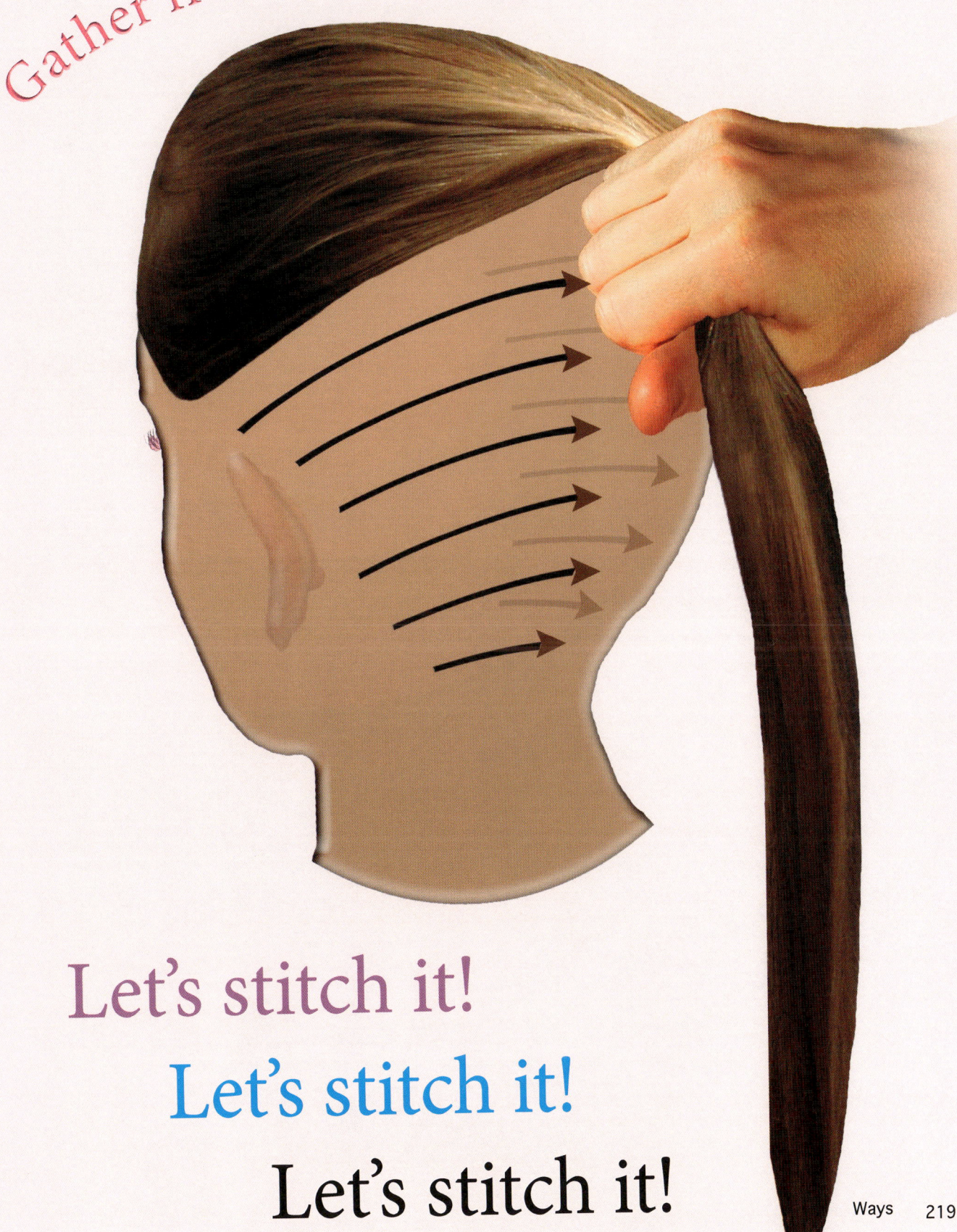

Gather from both sides

Let's stitch it!
Let's stitch it!
Let's stitch it!

5 Five-Strand French Stitch

You can always do more than you think you can. -John Wooden

1. Begin with clean, brushed hair.

2. Take a section of hair as illustrated.

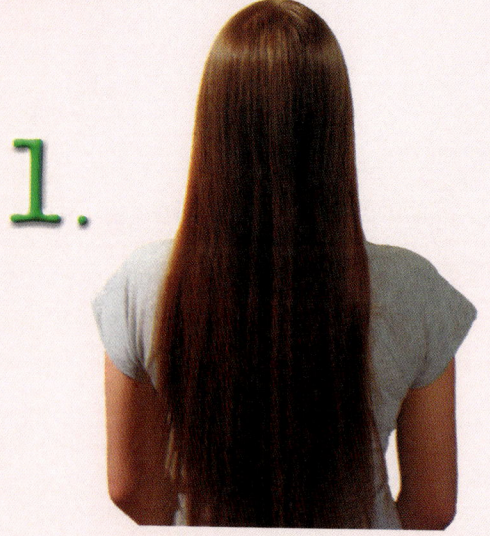

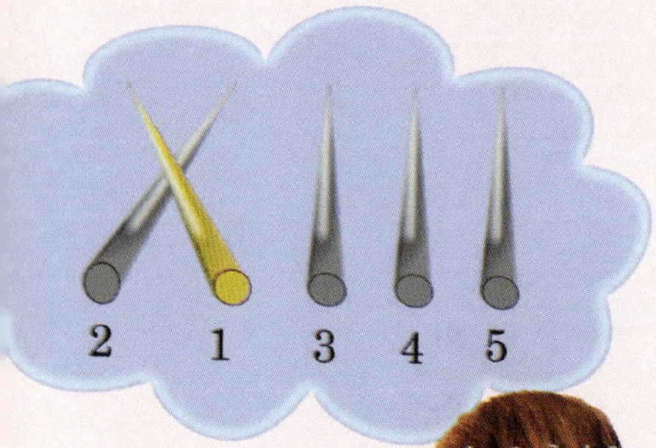

5. 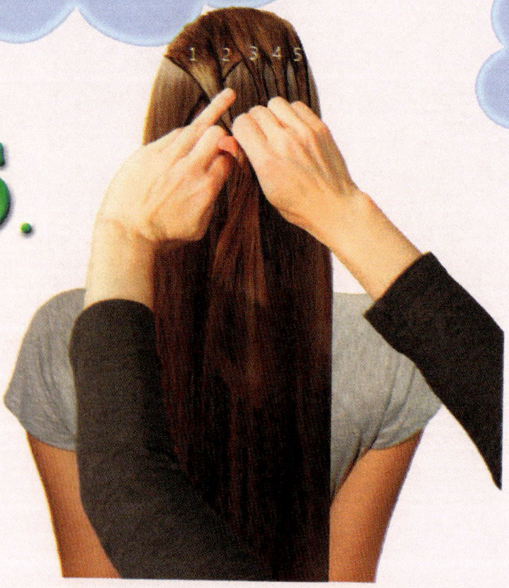 Grab strand 1 with the ring finger.

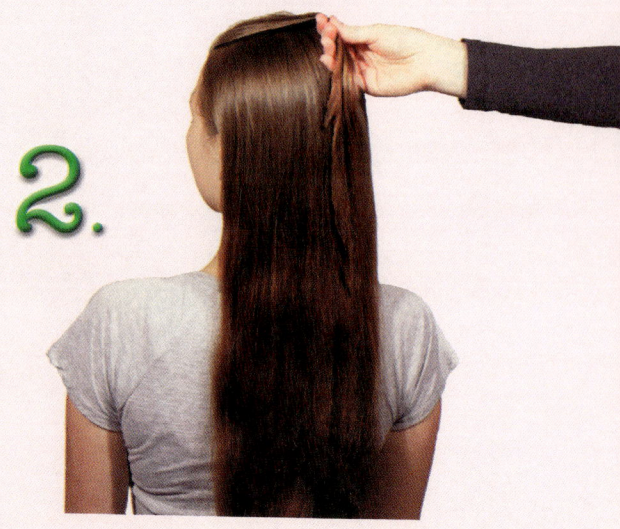

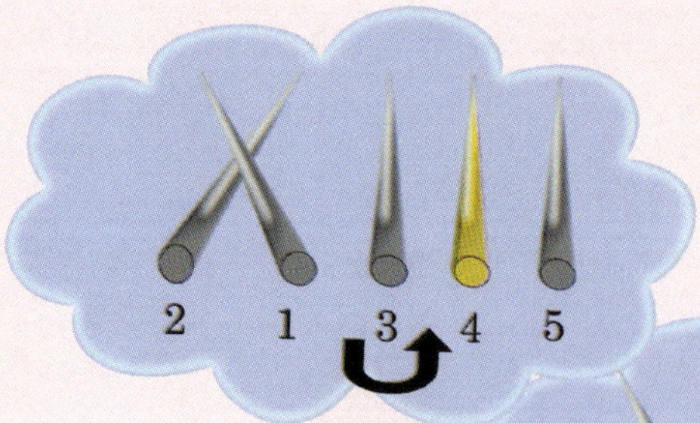

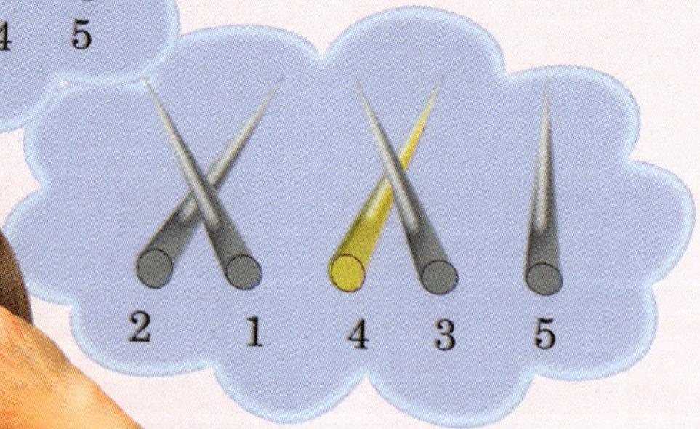

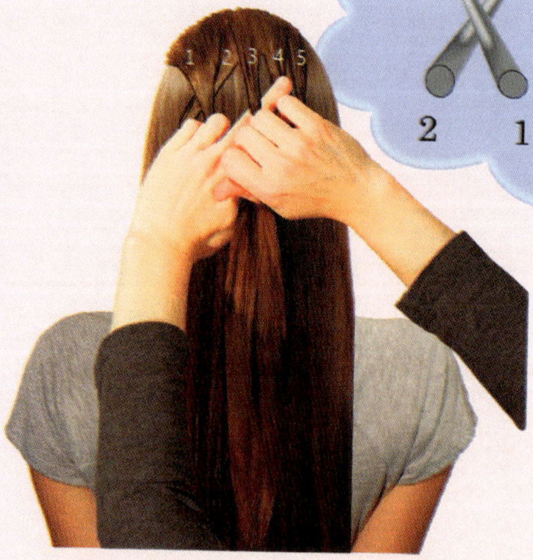

6. Reach under strand 3 and hook strand 4 with the middle finger.

Five-Strand French Stitch

5

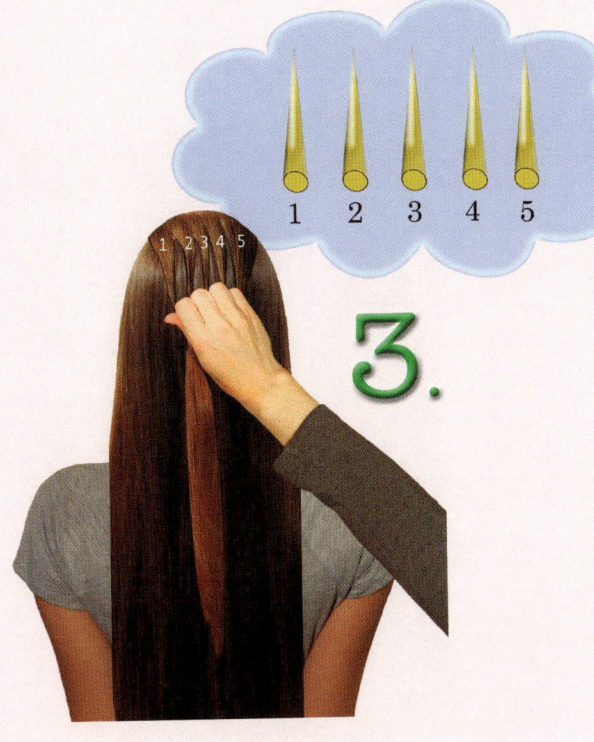

3.

Divide the section into five strands.

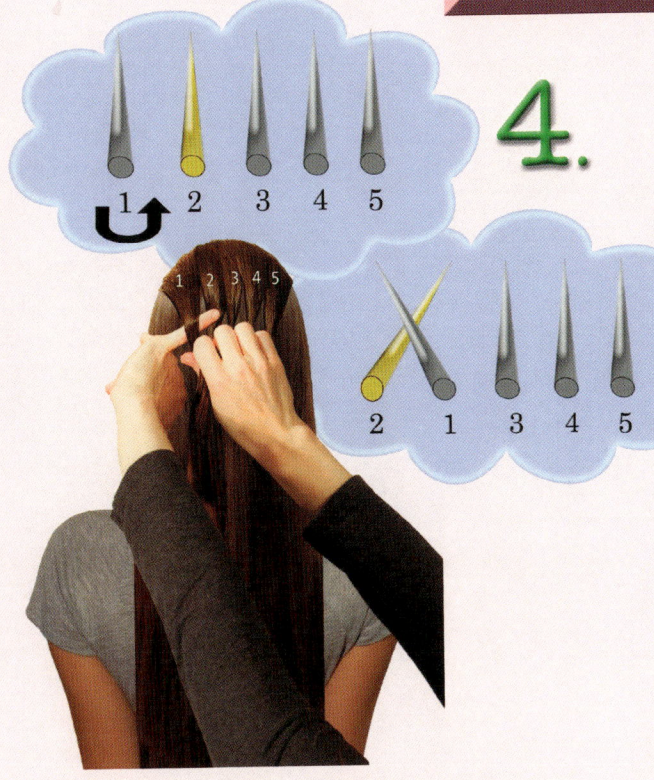

4.

Reach under strand 1 and hook strand 2 with the pinky finger.

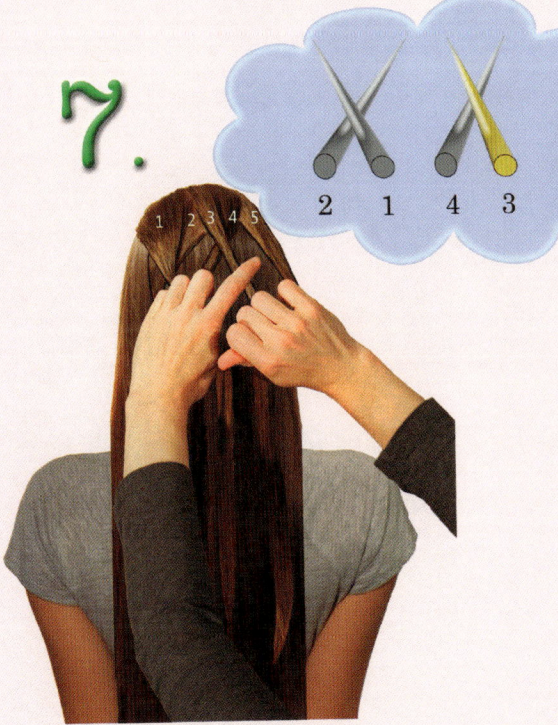

7.

Grab strand 3 with the pointer finger.

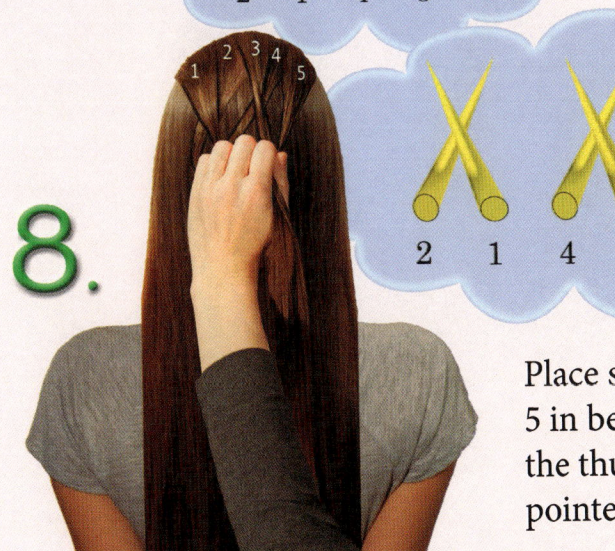

8.

Place strand 5 in between the thumb and pointer finger.

Ways

5. Continuing

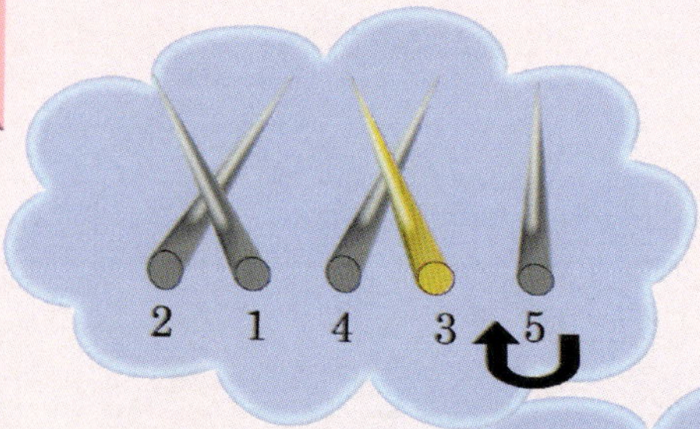

9. Reach under strand 5 and hook strand 3 with the pinky finger.

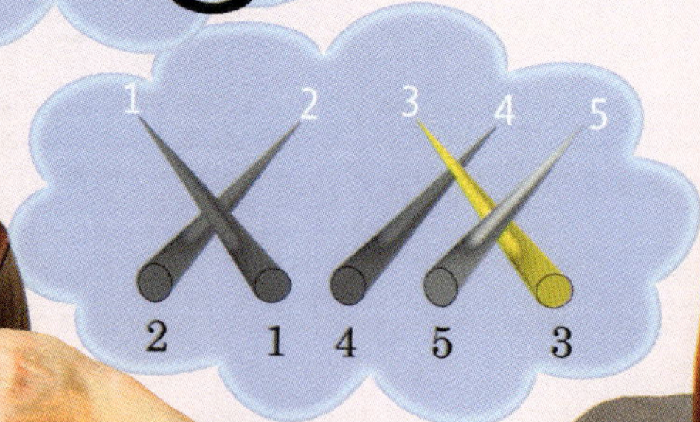

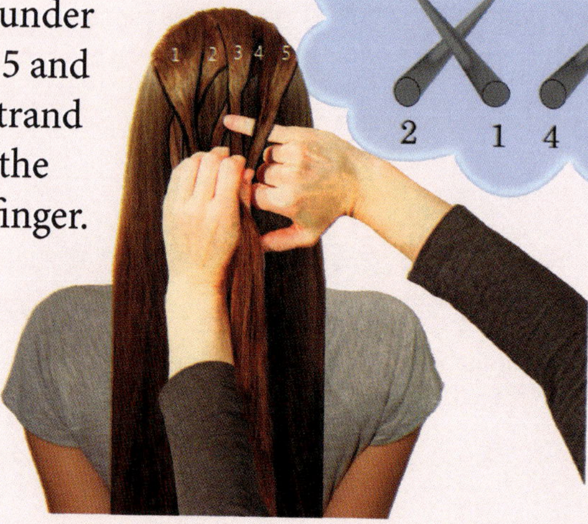

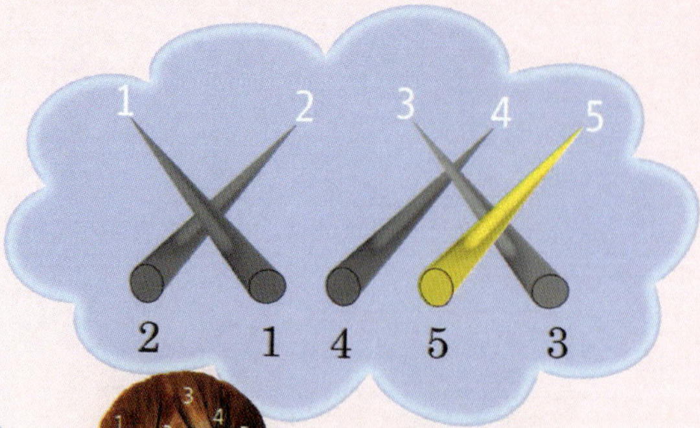

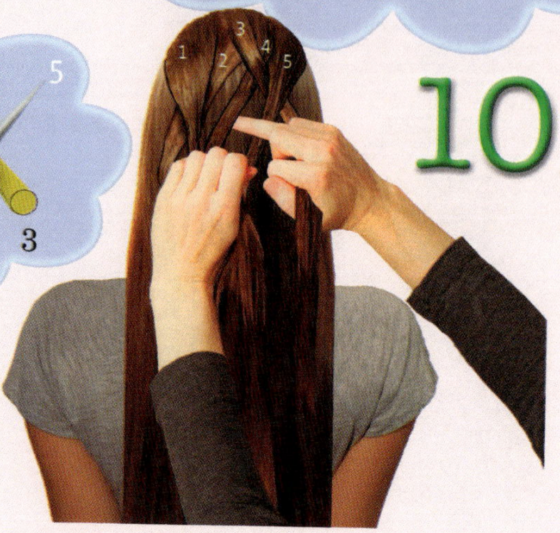

10. Grab strand 5 with the ring finger.

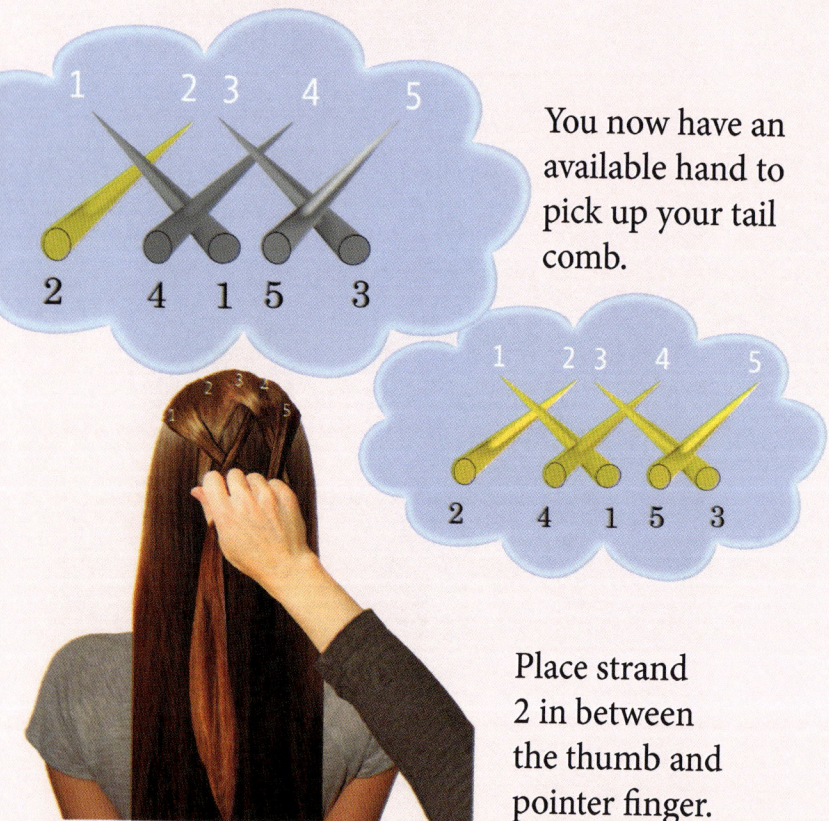

You now have an available hand to pick up your tail comb.

13. Place strand 2 in between the thumb and pointer finger.

14. Number your strands at your knuckles now. Sliver off a gather from the face all the way back to the braid.

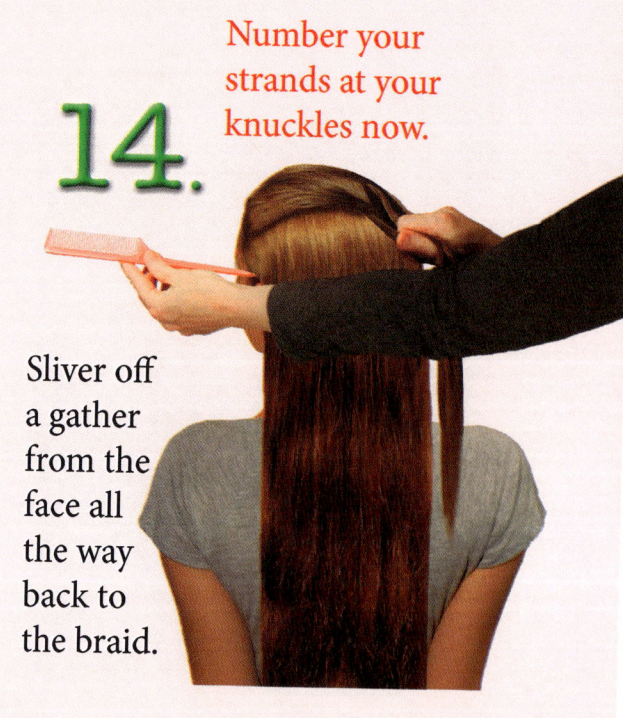

part 2. Five-Strand French Stitch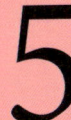

11. Reach under strand 4 and hook strand 1 with the middle finger.

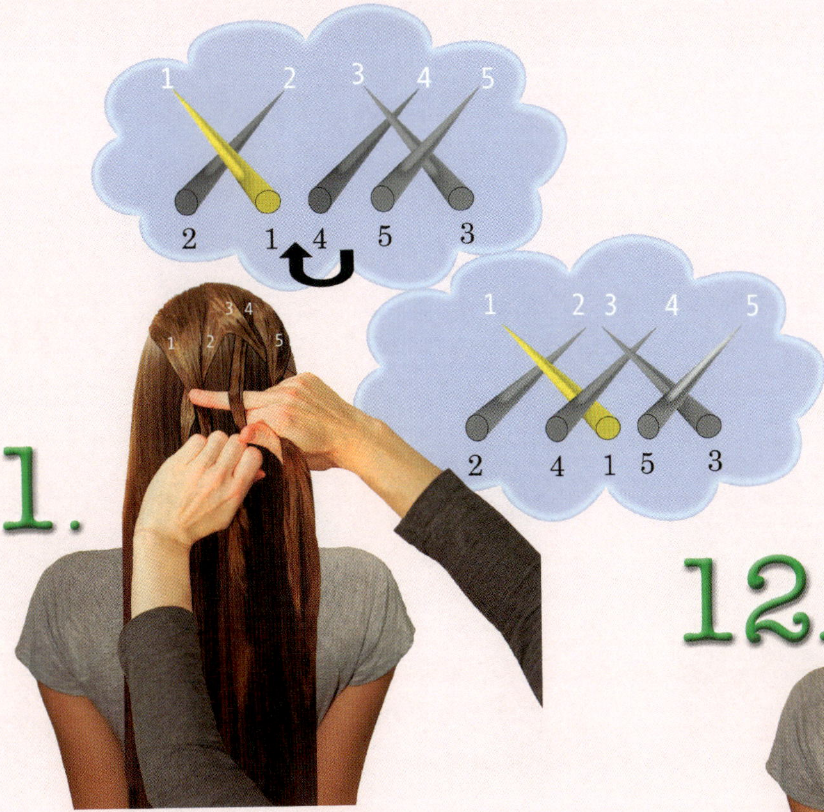

12. Grab strand 4 with the pointer finger.

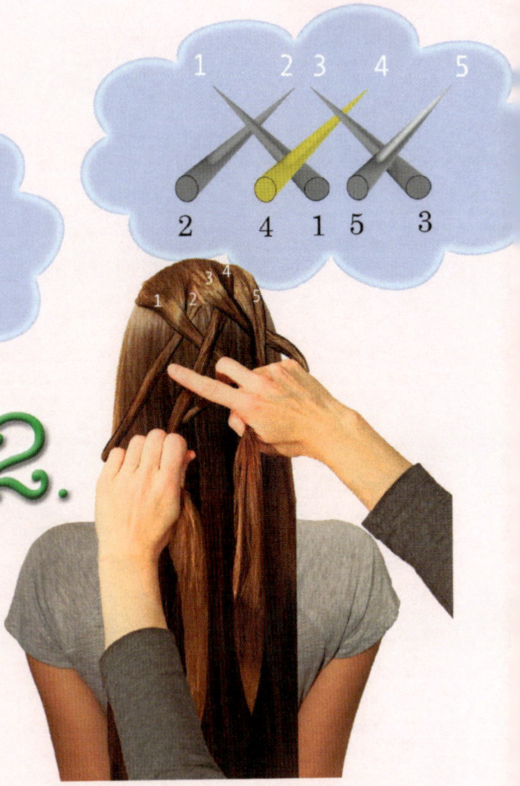

15. French gathers are placed in strand 1.

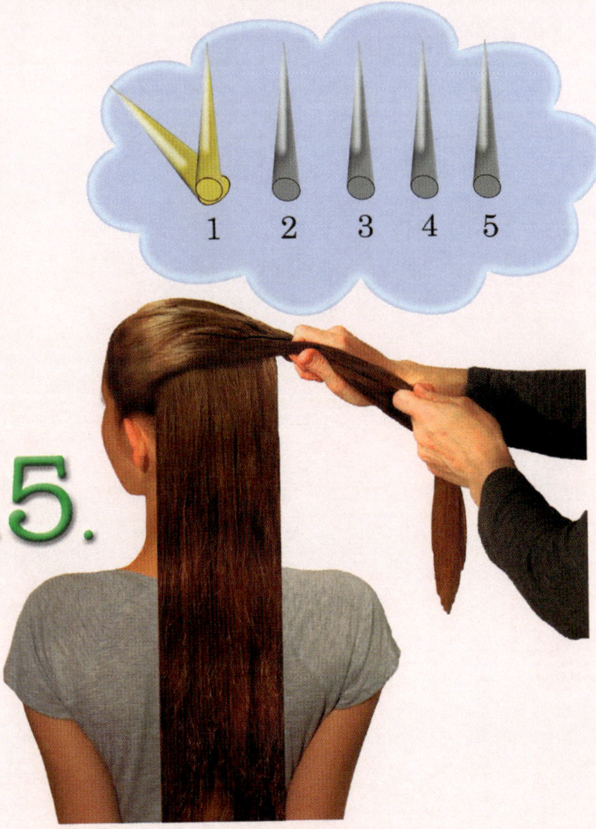

16. Weave back the other direction.

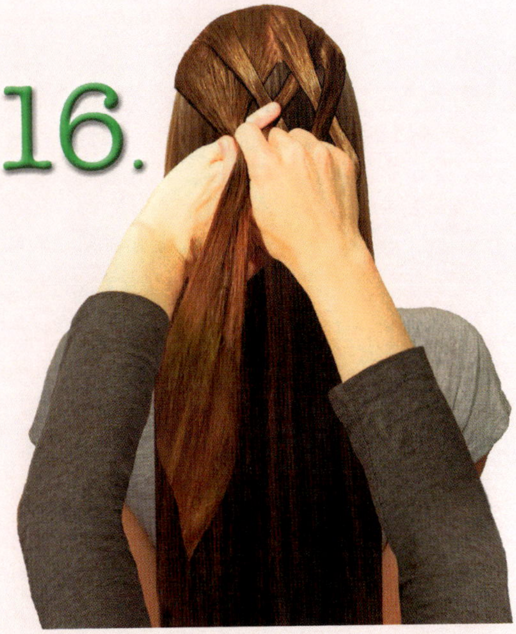

5 part 3. Five-Strand French Stitch

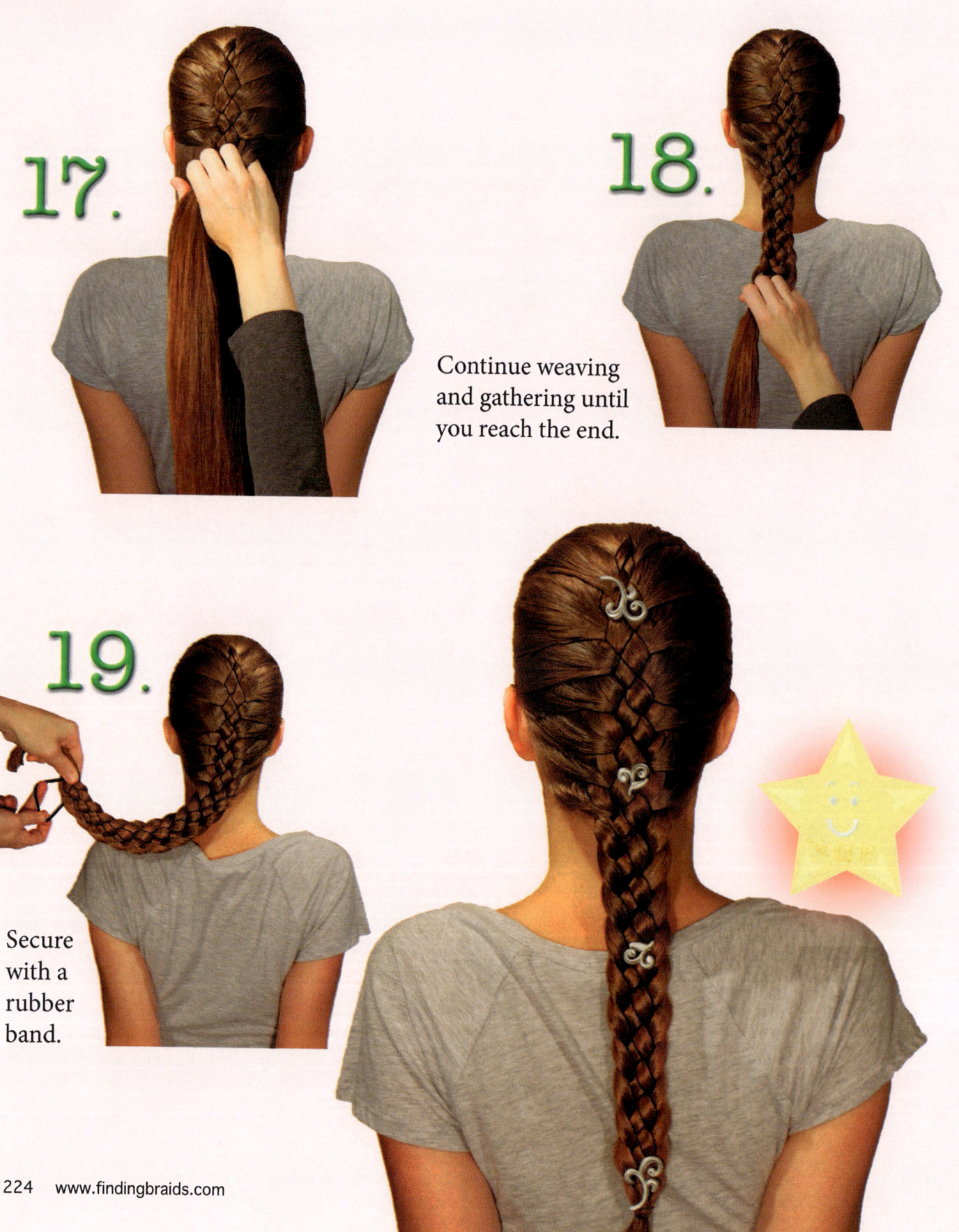

17.

18. Continue weaving and gathering until you reach the end.

19. Secure with a rubber band.

Five-Strand

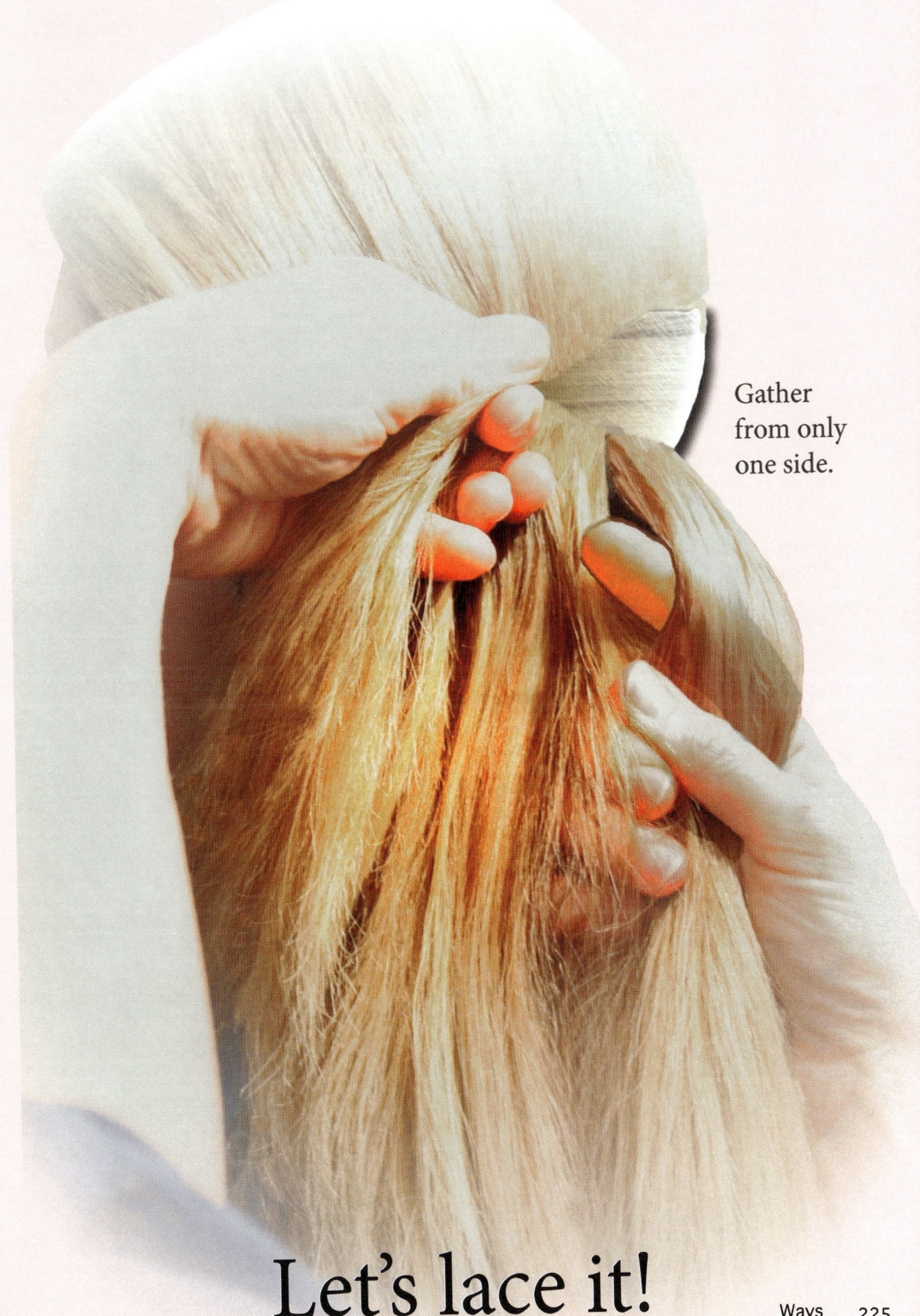

Gather from only one side.

Let's lace it!

5 Five-Strand French Lace

Every accomplishment starts with the decision to keep trying.

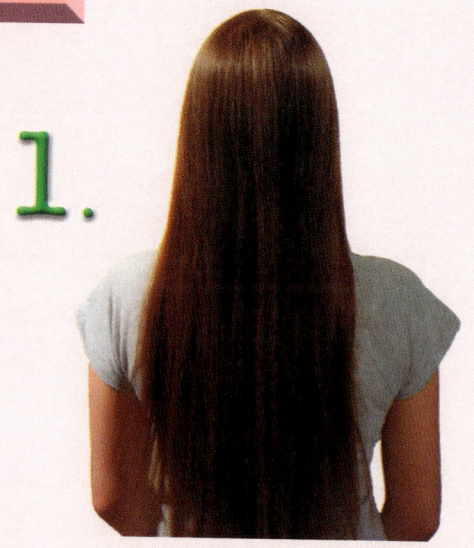

1. Begin with clean, brushed hair.

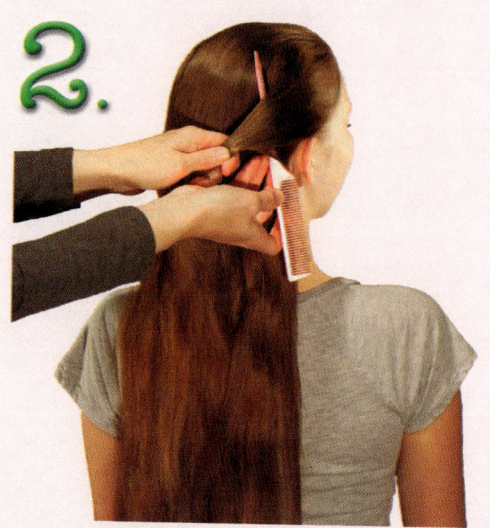

2. Take a section of hair as illustrated.

5. Grab strand 1 with the ring finger.

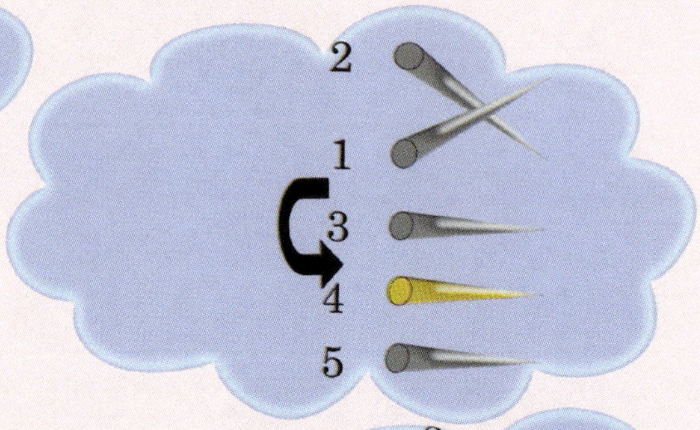

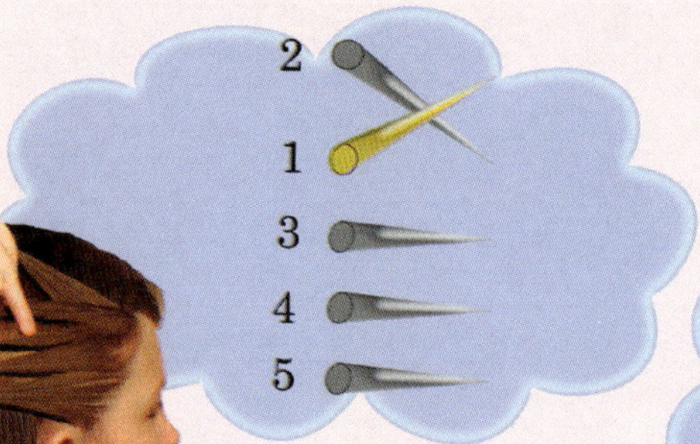

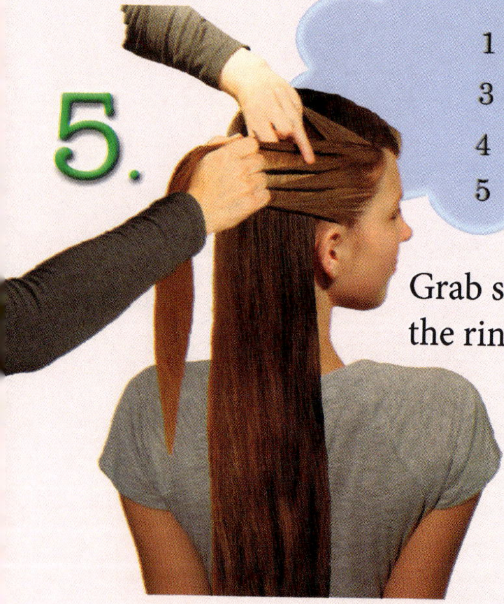

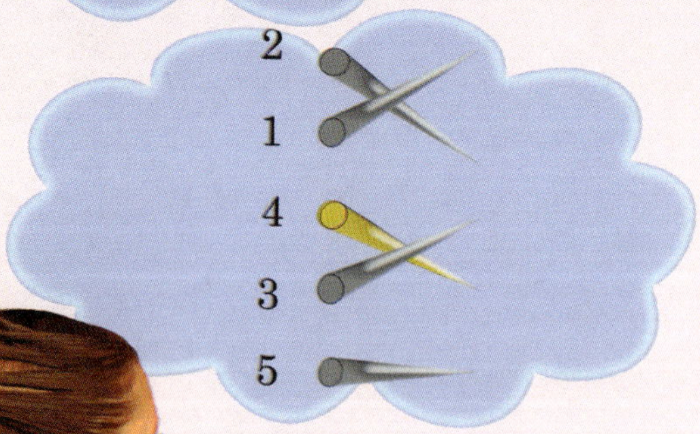

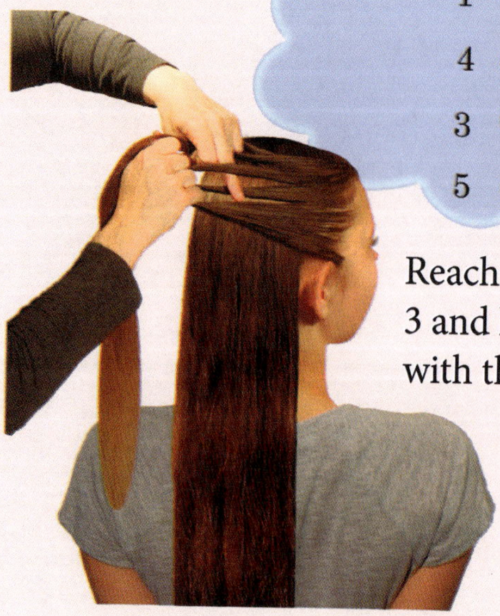

6. Reach under strand 3 and hook strand 4 with the middle finger.

226   www.findingbraids.com

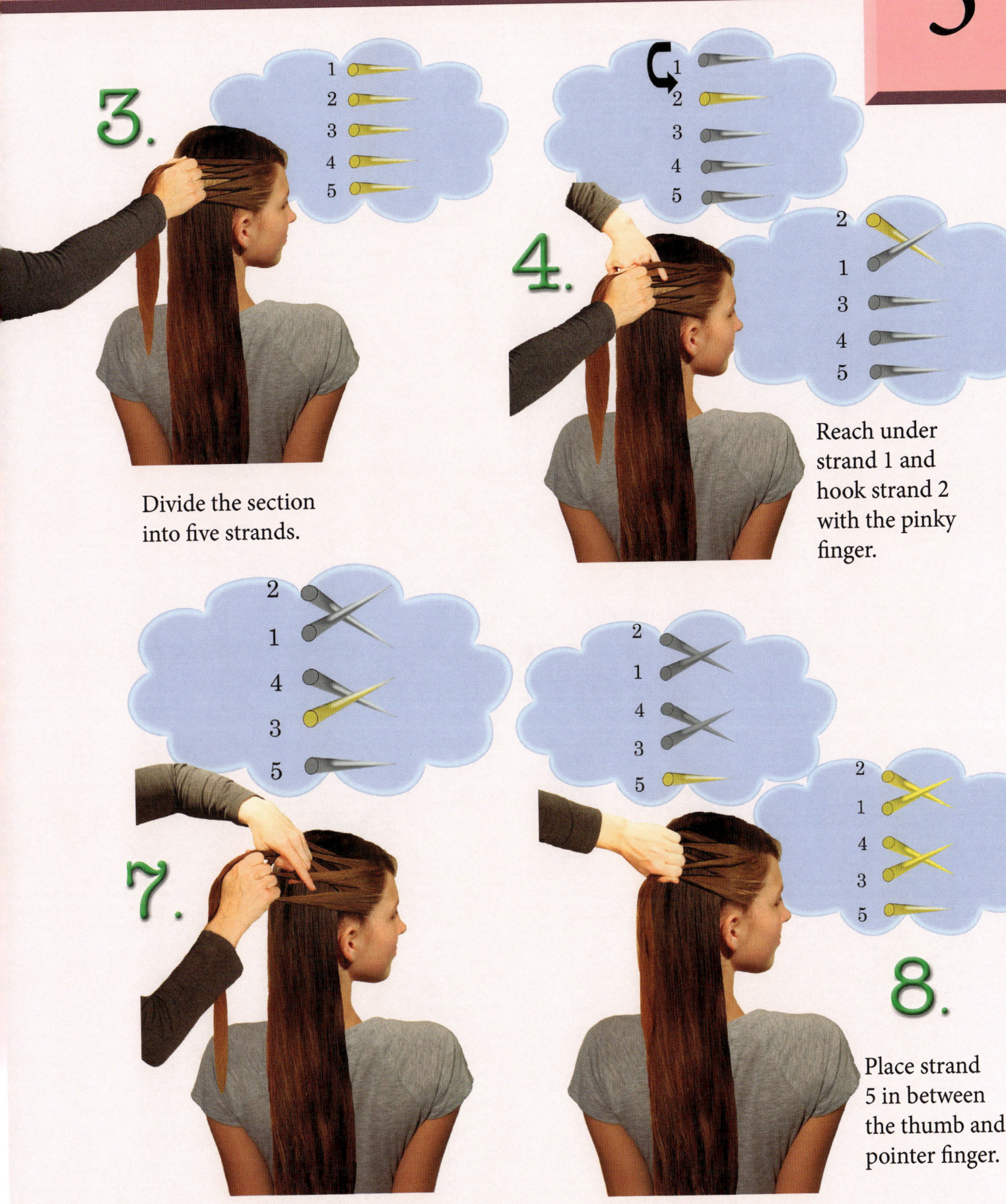

5 Continuing

9. Repeat the weave going the opposite direction as well. Then, repeat again and you will be ready to gather.

10. Sliver off a gather from the face all the way back to the braid.

French gathers are placed in strand 1.

13. Secure with a rubber band.

14. Fix the end of the tail with bobby pins to hold the braid in place.

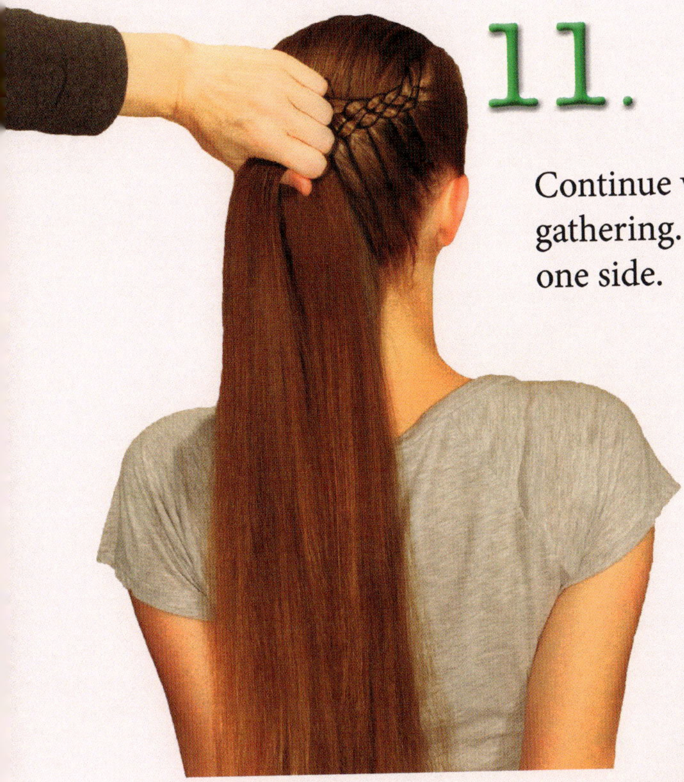

part 2. Five-Strand French Lace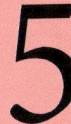

11.

Continue weaving and gathering. Gather from only one side.

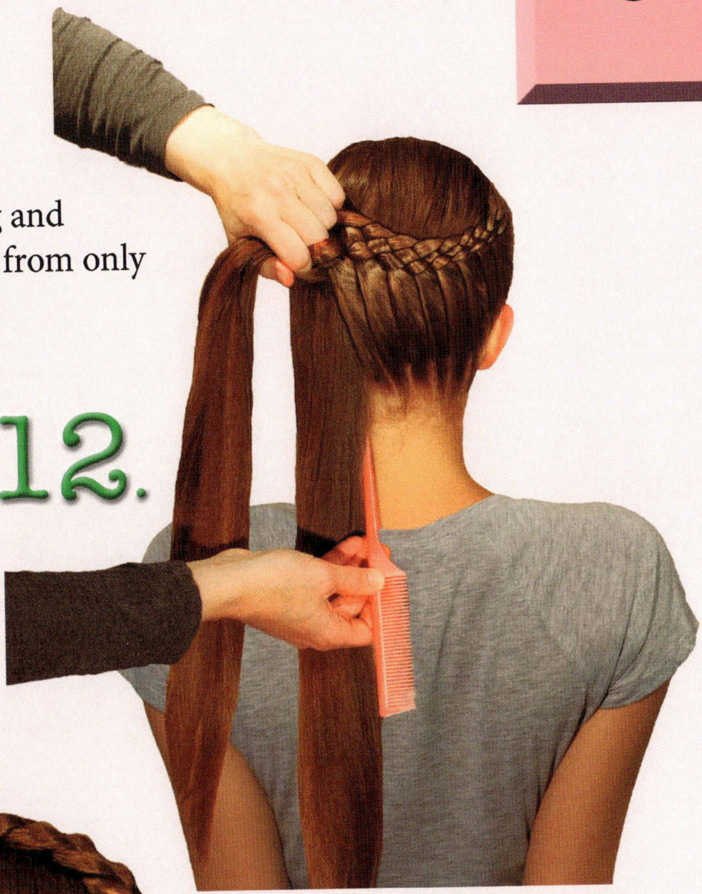

12.

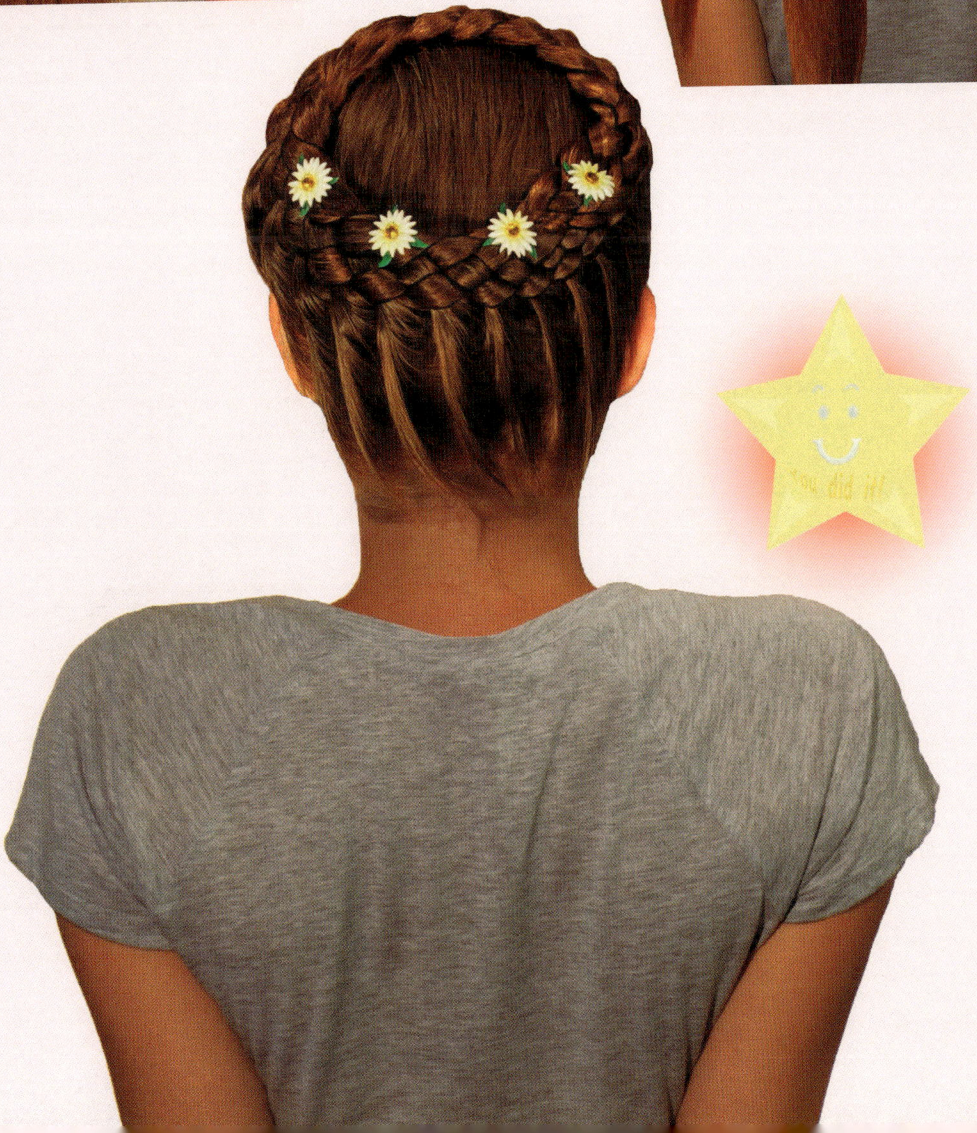

Five-Strand

Notes

Five-Strand

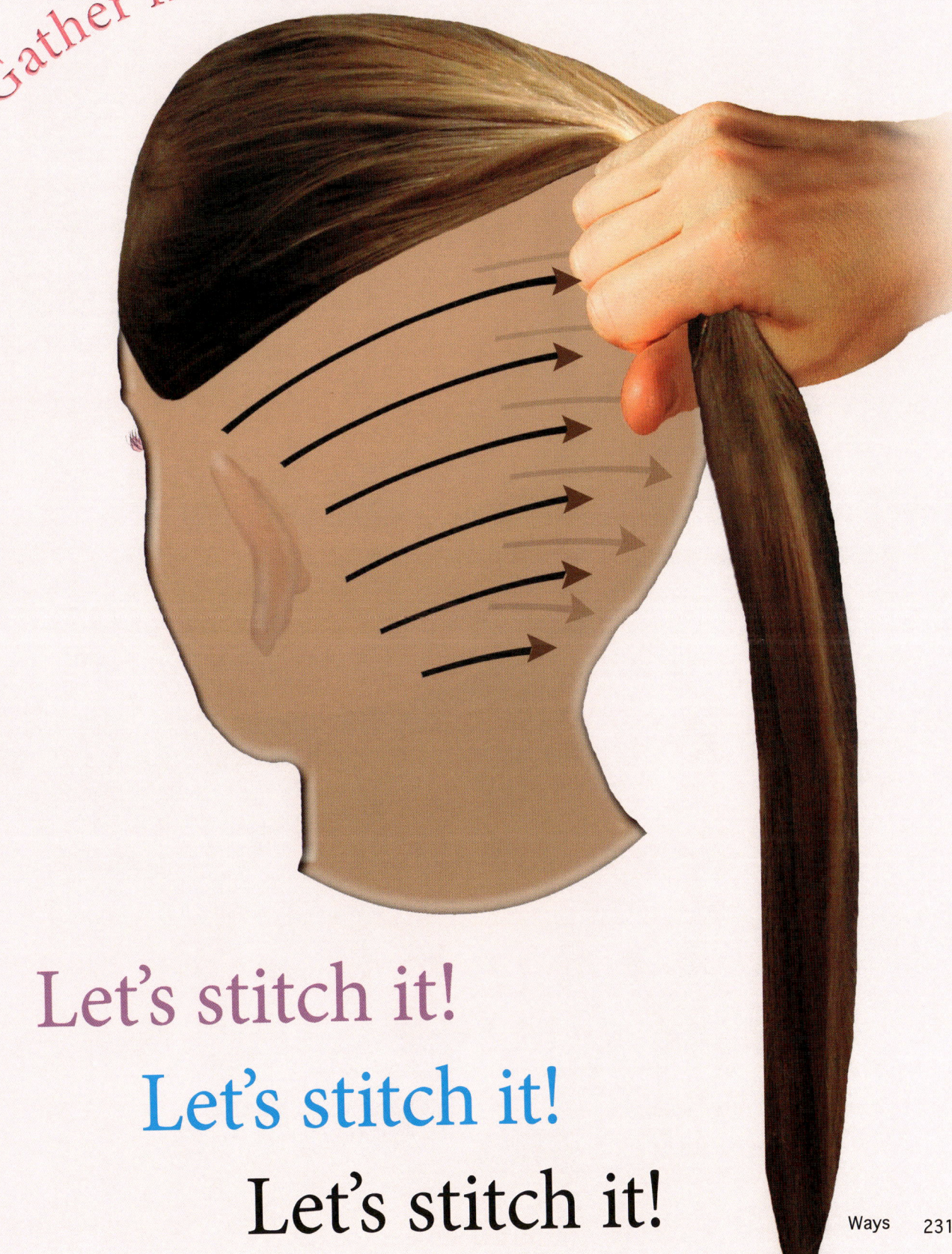

Gather from both sides

Let's stitch it!

Let's stitch it!

Let's stitch it!

5 Five-Strand Dutch Stitch

Make mistakes, but don't quit. - Conrad Hilton

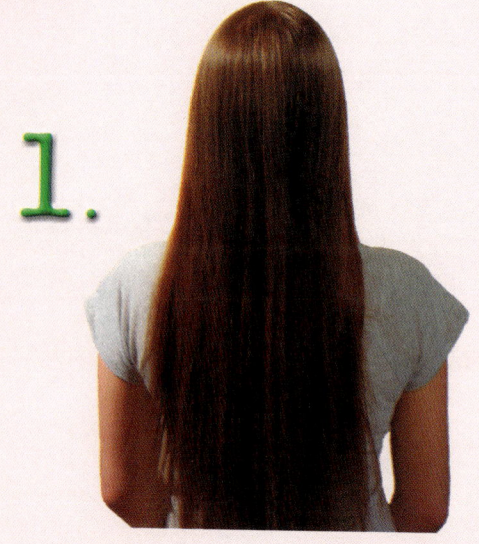

1. Begin with clean, brushed hair.

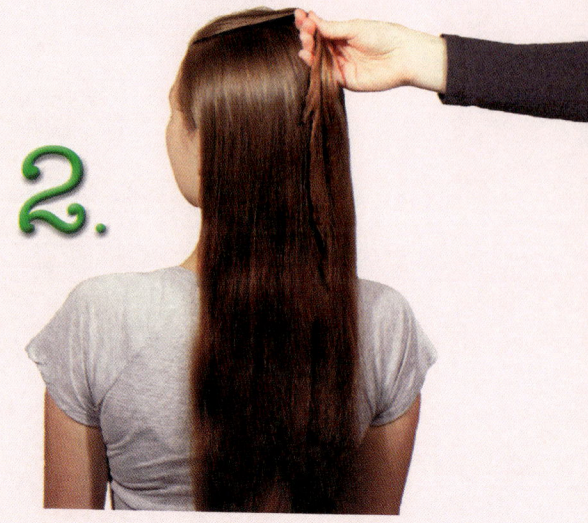

2. Take a section of hair as illustrated.

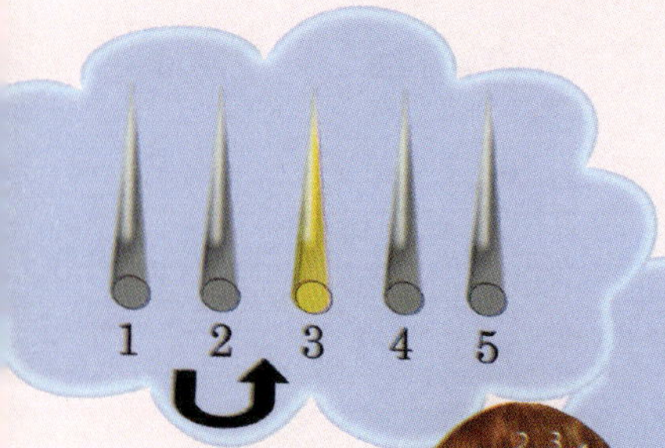

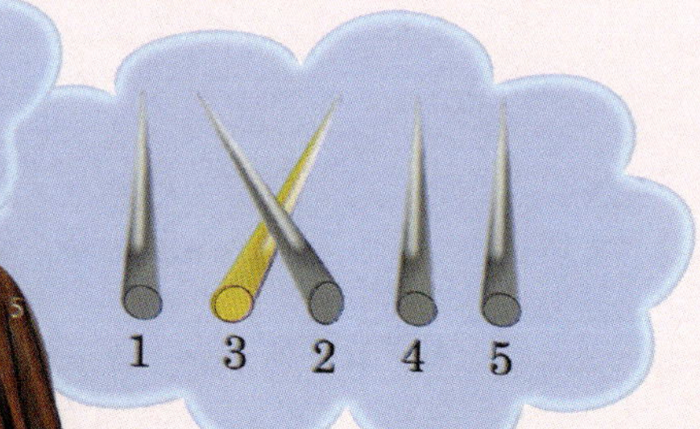

5. 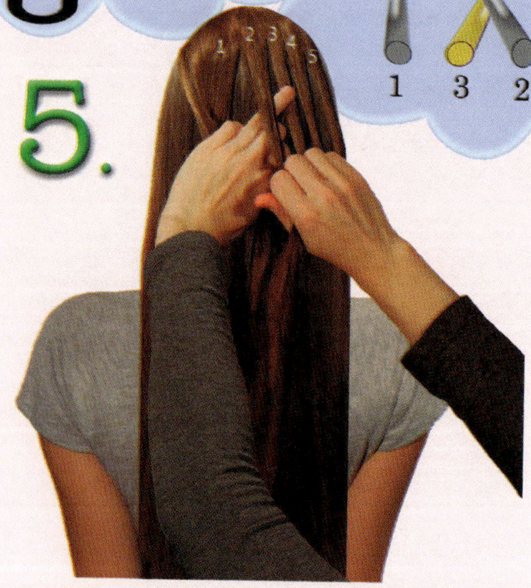 Reach under strand 2 and hook strand 3 with the ring finger.

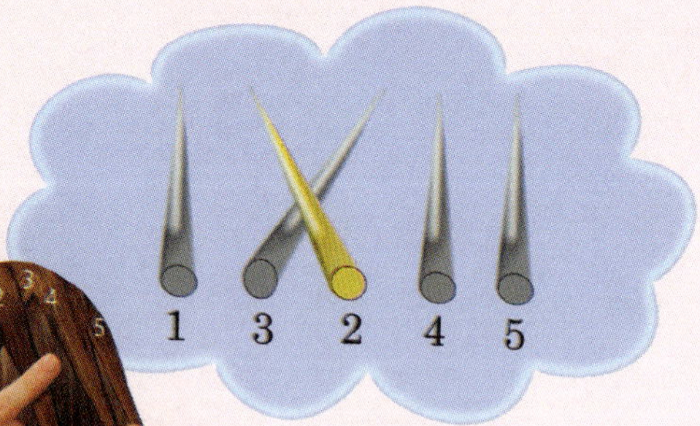

6. 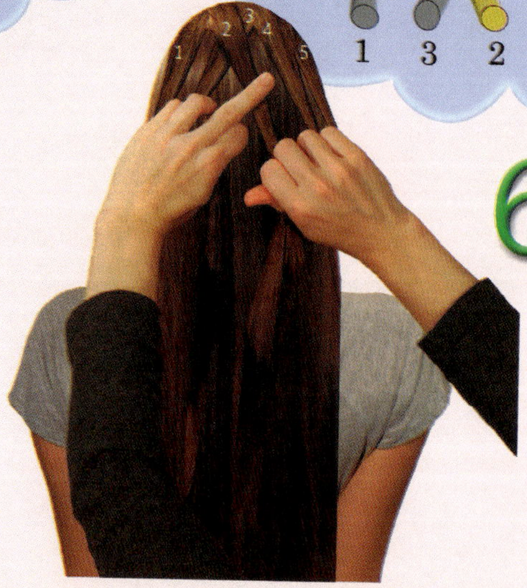 Grab strand 2 with the middle finger.

Five-Strand Dutch Stitch

5

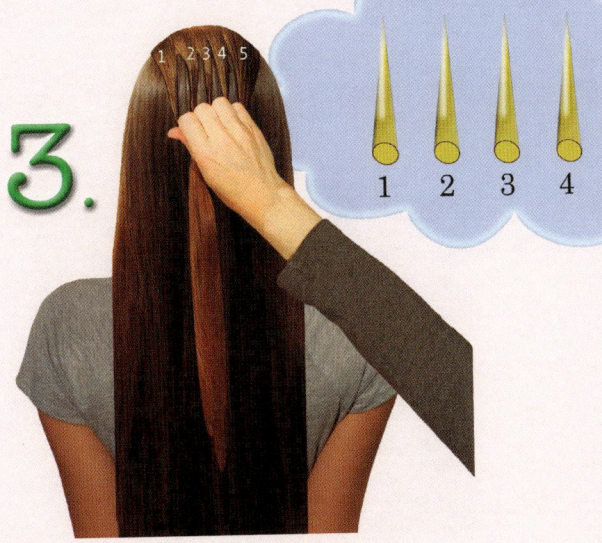

3. Divide the section into five strands.

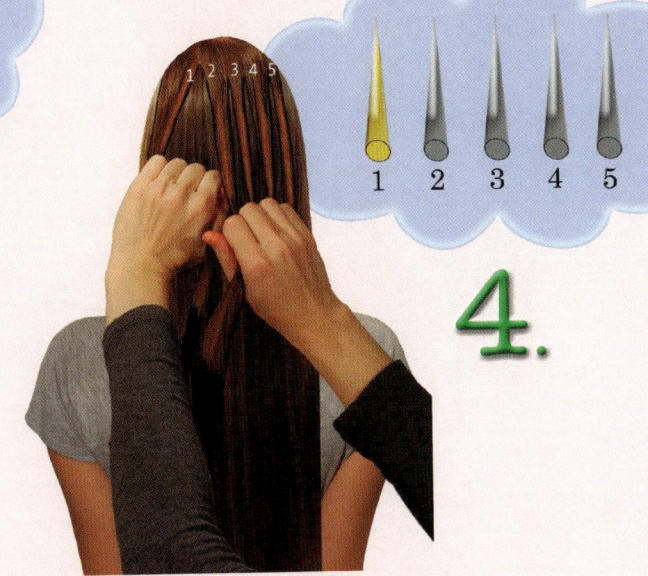

4. Start braiding by grabbing strand 1 with your palm down and your thumb facing your belly button.

7. Reach under strand 4 and hook strand 5 with the pointer finger.

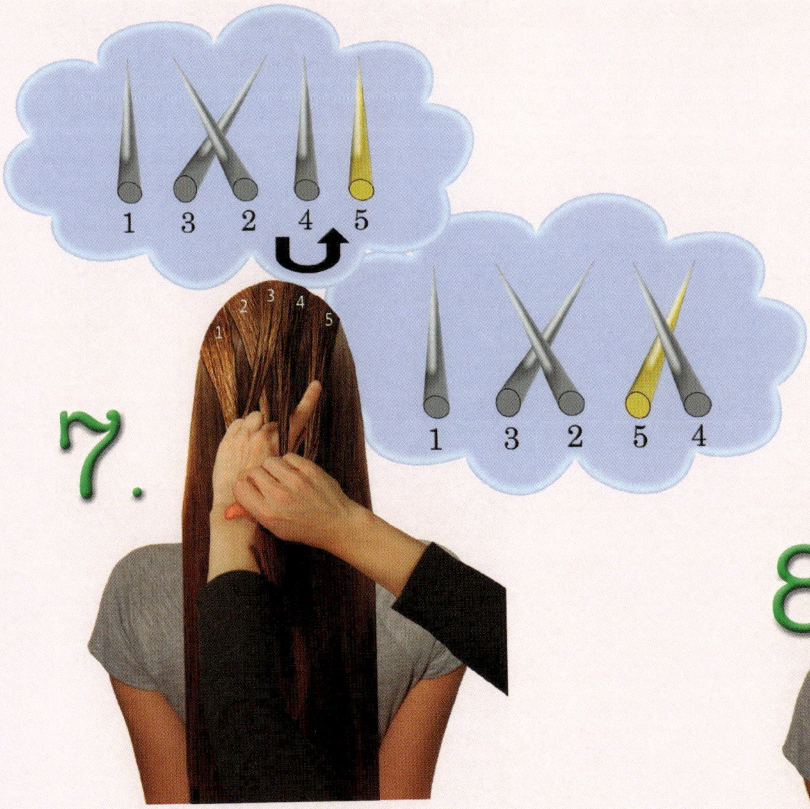

8. Place strand 4 in between the thumb and pointer finger.

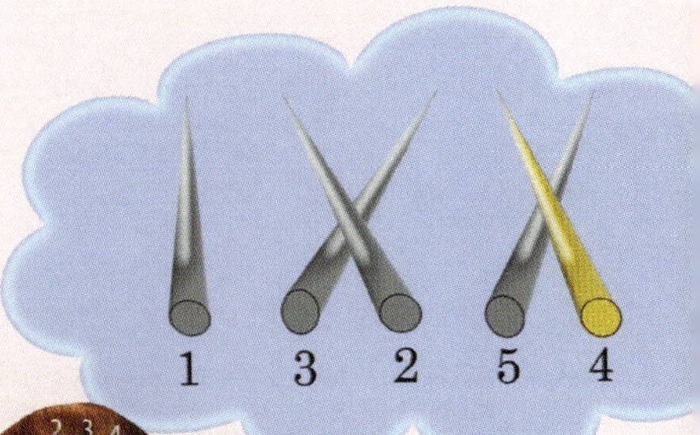

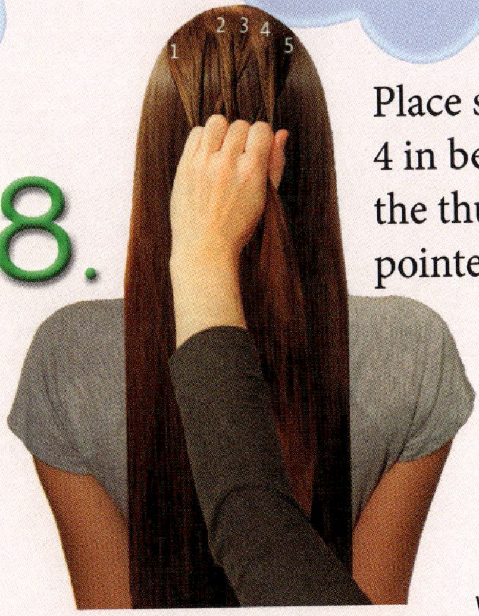

Ways 233

5 Continuing

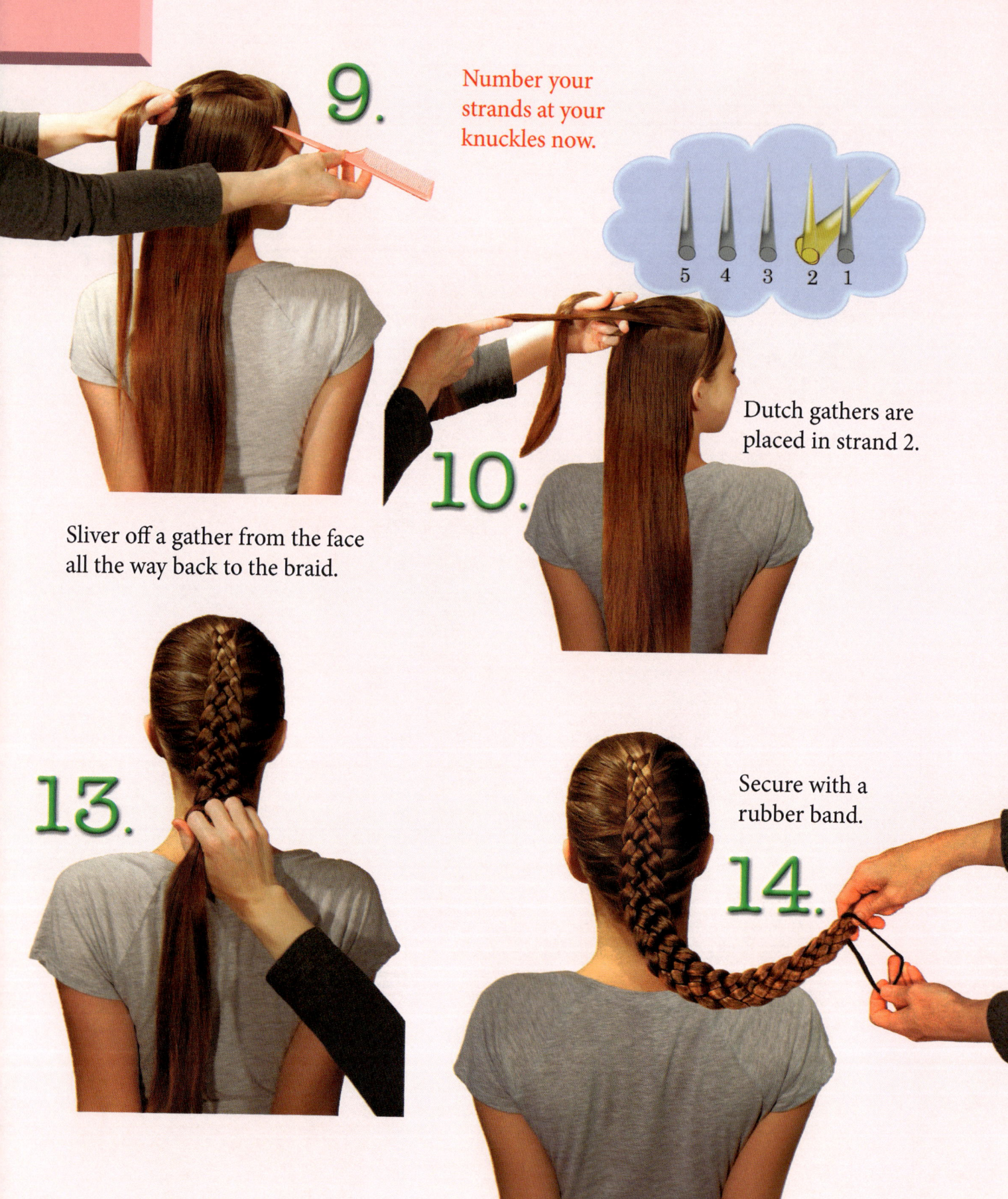

9. Sliver off a gather from the face all the way back to the braid.

Number your strands at your knuckles now.

10. Dutch gathers are placed in strand 2.

13.

14. Secure with a rubber band.

part 2. Five-Strand Dutch Stitch

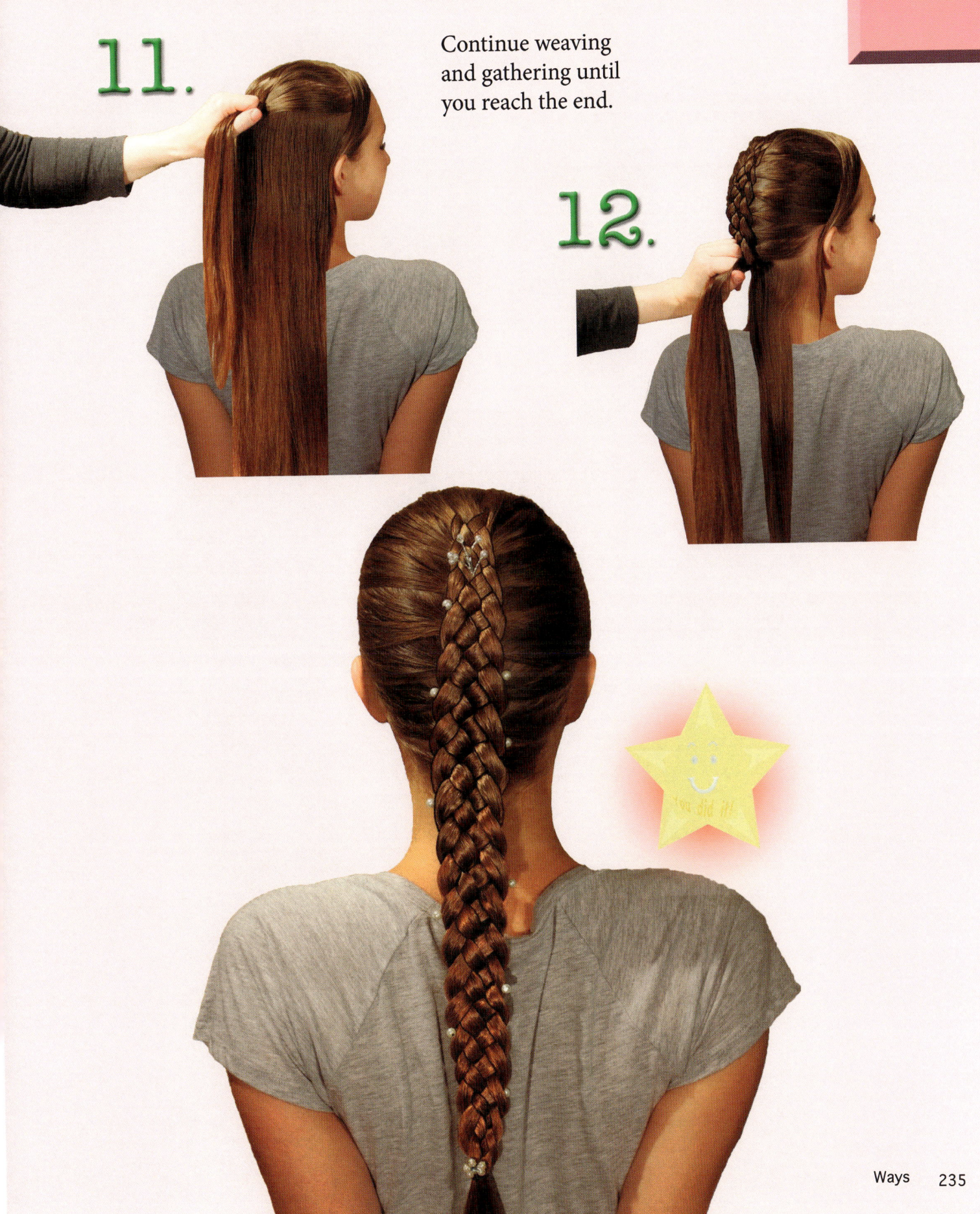

11.

Continue weaving and gathering until you reach the end.

12.

Five-Strand

Notes

Five-Strand

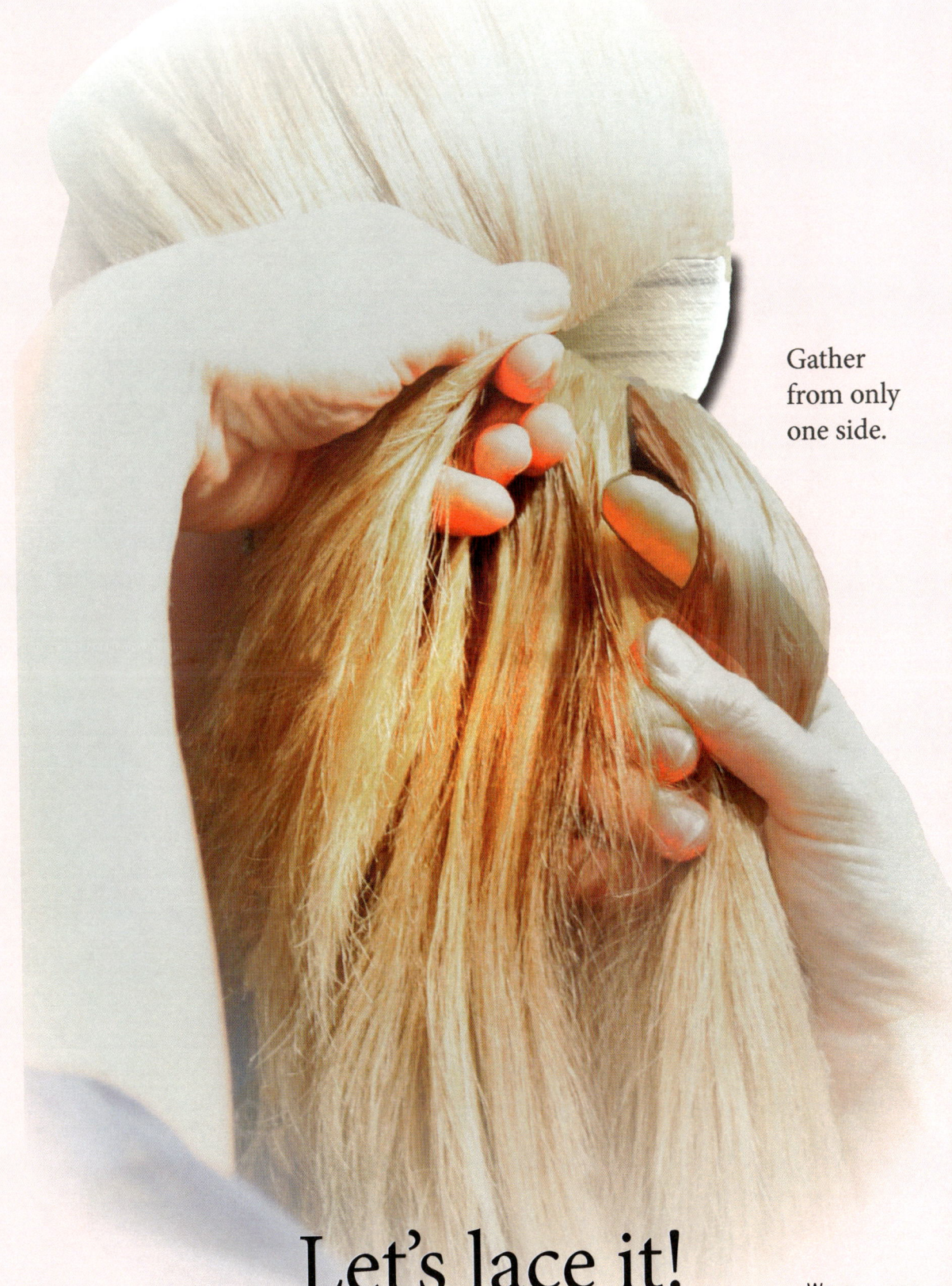

Gather from only one side.

Let's lace it!

Five-Strand Dutch Lace

5

The impossible can always be broken down into possibilities.

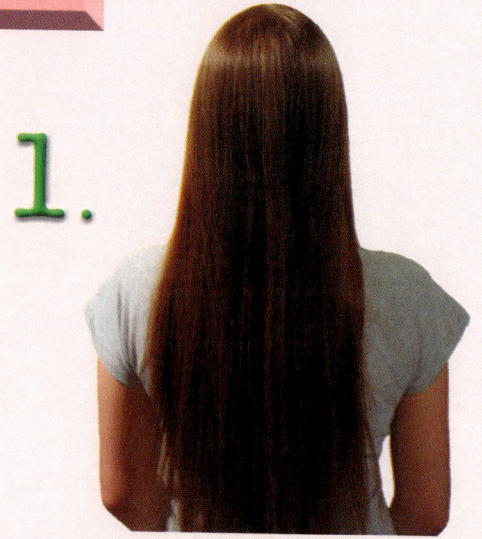

1. Begin with clean, brushed hair.

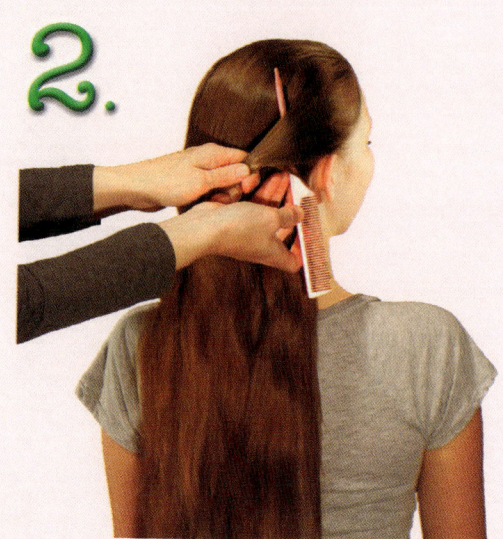

2. Take a section of hair as illustrated.

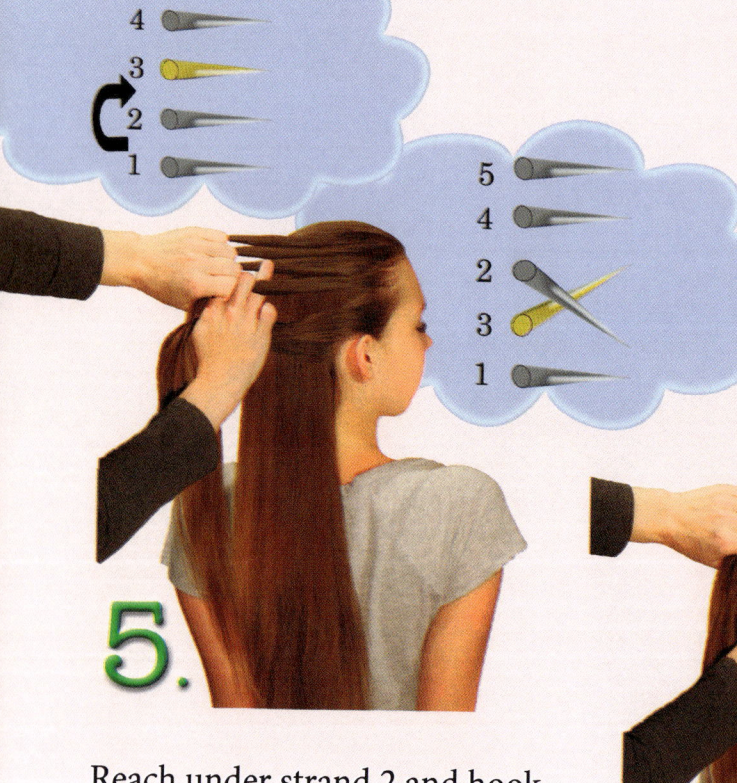

5. Reach under strand 2 and hook strand 3 with the ring finger.

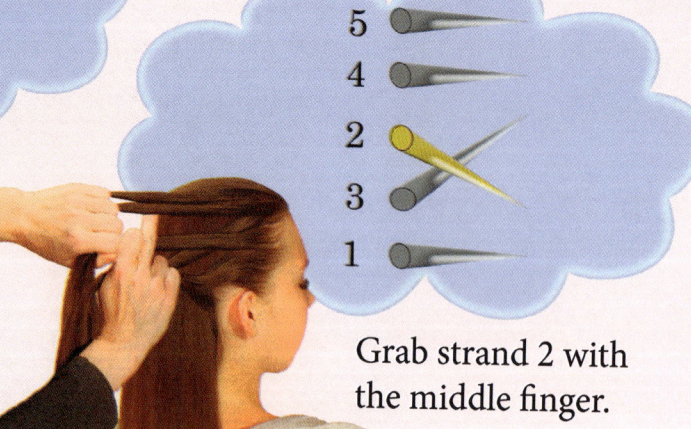

6. Grab strand 2 with the middle finger.

238 www.findingbraids.com

Five-Strand Dutch Lace

5

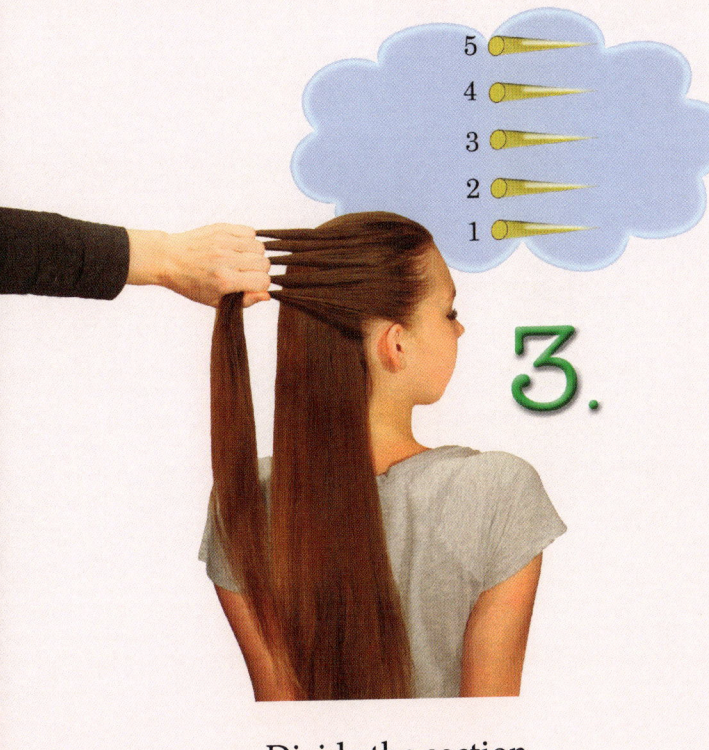

3.

Divide the section into five strands.

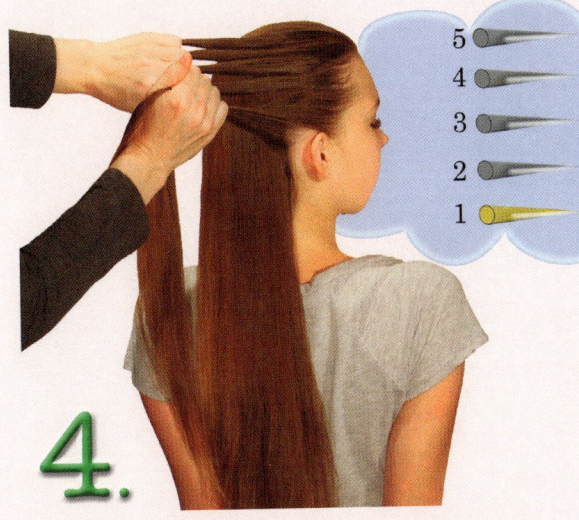

4.

Start braiding by grabbing strand 1 with your palm down and your thumb facing your belly button.

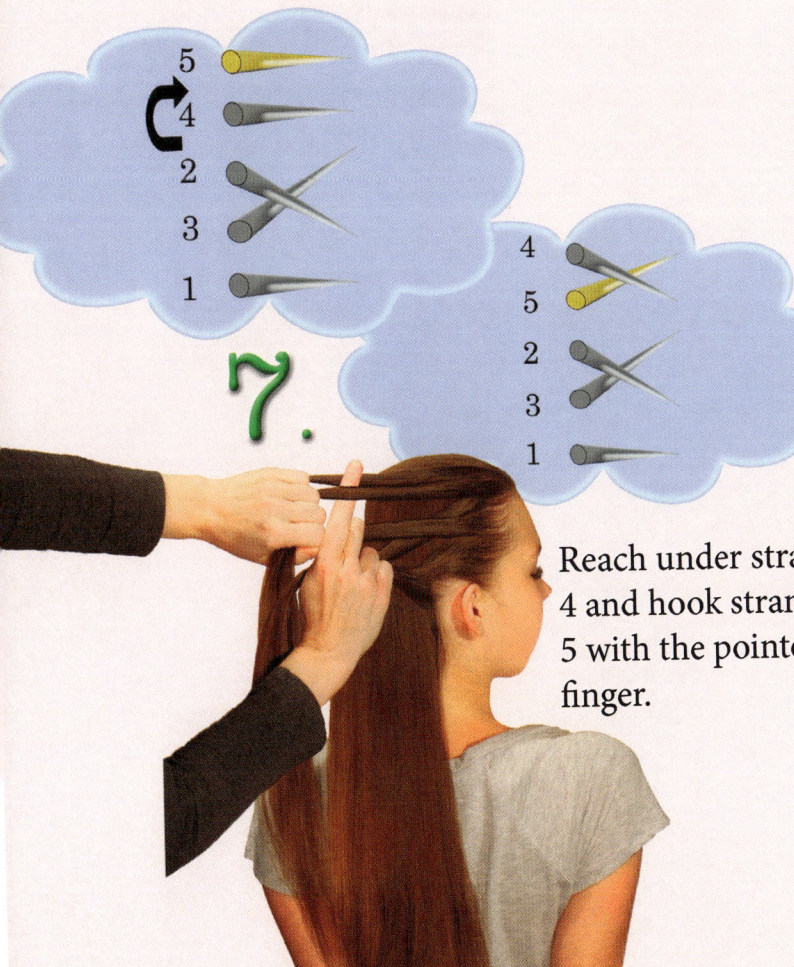

7.

Reach under strand 4 and hook strand 5 with the pointer finger.

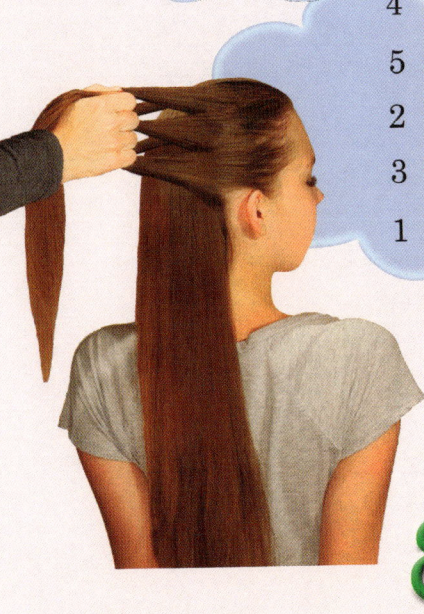

8.

Place strand 4 in between the thumb and pointer finger.

Ways 239

5 Continuing

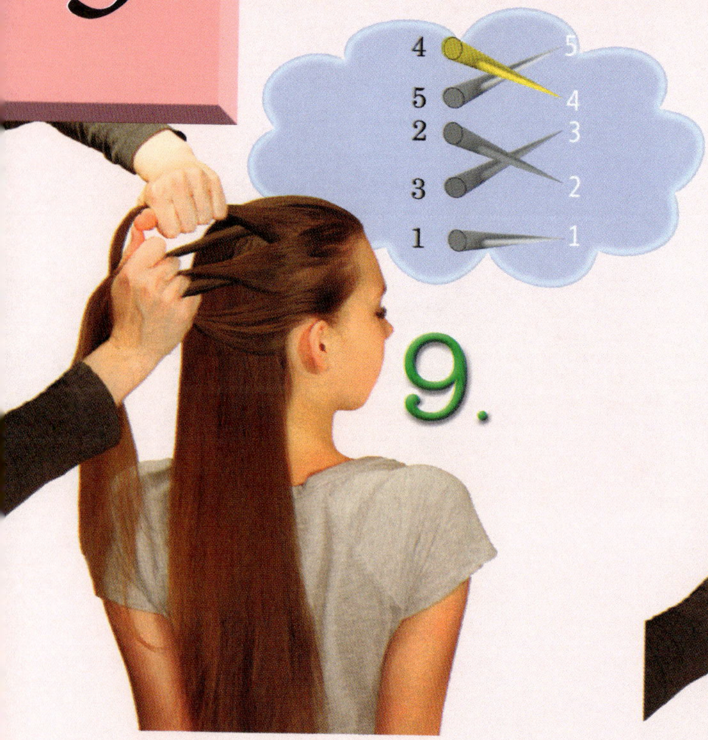

9.
Start braiding by grabbing strand 4 with your palm down and your thumb facing your belly button.

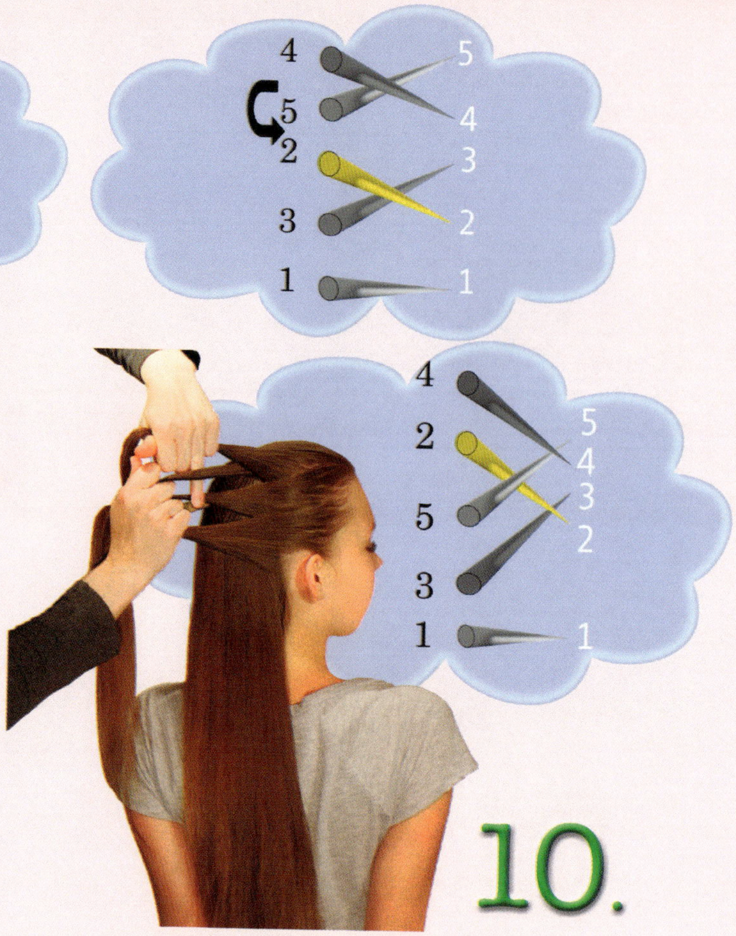

10.
Reach under strand 5 and hook strand 2 with the ring finger.

13.
Place strand 3 in between the thumb and pointer finger.

14.

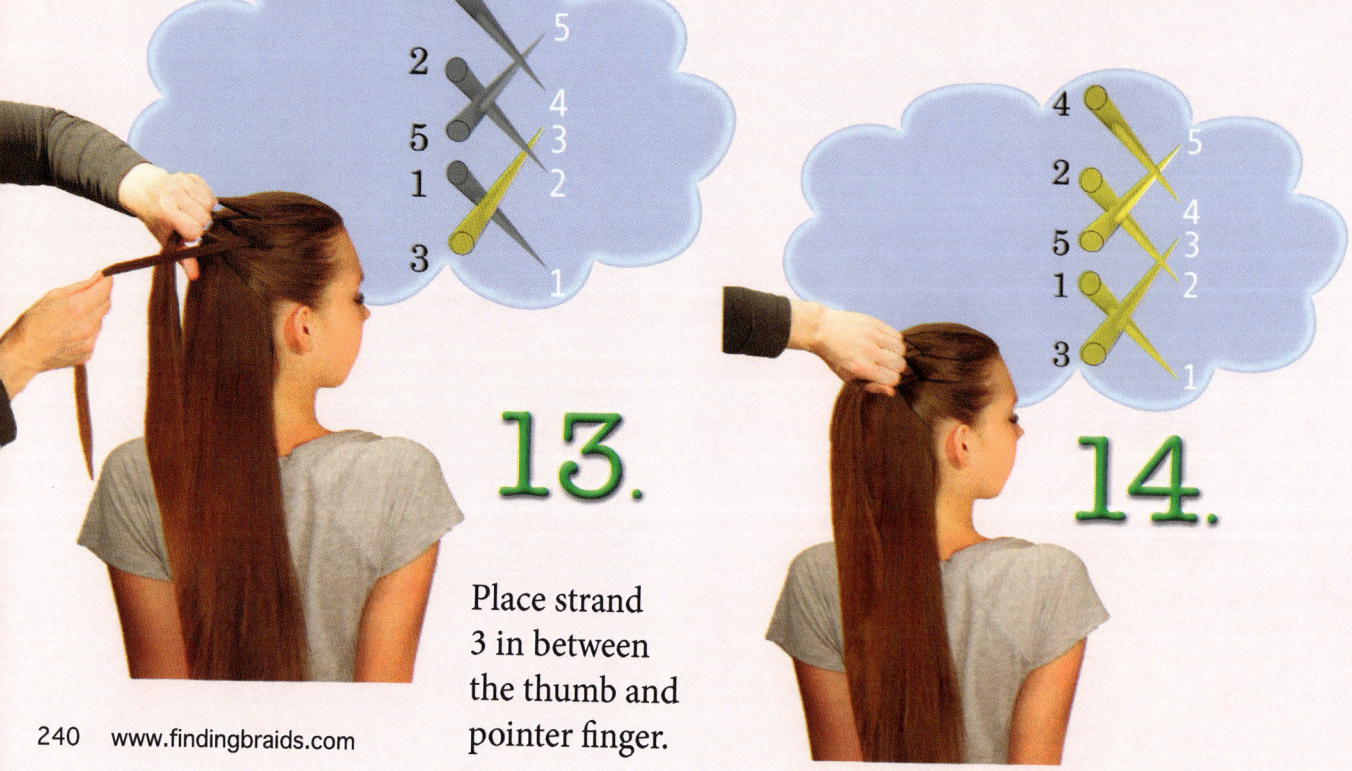

part 2. Five-Strand Dutch Lace

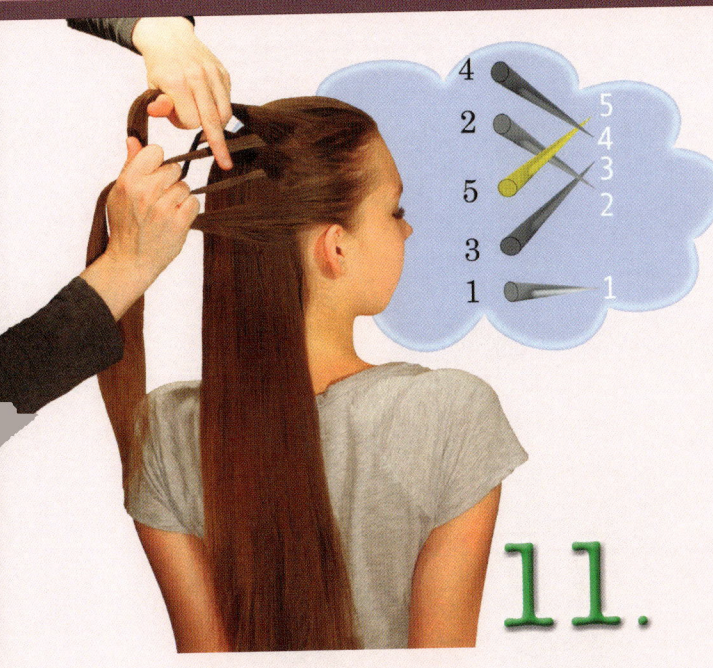

11.

Grab strand 5 with the middle finger.

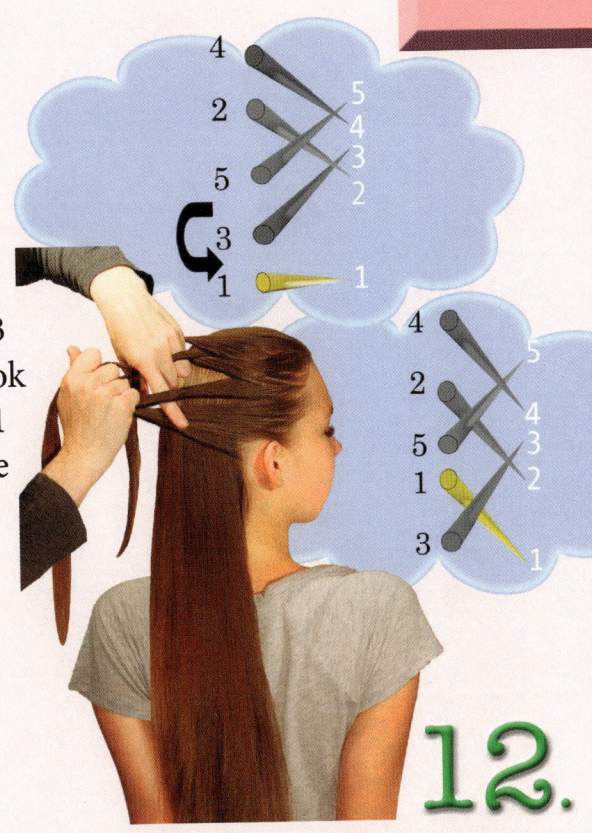

Reach under strand 3 and hook strand 1 with the pointer finger.

12.

Number your strands at your knuckles now.

15.

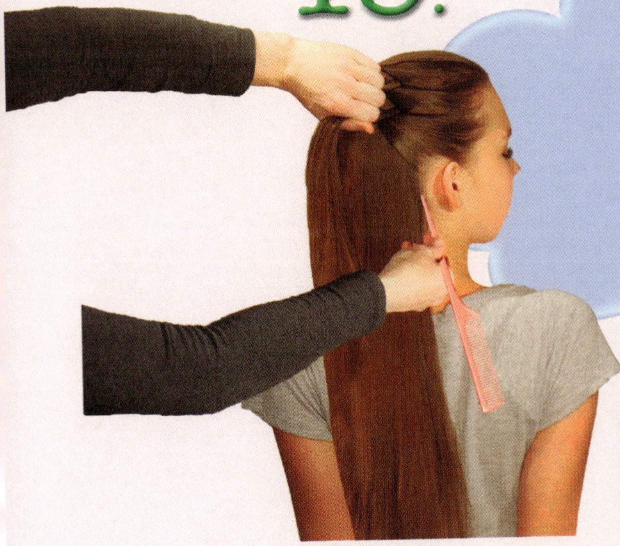

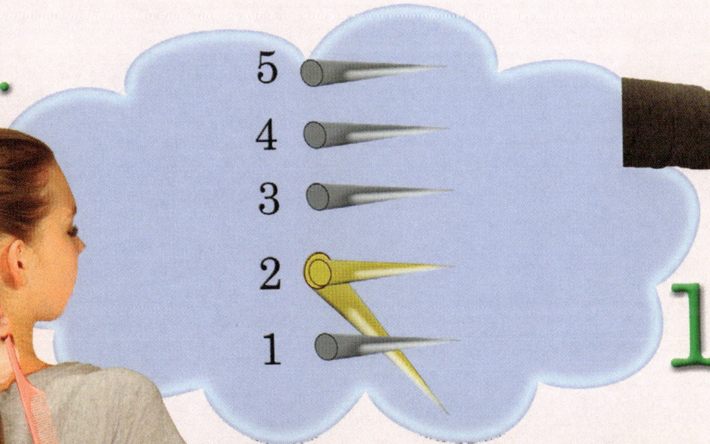

Sliver off a gather from the face all the way back to the braid.

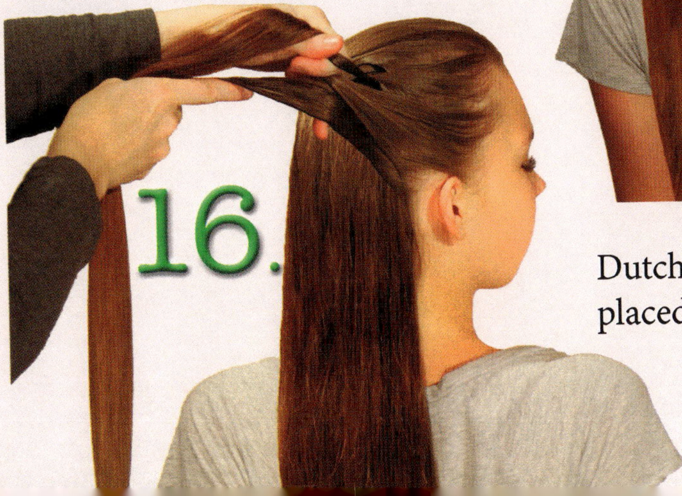

16.

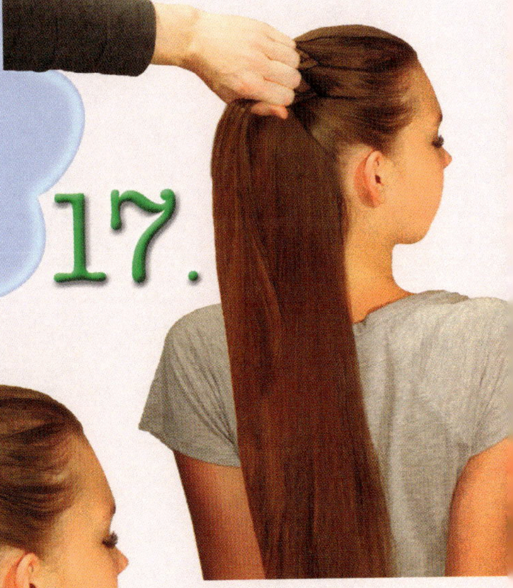

17.

Dutch gathers are placed in strand 2.

Ways 241

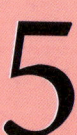

part 3. Five-Strand Dutch Lace

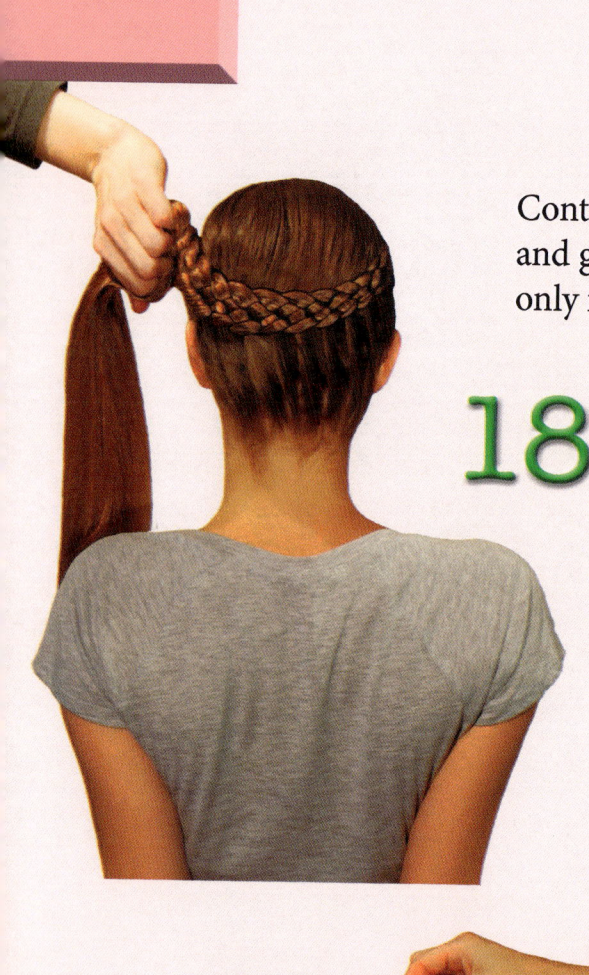

18. Continue weaving and gathering. Gather only from one side.

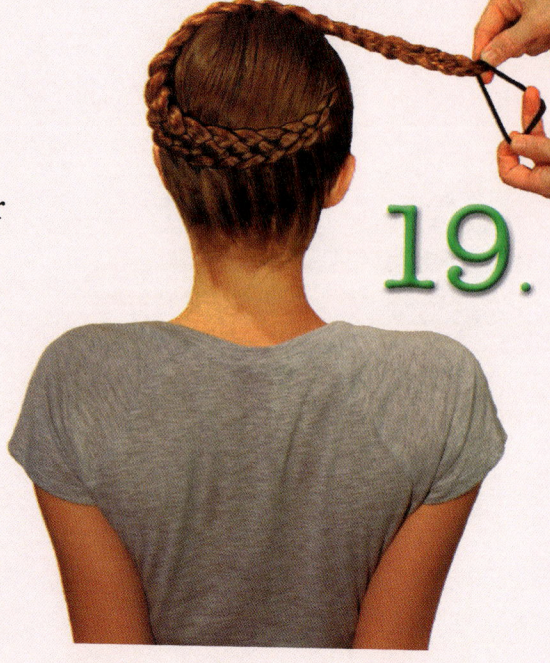

19. Secure with a rubber band.

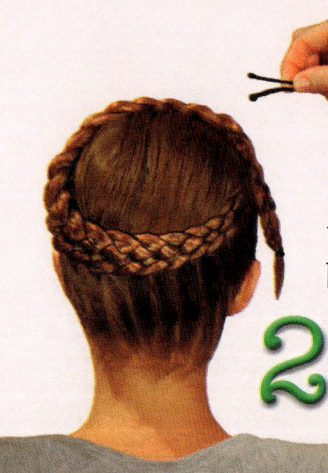

20. Fix the end of the tail with bobby pins.

Examples of Five-Strand

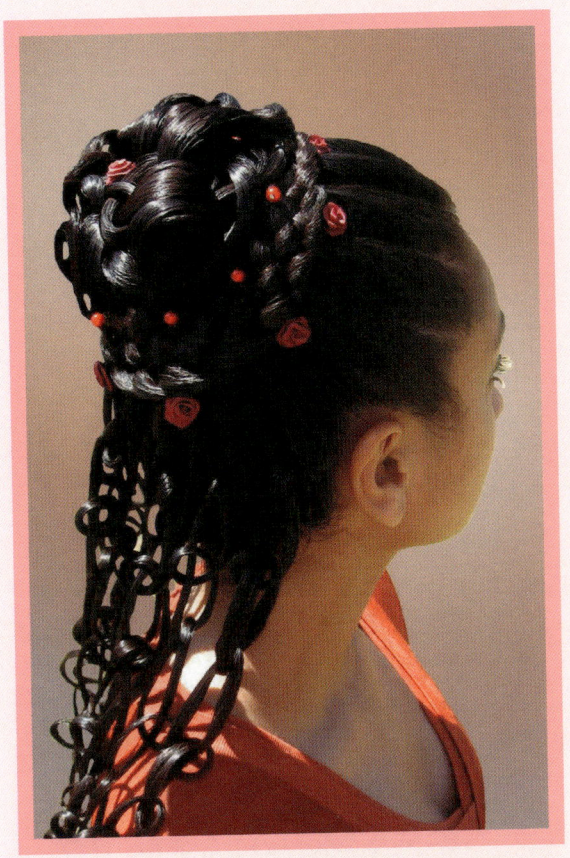
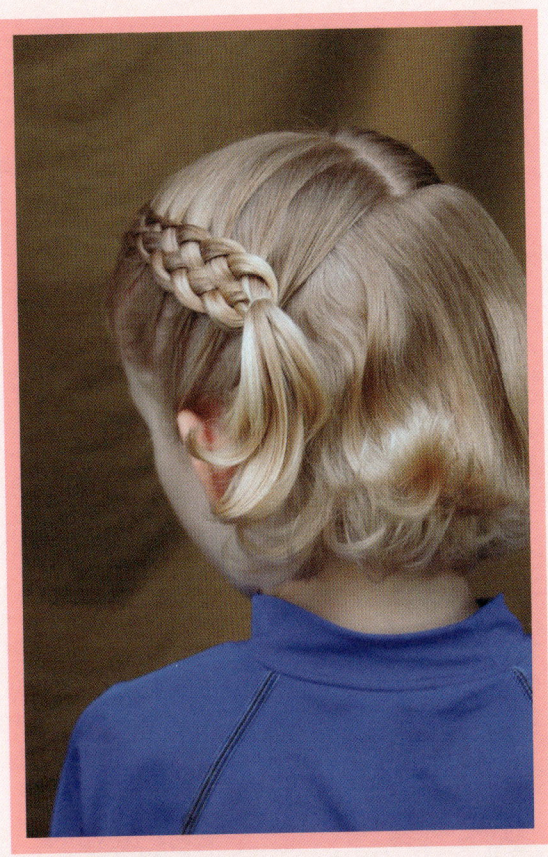
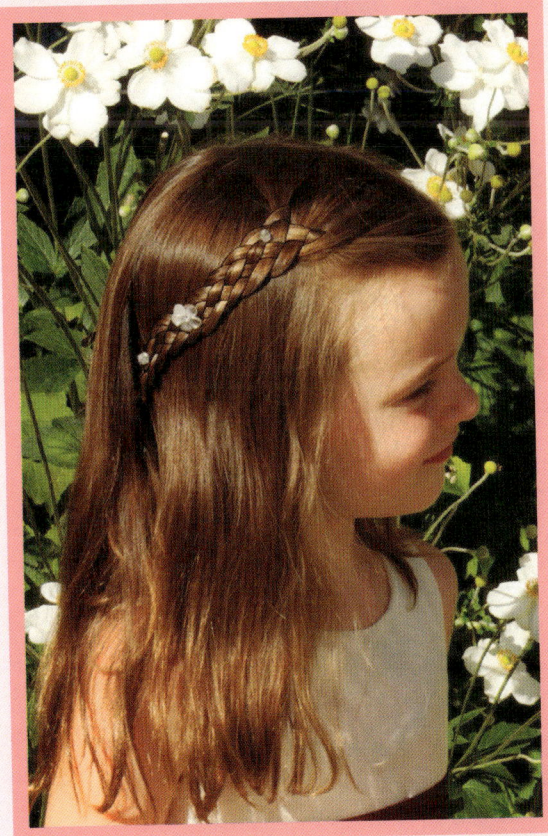
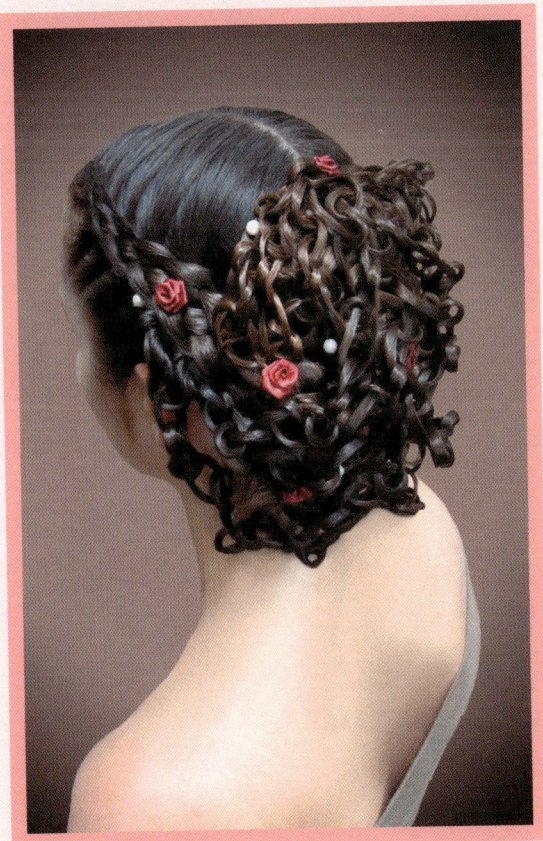

Visit my website to see more examples of the Five-Strand

Six-Strand

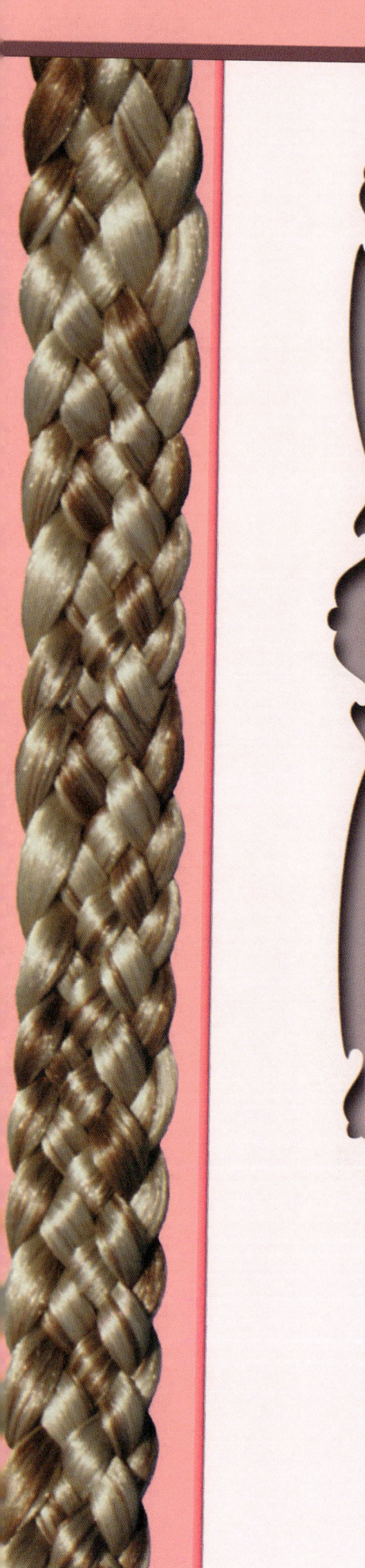

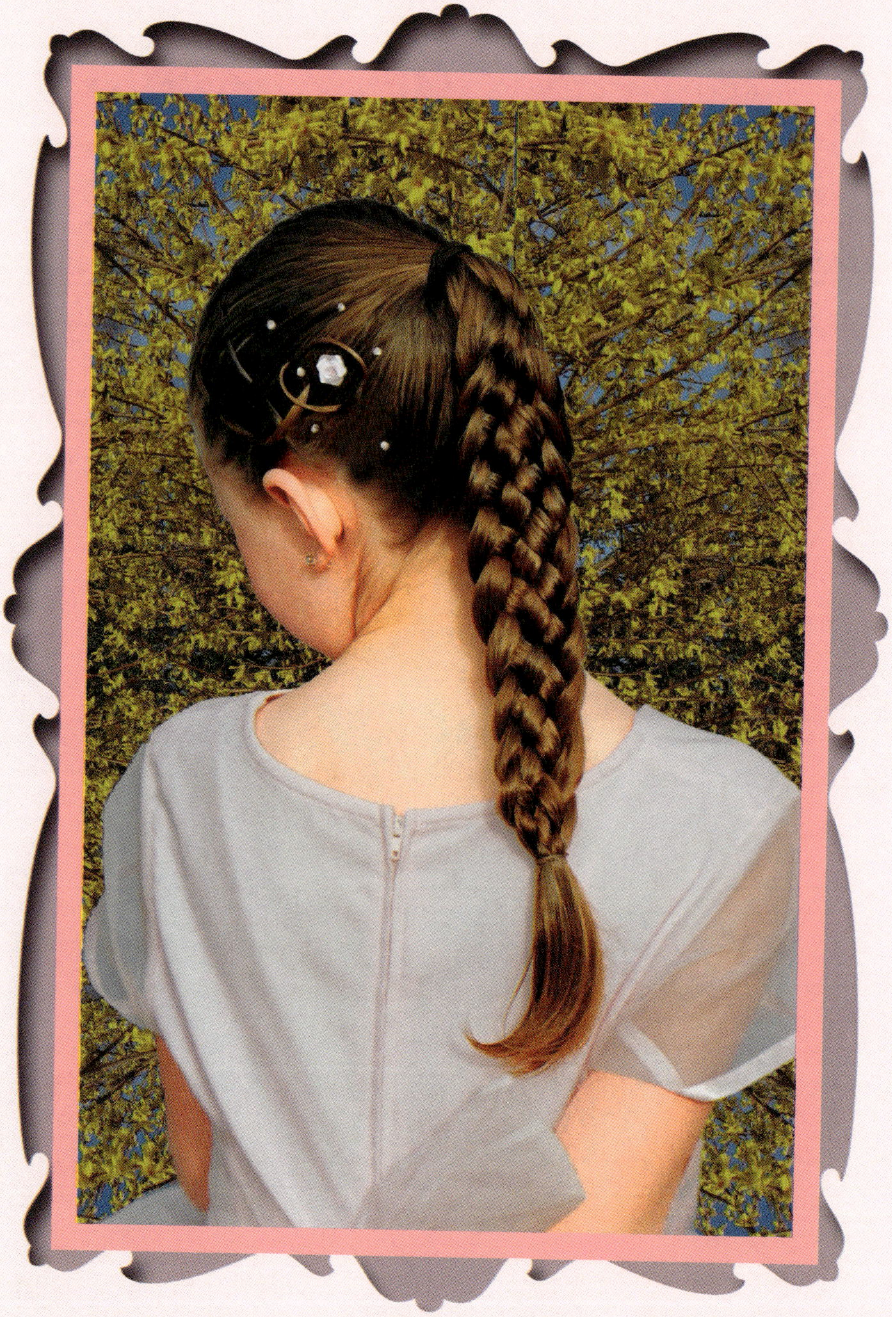

A braid for enthusiasts. Keep an eye on that sixth strand so it doesn't get away. You will be pleased with the comments you get from this braid.

Six-Strand

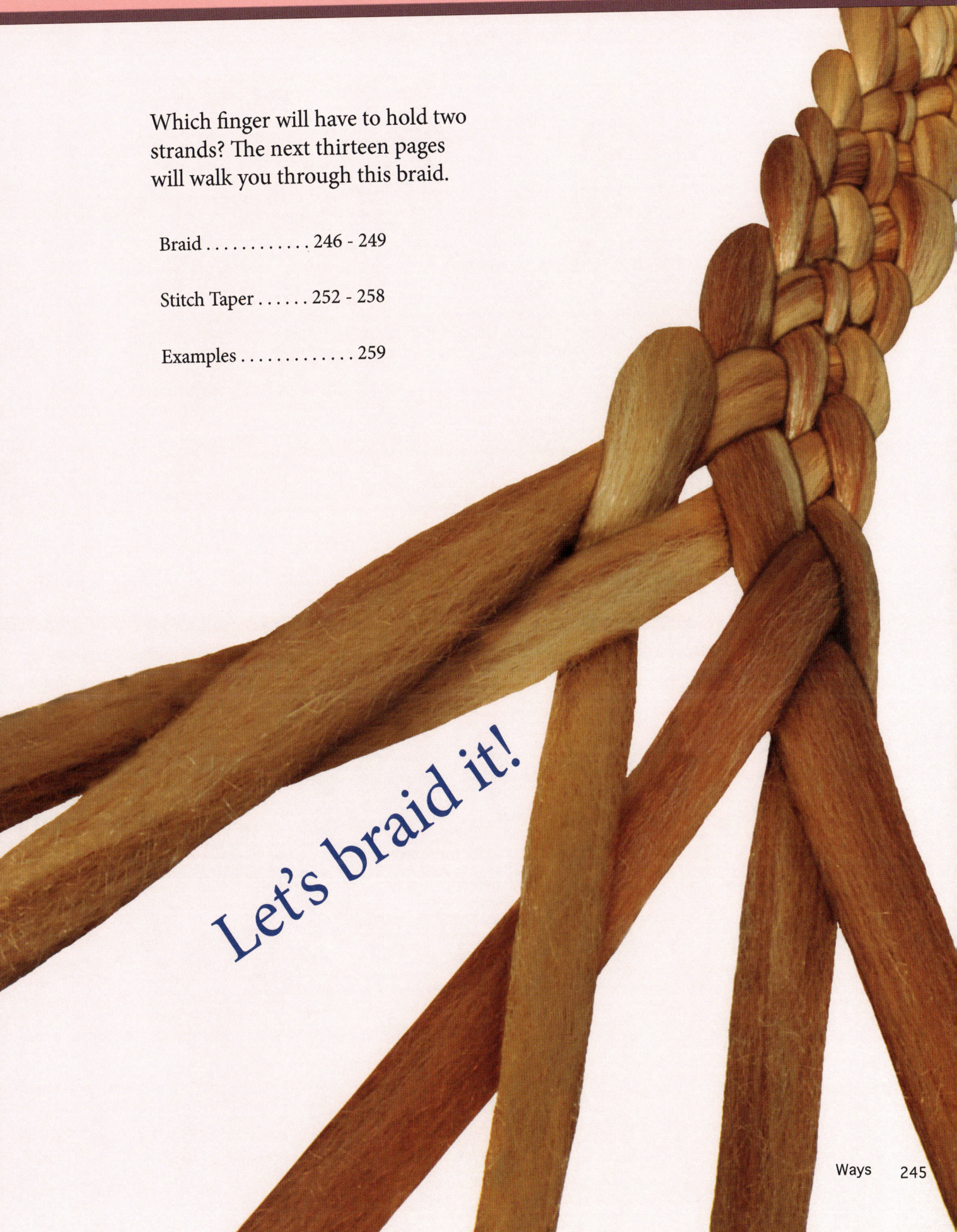

Which finger will have to hold two strands? The next thirteen pages will walk you through this braid.

Braid . . . . 246 - 249

Stitch Taper . . . . . . 252 - 258

Examples 259

Let's braid it!

Ways

Six-Strand Braid

6

Difficulties help you realize your potential.

1.
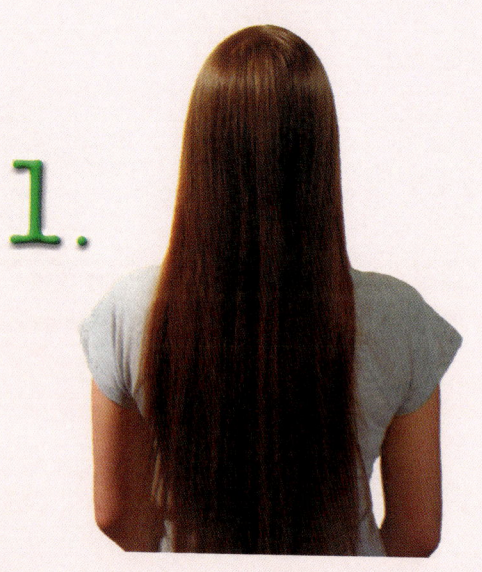
Begin with clean, brushed hair.

2.
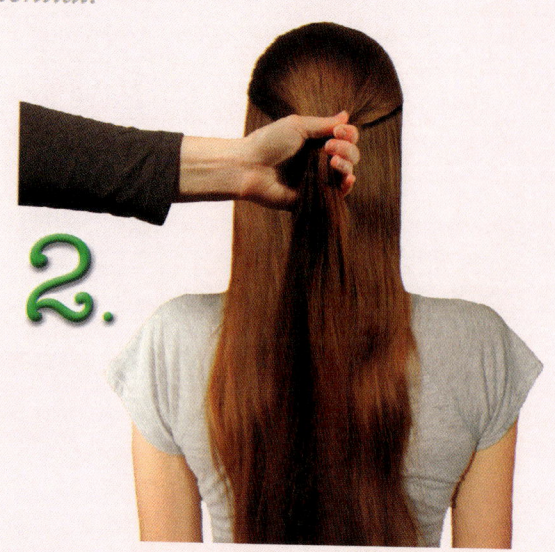
Take a section of hair.

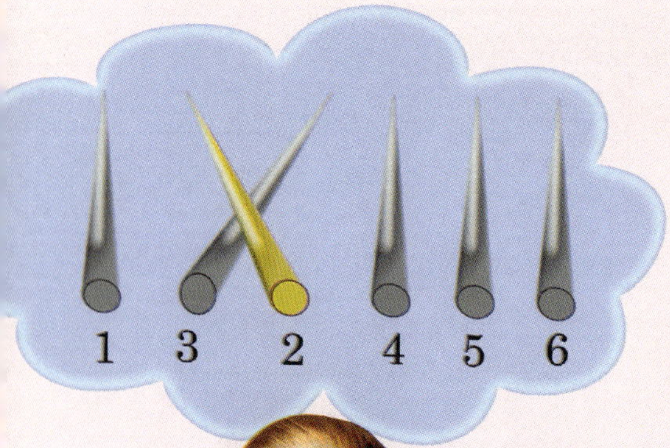

5.
Grab strand 2 with the ring finger.

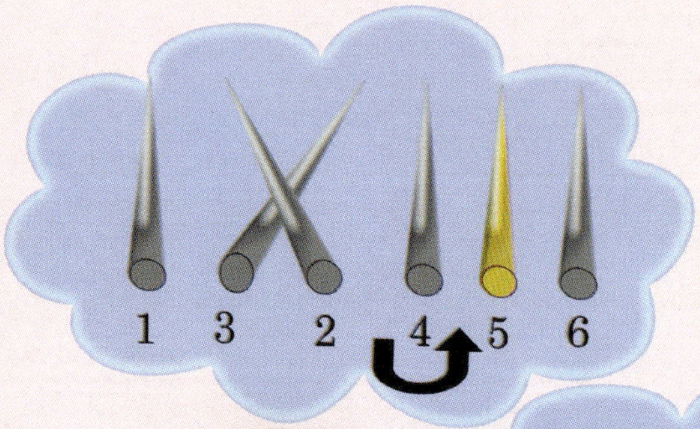

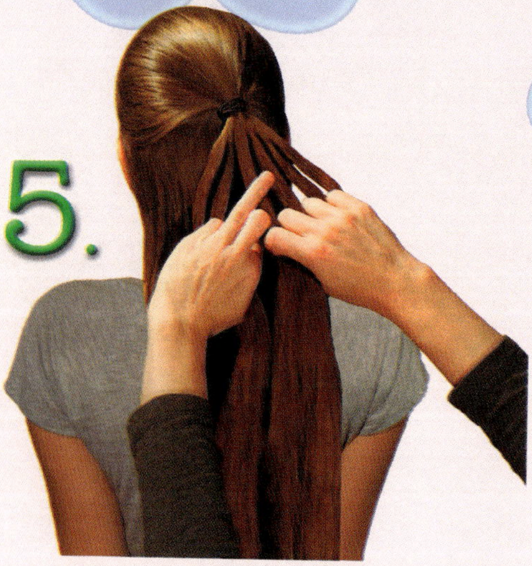

6.
Reach under strand 4 and hook strand 5 with the middle finger. 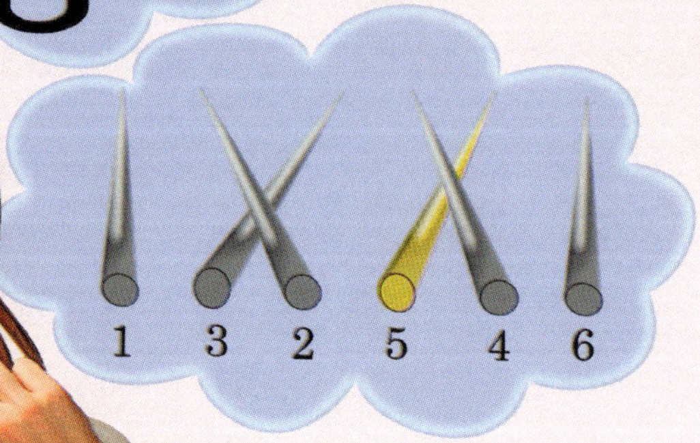 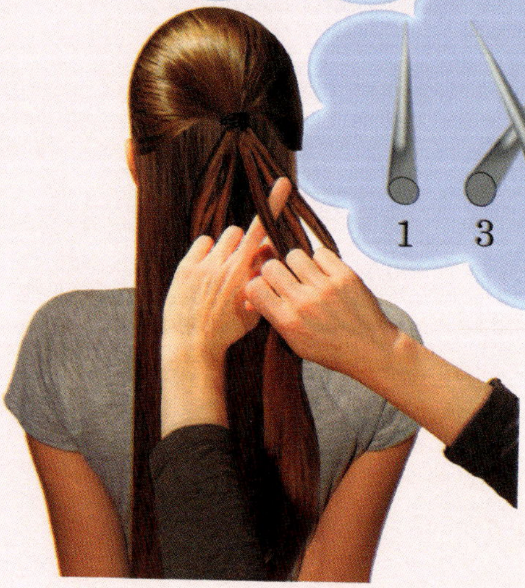

246   www.findingbraids.com

Six-Strand Braid

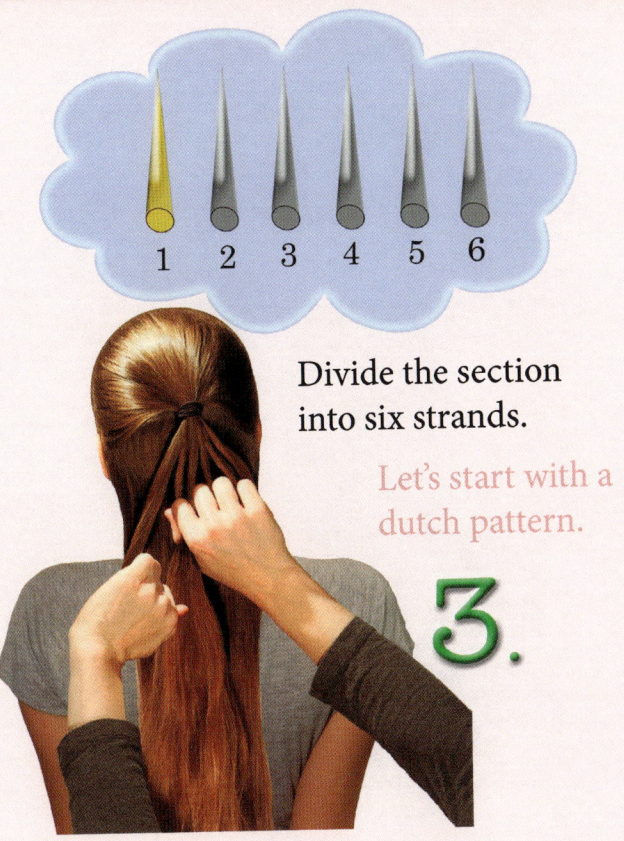

Divide the section into six strands.

Let's start with a dutch pattern.

3.

Take strand 1 with your palm down and your thumb facing your belly button.

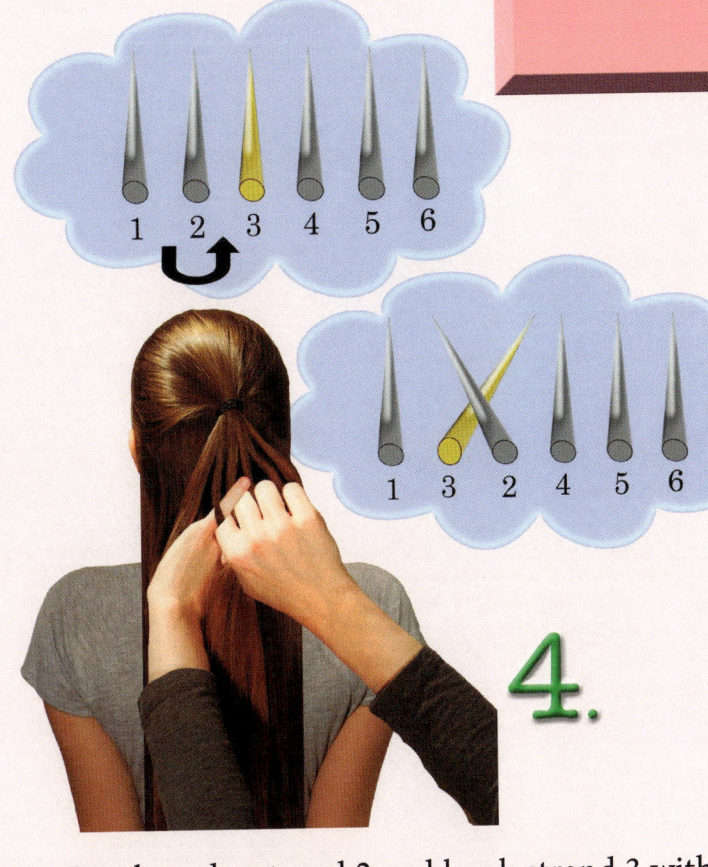

4.

Reach under strand 2 and hook strand 3 with the pinky finger. You're now holding two strands in your pinky finger.

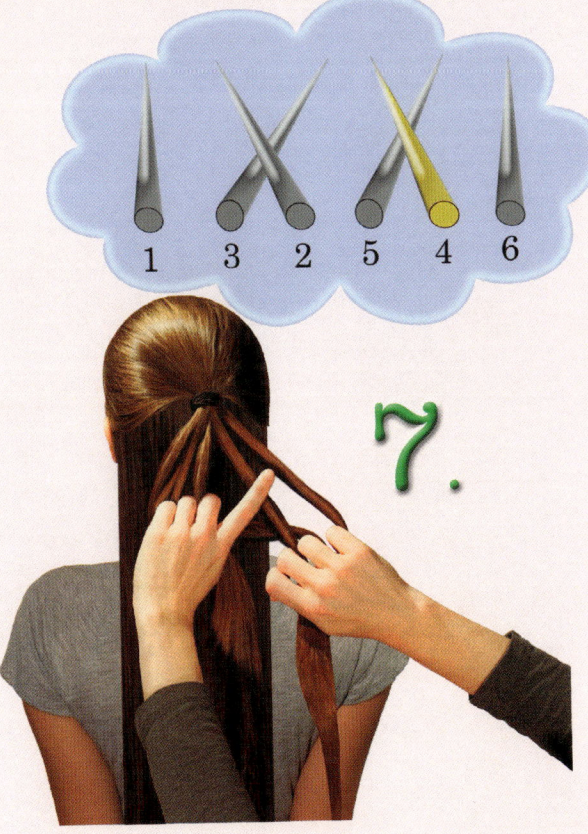

7.

Grab strand 4 with the pointer finger.

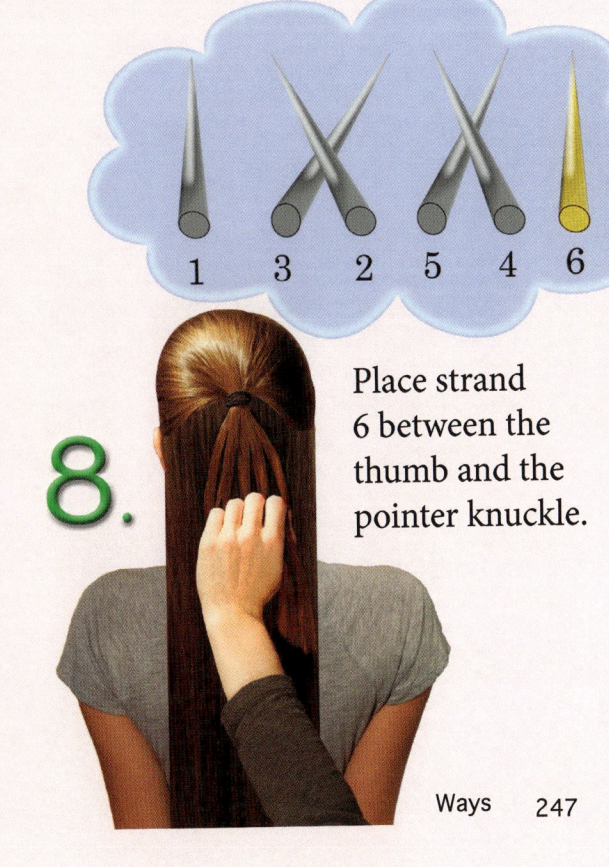

8.

Place strand 6 between the thumb and the pointer knuckle.

Ways 247

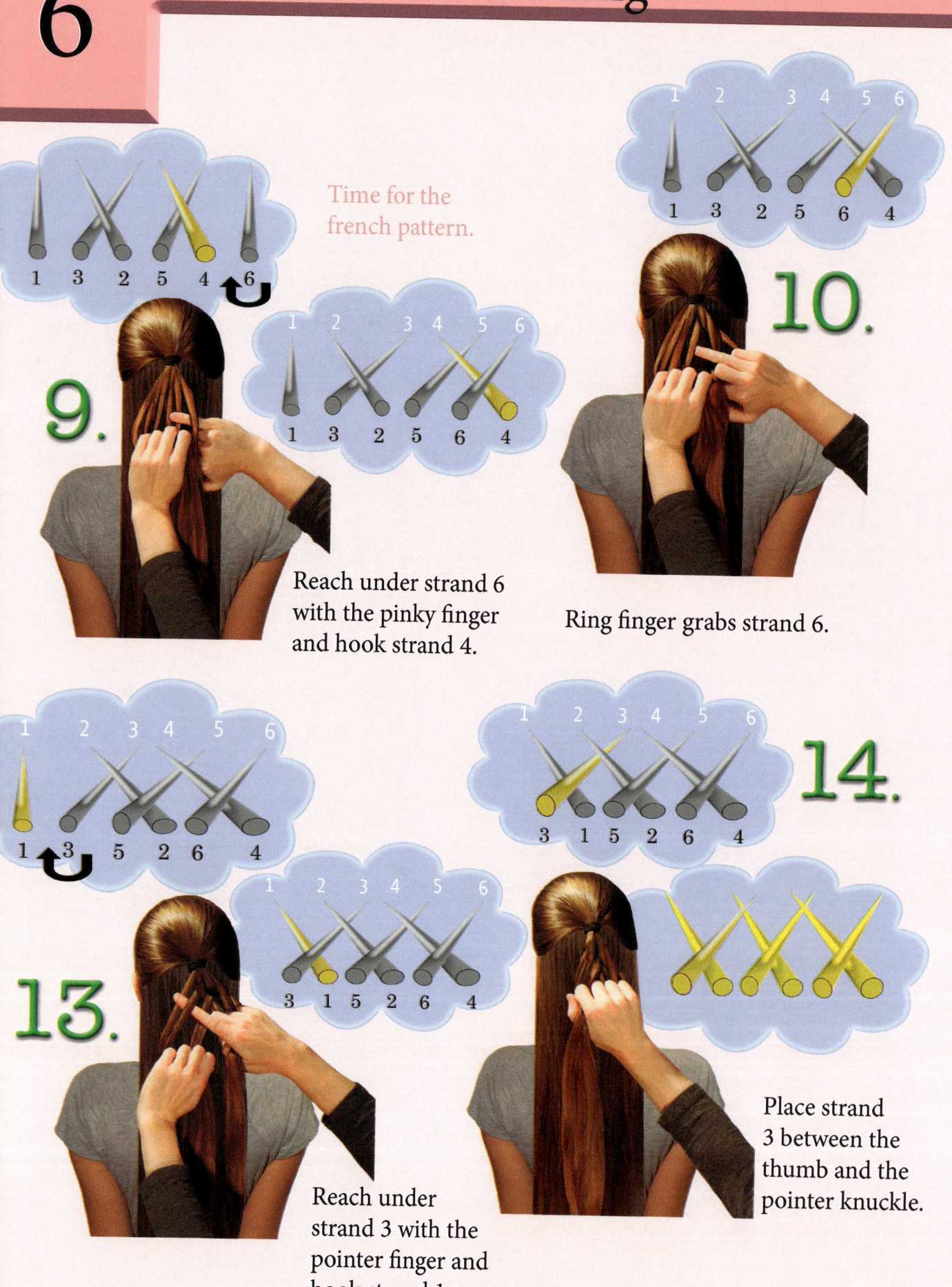

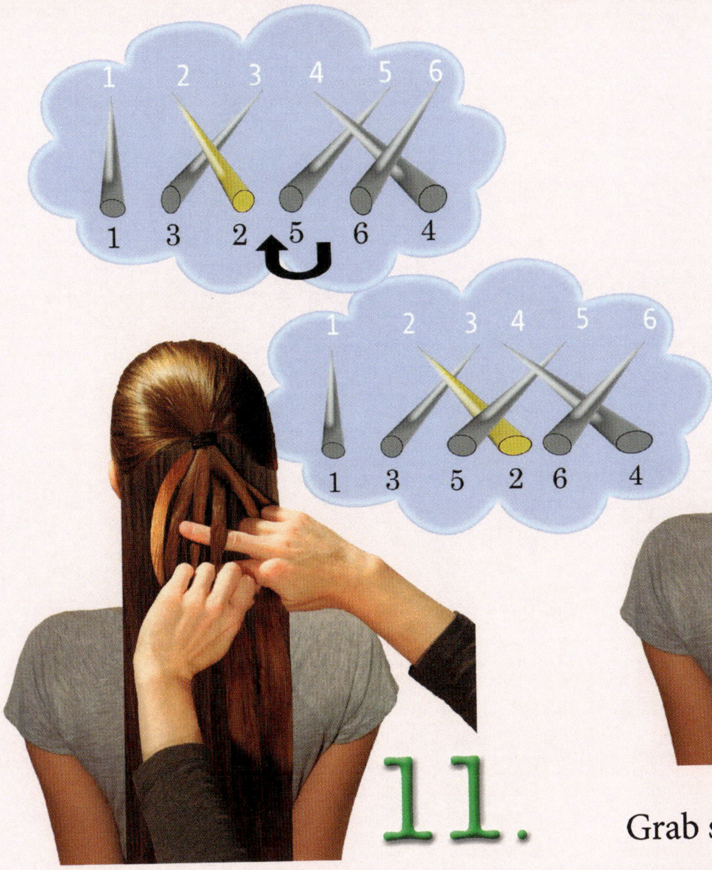

part 2. Six-Strand Braid

6

11.
Reach under strand 5 with the middle finger and hook strand 2.

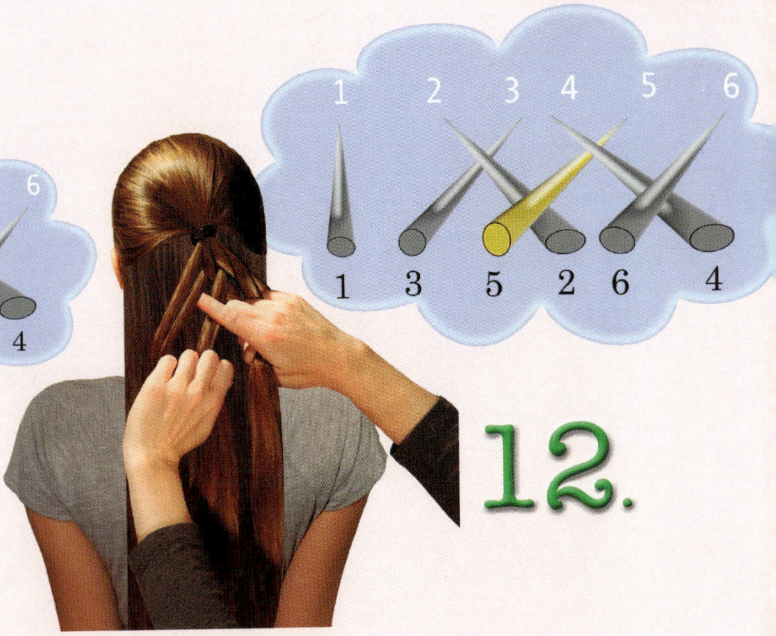

12.
Grab strand 5 with the pointer finger.

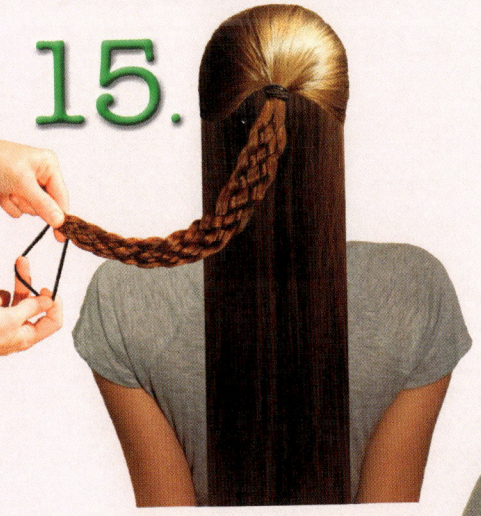

15.
Continue weaving, keep track of which hand weaves what pattern. Secure with a rubber band.

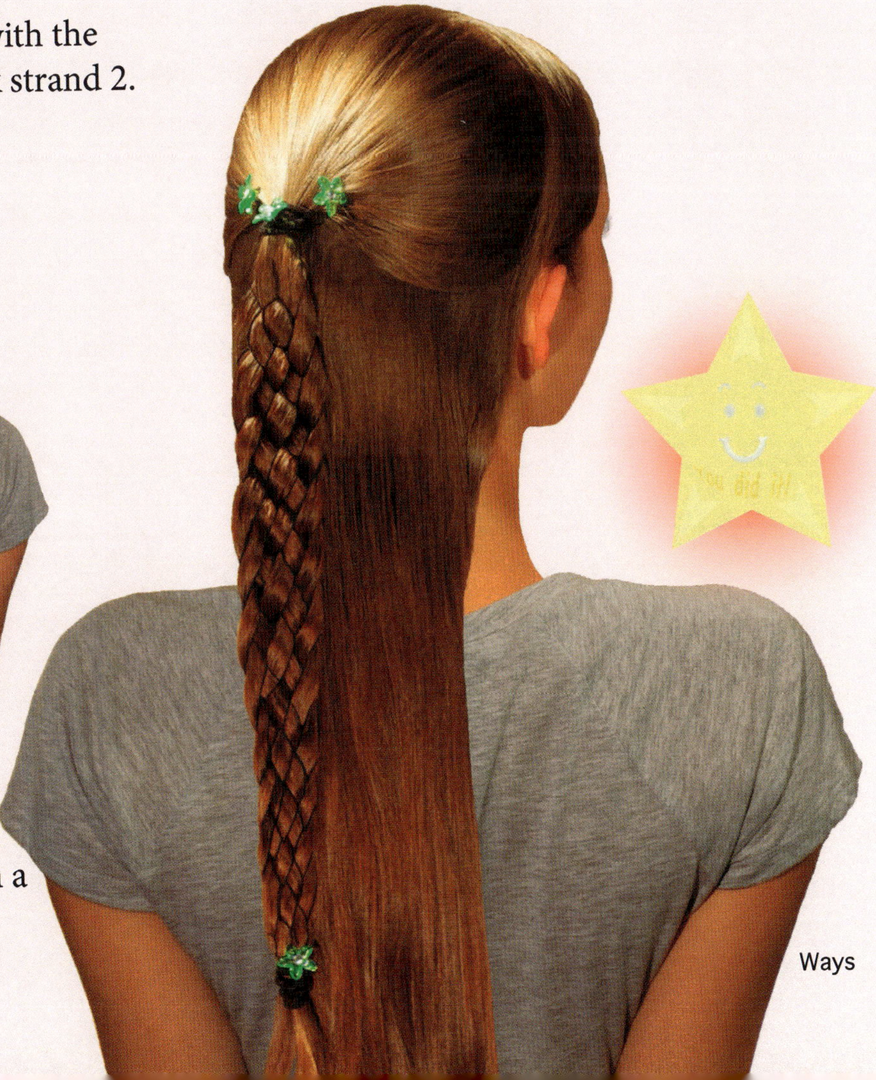

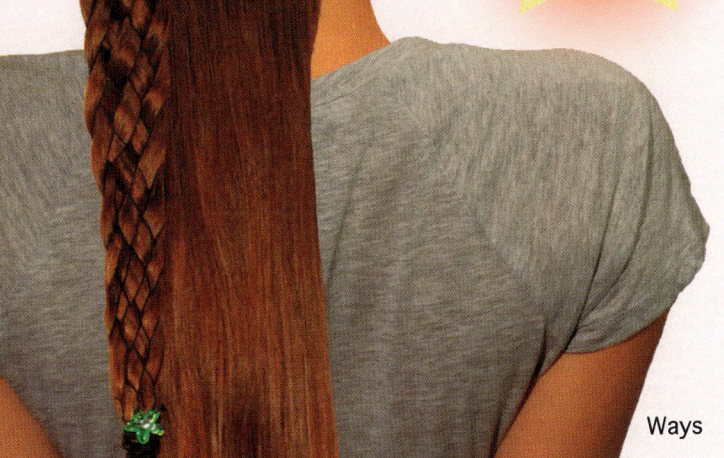

Ways 249

Six-Strand

Notes

_____

_____

_____

_____

_____

_____

_____

Which finger will hold two strands? When weaving the french pattern the pointer finger holds two strands. When weaving the dutch pattern the pinky finger holds two strands.

Six-Strand

Gather from both sides

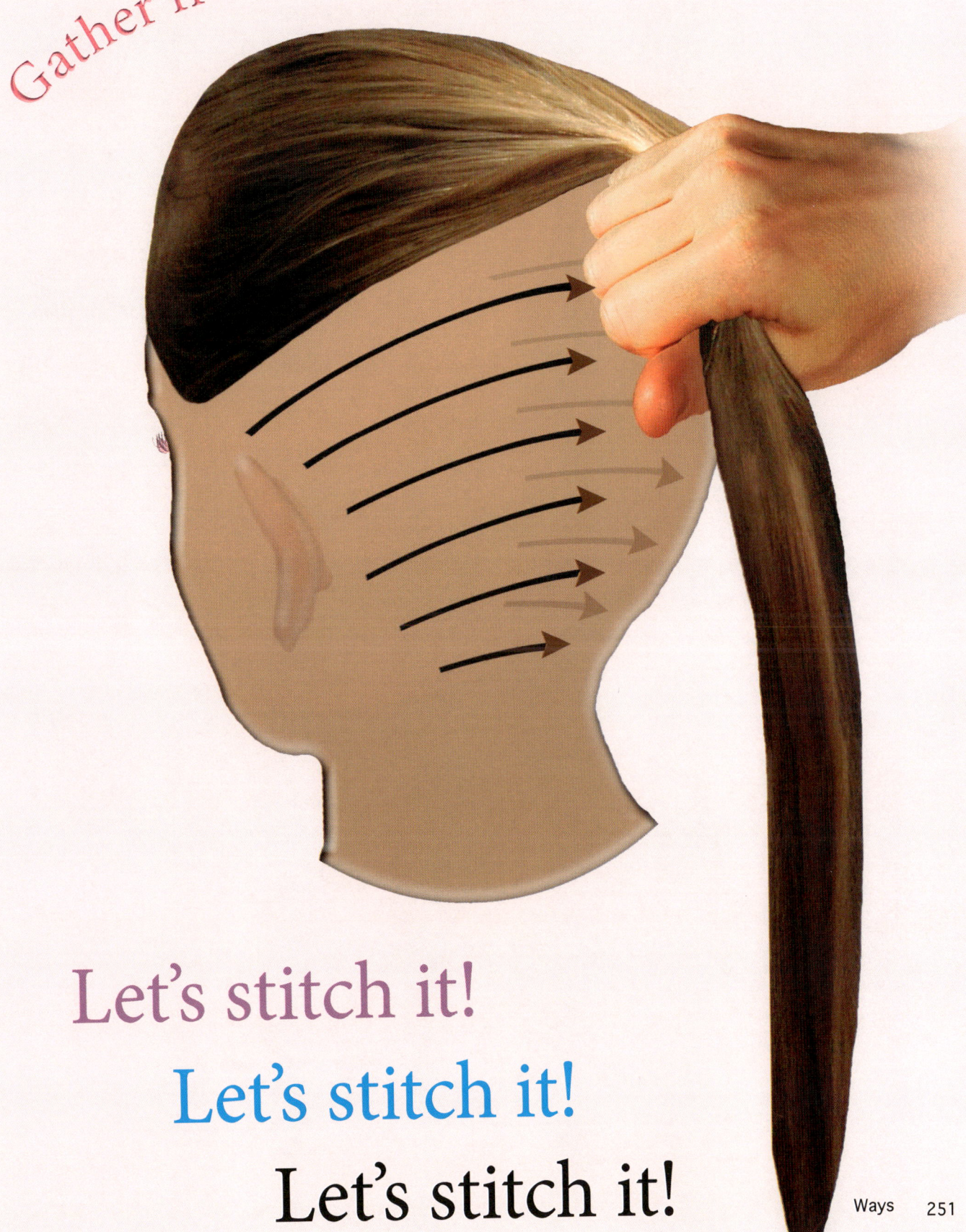

Let's stitch it!
Let's stitch it!
Let's stitch it!

6 Six-Strand Taper Stitch

Only those who are firmly determined to achieve their goals attain the accomplishment.
- Elmo Darcy

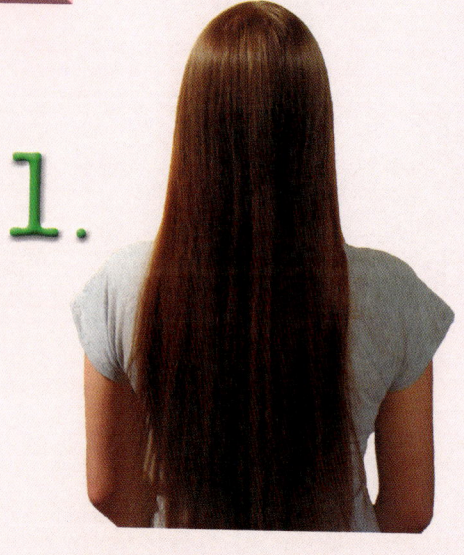

1. Begin with clean, brushed hair.

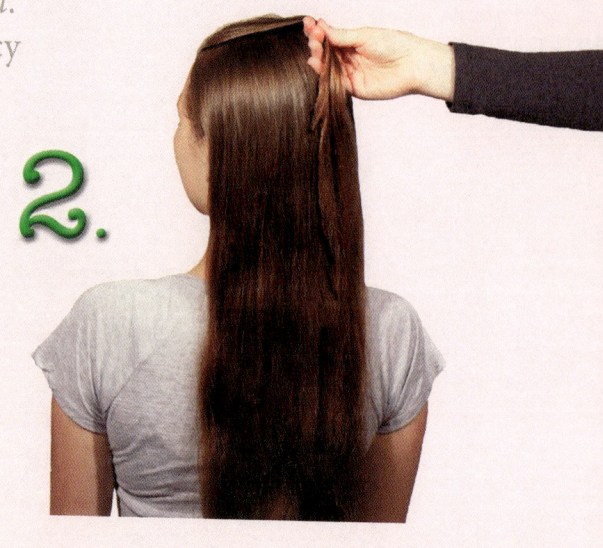

2. Take a section of hair as illustrated.

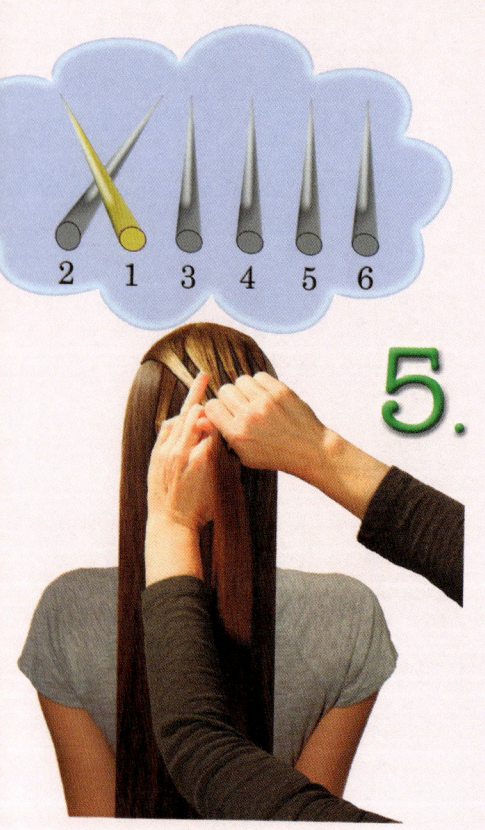

5. Grab strand 1 with the ring finger.

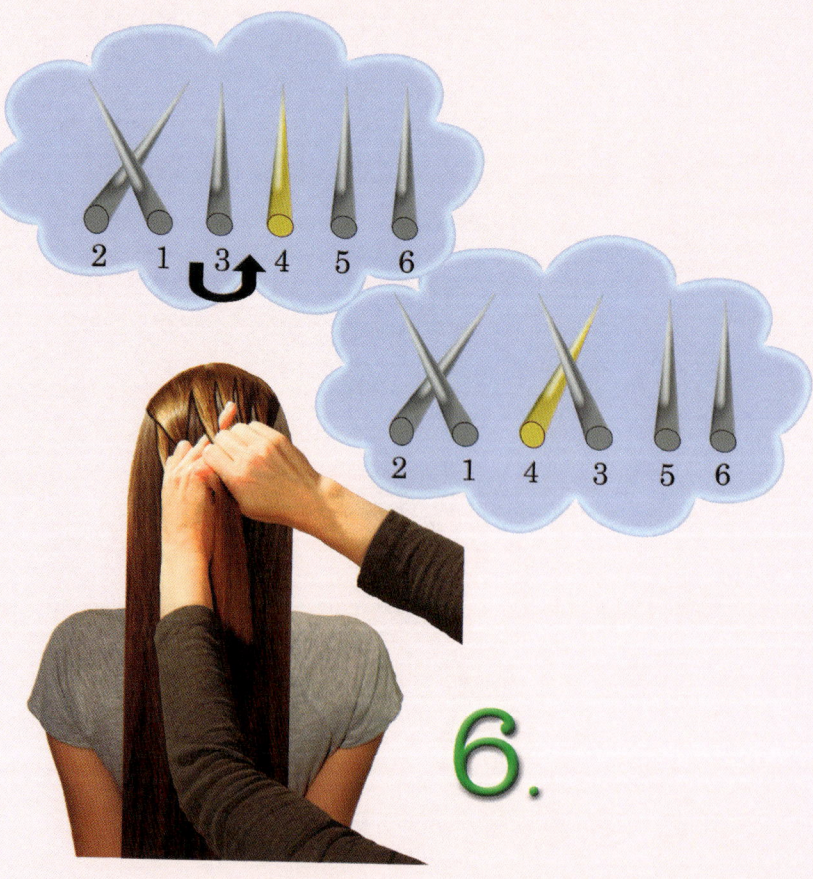

6. Reach under strand 3 with the middle finger and hook strand 4.

252 www.findingbraids.com

Six-Strand Taper Stitch

6

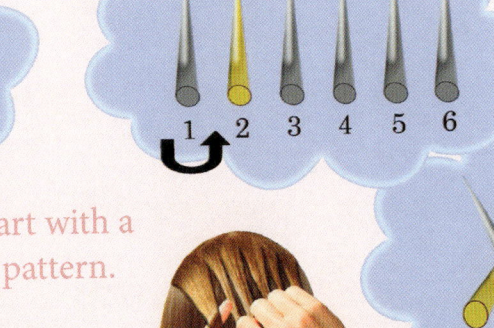

Let's start with a french pattern.

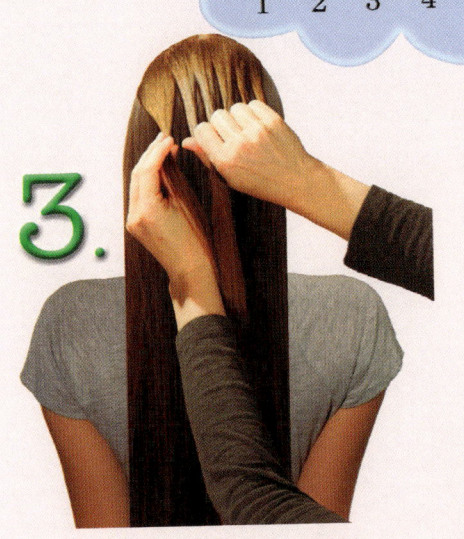

3.

Divide the section into six strands.

4.

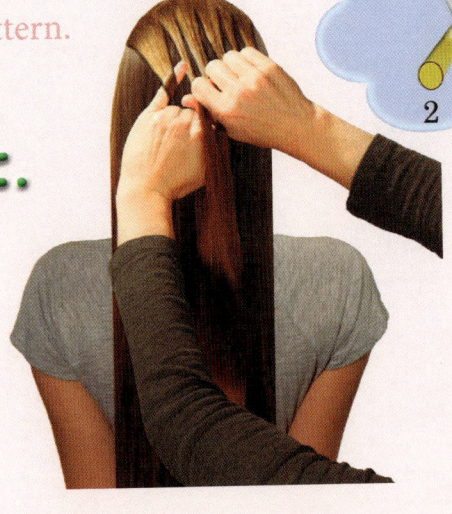

Reach under strand 1 with the pinky finger and hook strand 2.

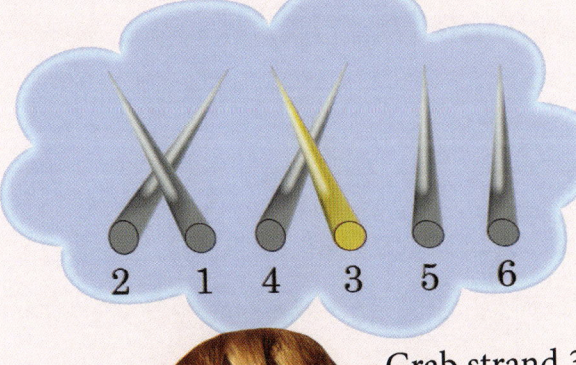

Grab strand 3 with the pointer finger.

7.

8.

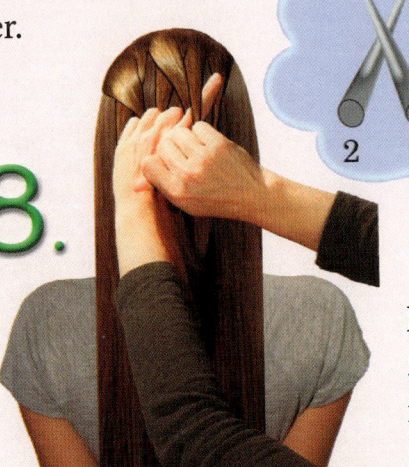

Reach under strand 5 with the pointer finger and hook strand 6.

Ways 253

6 Continuing

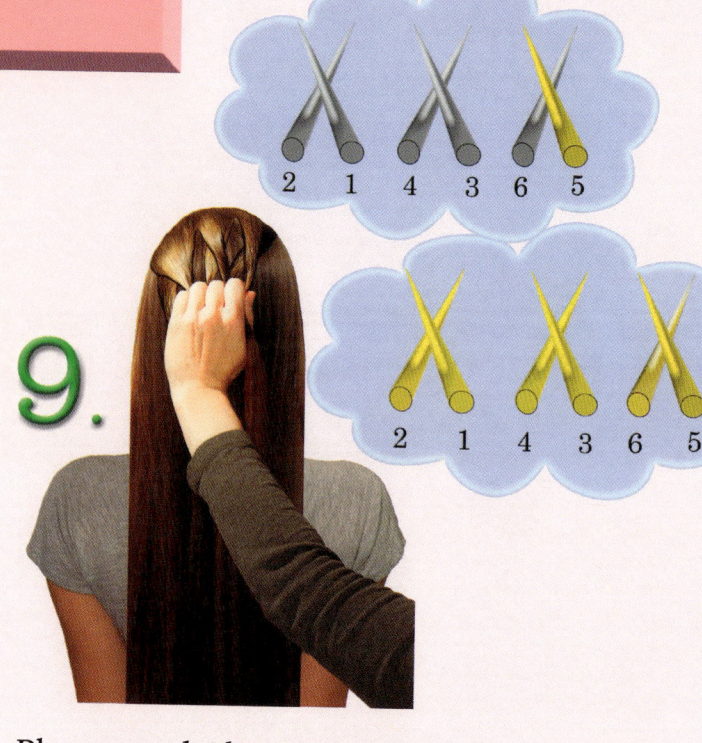

9. Place strand 5 between the thumb and the pointer knuckle.

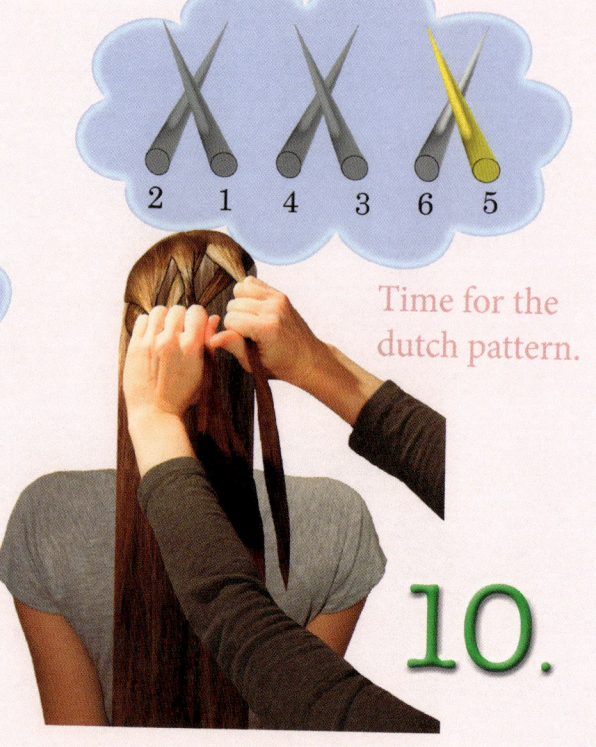

Time for the dutch pattern.

10. Take strand 5 with your palm down and your thumb facing your belly button.

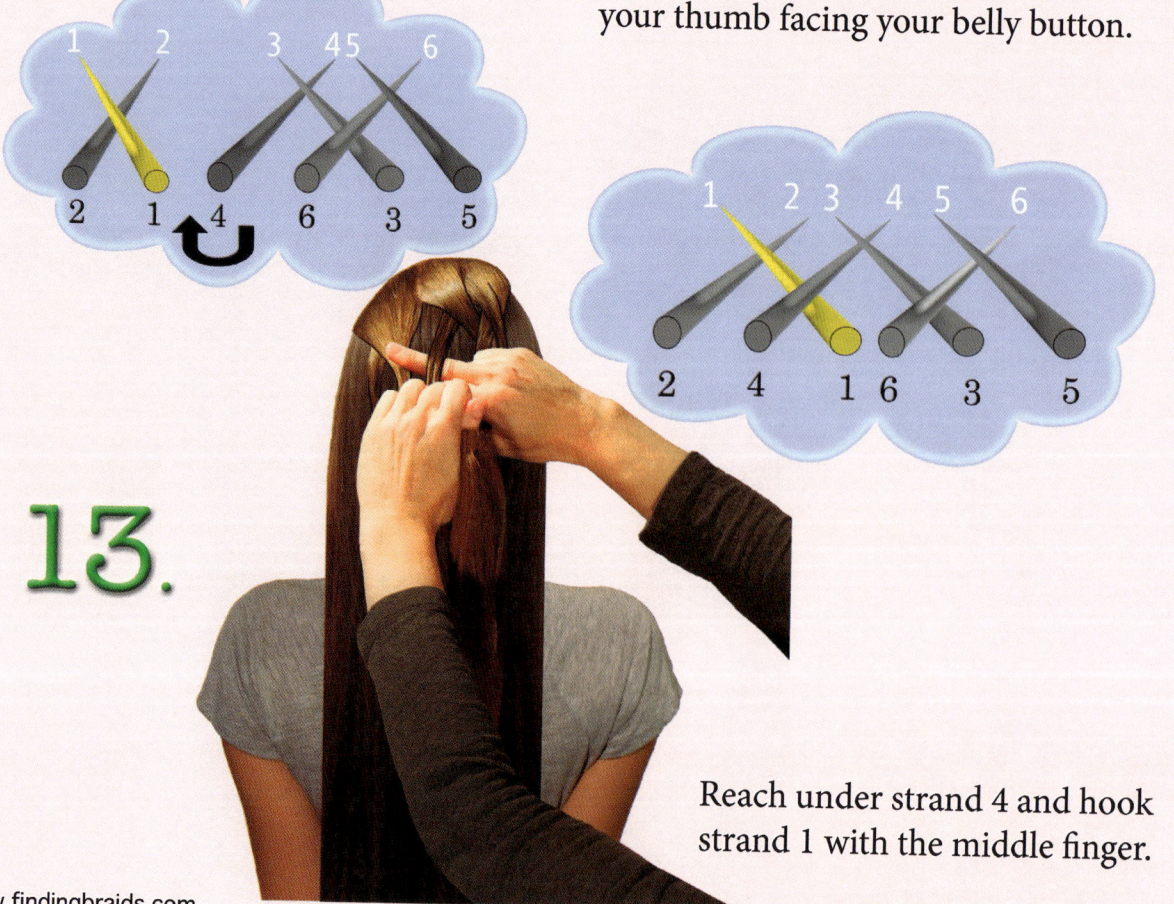

13. Reach under strand 4 and hook strand 1 with the middle finger.

part 2. Six-Strand Taper Stitch

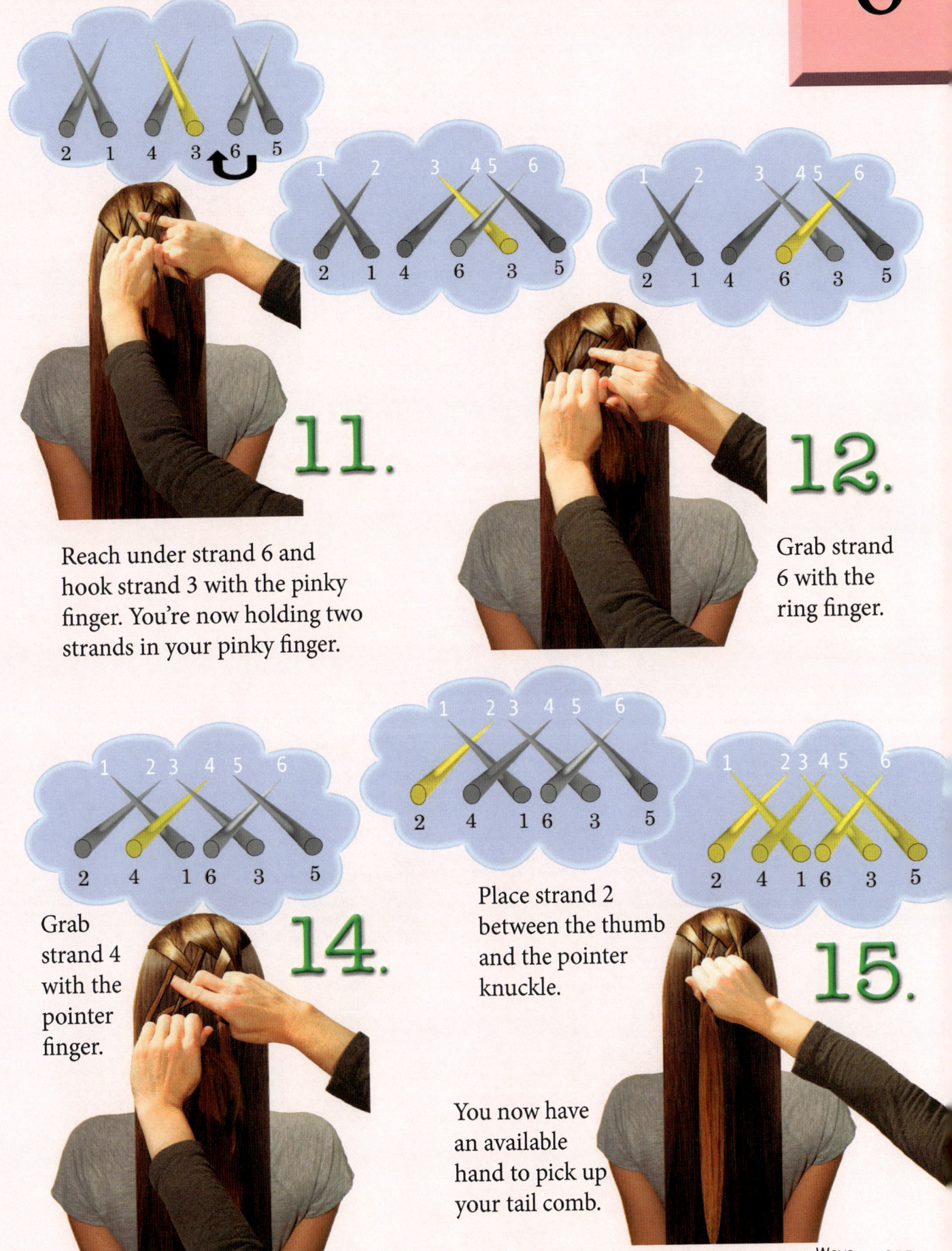

11. Reach under strand 6 and hook strand 3 with the pinky finger. You're now holding two strands in your pinky finger.

12. Grab strand 6 with the ring finger.

14. Grab strand 4 with the pointer finger.

15. Place strand 2 between the thumb and the pointer knuckle.

You now have an available hand to pick up your tail comb.

6 Continuing

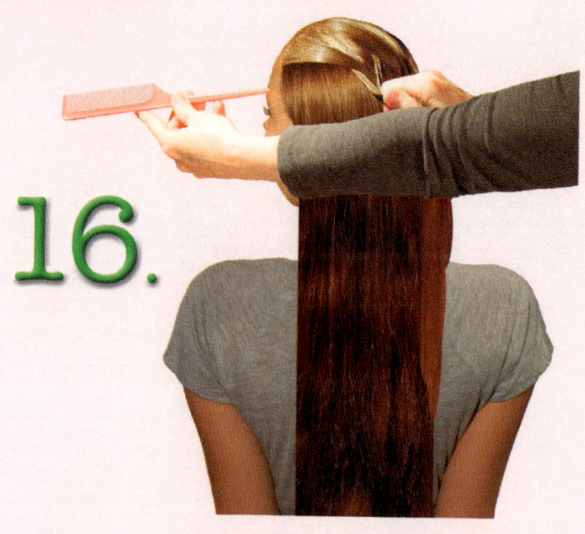

Sliver off a gather from the face back to the braid.

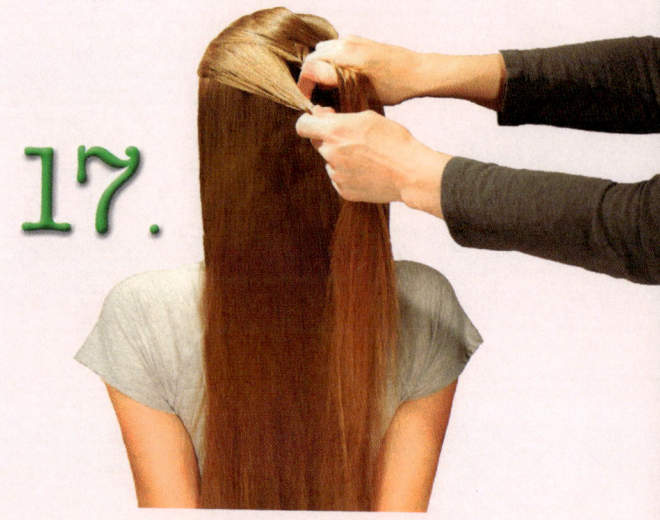

French gathers are placed in strand 1.

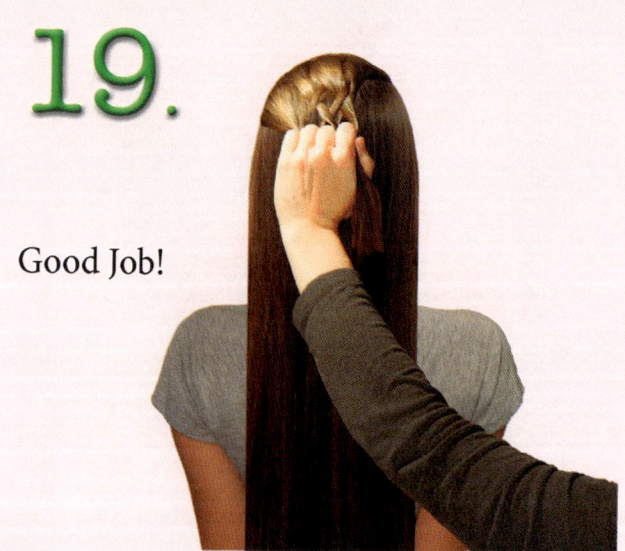

Good Job!

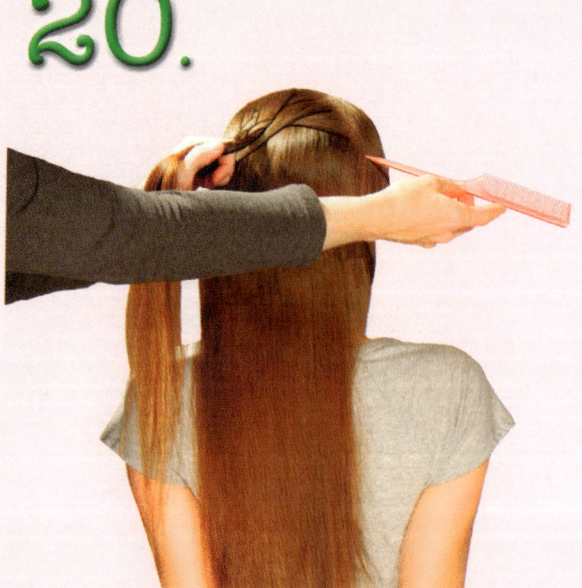

Sliver off a gather from the face back to the braid.

part 3. Six-Strand Taper Stitch

6

18.

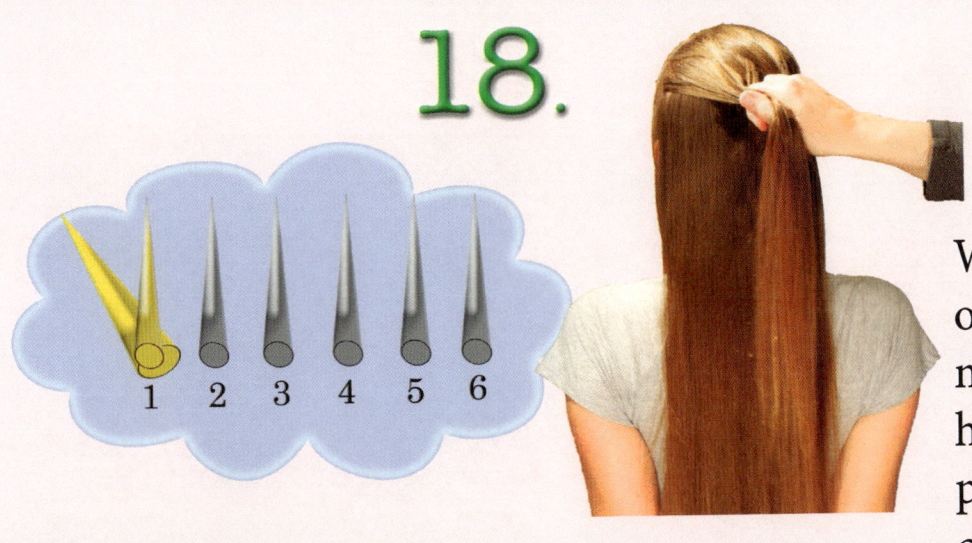

Weave back the other direction making sure you have the correct pattern with the correct hand.

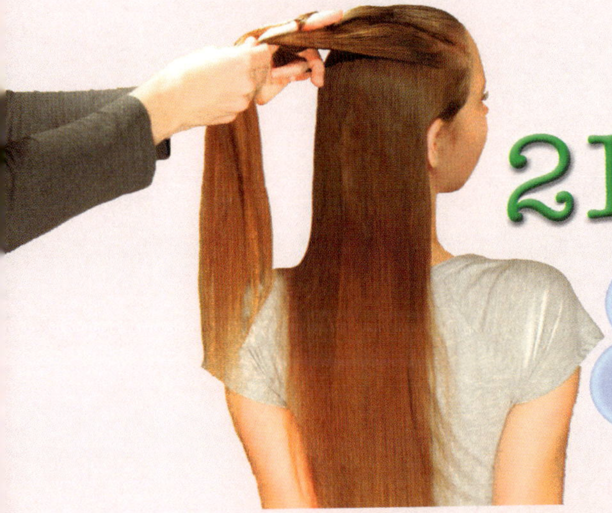

21.

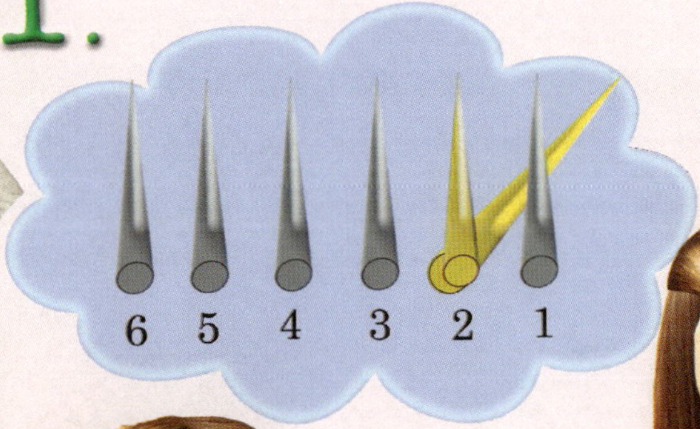

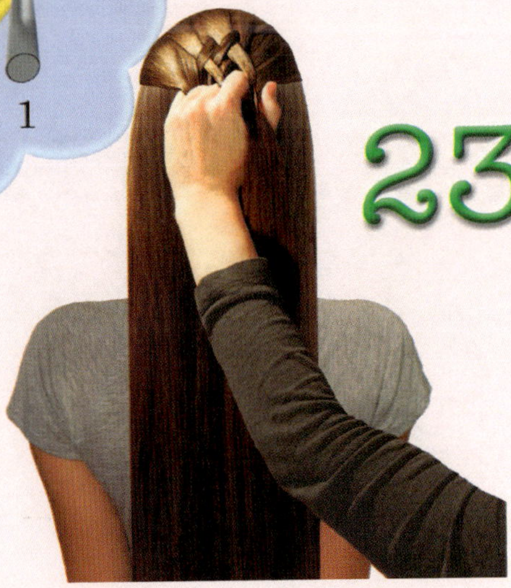

23.

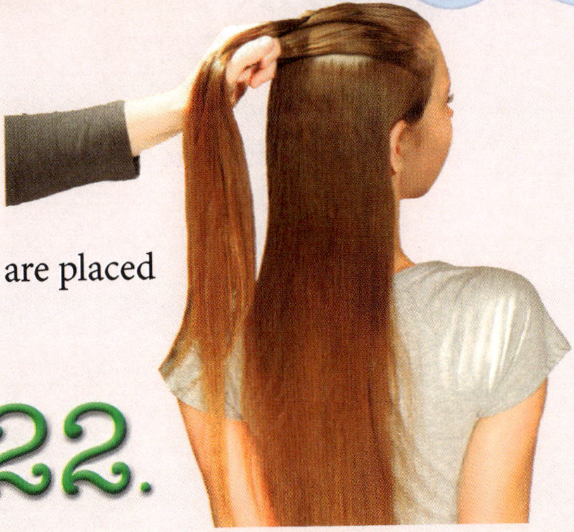

Dutch gathers are placed in strand 2.

22.

And you are ready to weave again. Do you know the pattern for this side?

Ways 257

6 part 4. Six-Strand Taper Stitch

24.

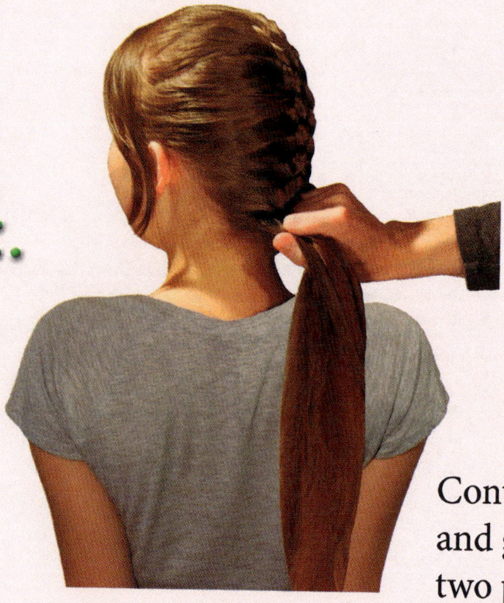

25. 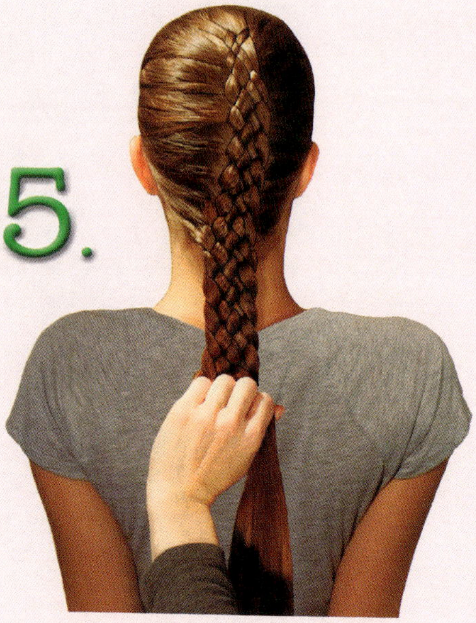 Continue weaving and gathering these two patterns until you reach the end of the hair.

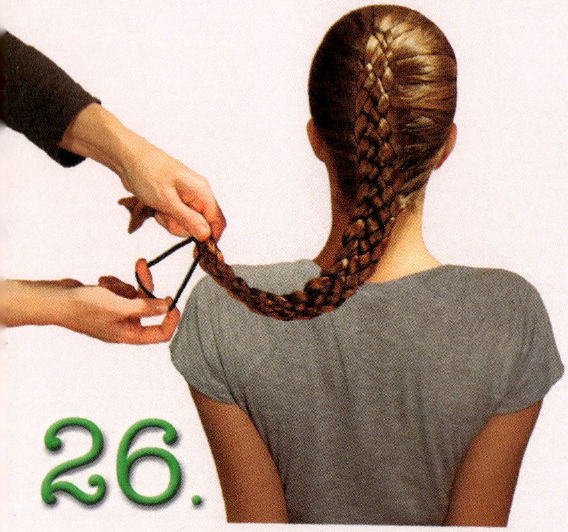

26. Secure with a rubber band.

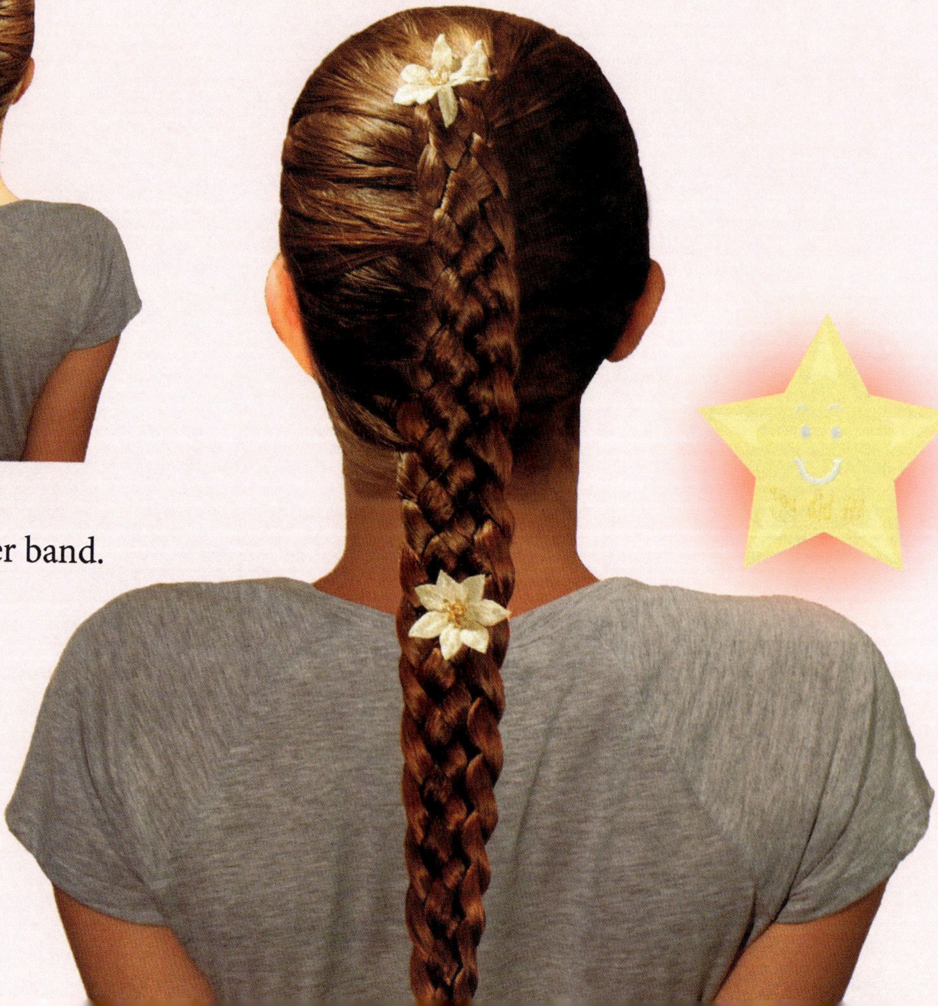

258   www.findingbraids.com

Examples of Six-Strand

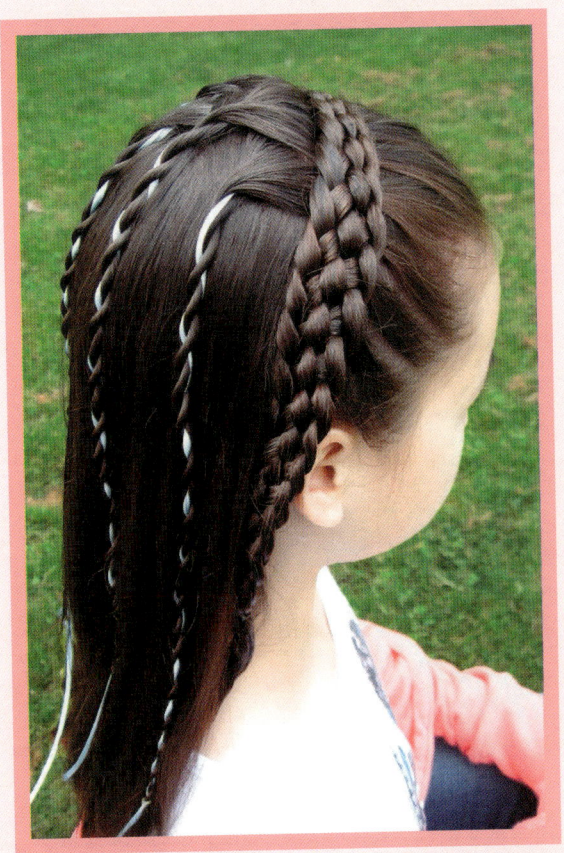
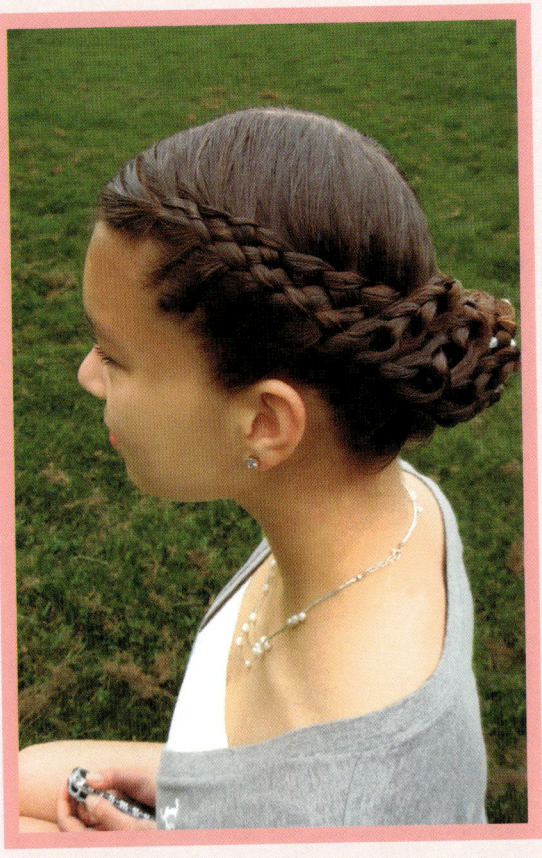
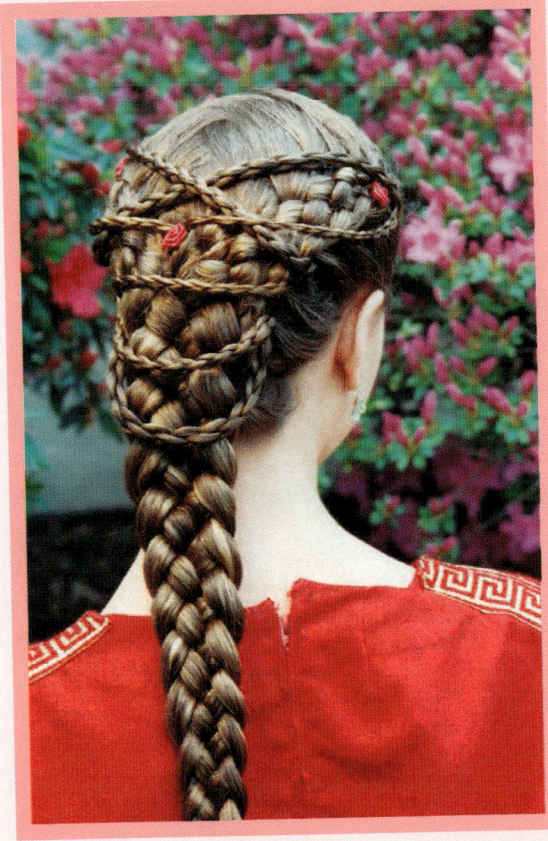
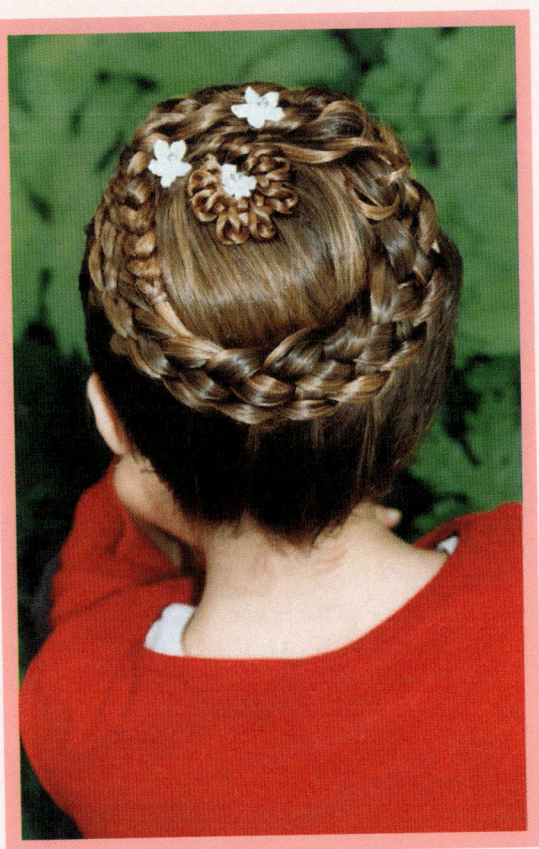

Visit my website to see more examples of the Six-Strand

Notes

How do you know what finger holds more than one strand? Just make a mental note about which finger grabbed two strands. Or choose to always assign certain fingers. It is this very reason that I find the nine-strand easier to do than the seven or eight. In the nine-strand all the fingers hold two strands and you don't have to remember.

A word on starting 7, 8 & 9s

So far we have been able to presection the strands before we start weaving our braids. Now, we will learn to weave without presectioning the strands. This is the last photo to show the strands presectioned. I am only showing it to demonstrate why we are changing our strategy. Notice how impossible it would be to start braiding while holding all of those strands seperate. This problem increases as the numbers of strands increase.

I also need you to calculate the total amount of hair versus how thick each strand is after sectioning. The size of each strand here is the size you will strive to make each strand in the following pages.

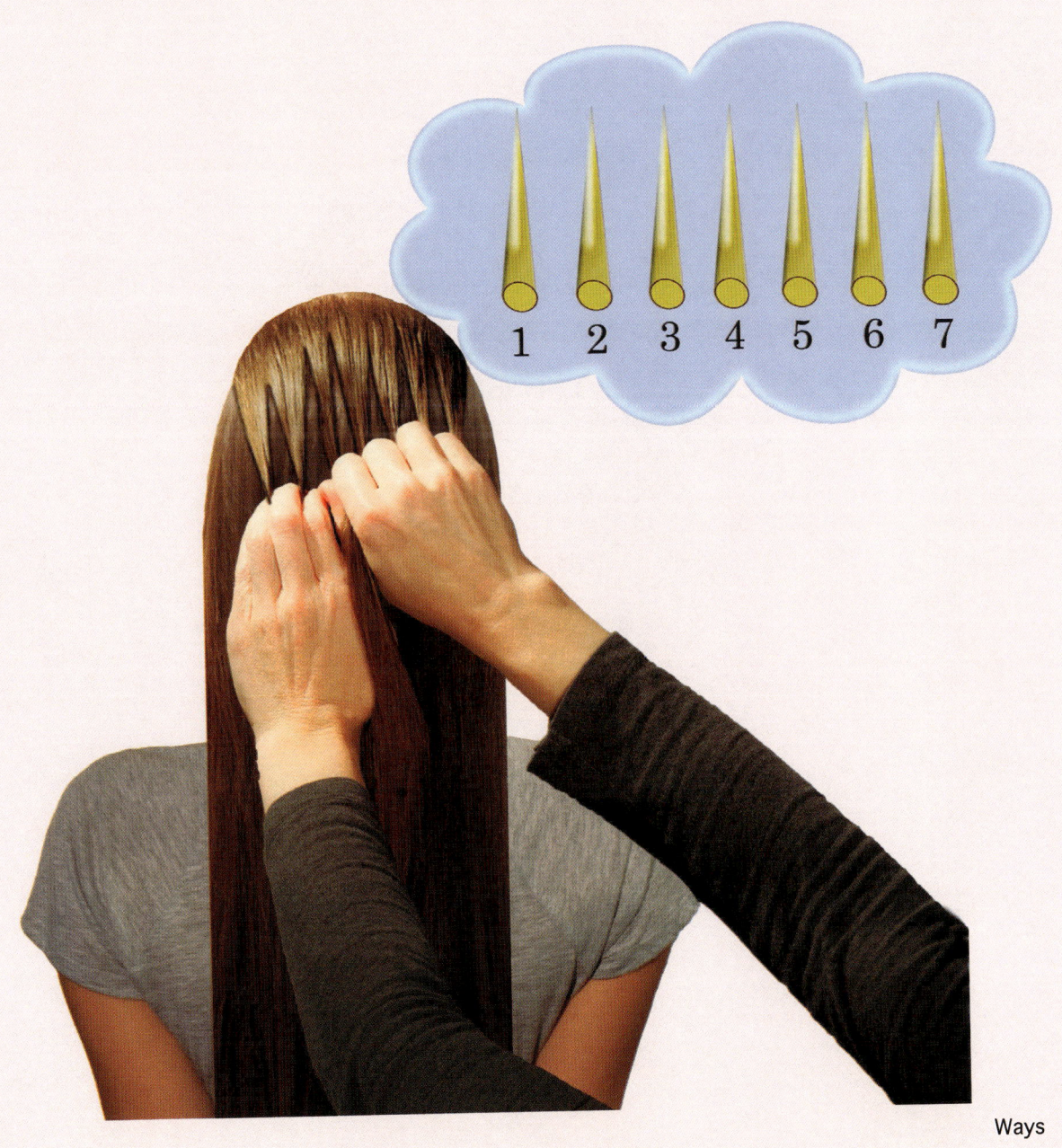

Ways

Seven-Strand

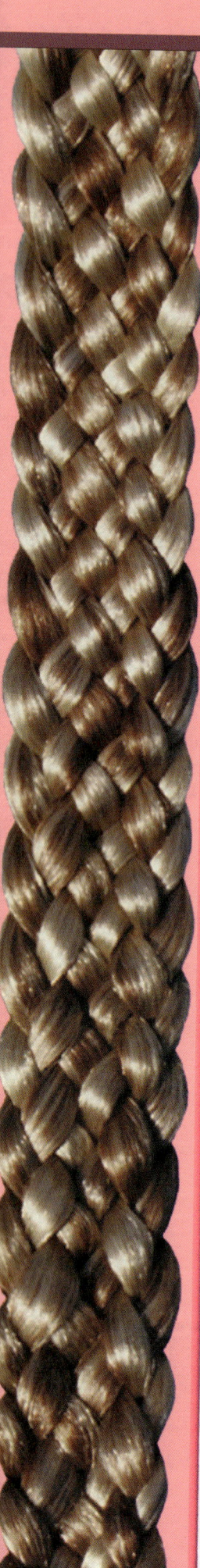

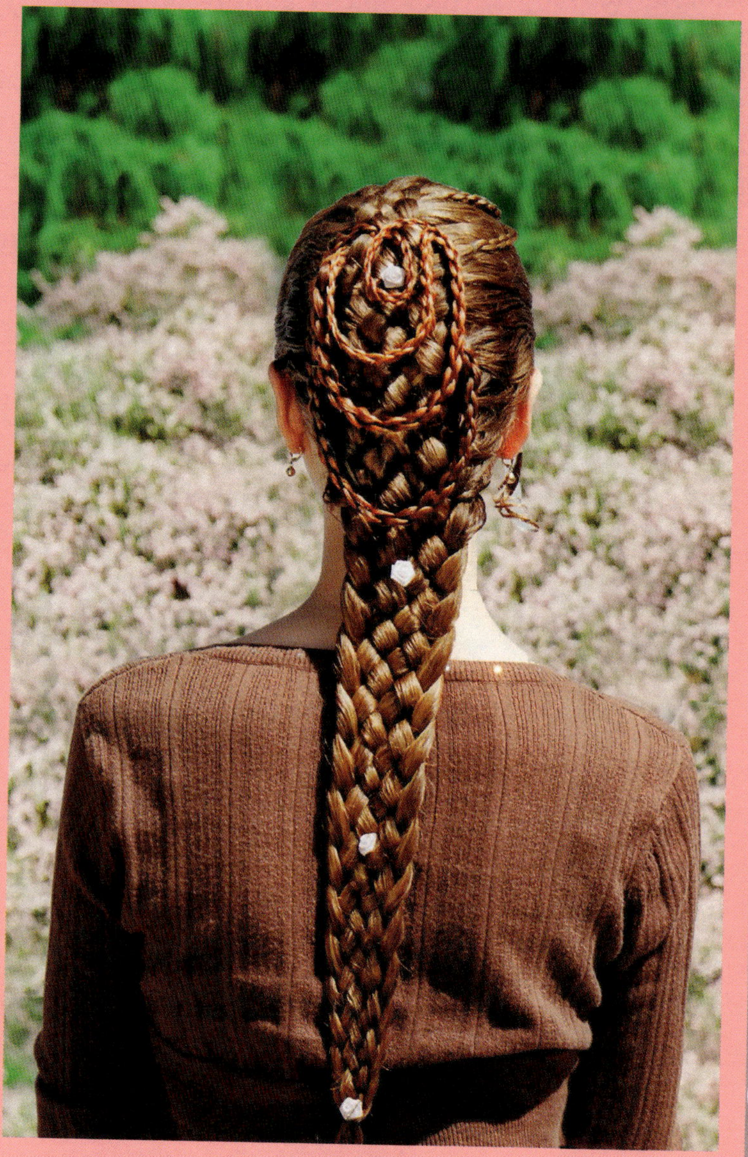

Visually compelling, it is hard to miss this braid in a crowd. Apply effort and patience while learning this and you will have it in no time!

Seven-Strand

Learn this distinctive braid. The next eighteen pages will walk you through this braid.

Braid . . . . 264 - 268

Stitch French . . 270 - 273

Stitch Dutch . . . 276 - 279

Examples 281

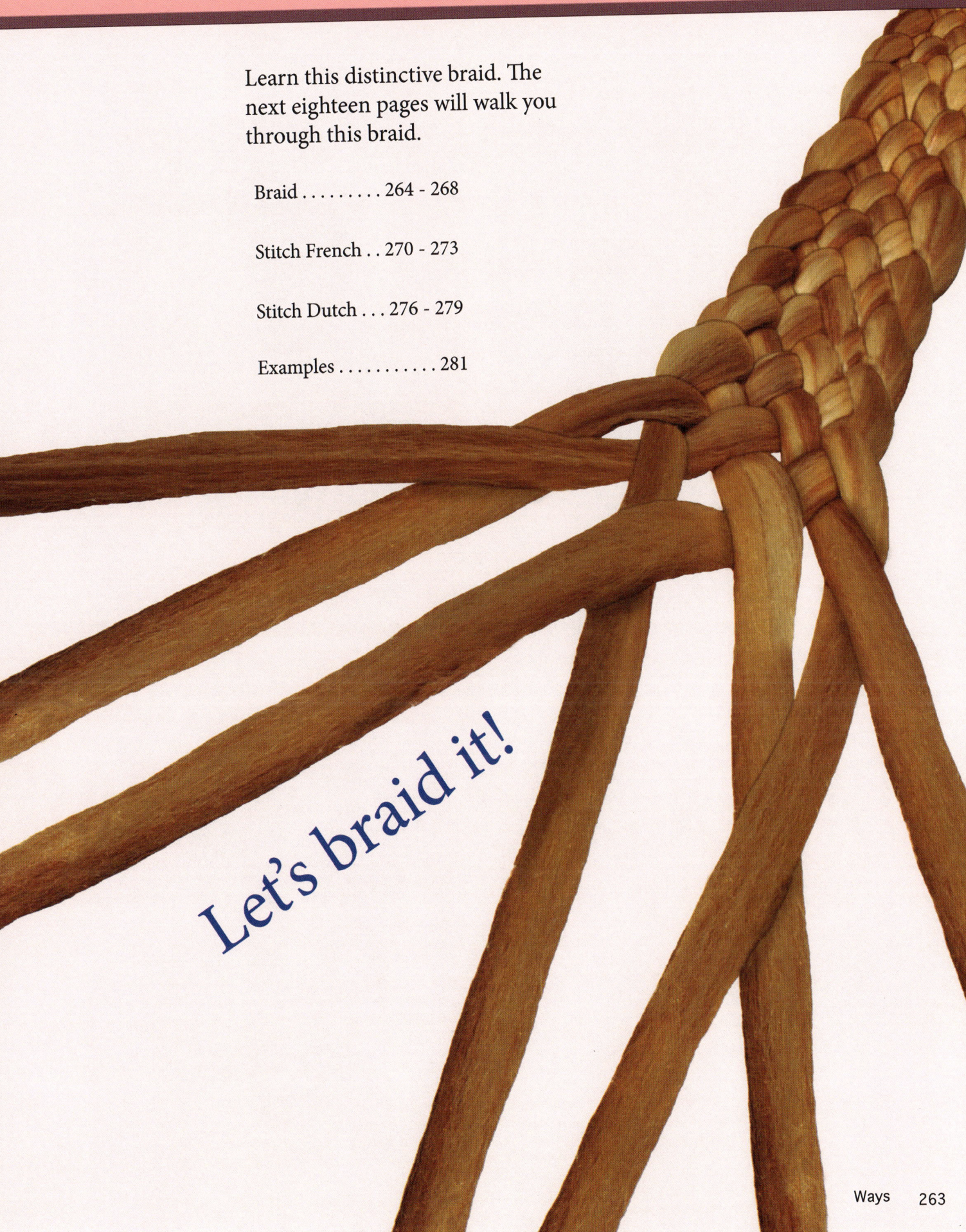

Let's braid it!

Seven-Strand Braid

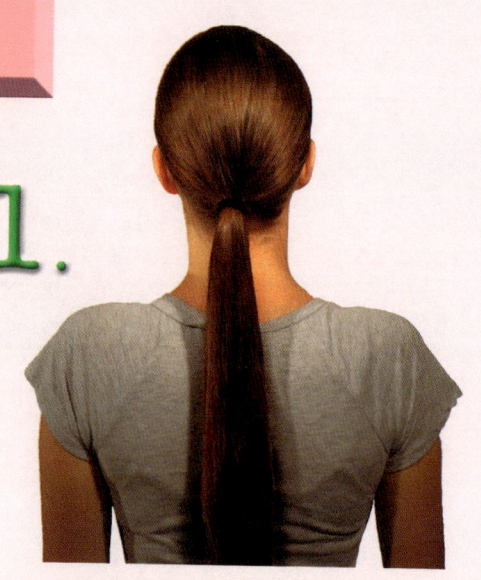

1. Take a section of hair.

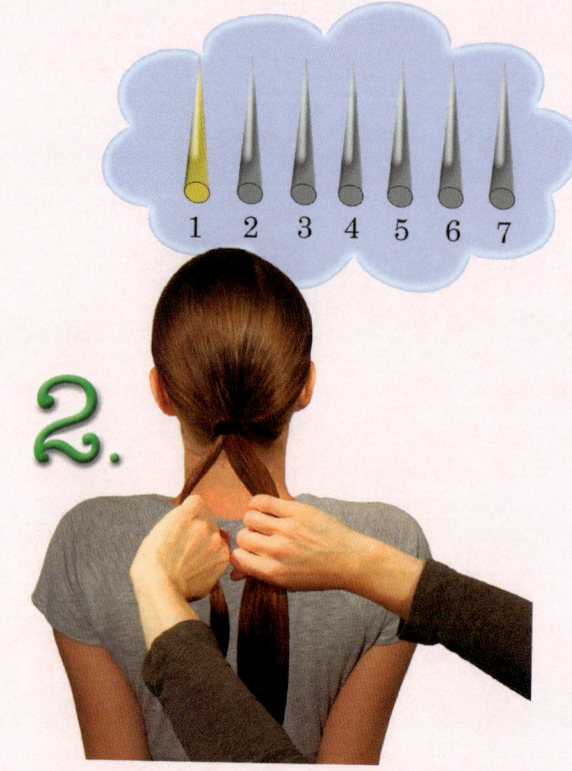

2. In your mind you will visualize the seven strands. Think about how thick they will each be and take the amount of one strand.

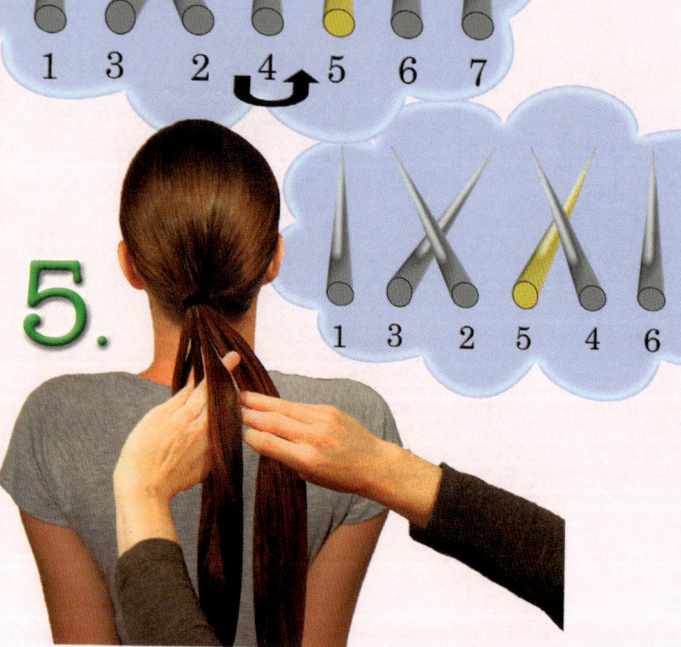

5. Reach under strand 4 and hook strand 5 with the ring finger.

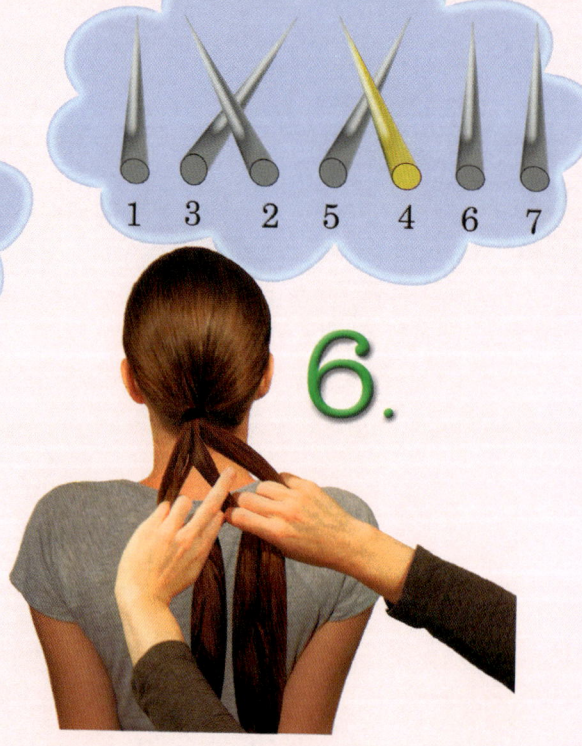

6. Grab strand 4 with the middle finger.

Seven-Strand Braid

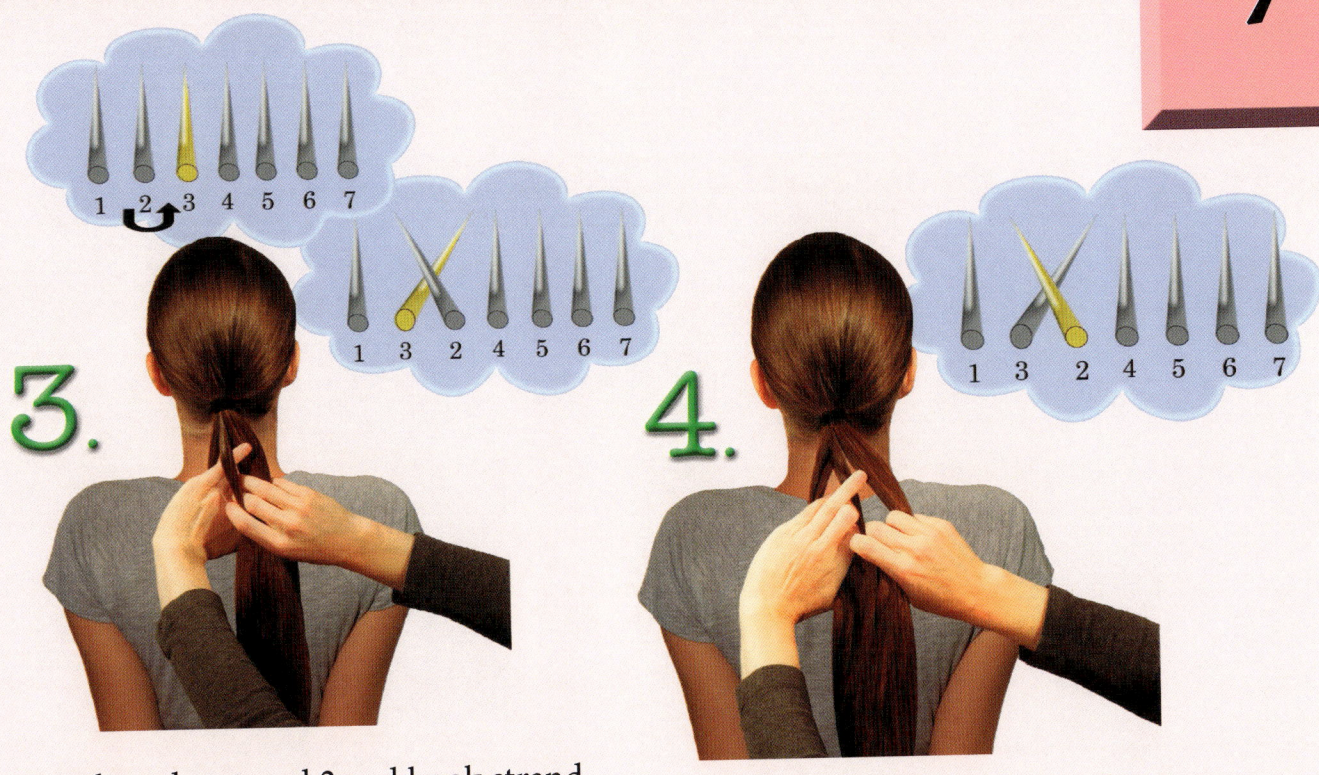

3. Reach under strand 2 and hook strand 3 with the pinky finger. You now have two strands in the pinky finger.

4. Grab strand 2 with the ring finger.

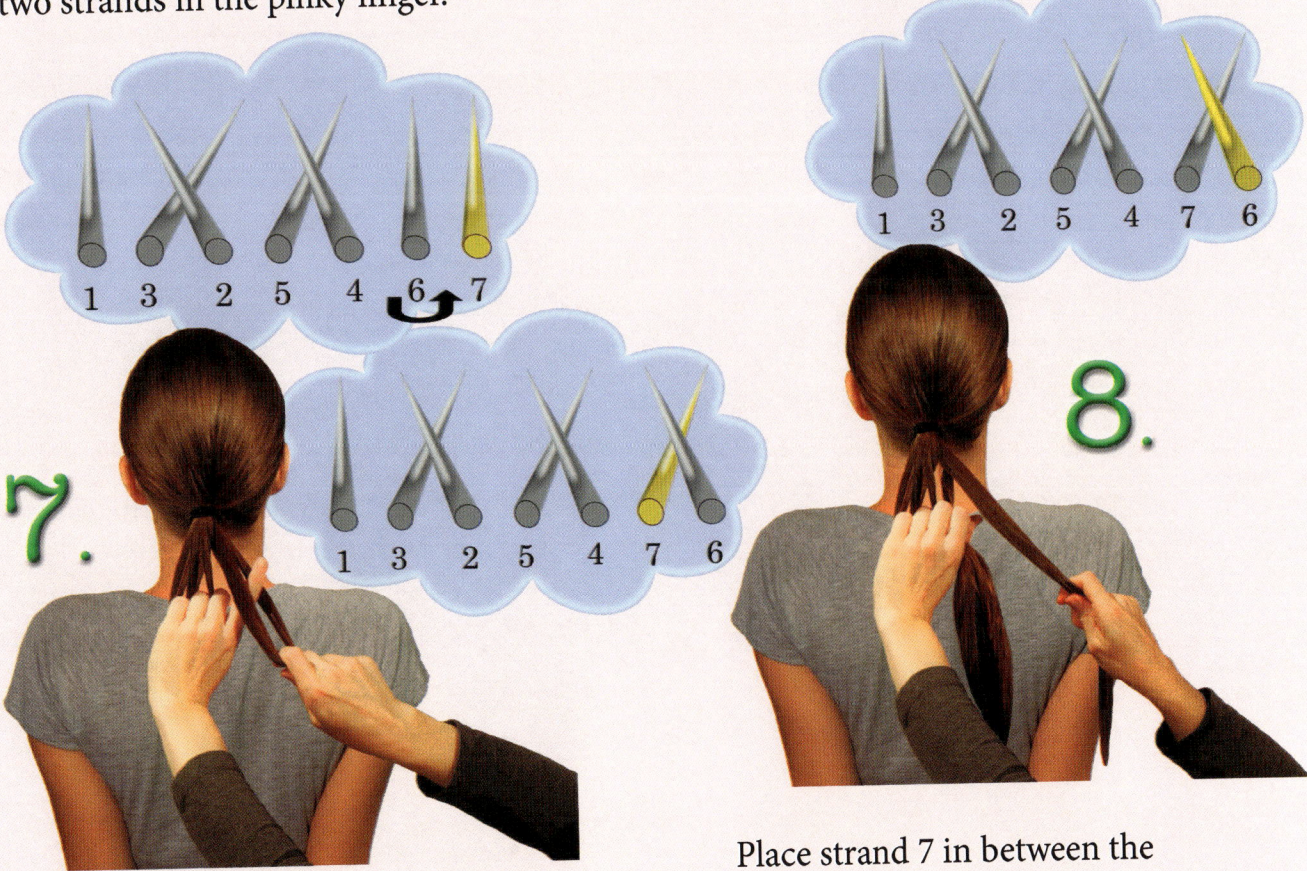

7. Reach under strand 6 and hook strand 7 with the pointer finger.

8. Place strand 7 in between the thumb and pointer finger.

7 Continuing

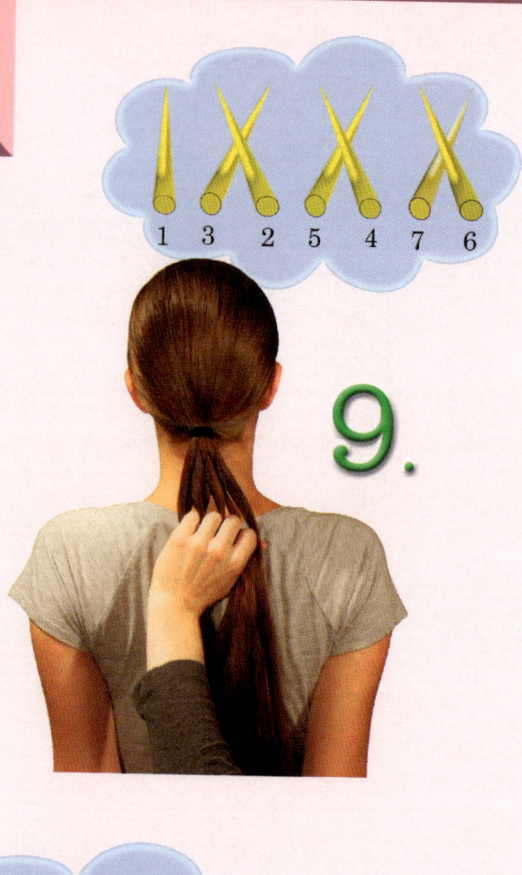

9.

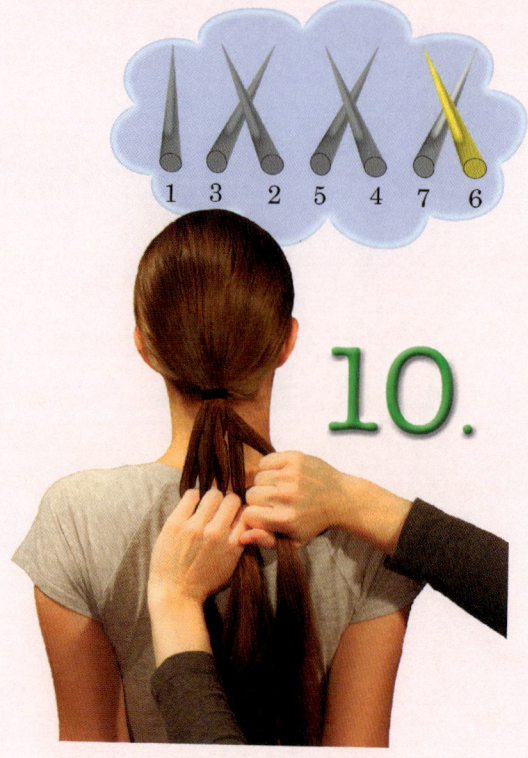

10.

Take strand 6 with your palm down and your thumb facing your belly button.

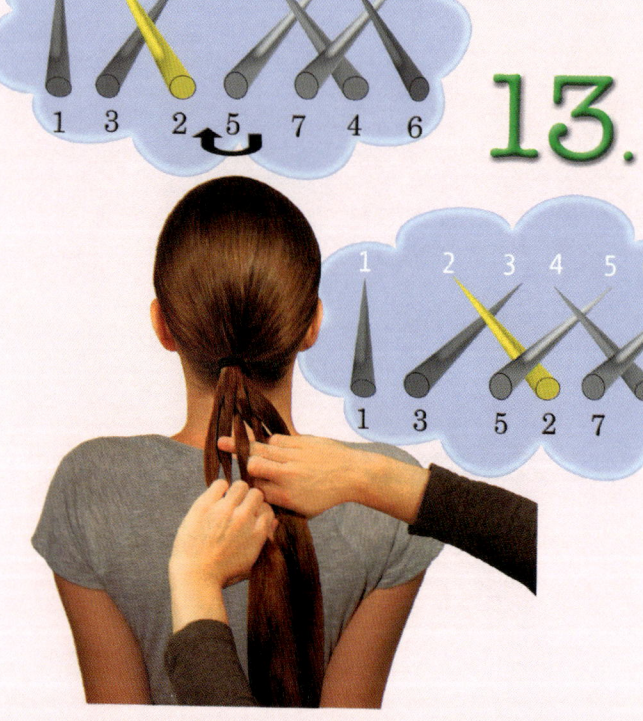

13.

Reach under strand 5 and hook strand 2 with the ring finger.

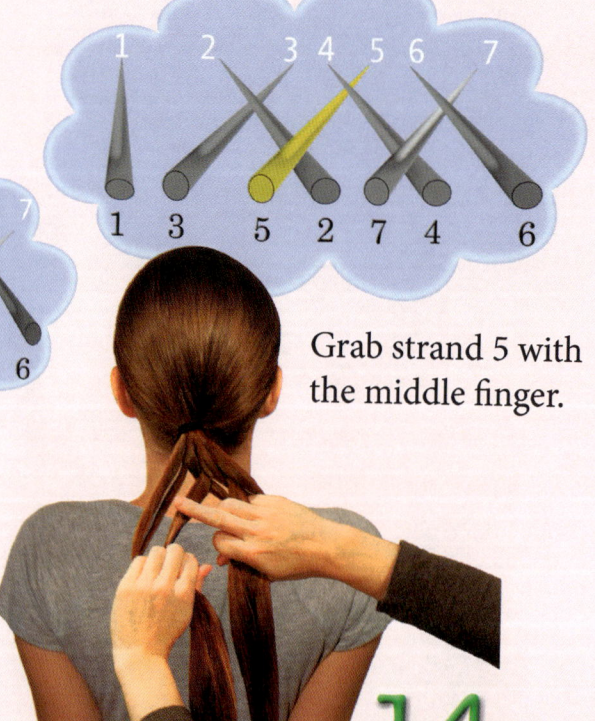

14.

Grab strand 5 with the middle finger.

part 2. Seven-Strand Braid

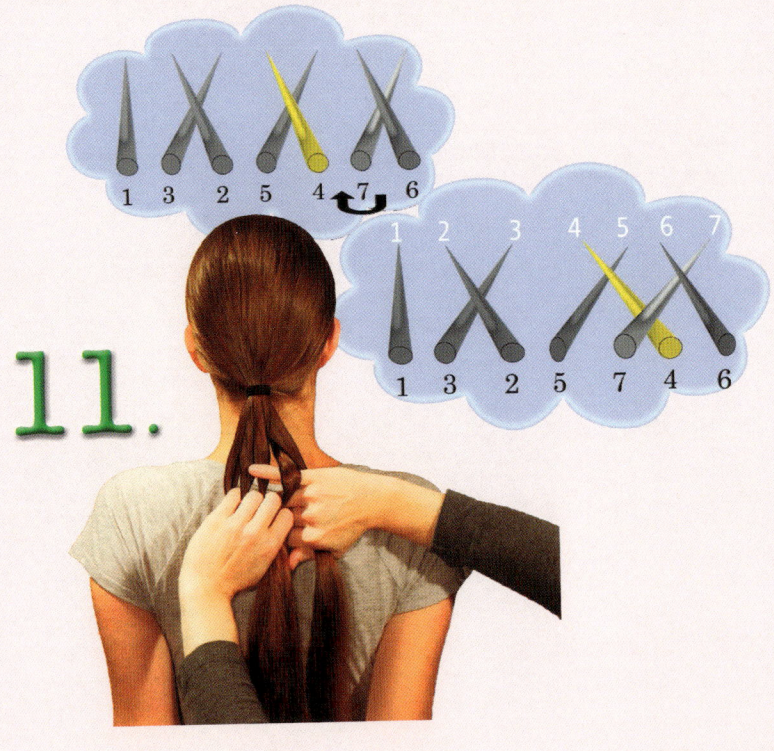

11. Reach under strand 7 and hook strand 4 with the pinky finger.

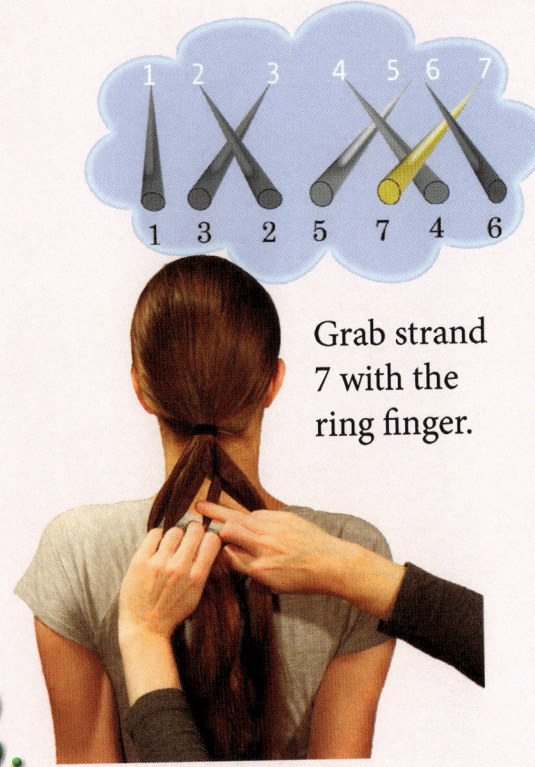

12. Grab strand 7 with the ring finger.

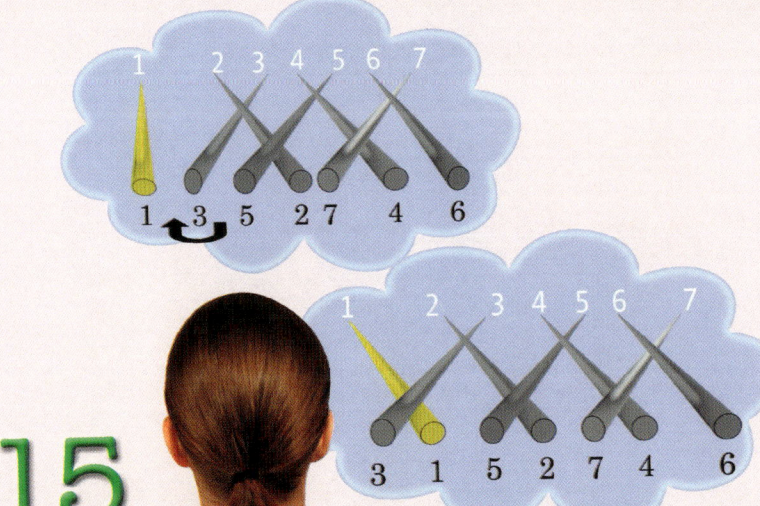

15. Reach under strand 3 and hook strand 1 with the pointer finger.

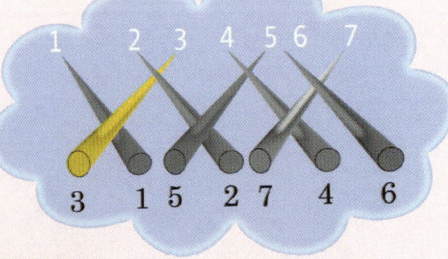

16. Place strand 3 in between the thumb and pointer finger.

part 3. Seven-Strand Braid

Nobody said that it would be easy...they just promised it would be worth it.
- Harvey Mackay

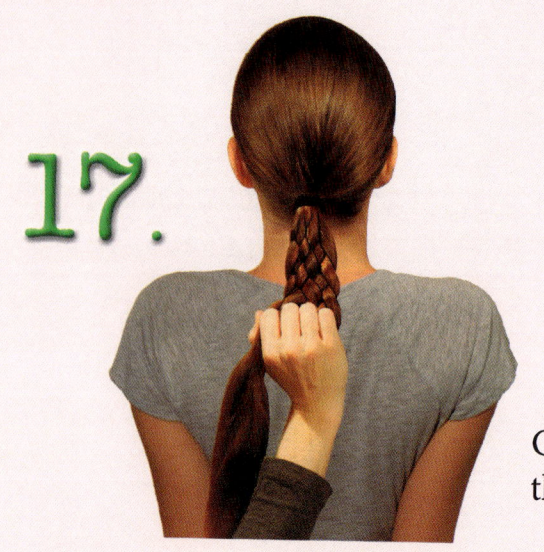

17.

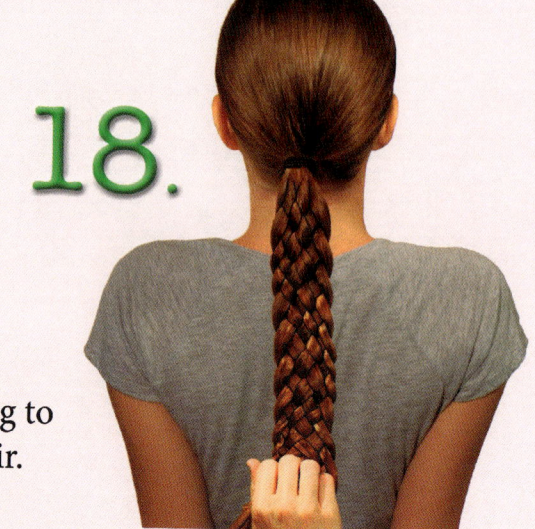

18. Continue weaving to the end of the hair.

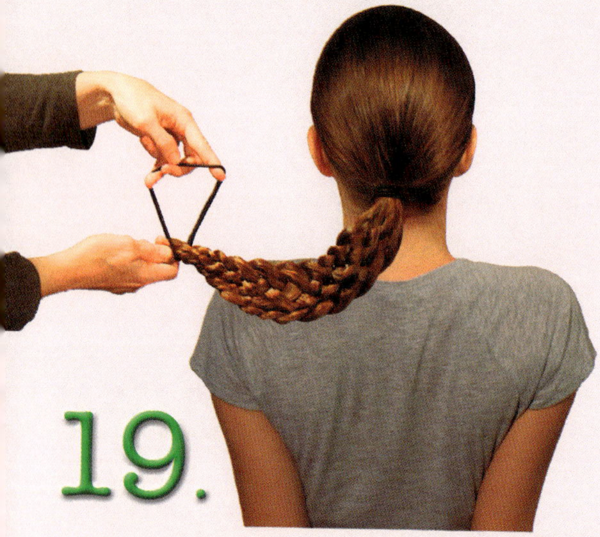

19. Secure with a rubber band.

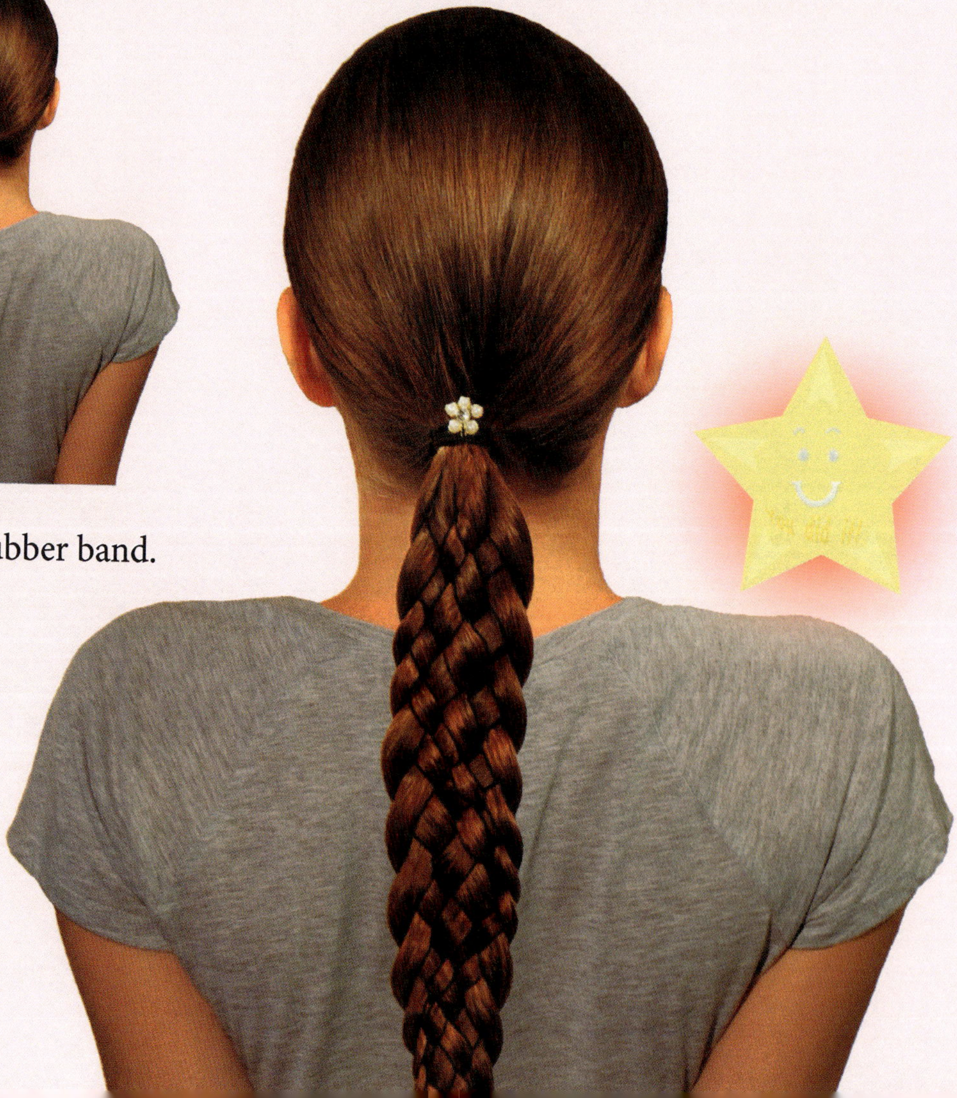

Seven-Strand

Gather from both sides

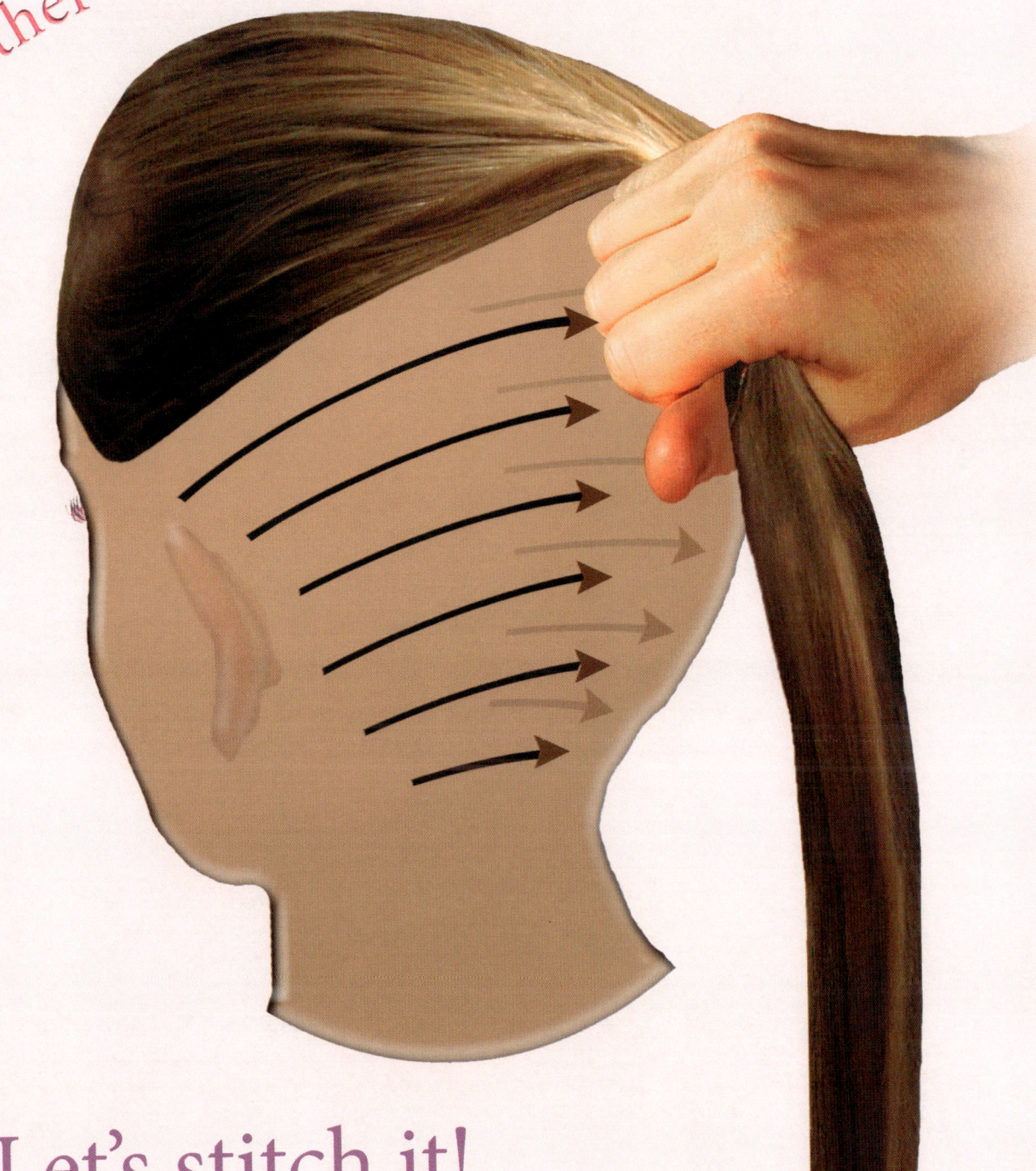

Let's stitch it!

Let's stitch it!

Let's stitch it!

7 Seven-Strand French Stitch

1.

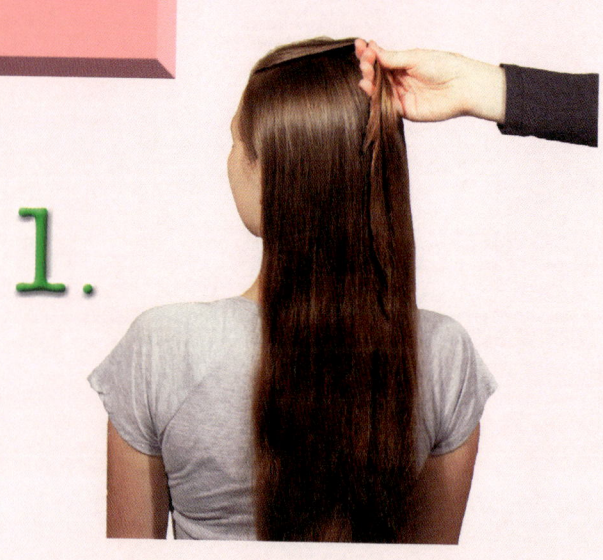

Take a section of hair as illustrated. In your mind you will visualize the seven strands. Think about how thick they will each be.

2.

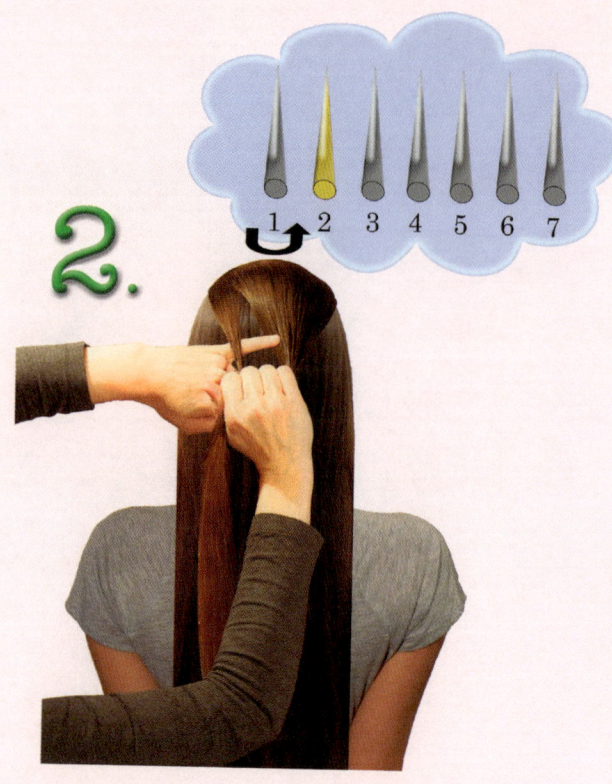

Reach under strand 1 and hook strand 2 with the pinky finger.

5.

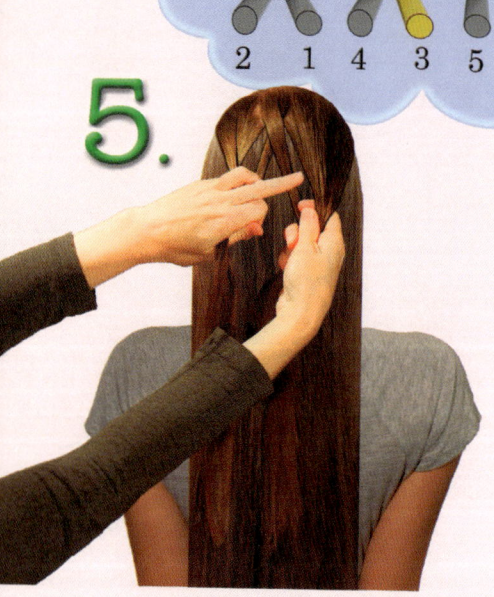

Grab strand 3 with the middle finger.

6.

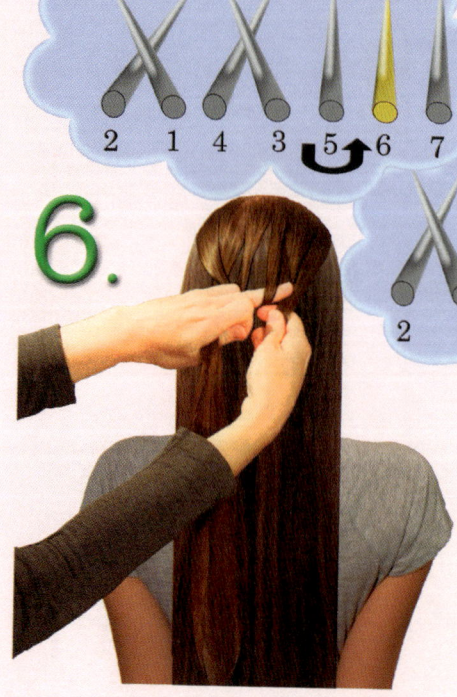

Reach under strand 5 and hook strand 6 with the middle finger.

270 www.findingbraids.com

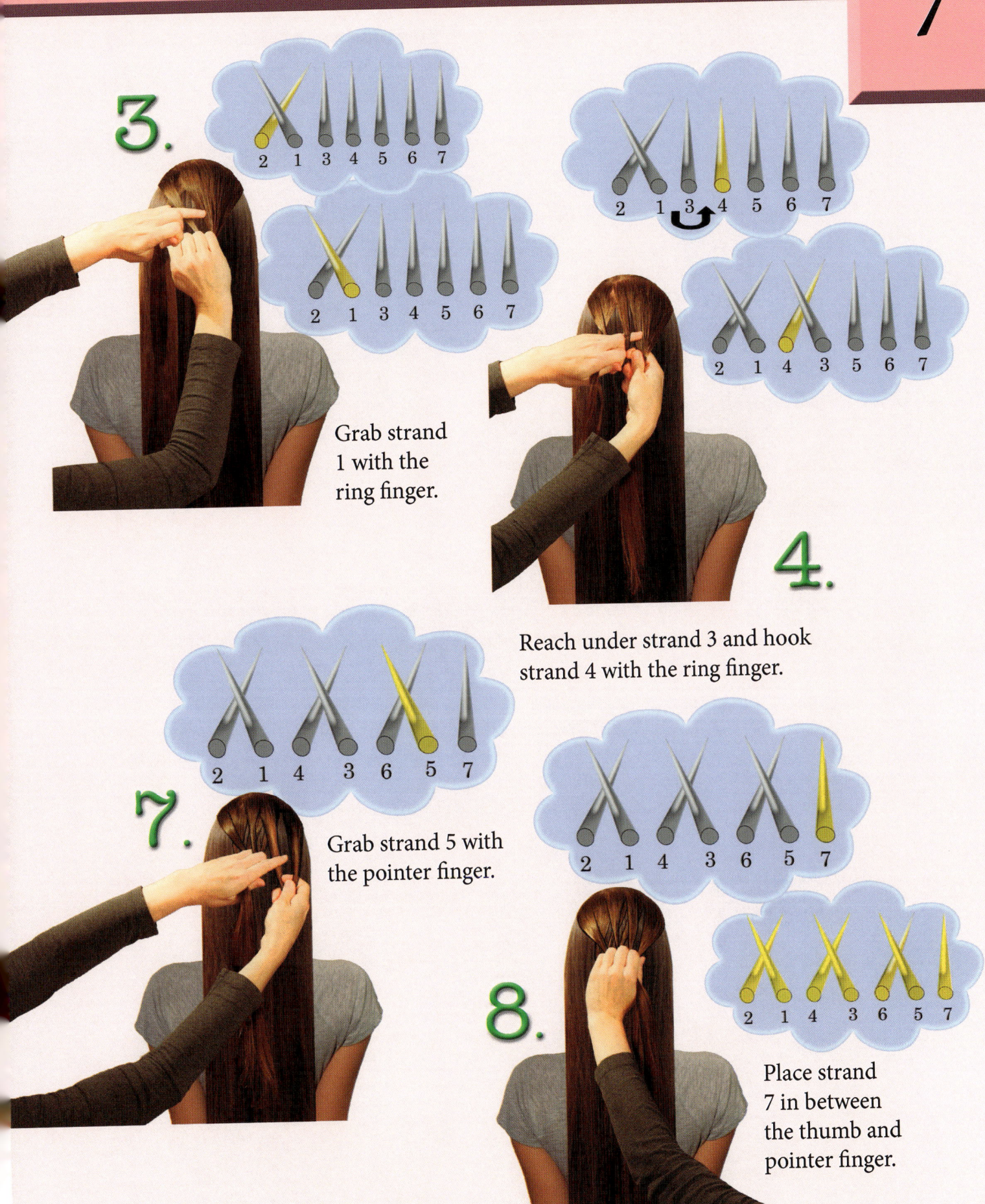

7 Continuing

Success seems to be connected with action. - Conrad Hilton

You now have an available hand to pick up your tail comb.

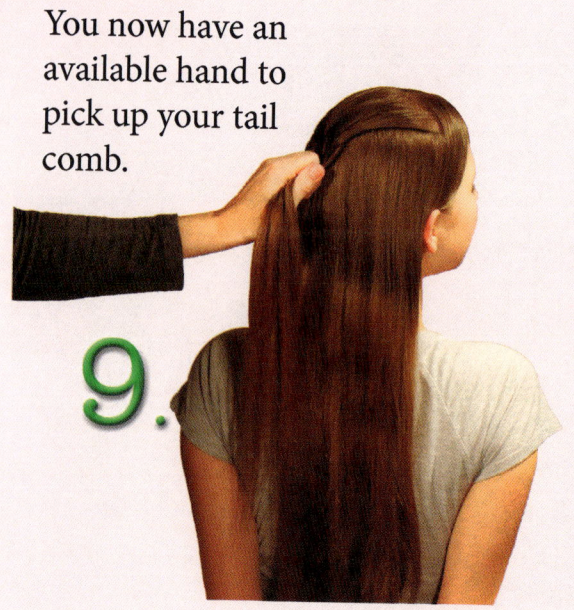

9.

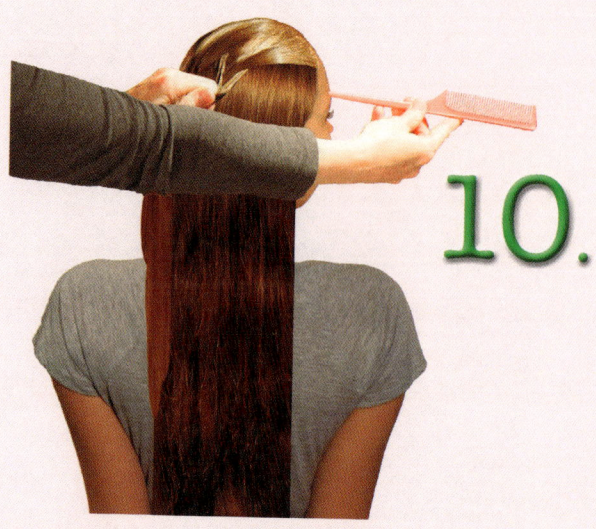

10.

Sliver off a gather from the face back to the braid.

To gather or not to gather? When is it time to gather? Look at number 9. If you gather with your right hand on the right side, you will only make strand 1 larger. Which is not a bad thing, but there isn't any point to it. Weave back the other direction to see if it is time to gather yet. You may still notice the original strand getting larger.

So when and why does a braider gather? There is no correct answer. You may gather from the get-go, as it does not hurt anything. I always gather on the third pass. That is when the gather stitches the braid to the head. Yes, it also makes the strand it is being added to larger; but the point of gathers...is to stitch the braid to the head. You should do what is easiest for you.

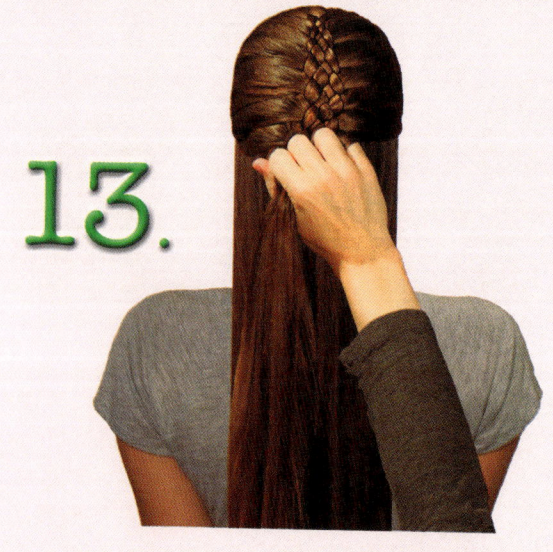

13.

Continue weaving and gathering until you reach the end of the hair.

14.

272 www.findingbraids.com

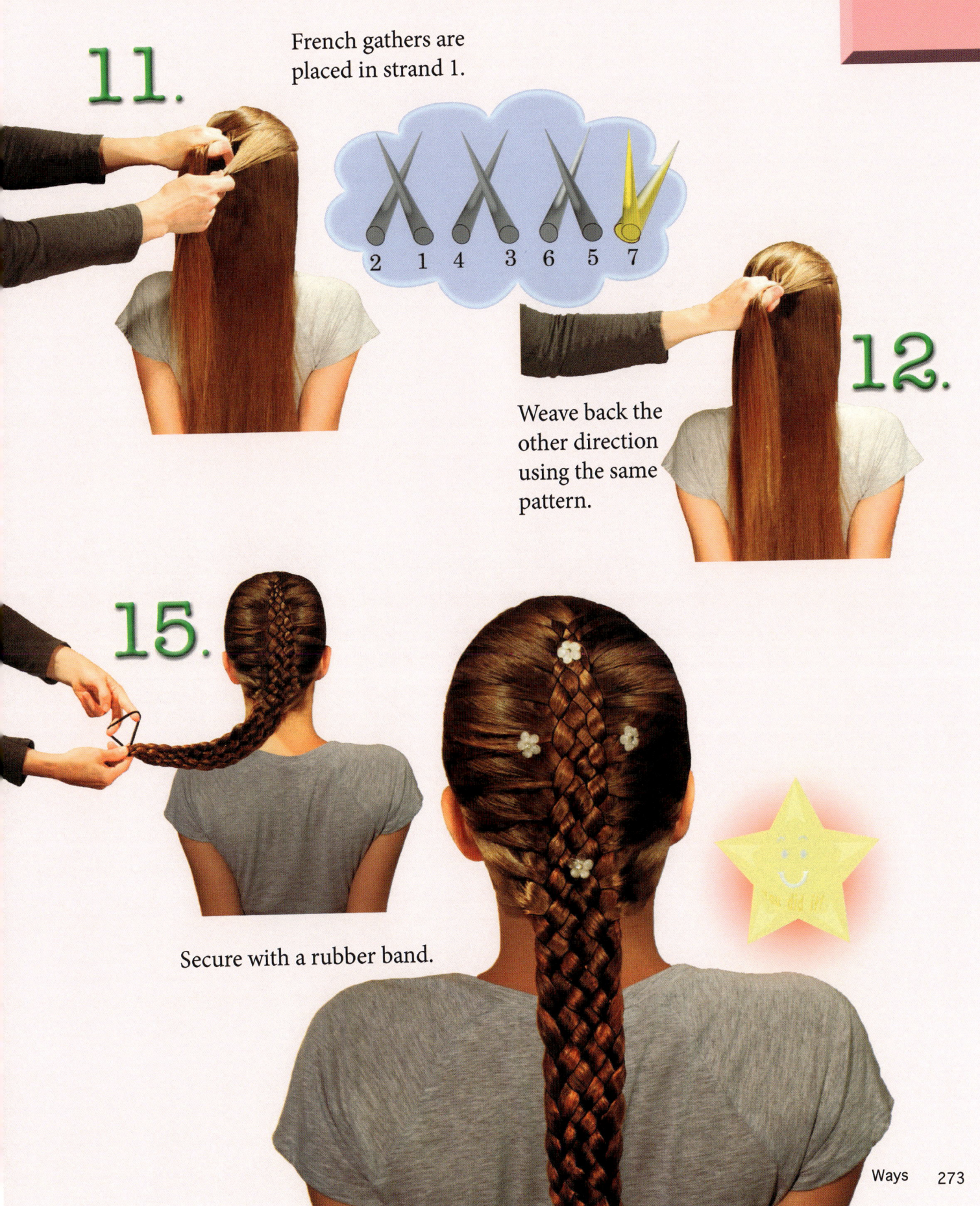

Seven-Strand

Notes

_____

_____

_____

_____

_____

_____

Does the logic in the background whisper to you about two strands in a finger? With the six, seven and eight strand braid patterns, which fingers grab two strands is up to the pattern and you. Yes, I specify what to do. I have to. It is a book. Let the words "take, under, take" bounce around your head when you braid and see if a rhythm develops.

Seven-Strand

Gather from both sides

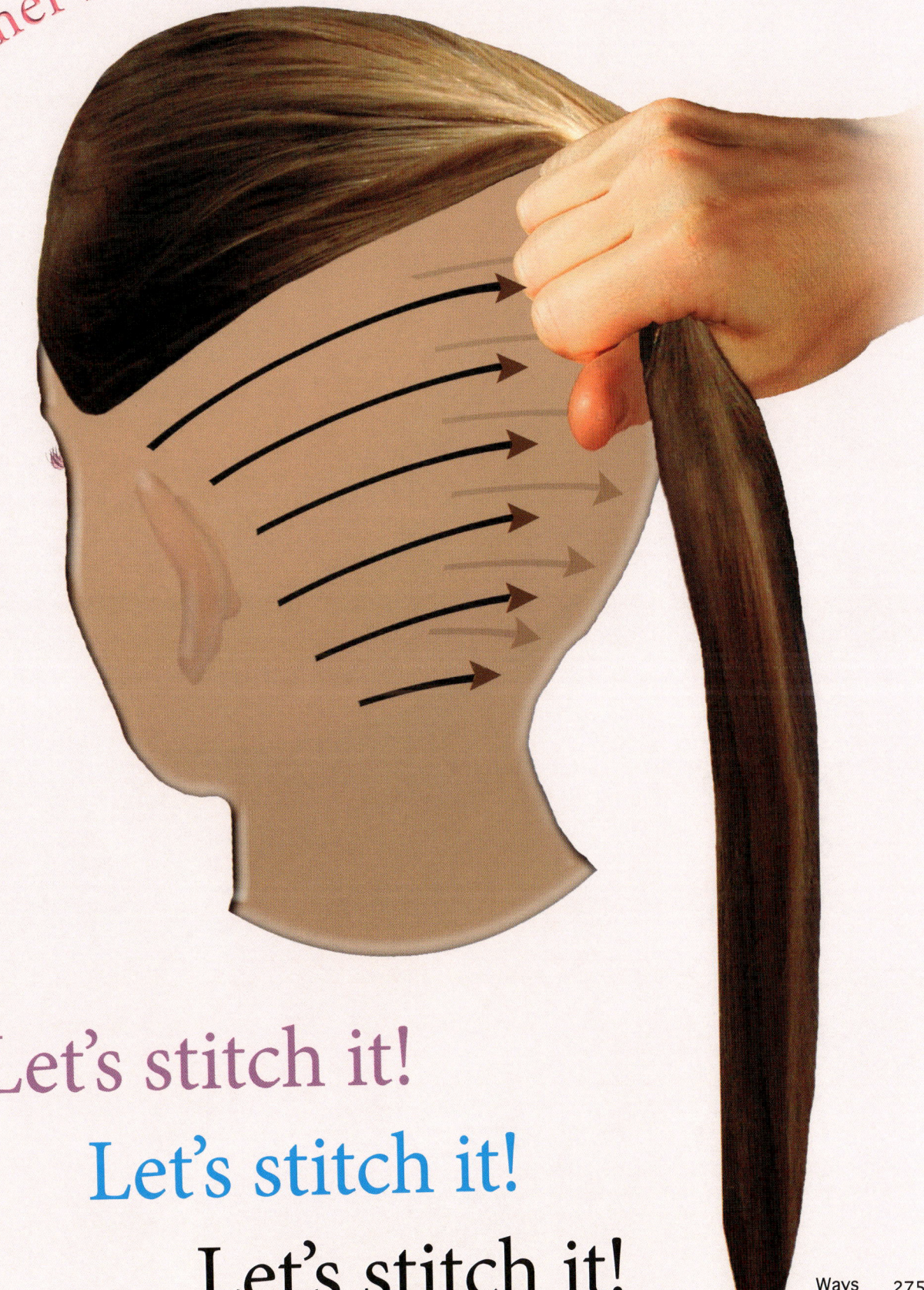

Let's stitch it!

Let's stitch it!

Let's stitch it!

7 Seven-Strand Dutch Stitch

Turn your can'ts into cans. - Yobi Yamada

1.
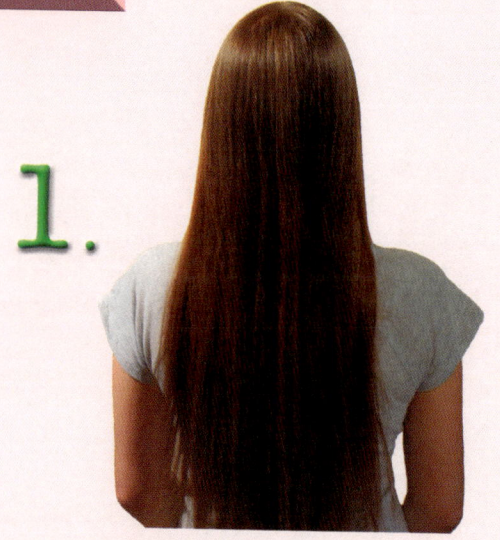

Begin with clean, brushed hair.

2.
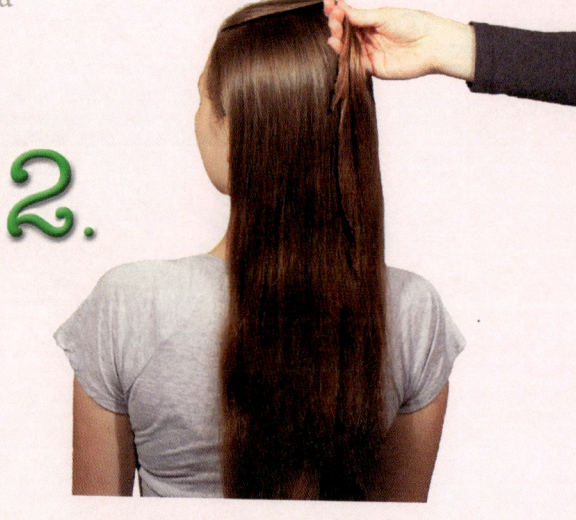

Take a section of hair as illustrated. In your mind you will visualize the seven strands. Think about how thick they will each be.

5.
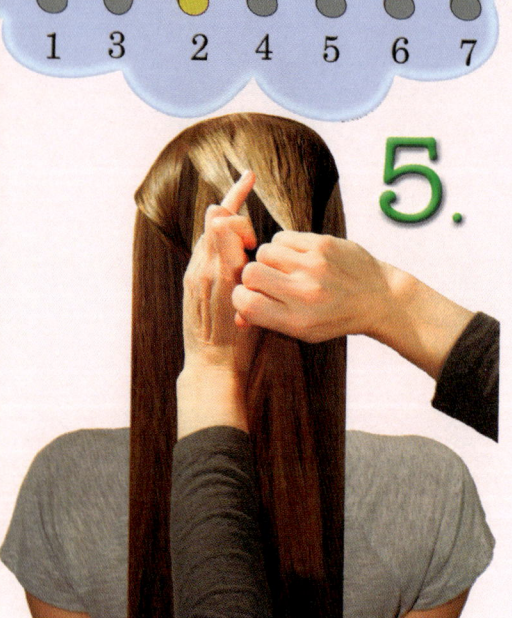

Grab strand 2 with the ring finger.

6.
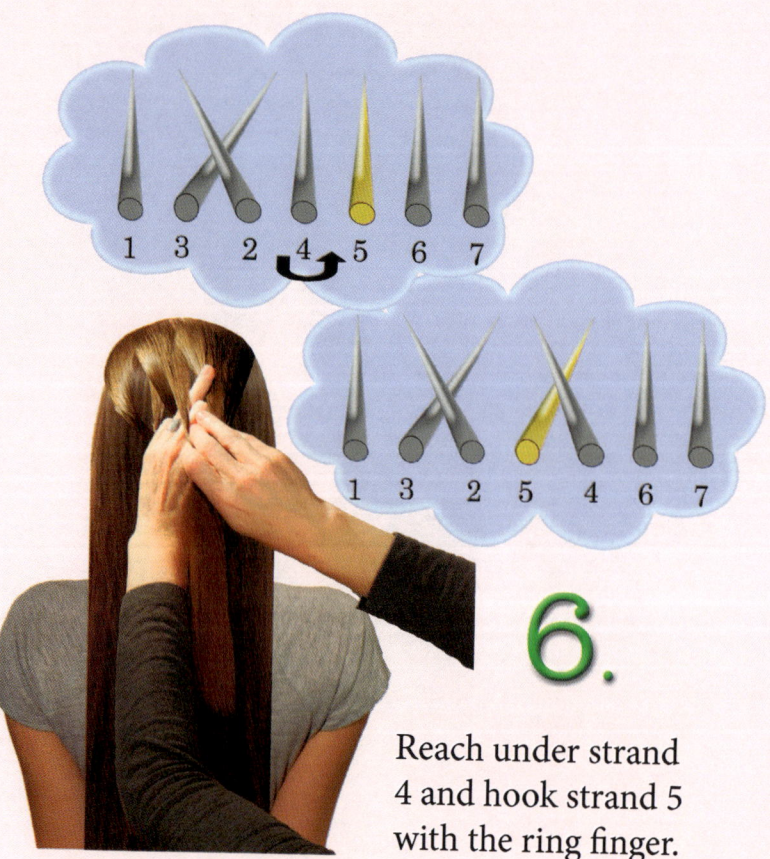

Reach under strand 4 and hook strand 5 with the ring finger.

www.findingbraids.com

Seven-Strand Dutch Stitch

7

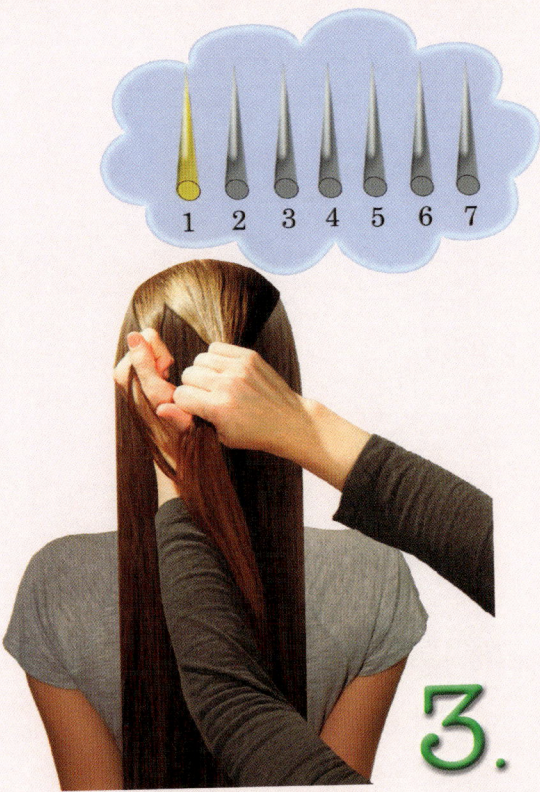

3.

Take strand 1 with your palm down and your thumb facing your belly button.

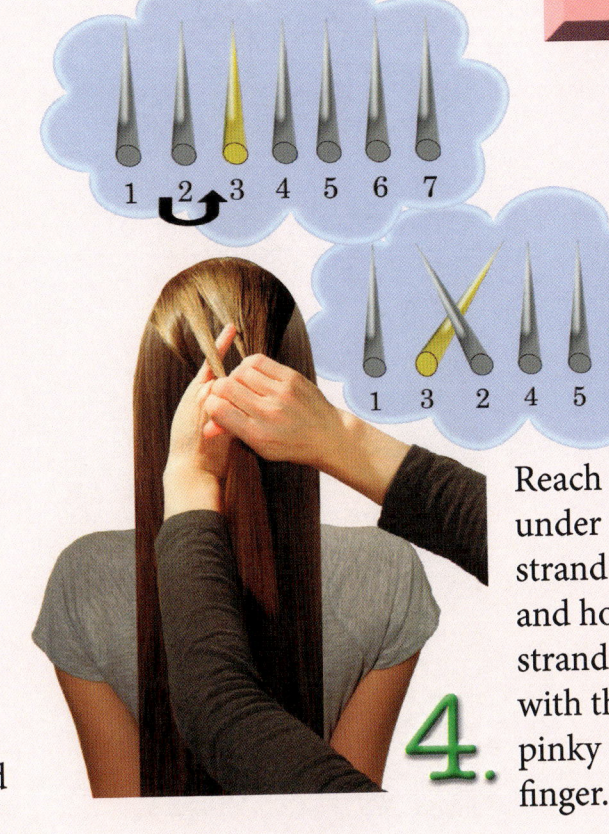

4.

Reach under strand 2 and hook strand 3 with the pinky finger.

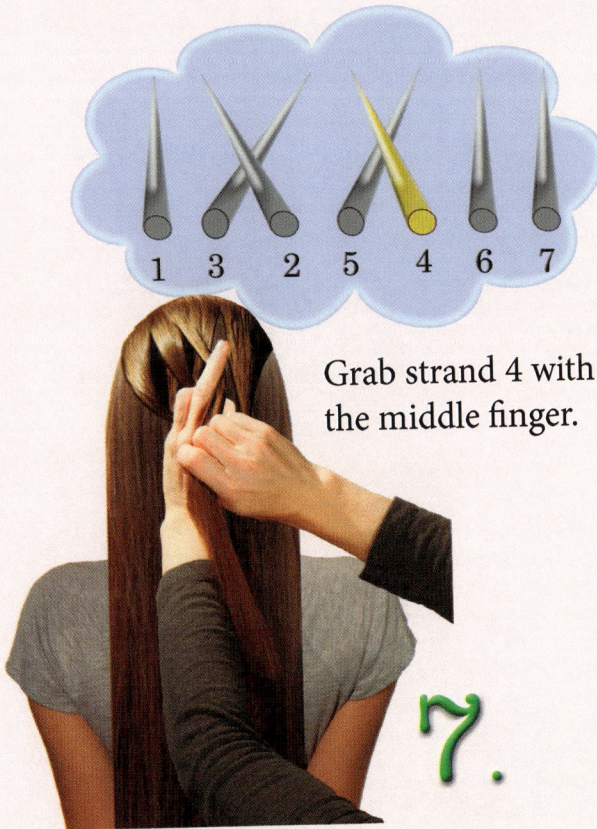

7.

Grab strand 4 with the middle finger.

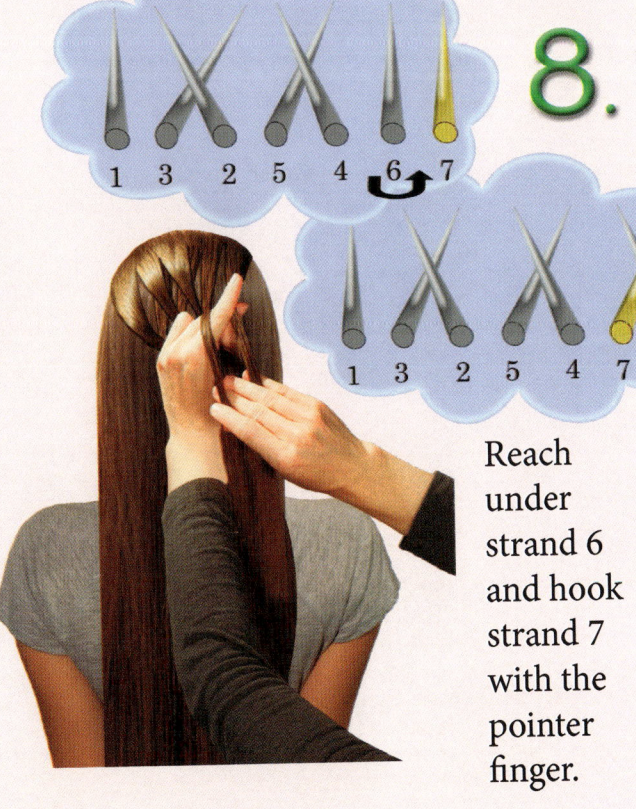

8.

Reach under strand 6 and hook strand 7 with the pointer finger.

Ways

7 Continuing

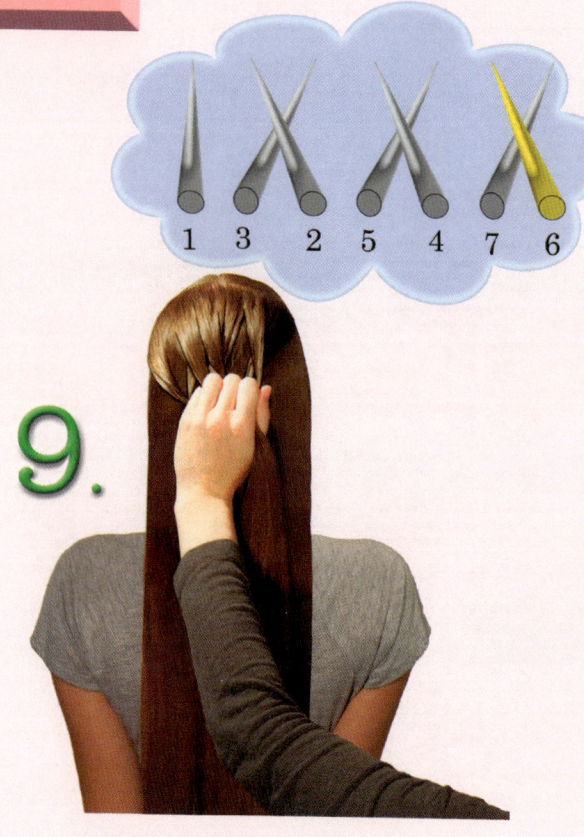

9. Place strand 6 in between the thumb and pointer finger.

To gather or not to gather?

When is it time to gather? Look at number 9. If you gather with your right hand on the right side, you will only make strand 1 larger. Which is not a bad thing, but there isn't any point to it. Weave back the other direction to see if it is time to gather yet. You may still notice the original strand getting larger.

So when and why does a braider gather? You may gather from the get go, as it does not hurt anything. I always gather on the third pass. That is when the gather stitches the braid to the head. Yes, it also makes the strand it is being added to larger; but the point of gathers…is to stitch the braid to the head. You should do what is easiest for you.

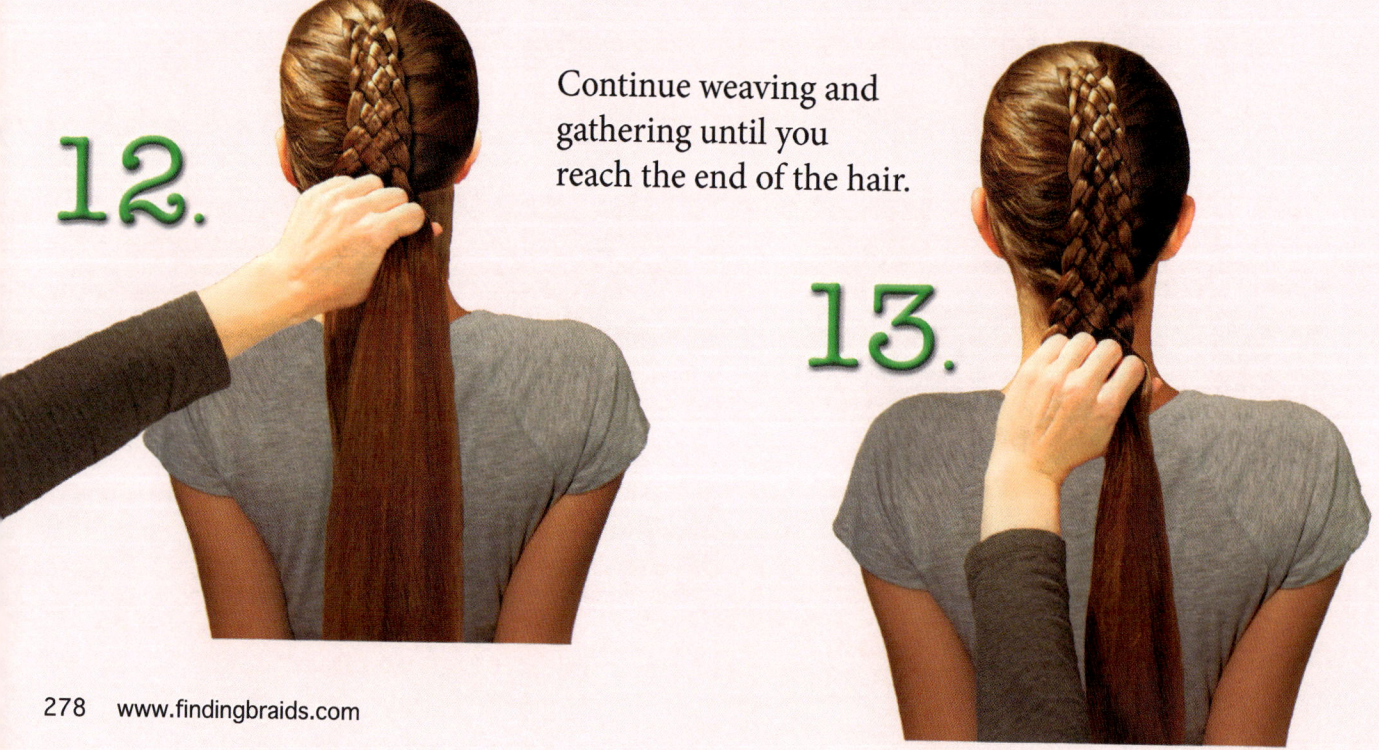

Continue weaving and gathering until you reach the end of the hair.

278 www.findingbraids.com

part 2. Seven-Strand Dutch Stitch

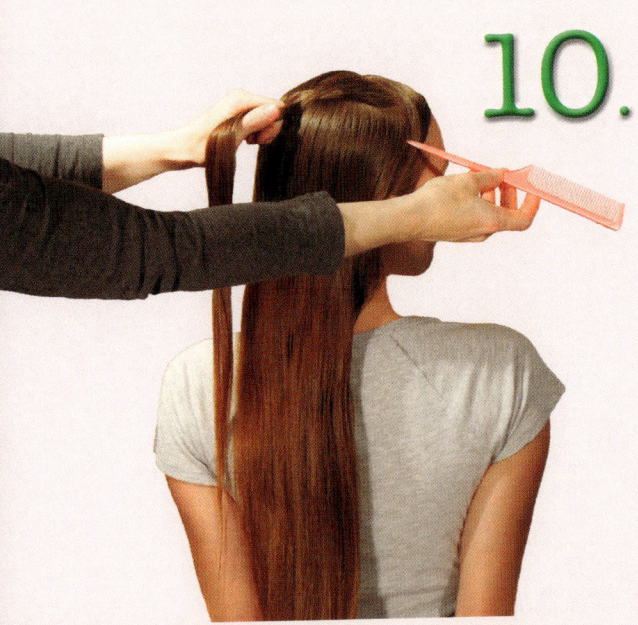

10.

Sliver off a gather from the face back to the braid.

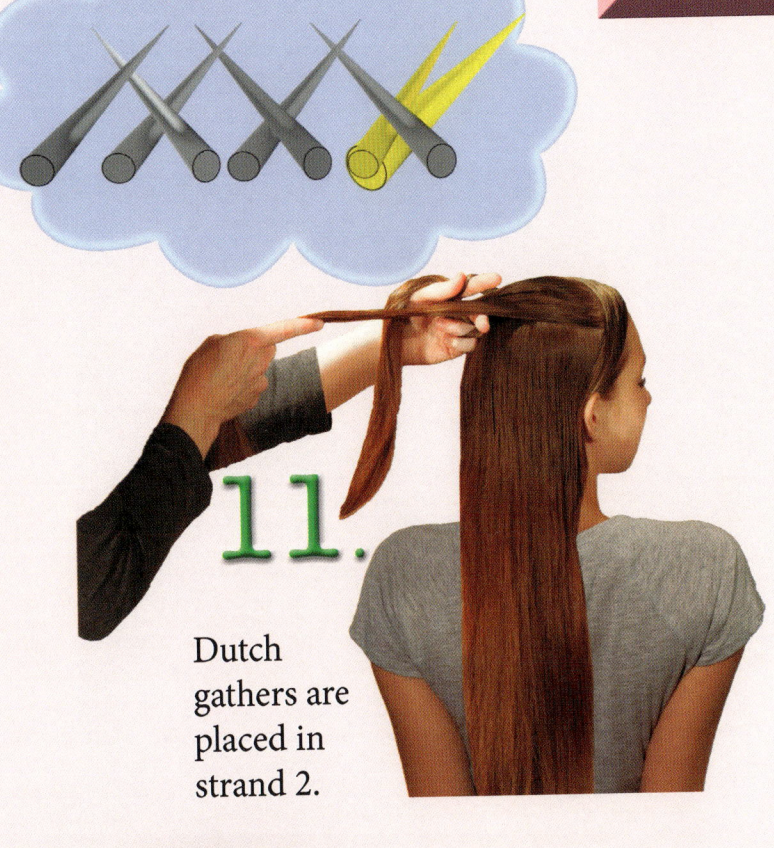

11.

Dutch gathers are placed in strand 2.

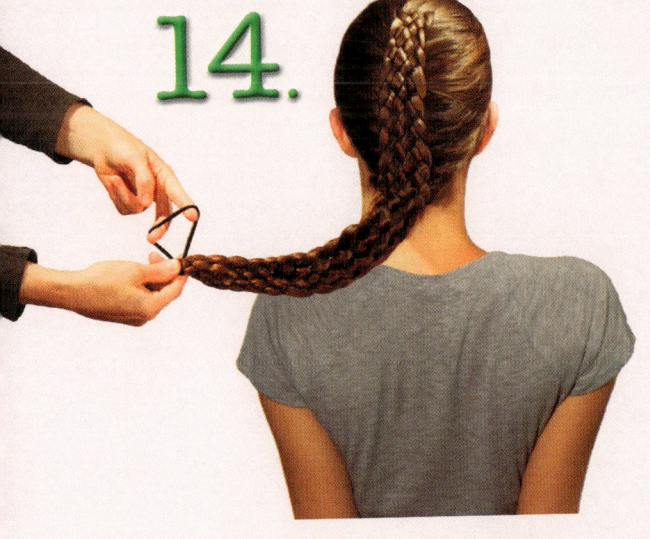

14.

Secure with a rubber band.

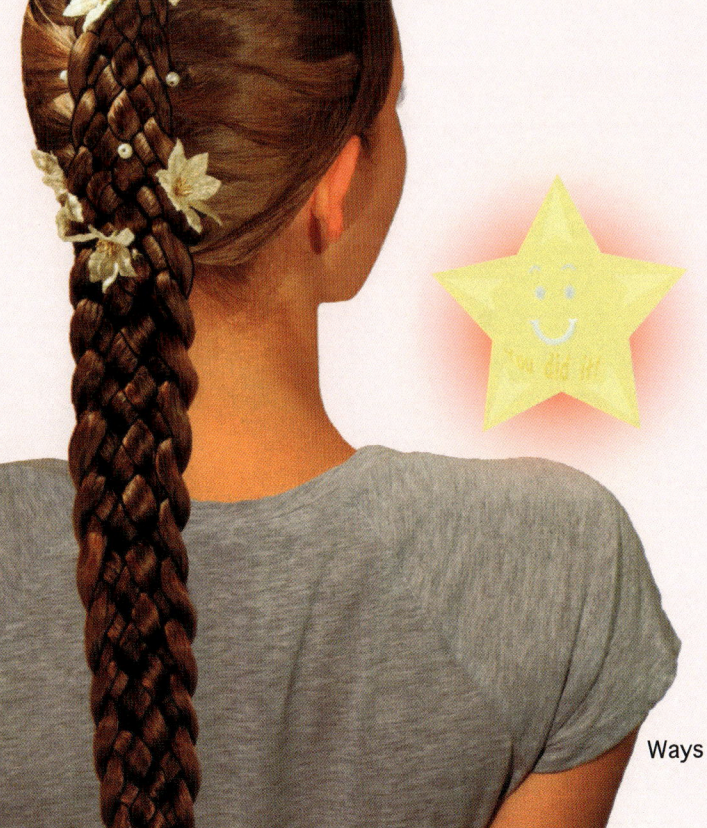

Seven-Strand

Notes

Try these examples on yourself or a friend!

Examples of Seven-Strand

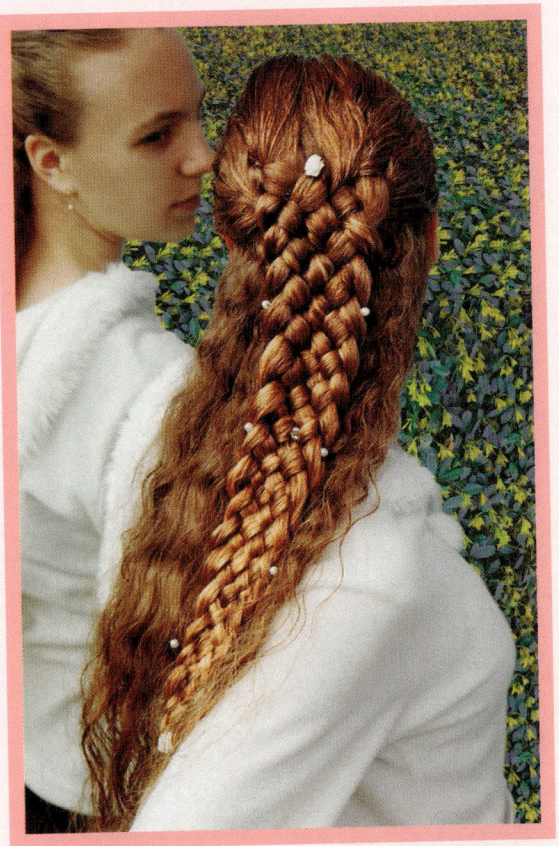
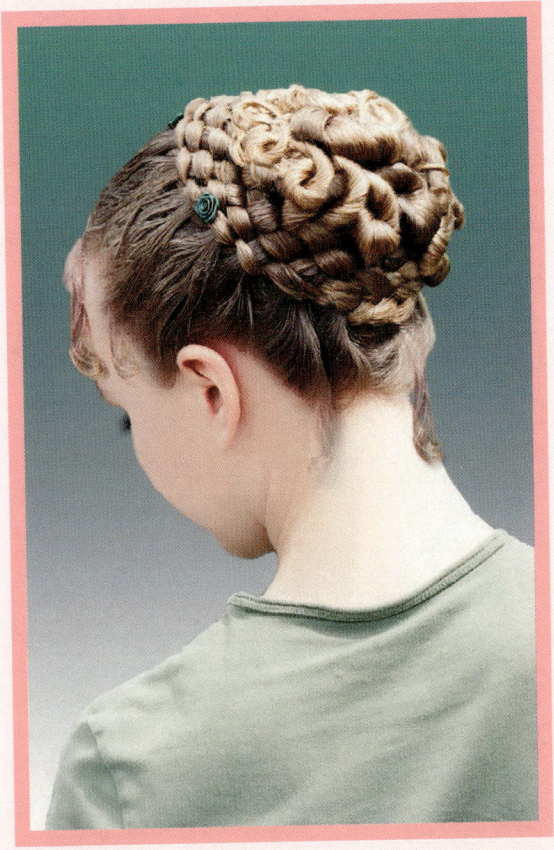
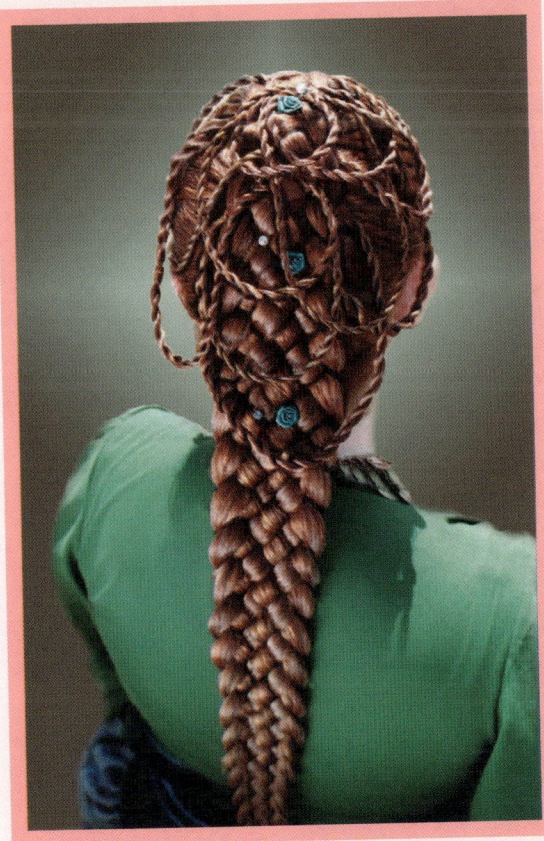
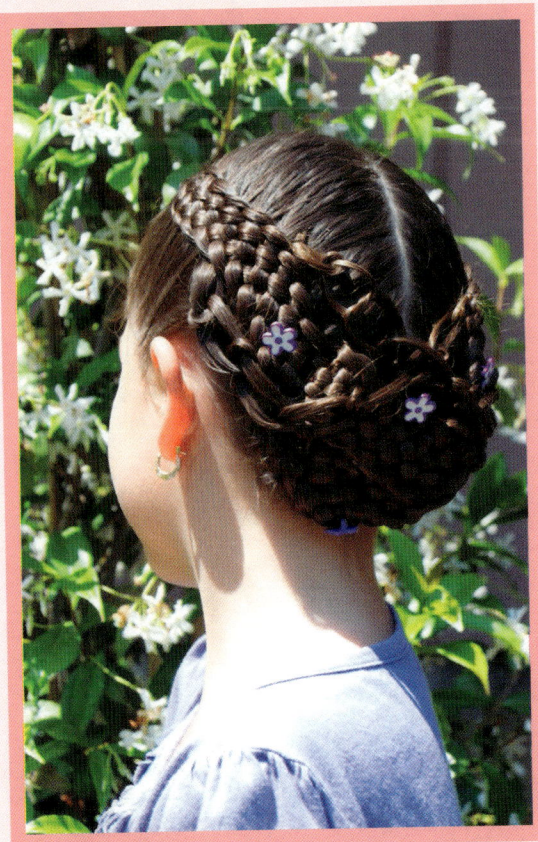

Visit my website to see more examples of the Seven-Strand Ways

Eight-Strand

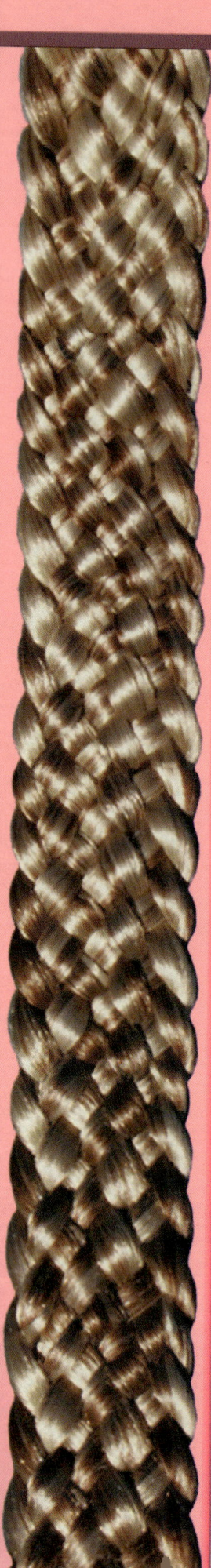

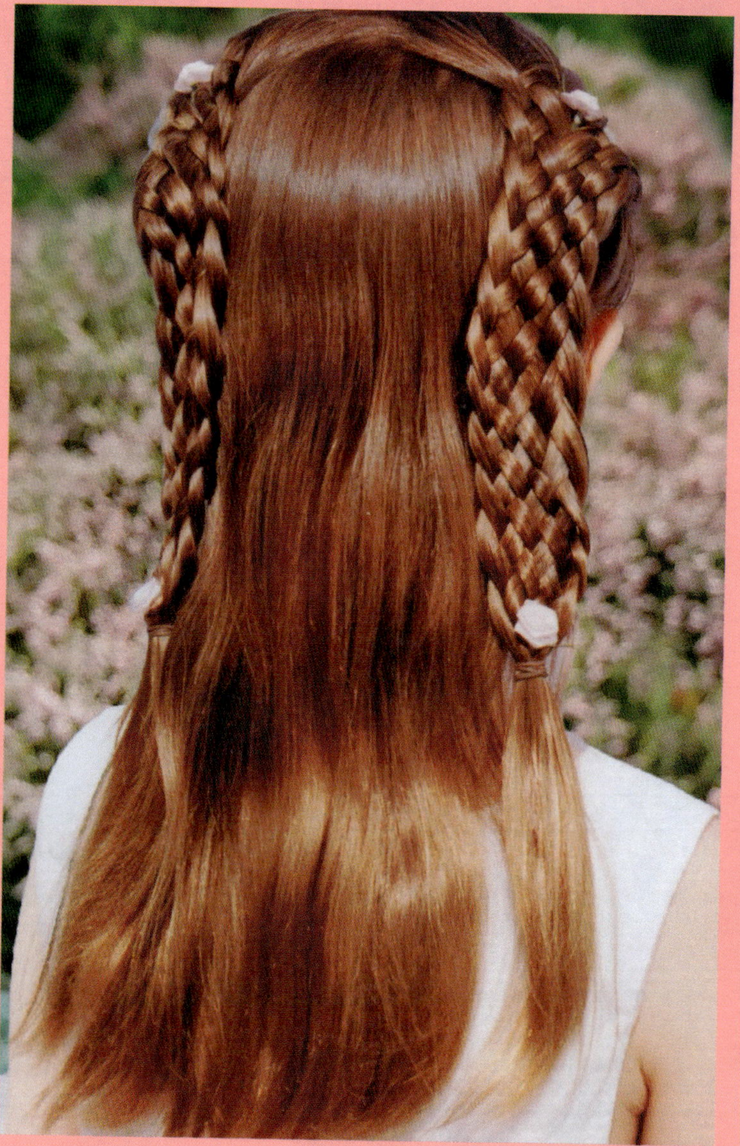

Mezmerizing as a tail braid, the potential to dazzle is instant. Applying this way to braid in more complicated forms just adds to the genius of it all.

Eight-Strand

Sure to wow. The next fourteen pages will walk you through this braid.

Braid . . . . 284 - 288

Stitch Taper . . . . 290 - 295

Examples 297

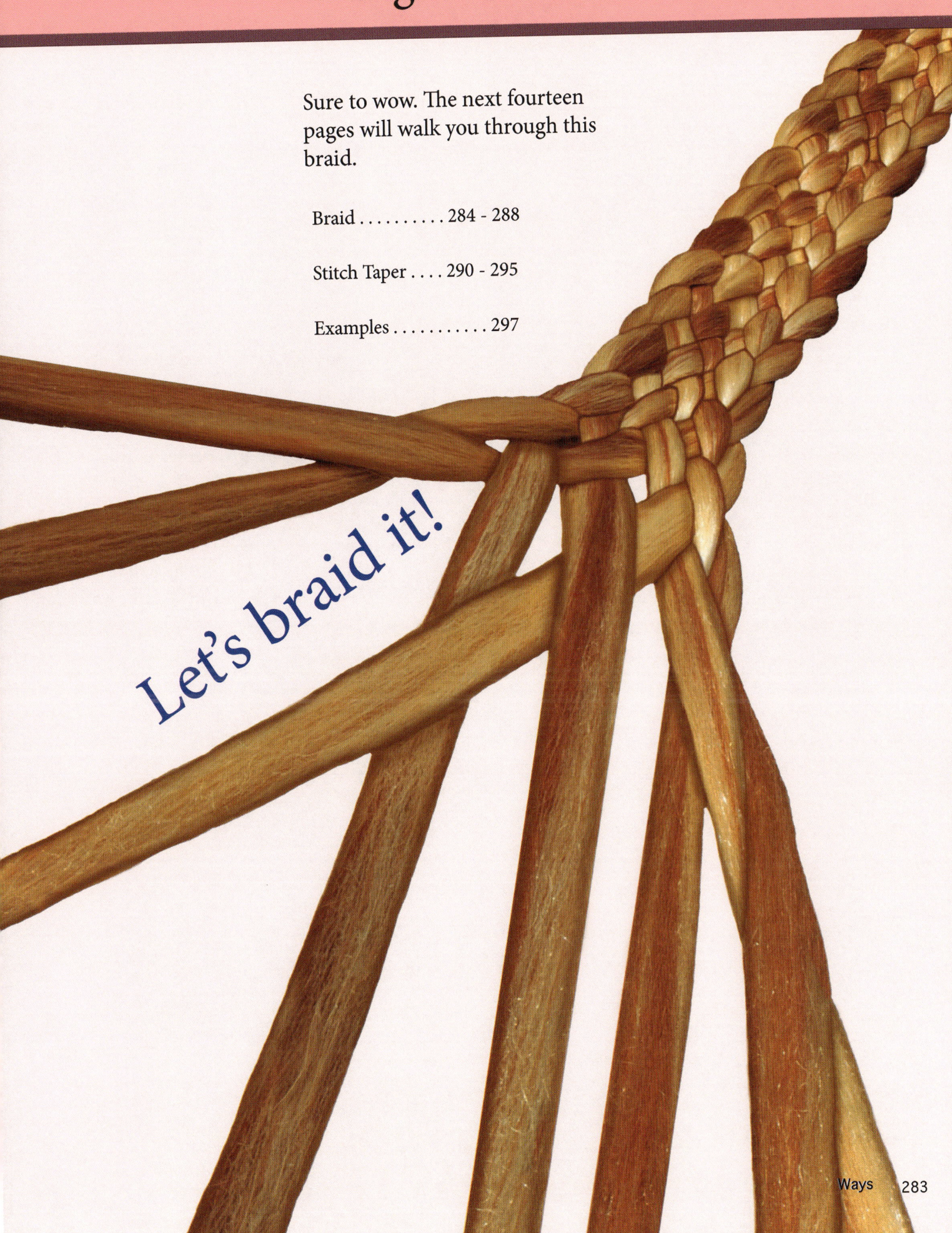

Let's braid it!

Eight-Strand Braid

Find your joy and share it with others.

1.

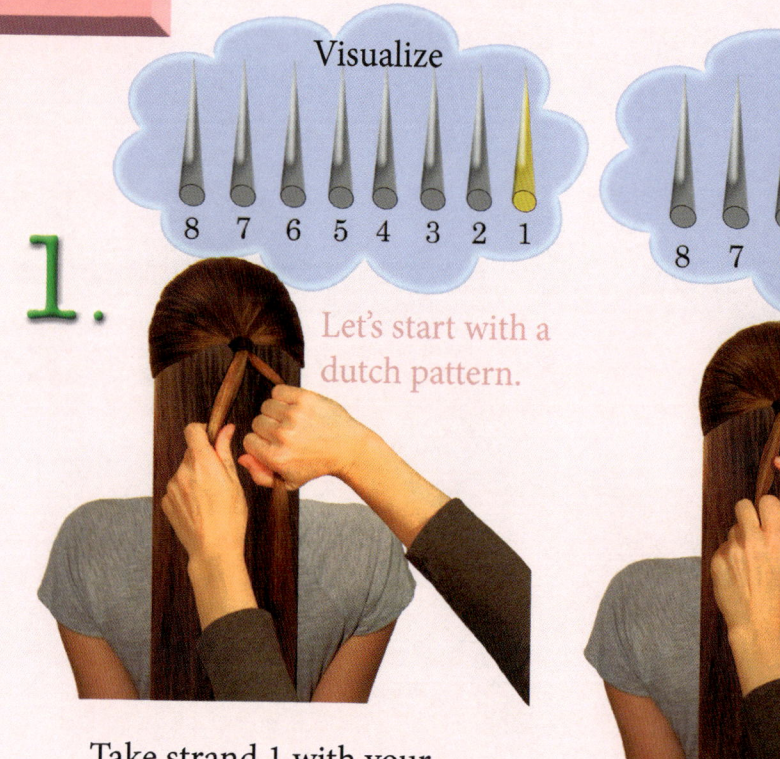

Take strand 1 with your palm down and your thumb facing your belly button.

Let's start with a dutch pattern.

2.

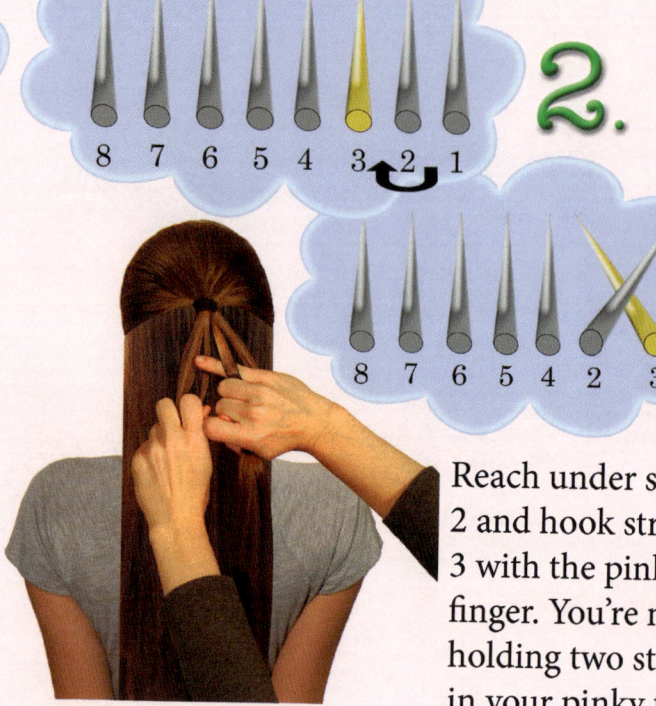

Reach under strand 2 and hook strand 3 with the pinky finger. You're now holding two strands in your pinky finger.

5.

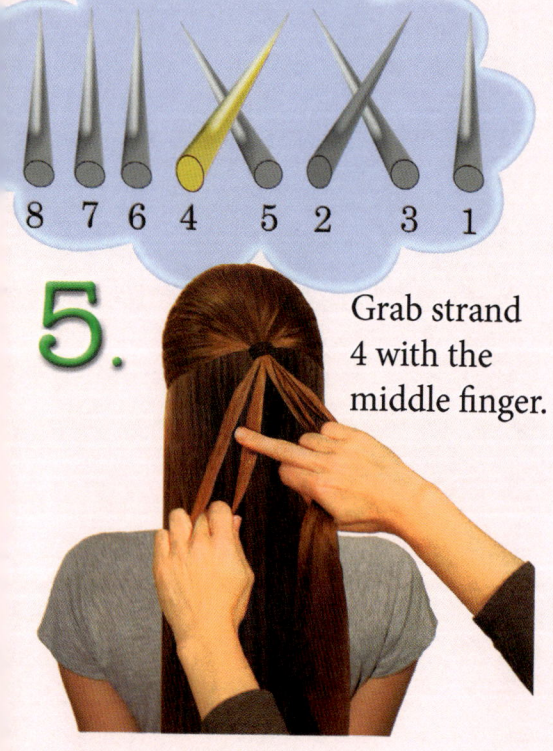

Grab strand 4 with the middle finger.

6.

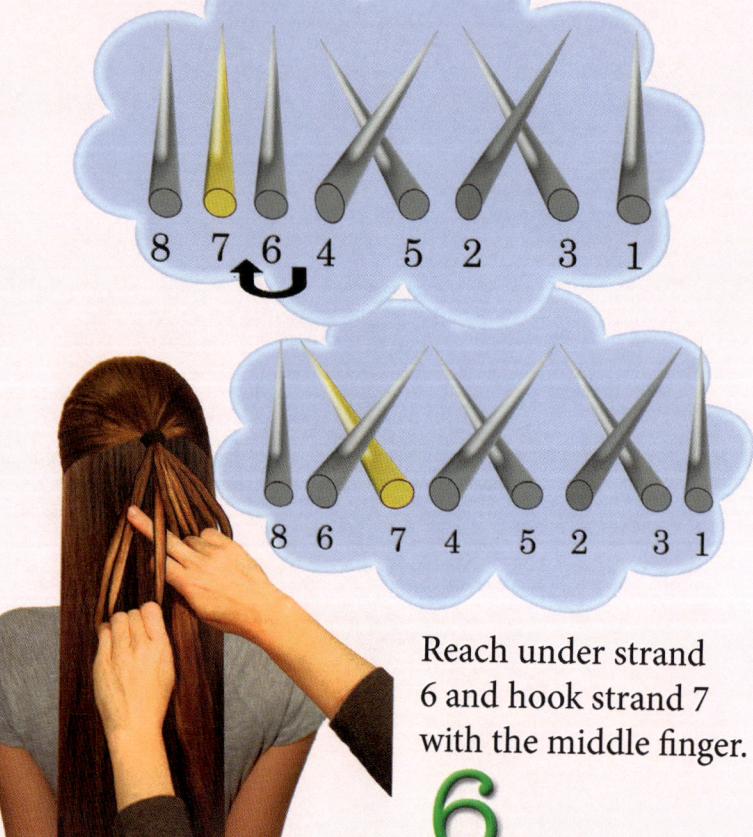

Reach under strand 6 and hook strand 7 with the middle finger.

284 www.findingbraids.com

Eight-Strand Braid

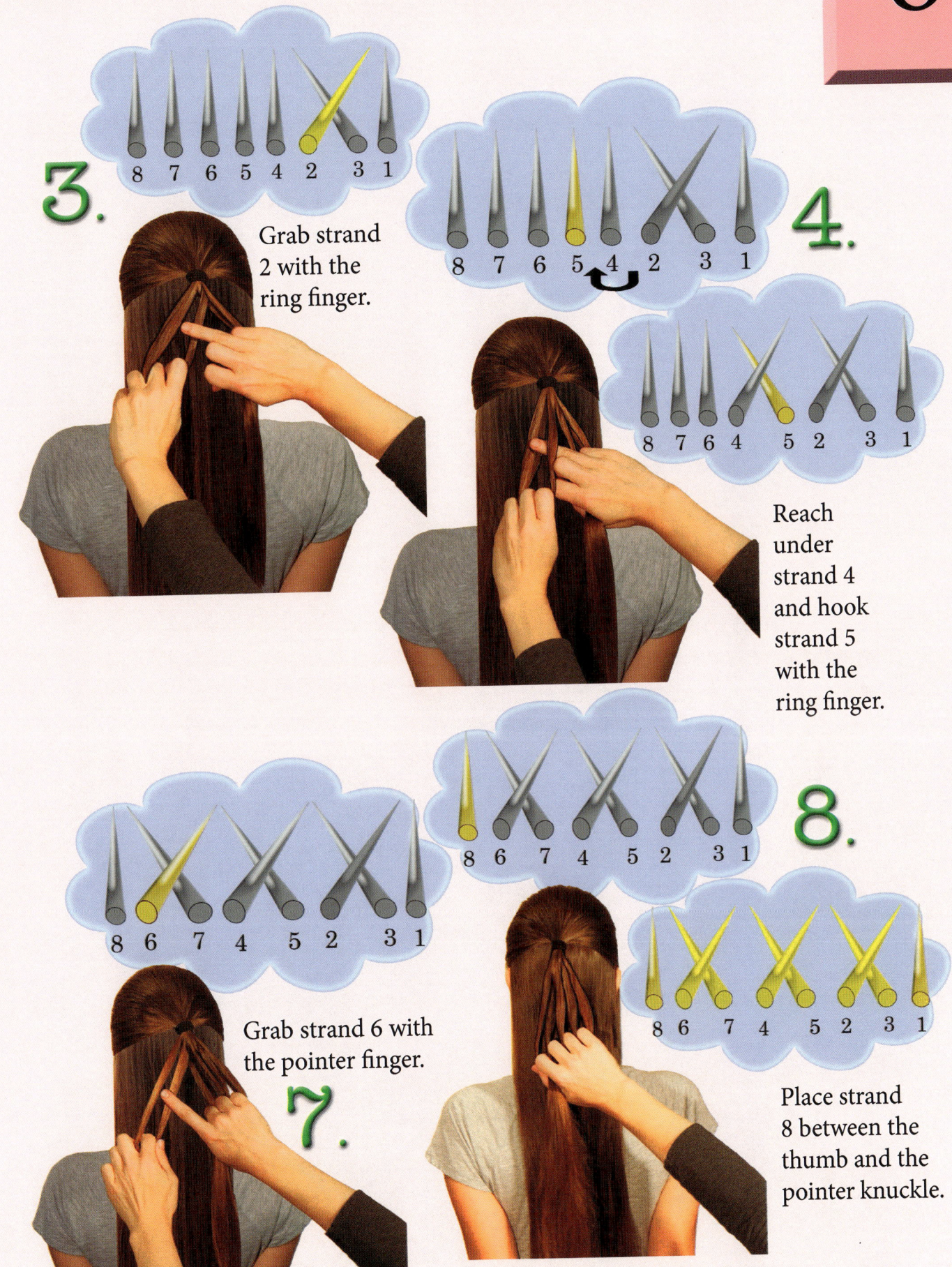

8 Continuing

Time for the french pattern.

Number your strands at your knuckles now.

Reach under strand 1 with the pinky finger and hook strand 2.

9.

Ring finger grabs strand 1.

10.

Reach under strand 5 with the middle finger and hook strand 6.

13.

14.

Grab strand 5 with the pointer finger.

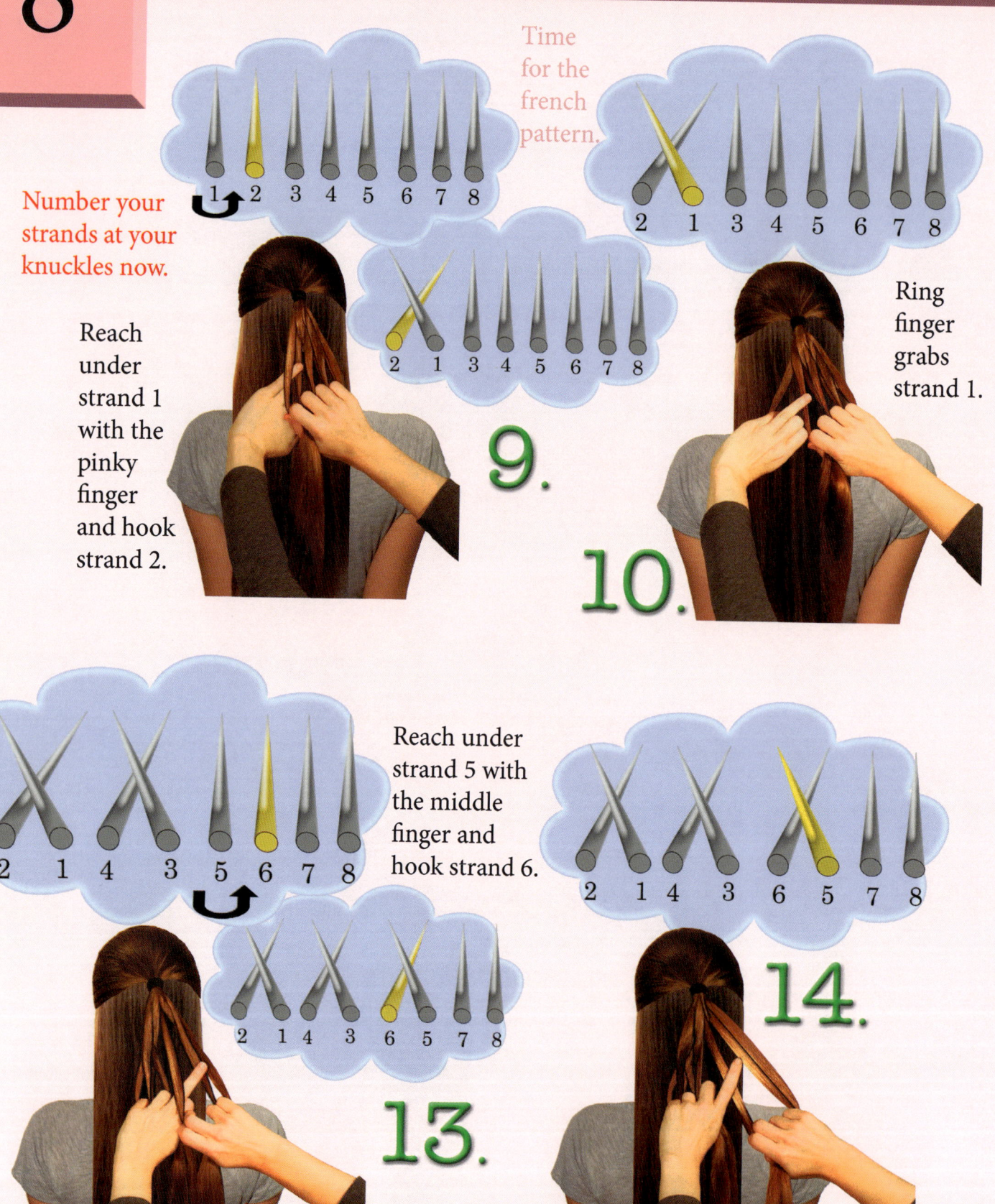

part 2. Eight-Strand Braid

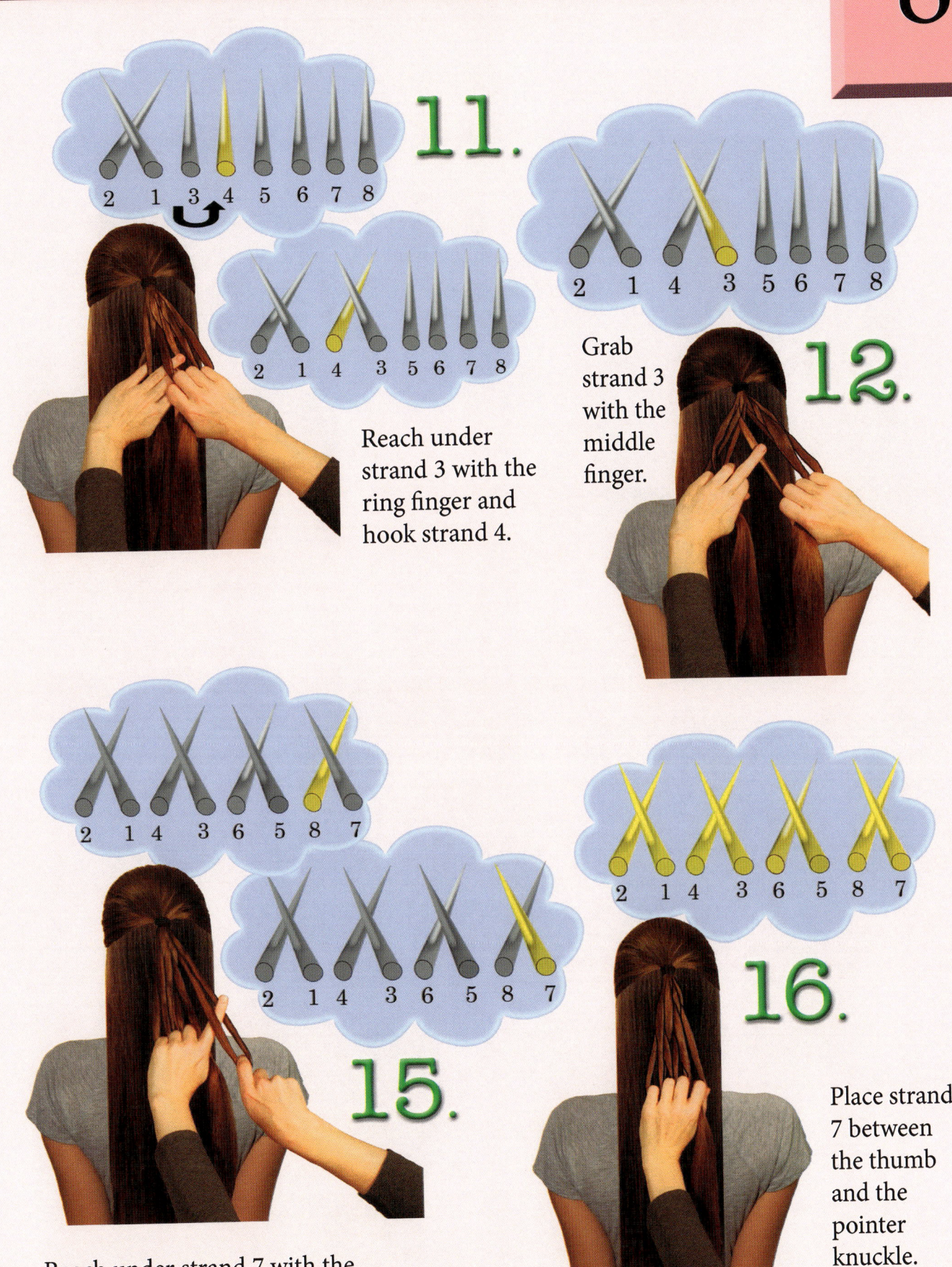

Eight-Strand Braid

8

17.

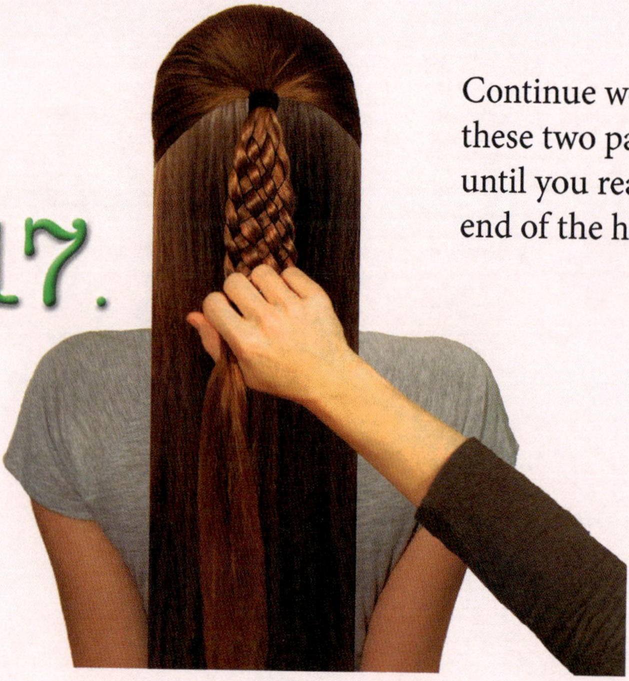

18. Continue weaving these two patterns until you reach the end of the hair.

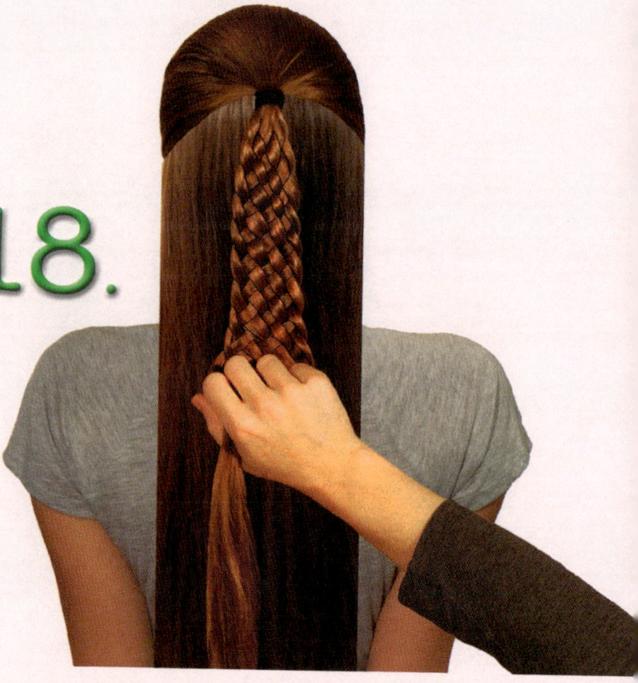

19. 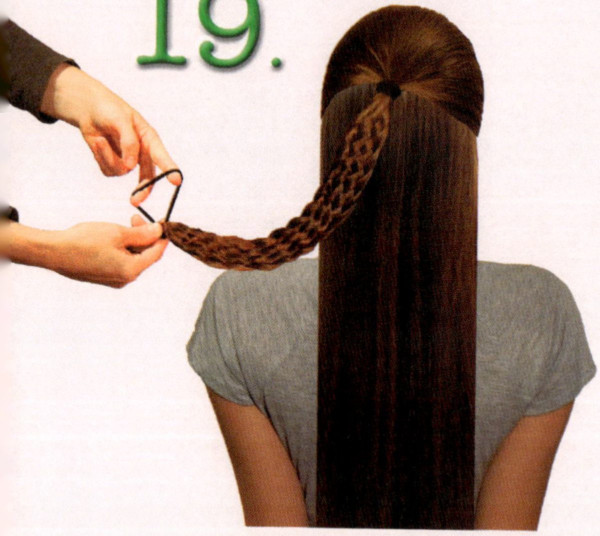 Secure with a rubber band.

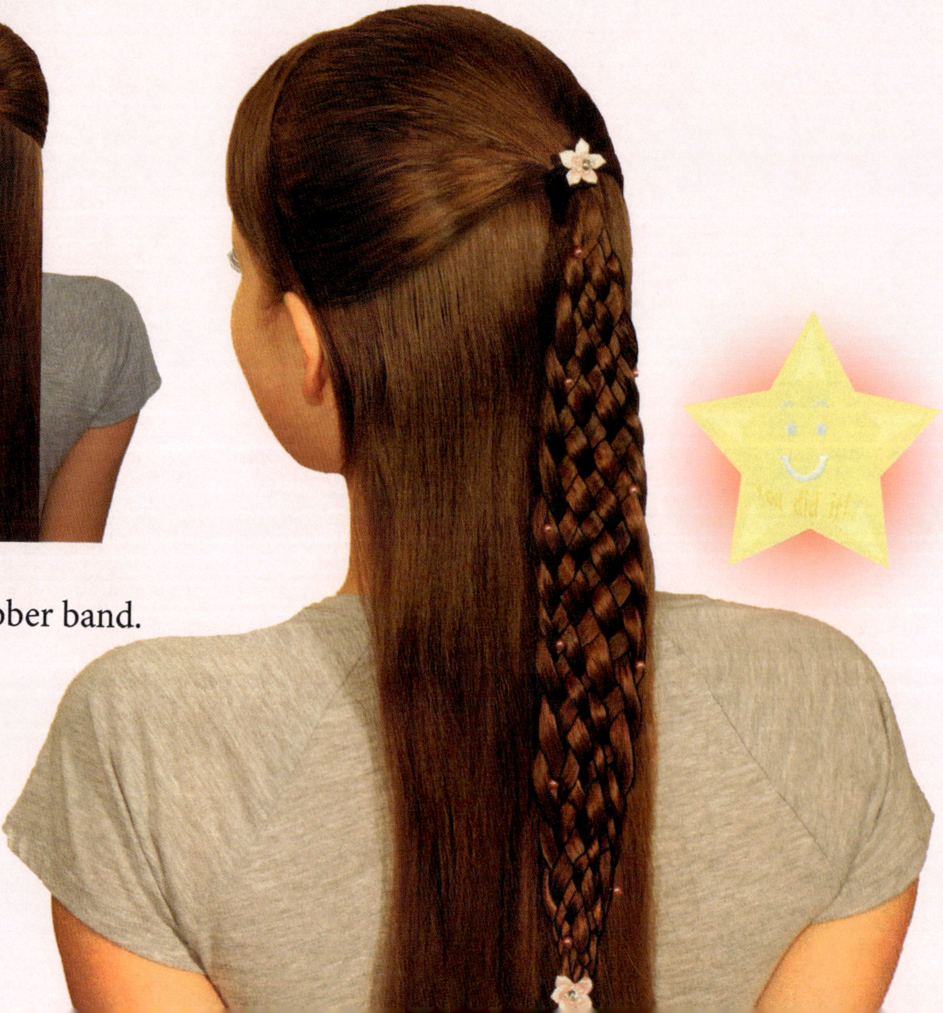

288 www.findingbraids.com

Eight-Strand

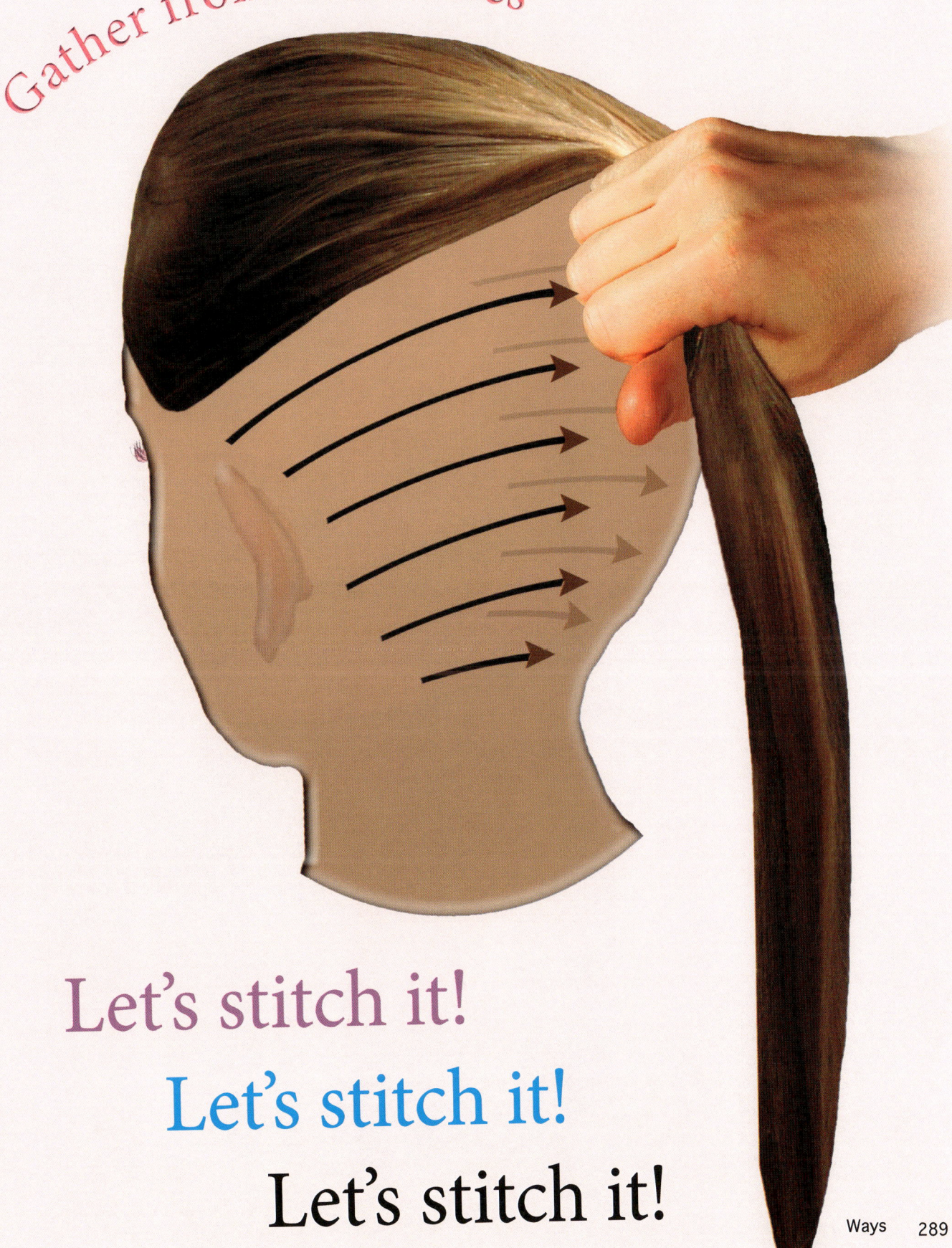

Gather from both sides

Let's stitch it!

Let's stitch it!

Let's stitch it!

Eight-Strand Taper Stitch

Only those who dare to fail greatly...can ever achieve greatly.
— Robert F. Kennedy

Let's start with a dutch pattern.

1. Visualize

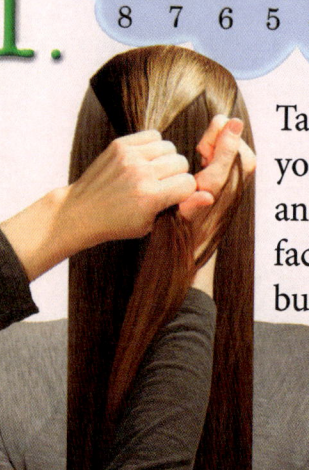

Take strand 1 with your palm down and your thumb facing your belly button.

2.

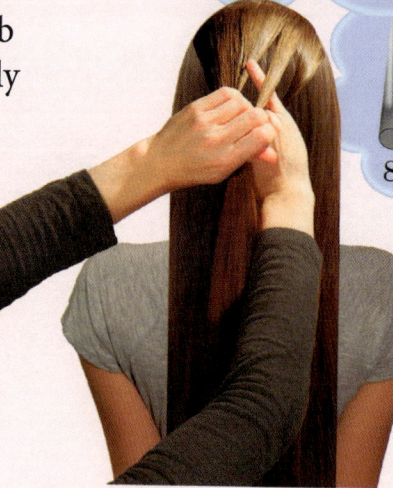

Reach under strand 2 and hook strand 3 with the pinky finger. You're now holding two strands in your pinky finger.

5.

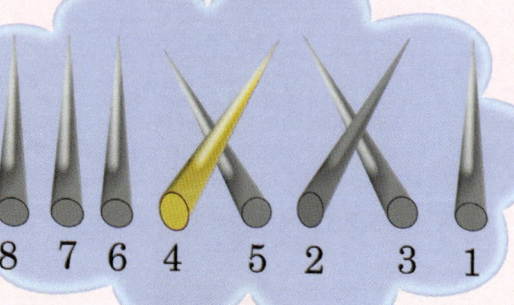

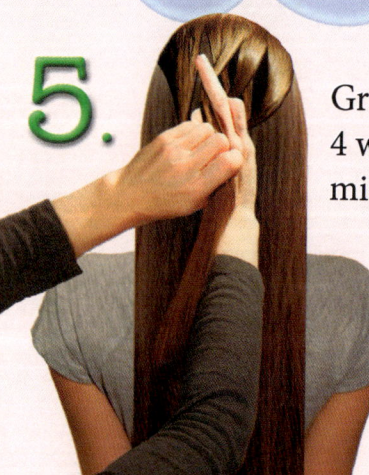

Grab strand 4 with the middle finger.

6.

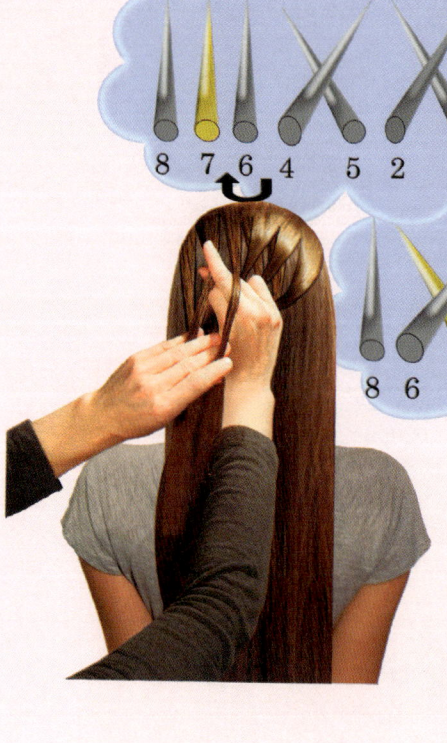

Reach under strand 6 and hook strand 7 with the middle finger.

Eight-Strand Taper Stitch

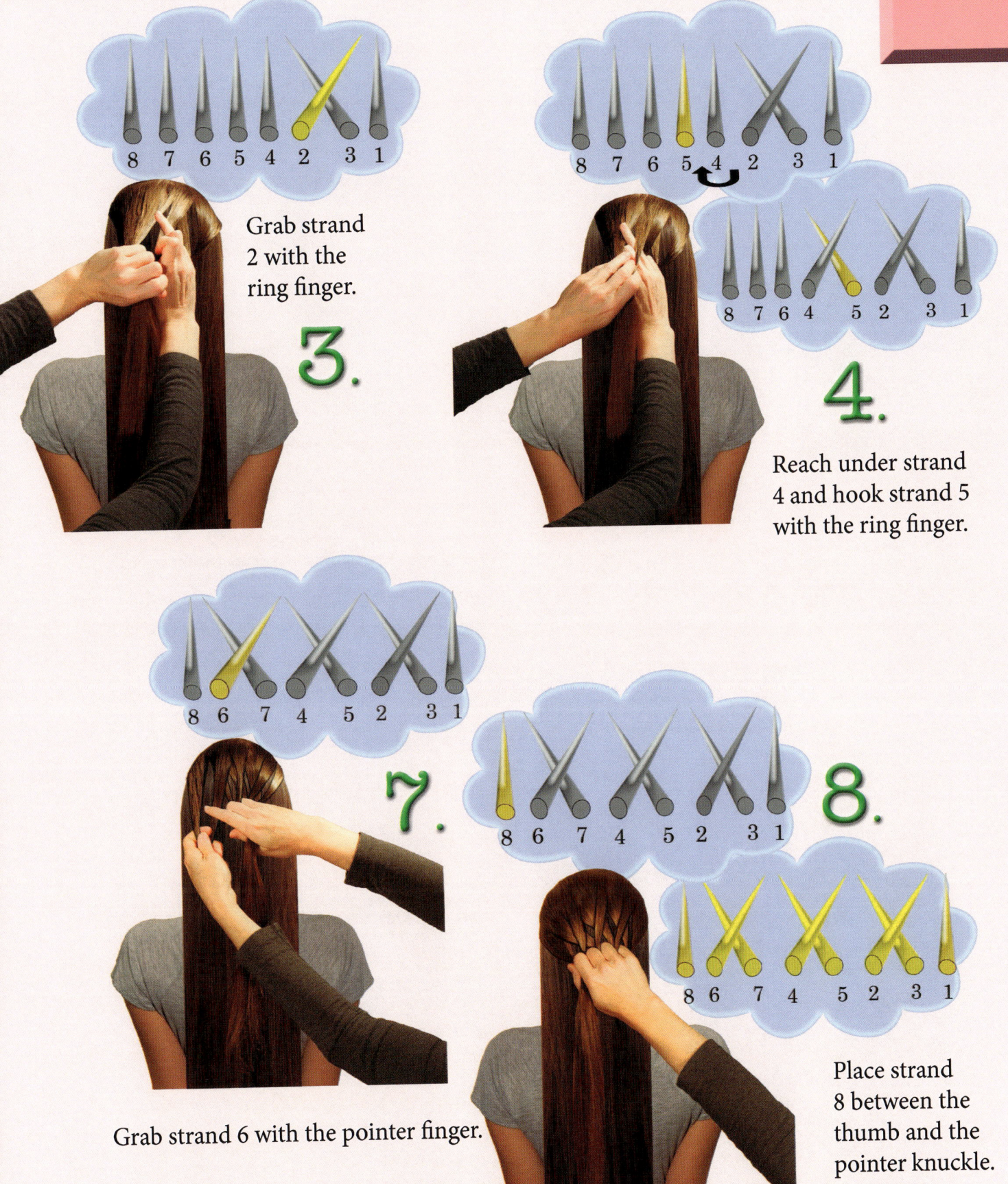

3. Grab strand 2 with the ring finger.

4. Reach under strand 4 and hook strand 5 with the ring finger.

7. Grab strand 6 with the pointer finger.

8. Place strand 8 between the thumb and the pointer knuckle.

8 Continuing

Number your strands at your knuckles now.

Time for the french pattern.

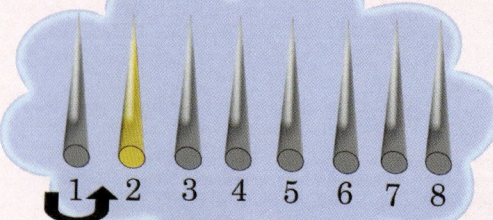

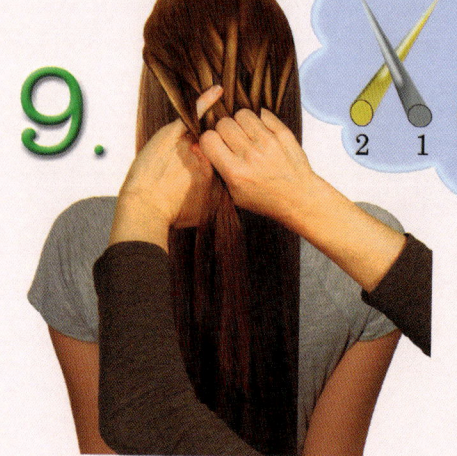

9.
Reach under strand 1 with the pinky finger and hook strand 2.

10.
Ring finger grabs strand 1.

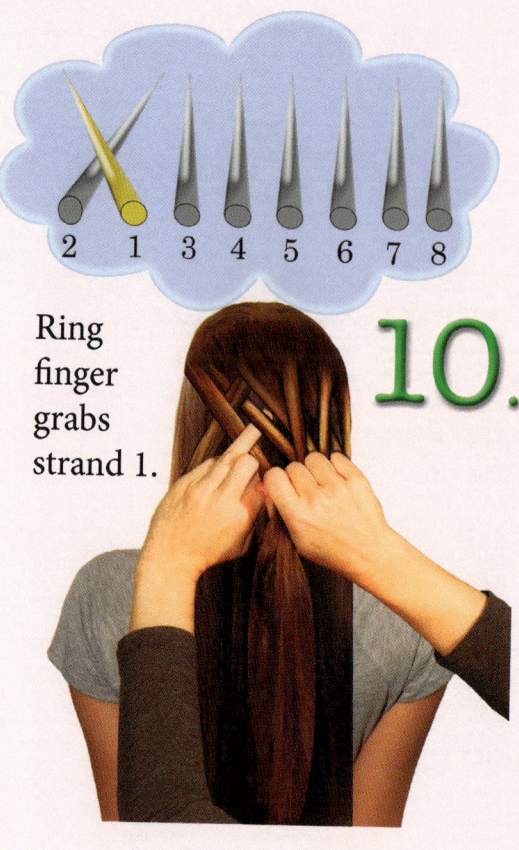

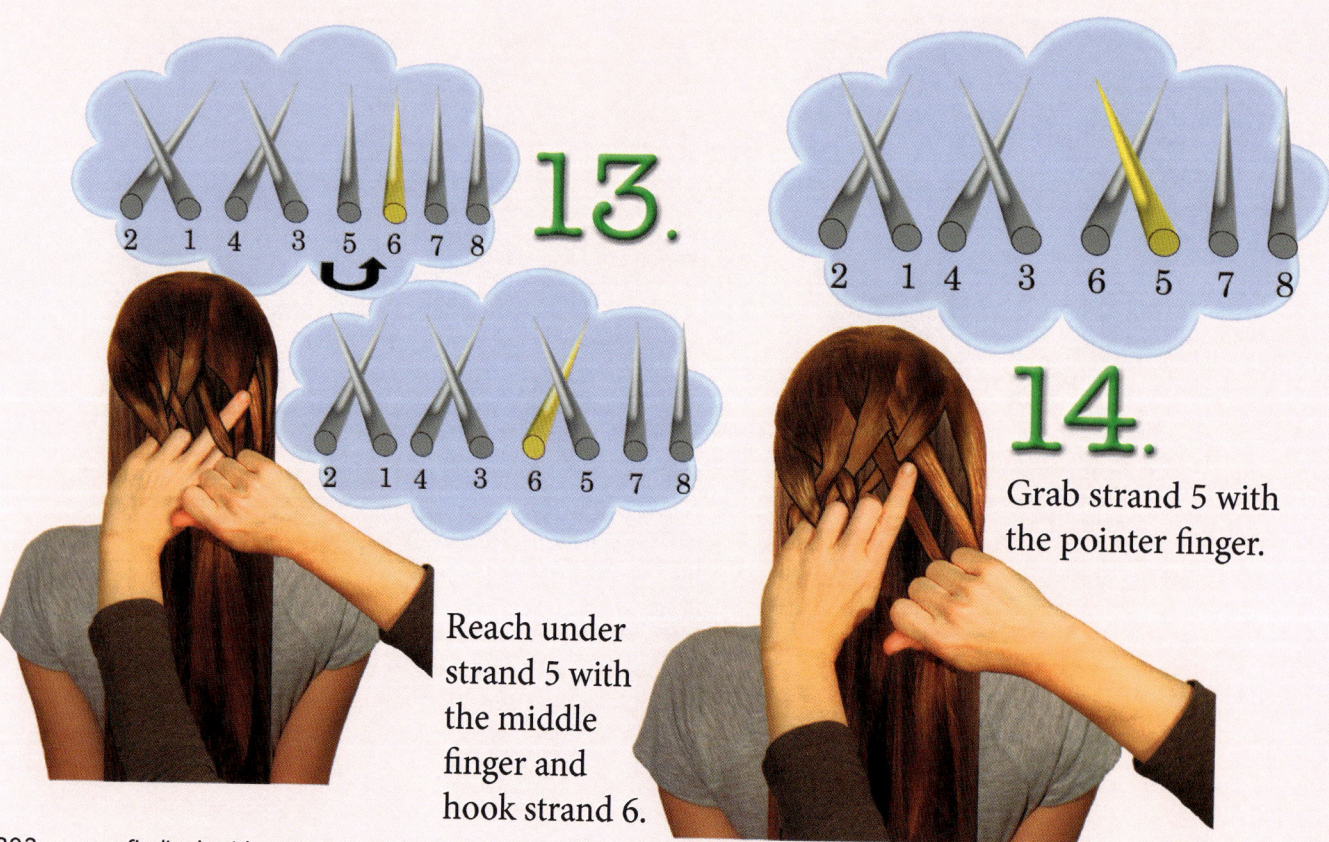

13.
Reach under strand 5 with the middle finger and hook strand 6.

14.
Grab strand 5 with the pointer finger.

part 2. Eight-Strand Taper Stitch

11.

2 1 3 4 5 6 7 8

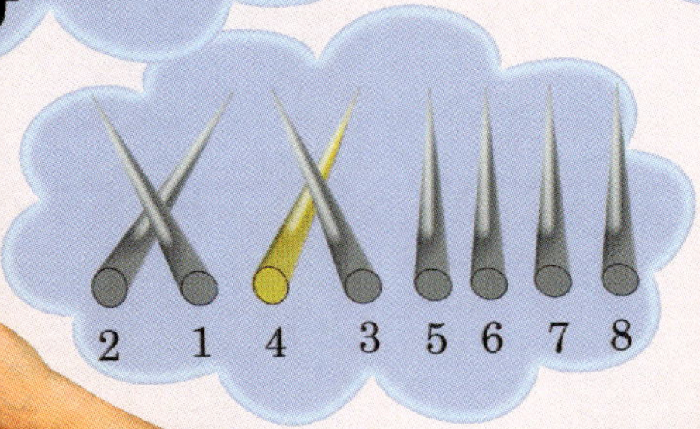

2 1 4 3 5 6 7 8

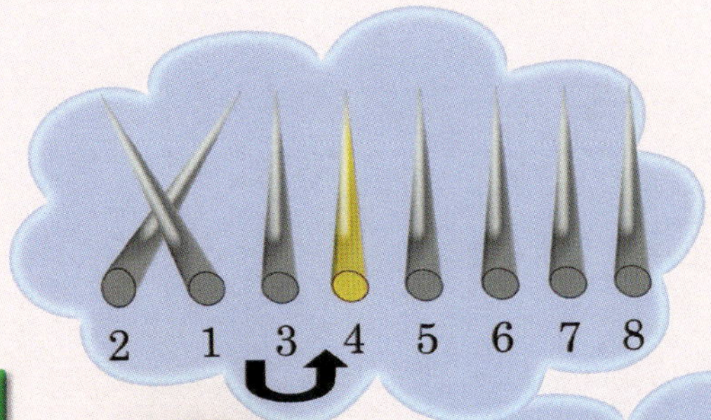

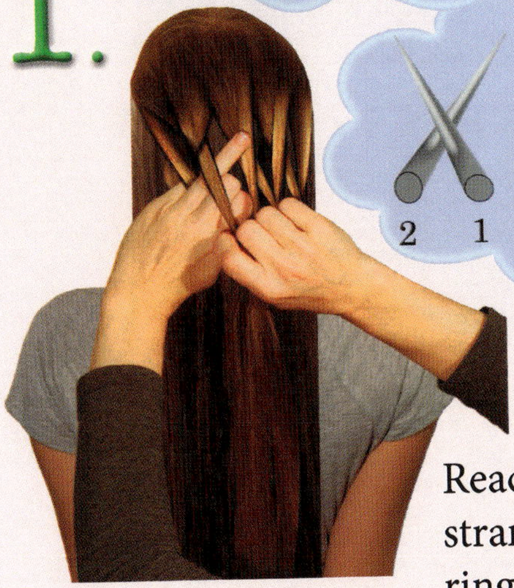

Reach under strand 3 with the ring finger and hook strand 4.

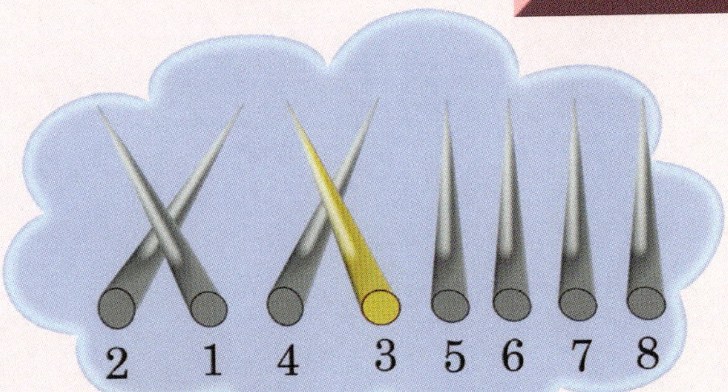

2 1 4 3 5 6 7 8

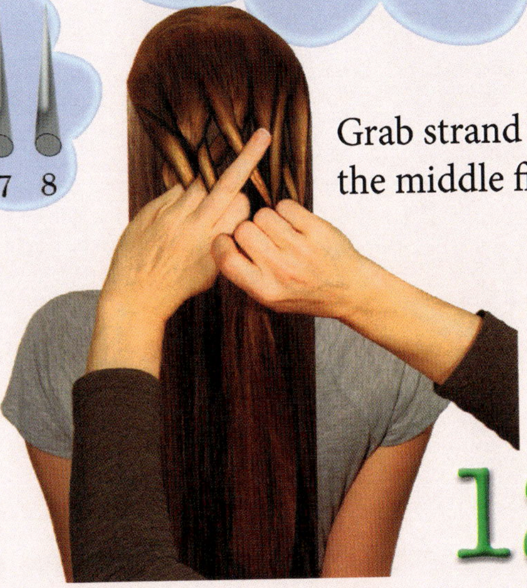

Grab strand 3 with the middle finger.

12.

15.

2 1 4 3 6 5 8 7

2 1 4 3 6 5 8 7

Reach under strand 7 with the middle finger and hook strand 8.

2 1 4 3 6 5 8 7

Place strand 7 between the thumb and the pointer knuckle.

16.

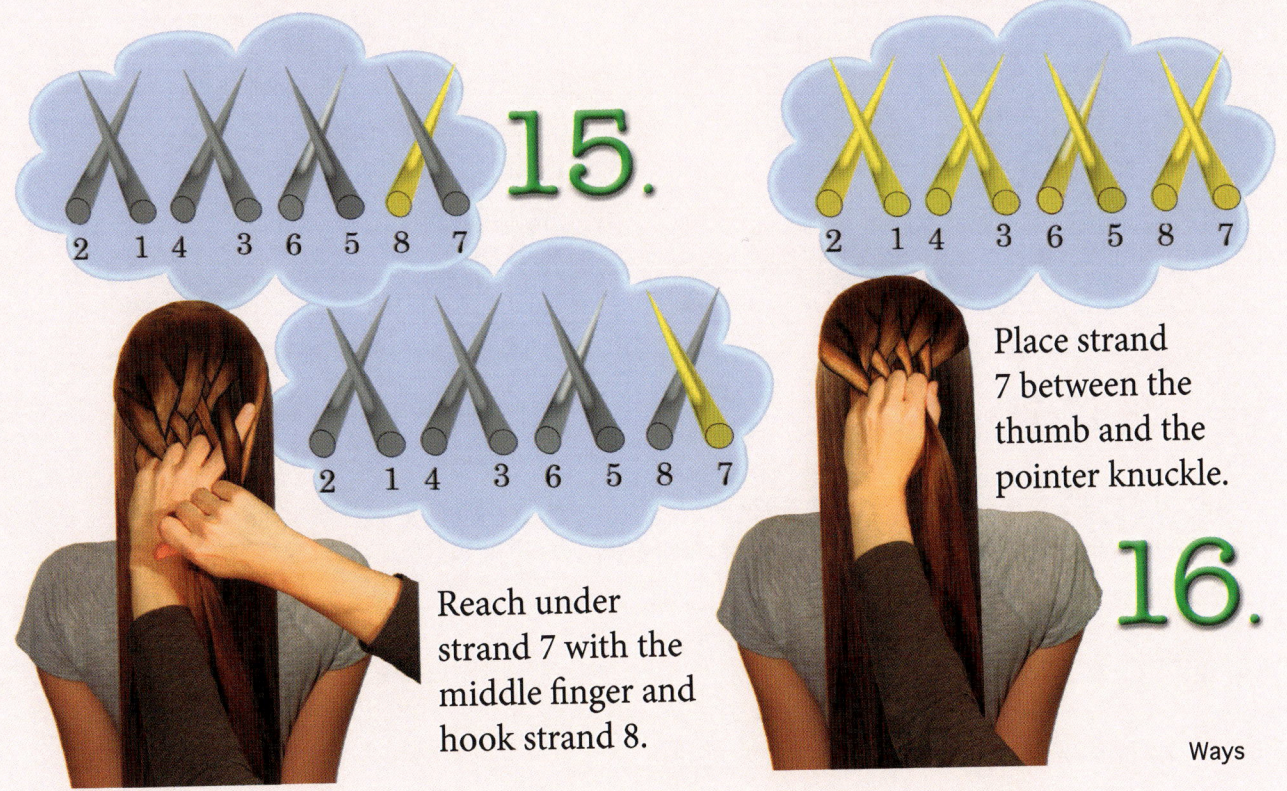

Ways   293

8 Continuing

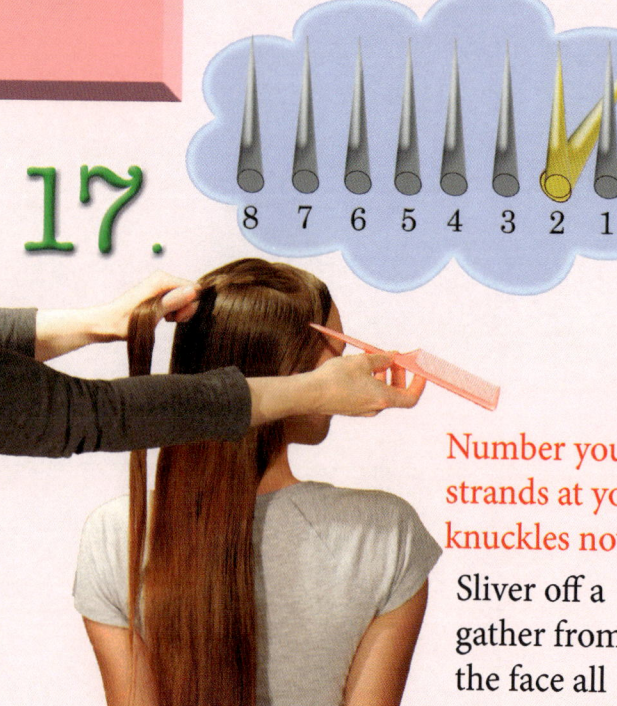

17.

Number your strands at your knuckles now.

Sliver off a gather from the face all the way back to the braid.

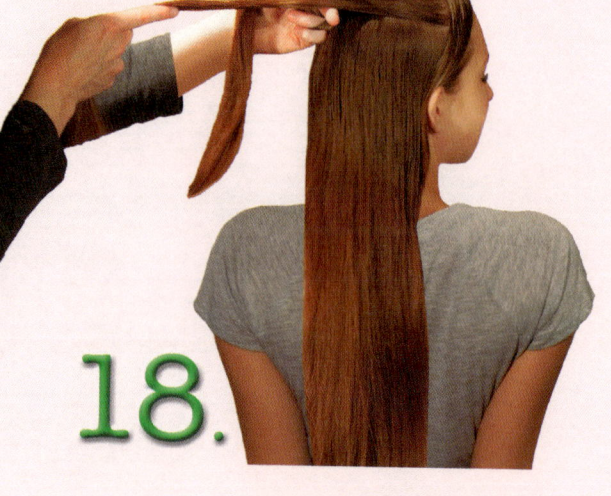

18.

Dutch gathers are placed in the second strand.

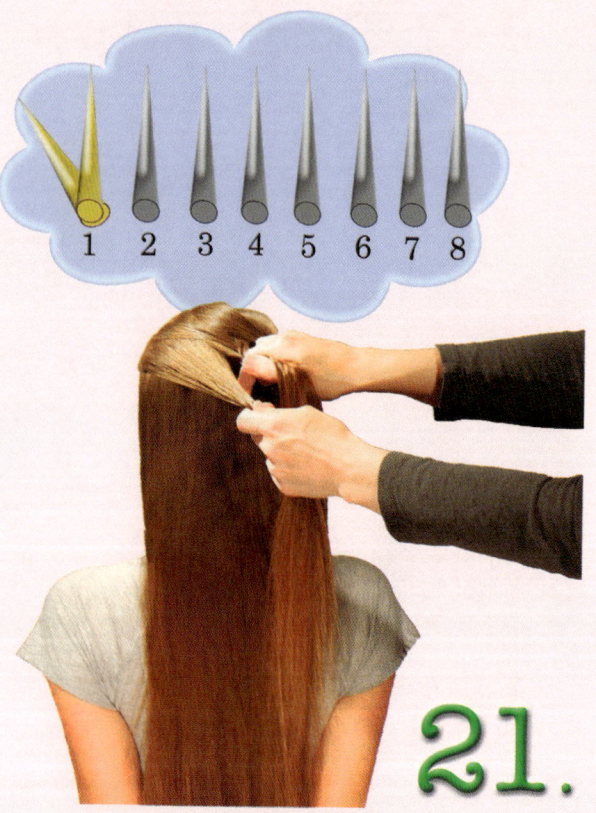

21.

French gathers are placed in the first strand.

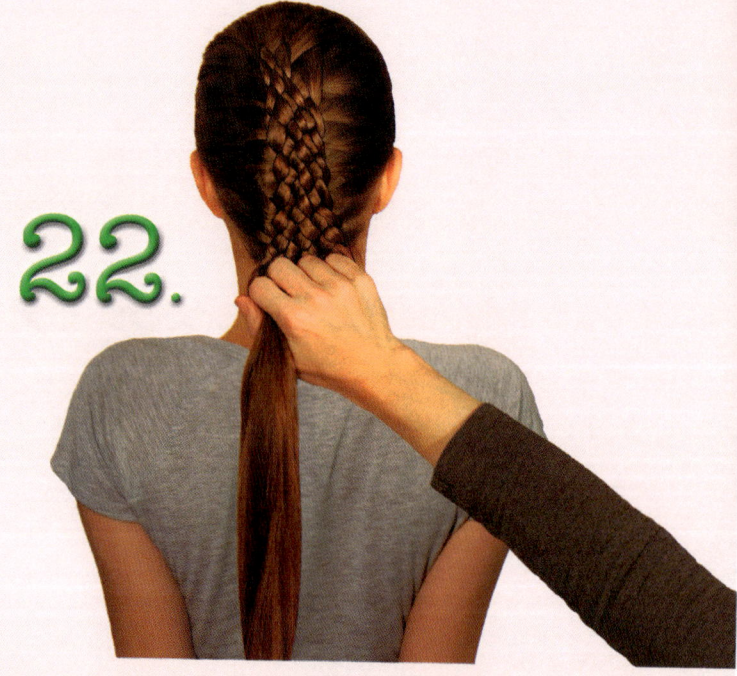

22.

Continue weaving and gathering these two patterns until you reach the end of the hair.

part 3. Eight-Strand Taper Stitch

19.

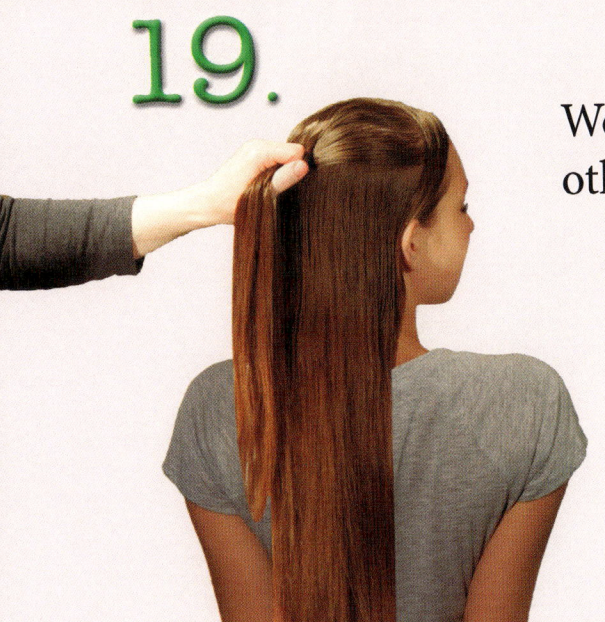

Weave back the other direction.

20.

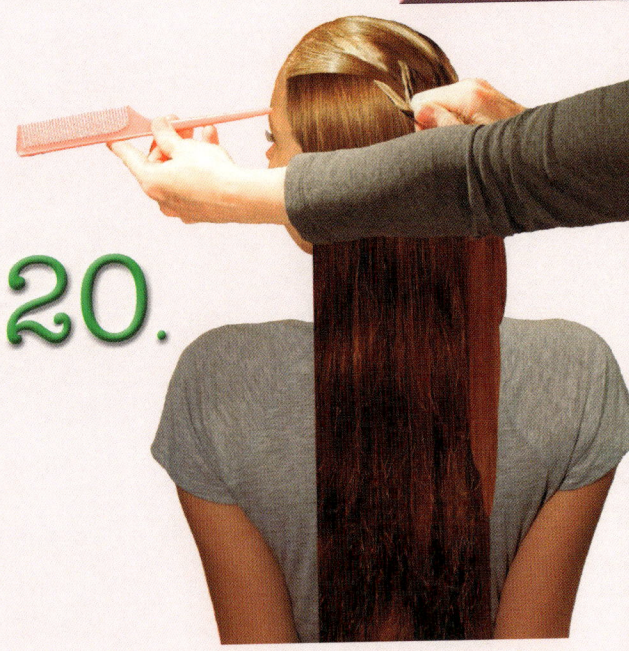

Sliver off a gather from the face all the way back to the braid.

23.

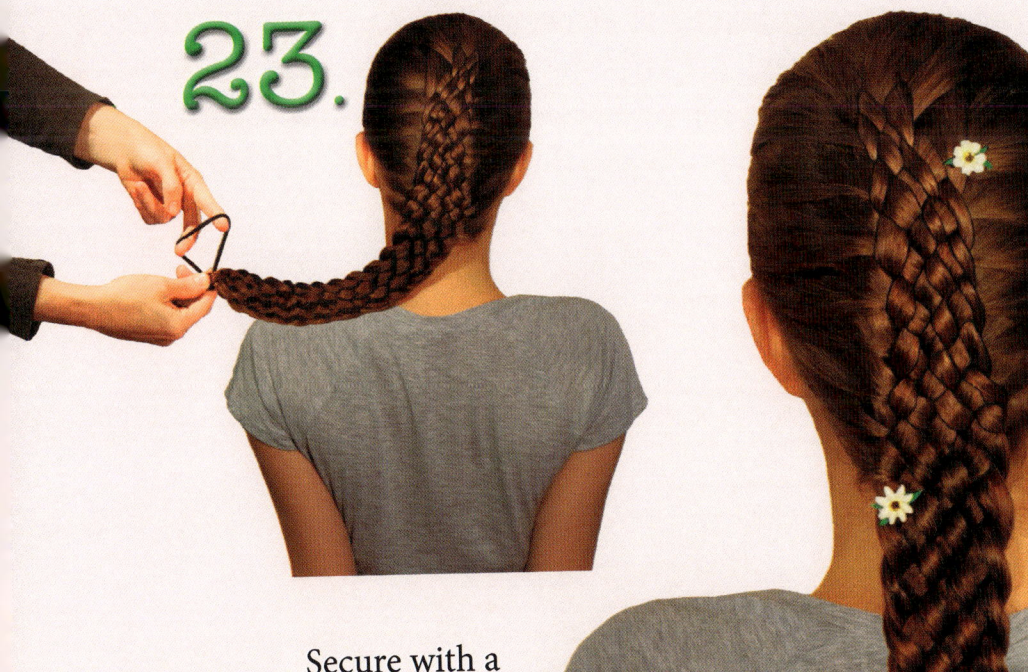

Secure with a rubber band.

Eight-Strand

Notes

_____

_____

_____

_____

_____

_____

_____

Go through the entire book examples and do them all with eight-strands!

Examples of Eight-Strand

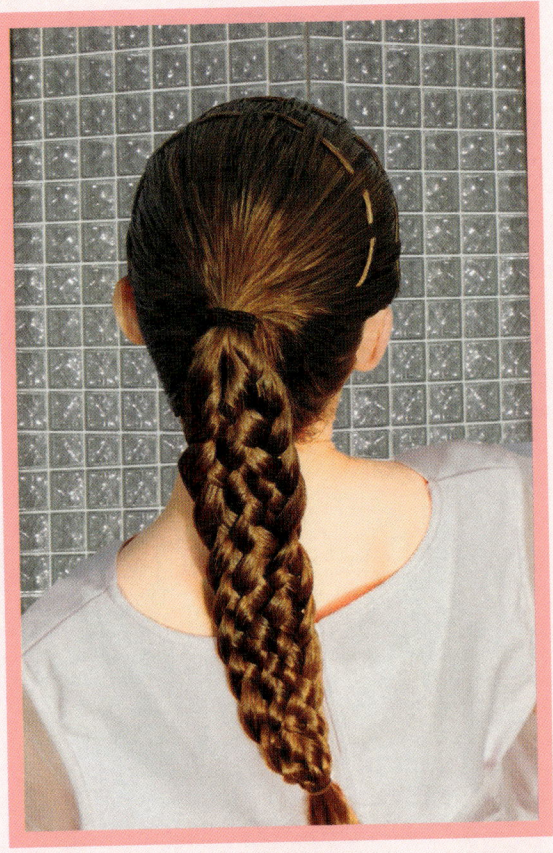
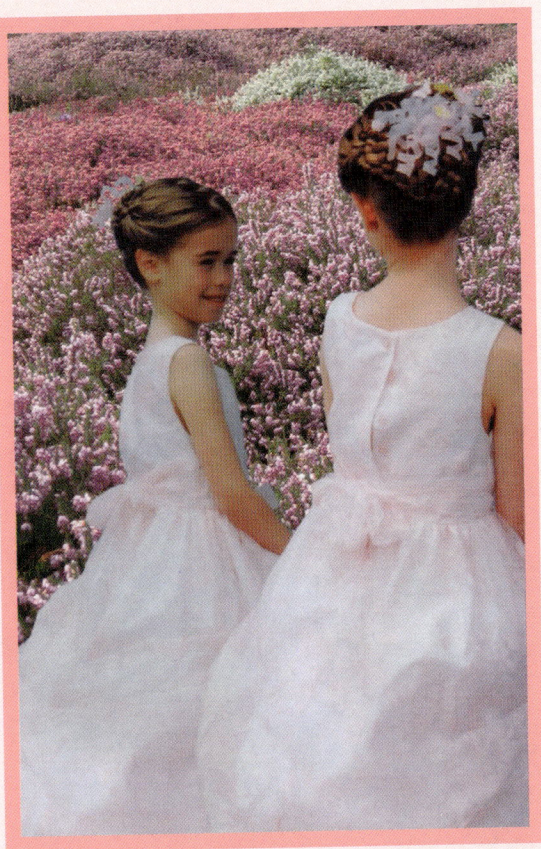
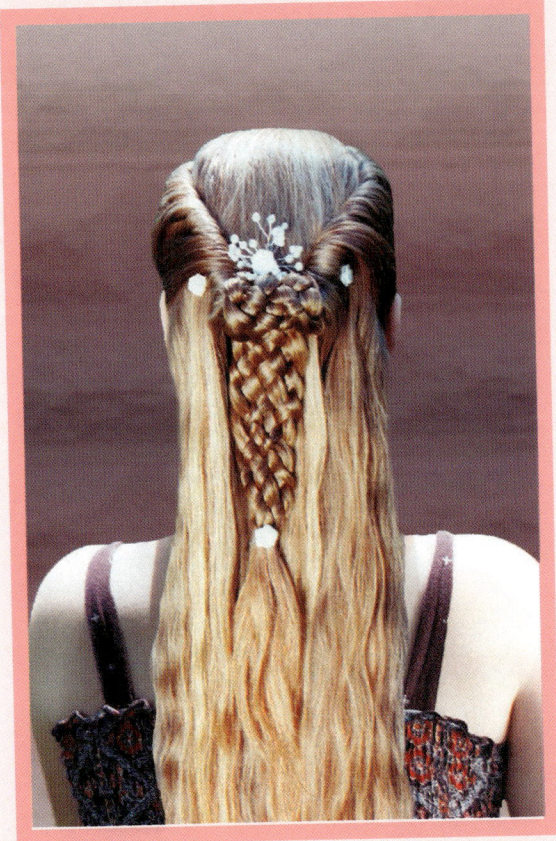
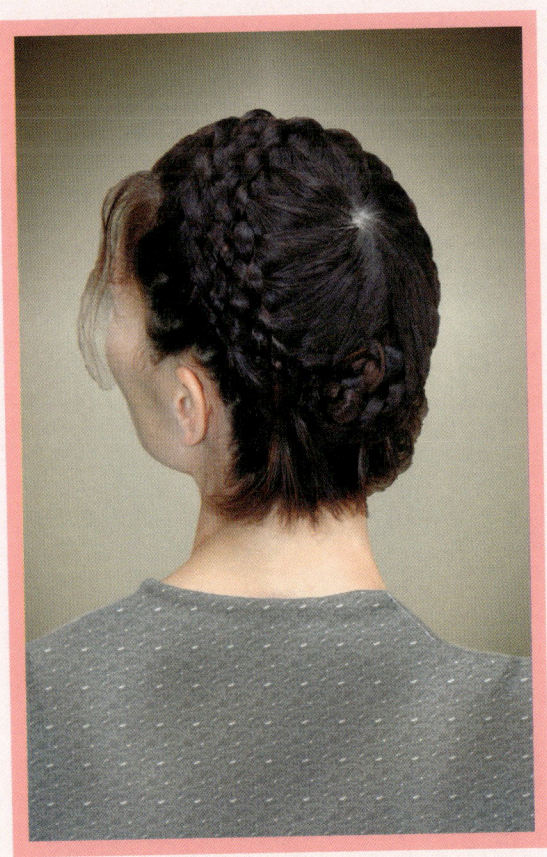

Visit my website to see more examples of the Eight-Strand

Nine-Strand

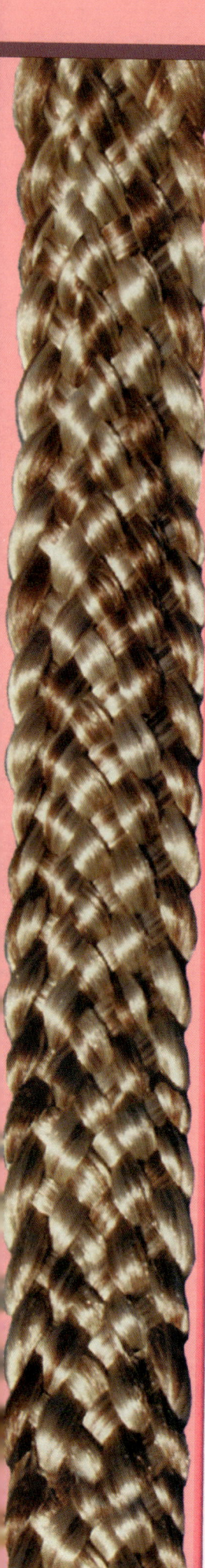

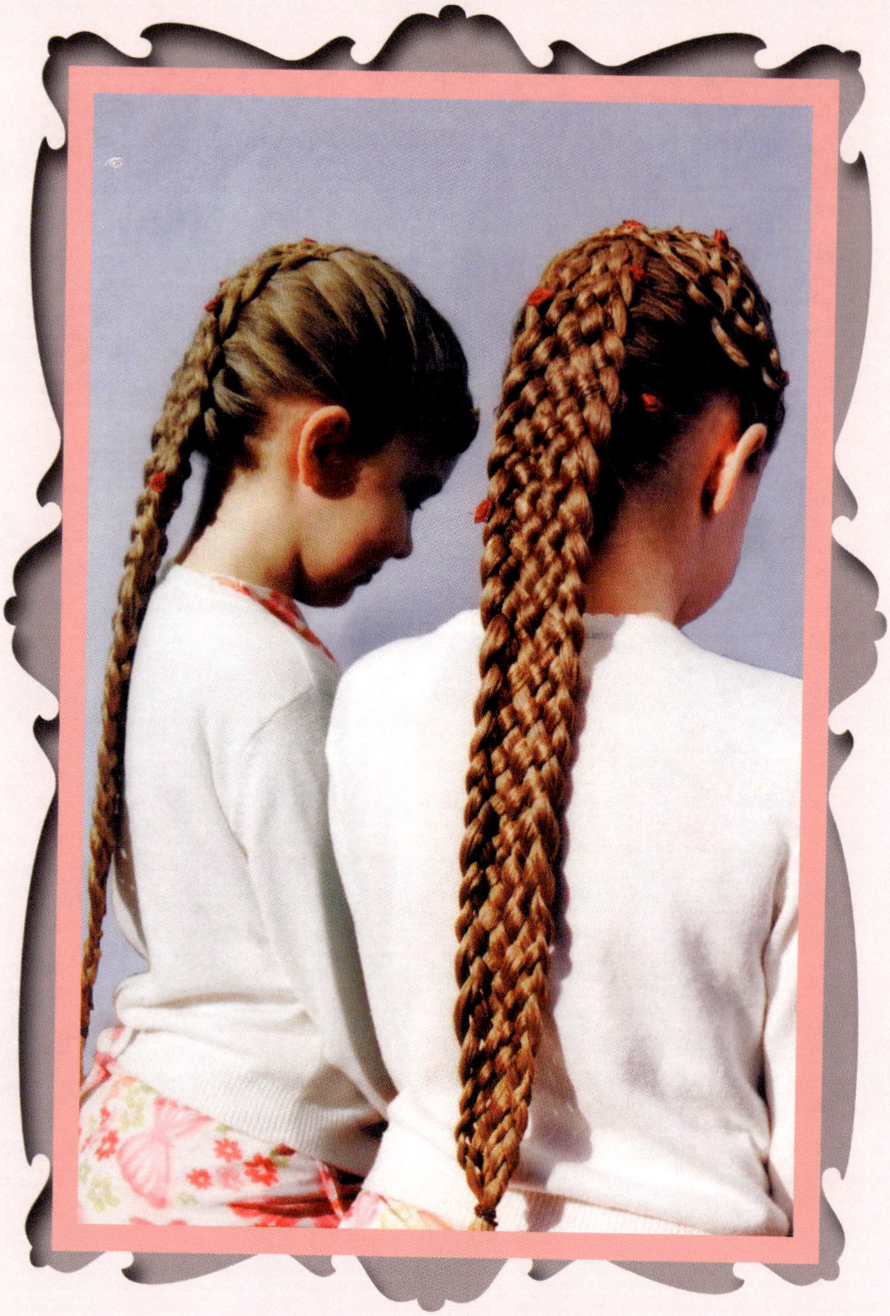

I invite you to one last challenge. After mastering this braid you are welcome to experiment on your own with larger numbers. I have only done up to eleven strands.

Nine-Strand

Any more strands than this and it would start to get difficult. The next fourteen pages will walk you through this braid.

Braid . . . . 300 - 302

Stitch dutch . . . . . . 304 - 309

Examples 311

Let's braid it!

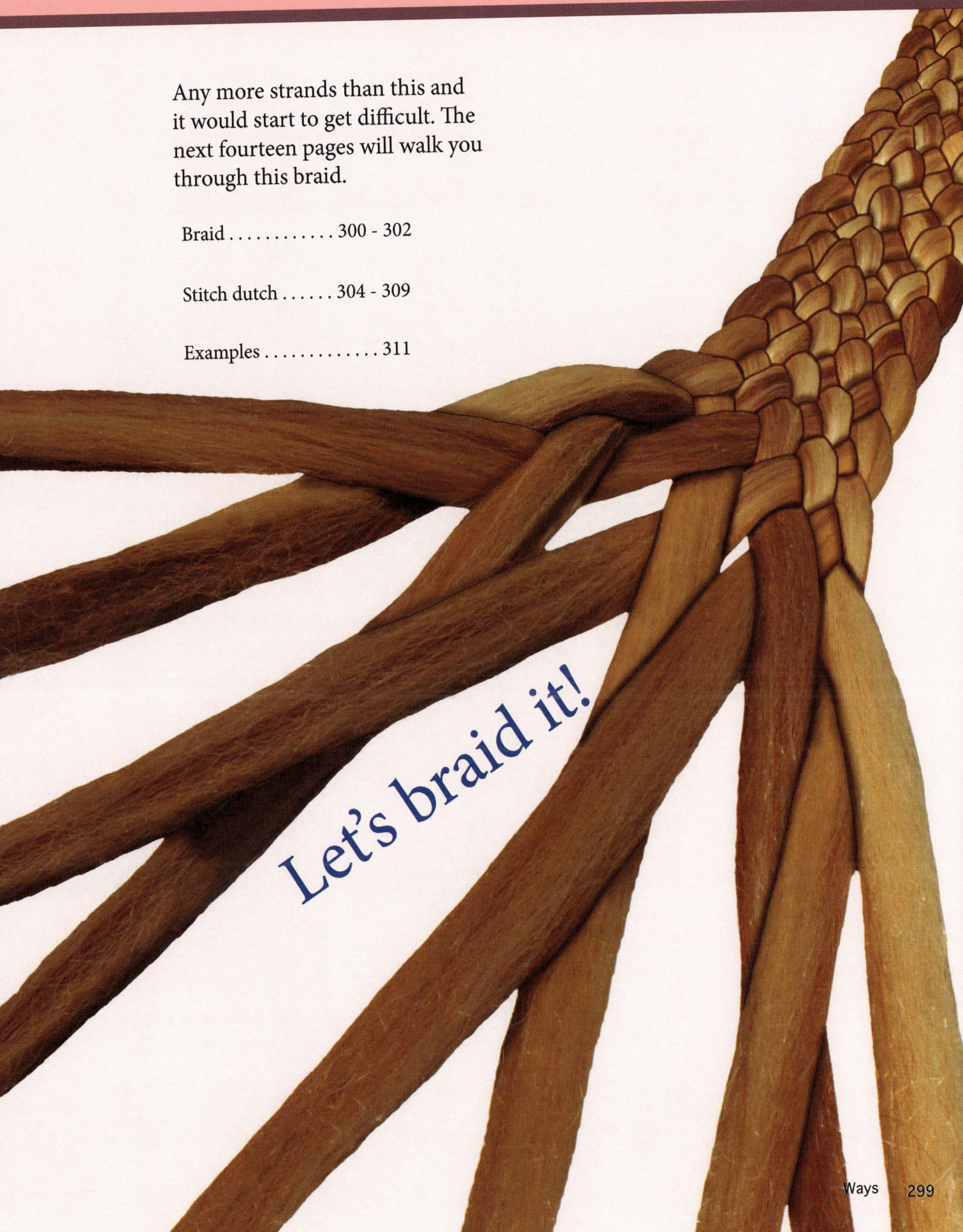

9 Nine-Strand Braid

We may be dissappointed if we fail, but we are doomed if we don't try.
— Beverly Sills

1.
Take strand 1 with your palm down and your thumb facing your belly button.

2.
Reach under strand 2 and hook strand 3 with the pinky finger.

5.
Grab strand 4 with the middle finger.

6.
Reach under strand 6 and hook strand 7 with the middle finger.

300 www.findingbraids.com

Nine-Strand Braid

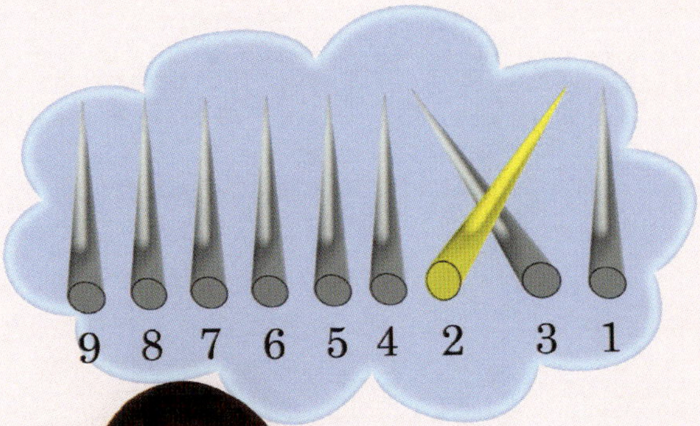

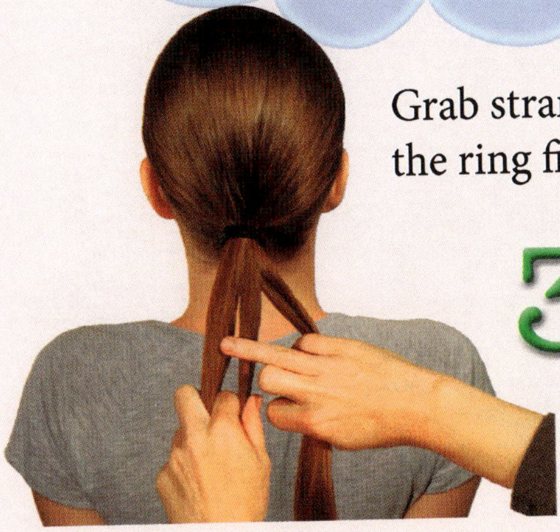

3. Grab strand 2 with the ring finger.

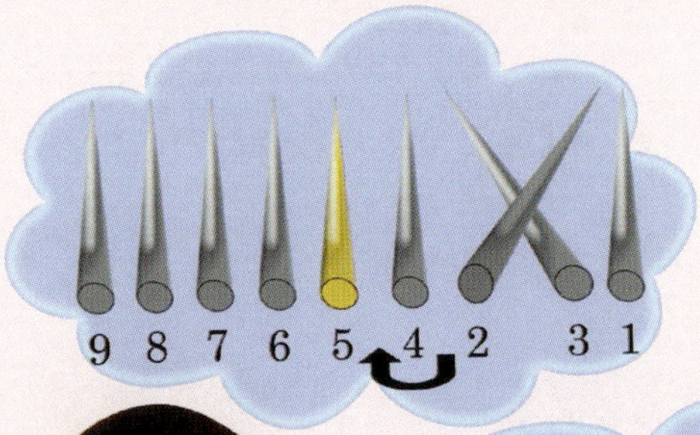

4. 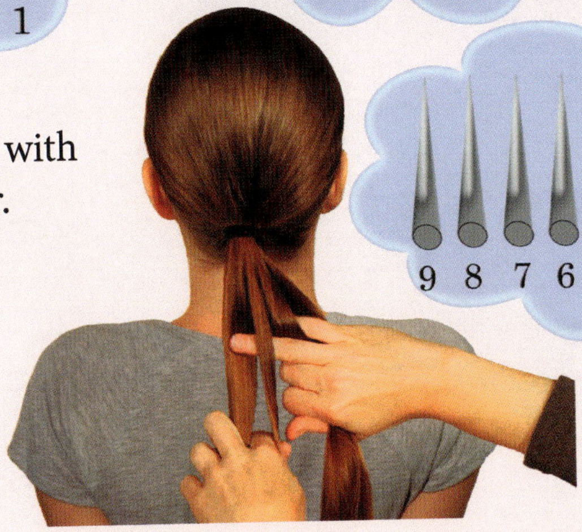 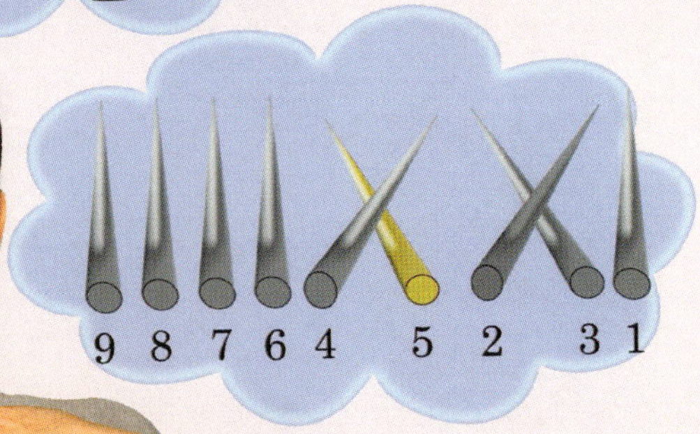 Reach under strand 4 and hook strand 5 with the ring finger.

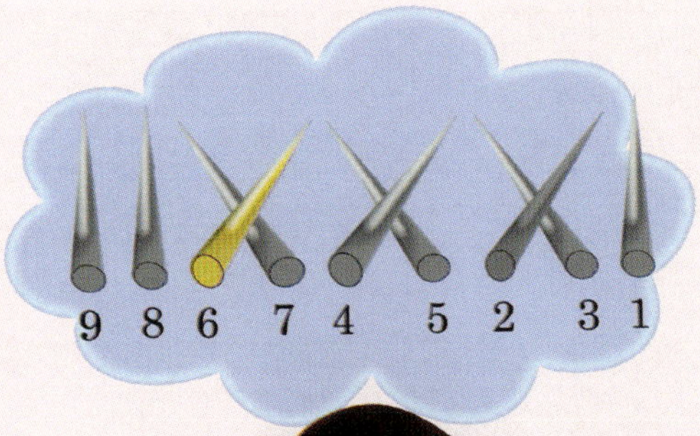

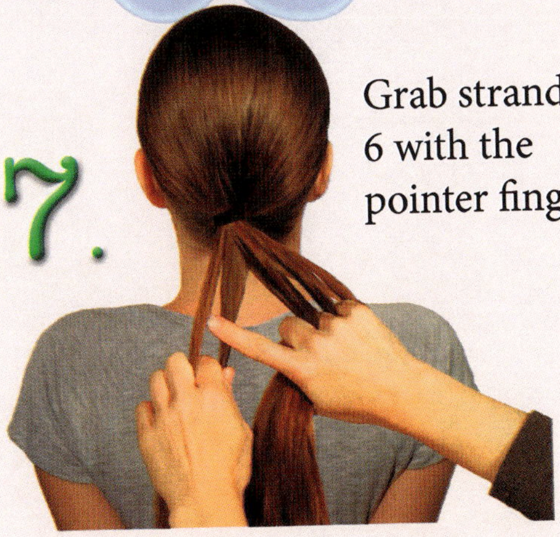

7. Grab strand 6 with the pointer finger.

8. Reach under strand 8 and hook strand 9 with the pointer finger.

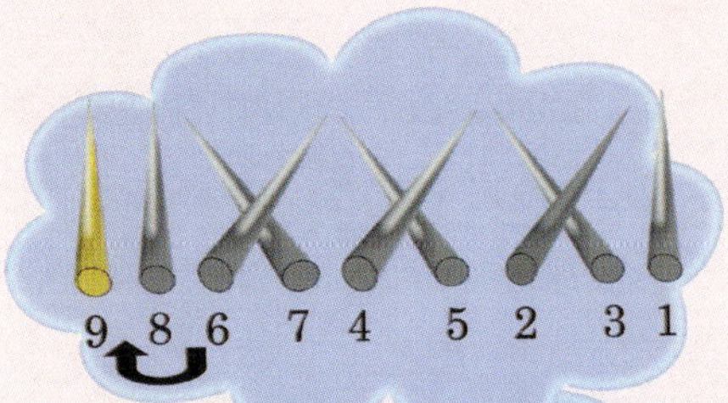

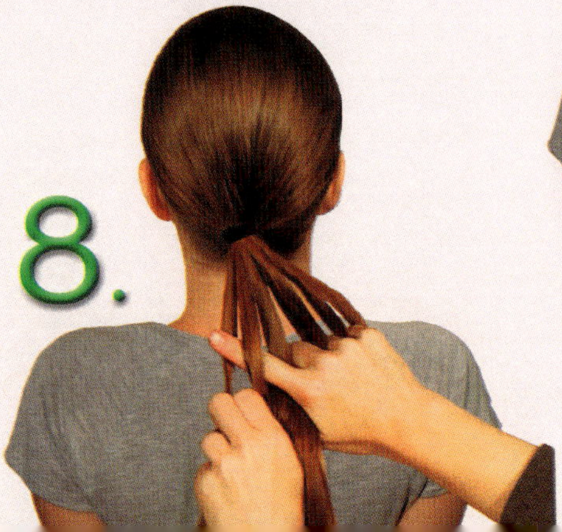

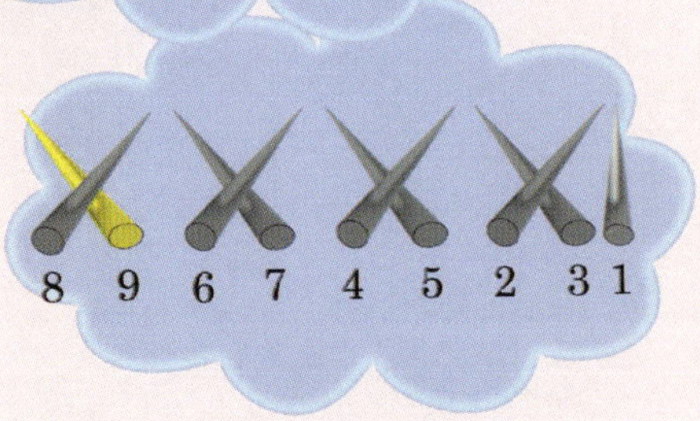

9. Place strand 8 in between the thumb and pointer finger.

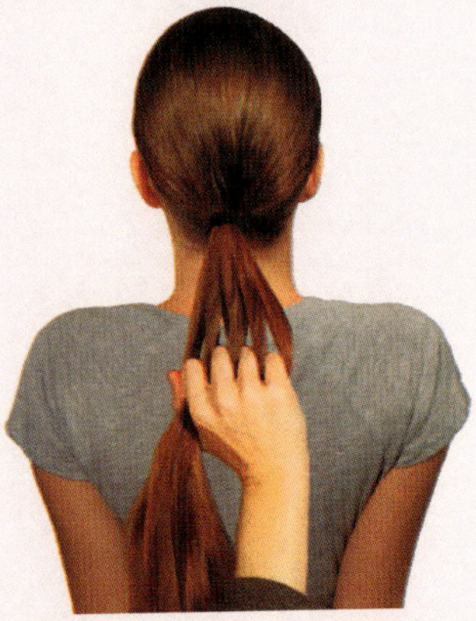

part 2. Nine-Strand Braid

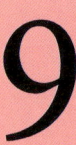

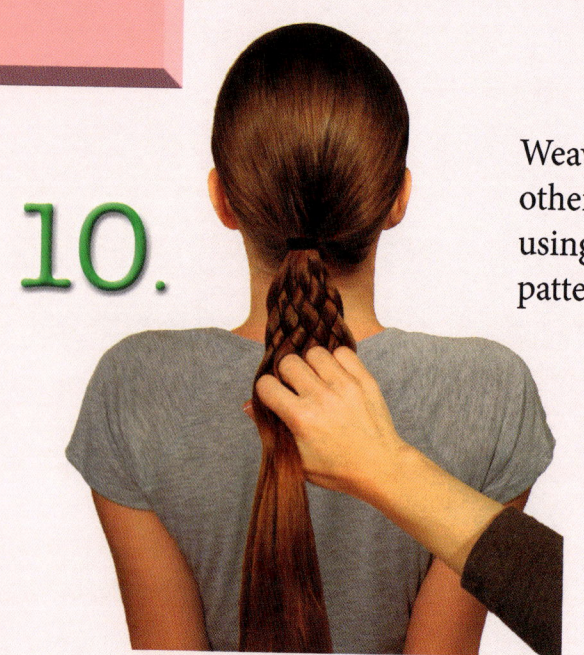

Weave back the other direction using the same pattern.

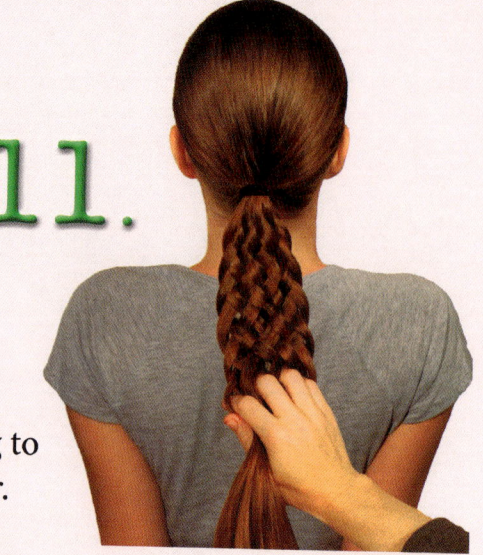

Continue weaving to the end of the hair.

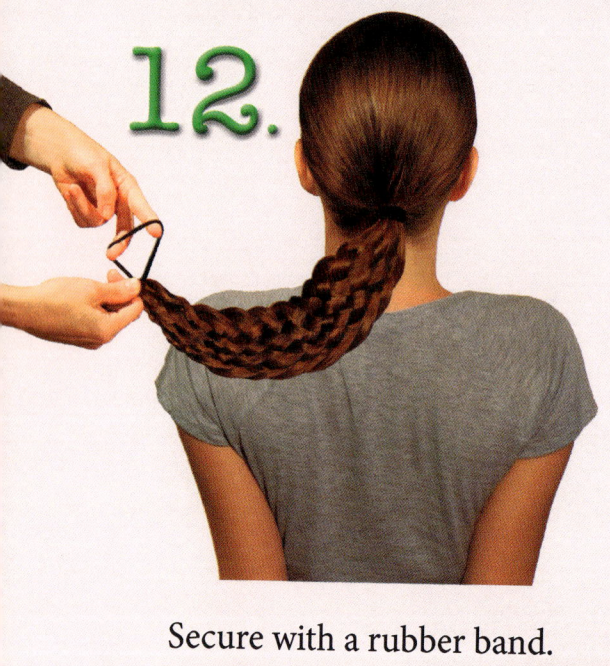

Secure with a rubber band.

Nine-Strand

Gather from both sides

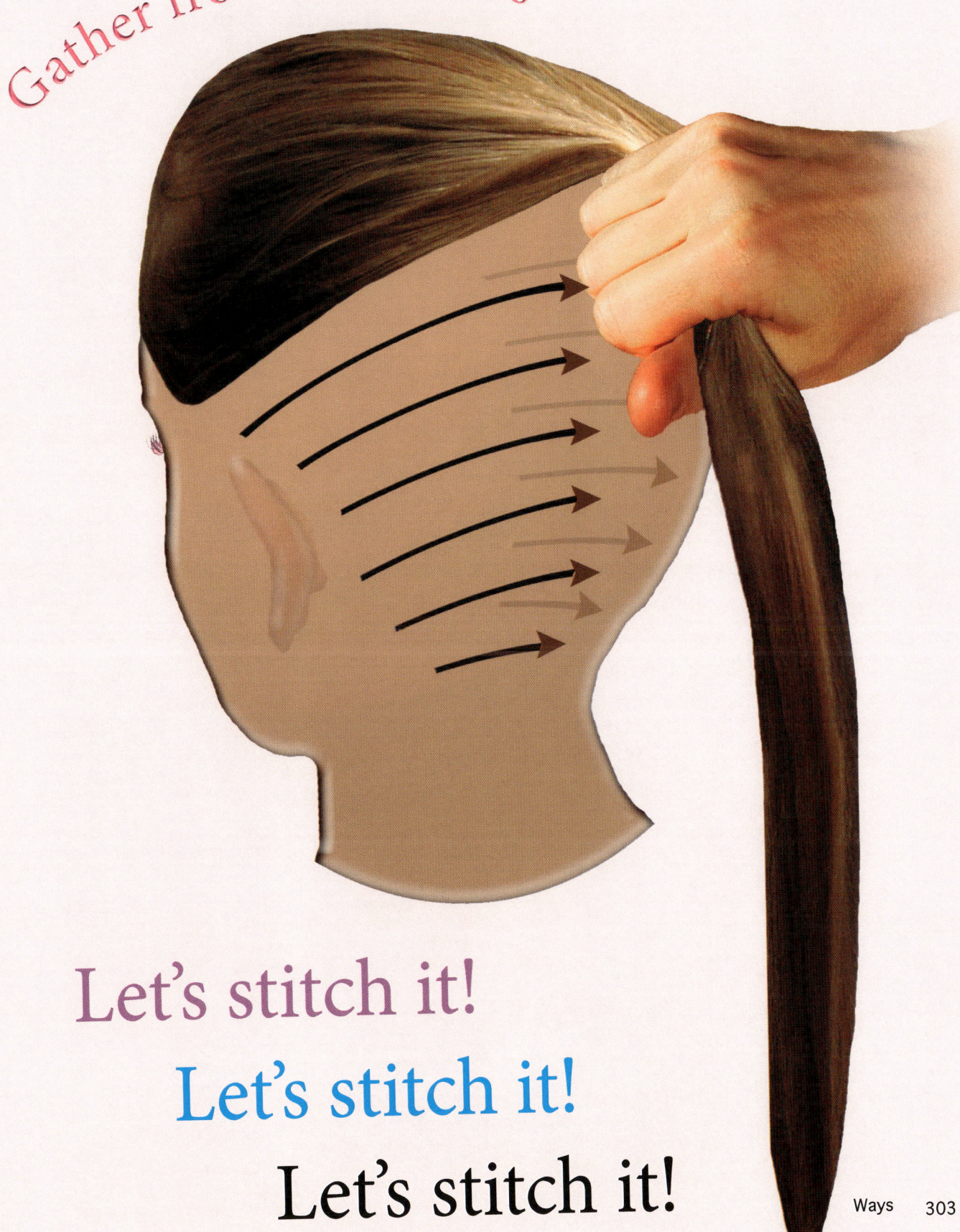

Let's stitch it!

Let's stitch it!

Let's stitch it!

9 Nine-Strand Dutch Stitch

Ships in harbor are safe, but that is not what ships are built for. - John A. Shedd

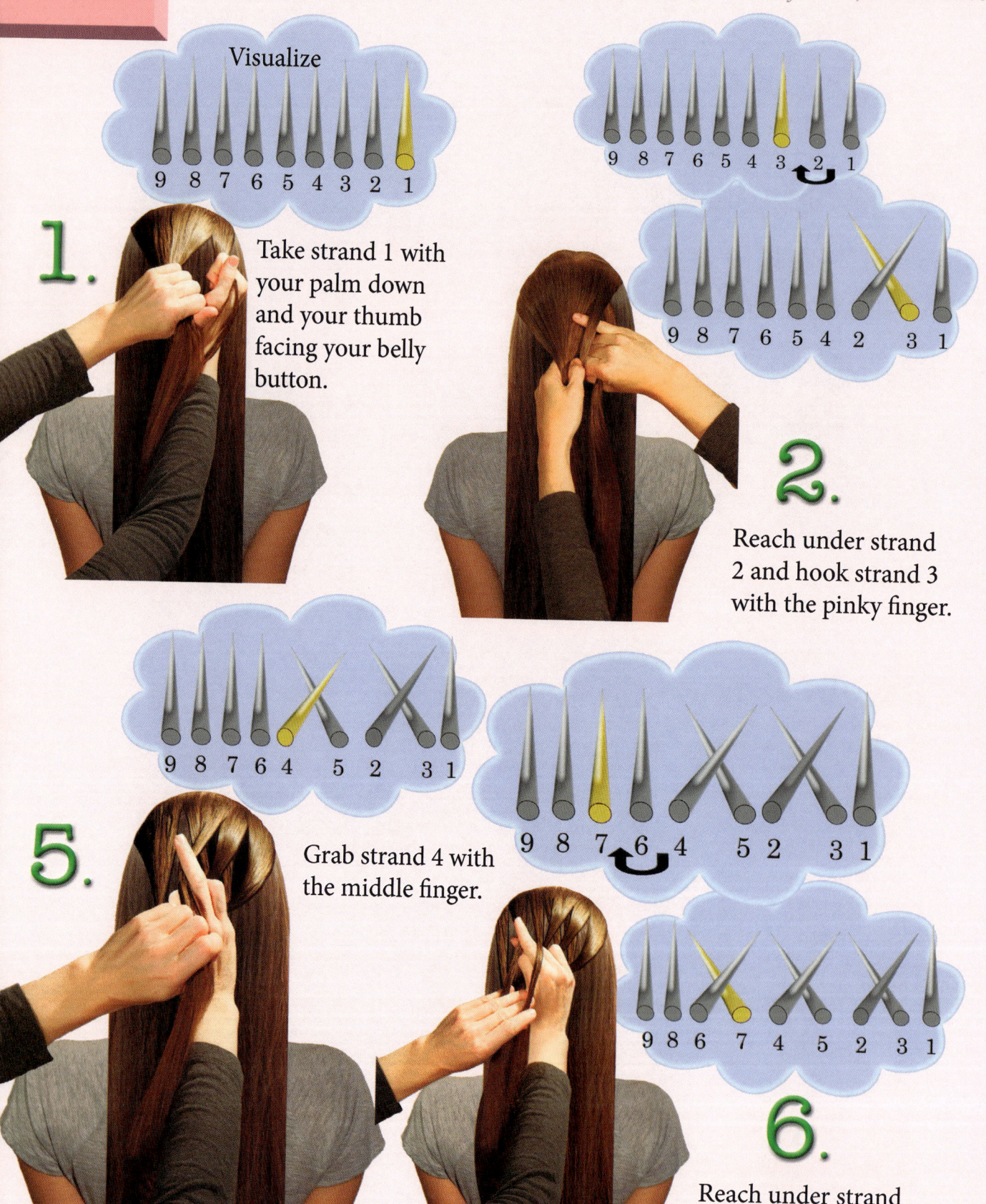

1. Take strand 1 with your palm down and your thumb facing your belly button.

2. Reach under strand 2 and hook strand 3 with the pinky finger.

5. Grab strand 4 with the middle finger.

6. Reach under strand 6 and hook strand 7 with the middle finger.

Nine-Strand Dutch Stitch

9

3. Grab strand 2 with the ring finger.

4. Reach under strand 4 and hook strand 5 with the ring finger.

7. Grab strand 6 with the pointer finger.

8. Reach under strand 8 and hook strand 9 with the pointer finger.

9. Place strand 8 in between the thumb and pointer finger.

Ways 305

9 Continuing

Number your strands at your knuckles now.

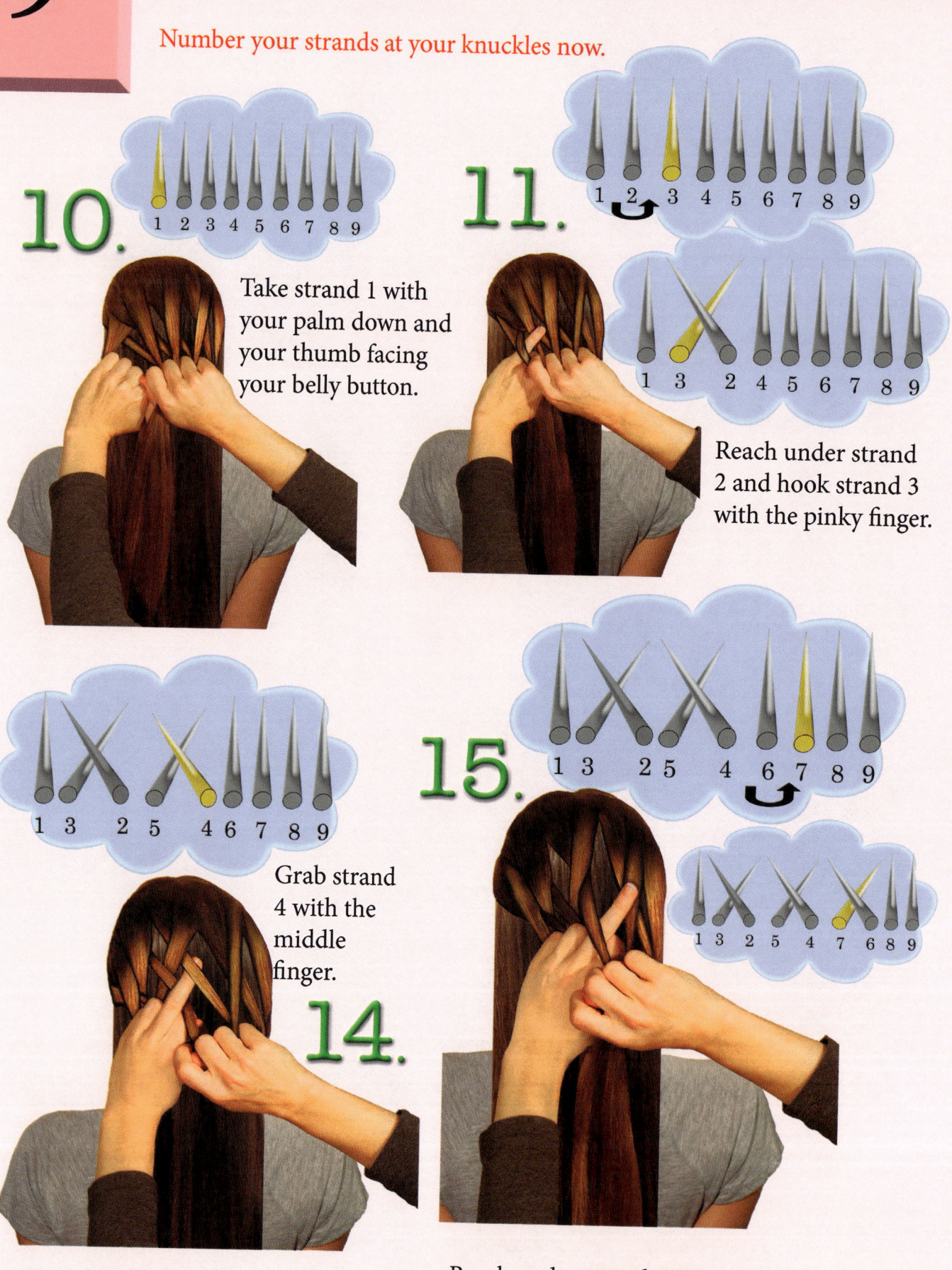

10. Take strand 1 with your palm down and your thumb facing your belly button.

11. Reach under strand 2 and hook strand 3 with the pinky finger.

14. Grab strand 4 with the middle finger.

15. Reach under strand 6 and hook strand 7 with the middle finger.

306   www.findingbraids.com

part 2. Nine-Strand Dutch Stitch

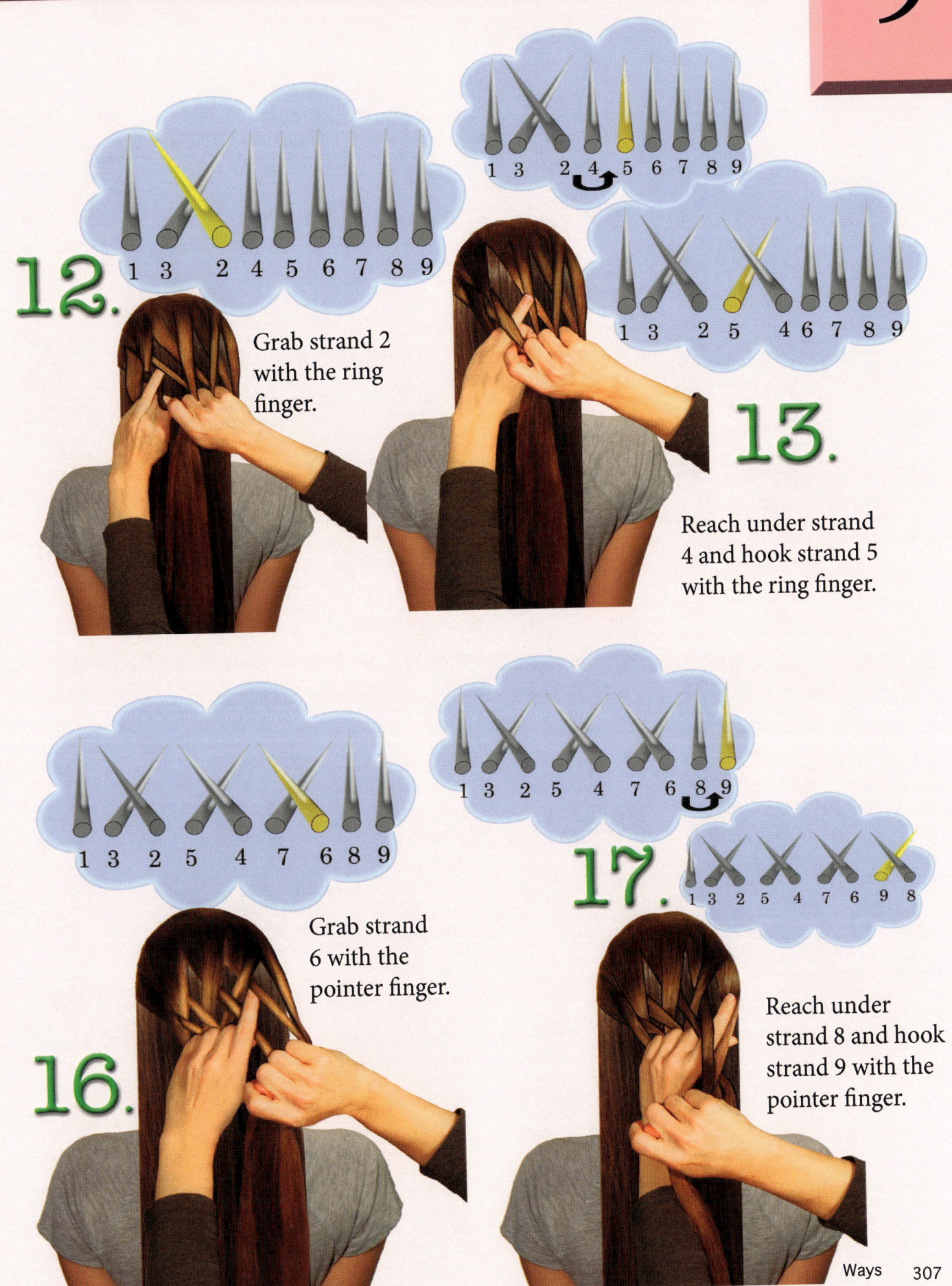

9 Continuing

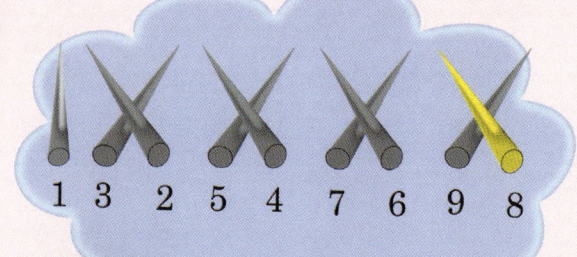

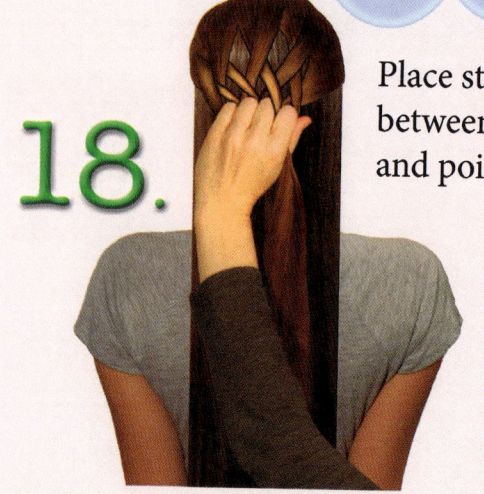

18.

Place strand 8 in between the thumb and pointer finger.

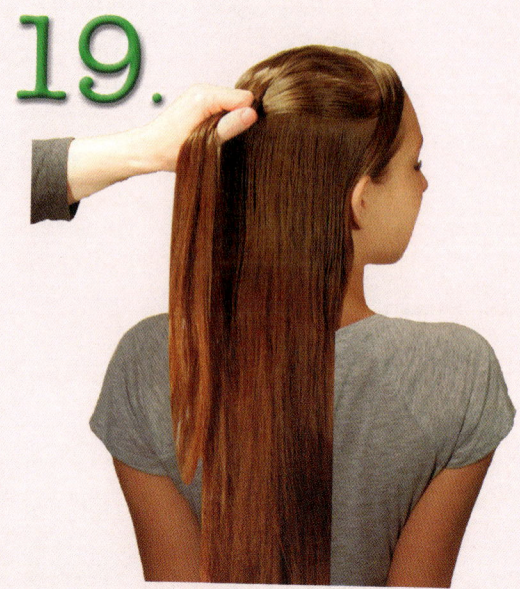

19.

You now have an available hand to pick up your tail comb.

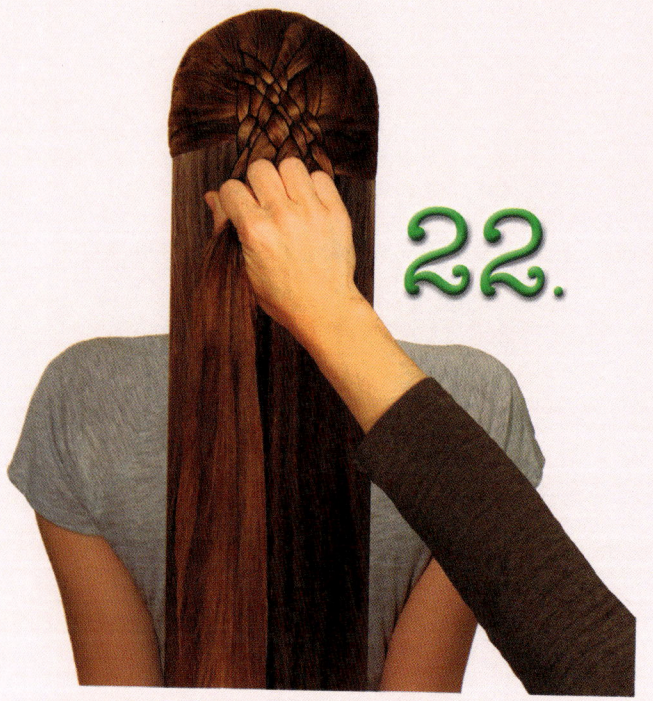

22.

Continue weaving and gathering until you reach the end of the hair.

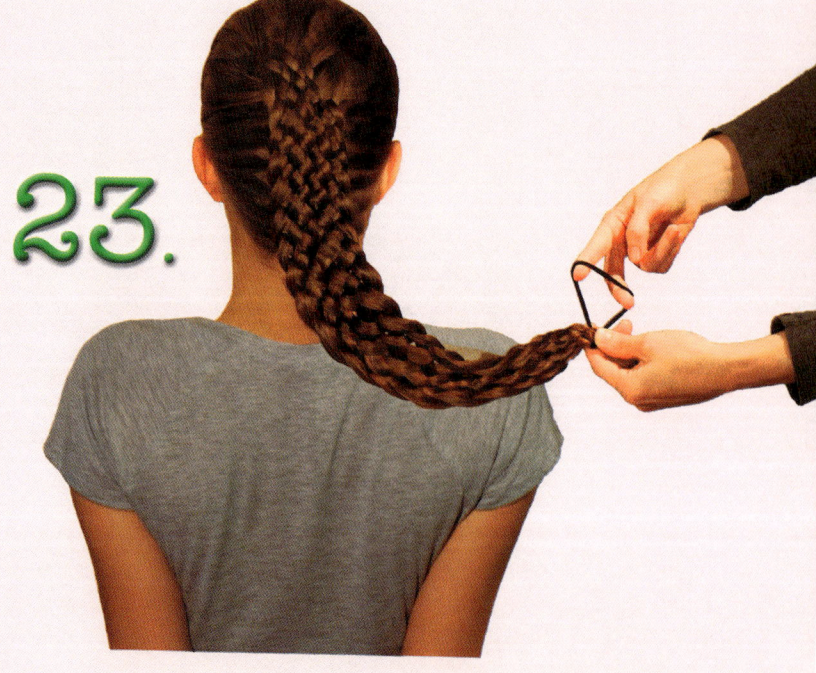

23.

Secure with a rubber band.

part 3. Nine-Strand Dutch Stitch

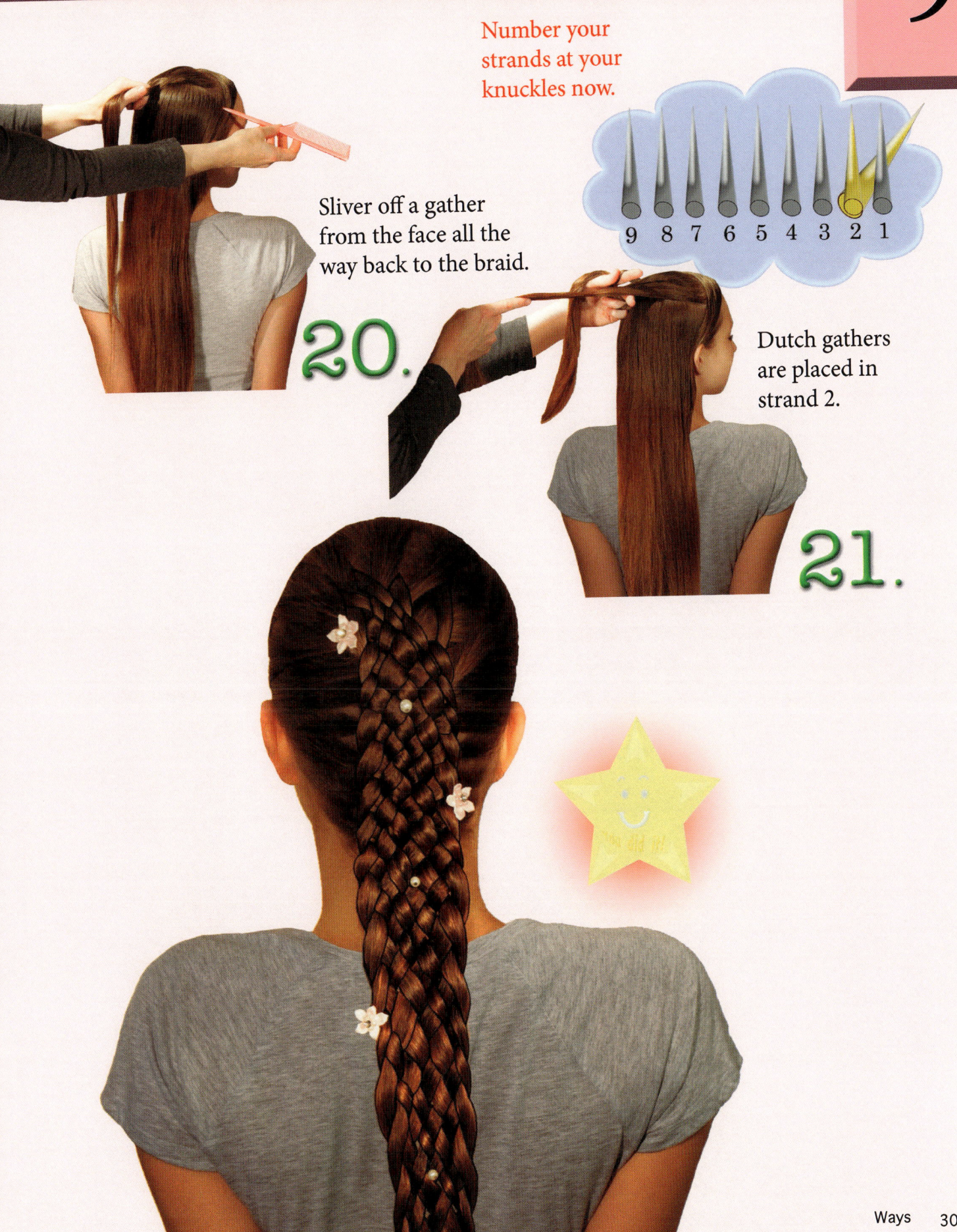

Number your strands at your knuckles now.

9 8 7 6 5 4 3 2 1

Sliver off a gather from the face all the way back to the braid.

20.

Dutch gathers are placed in strand 2.

21.

Nine-Strand

Notes

Examples of Nine-Strand

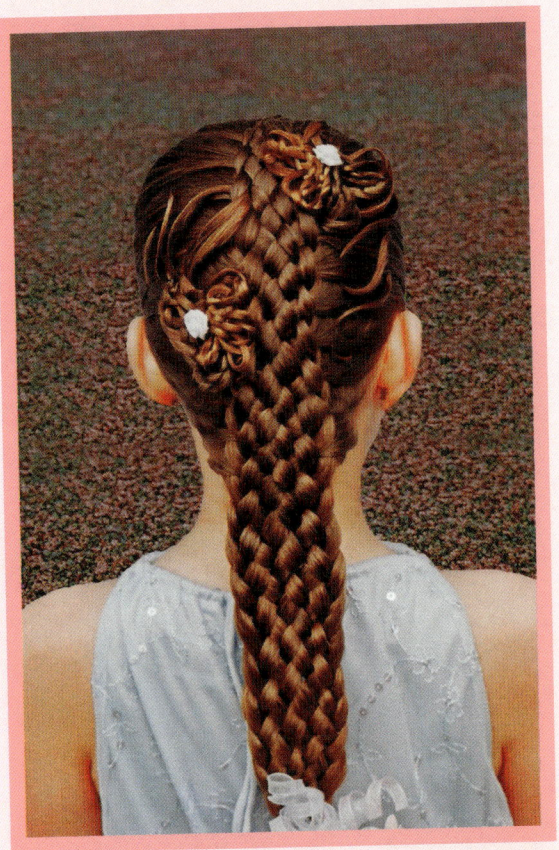
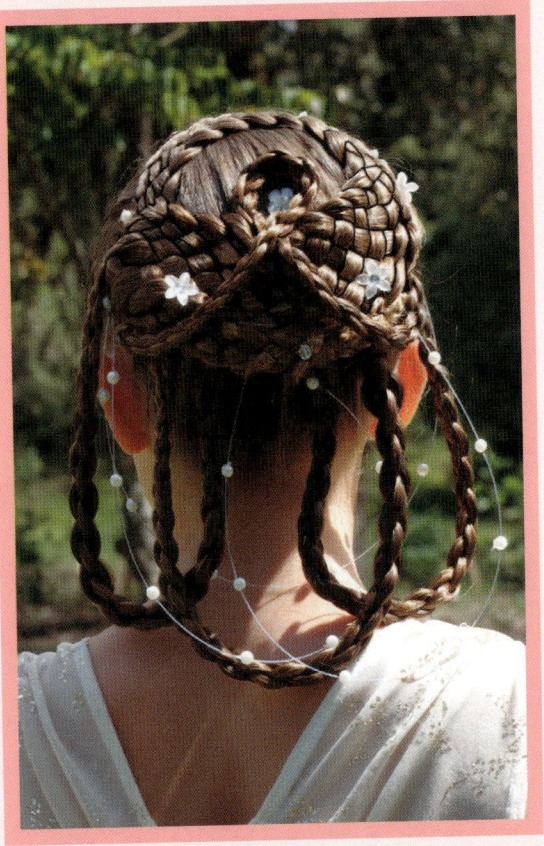
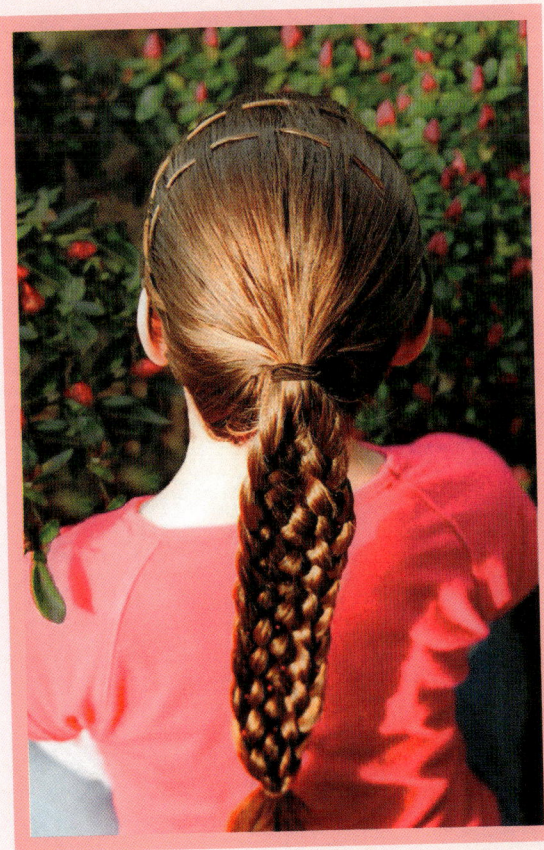
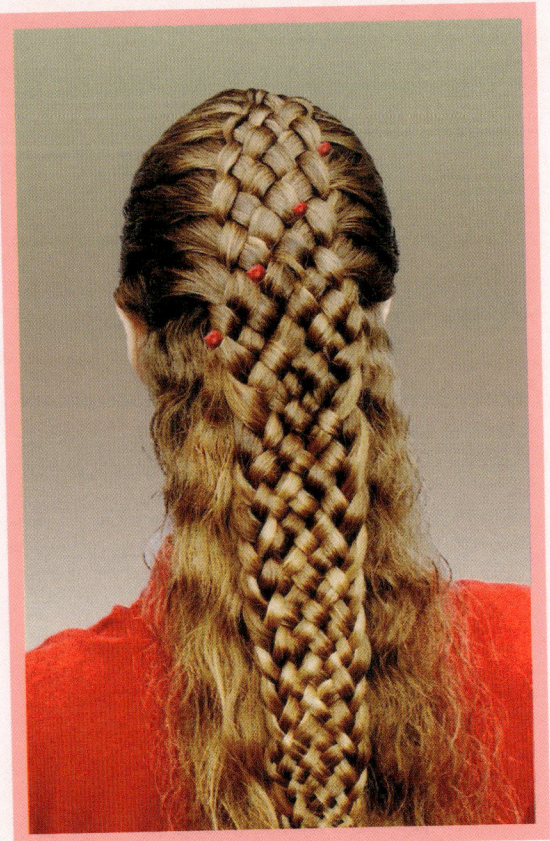

Visit my website to see more examples of the Nine-Strand

Merging

The point in a hairstyle when two seperate braids join together to become one braid.

Merging

M
E
R
G
I
N
G

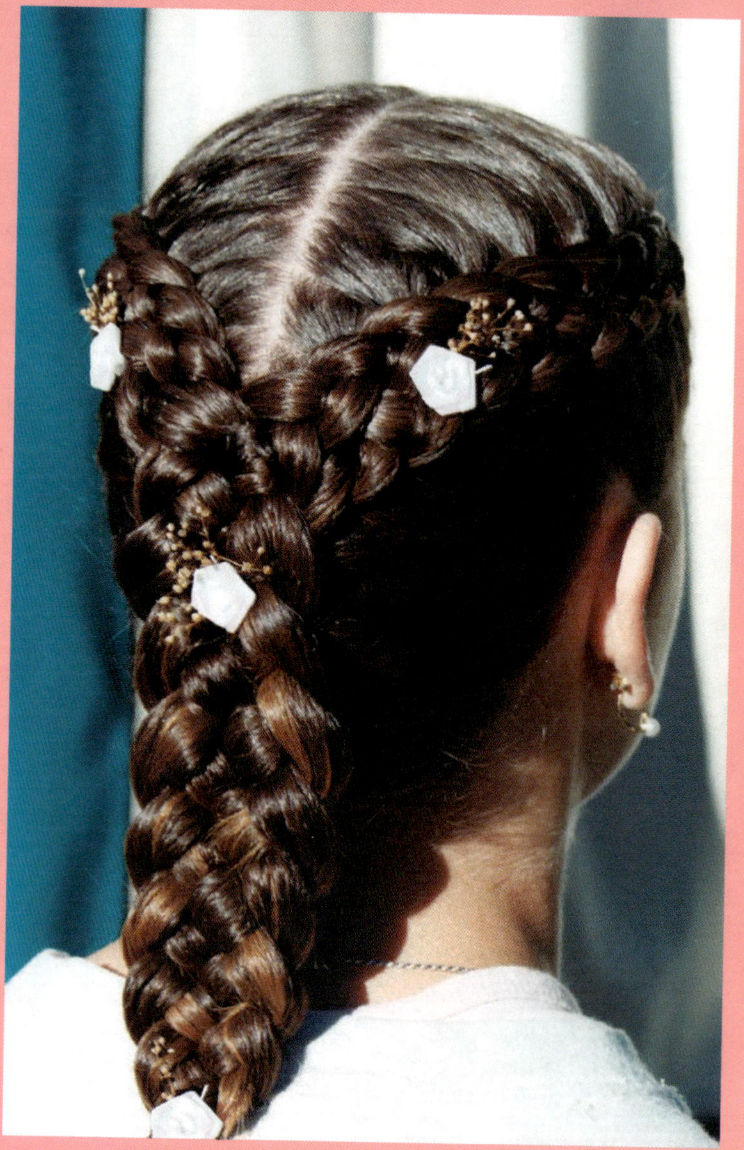

Bring two seperate braids together and bind them as one. Each strand follows its own path to finish the specific pattern, all working together in harmony.

When Two Come Together

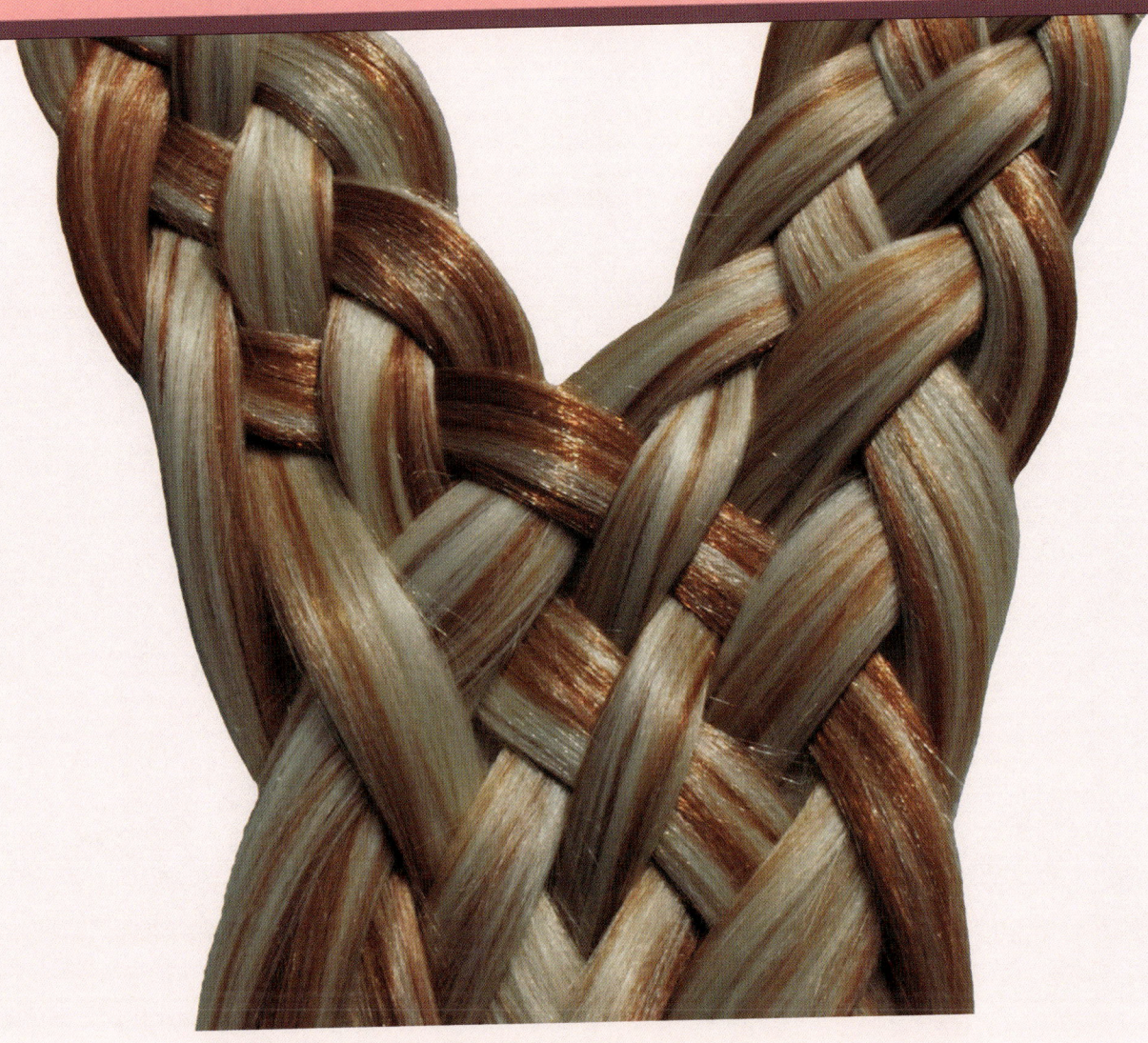

There is a pattern to merging. To be honest, I rarely find or use that pattern when I merge braids. I usually take one of these approaches. 1. Close my eyes and mash the two braids together and continue braiding. 2. Clump two strands near each other to make them one and continue braiding. 3. Overlap one side on top of the other side and continue braiding.

I decide which I will do the instant I do it. Factors that influence my desicion include the difficulty of the braid I am doing, the person's hair type, the occasion the person is attending, their role in said occasion, the amount of time I have and my patience that day.

Just breifly getting into it so you understand the level of knowledge needed to perfectly merge each possible braid type, this merge is a five into nine. If I had done five into ten I would have gone from odd number to even numbers and page 182 helps explain all that that entails. Feel free to self study all the ways to merge all the braid possibilities. Or, do what I do and cover up bad merges with flowers.

Ways

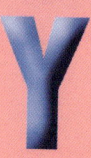

Merging

Success seems to be largely a matter of hanging on after others have let go.
— William Feather

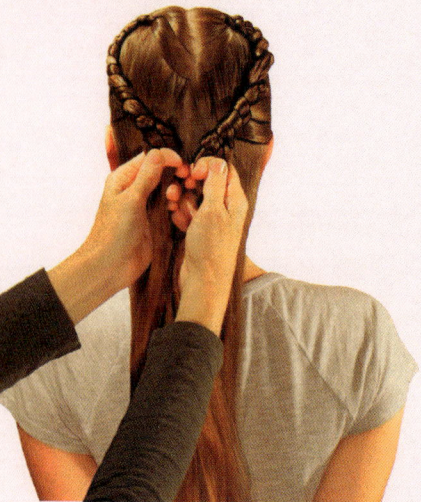 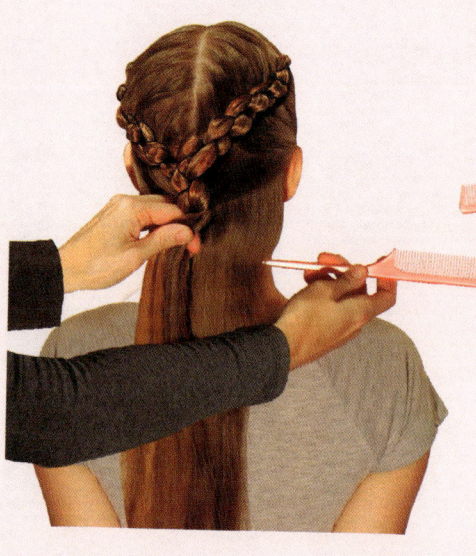 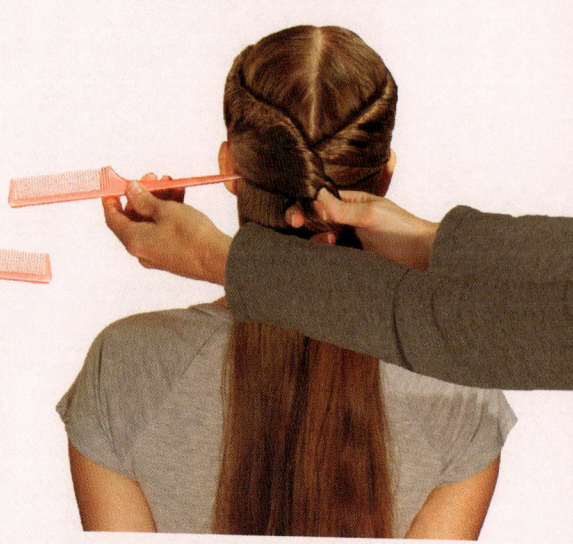

Each new number-of-strand set has it's own unique and correct merging pattern.

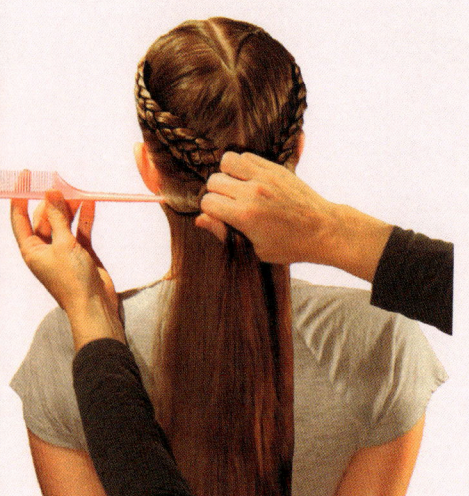 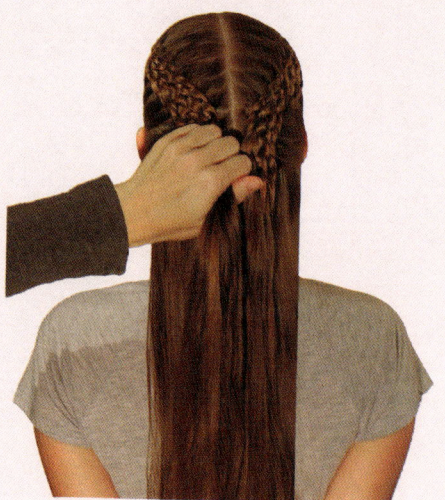 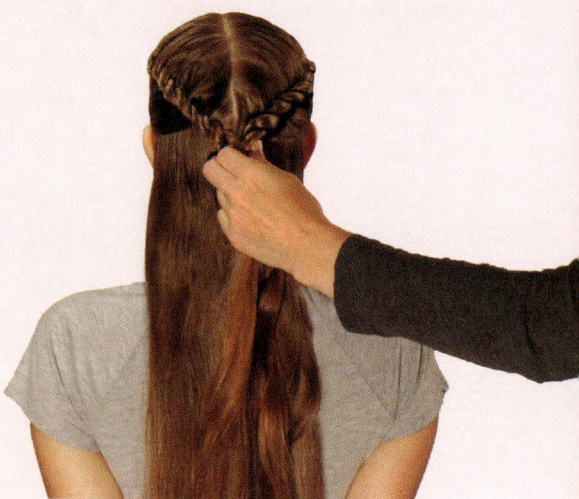

These are just a few of the vast possibilities for combinations with the number of strands.

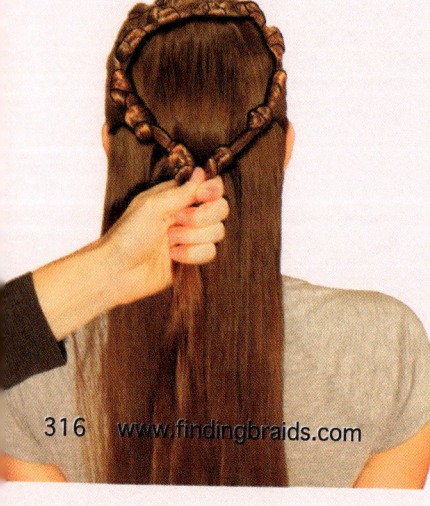 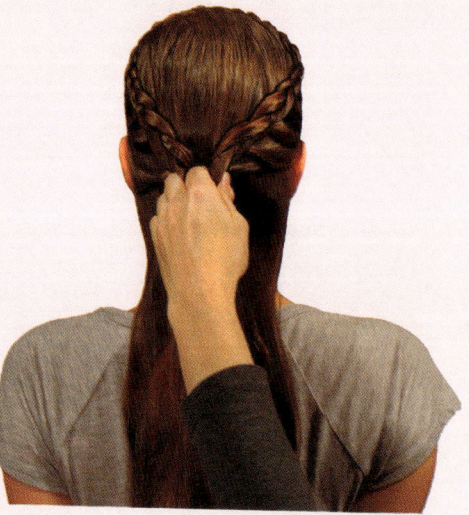 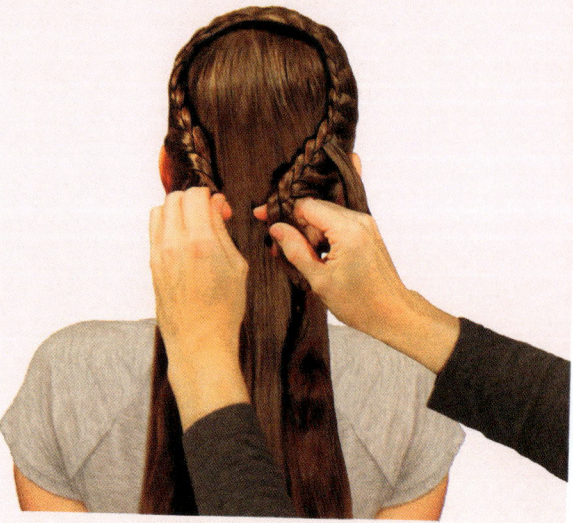

Examples of Merging

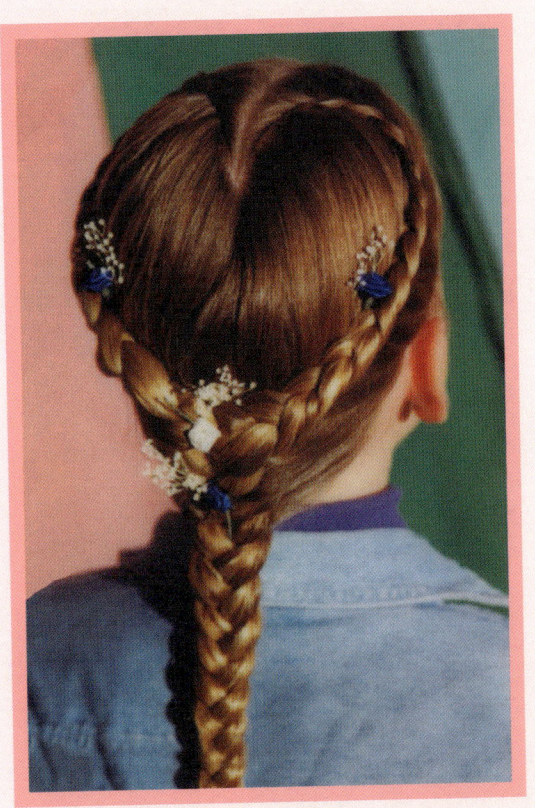
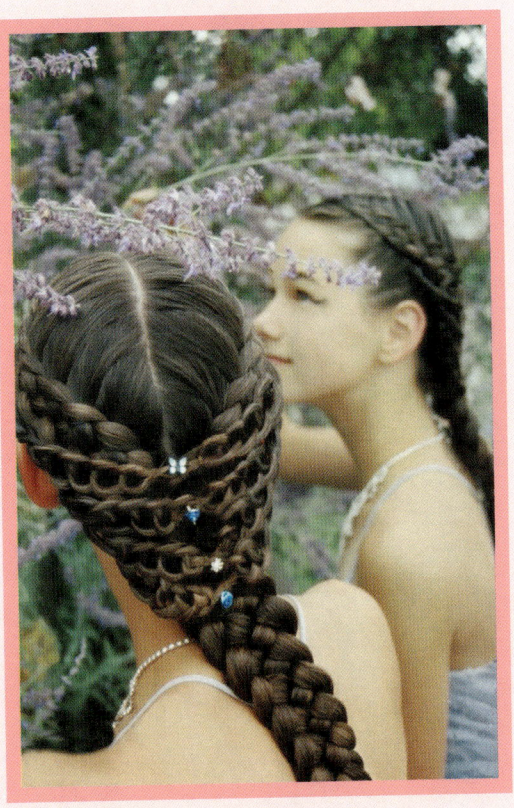
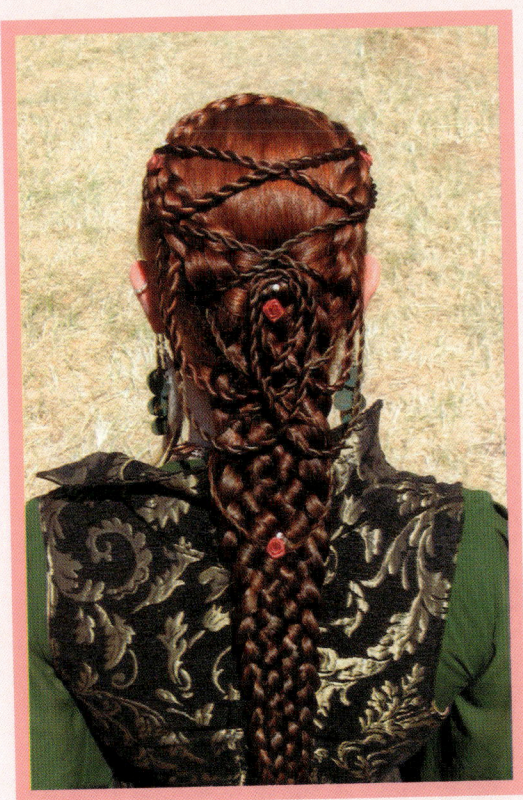
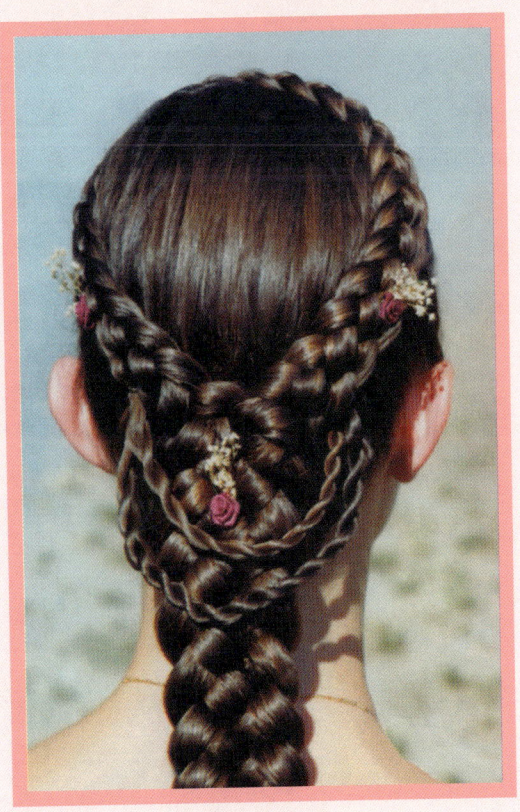

Visit my website to see more examples of braids that merge

Chapter Two

Tools needed for basic and cascaded forms:
- Brush
- Tail Comb
- Water Spray Bottle
- Hair Product
- 2 Rubber Bands
- Butterfly Clip
- 5 Bobby Pins

Tools needed for accented and accented cascade forms:
- Brush
- Tail Comb
- Water Spray Bottle
- Hair Product
- 2 Rubber Bands
- Tiny Rubber Bands
- Butterfly Clip
- 15 Bobby Pins
- Latch Hook
- Curling Iron
- Flat Iron
- Beads
- Fake hair

Chapter Two ~ Forms

Each form has two options right off the bat.

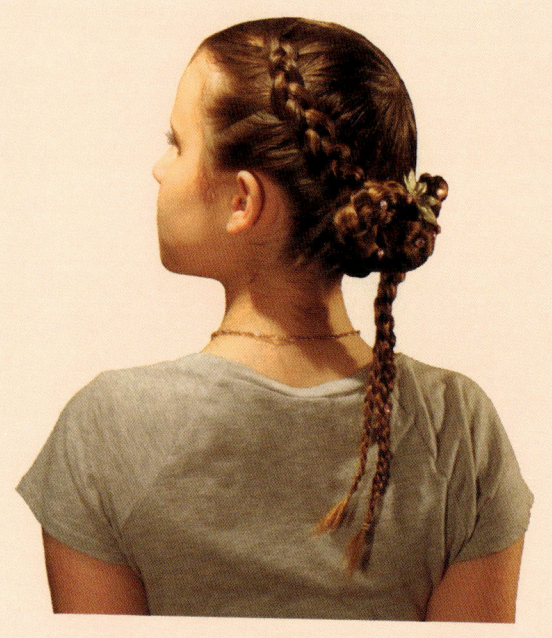

Basic
All hair is incorporated into the form.

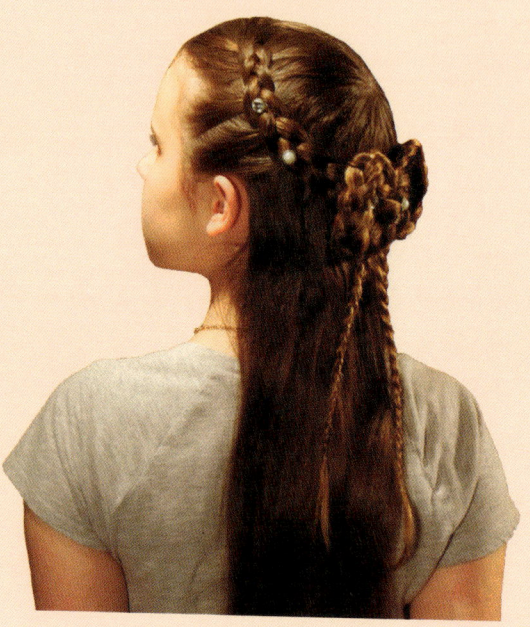

Cascade
Half of the hair is left down.

Cascading a form lends a less formal look and keeps your neck warm. Cascading also changes the length requirement. When half the hair is left down, the form can be done on shorter and/or thicker hair. Cascading thick hair can also save the aesthetically pleasing aspect of certain forms. Only practice and application can clarify these statements.

Knowing a lot ... is a springboard to creativity. – Charlie Rose

What's the difference?

For the next hundred and fifty pages we will be delving into four options that each form offers and finishing with the topic of variations. Why are there so many options?

Many people will not wear all of there hair up, hence the basic and cascade options. Those two options also have the option to be accented. The four options are thus labeled:

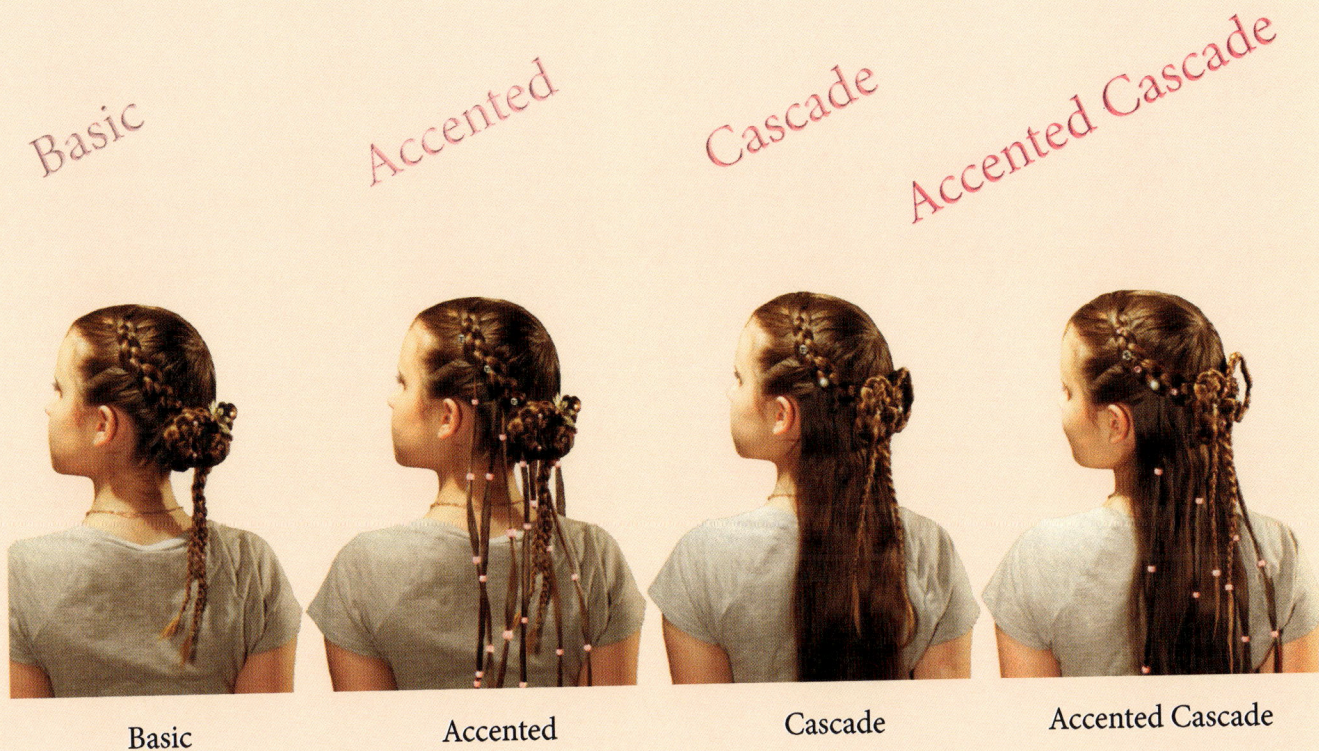

Basic   Accented   Cascade   Accented Cascade

How should you use Chapter Two? I invite you to use it as a suggestion. Scan the how-to photos of all four options of each form. It will give you a good overveiw of the nature of each form and you will be able to execute lovely styles based on what you learn there.

This book has limited room to show you in-depth details of each form and their options. Please purchase the mini series for more instructions. Each form has its own book dedicated to educating you in the art of that form.

Chapter Two ~ Forms

Introducing the twelve forms we will be working with

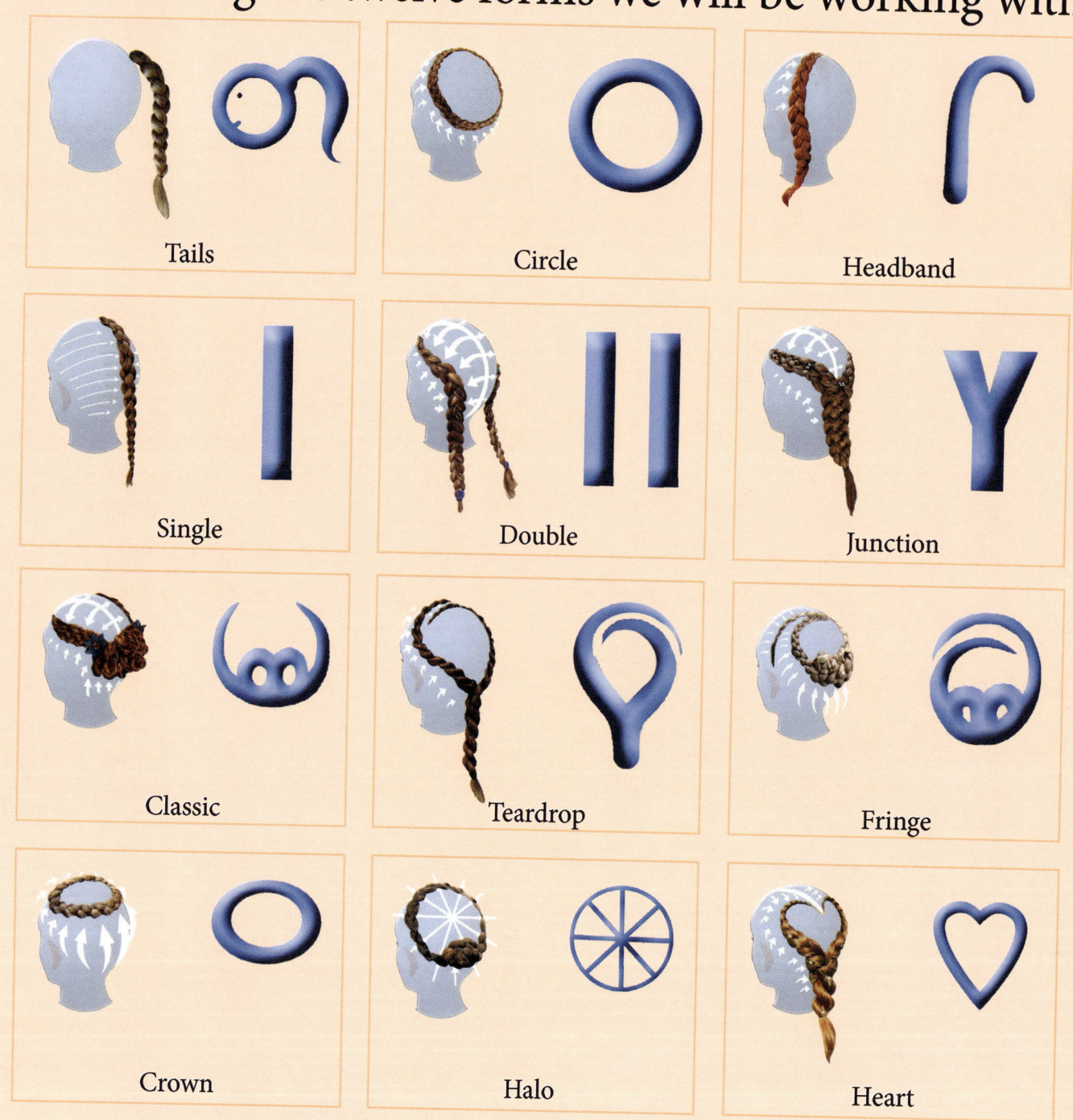

There are probably hundreds of other forms. I picked my favorites to show what forms are capable of. I encourage you to transfer the concepts shown on these pages to all the forms in the world that cross your path. This is an organized system for mixing-it-up a bit.

Adventure out with your own creativity

Let's take what we learned from Chapter One and apply it here in Chapter Two. Each form may be constructed using any number of strands. Truly! You may braid, stitch or lace any form. Experiment to find your favorite construction process for each form. Please do not get frustrated as you see me changing where I start and end each form. And remain open-minded if I change from stitching a form to lacing a form. The point of forms is not where you start and end it, or if you braid, stitch or lace it; the point is: the shape you create while you braid.

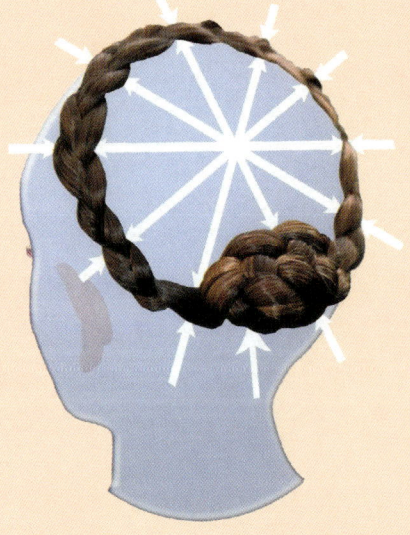

Let's use the Halo as an example. A person might concern themselves with where this form should start and end. I would like you to notice the starburst pattern. This pattern also resembles a cut pie. You may start at any arrowhead. The Halo generally starts and then ends in the same place. The bun indicates the ending and start point and is usually placed over the starting point, I am referring to the times you choose to incorporate a bun into your design, you may not choose to make a bun with the left over hair.

Chapter Two will be most useful if you study all four options of each form before you decide how that form works. Notice where I start each option. See how I end each option. Observe the entire process of the options involved in each form. Then formulate a conclusion about the basic structure of that form. Think about how you can change it up a bit to give it your signature.

Forms

Forms

TAILS

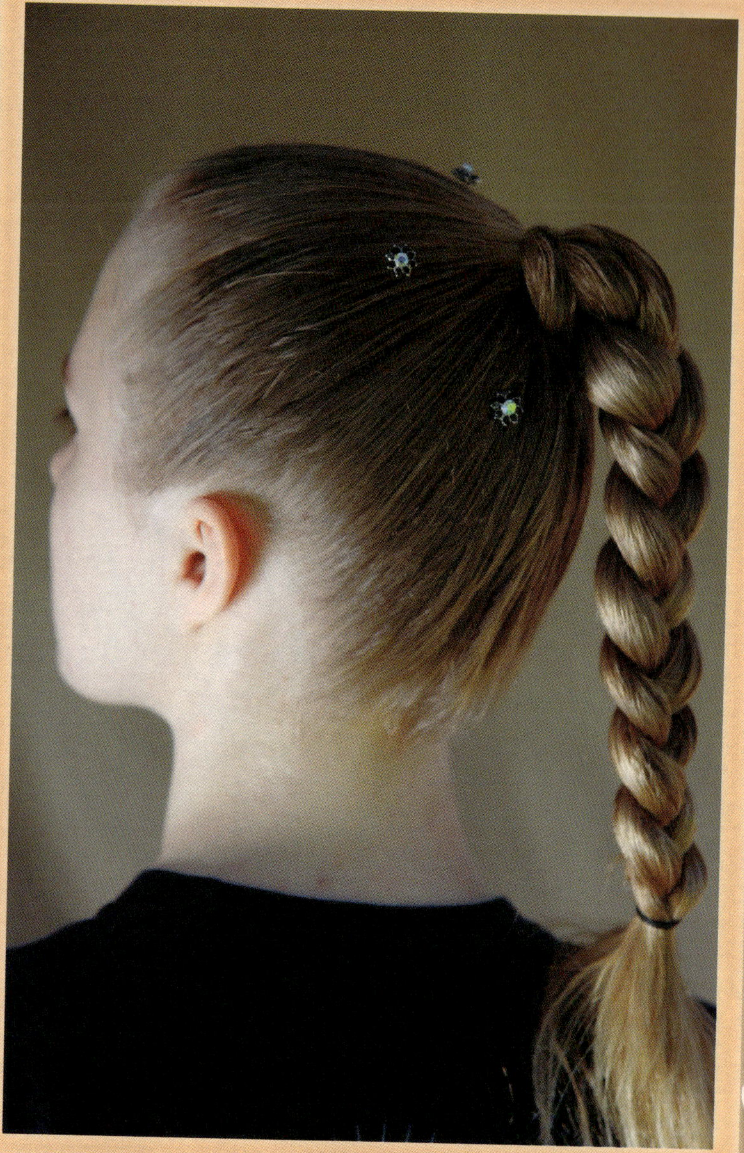

A form of ten thousand plus options. How will you make this uniquely yours? Use this form for your everyday look and spice it up for your formal needs.

Forms

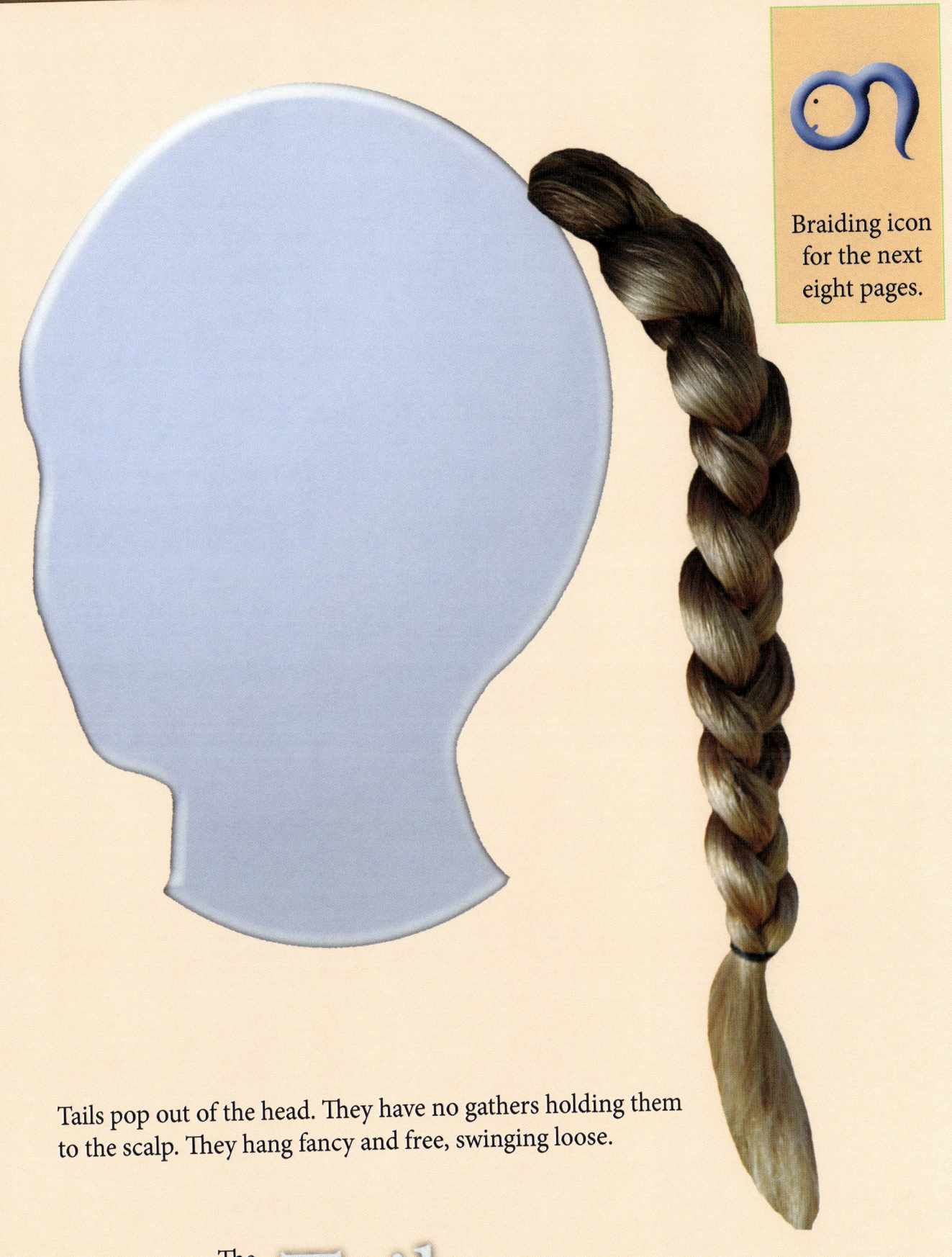

Braiding icon for the next eight pages.

Tails pop out of the head. They have no gathers holding them to the scalp. They hang fancy and free, swinging loose.

The **Tails** Form

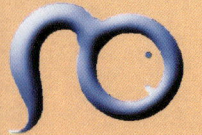

Basic Tails

1.

Begin with clean, brushed hair.

2.

Part the hair down the center.

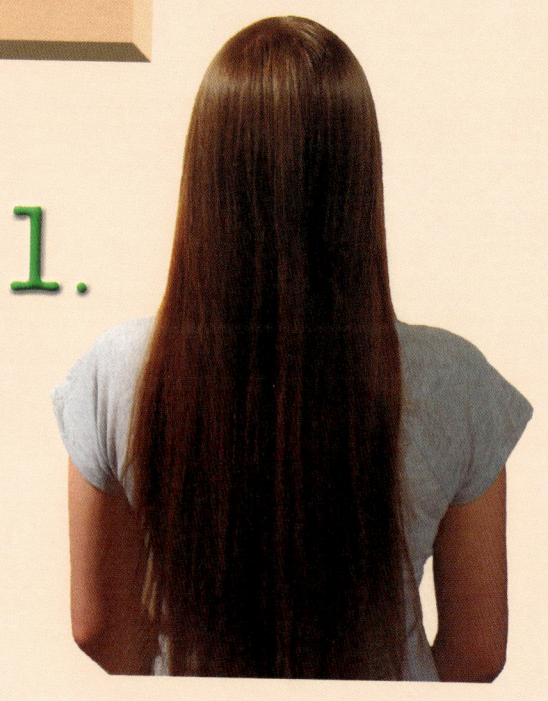

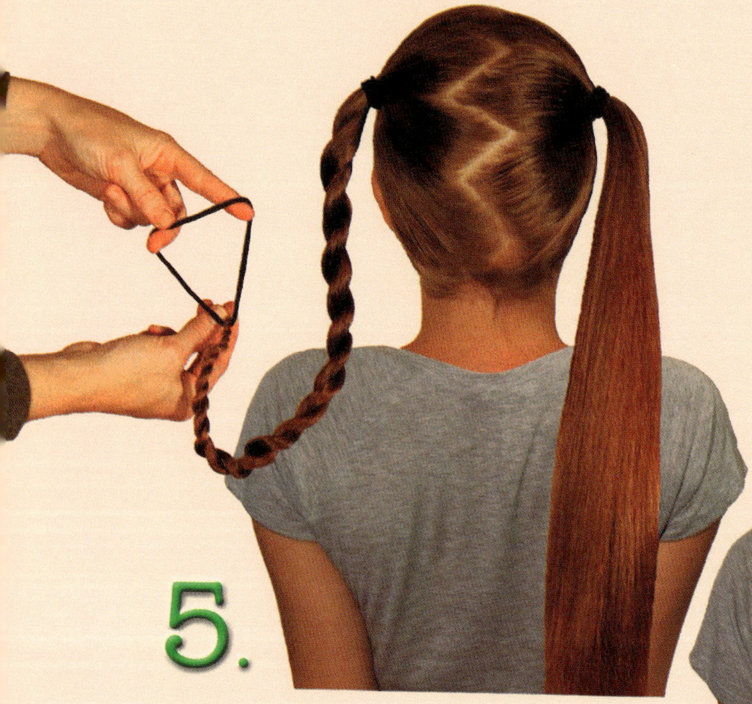

5.

This is a two-strand rope.

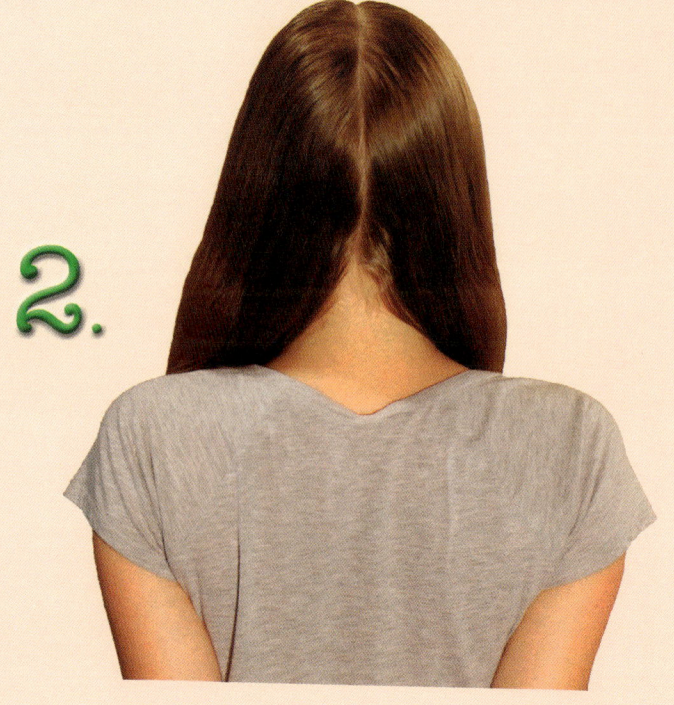

6.

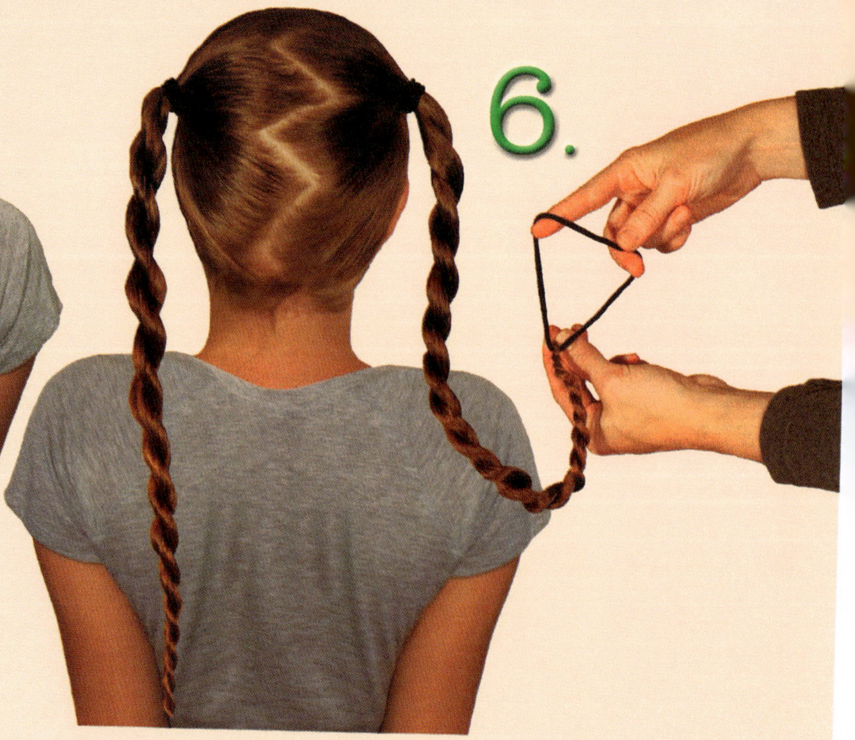

326   www.findingbraids.com

Basic Tails

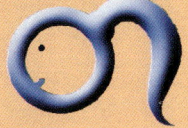

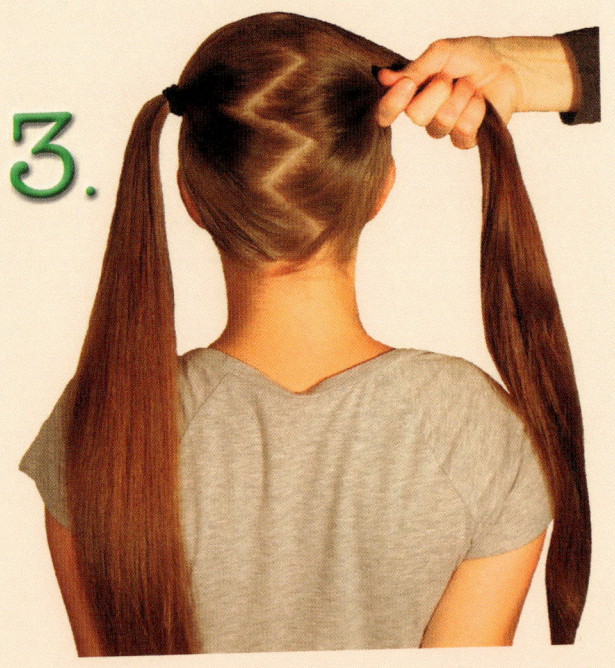

3.

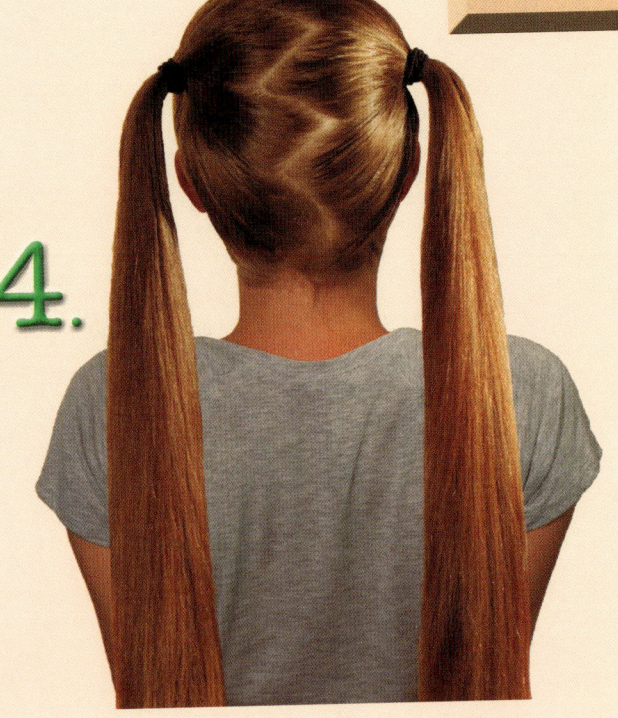

4.

Or, part the hair into a zig zag. Make pig tails using covered bands.

Choose the braid you will do. Choose the sweet style you will create with those two braids.

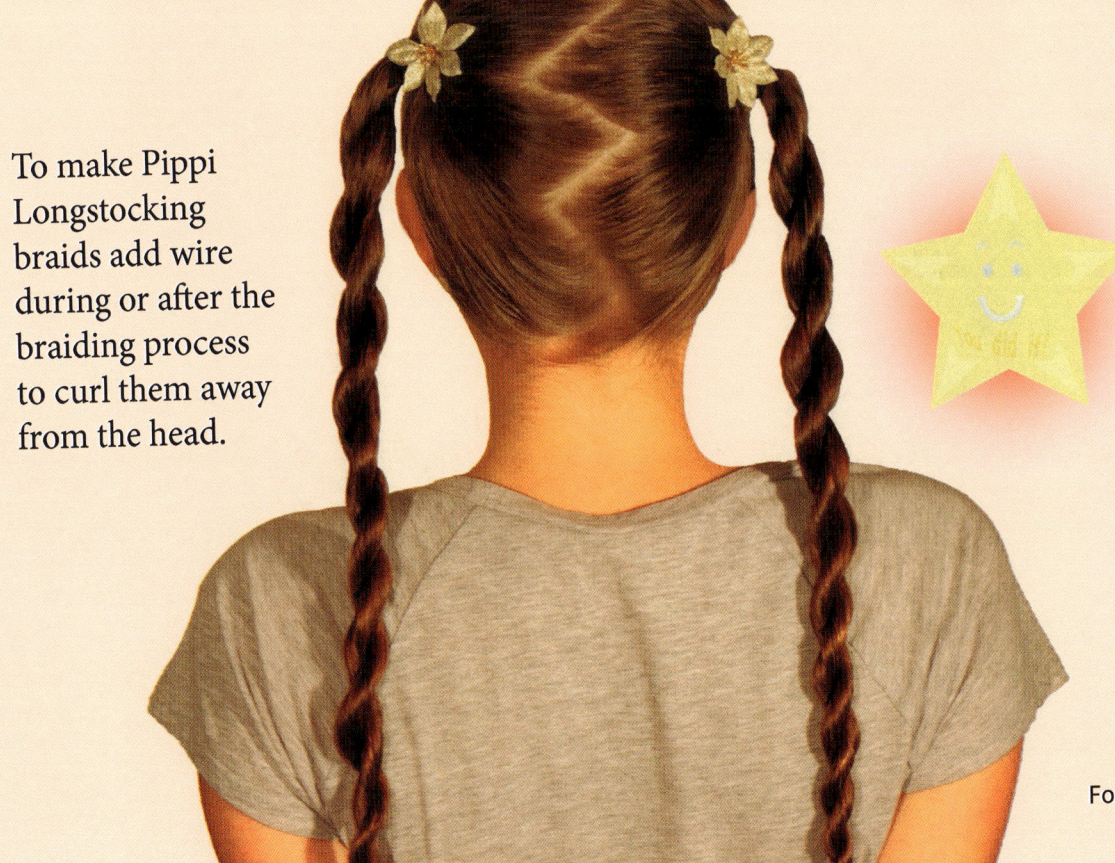

To make Pippi Longstocking braids add wire during or after the braiding process to curl them away from the head.

Forms 327

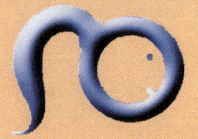

Accented Tails

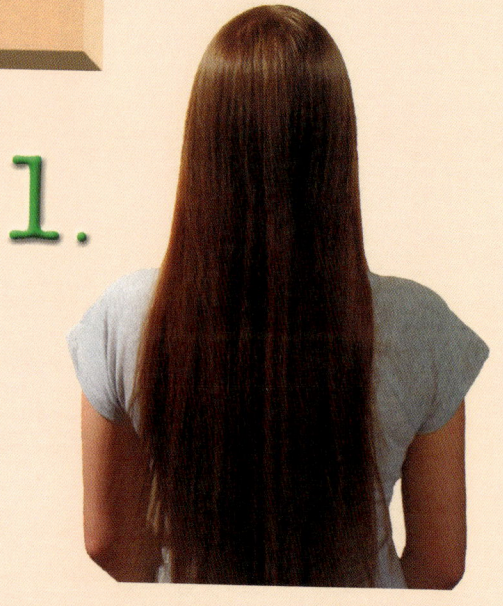

1.

Begin with clean, brushed hair.

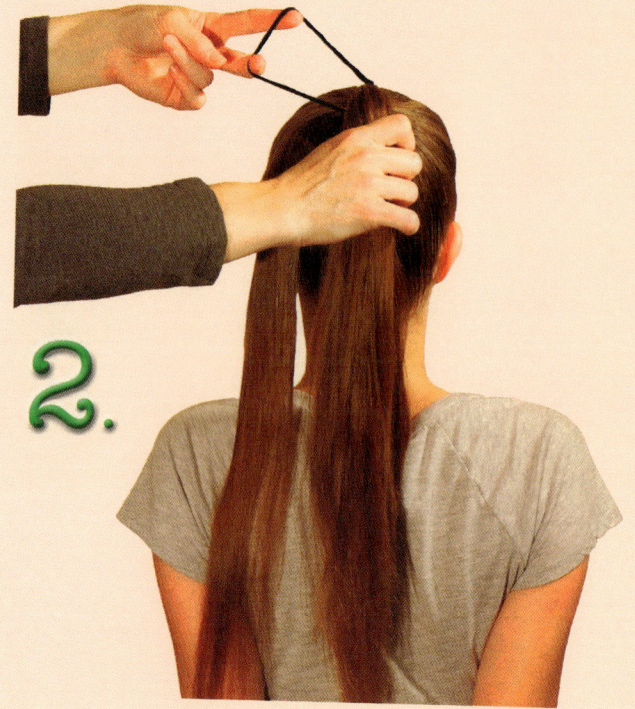

2.

The pony tail can be left plain and have an accent. Or, the pony tail can be braided and have an accent. Let's get fancy.

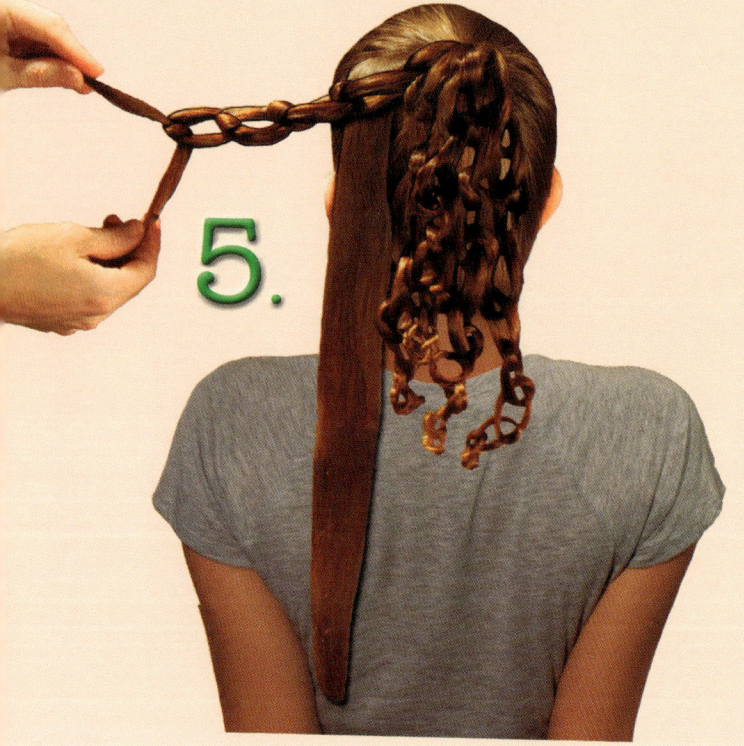

5.

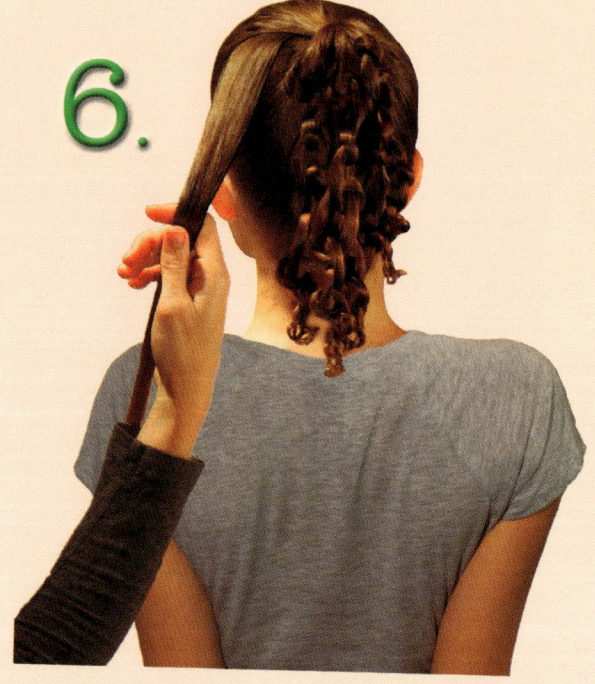

6.

Oh, the styles you can make. Of all the accents I could use to decorate this braid, I chose the loose accent. Latch hook it in a design of your making.

328 www.findingbraids.com

Accented Tails

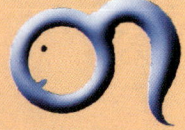

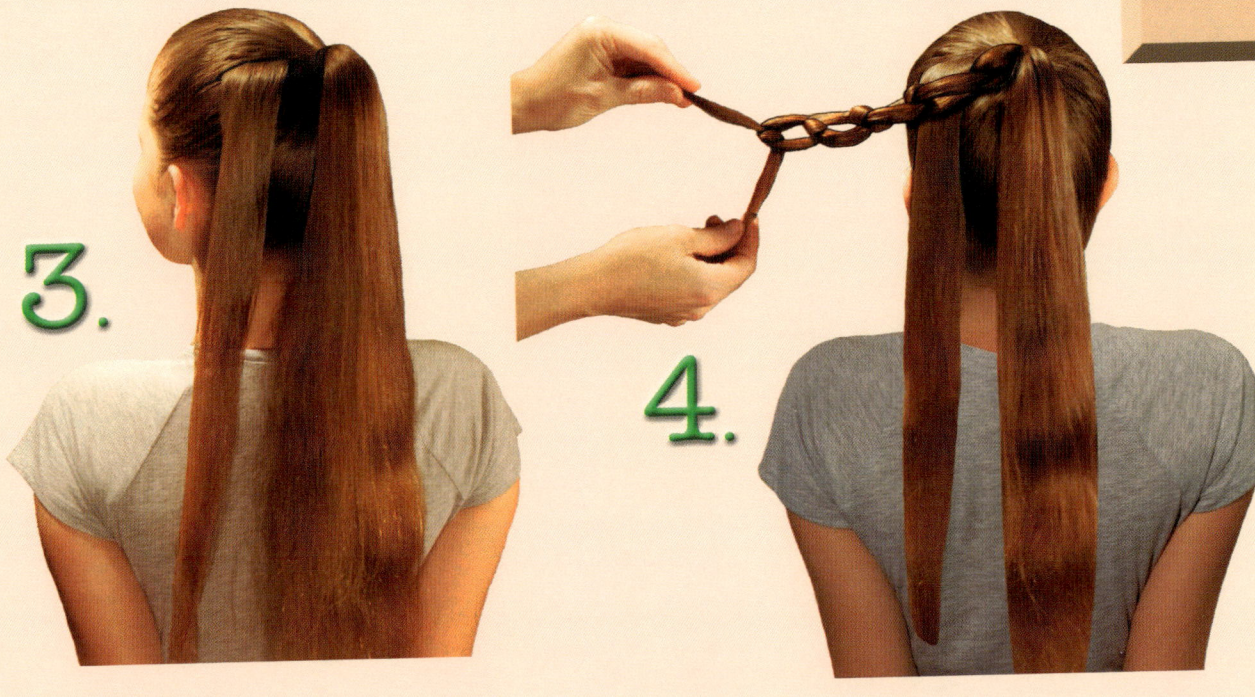

3. Choose the number of stands you will work with and create your style.

4. I am making lots of two-strand knot braids. Tie off the ends of the tails with small bands.

7.

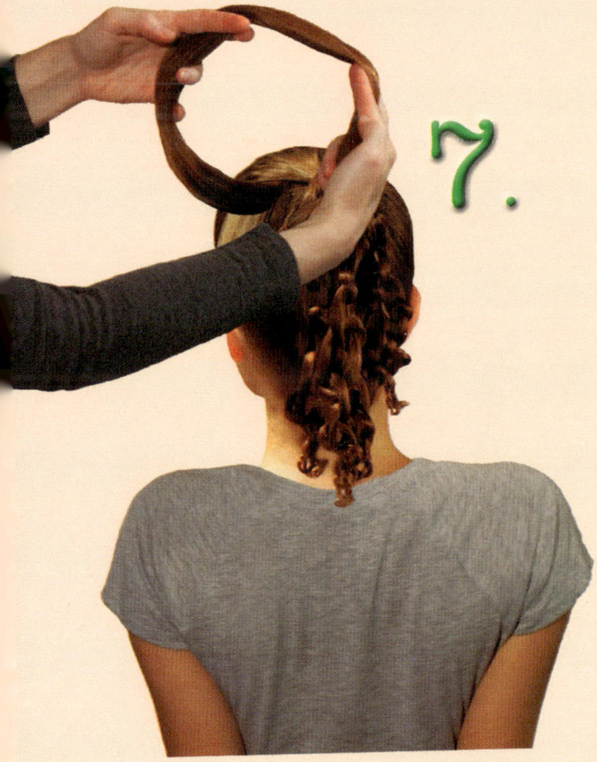

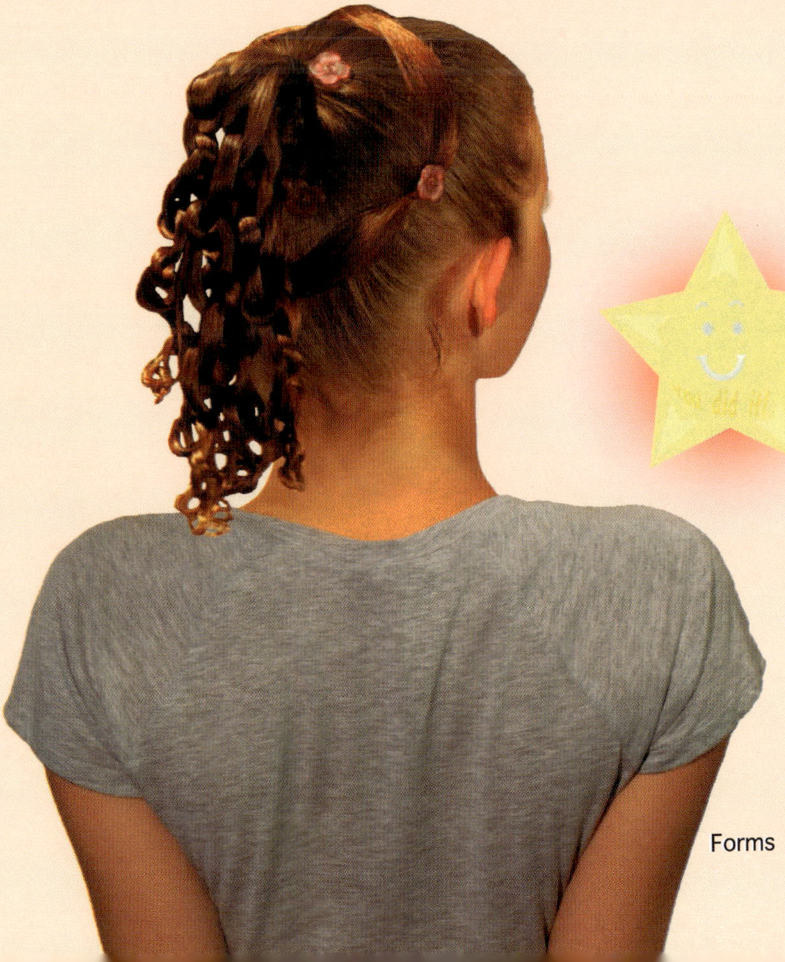

Forms 329

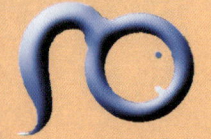

Tails Cascade

1.

Begin with clean, brushed hair.

2.

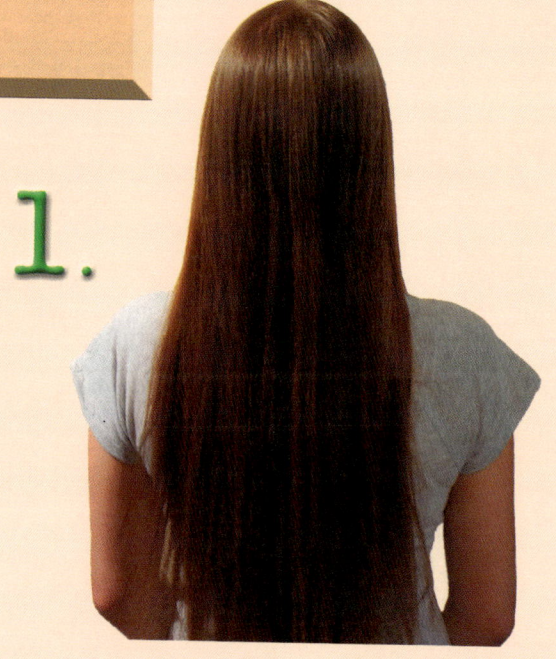

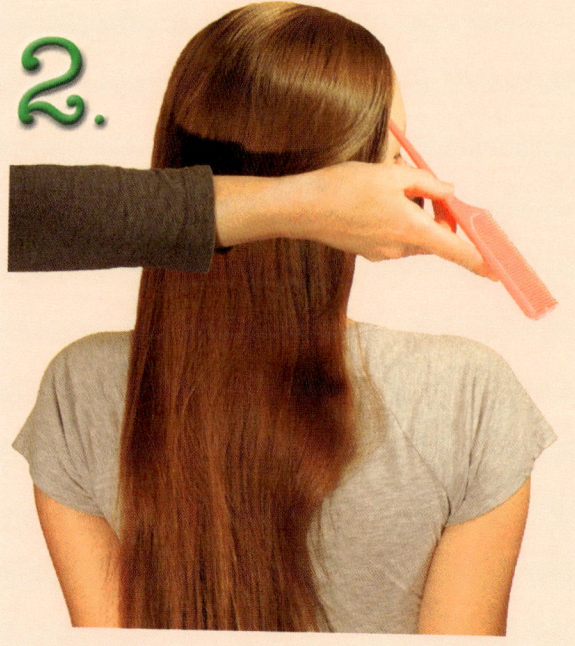

Cascades leave hair down to showcase the natural beautiy of your hair or to keep your neck warm. Choose the number of strands you will braid for this style.

5.

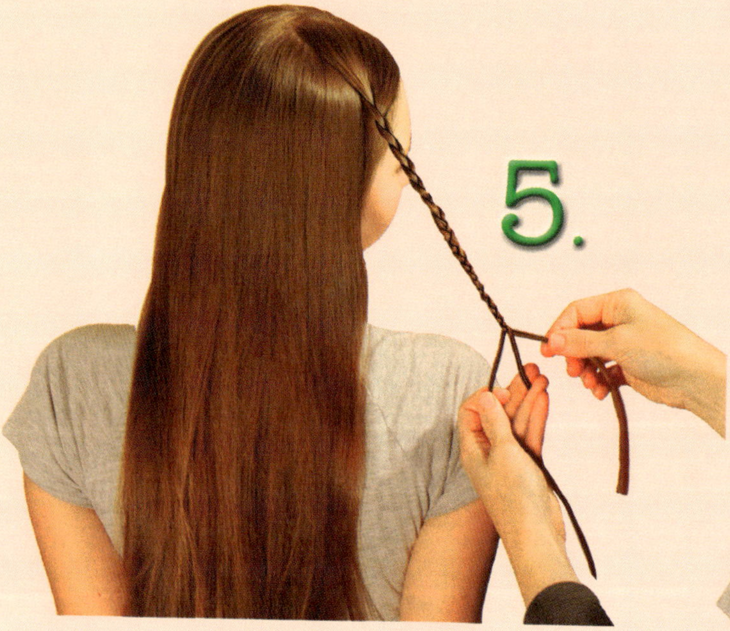

6.

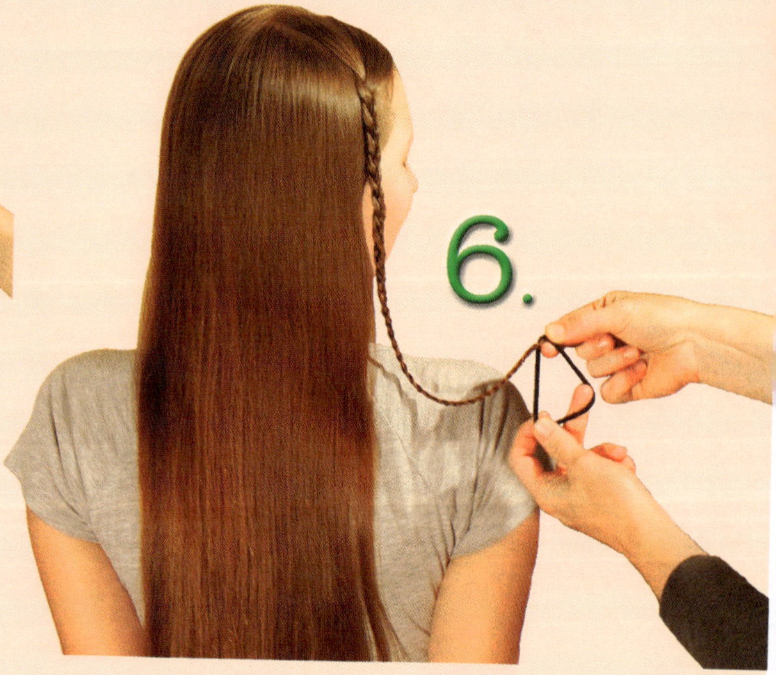

Secure with a rubber band.

www.findingbraids.com

Tails Cascade

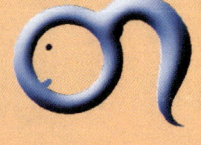

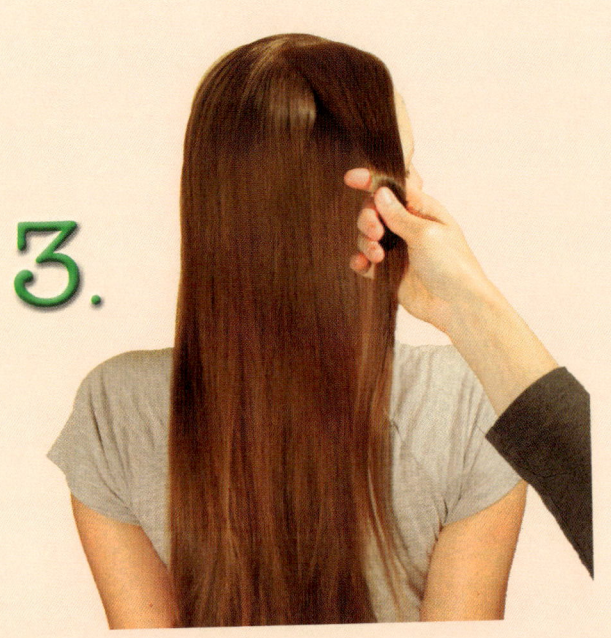

3.

Take a section of hair.

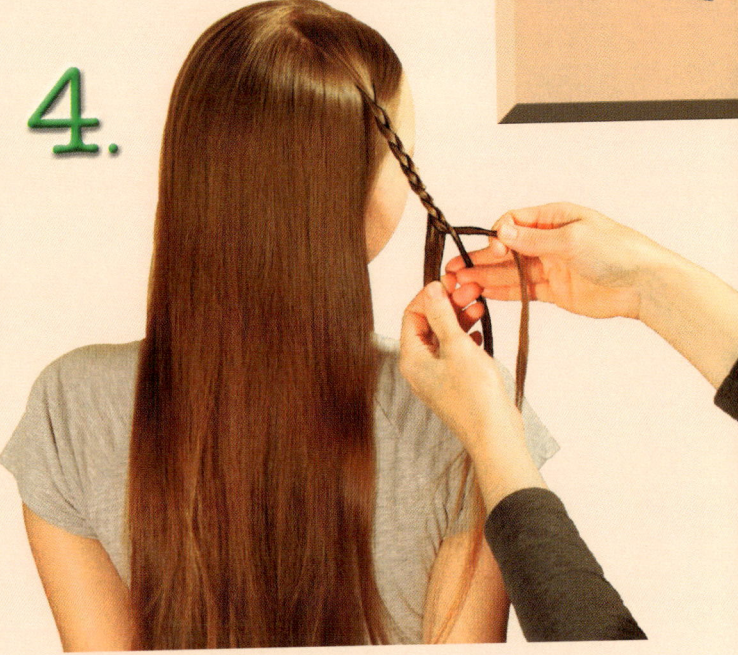

4.

Create your braid.

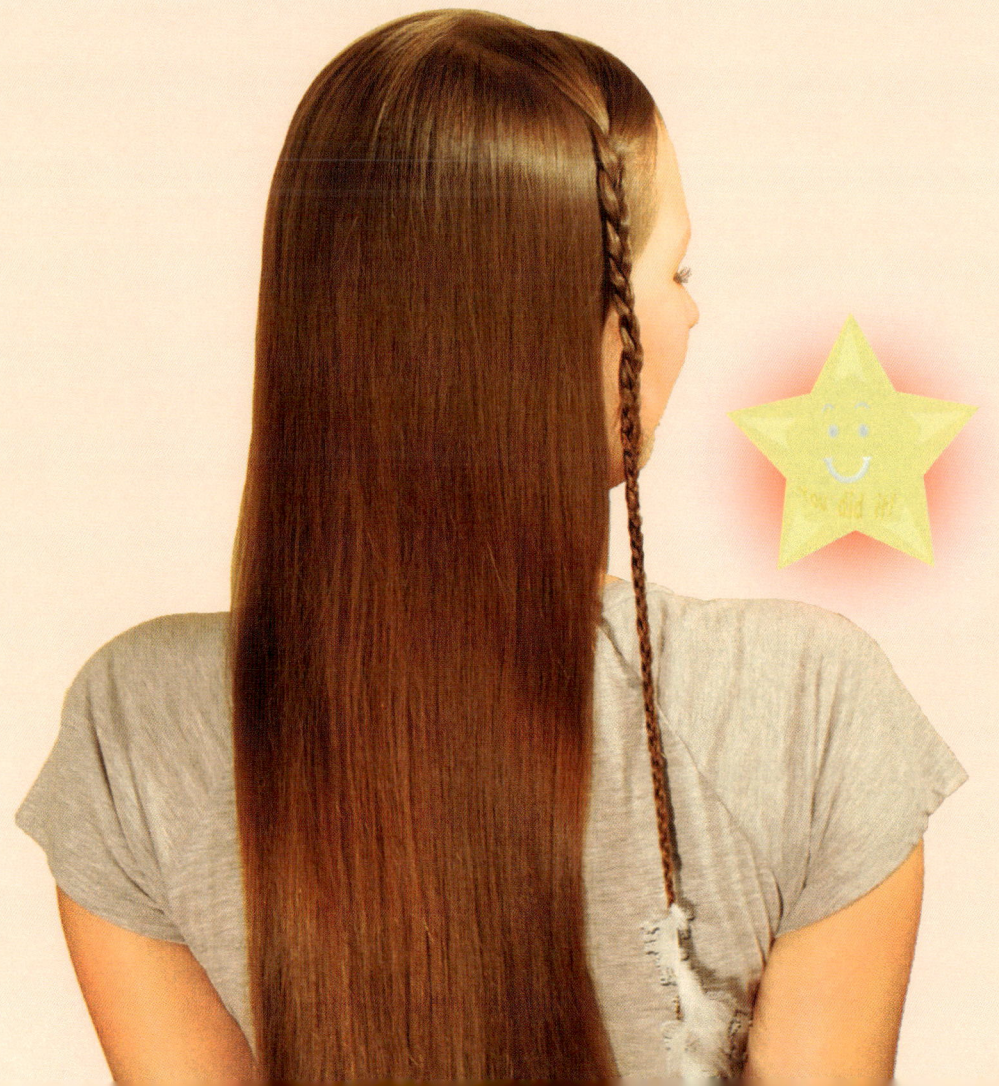

So many options. Use one braid or fifty, tiny braids or large bulk braids, repeat a braid or use a varied number of braids. Arrange the braids into the desired style. Use common styles or do something out of this world cool.

Accented Tails Cascade

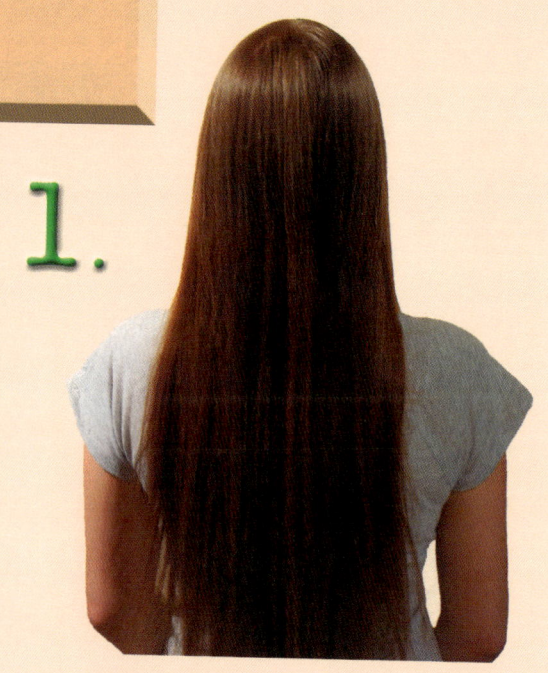

1. Begin with clean, brushed hair.

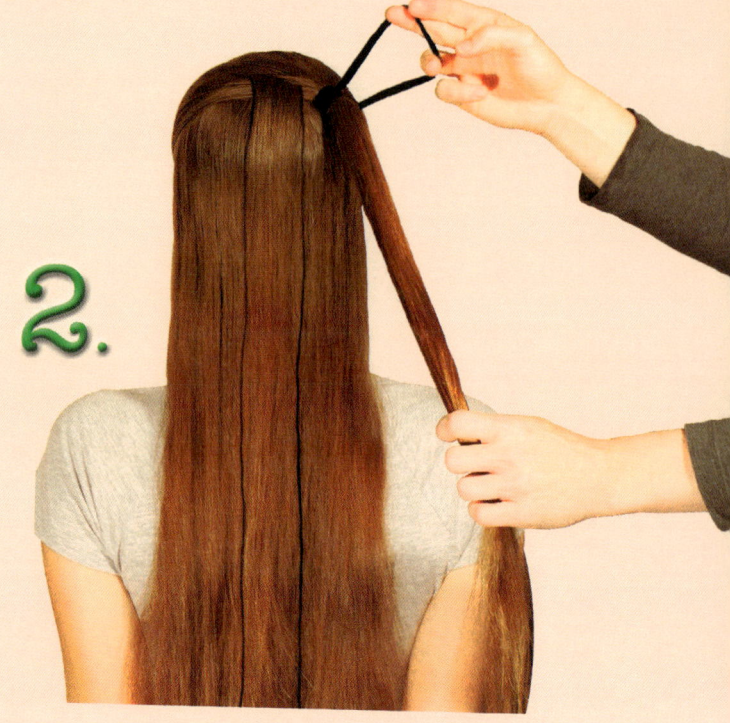

2. Create the desired pony tail placement. Leave out a strand of hair for an accent. This style is cascaded so leave hair down.

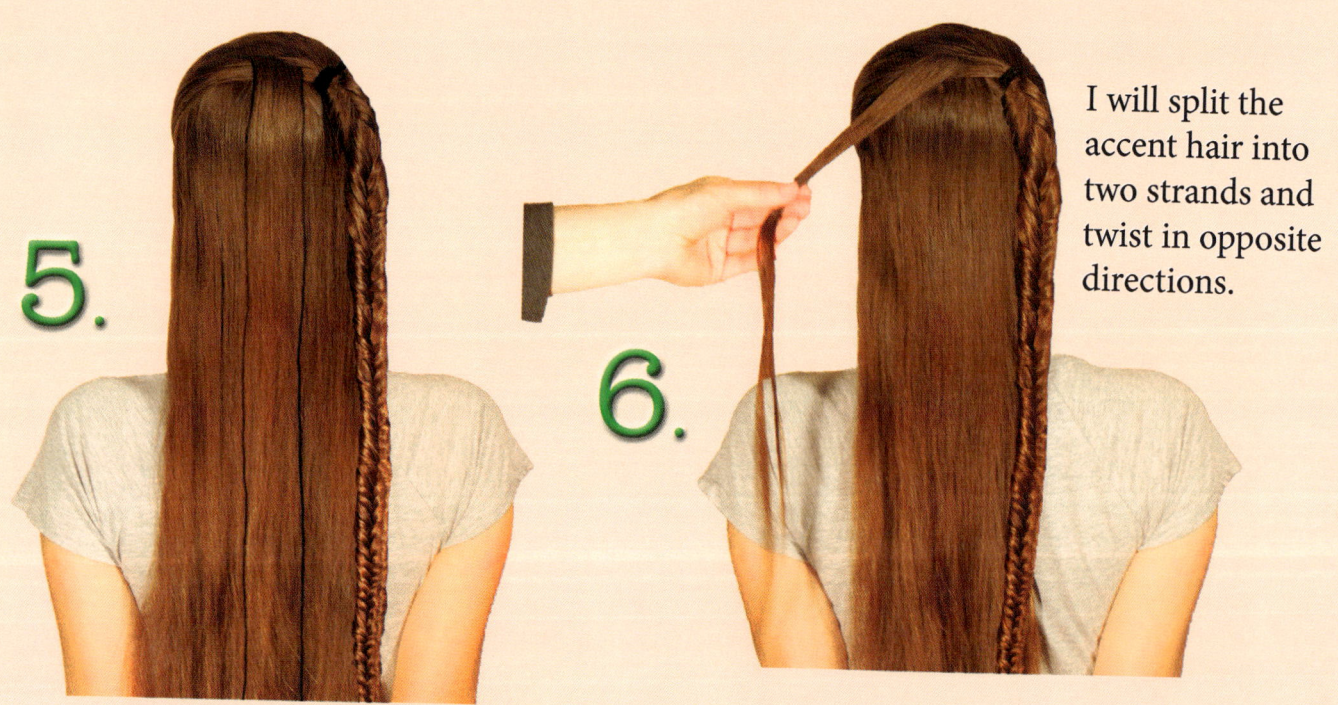

5.

6. I will split the accent hair into two strands and twist in opposite directions.

Choose an accent you will work with and finish the hairstyle.

Accented Tails Cascade

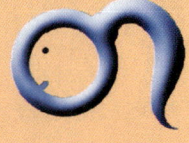

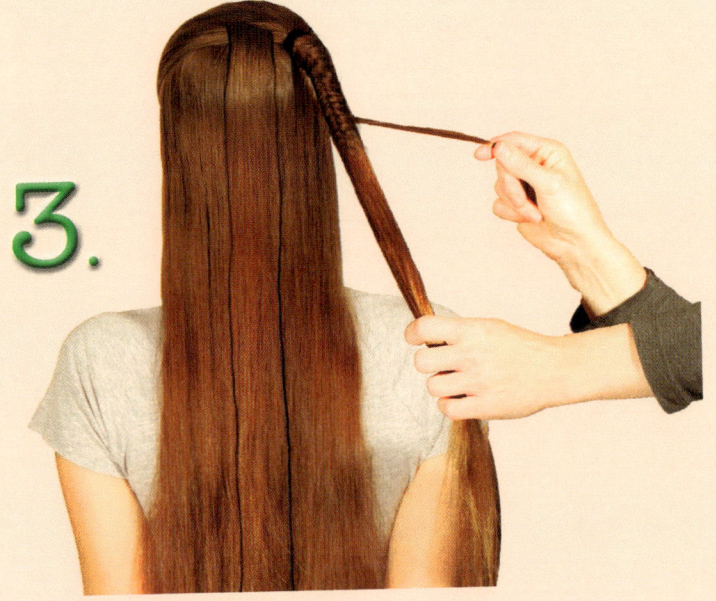

3.

Choose the number of strands you will work with and create a braid.

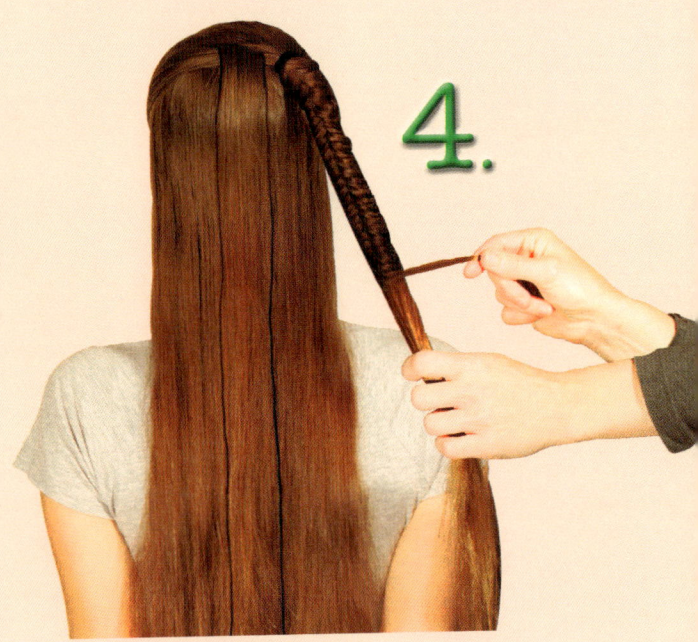

4.

Have your client hold one of the strands while you twist the other.

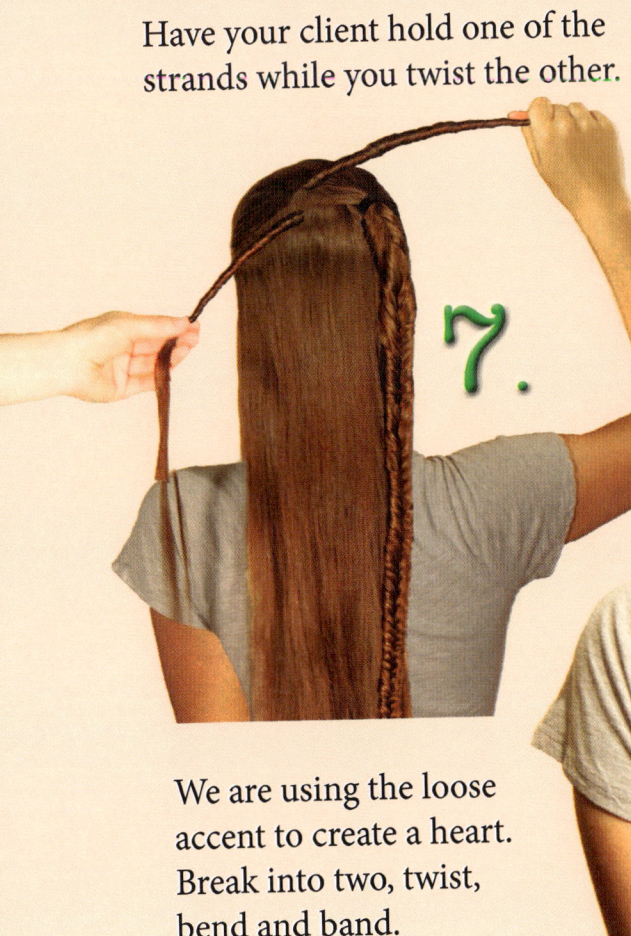

7.

We are using the loose accent to create a heart. Break into two, twist, bend and band.

Forms   333

Forms

Notes

Examples of Tails

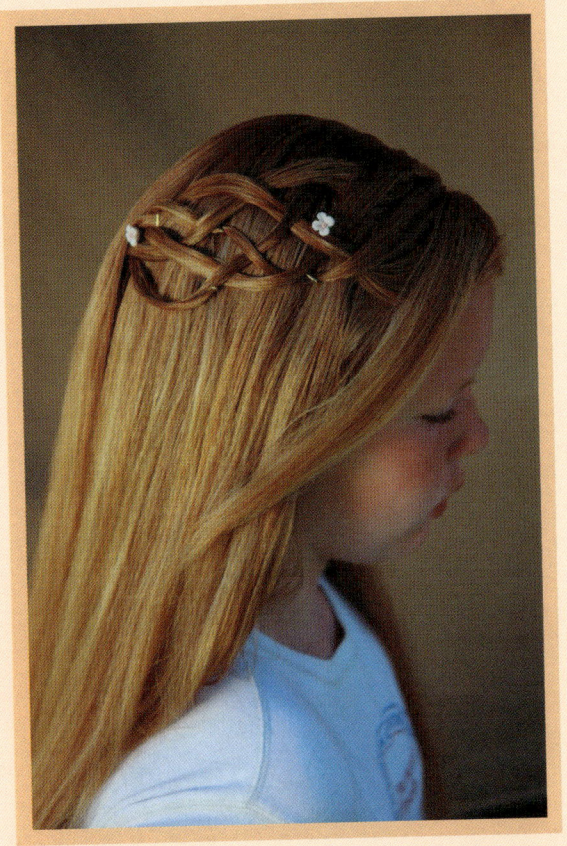
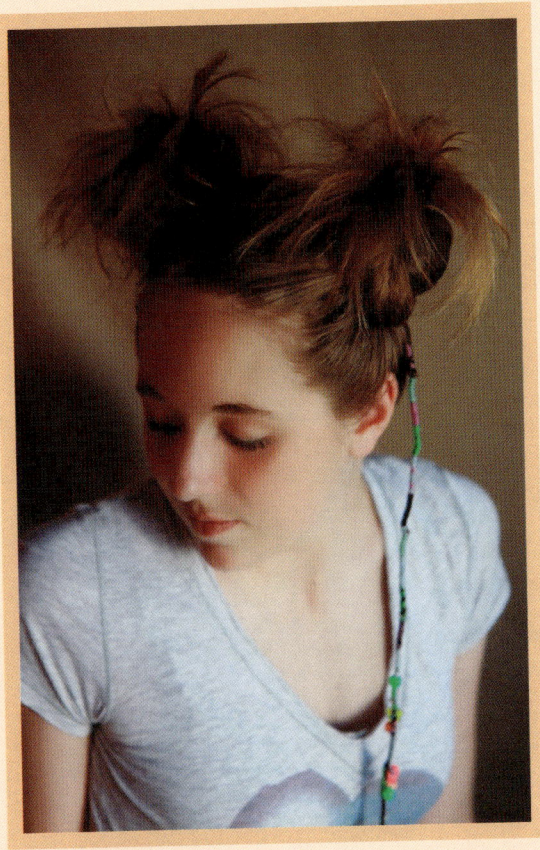
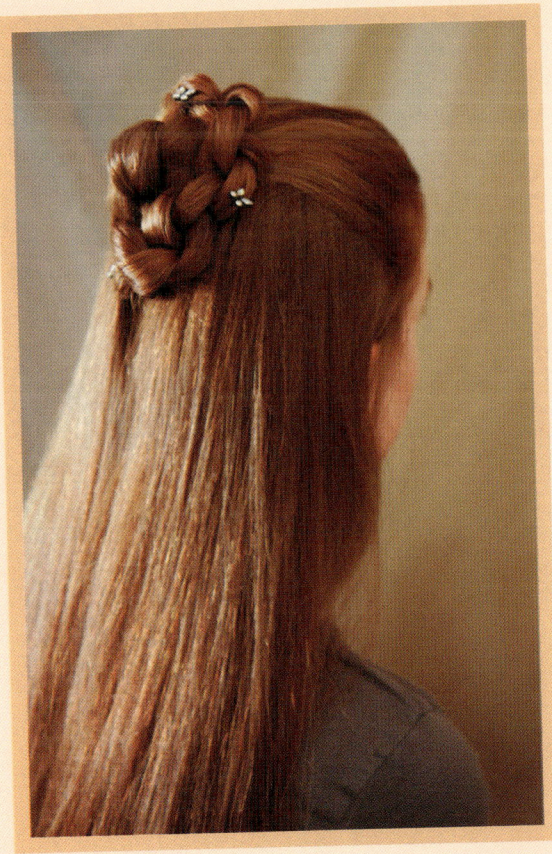
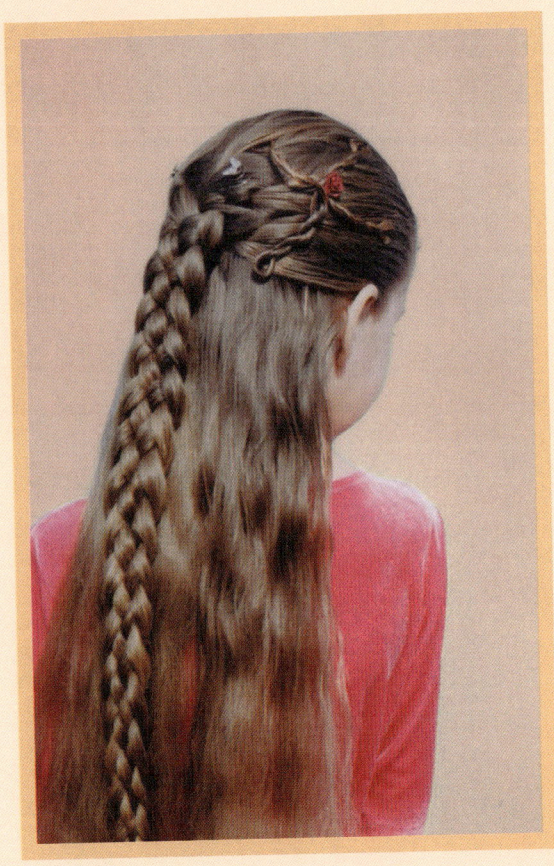

Visit my website to see more examples of Tails

Forms

HEADBAND

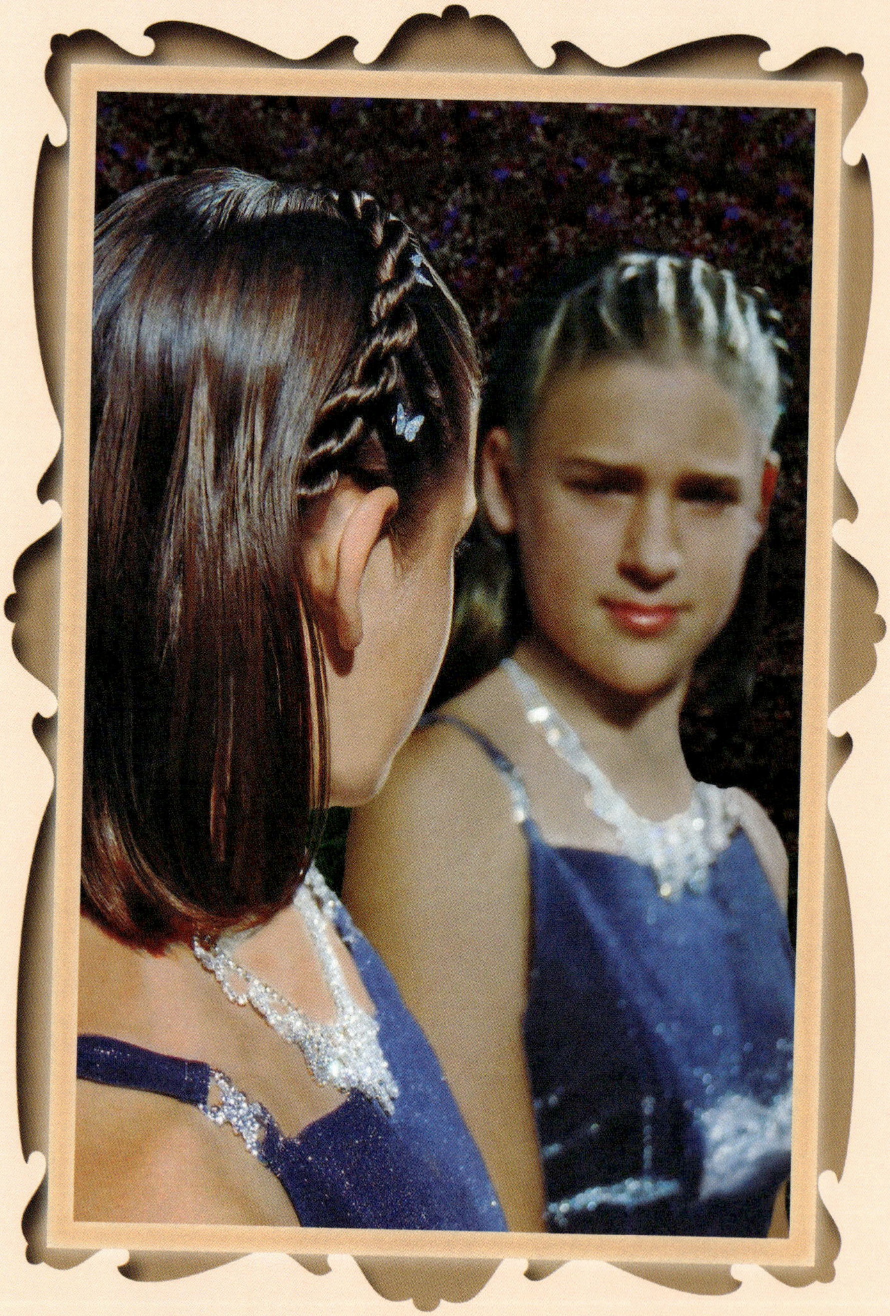

The headband form is a practical and beautiful way to showcase almost any braid. What a great hairstyle for keeping your hair out of your face.

Forms

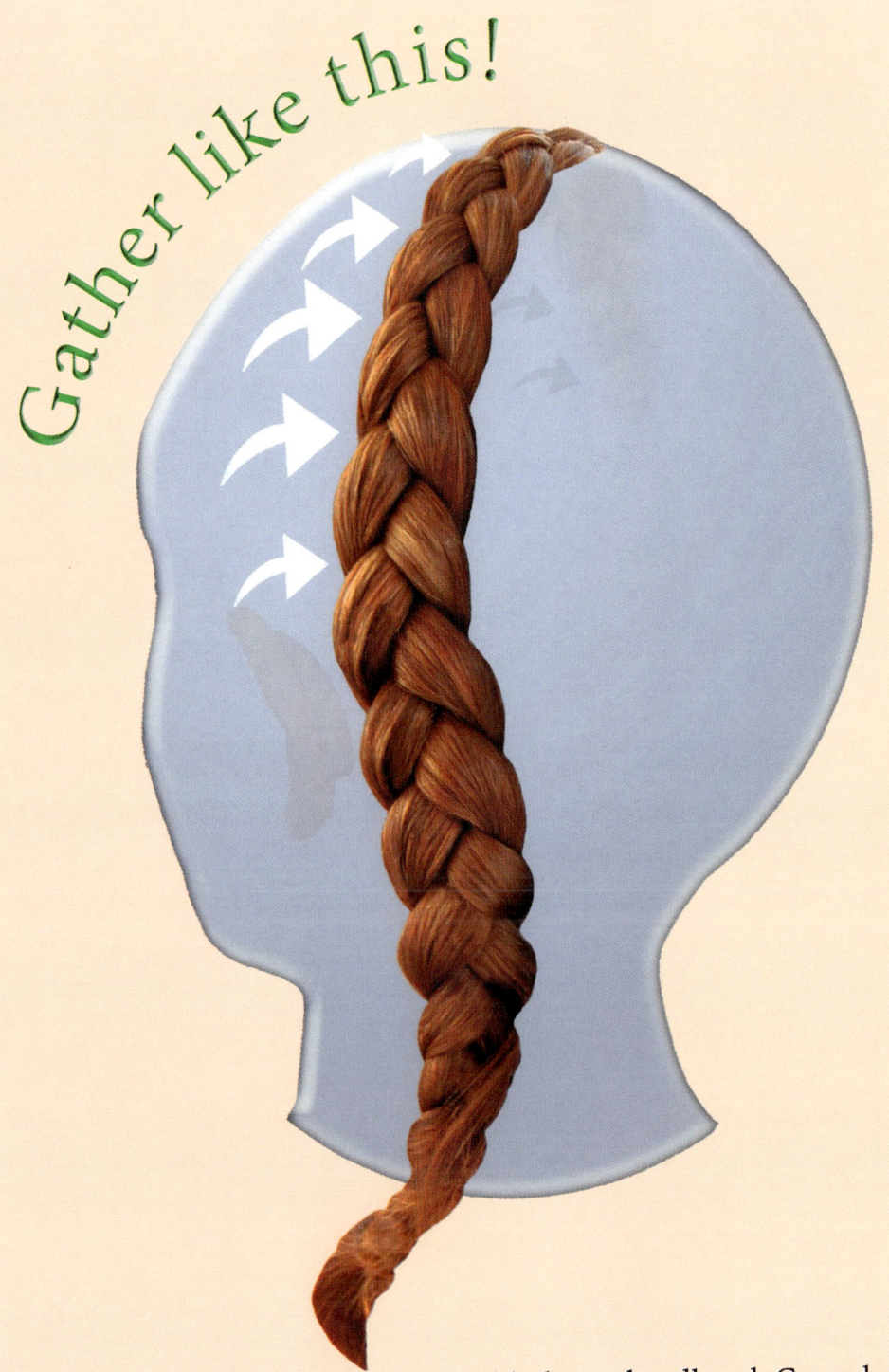

Gather like this!

Braiding icon for the next eight pages.

Headbands sit exactly where you would place a headband. Cascade headbands are the most enchanting when lace braided. Braid from ear to ear.

The **Headband** Form

Basic Headband

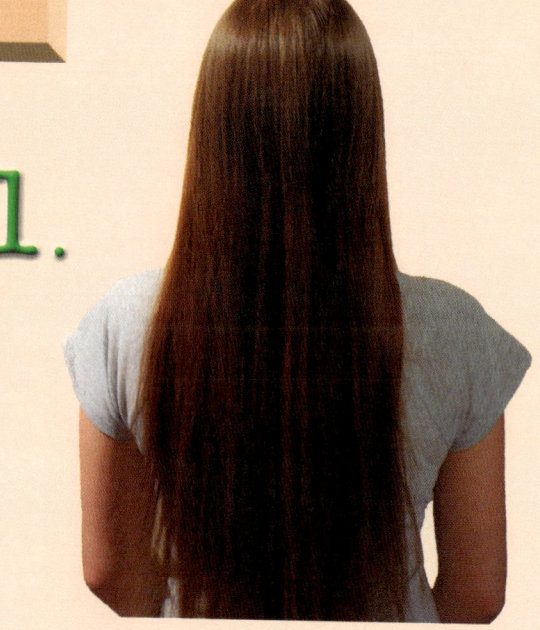

1.

Begin with clean, brushed hair.

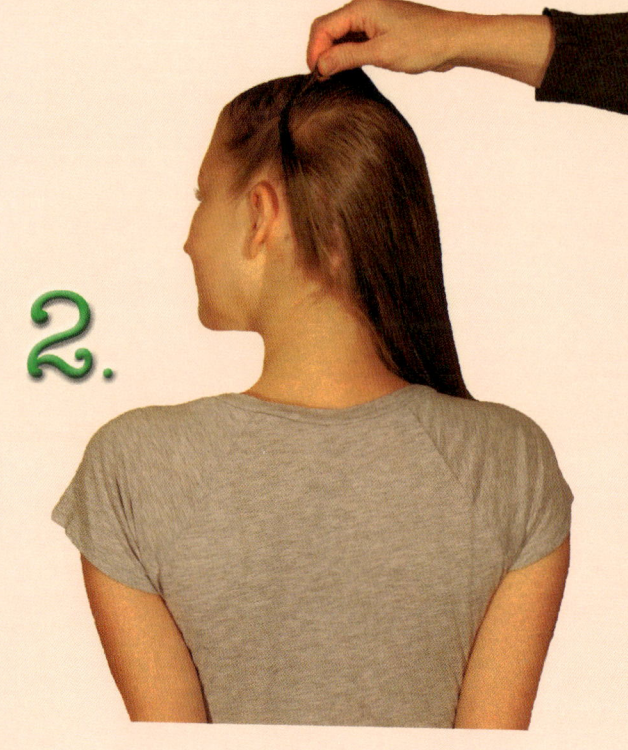

2.

Take the first section from around the ear.

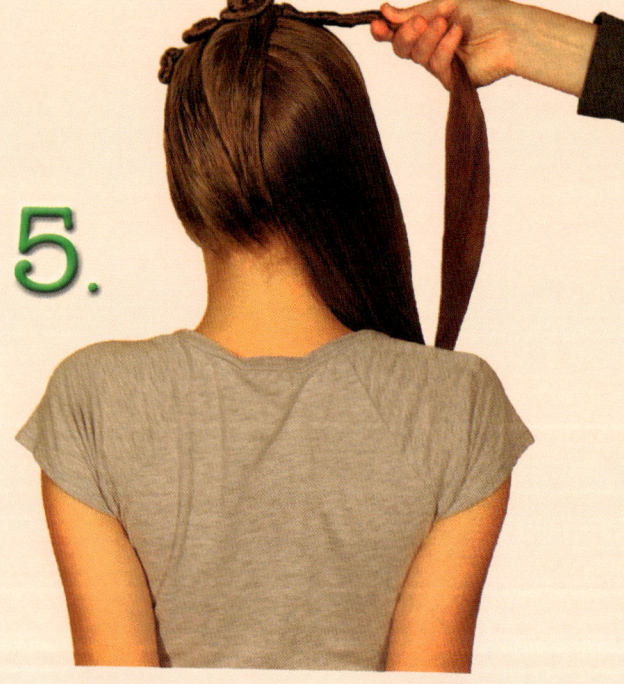

5.

This is a one-strand rosette.

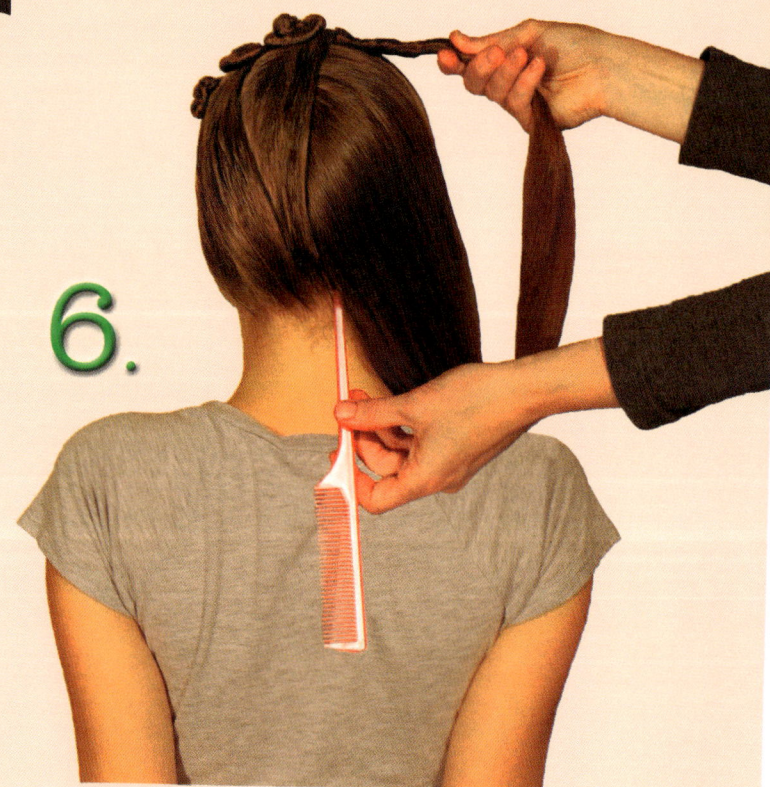

6.

Basic Headband

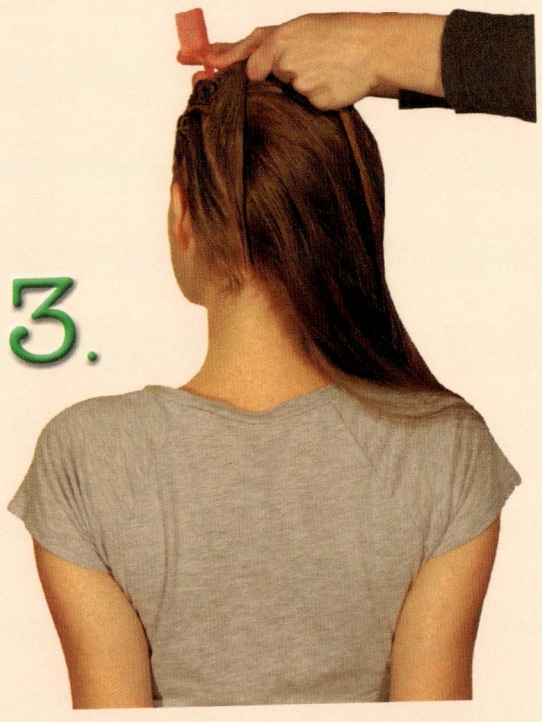

3.

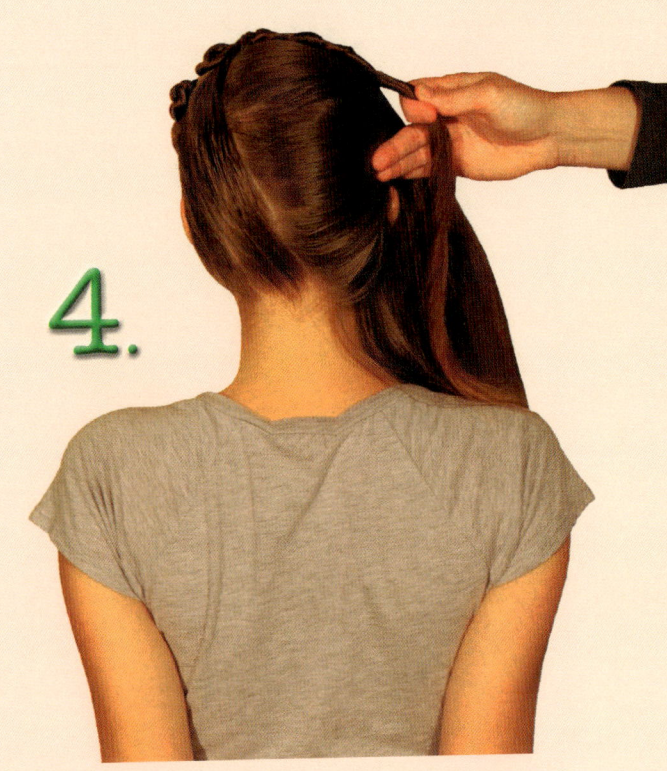

4.

Choose the number of strands you will braid with. Gather into both sides while working your way across the head to the other ear.

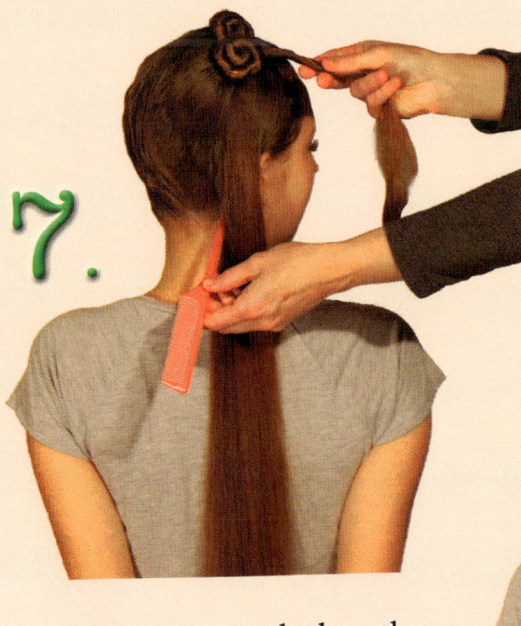

7.

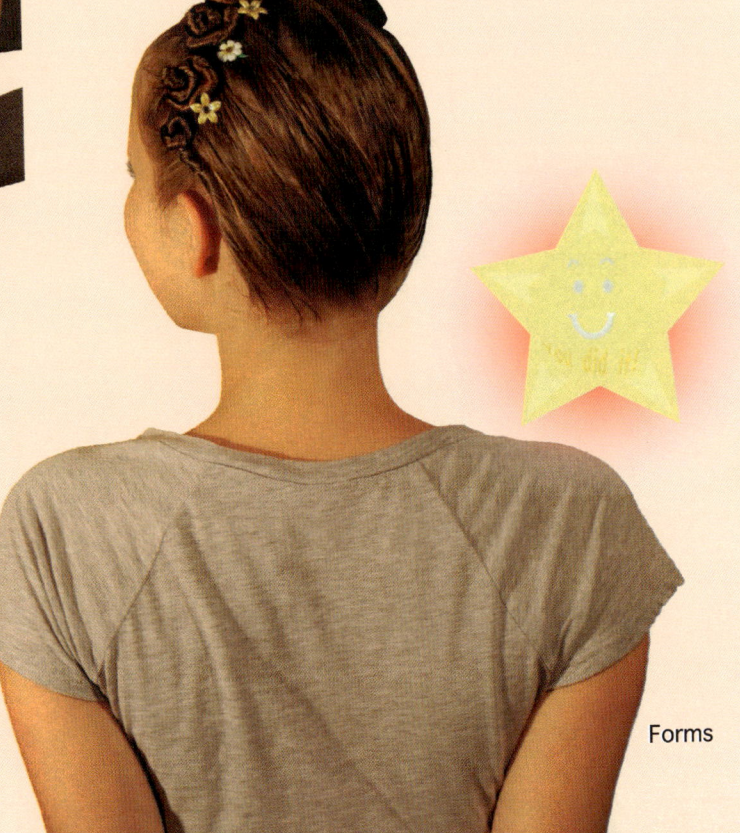

When you reach the other ear, decide if you will bun the tail, leave it down or wrap it around the back of the head to the other ear.

Accented Headband

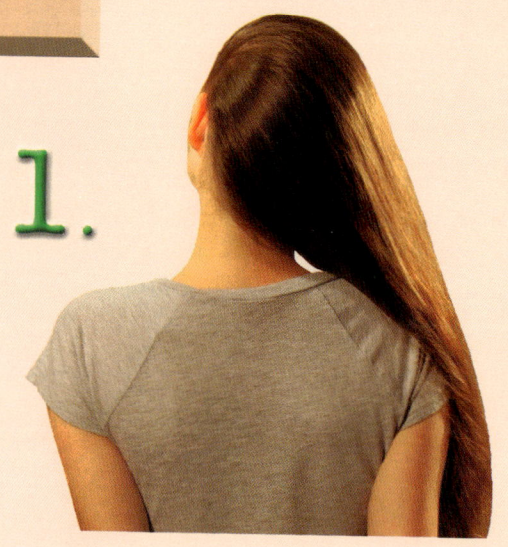

1. Brush the hair in the direction you will be braiding this form. Choose a number of strands you will be working with.

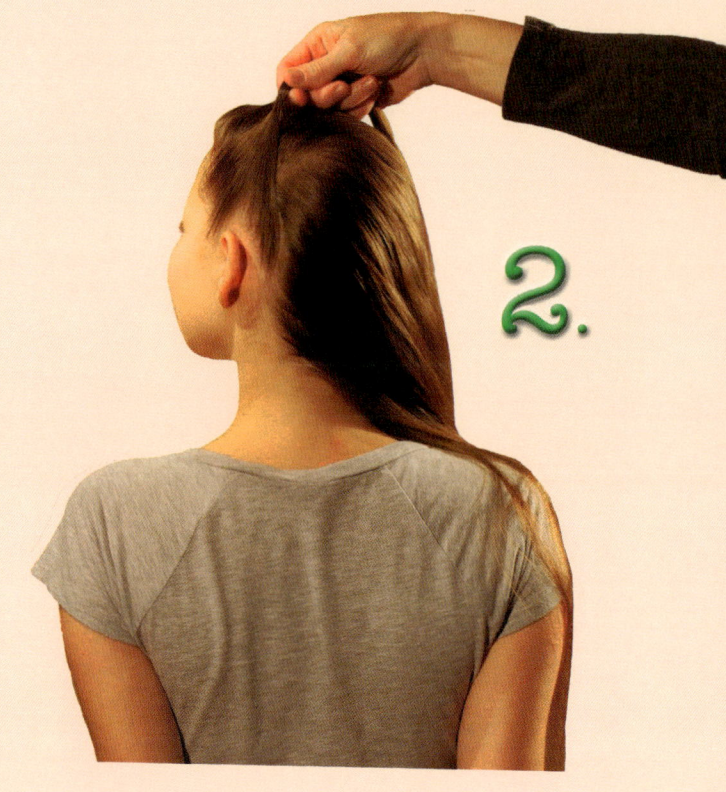

2. Take the first section from around the ear.

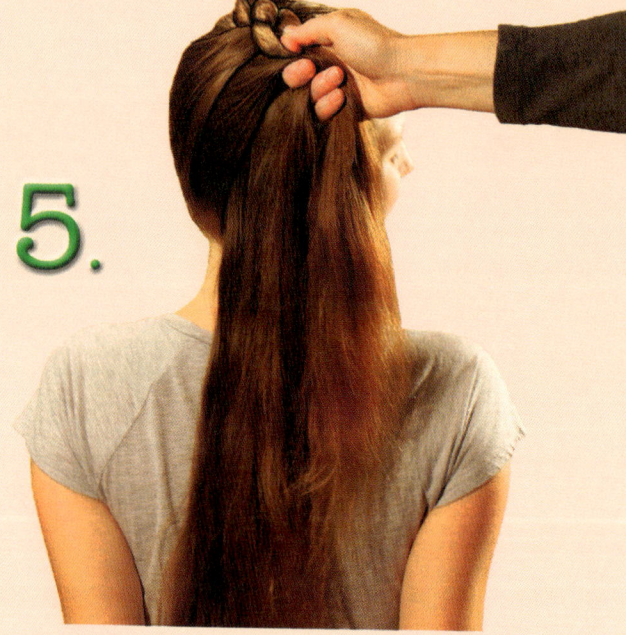

5. When you reach the other ear, decide if you will bun the tail, leave it down or wrap it around the back of the head to the other ear and the begining of the braid.

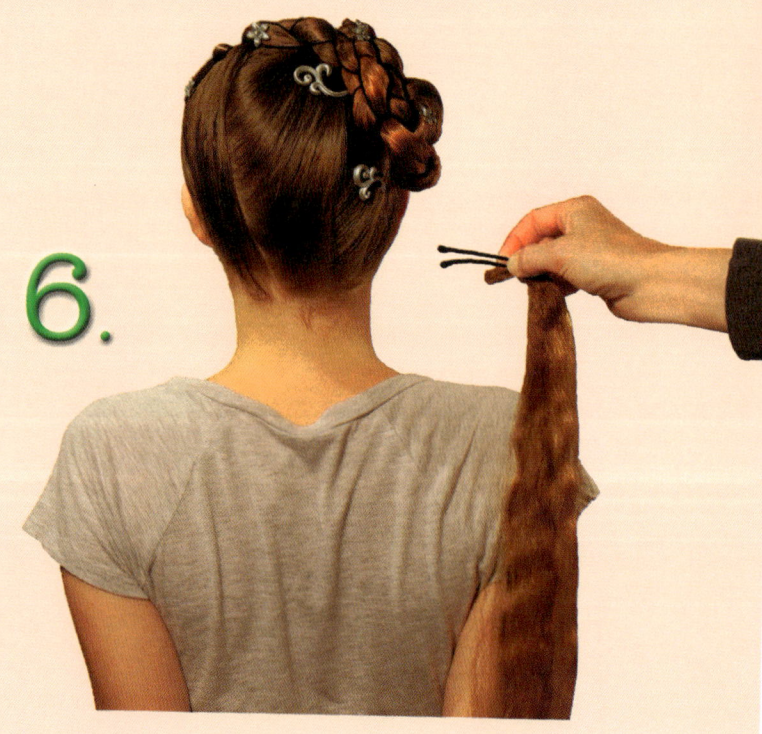

6.

340 www.findingbraids.com

Accented Headband

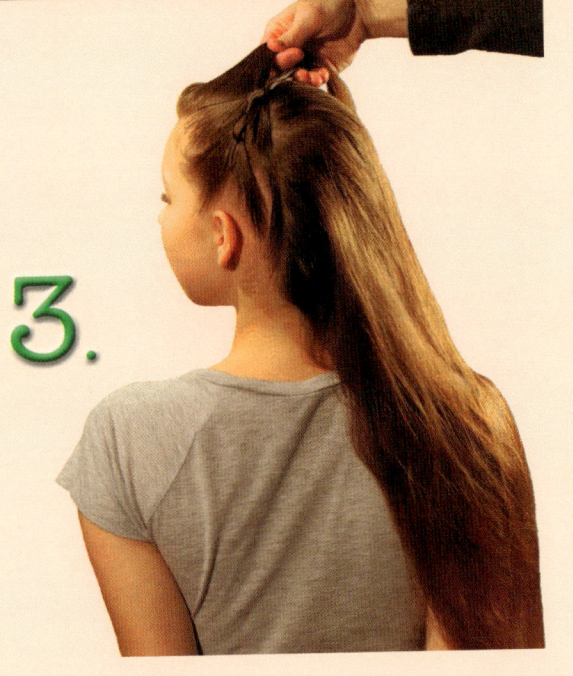

3. Gather into both sides while working your way across the head to the other ear.

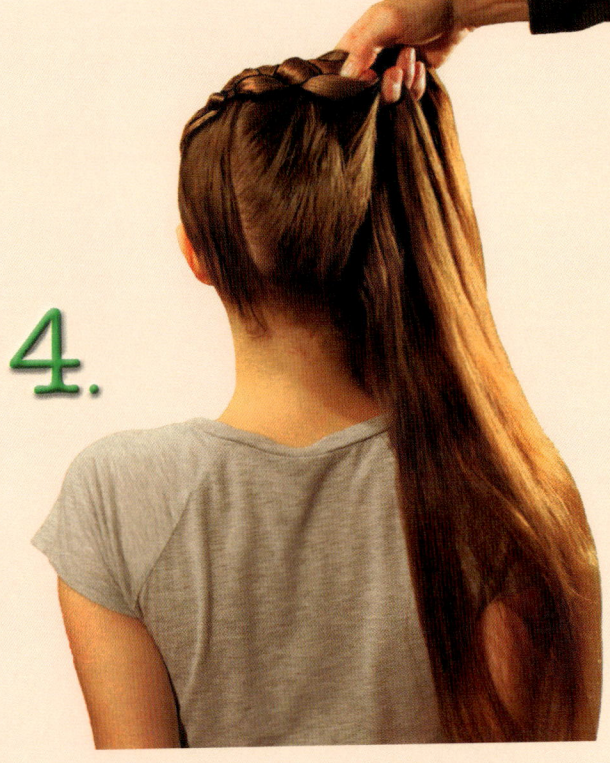

4. This is a two-strand knot.

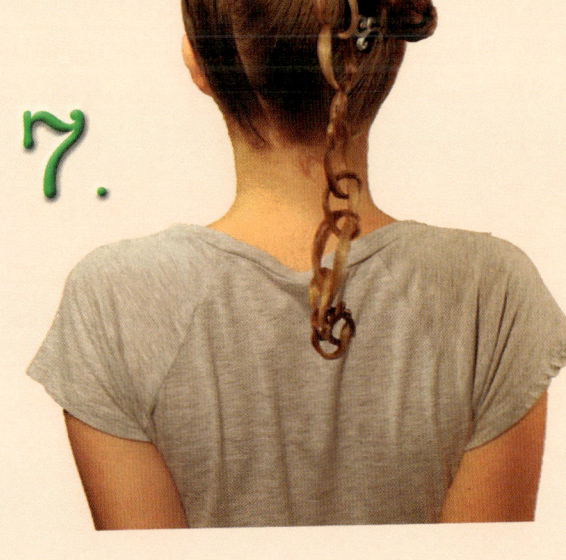

7. Add fake hair with a bobby pin. It can be natural colored hair or neon. Choose an accent and execute it. This is a two-strand knot braid made of fake hair.

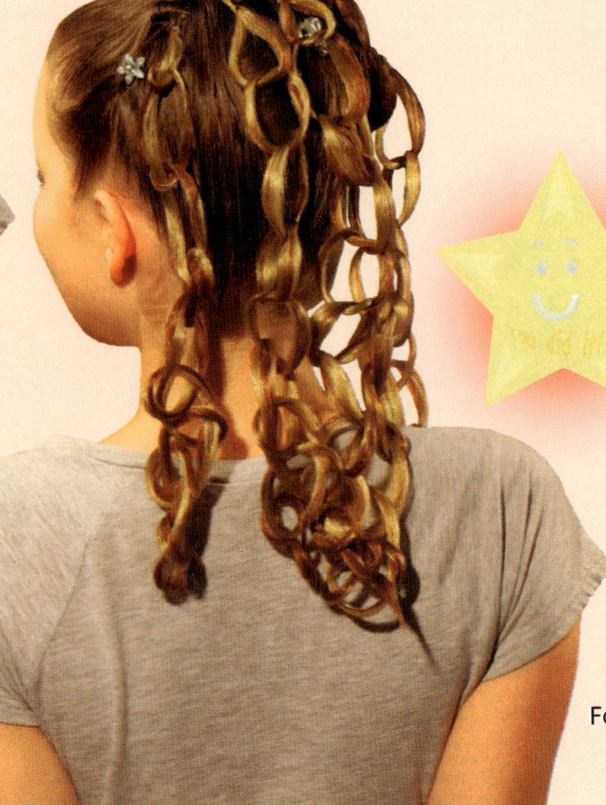

Forms 341

Headband Cascade

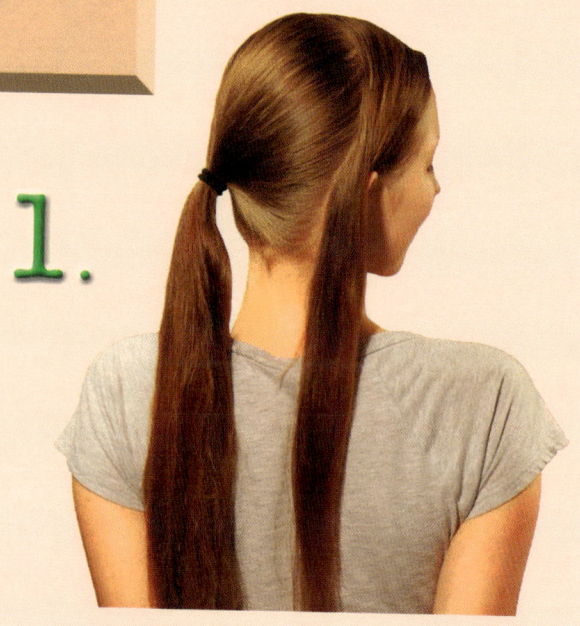

1.

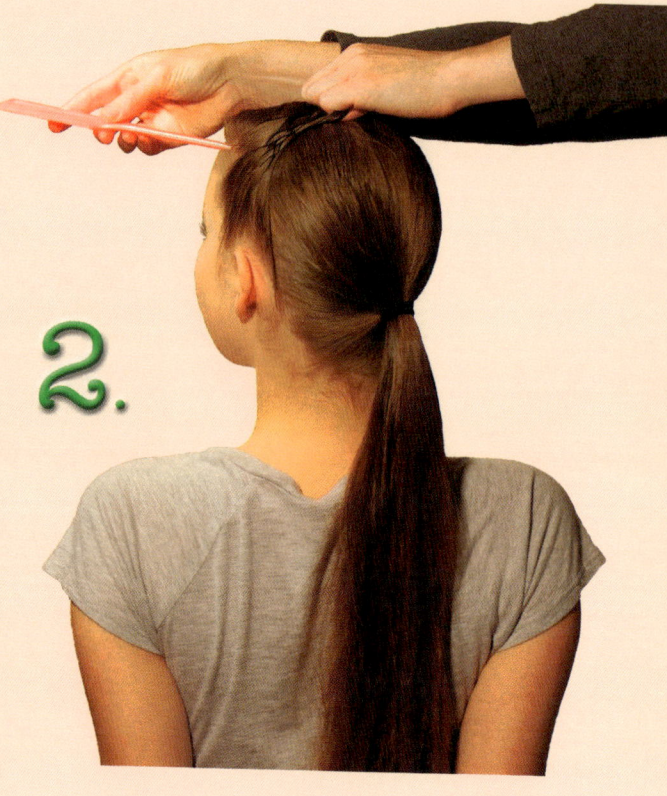

2.

This is a cascade form and the cascade is sectioned off immediately and set aside. Comb the loose hair that will be braided in the direction you will be braiding it.

Take the first section from around the ear.

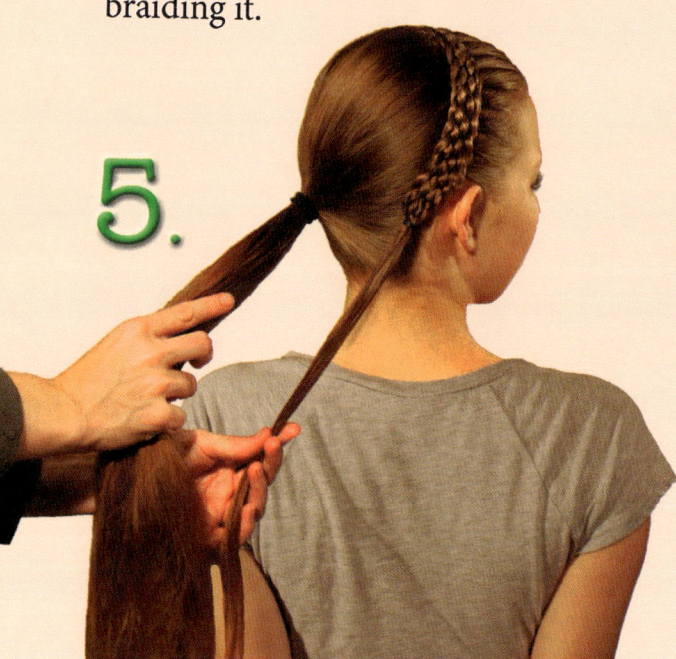

5.

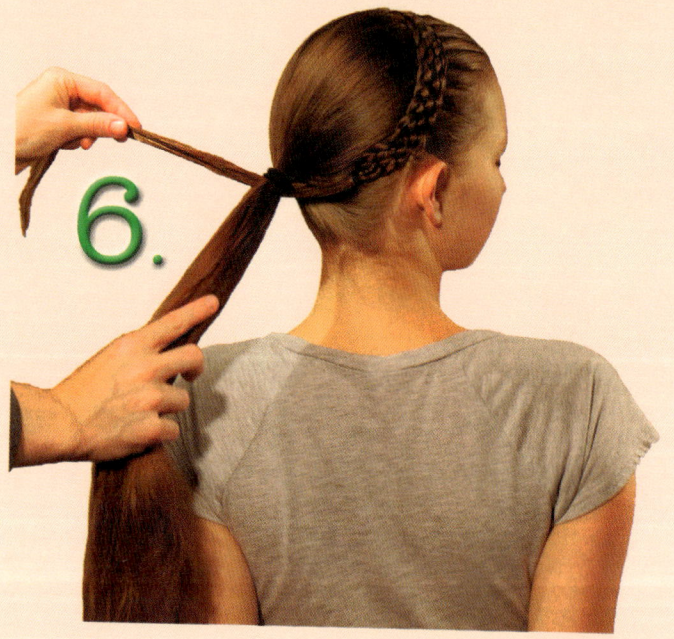

6.

Use the tail of the headband to cover the band when the cascade is left in a pony tail.

Headband Cascade

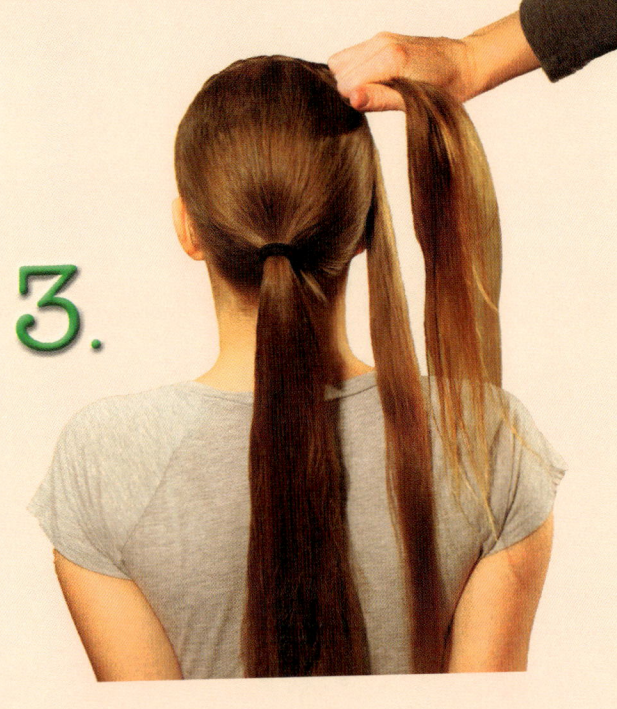

3. Choose the number of strands to braid with. Lace this braid while working your way across the head to the other ear. This is seven stands.

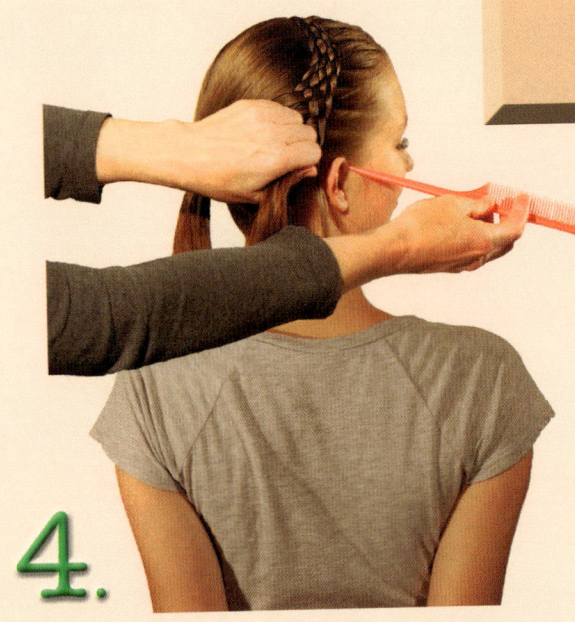

4. When you reach the other ear, decide if you will bun the tail, leave it down or wrap it around the back of the head to the other ear and the begining of the braid.

7. After the tail is wrapped completely around the band use a bobby pin to keep it bound in place.

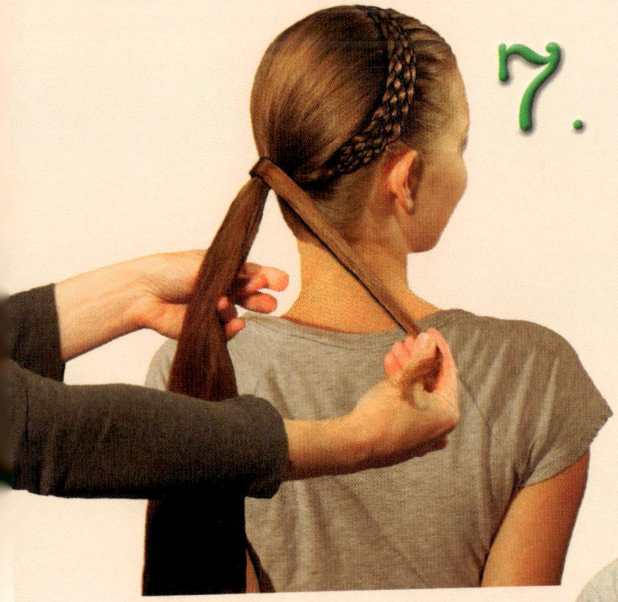

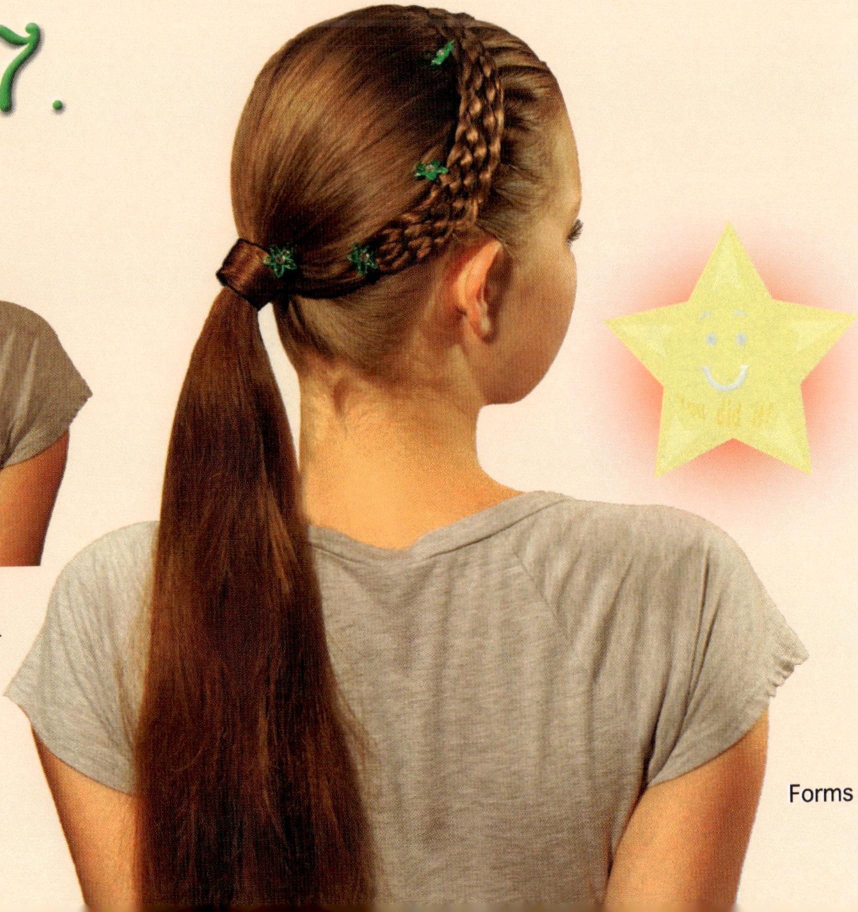

Forms 343

Accented Headband Cascade

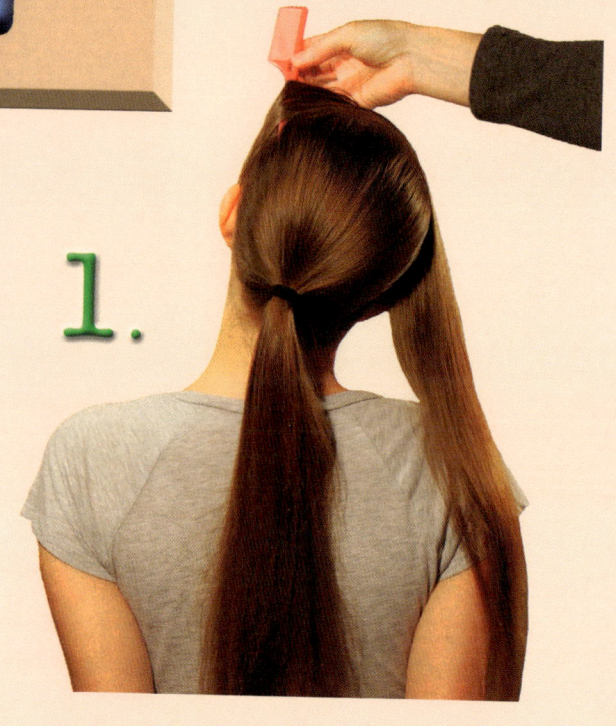

Take the first section near the ear.

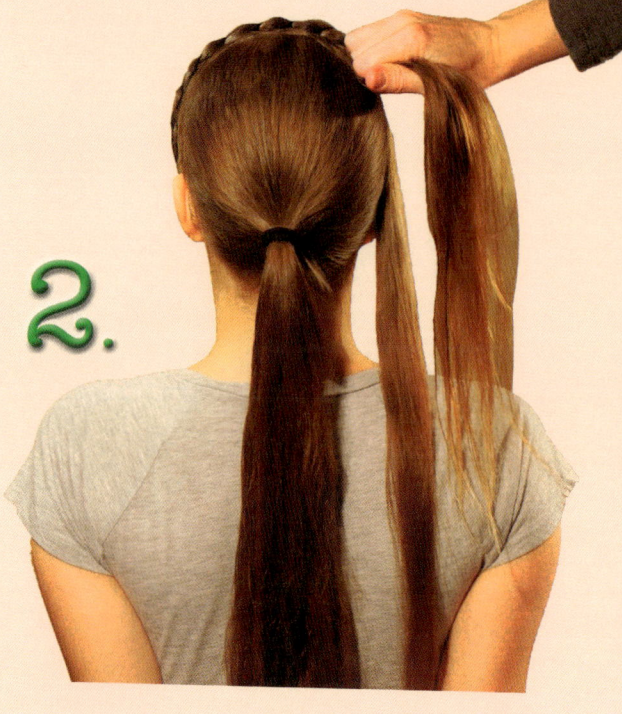

Choose the number of strands to braid with. Lace this braid while working your way across the head to the other ear. This is five stands.

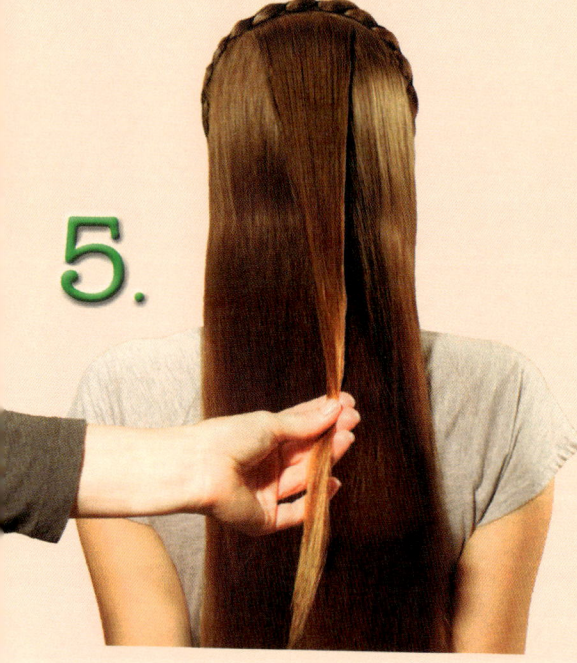

The accent we are using here is the headdress. Please try this style with all the other accents to see how beautiful it is. Do not limit yourself.

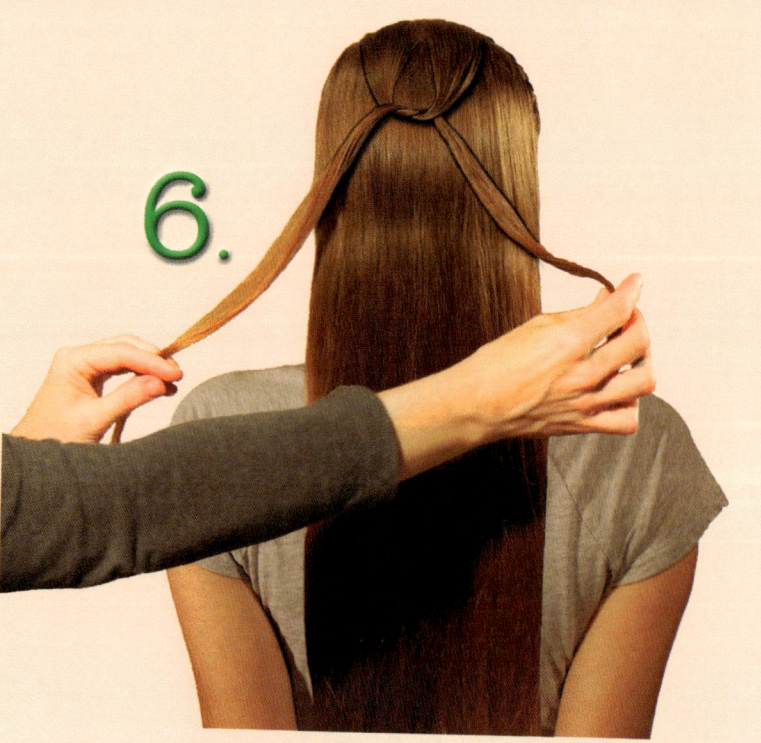

www.findingbraids.com

Accented Headband Cascade

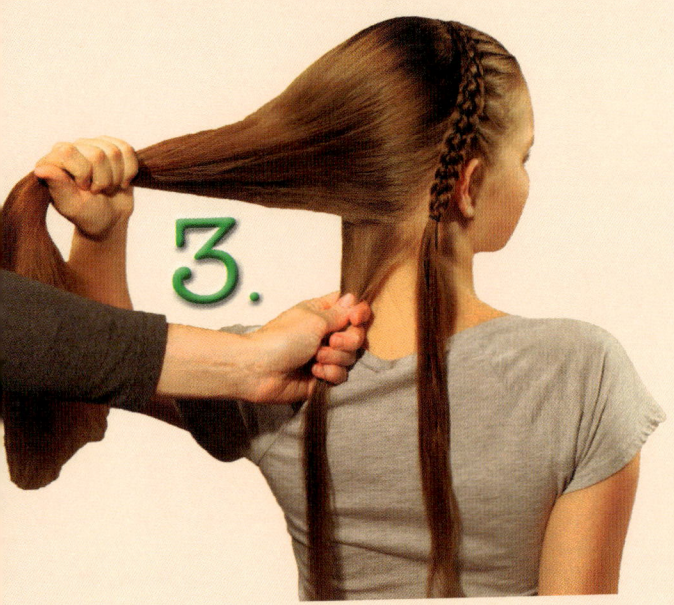

3. Finish your headband behind the ear. To hide the tail of the headband take a section of hair from underneath the remaining cascade.

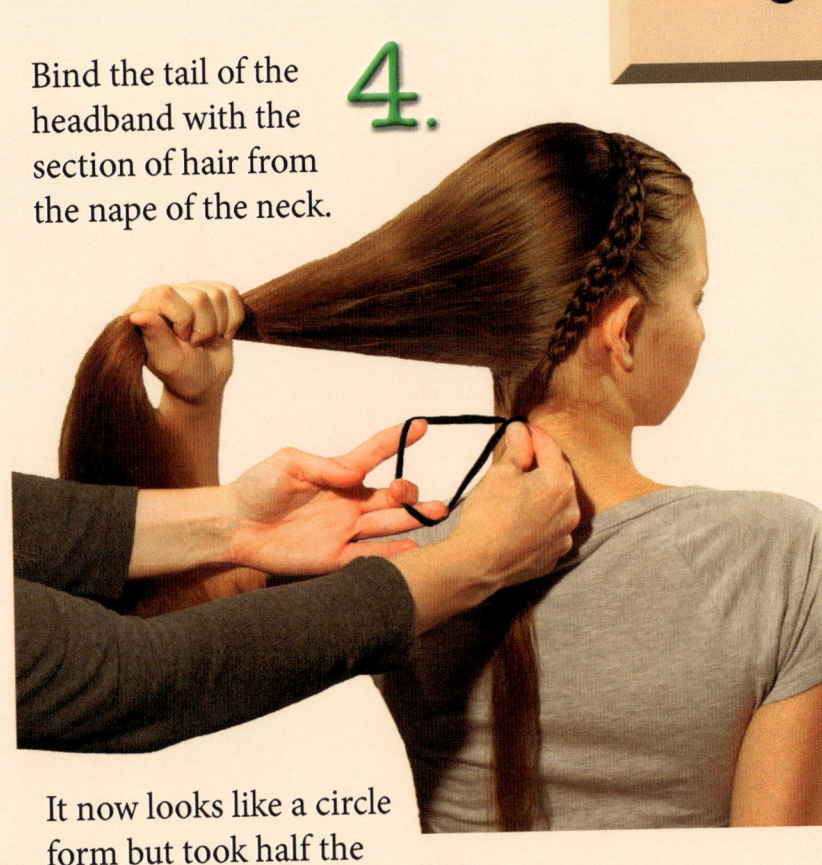

4. Bind the tail of the headband with the section of hair from the nape of the neck.

It now looks like a circle form but took half the time to create. Sweet!

7. I secure the headdress behind the cascade with a band and I add pearl pins to make the accent jump out and dazzle the eye.

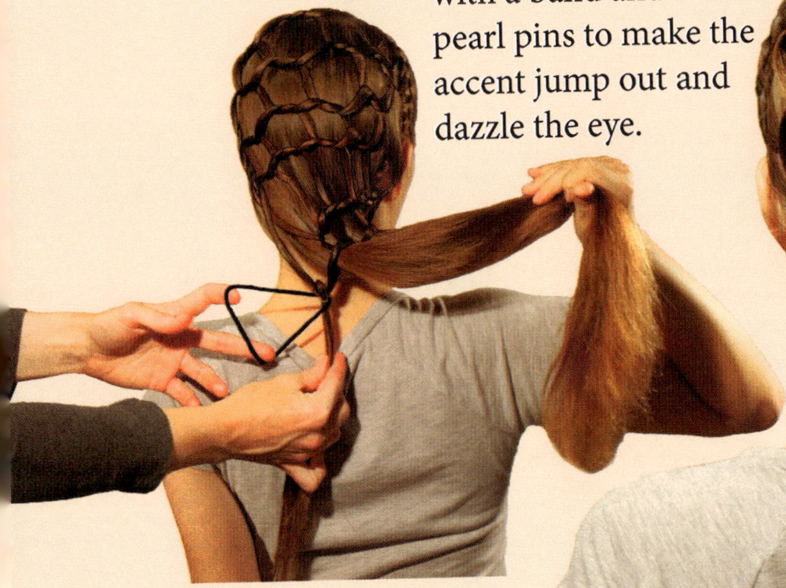

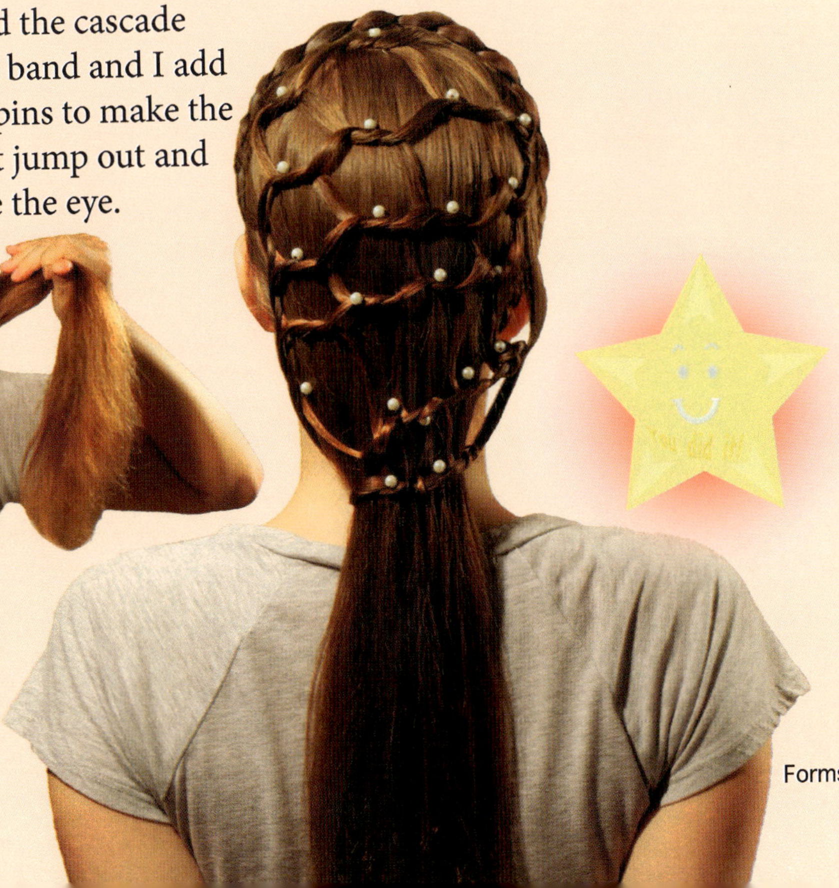

Forms 345

Forms

Notes

Examples of Headbands

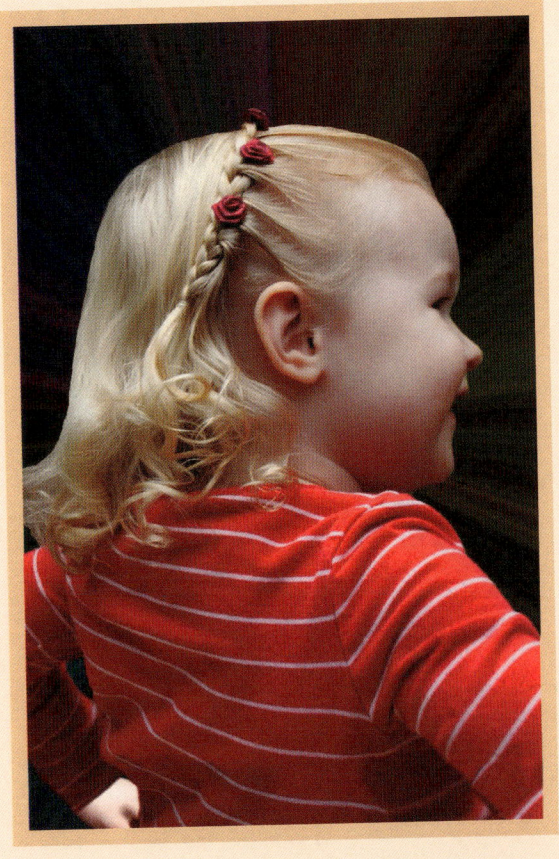
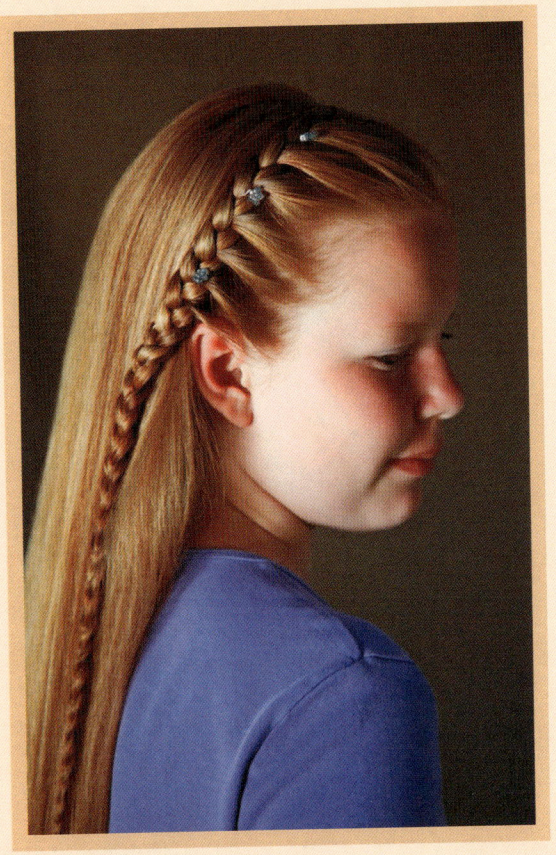
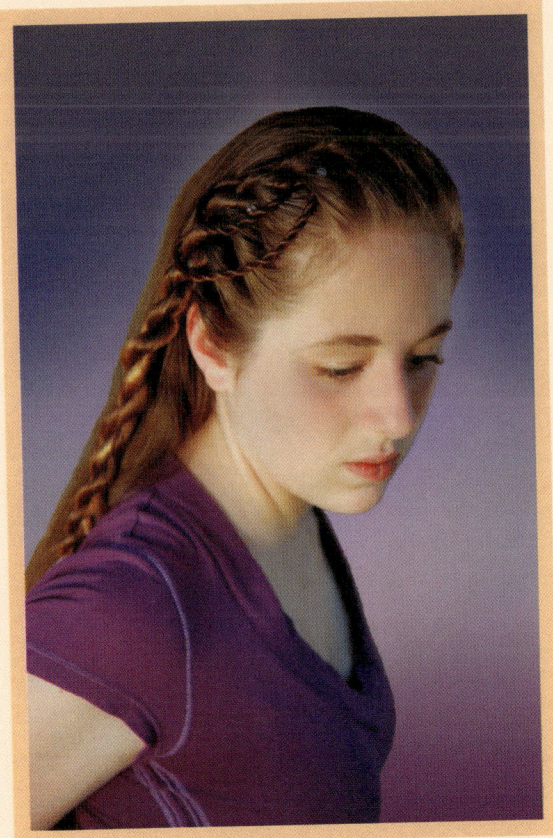
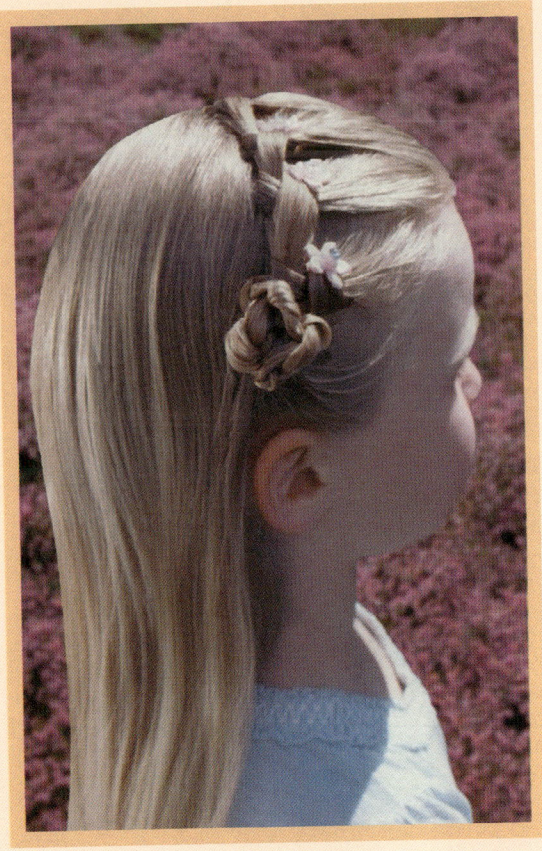

Visit my website to see more examples of Headbands

Forms

CIRCLE

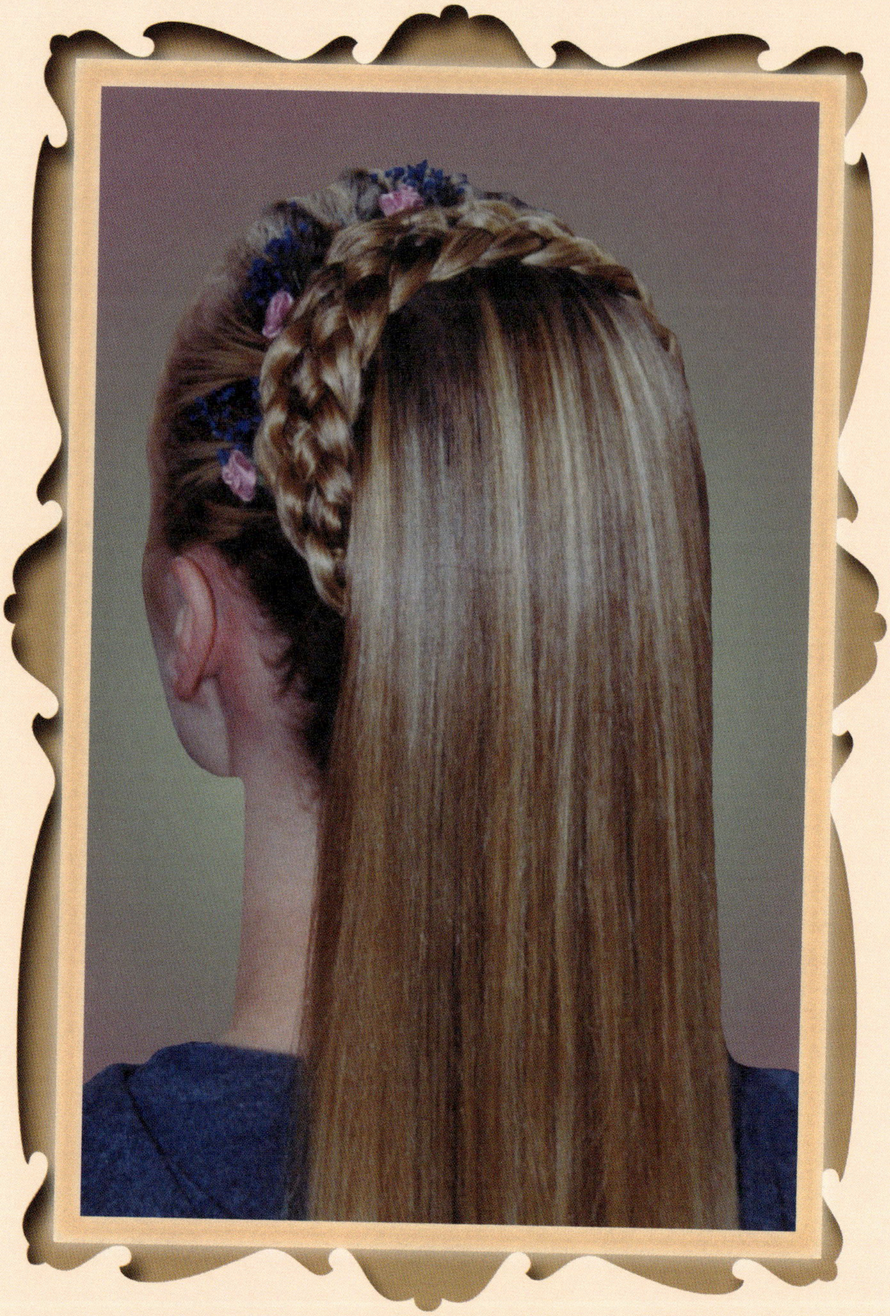

For aspiring princesses. The circle is one of the most feminine, graceful forms. With a little bit of imagination this form is incredibly versatile.

Forms

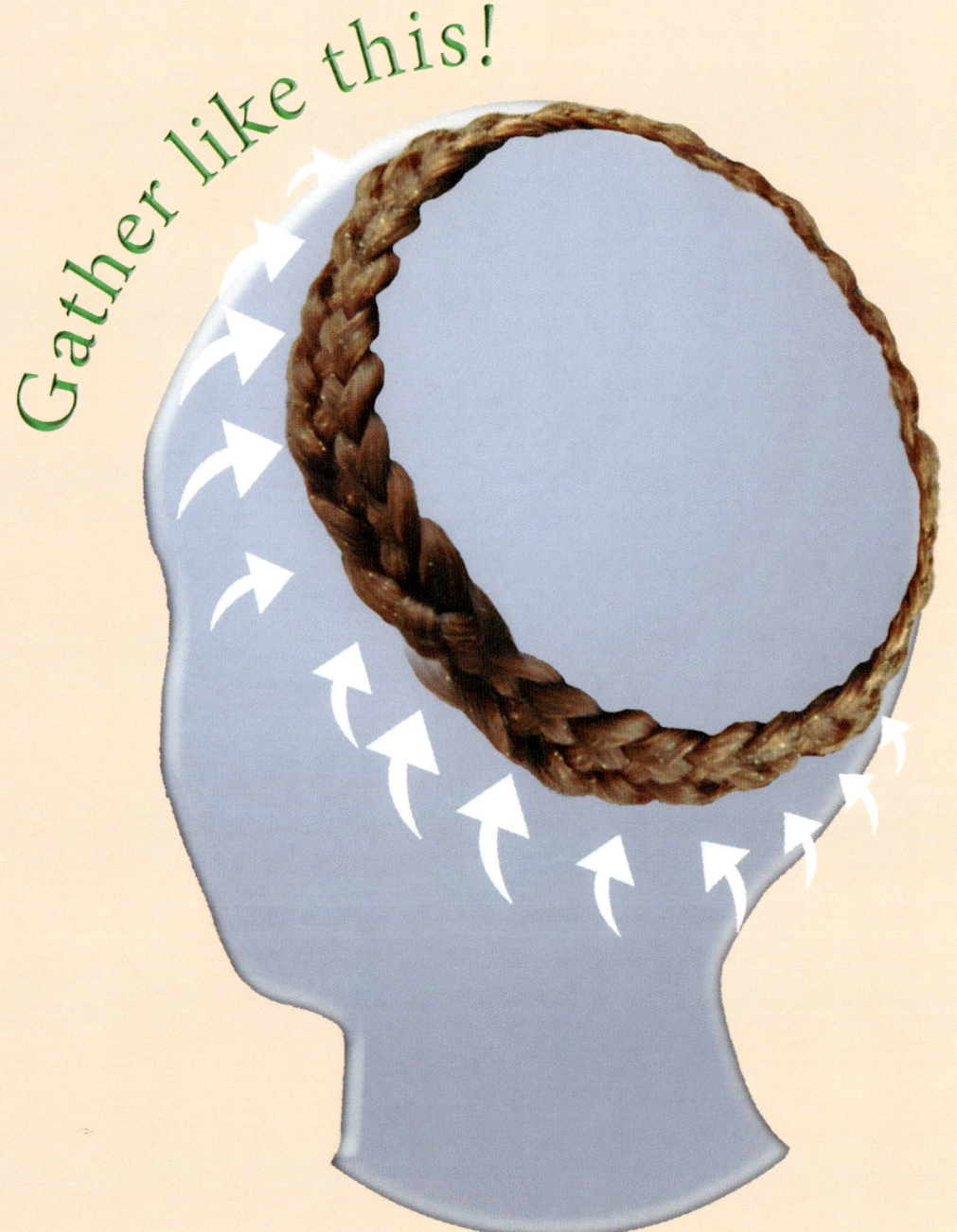

Gather like this!

Start the circle at the nape of the neck. Braid your way around the head. Lace the braid, gathering only from the outside. The inside stays smooth without any visible parts. This braid exudes sophistication.

Braiding icon for the next eight pages.

The **Circle** Form

Basic Circle

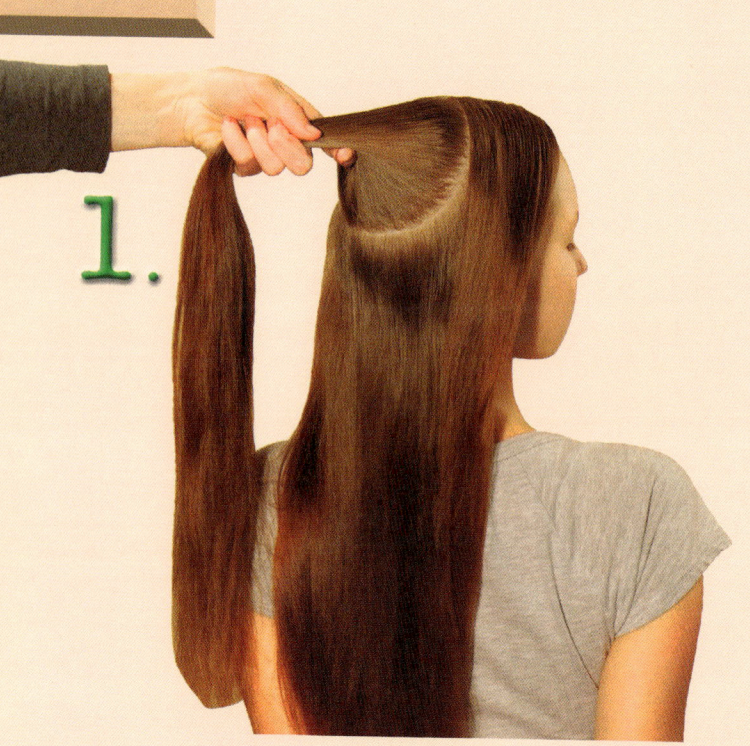

1.

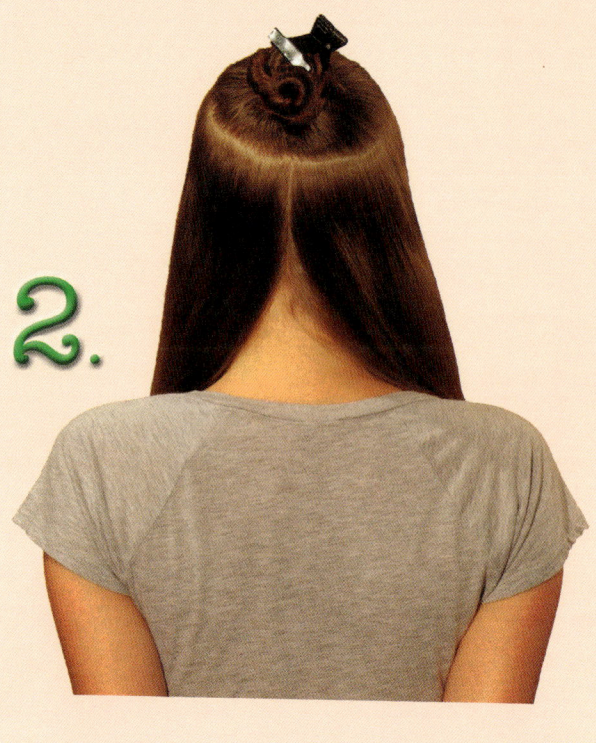

2.

Part out the center of the hair and clip it out of the way while you work.

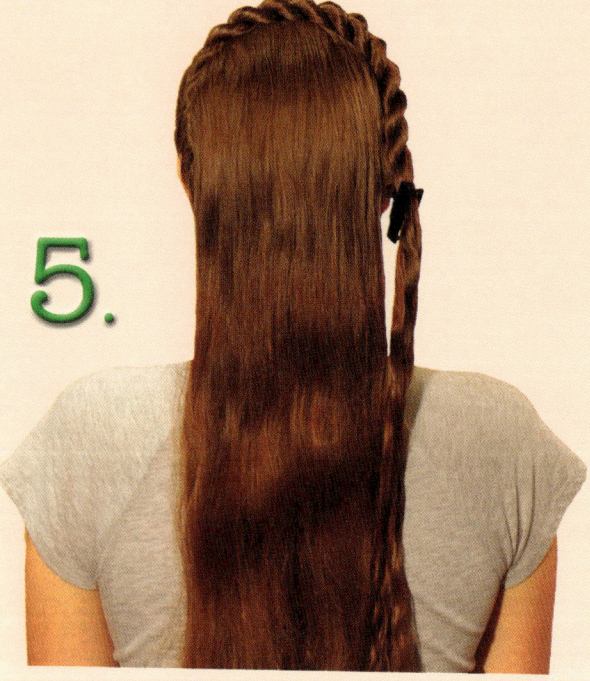

5.

At the other ear, let down the hair from the clip.

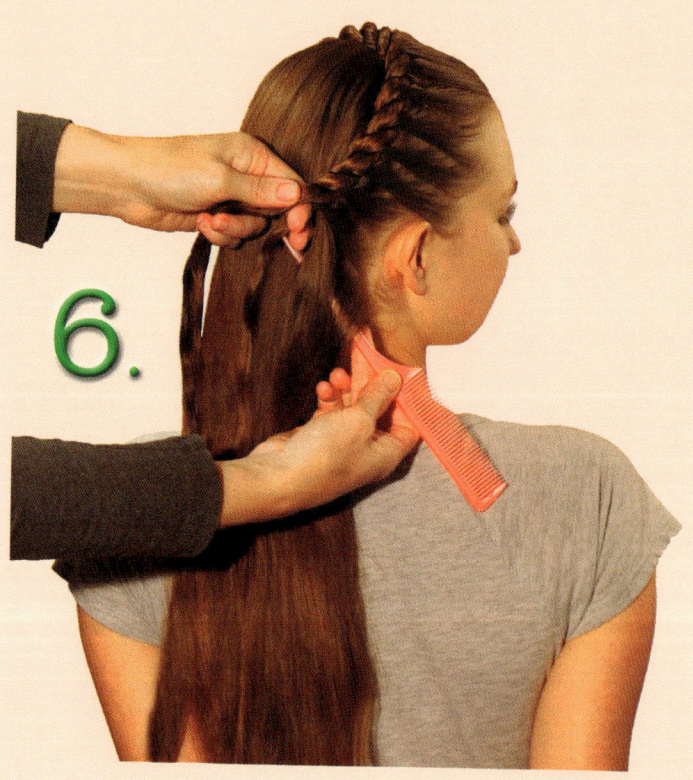

6.

Braid the newly released hair into the style.

350   www.findingbraids.com

Basic Circle

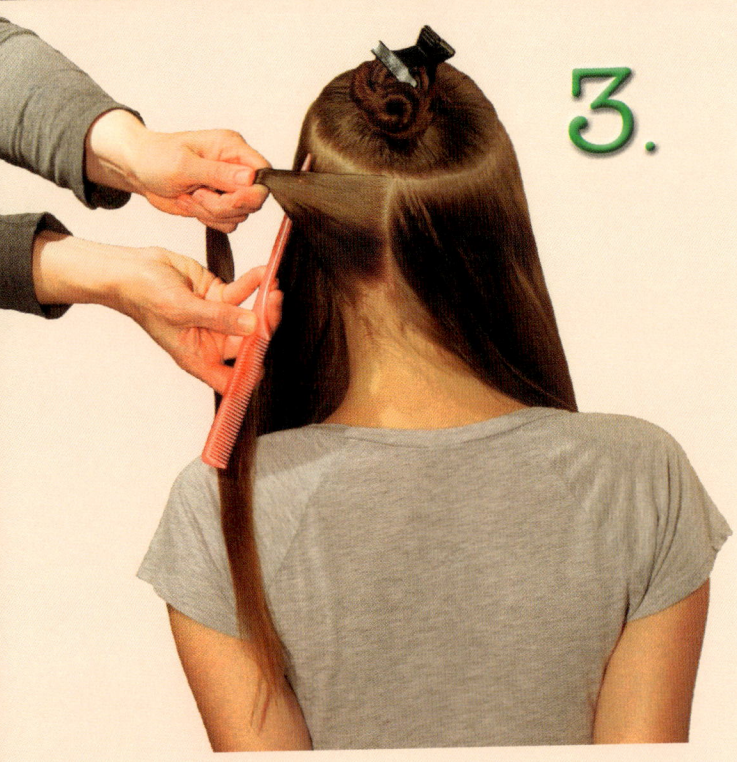

3. Take the first section from the nape of the neck and braid around the head.

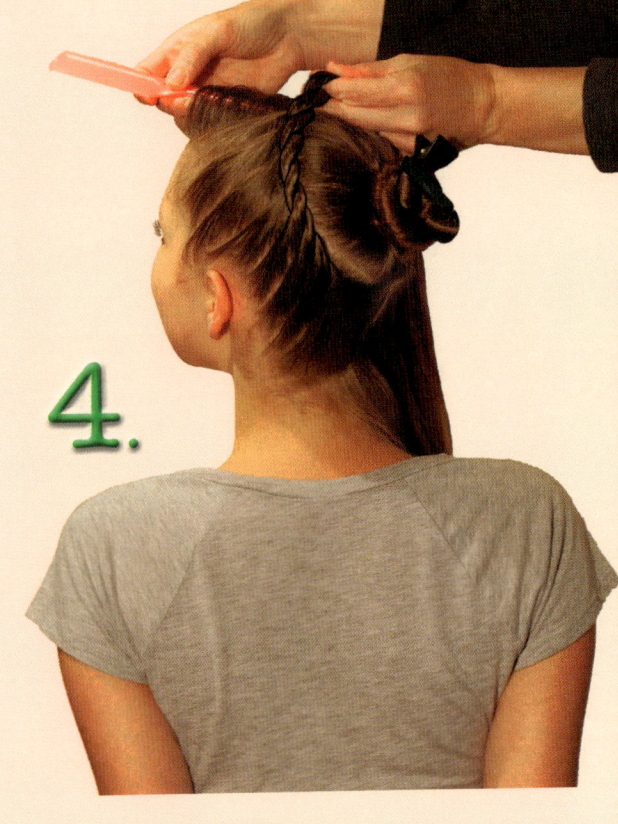

4. This is a two-strand rope.

Create a beautiful bun with the tail of the braid. Buns come in all shapes and sizes. They can be circle buns, heart buns, eternity symbols and flower shaped.

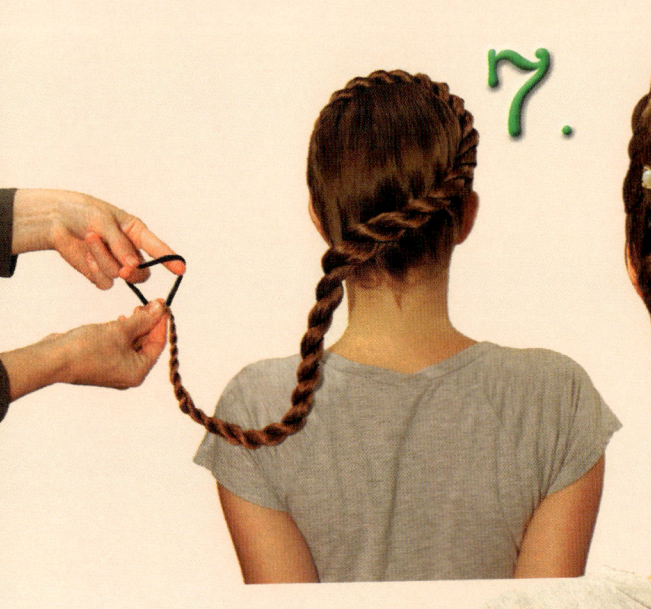

7. Secure the end of the braid with a band.

Forms 351

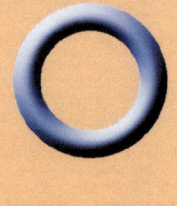

Accented Circle

1.

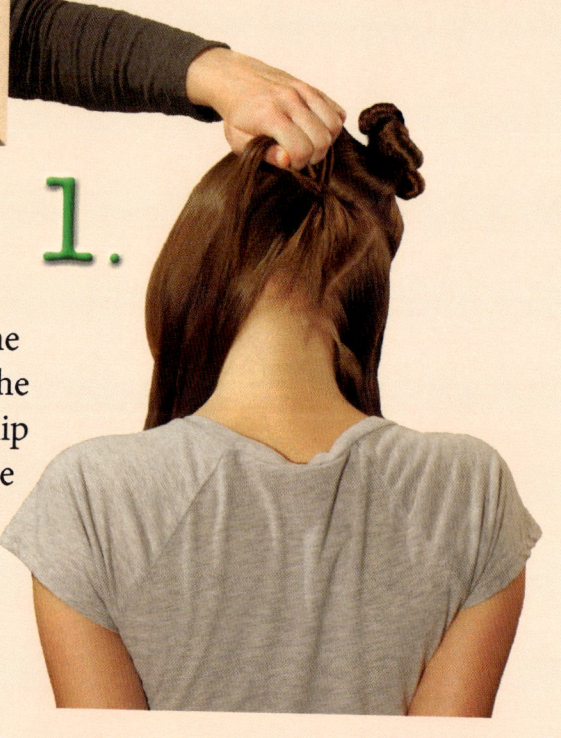

Part out the center of the hair and clip it out of the way while you work.

Take the first section from the nape of the neck and braid around the head. When braiding from ear to ear place the braid at the headband area of the head.

2.

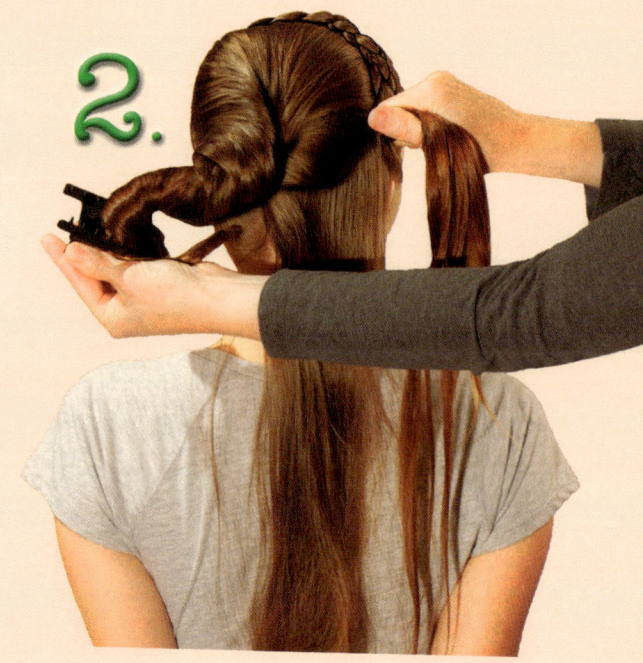

At the second ear, let down the center hair from the clip and braid it into the style. This style has accents.

5.

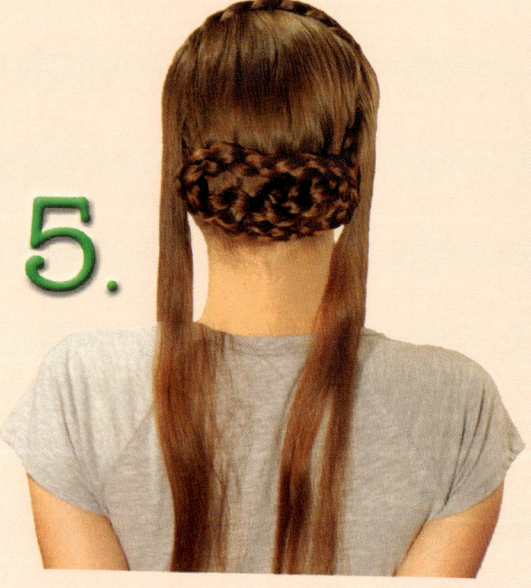

Buns come in all shapes and sizes. They can be circle buns, heart buns, eternity symbols and flower shaped. Let your intuition guide you while you design the styles you create.

6.

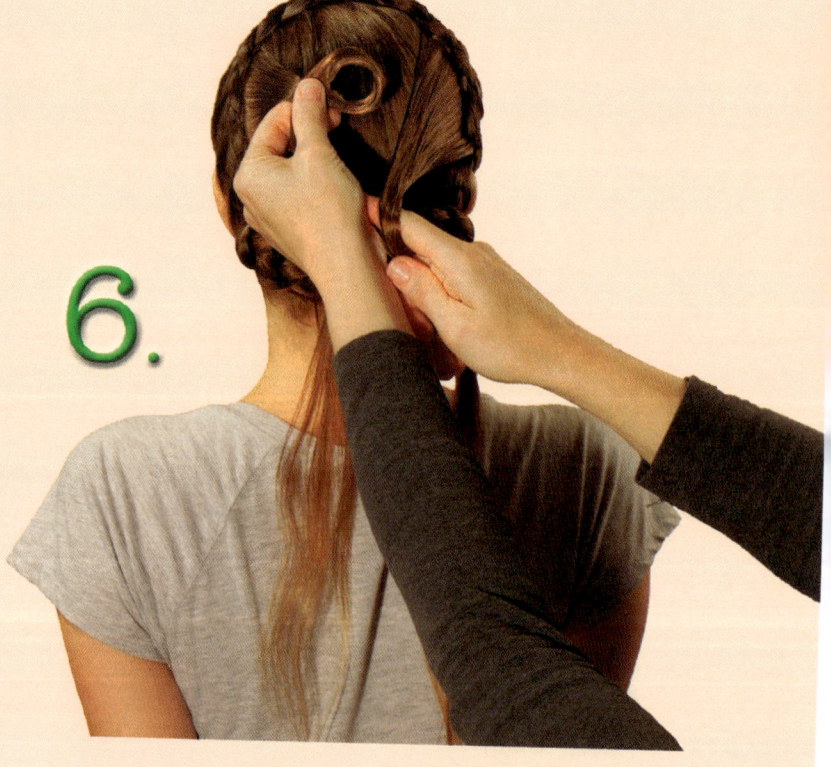

Create your accent and pin it securely when finished. Hairspray protects your hard work.

352   www.findingbraids.com

Accented Circle

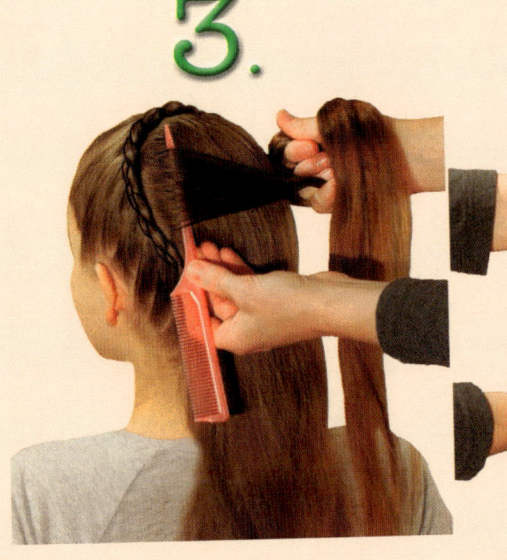

3.

Pull out accent strands where you need them.

Secure the end of the braid with a band and create a beautiful bun with the tail of the braid.

4.

This is a four-strand round.

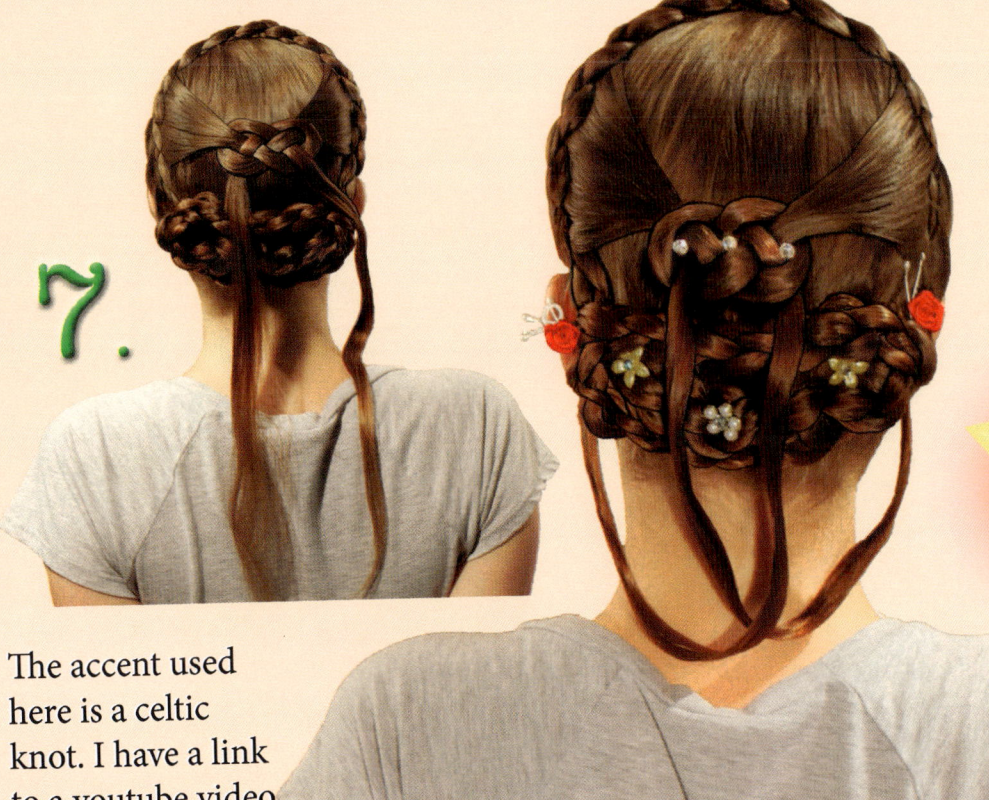

7.

The accent used here is a celtic knot. I have a link to a youtube video showing this at the back of the book.

Forms 353

Circle Cascade

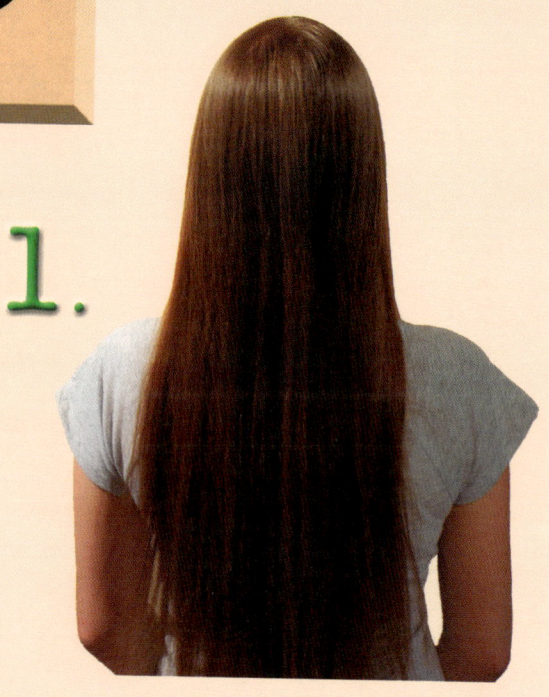

1. Begin with clean, brushed hair.

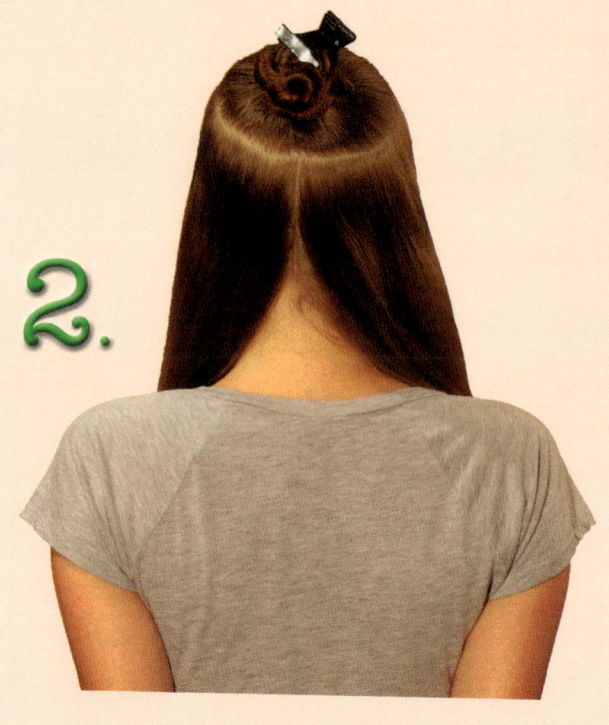

2. Part out the center of the hair and clip it out of the way while you work.

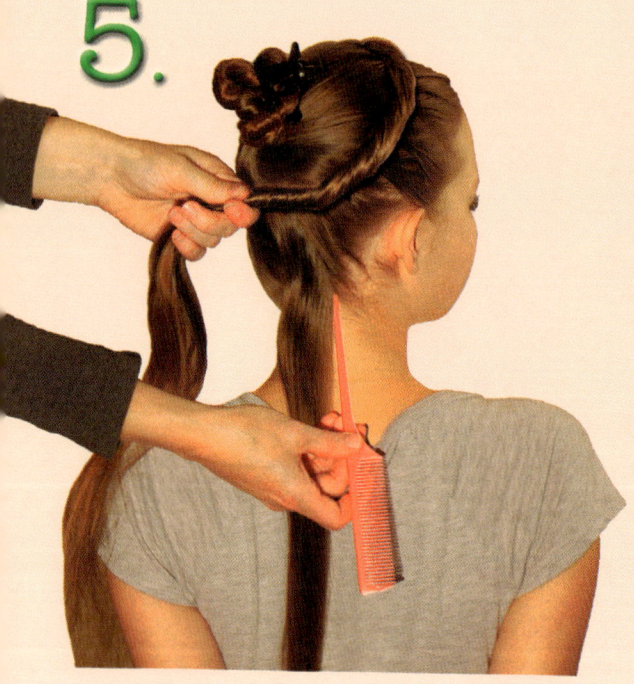

5. This is a cascading style so do not braid in the clipped off center hair.

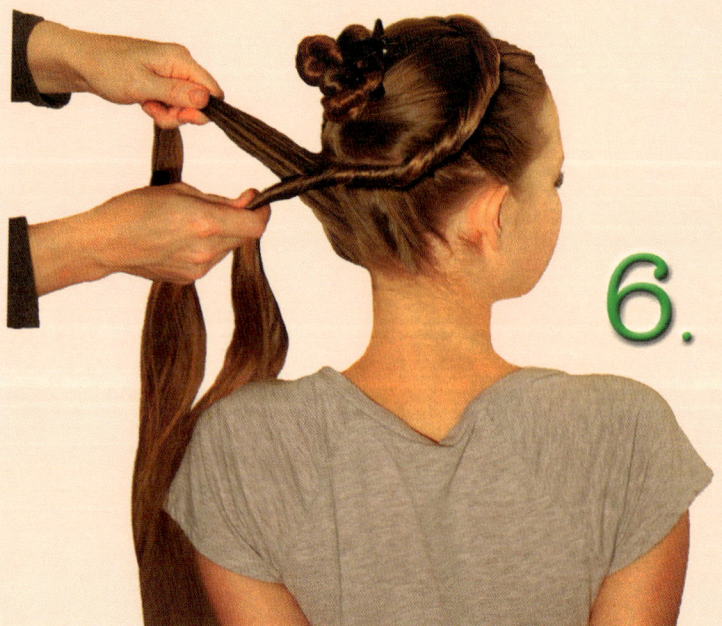

6.

Circle Cascade

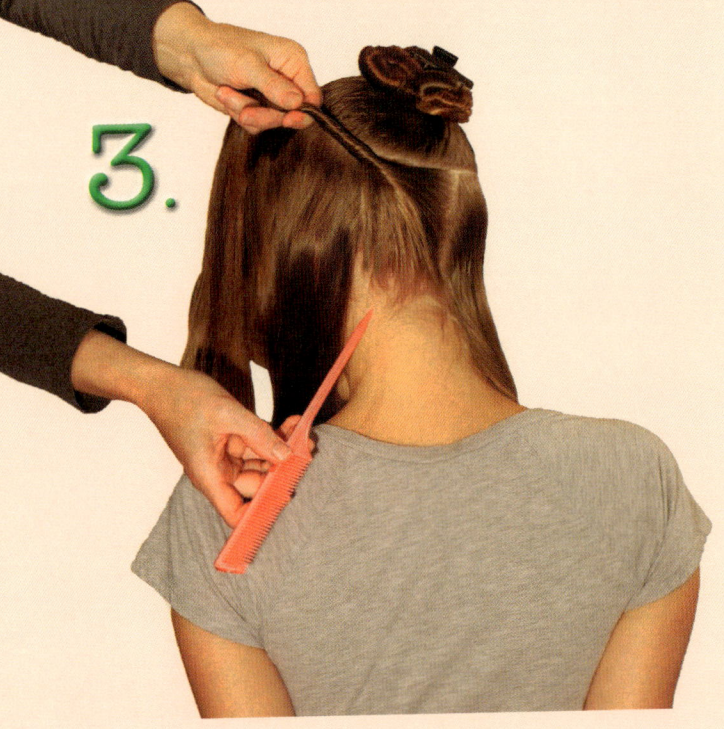

3. Take the first section from the nape of the neck and braid around the head. Going from ear to ear, place the braid where a headband would sit.

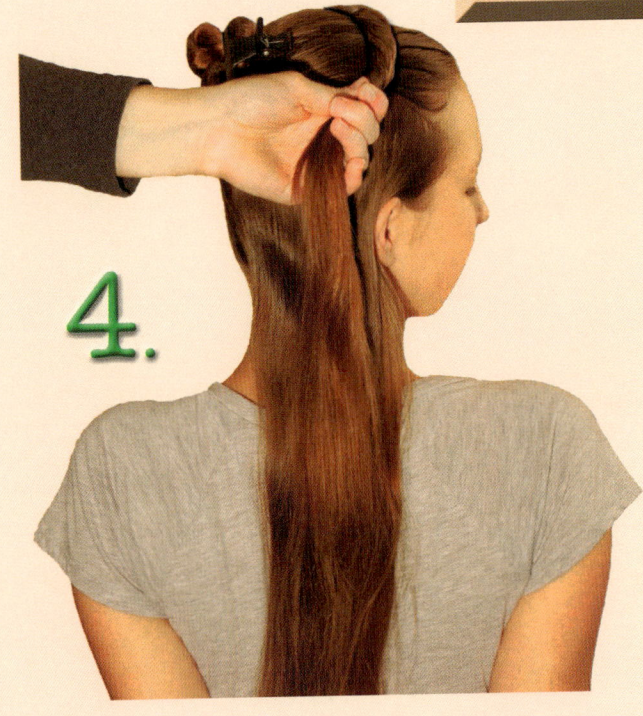

4. This is a one-strand twist.

7. Secure the end of the braid with a band and wrap it around the head pinning it to the first braid.

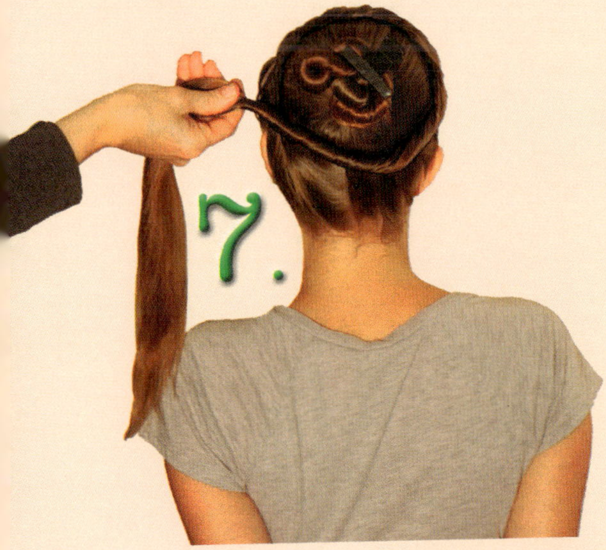

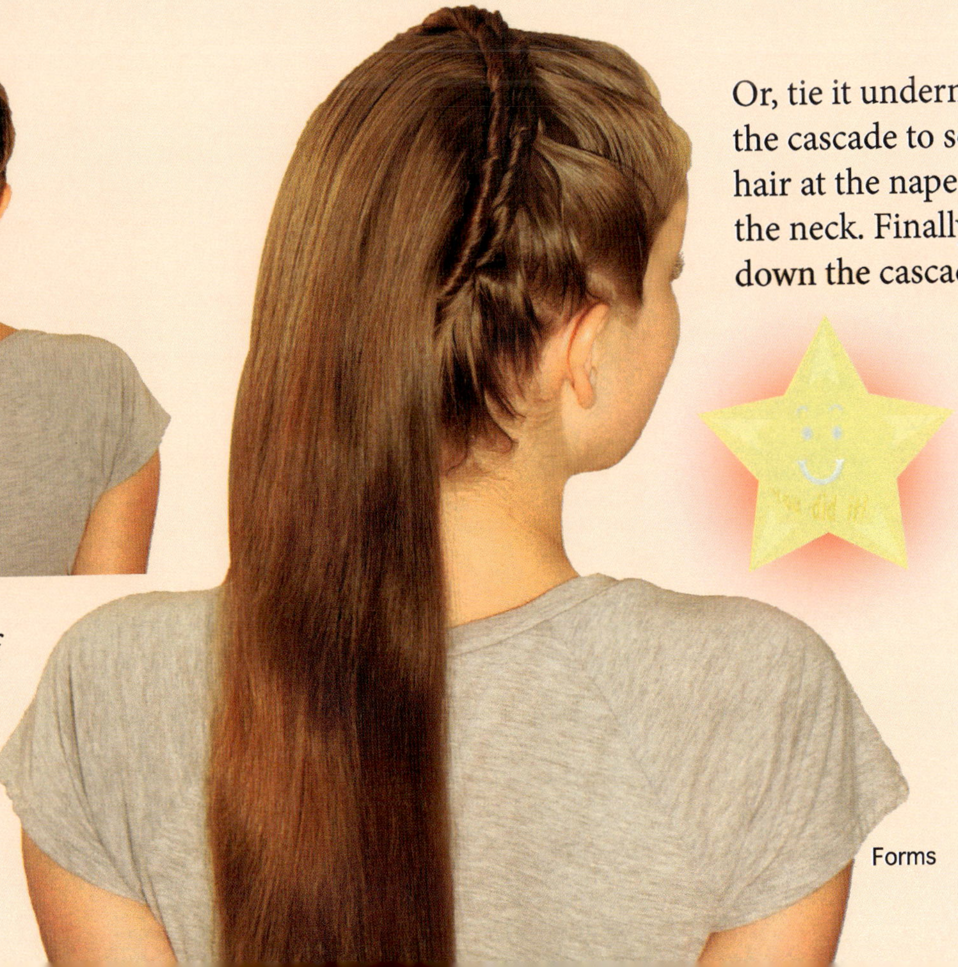

Or, tie it underneath the cascade to some hair at the nape of the neck. Finally, let down the cascade.

Forms 355

Accented Circle Cascade

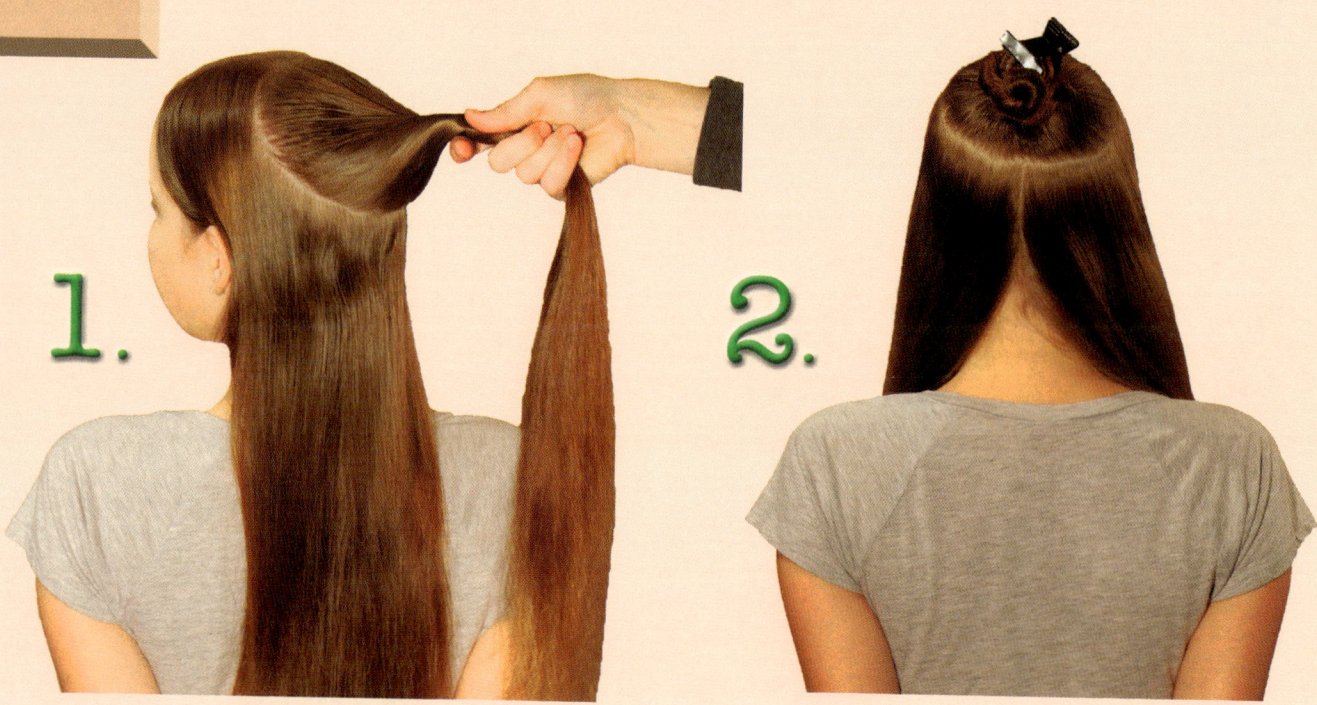

1. Part out the center of the hair and clip it out of the way while you work.

2. Make the circle as wide or narrow as you wish.

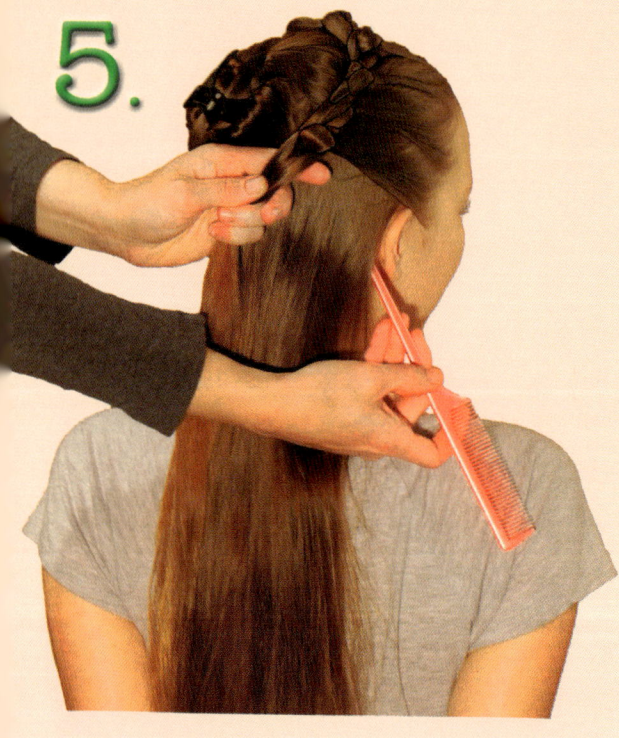

5.

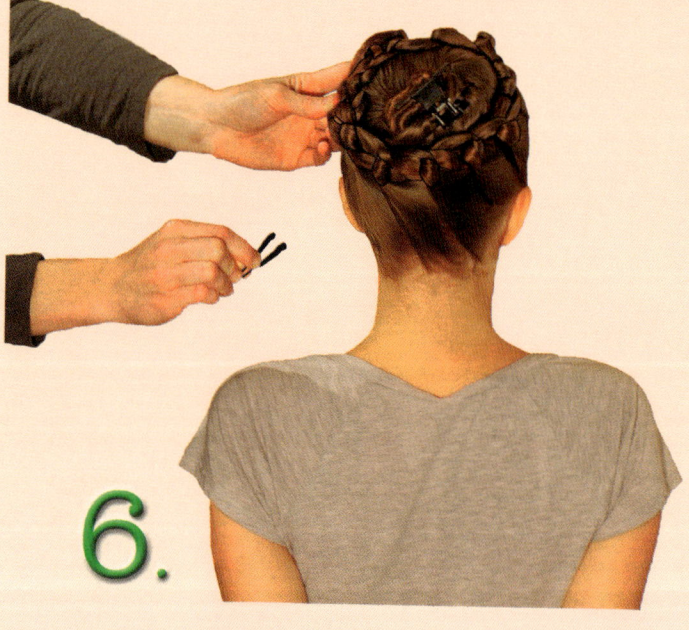

6. Secure the end of the braid with a band and wrap it around the head pinning it to the first braid or tie it underneath the cascade to some hair at the nape of the neck. Finally, let down the cascade.

Accented Circle Cascade

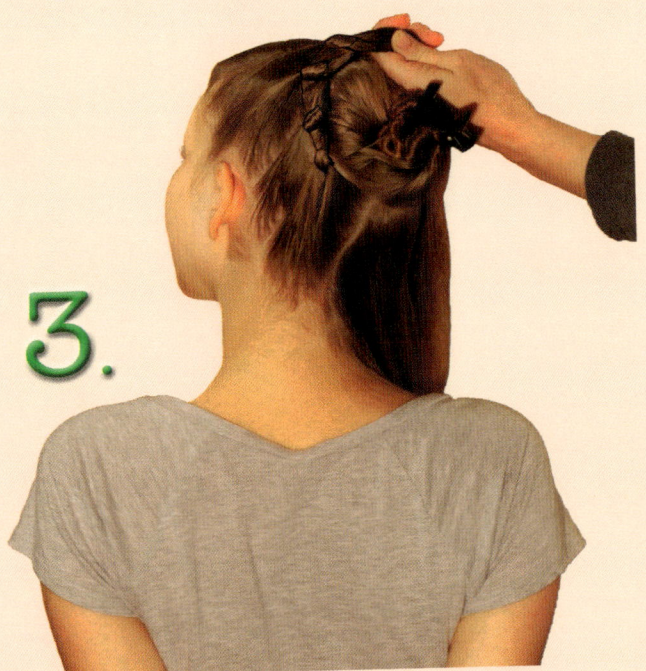

3.

Take the first section from the nape of the neck and braid around the head.

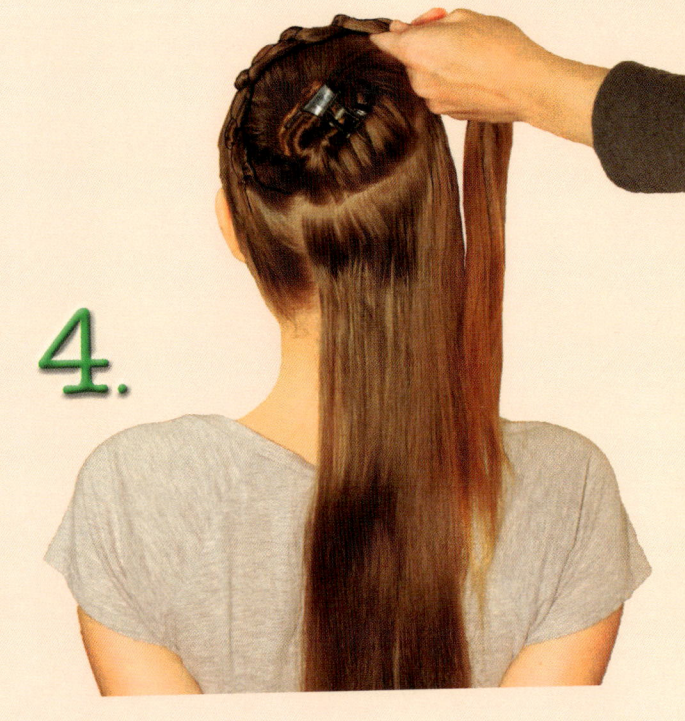

4.

This is a two-strand knot.

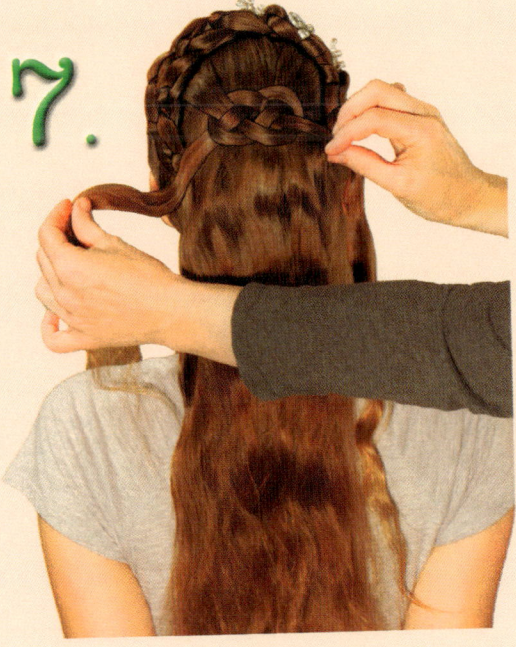

7.

Pull out accent strands where you need them.

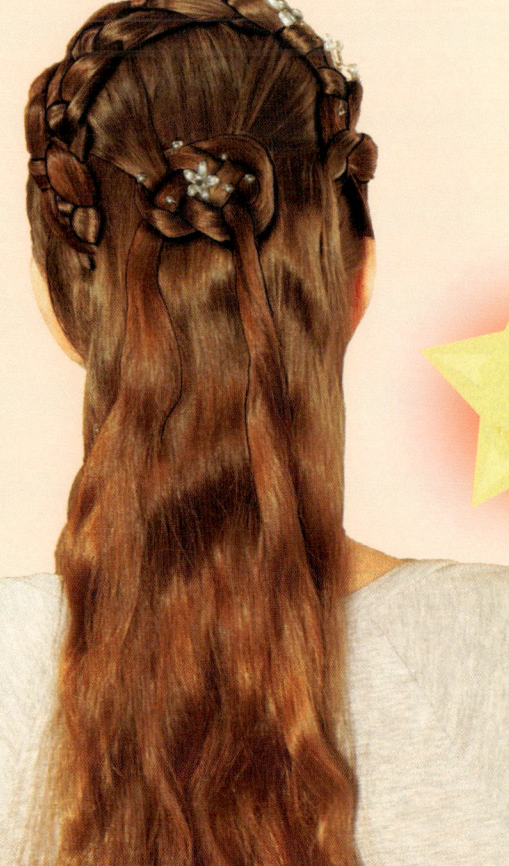

Forms

Forms

Notes

Examples of Circles

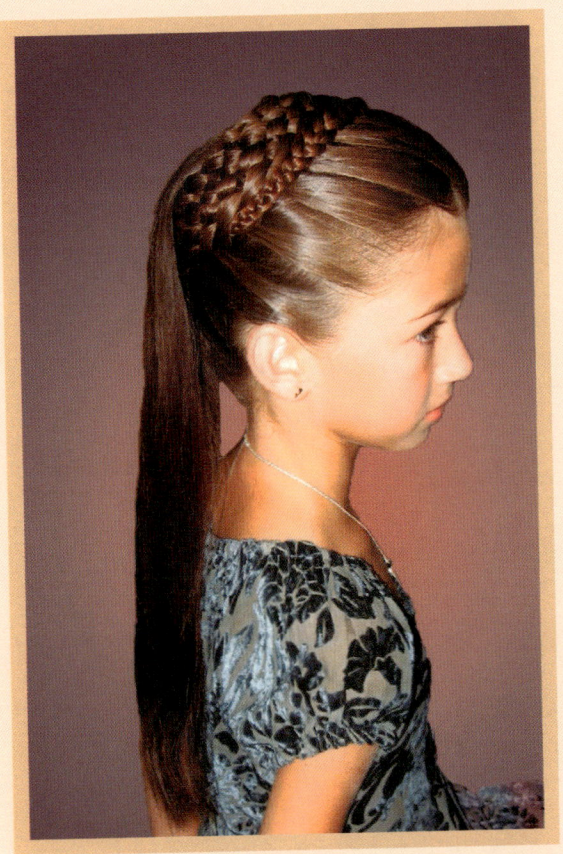
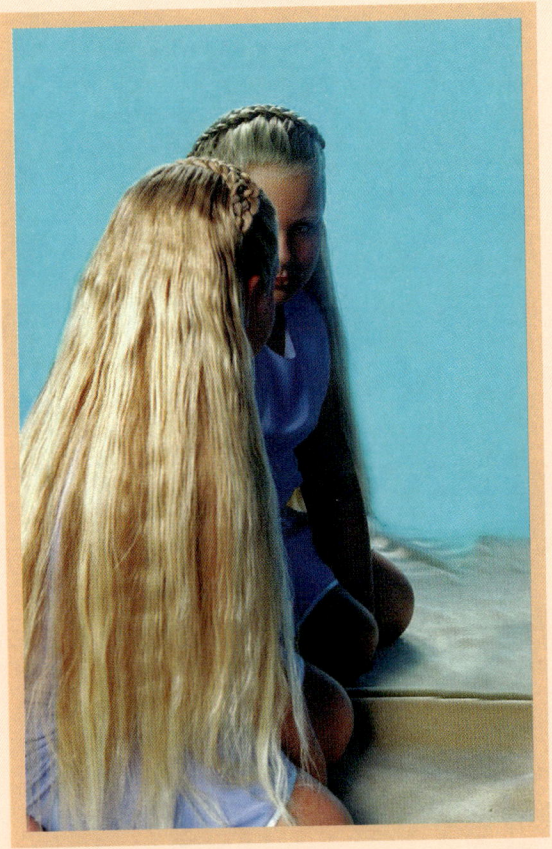
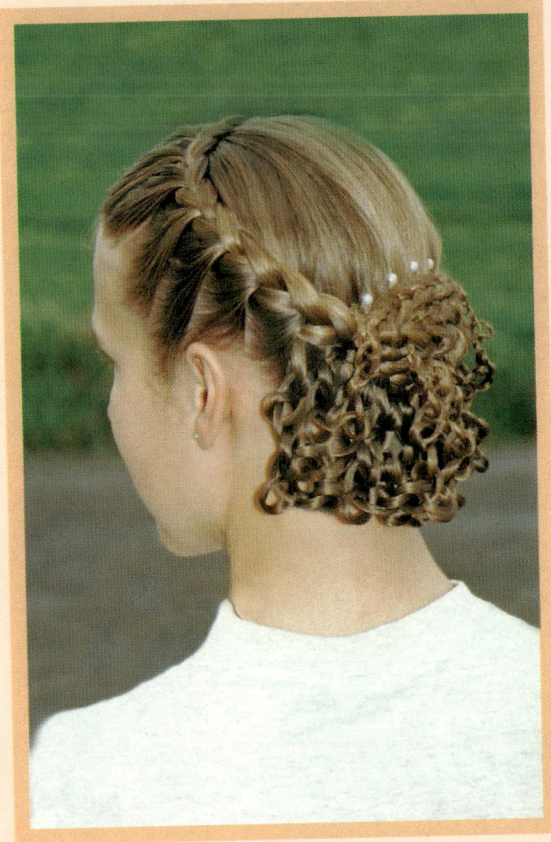
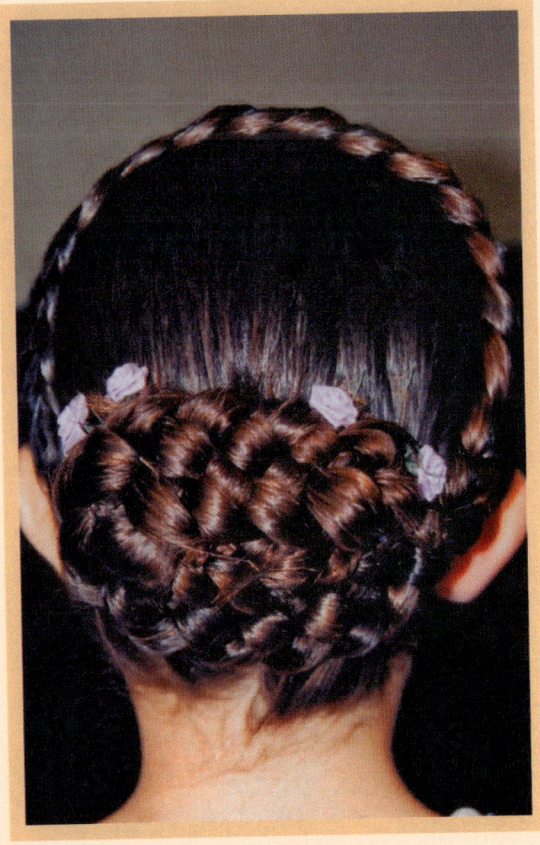

Visit my website to see more examples of Circles

Forms

S I N G L E

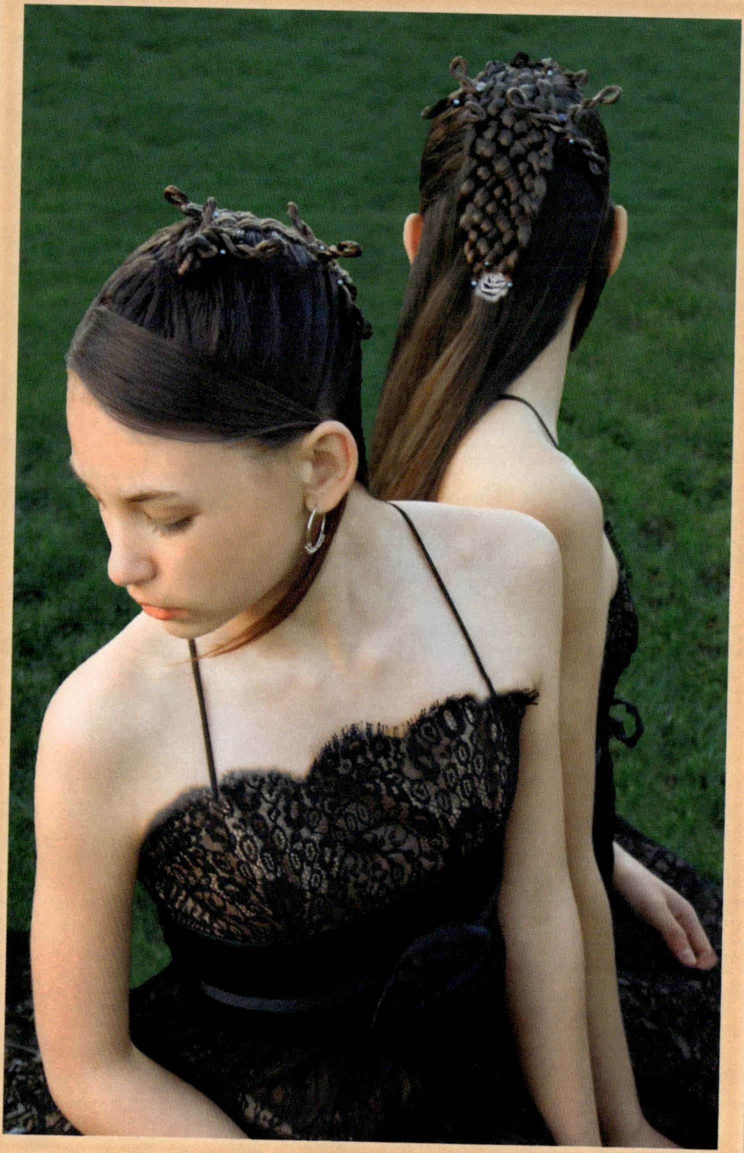

This form rapidly changes appearance as the number of strands being braided changes. Take this universal form and make it your own with fun accents.

Forms

Gather like this!

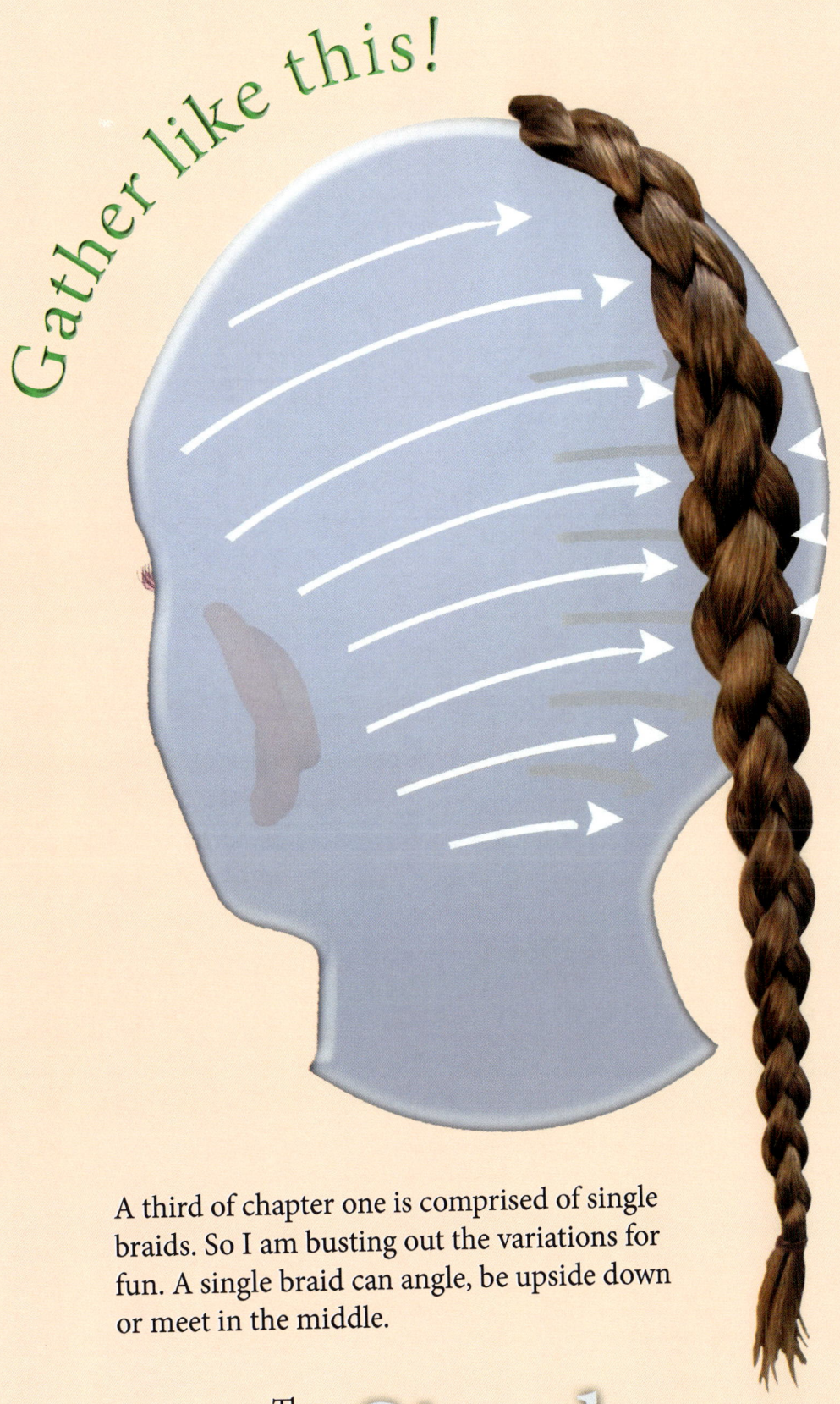

Braiding icon for the next eight pages.

A third of chapter one is comprised of single braids. So I am busting out the variations for fun. A single braid can angle, be upside down or meet in the middle.

The **Single** Form

Basic Single

1. 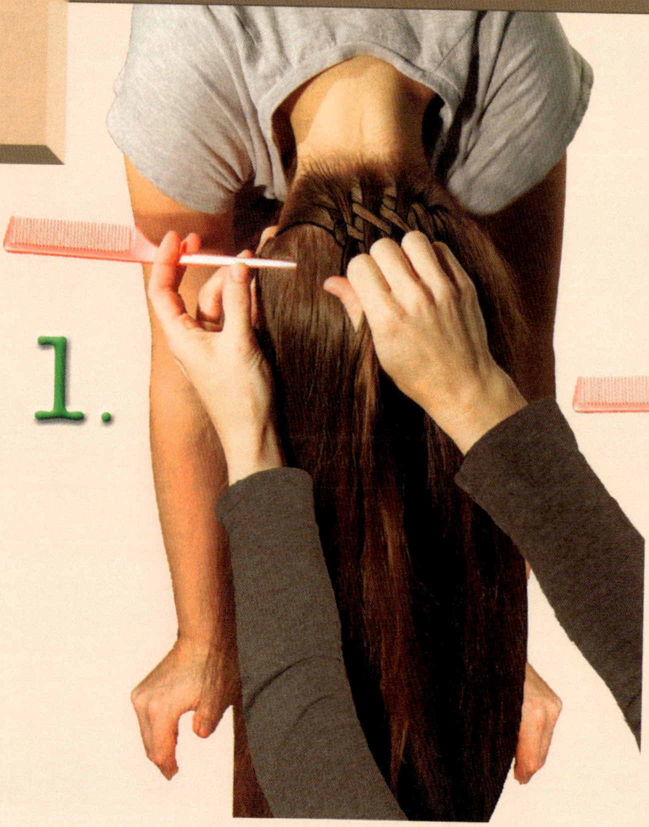
2.

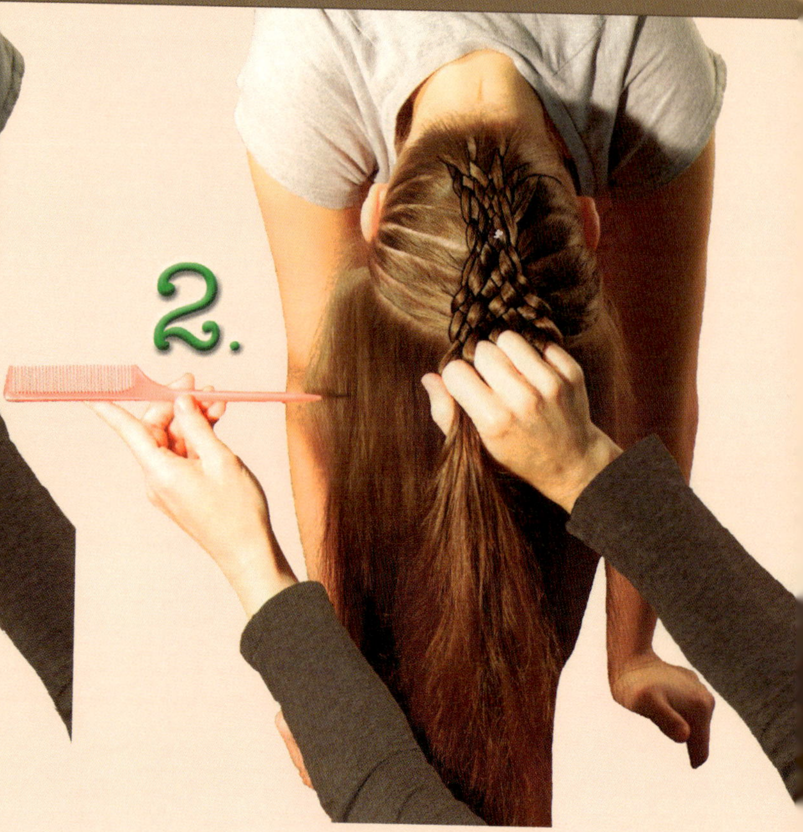

Create a single braid with any number of strands. This one is a nine-strand dutch braid. It is being done upside down.

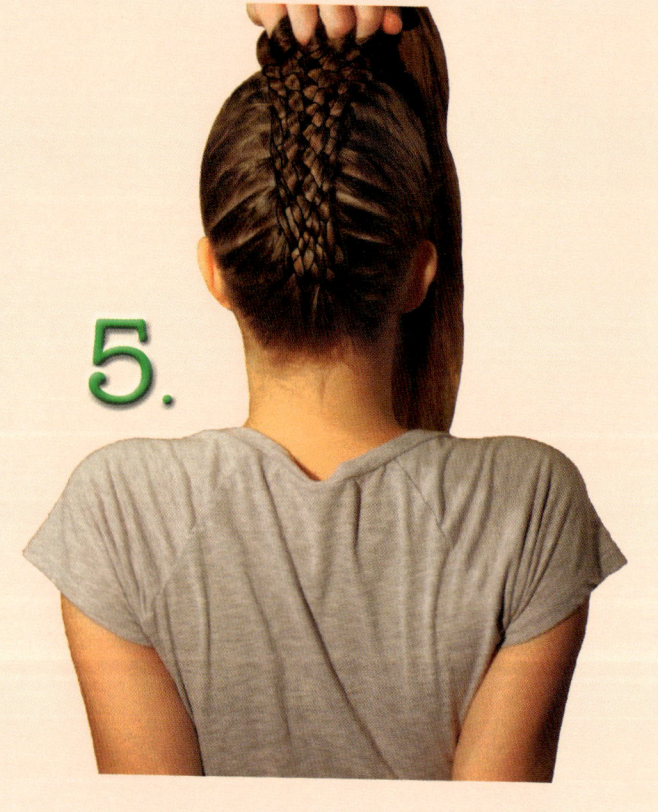

5.

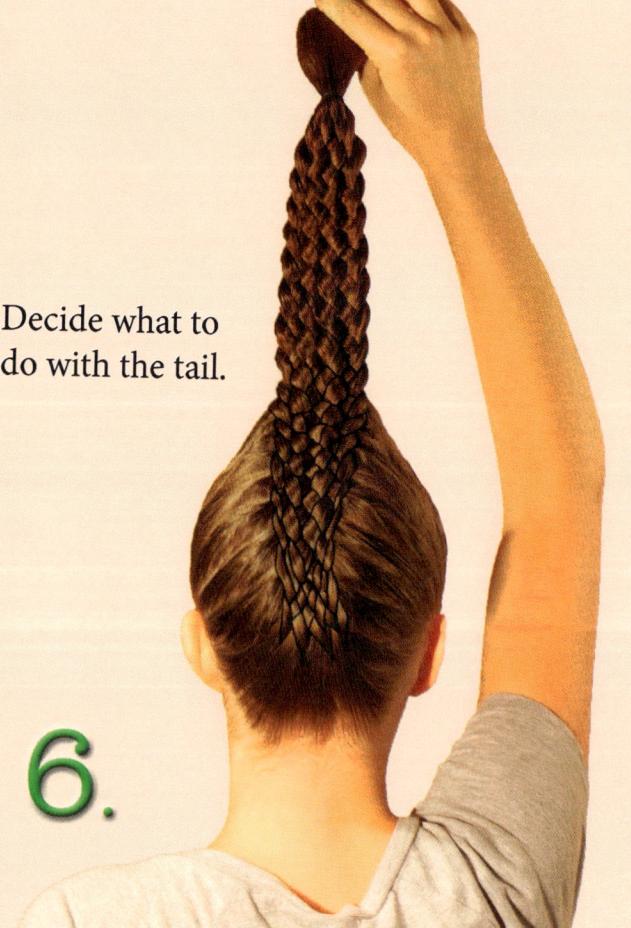

Decide what to do with the tail.

6.

Basic Single

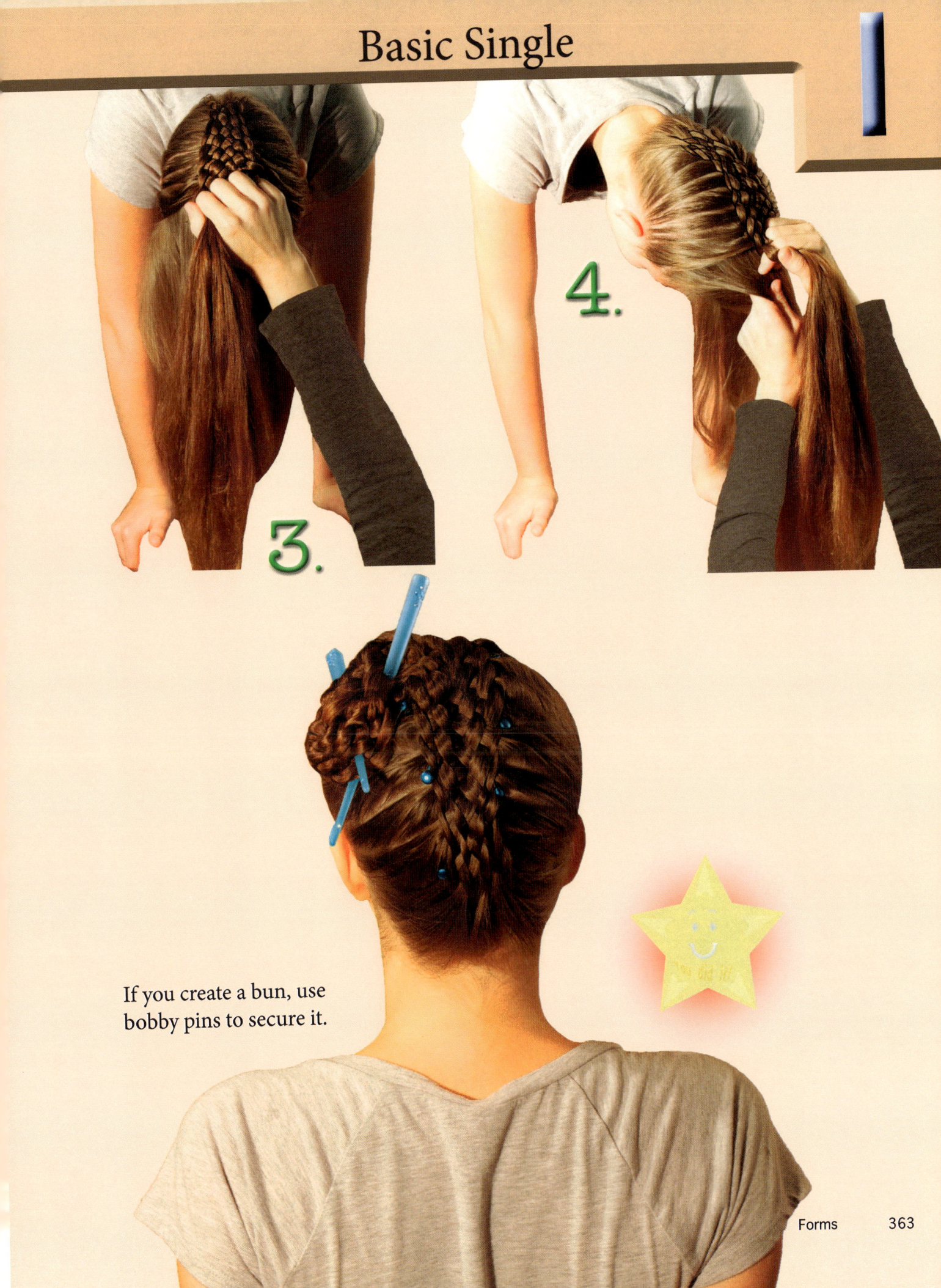

3.

4.

If you create a bun, use bobby pins to secure it.

Forms 363

Accented Single

1. Begin with clean, brushed hair.

In this example I take my accent section out first.

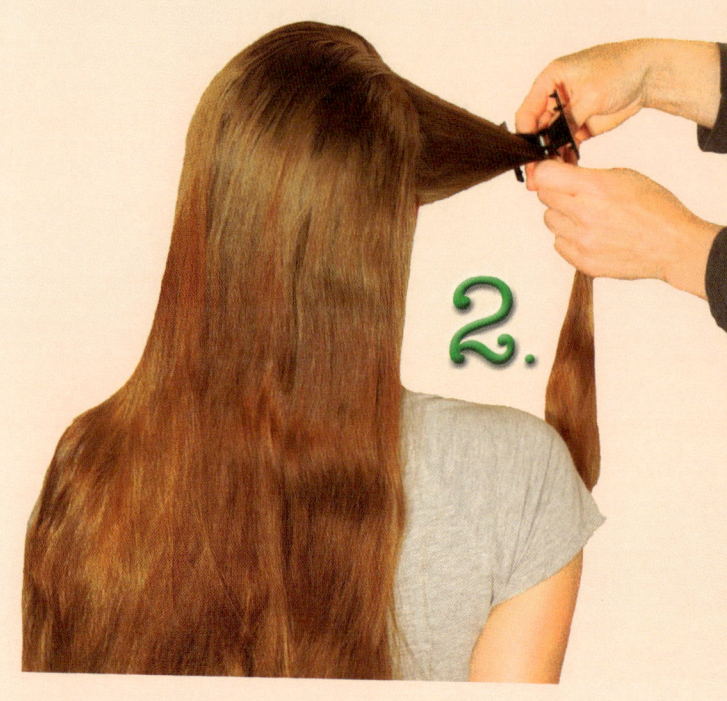

2. Pull out accent strands where you need them.

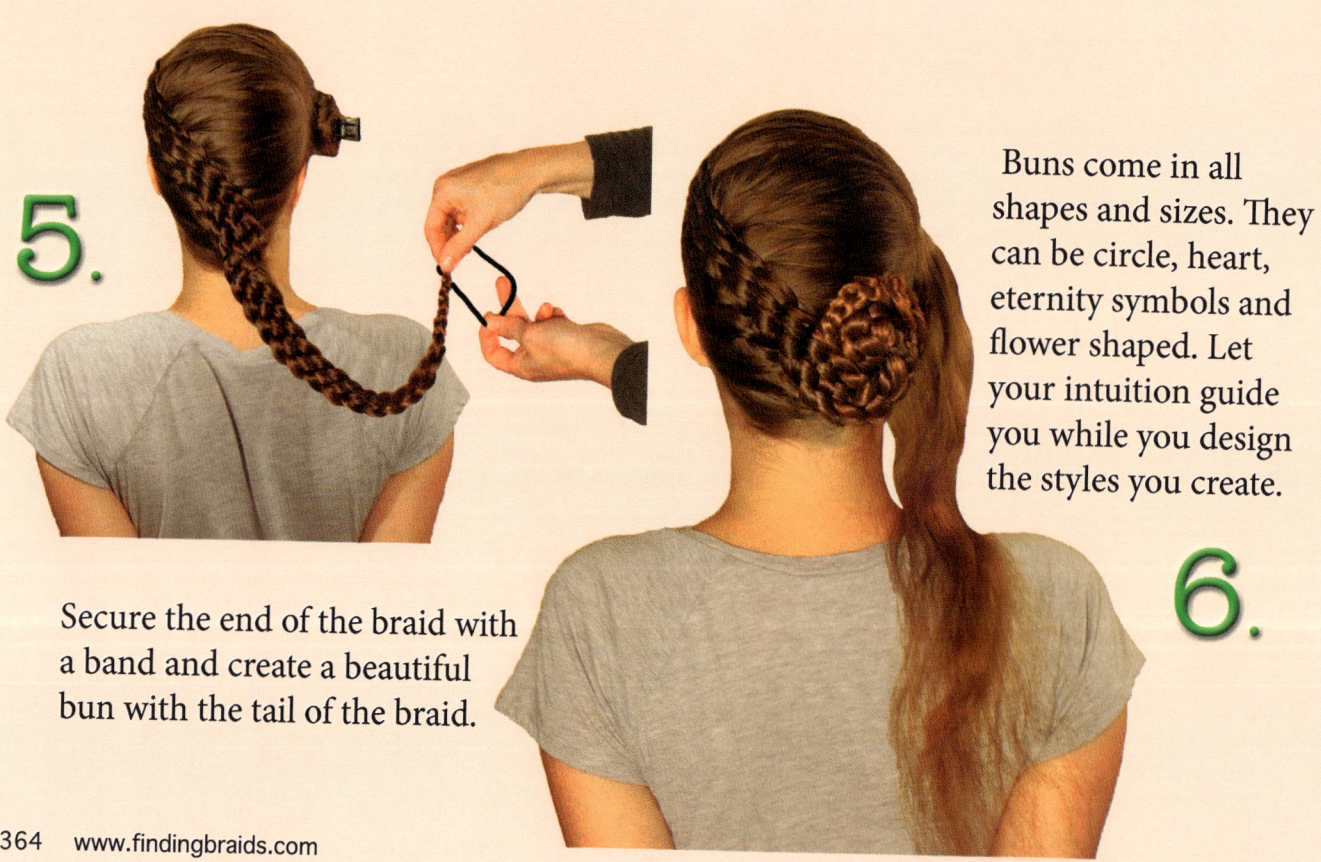

5. Secure the end of the braid with a band and create a beautiful bun with the tail of the braid.

6. Buns come in all shapes and sizes. They can be circle, heart, eternity symbols and flower shaped. Let your intuition guide you while you design the styles you create.

Accented Single

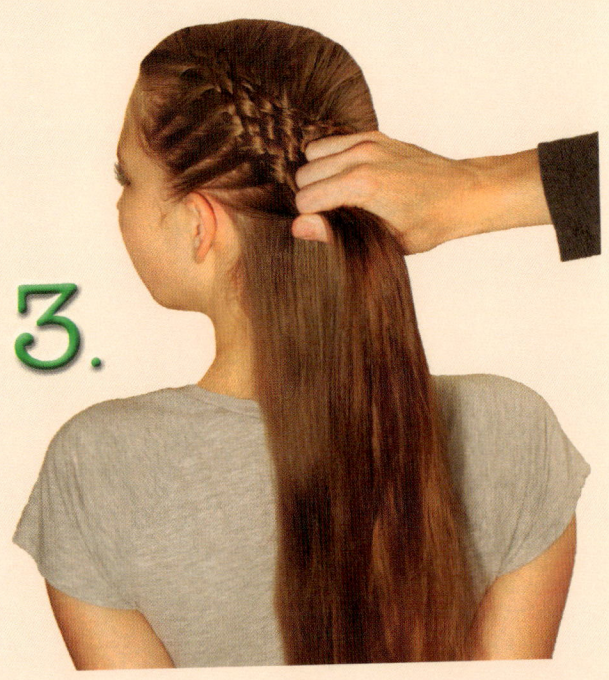

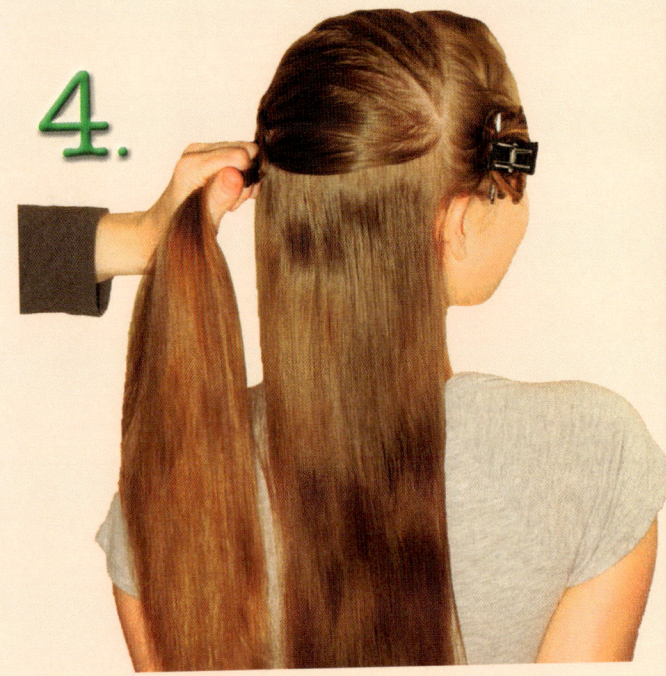

Create a single braid with any number of strands. This one is an eight-strand taper braid. It is being done at an angle.

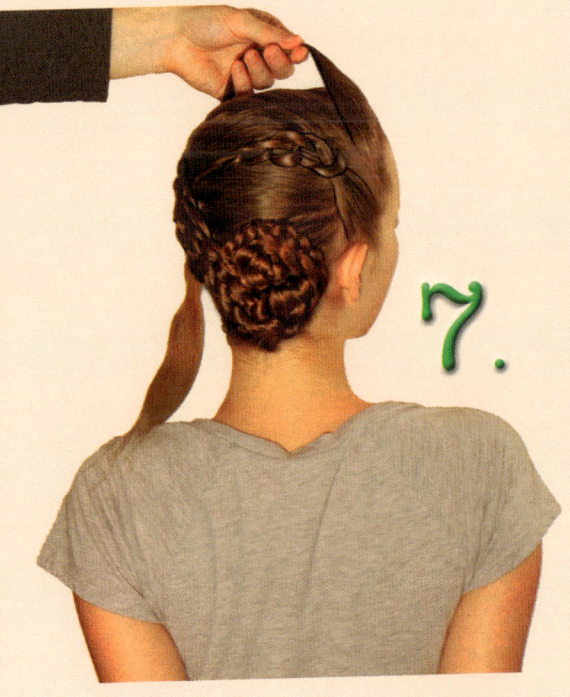

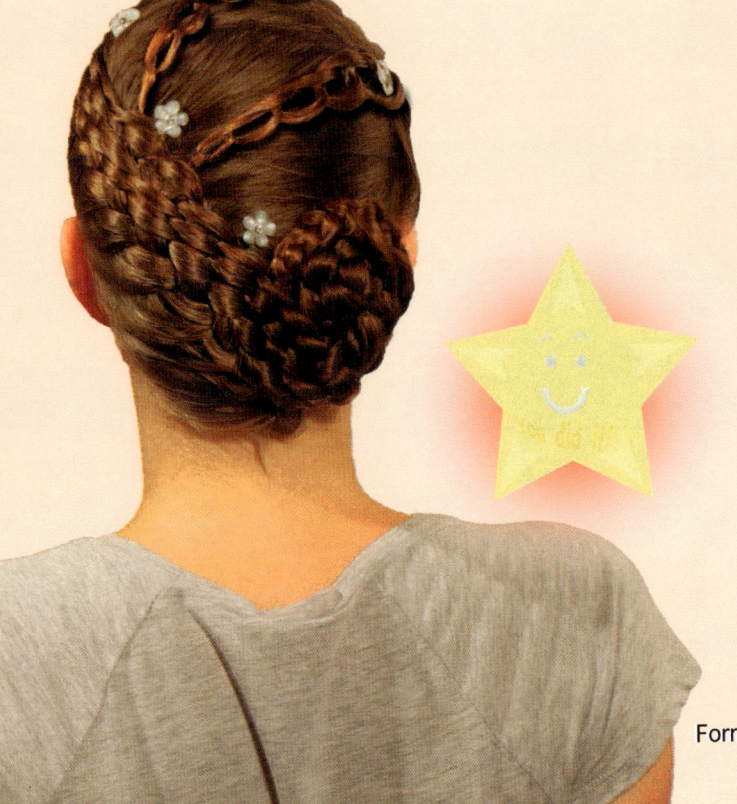

Create your accent and pin it securely when finished. Hairspray protects your hard work.

Forms

Single Cascade

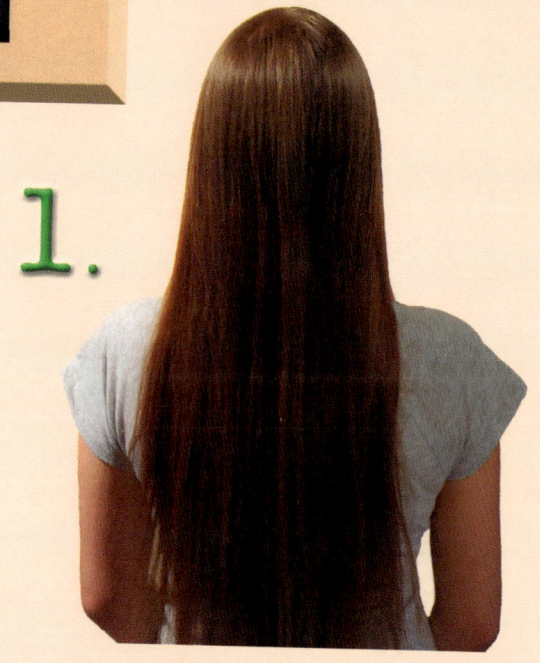

1. Begin with clean, brushed hair.

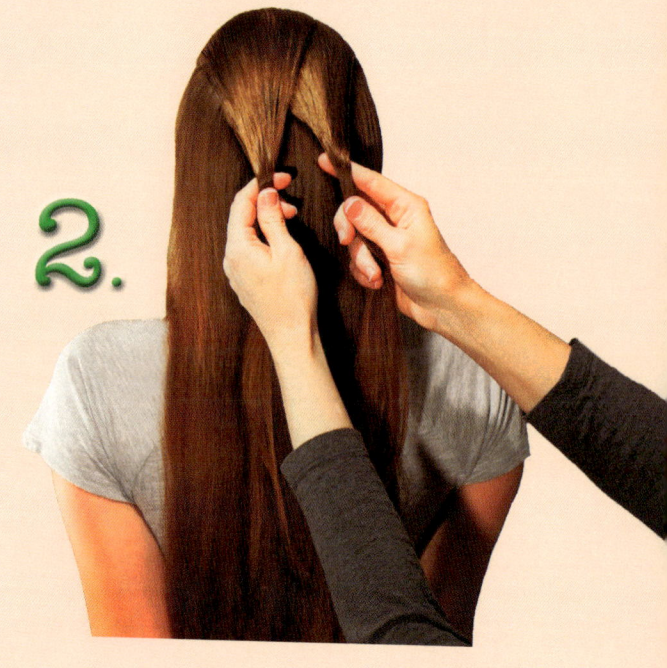

2. Create a single braid with any number of strands.

5.

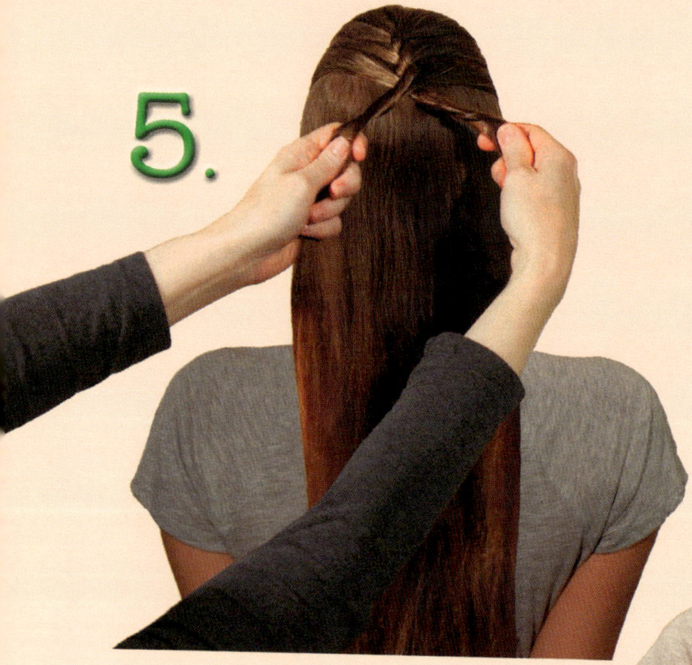

6.

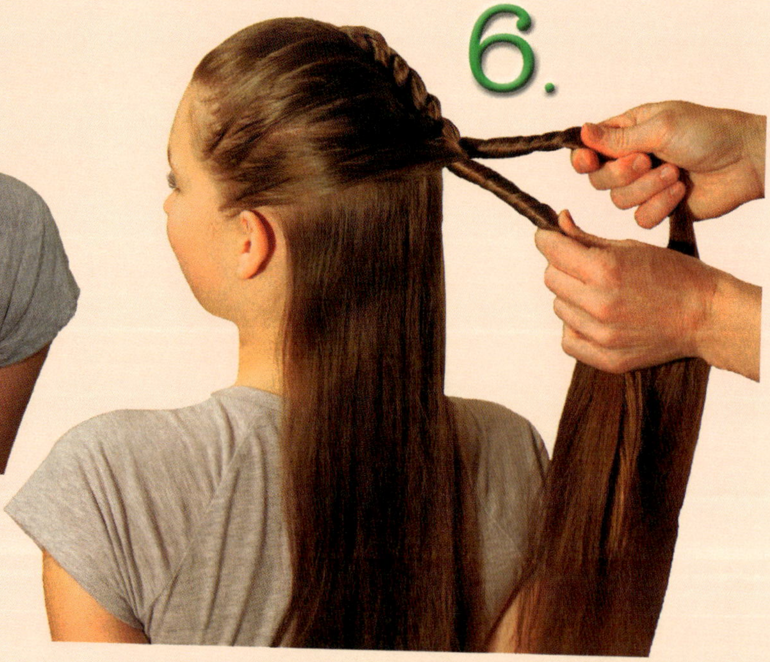

Then stop gathering while finishing the braid to the end of the tail.

www.findingbraids.com

Single Cascade

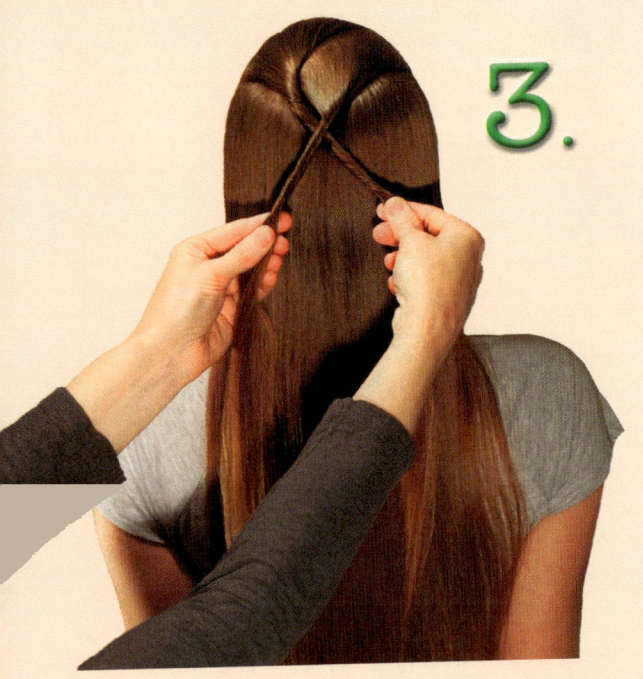

This one is a two-strand rope.

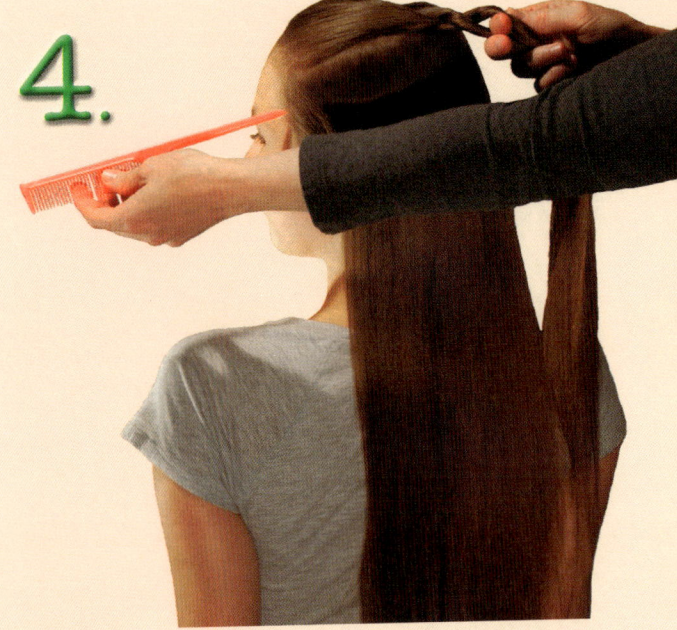

Braid while gathering until you reach the ears.

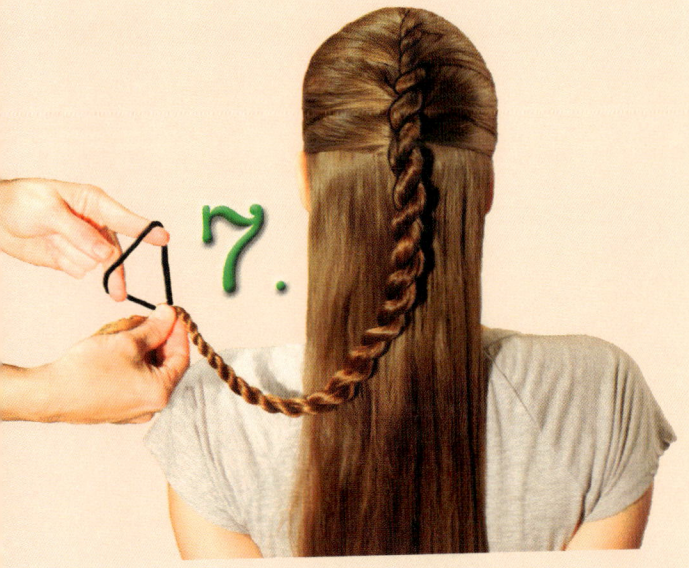

Secure the end with a band.

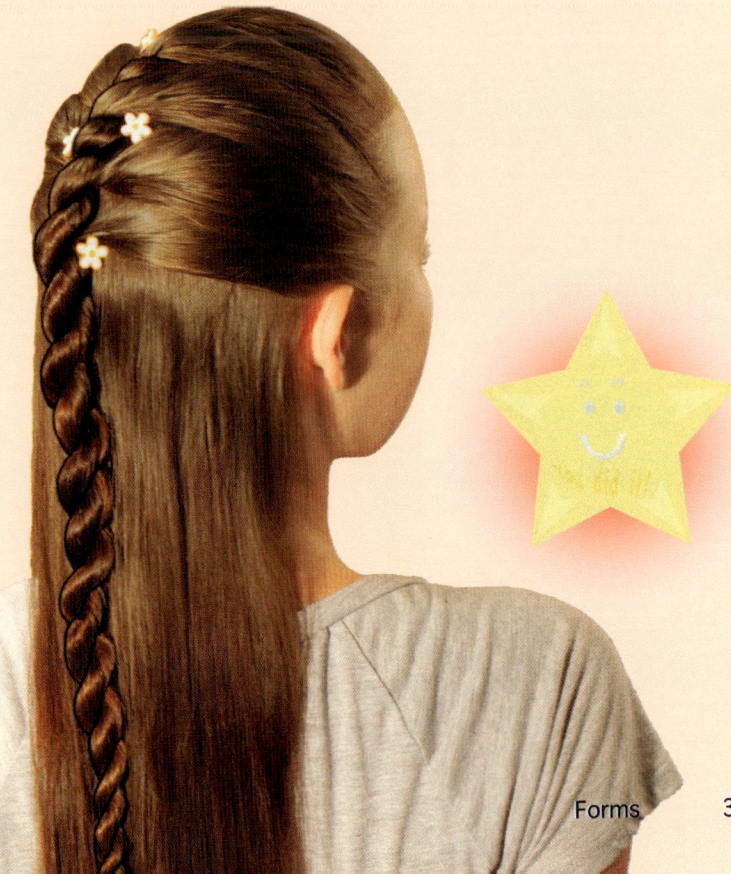

Accented Single Cascade

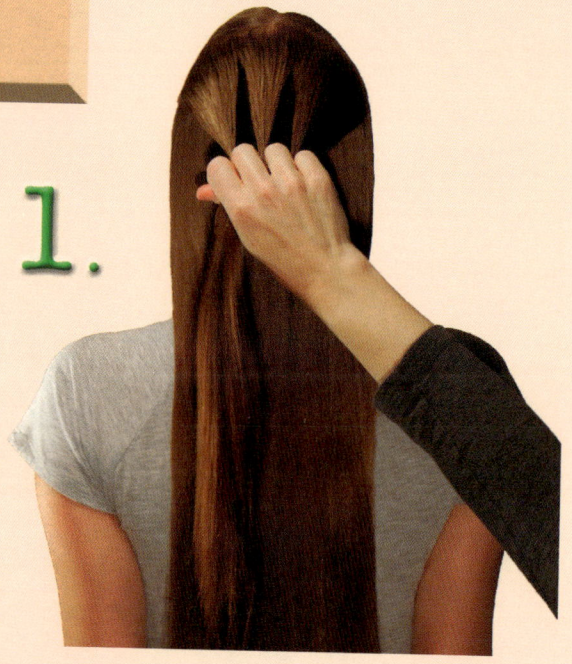

1. Single braids can go straight back, diagonal, upside down or in an "S" snake pattern.

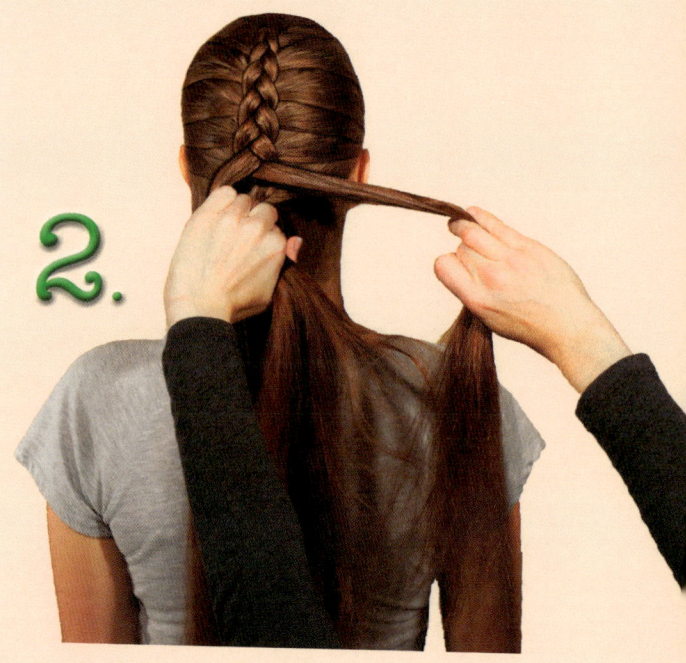

2. Create a single braid with any number of strands. This one is a three-strand dutch. This is also a cascade with accents.

5. Continue tugging out the sides of the braid all the way up each bump of the braid until you have done the entire braid.

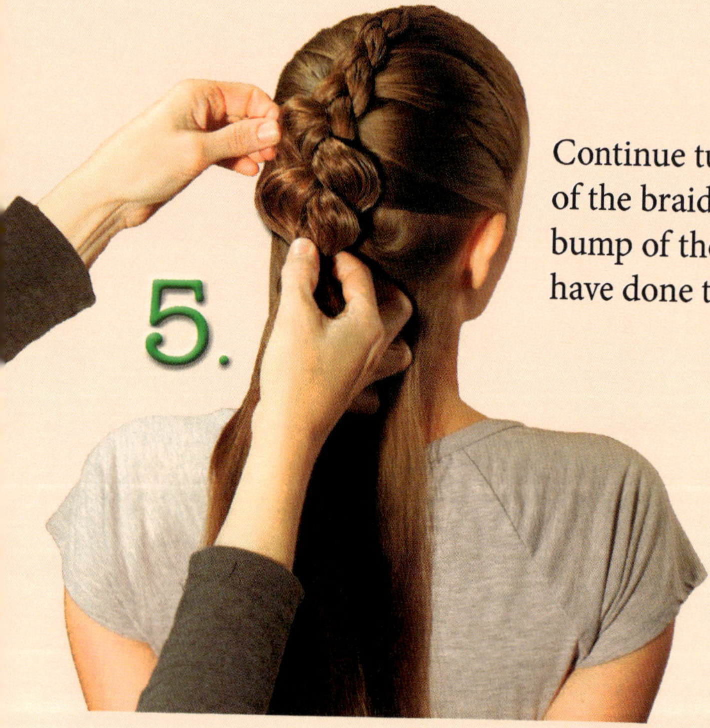

6. Pull out accent strands where you need them.

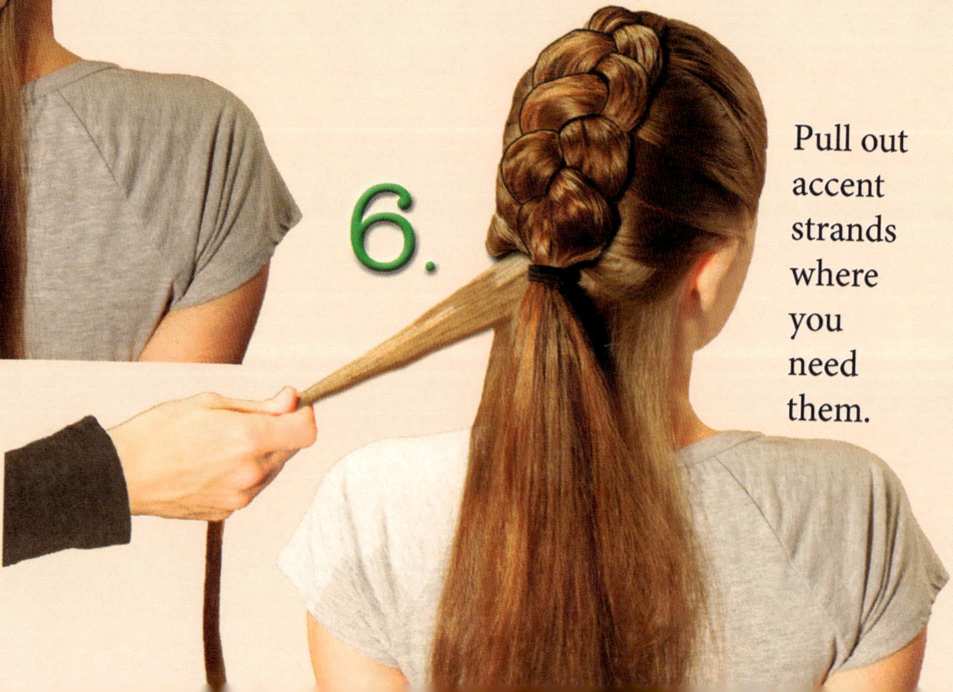

368   www.findingbraids.com

Accented Single Cascade

3.

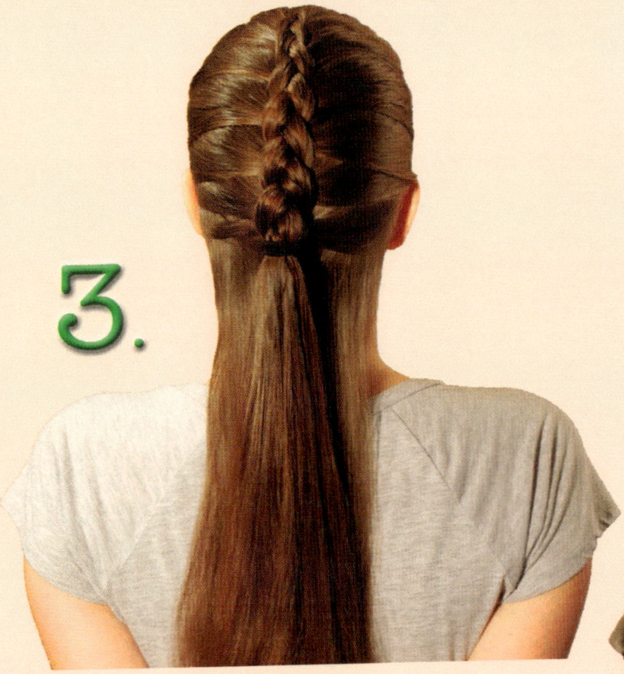

Braid until you reach the ears with your gathers and stop gathering. Here we will tie off the braid, level with the ears.

4. Tug out the sides of the braid itself.

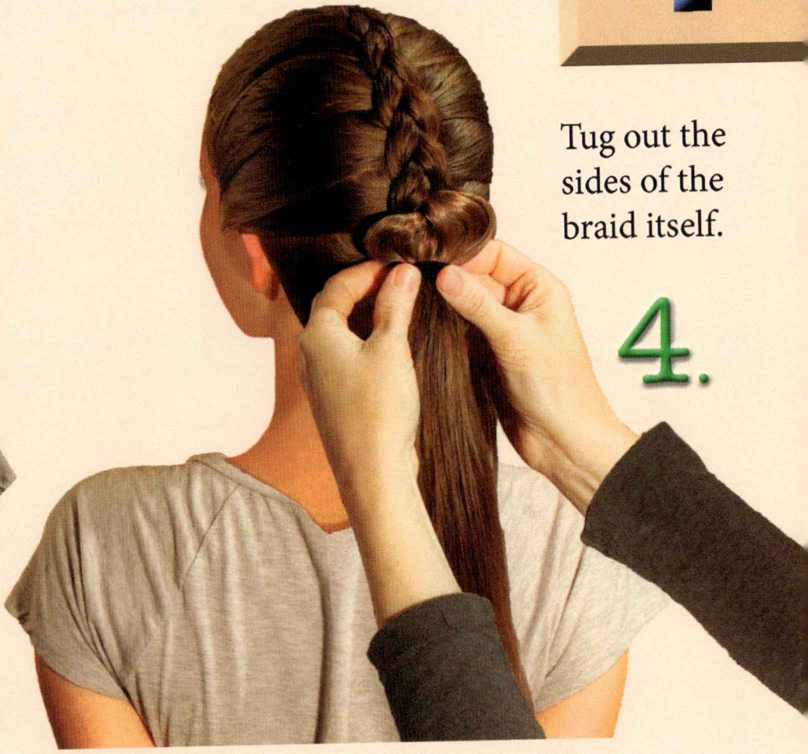

7.

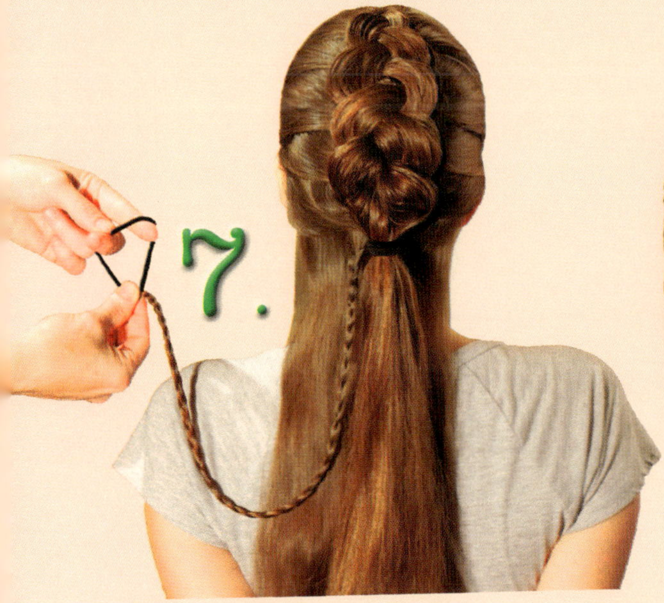

Create your accent. Pin it securely when finished.

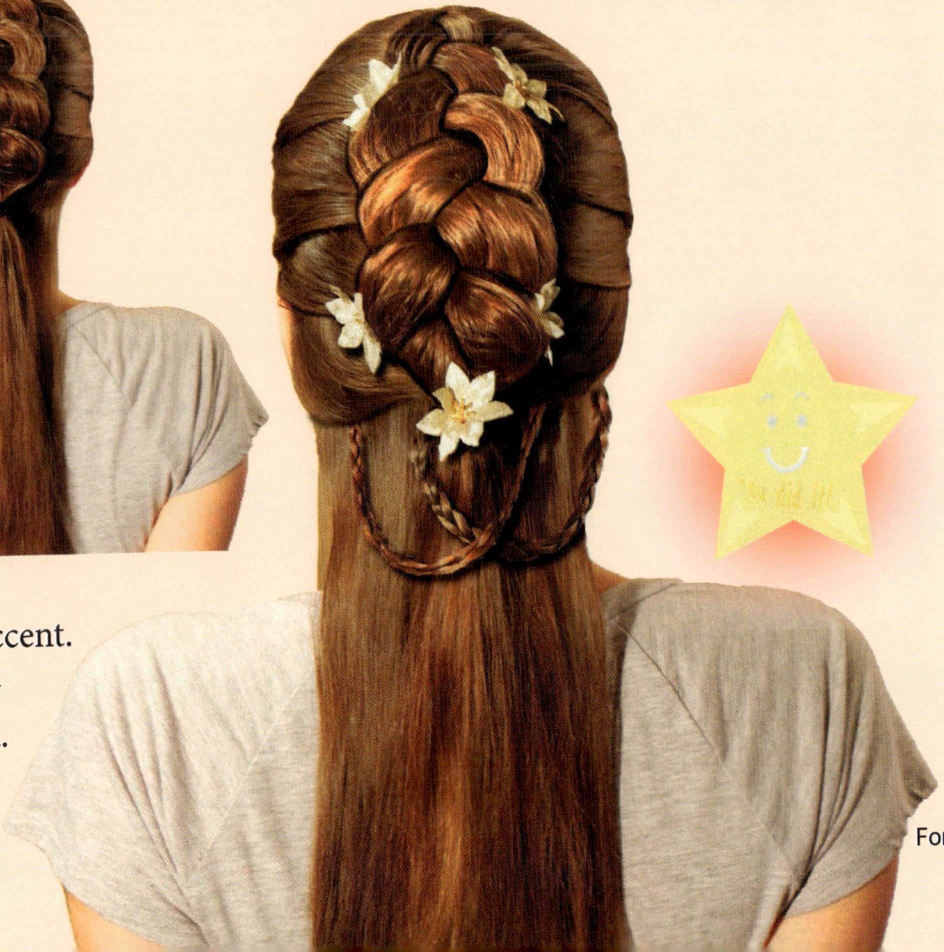

Forms 369

Forms

Notes

Examples of Singles

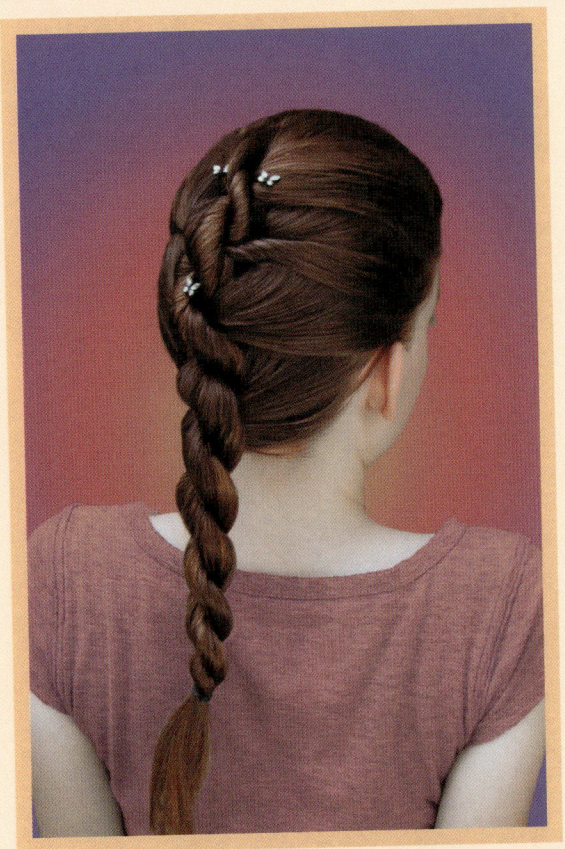
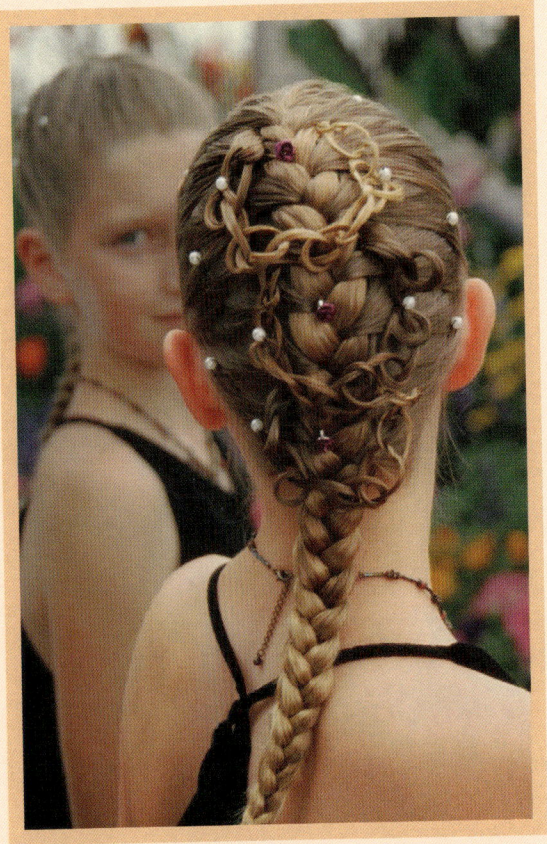
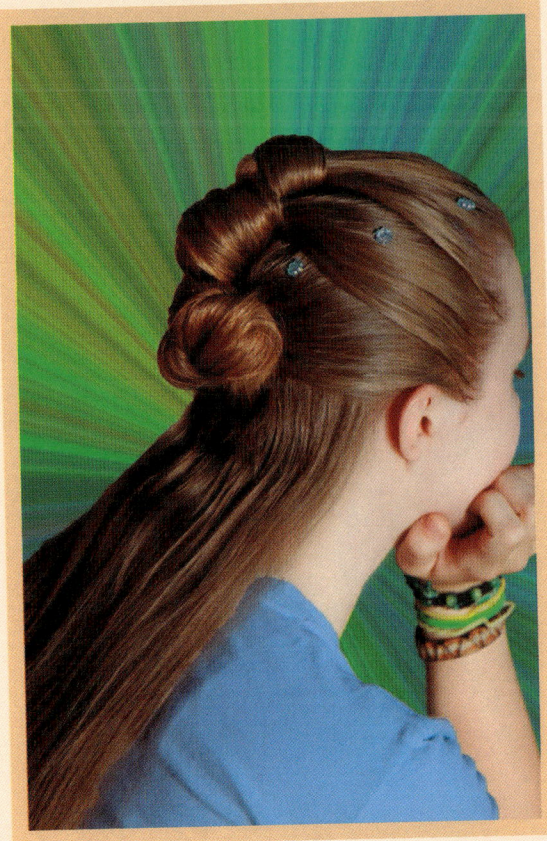
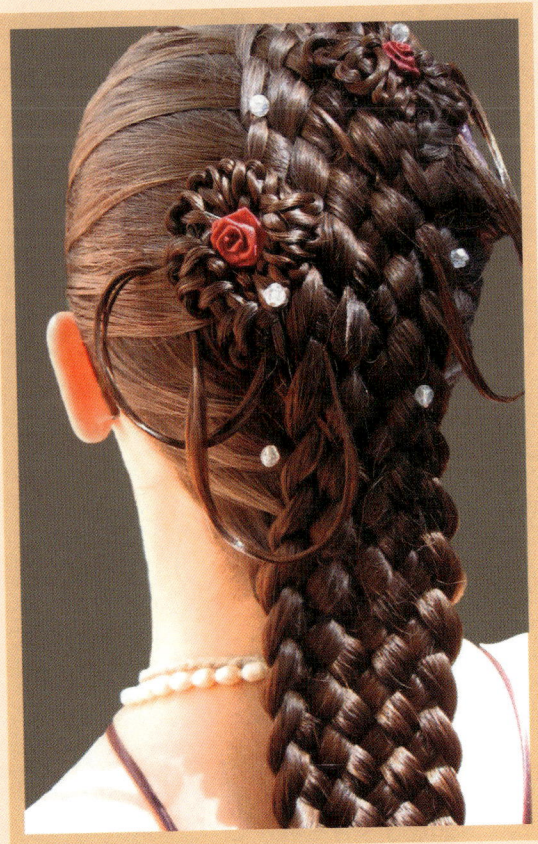

Visit my website to see more examples of Singles

Forms

DOUBLE

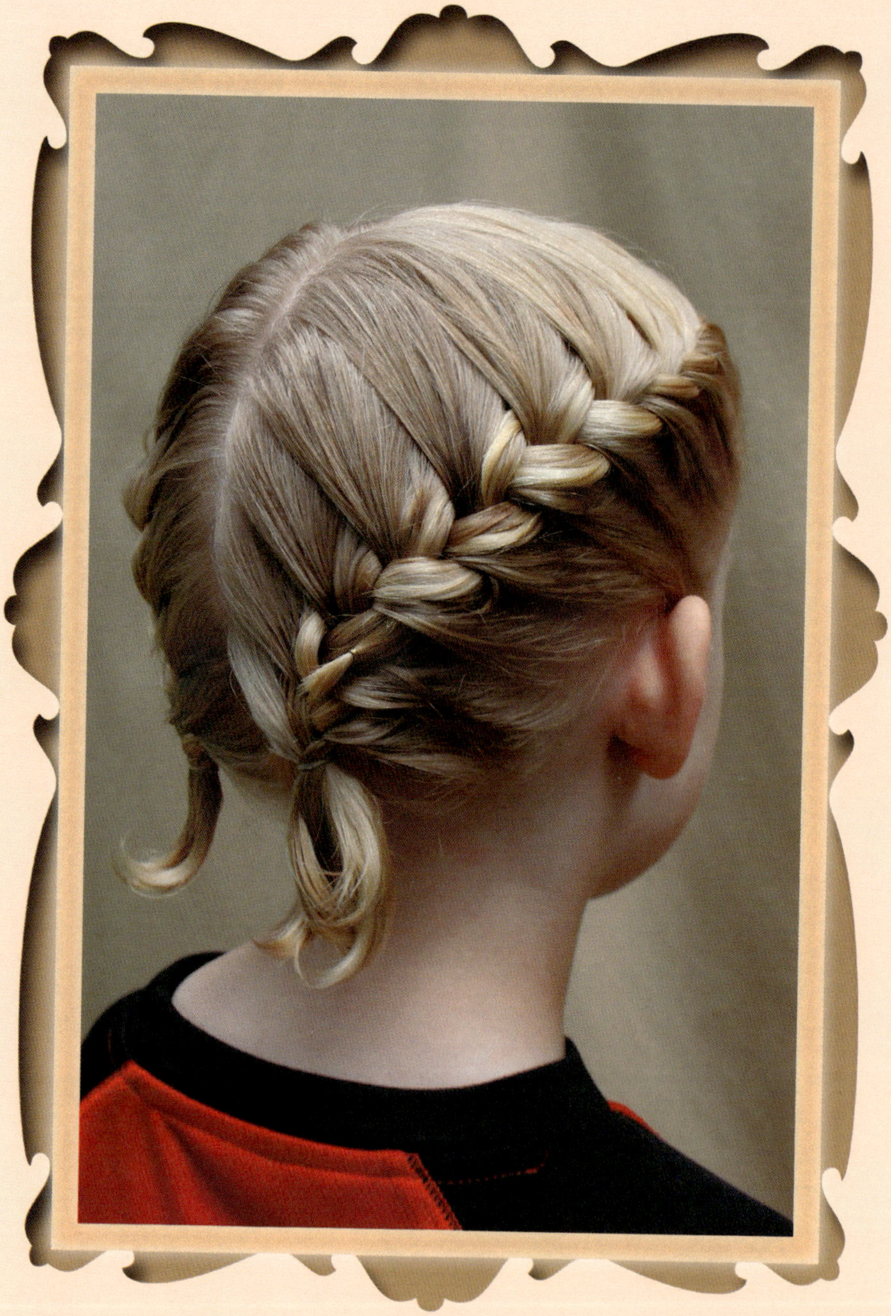

Ignite your imagination with the possibilities in this form. Perfect for practical use and with a bit more effort, extreme elegance at your disposal.

Forms

Gather like this!

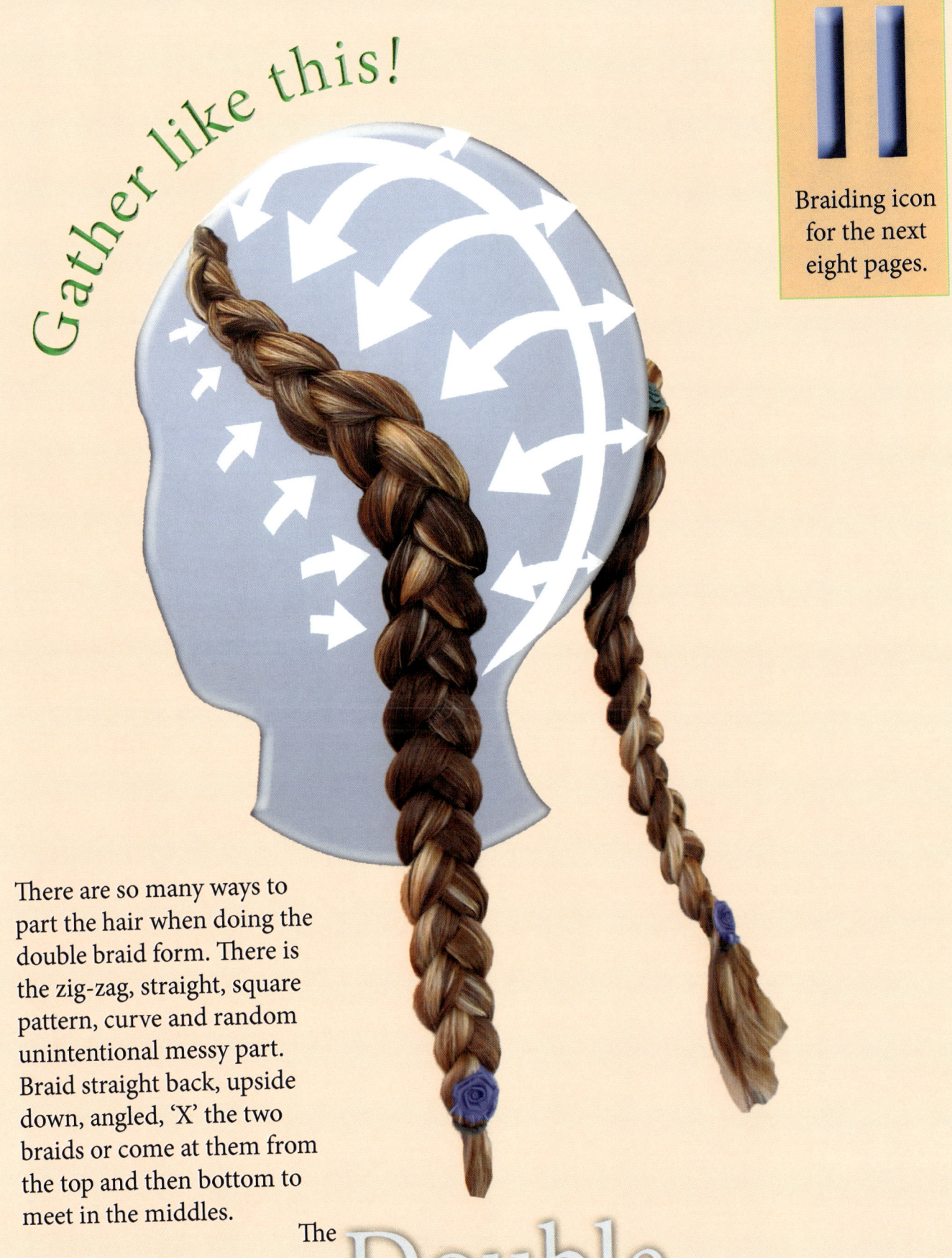

Braiding icon for the next eight pages.

There are so many ways to part the hair when doing the double braid form. There is the zig-zag, straight, square pattern, curve and random unintentional messy part. Braid straight back, upside down, angled, 'X' the two braids or come at them from the top and then bottom to meet in the middles.

The **Double** Form

Basic Double

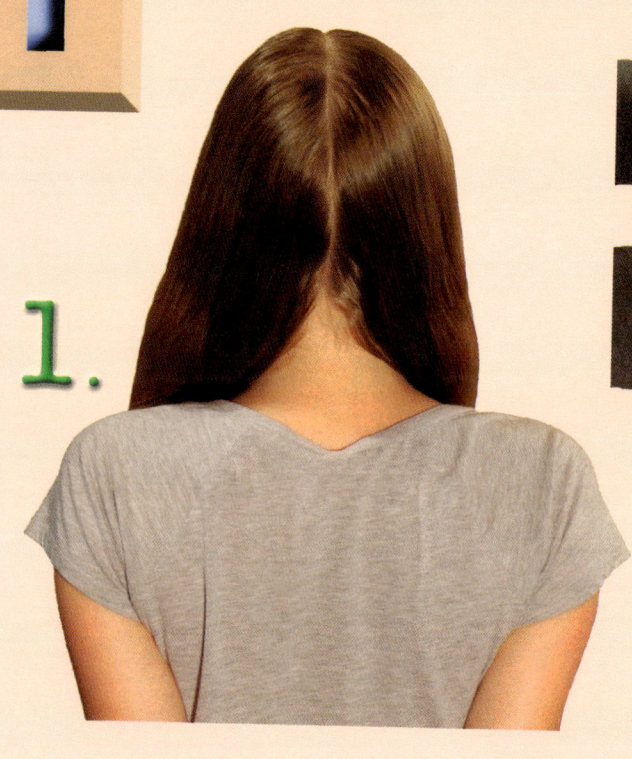

Part down the middle.

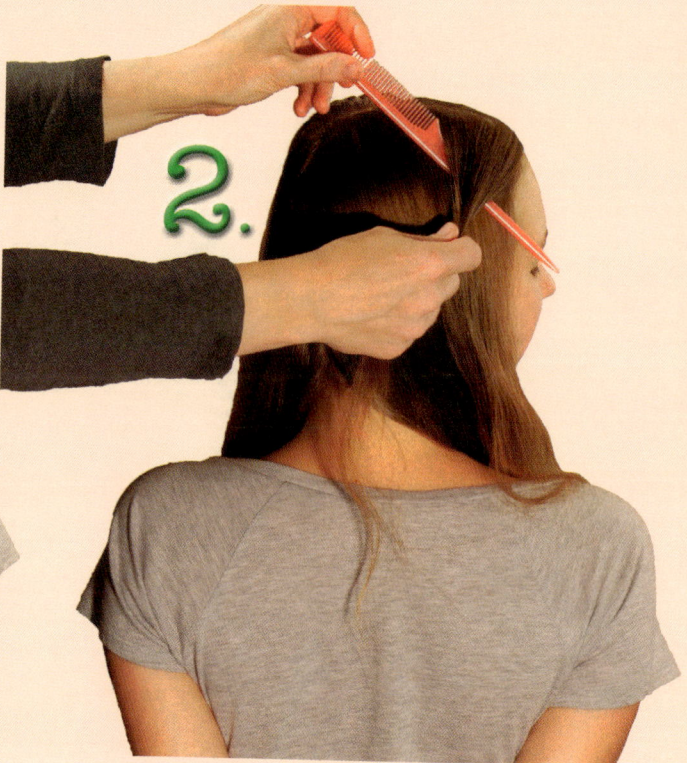

Choose the number of strands you will work with and start on one side of the head.

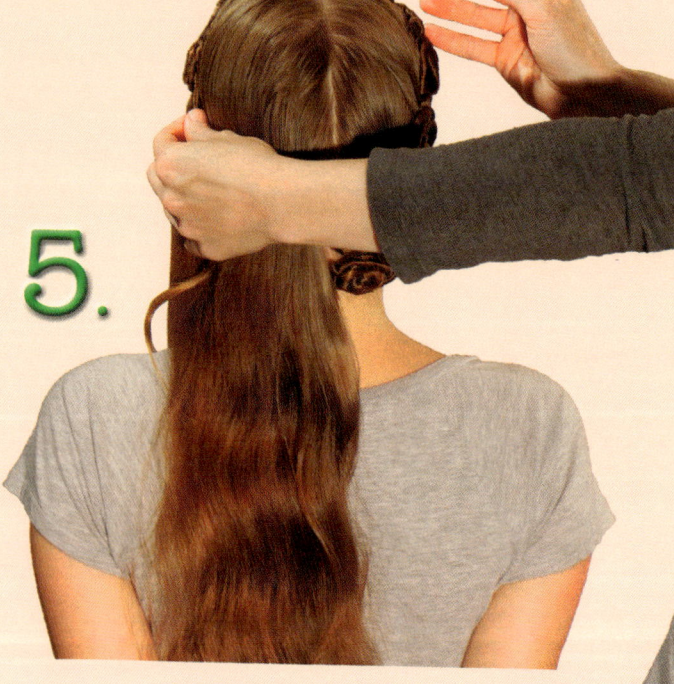

Do the same on the opposite side.

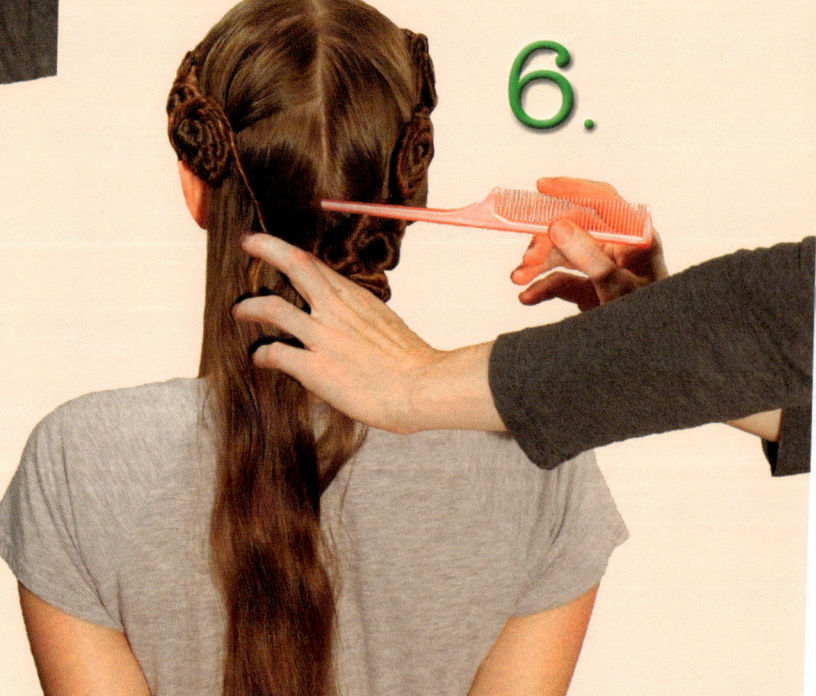

Basic Double

11

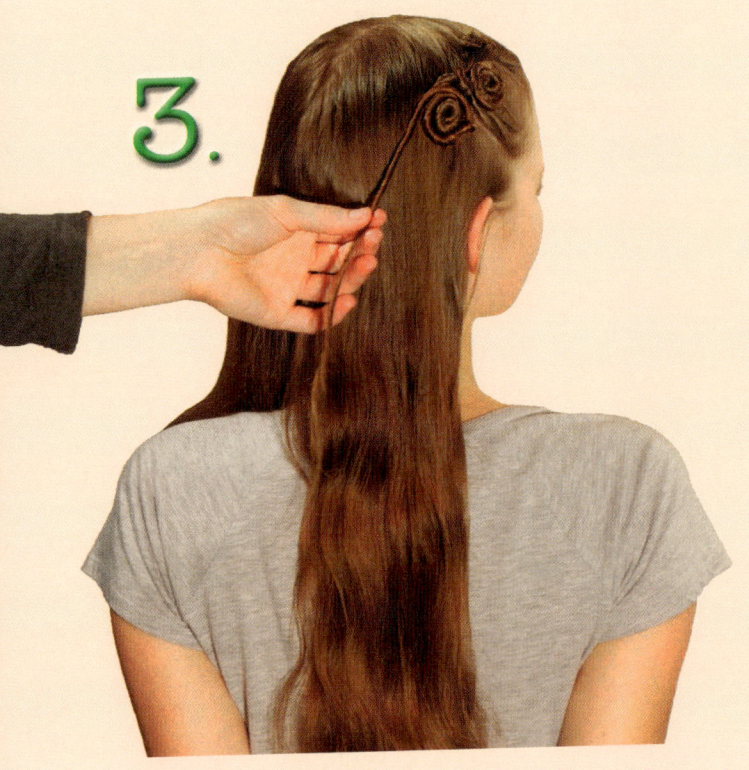

3.

Braid your way to the back of the head.

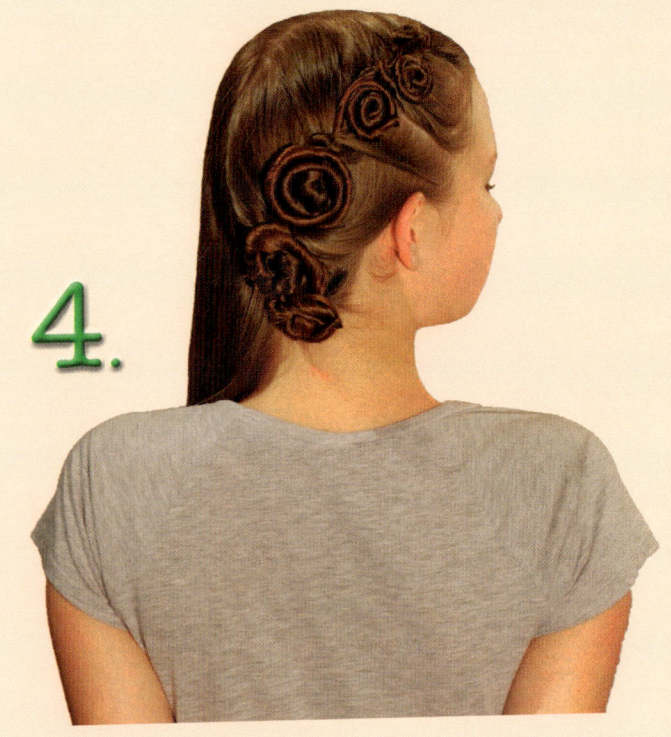

4.

This is a one-strand rosette.

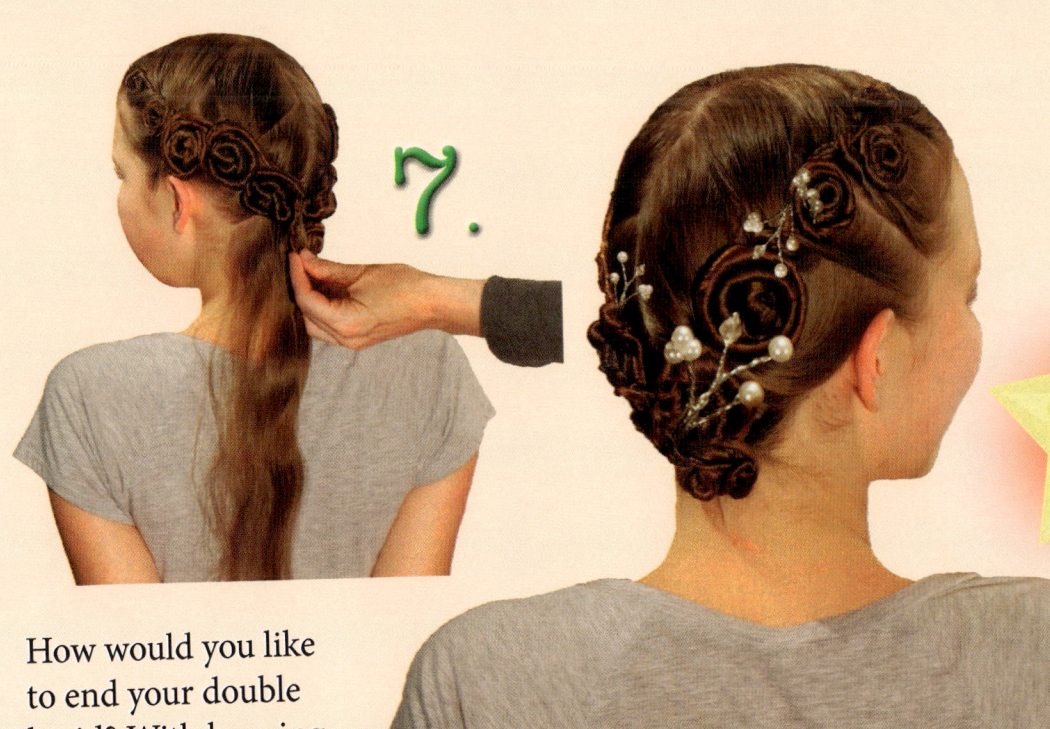

7.

How would you like to end your double braid? With hanging hair, a low bun or two braids down the back?

Forms 375

Accented Double

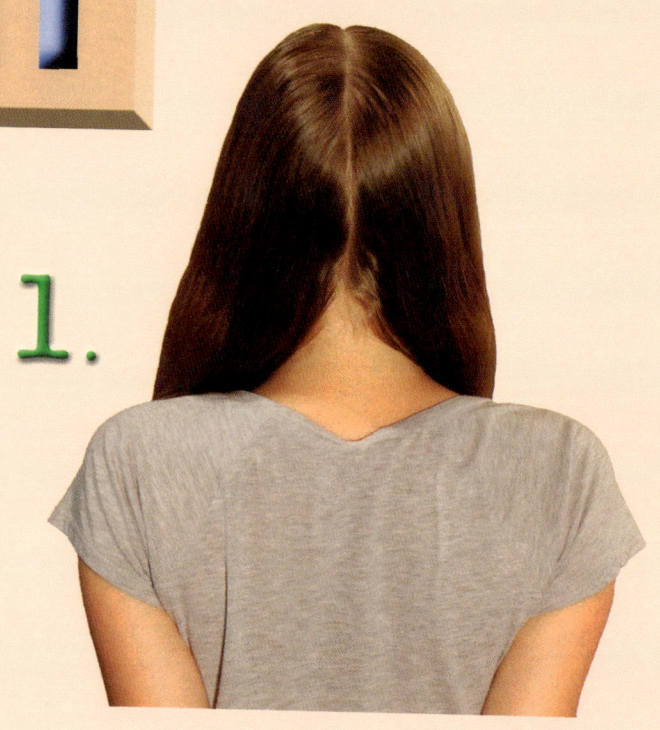

1. Part down the middle.

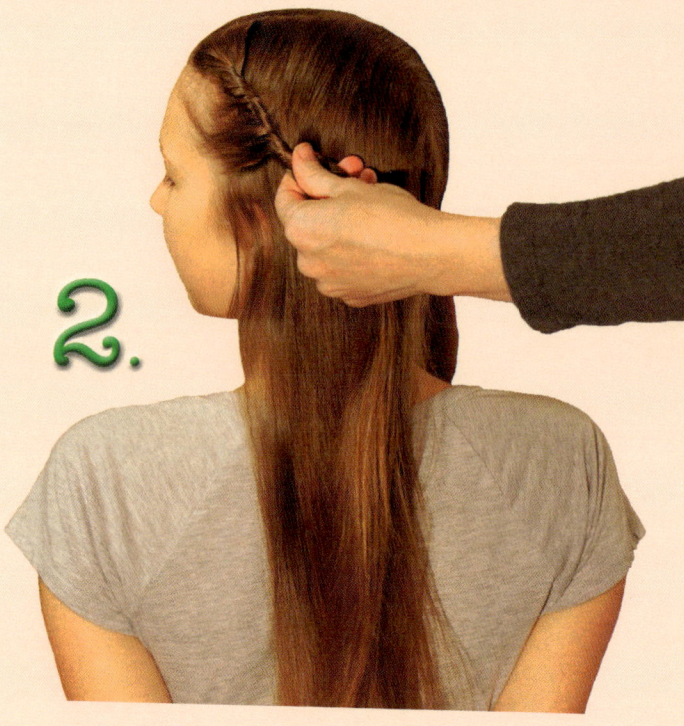

2. Choose the number of strands you will work with and start on one side of the head. Braid your way to the back of the head.

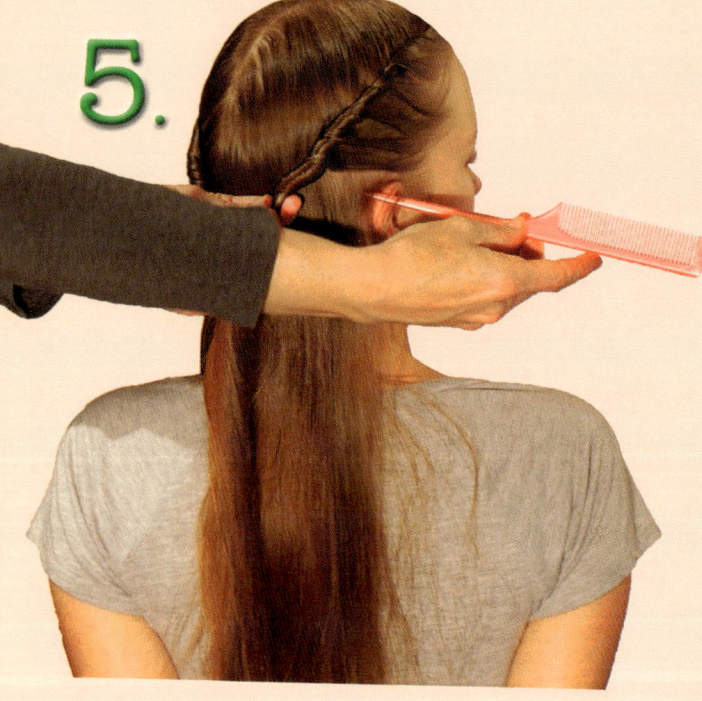

5. Do the same on the opposite side.

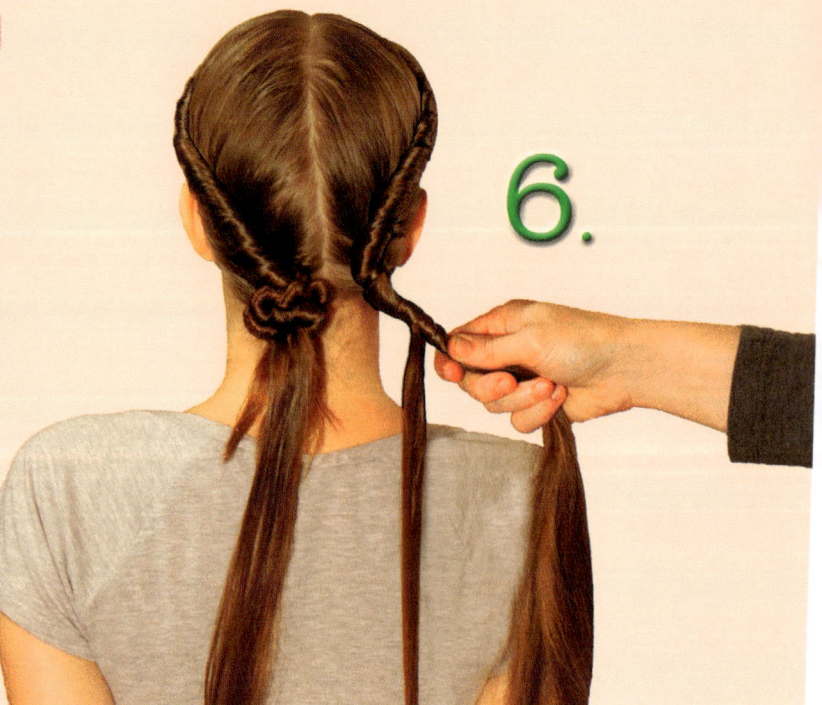

6.

www.findingbraids.com

Accented Double

3.

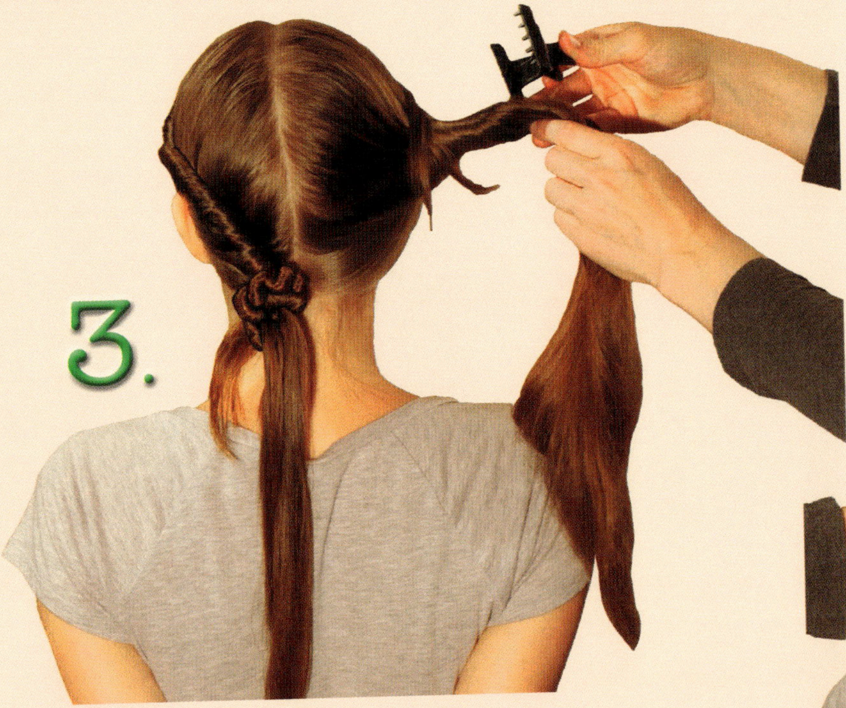

Do the same thing on the other side of the head assuming you are creating something symmetrical.

4.

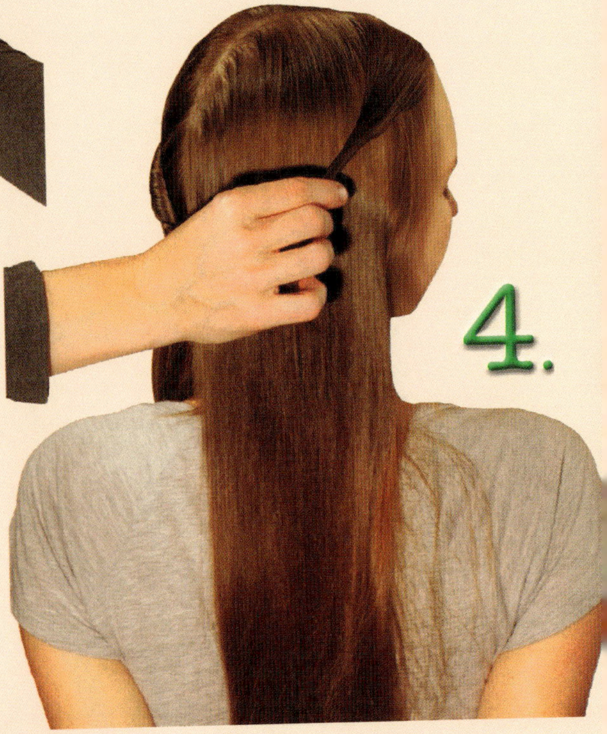

This is a one-strand twist.

7.

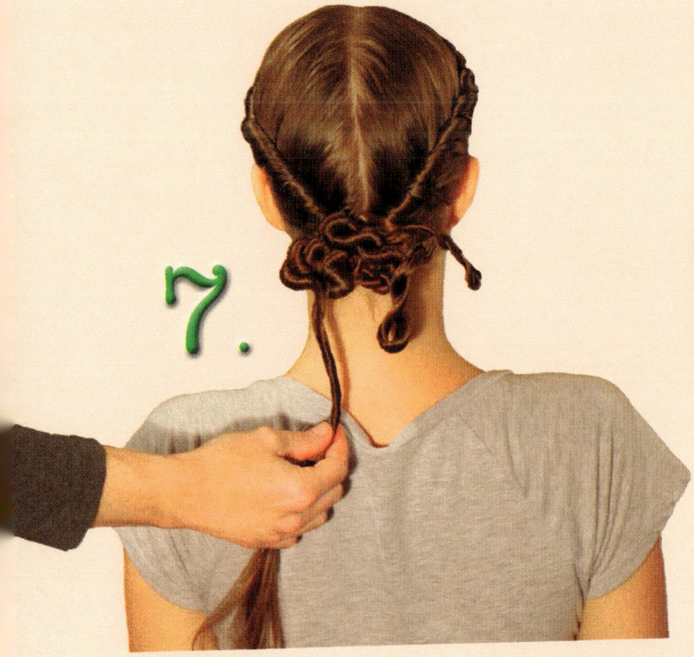

I use the tails to create a bunch of mini one-strand twist accents.

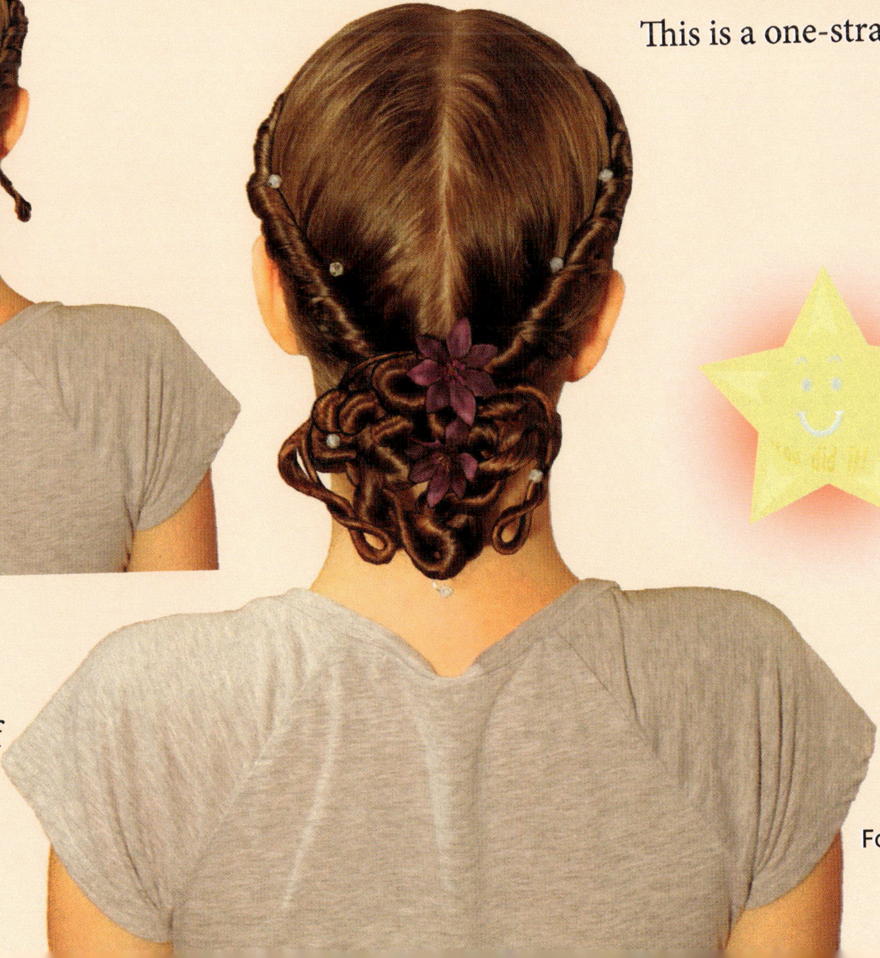

Double Cascade

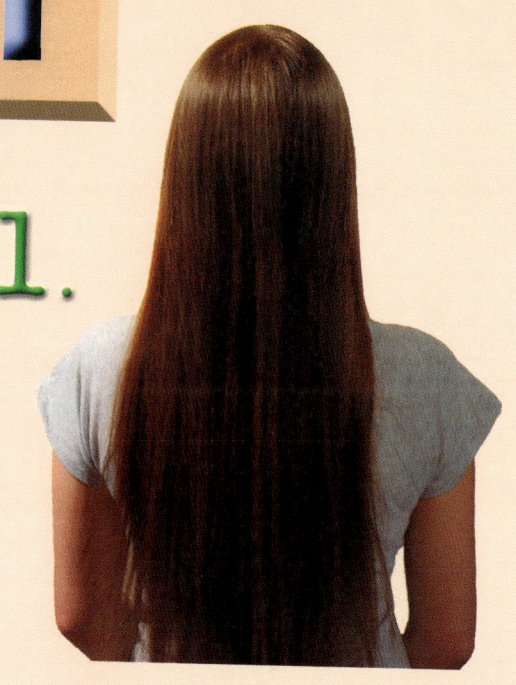

1. Begin with clean, brushed hair.

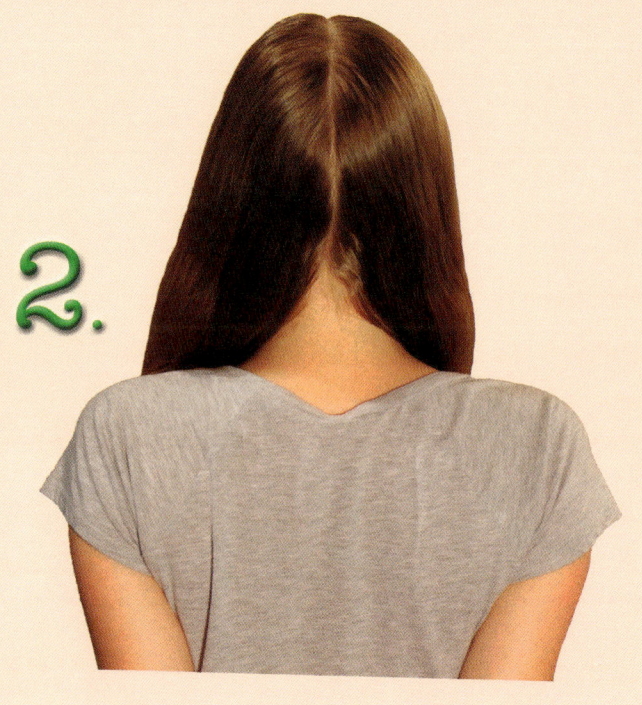

2. Part down the middle.

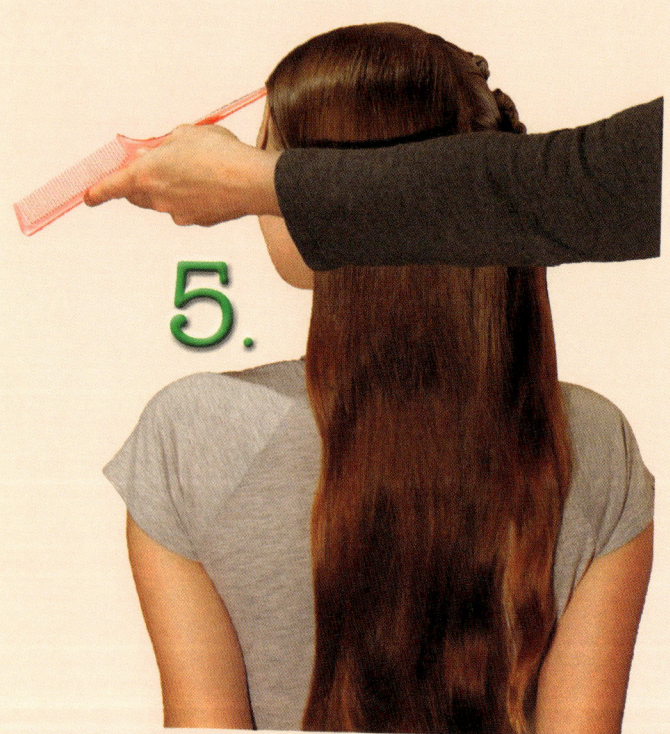

5. Do the same on the opposite side.

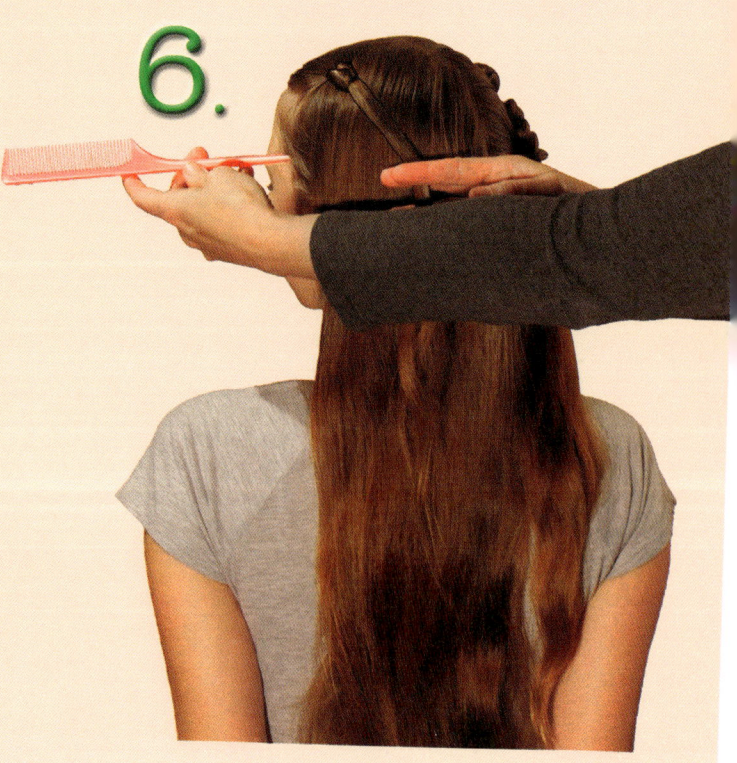

6.

Double Cascade

3.

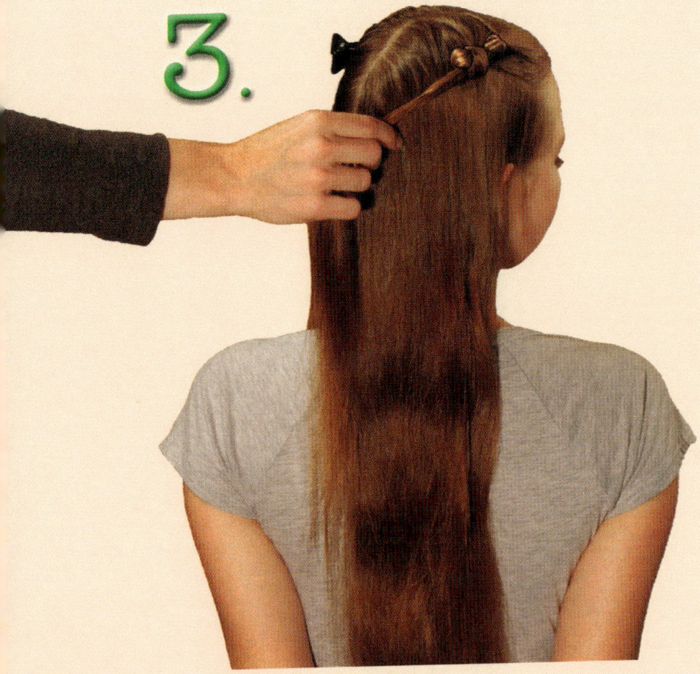

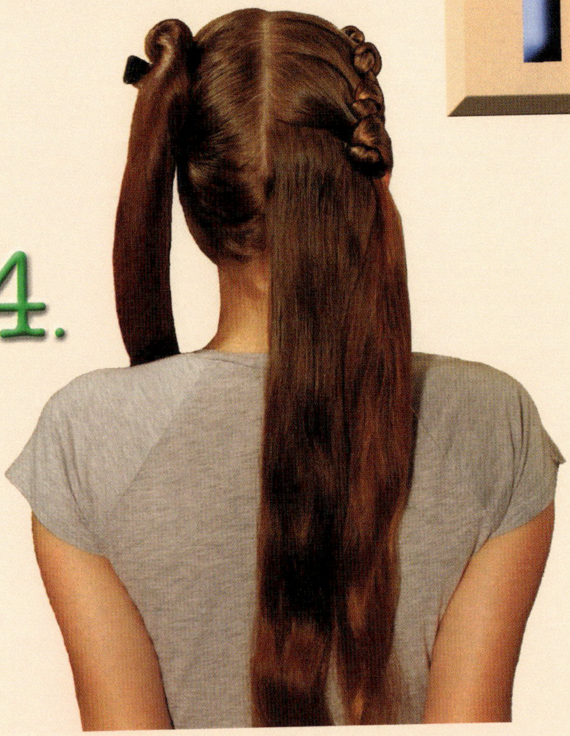

Choose the number of strands you will work with and start on one side of the head.

4.

Braid your way to the back of the head stopping just behind the ears to leave a cascade. This is a one-strand pretzel.

7.

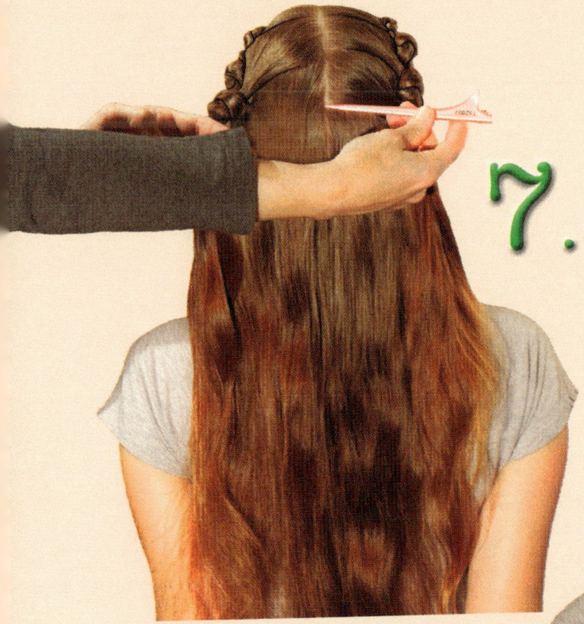

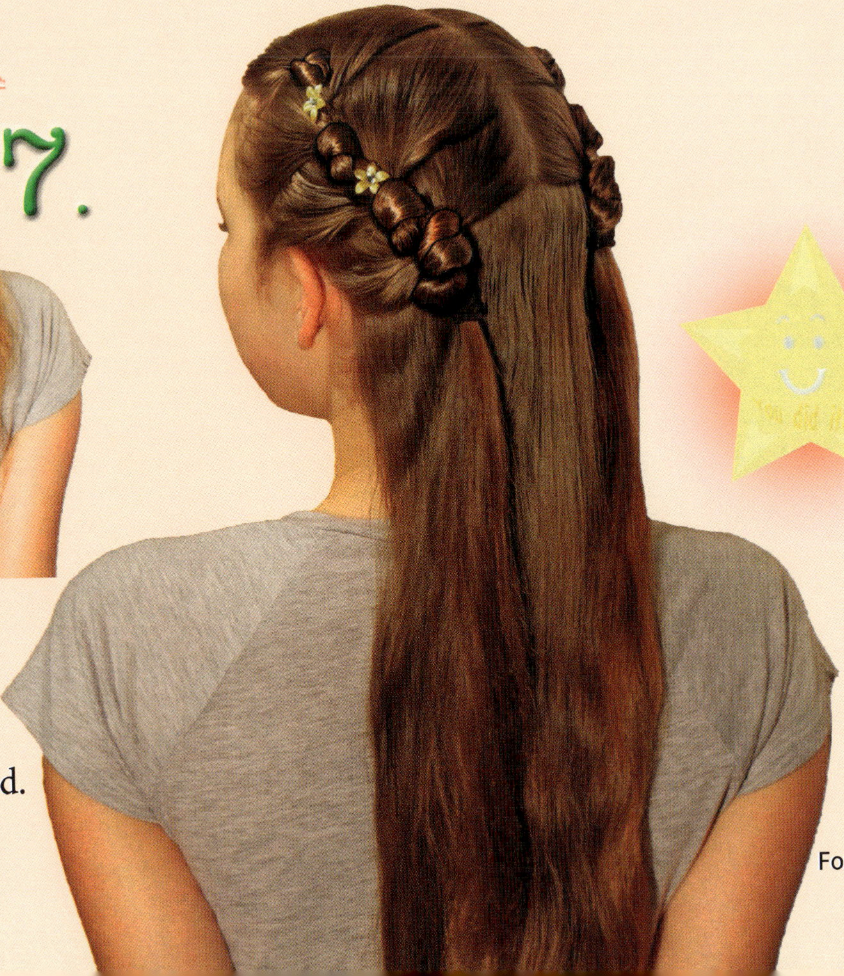

If you can match the gather lines opposite each other it makes a very tidy finished braid.

Forms 379

Accented Double Cascade

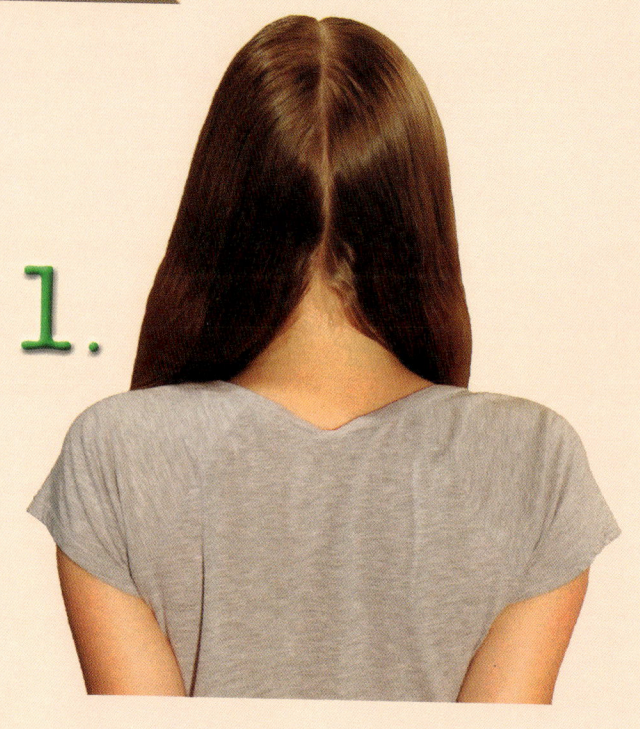

1. Part down the middle.

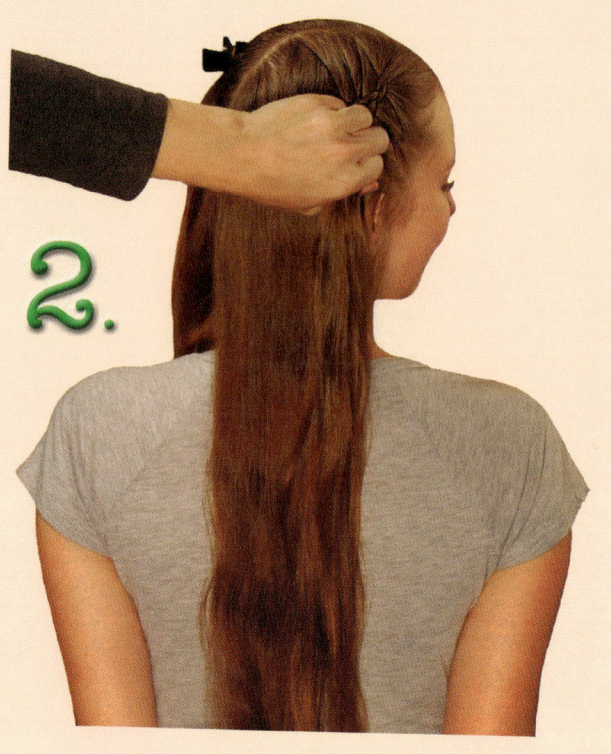

2. Choose the number of strands you will work with and start on one side of the head.

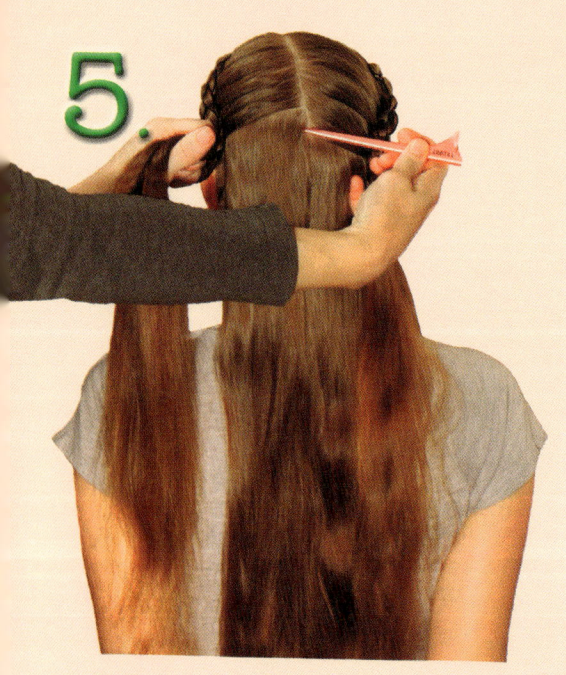

5.

6. Take your accent strands from an appropriate place, I am taking them from under the braid from the cascade.

Accented Double Cascade

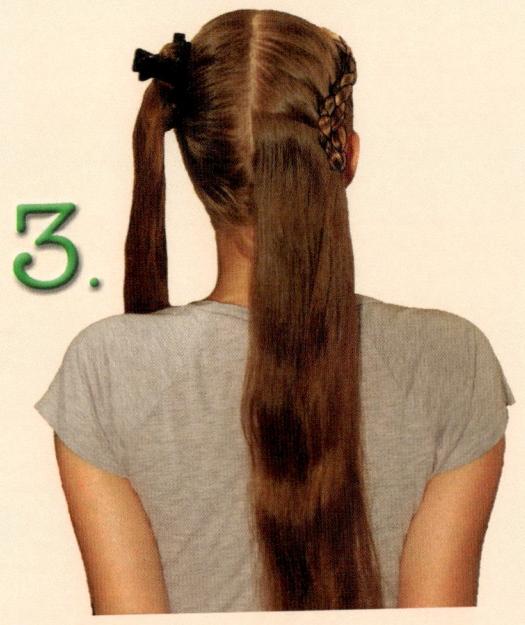

3.

Braid your way to the back of the head stopping just behind the ears to leave a cascade. This is a four-strand round.

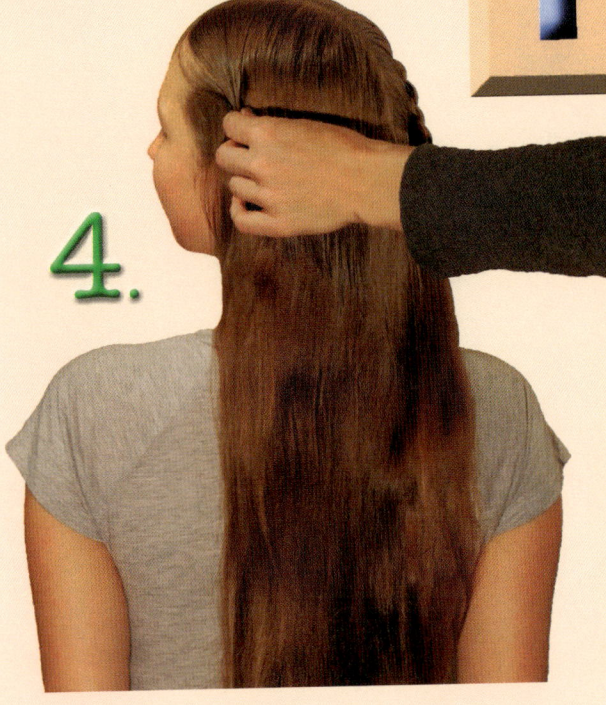

4.

Do the same on the opposite side.

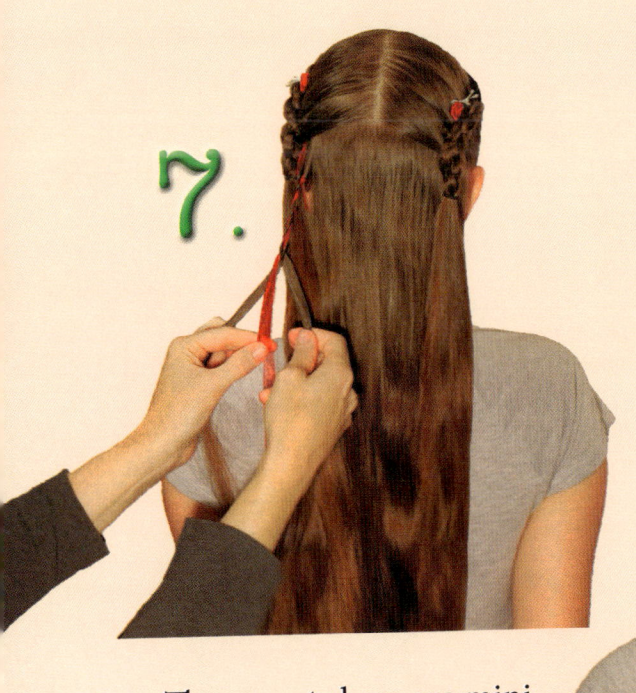

7.

The accents here are mini three-strands made with a ribbon and hair. Drape them in a fashion that is attractive.

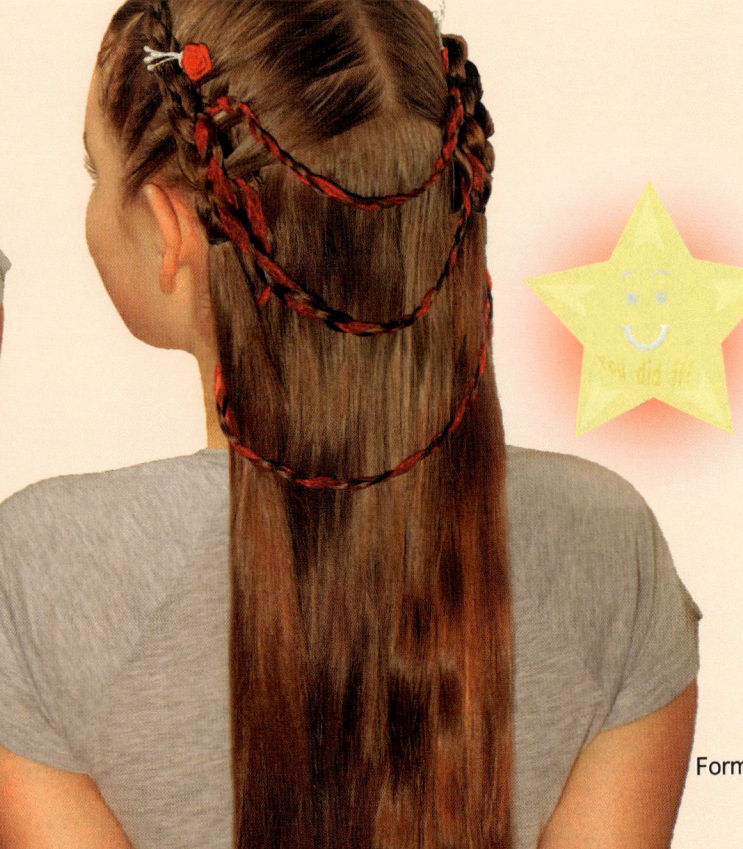

Forms

Notes

Examples of Doubles

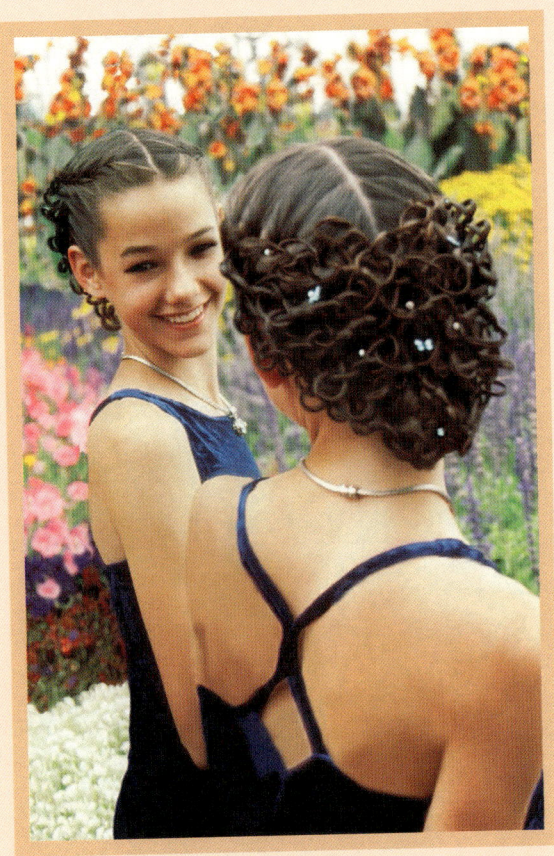
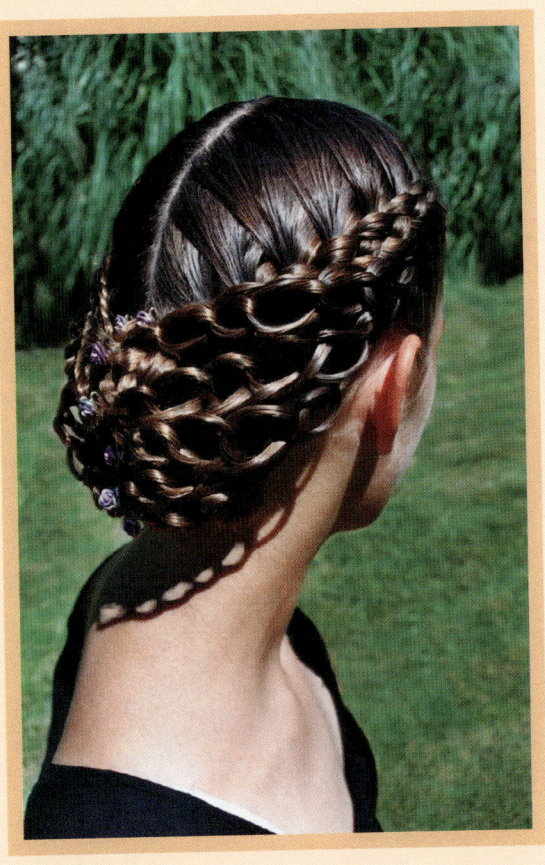
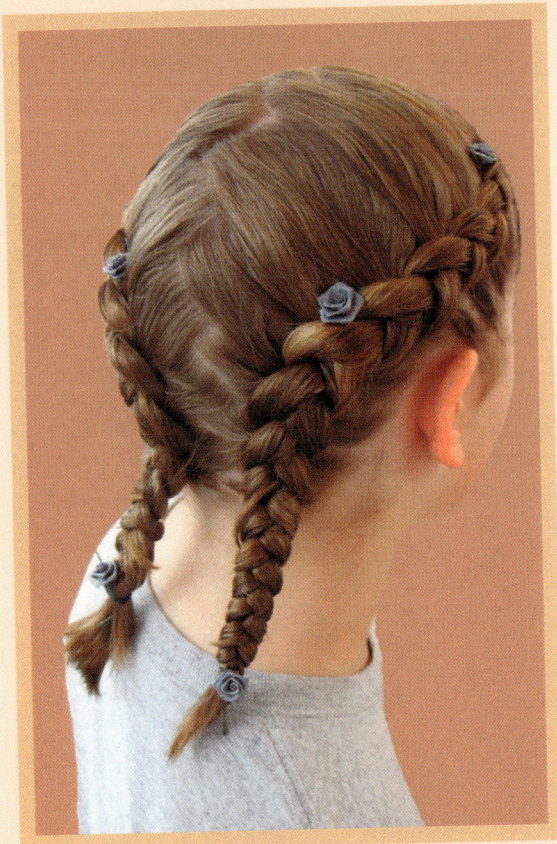
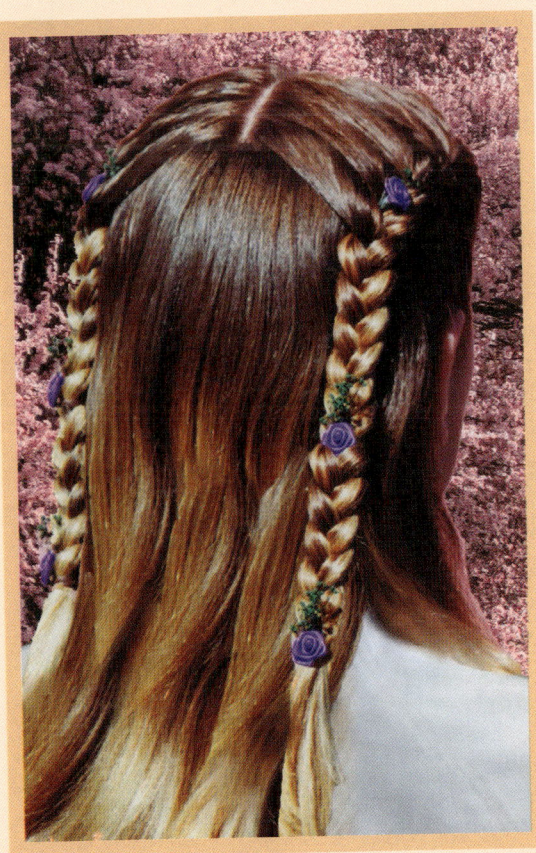

Visit my website to see more examples of Doubles

Forms

JUNCTION

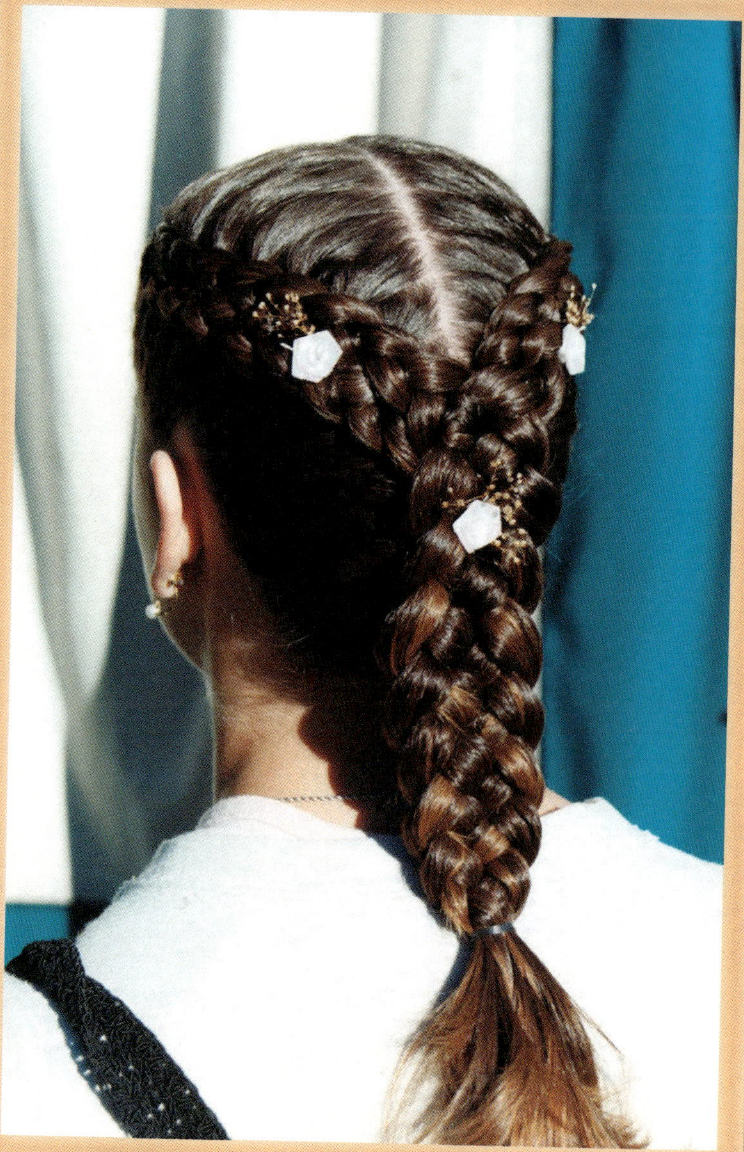

As your skill grows you will want this form in your bag of tricks. Utilitarian for a hard day's work or add a little flare to the form and you will leave an impression on the crowd.

Forms

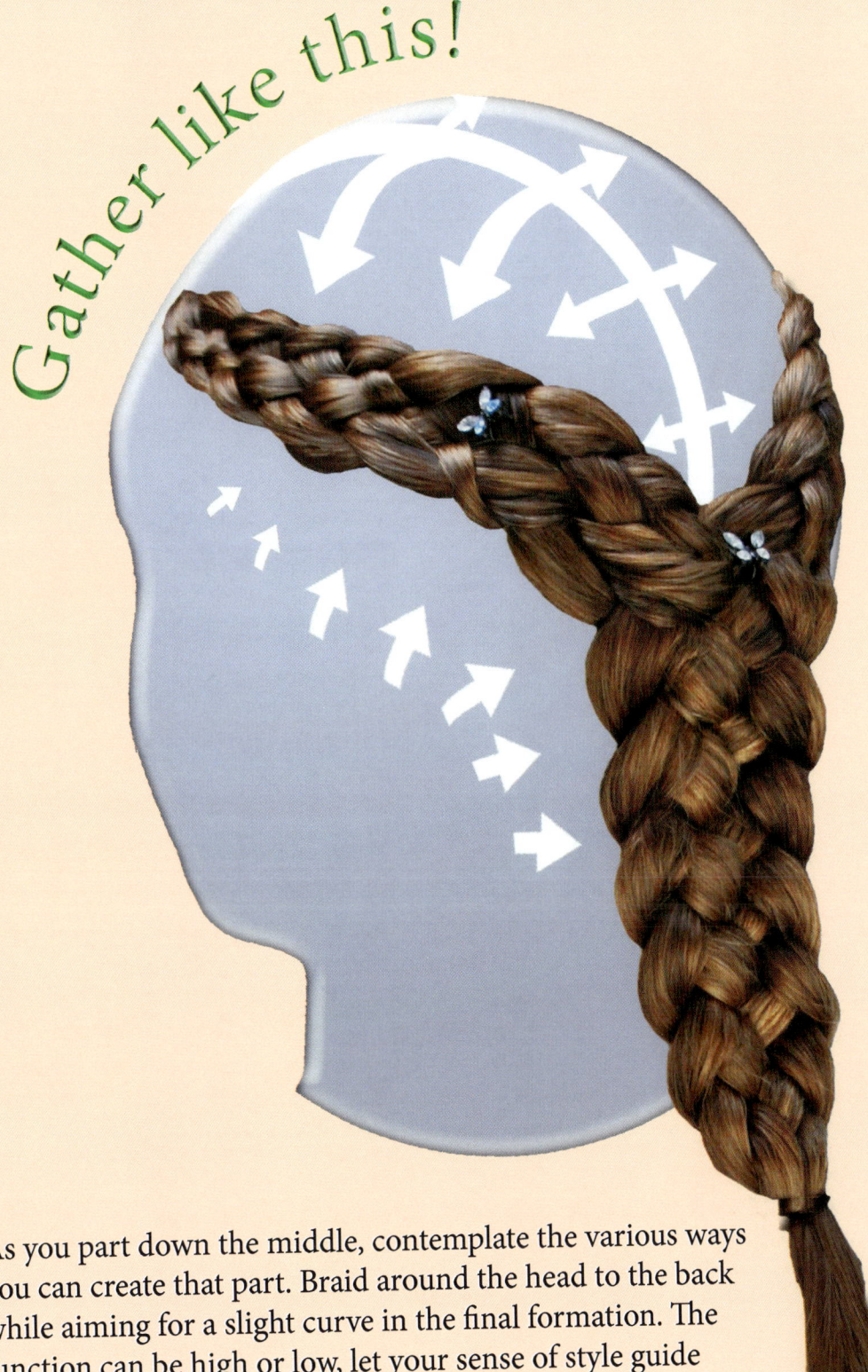

Gather like this!

Y — Braiding icon for the next eight pages.

As you part down the middle, contemplate the various ways you can create that part. Braid around the head to the back while aiming for a slight curve in the final formation. The junction can be high or low, let your sense of style guide you as you create each masterpiece.

The **Junction** Form

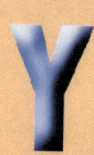

Basic Junction

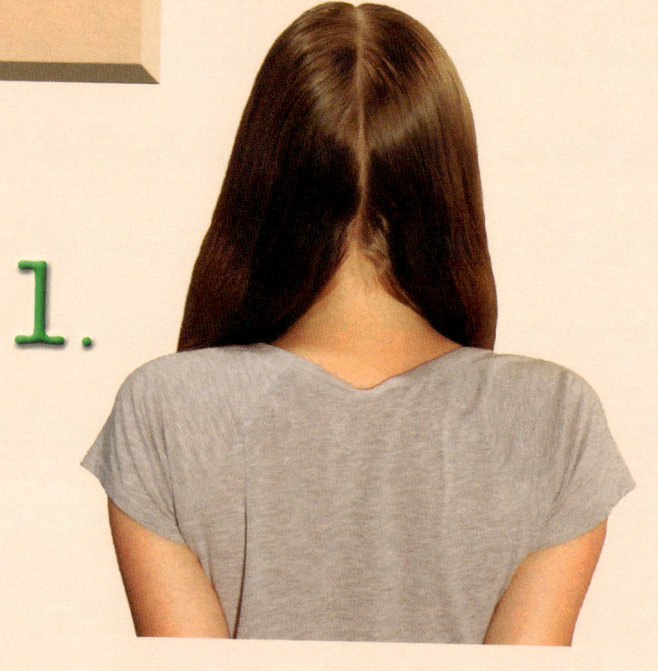

1. Part down the middle.

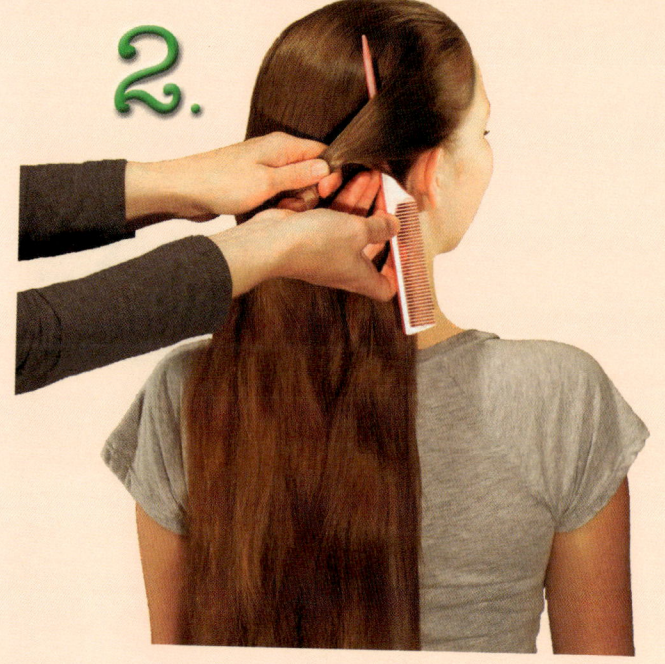

2. Choose the number of strands you will work with.

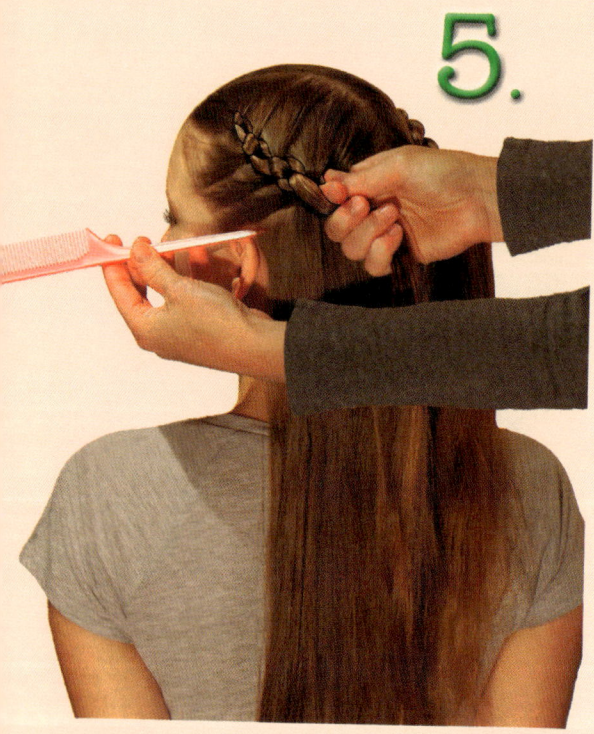

5. Do the same on the opposite side.

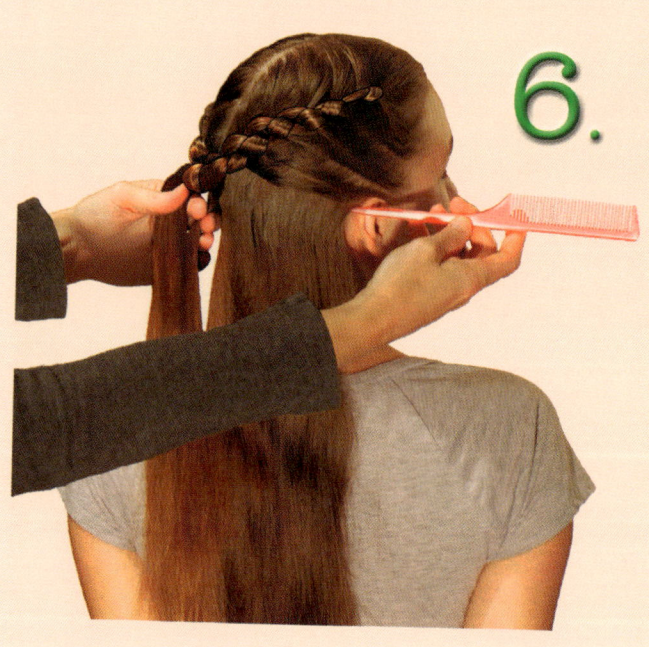

6. When you merge the tails you may use the same number of strands you have been braiding with or you can use all the strands from both sides to double the number of strands, or you can use a completely different number.

www.findingbraids.com

Basic Junction

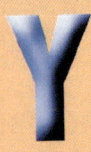

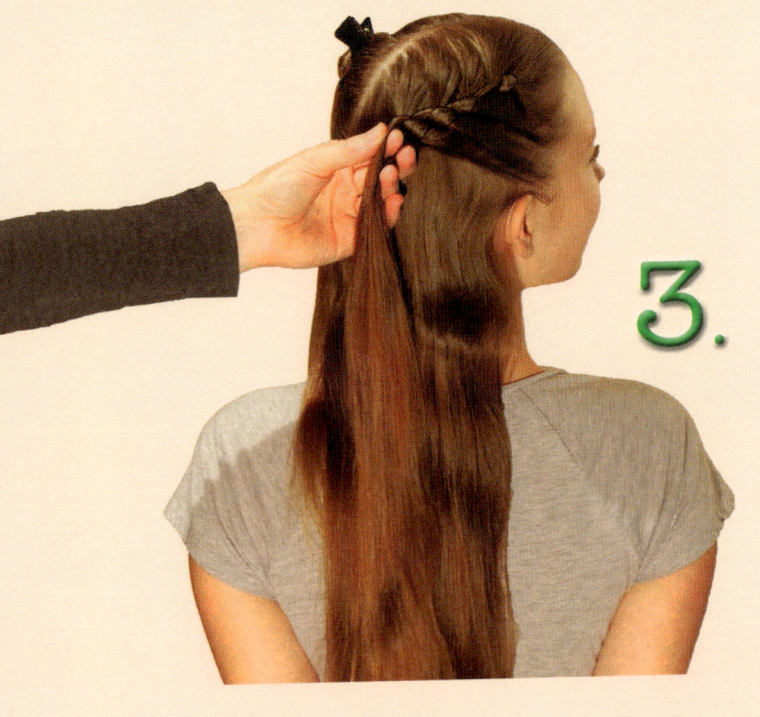

3.

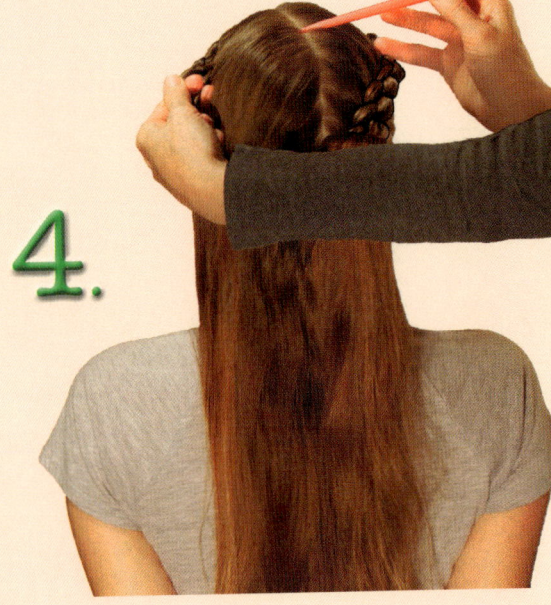

4.

This is a two-strand knot merging into a two-strand knot. Start of one side and braid your way to the back of the head.

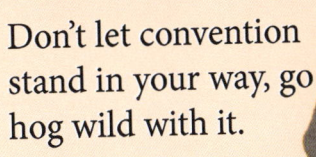

7.

Don't let convention stand in your way, go hog wild with it.

Accented Junction

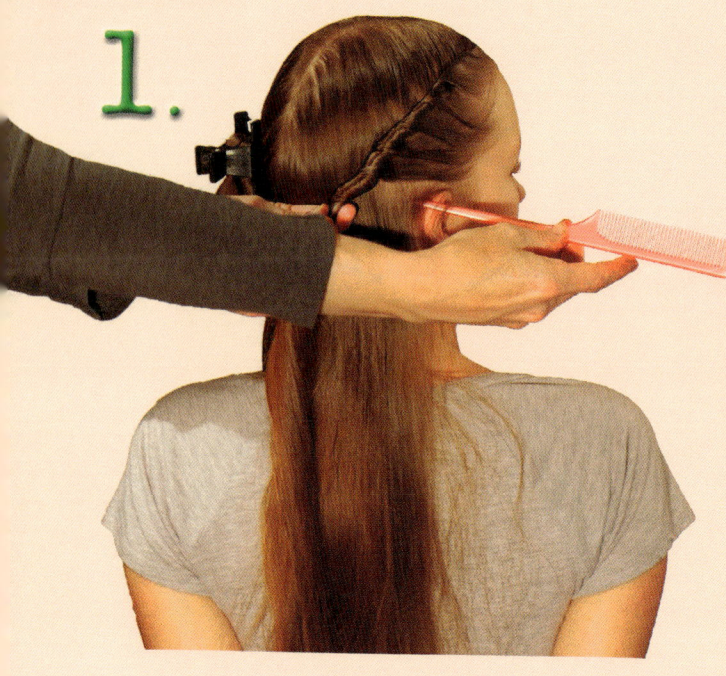

1. Choose the number of strands you will work with.

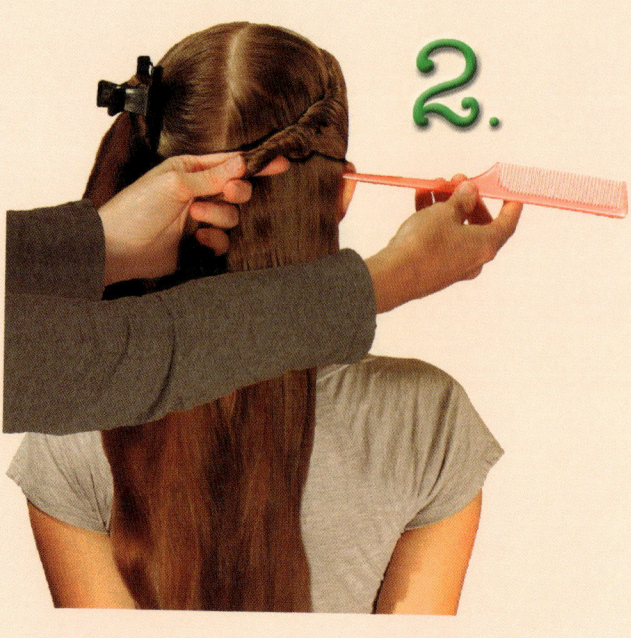

2. Junctions part down the middle and braid to the back of the head on each side. Try to make them symetrical and join the two braids in the back.

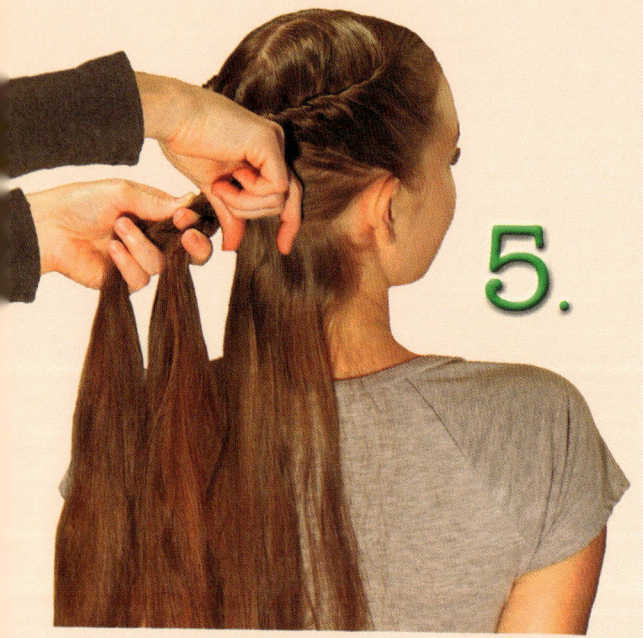

5. Take your accent from a location that will acheive the look you desire from the style.

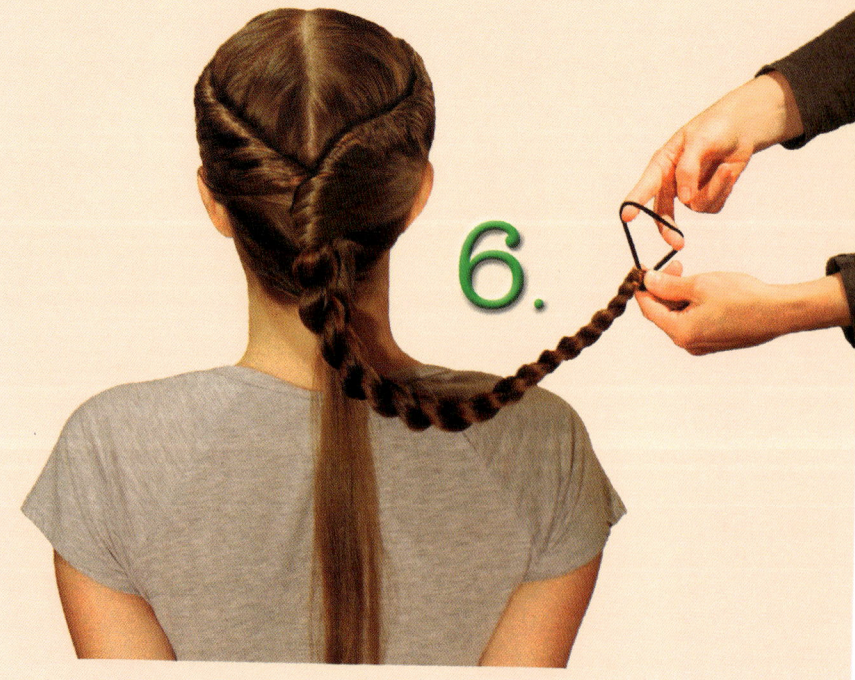

6.

Accented Junction

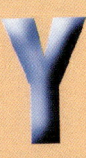

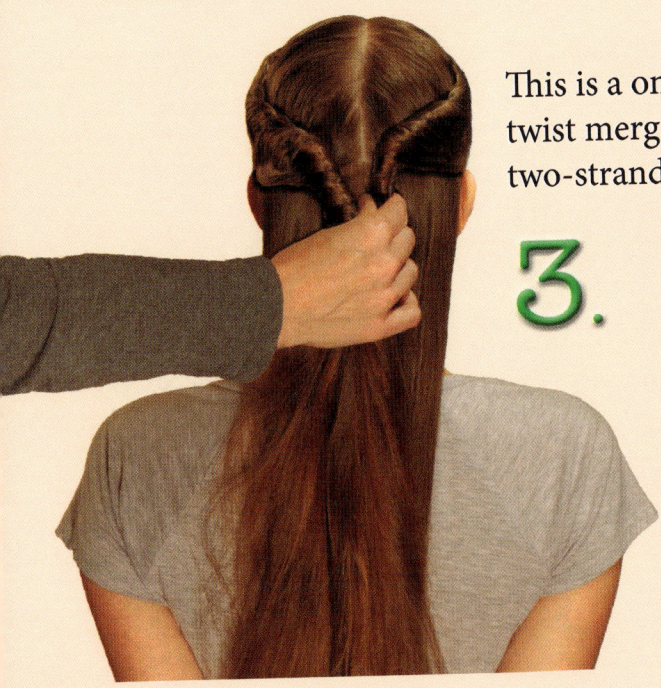

This is a one-strand twist merging into a two-strand rope.

3.

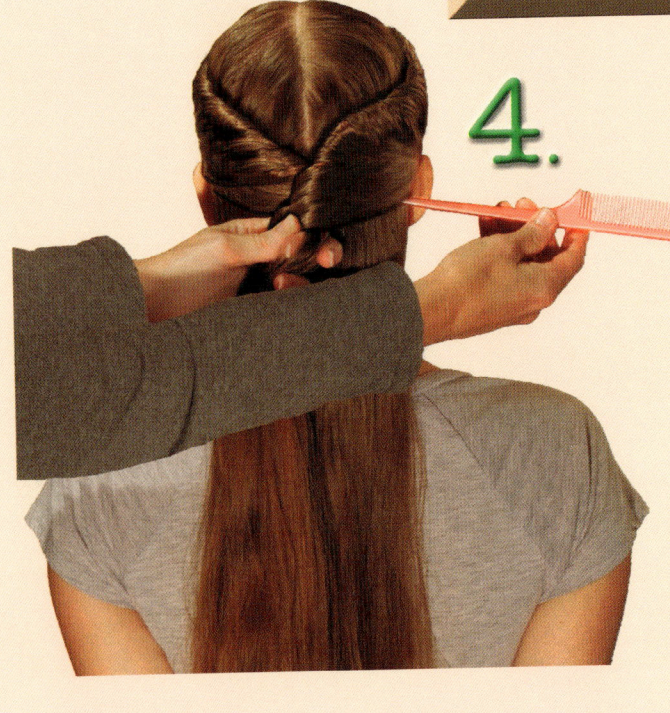

4.

Braid down the back to the ends of the hair.

The accents are two-strand rope made with hair and ribbon.

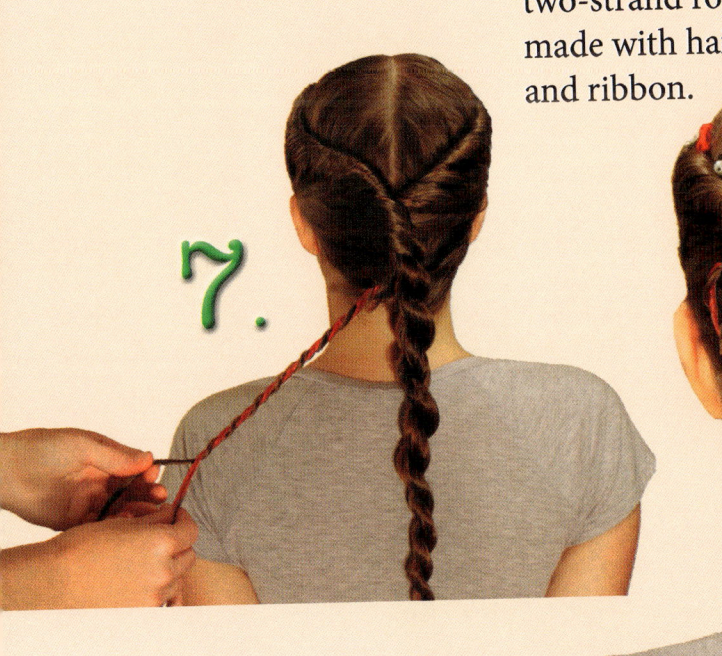

7.

Create the accents you have chosen for this style and place them in a pleasing manner.

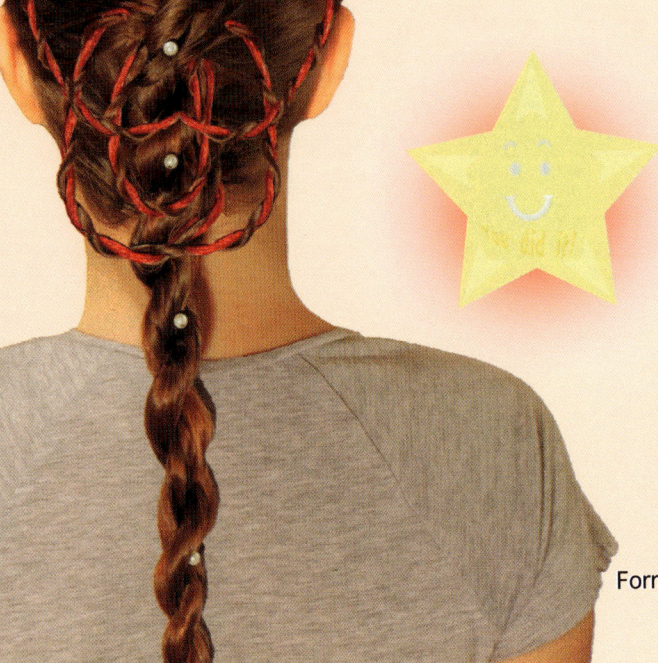

Forms   389

Junction Cascade

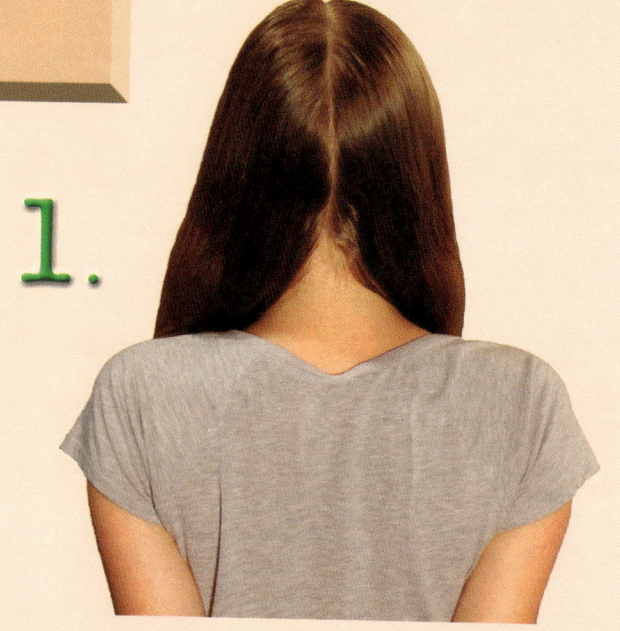

1. Part down the middle.

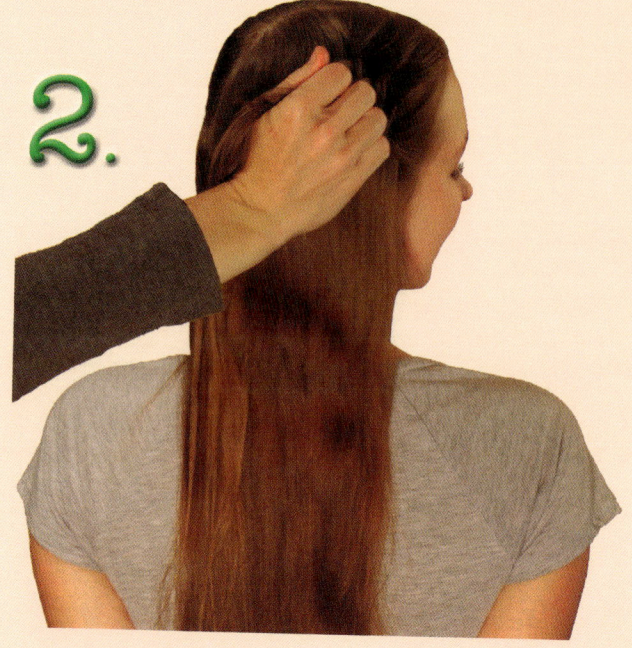

2. Choose the number of strands you will work with and start on one side of the head. Braid your way to the back of the head. This is a seven-strand merged into a nine-strand.

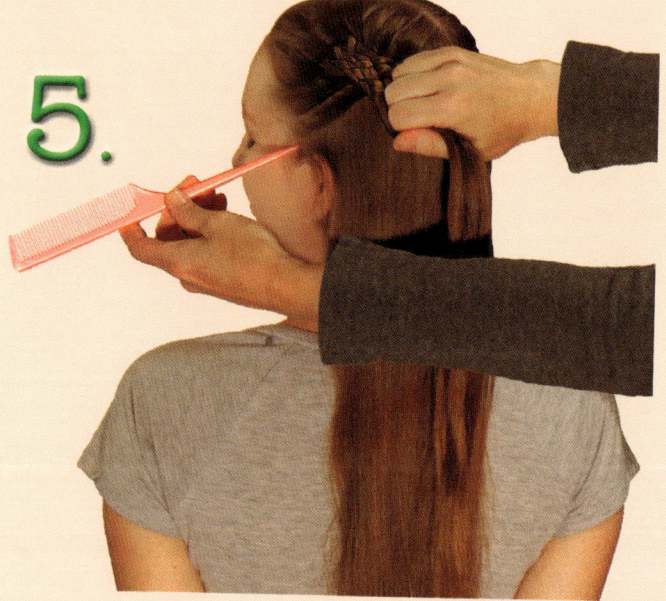

5. Or, braid loose and clumpy for that bed head braided look. You control the style. Let the hair be the material for your artwork.

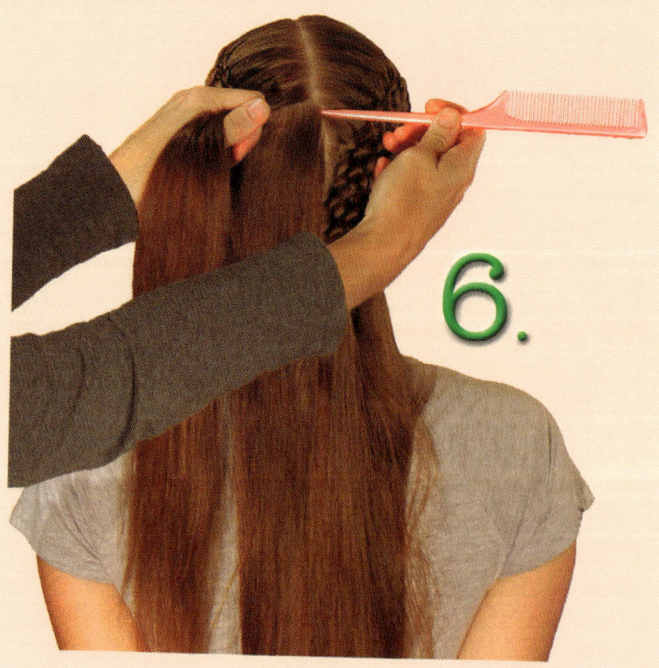

6.

Junction Cascade

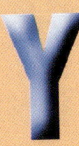

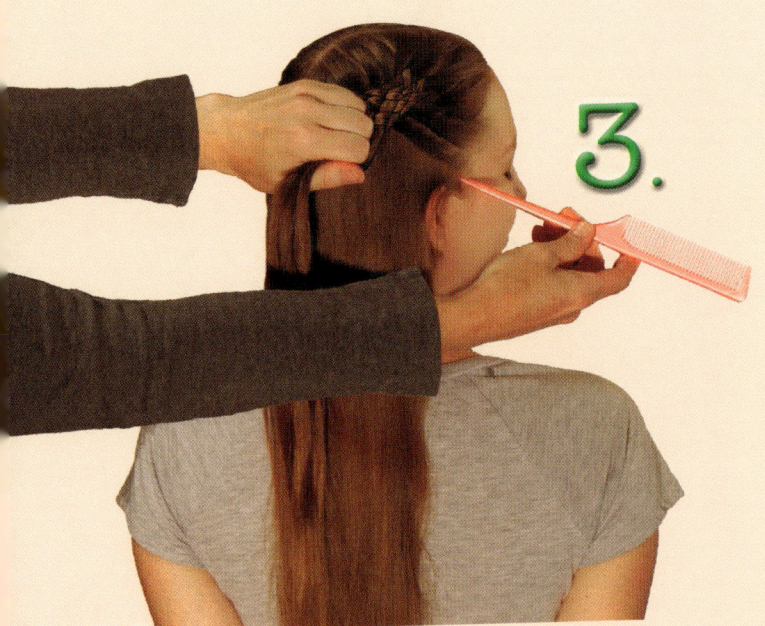

3.

Take the time to detangle as you braid.

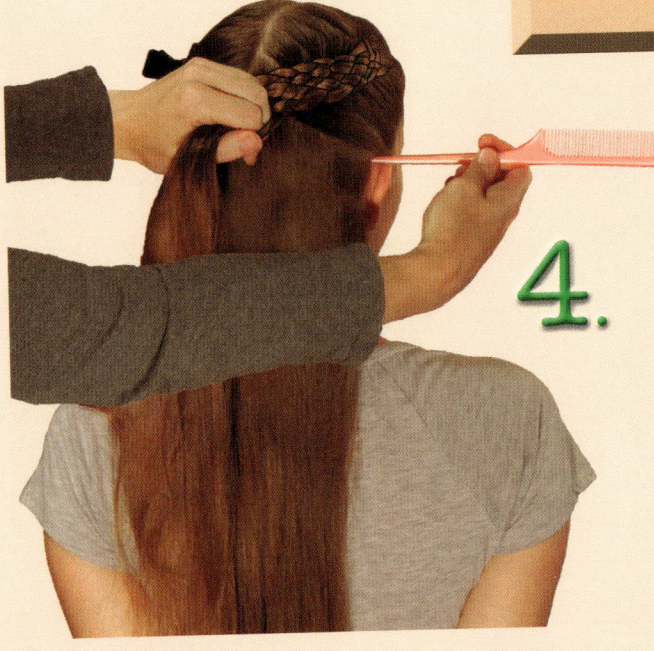

4.

Smooth each gather for a tidy polished look.

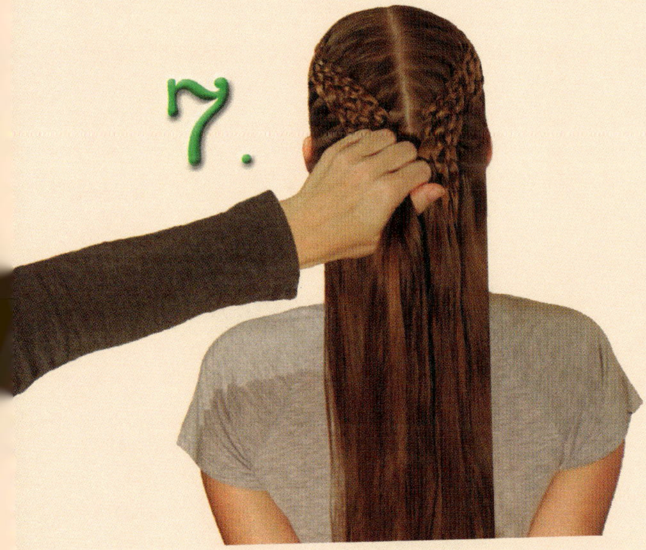

7.

Merge the braids leaving half of the hair down. Braid down the end of the tail or leave it loose as a ponytail.

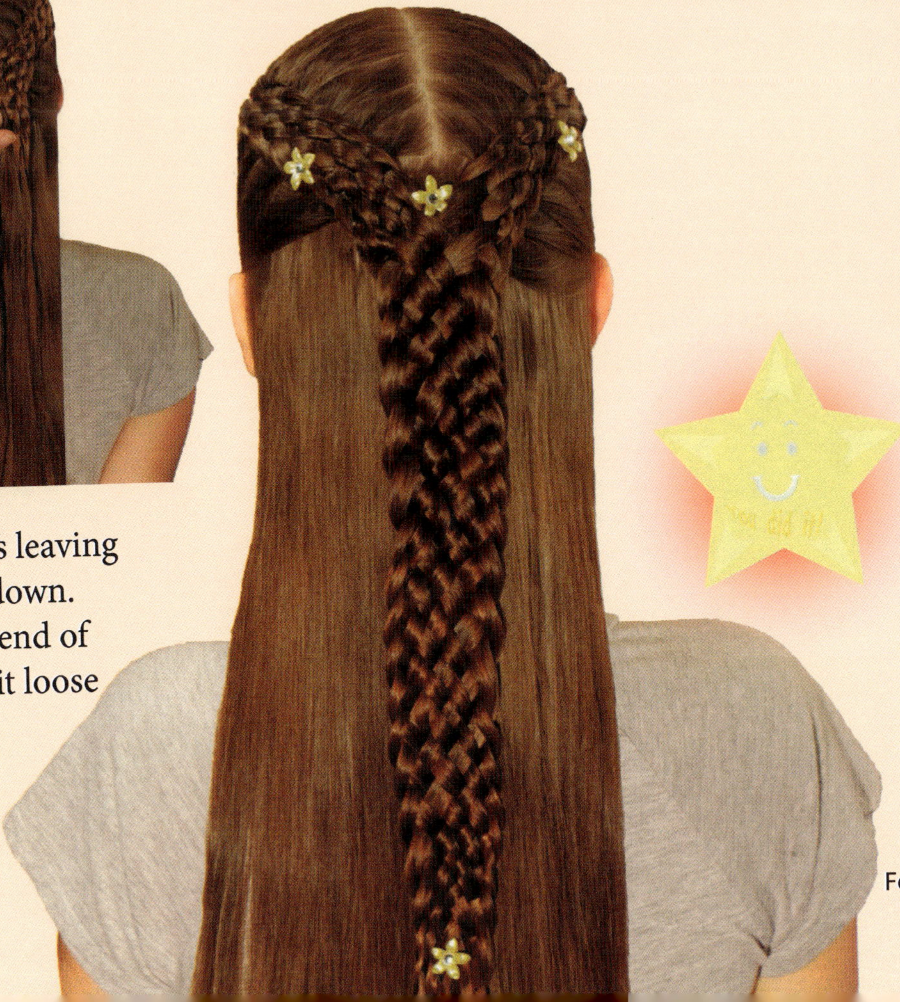

Accented Junction Cascade

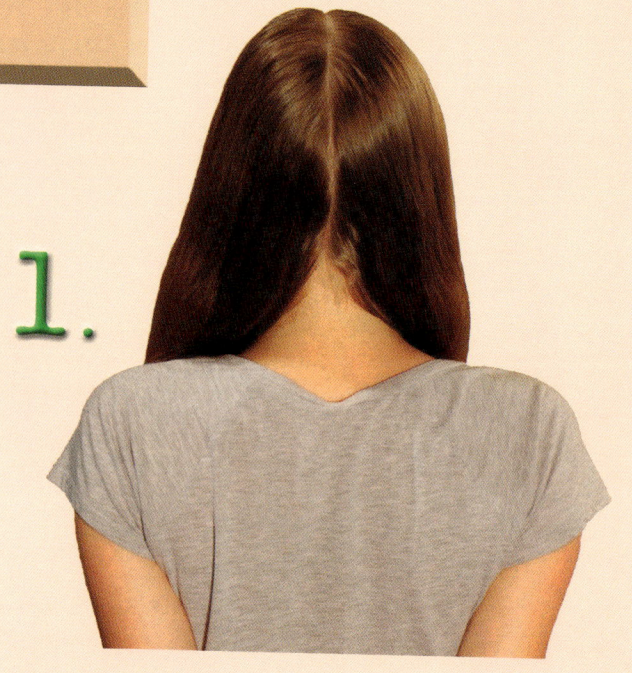

1\. Choose the number of strands you will work with.

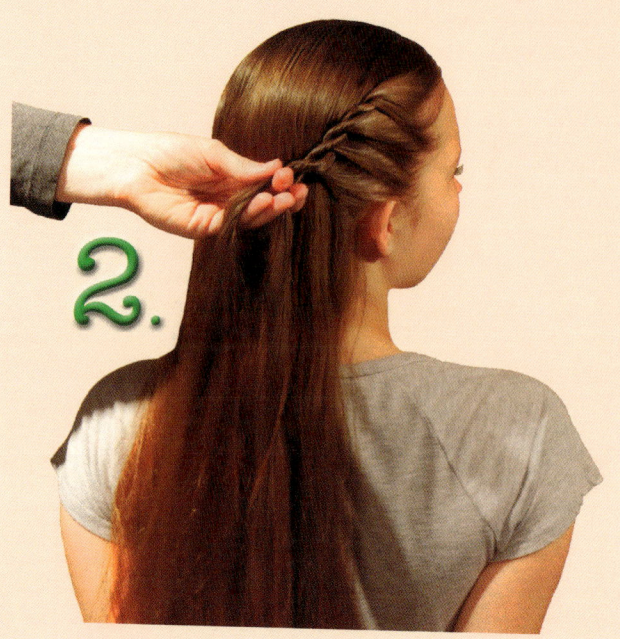

2\. Braid to the back of the head from each side.

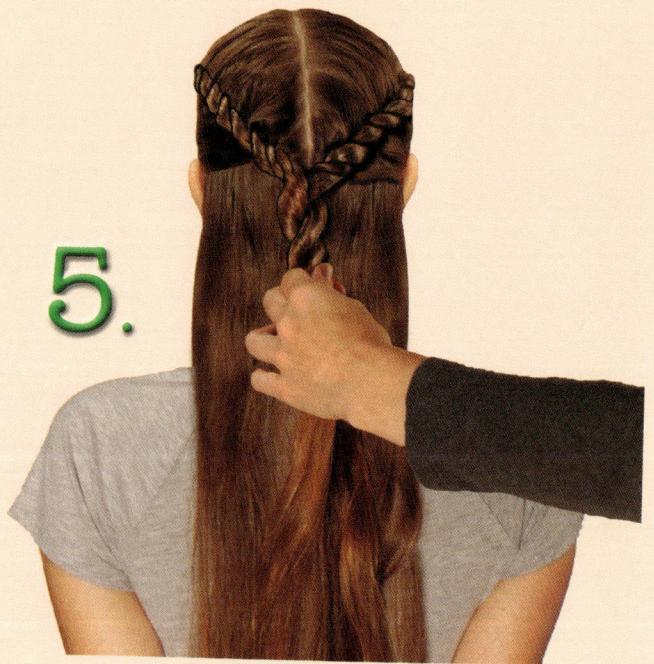

5\. The merged braid may be done with any number strand braid. Have fun.

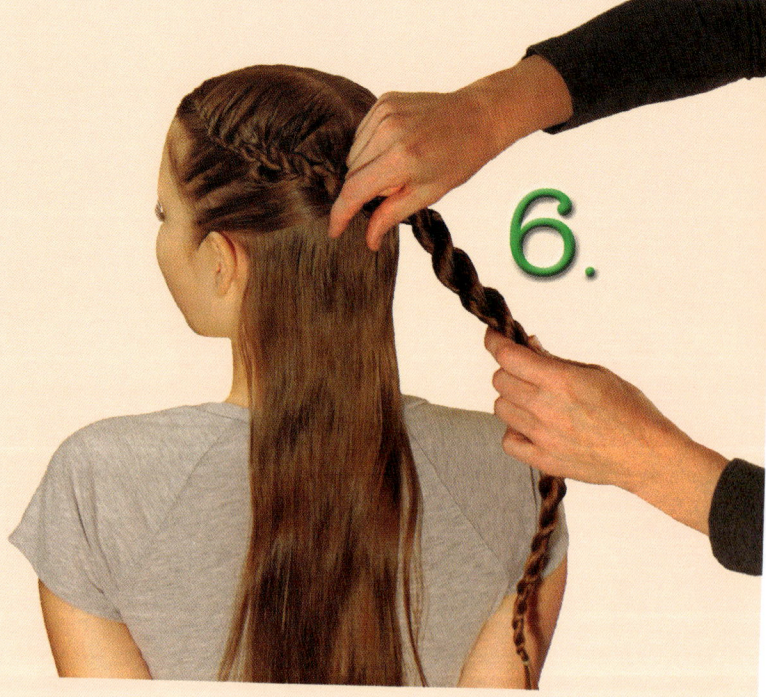

6\. Take your accents from a desirable location to help you acheive the look you are striving for. These are two-strand rope accents.

Accented Junction Cascade

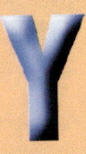

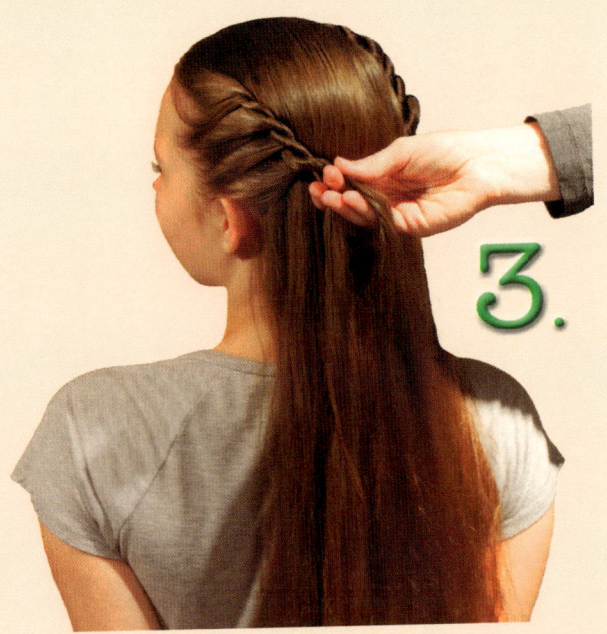

3.

This is a two-strand rope braid merged into a two-strand rope braid.

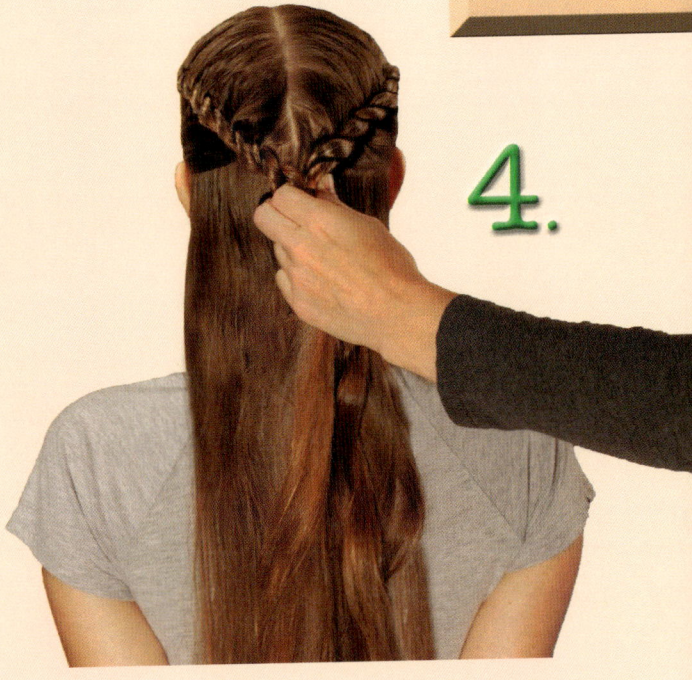

4.

Merge the two braids in the back leave down half the hair as the cascade.

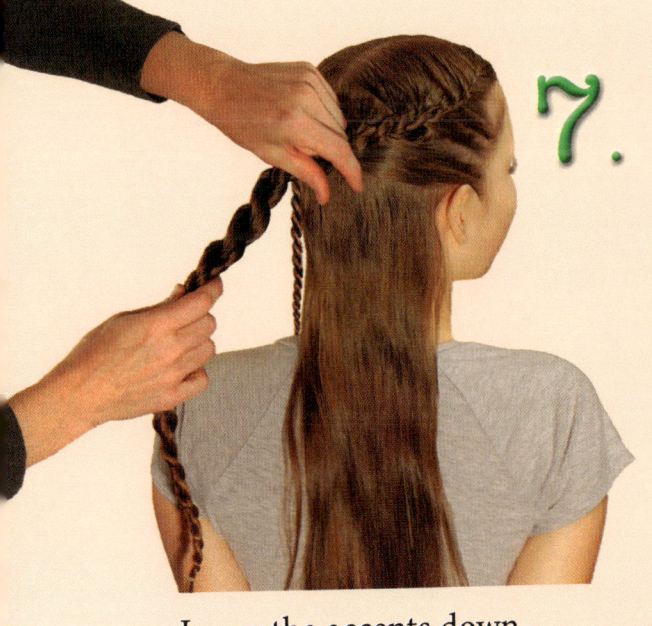

7.

Leave the accents down, pin them up, wrap them around, spray them with colors.

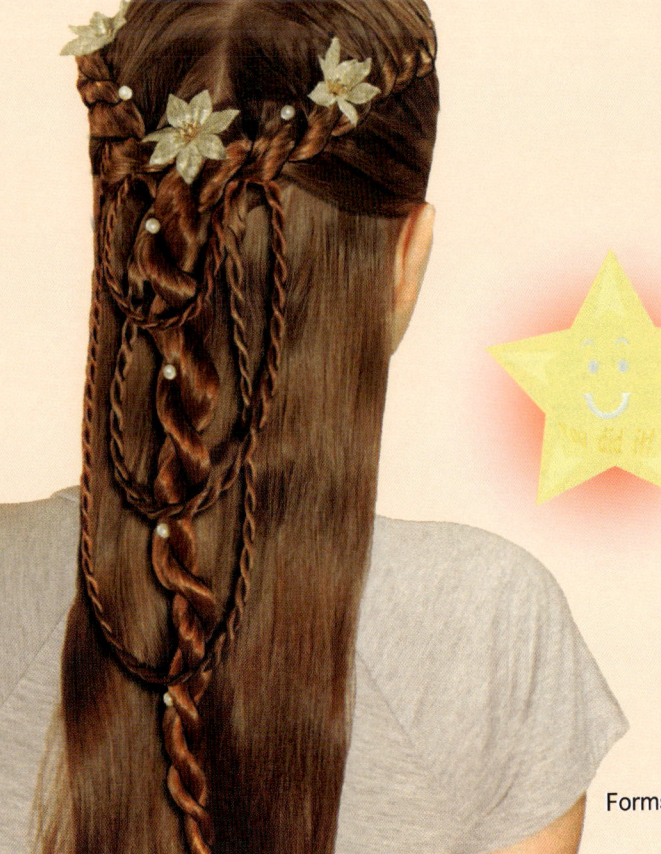

Forms

Notes

Examples of Junctions

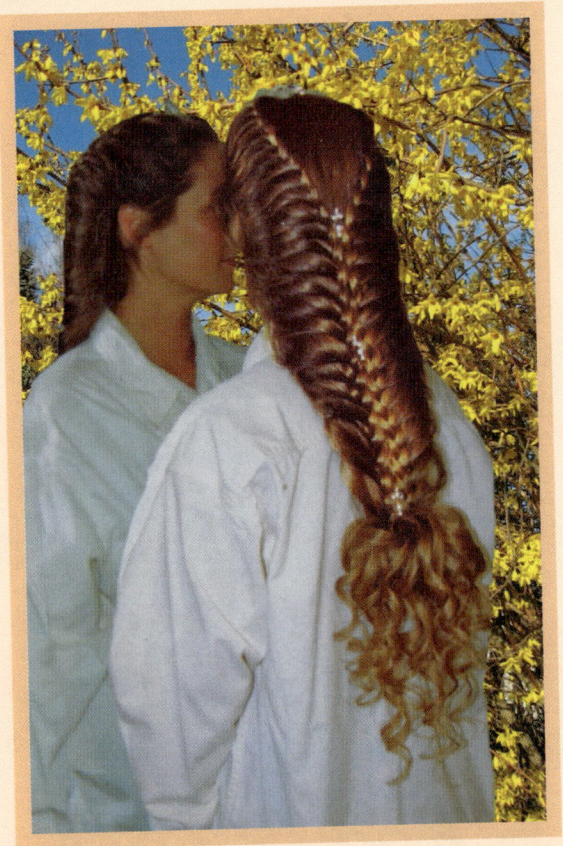
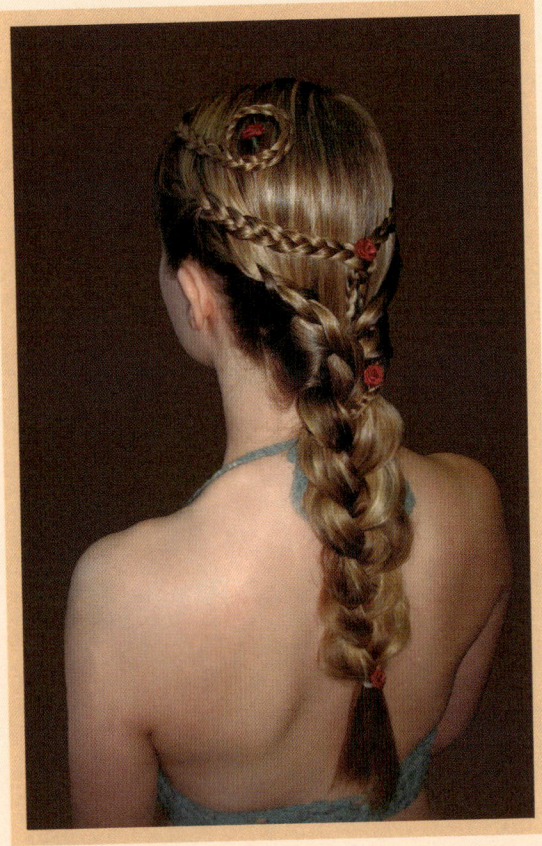
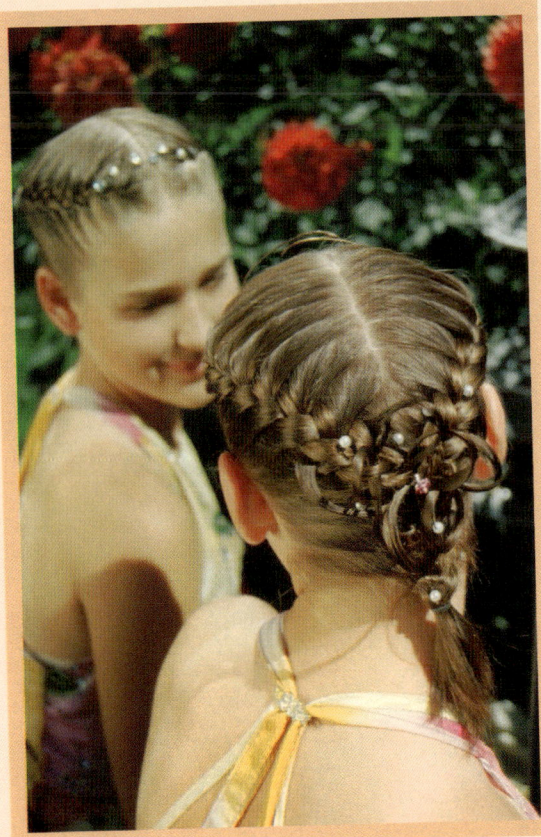
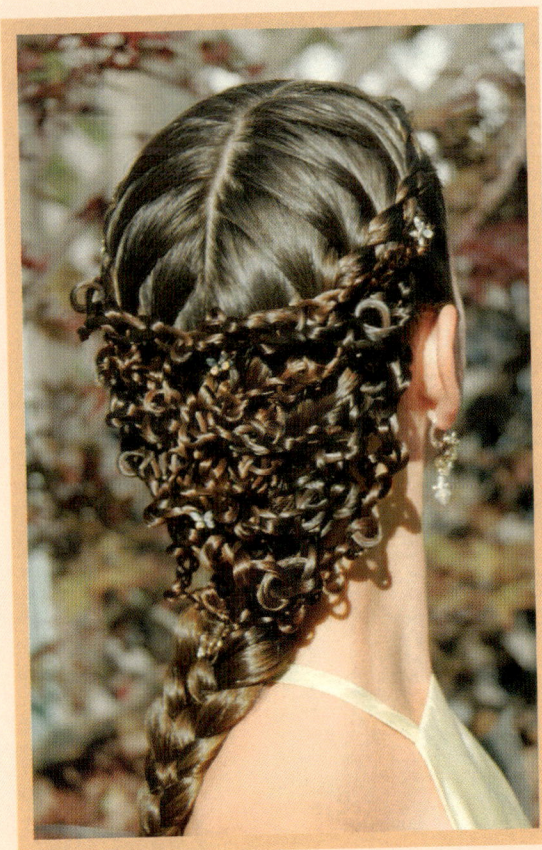

Visit my website to see more examples of Junctions

Forms

CLASSIC

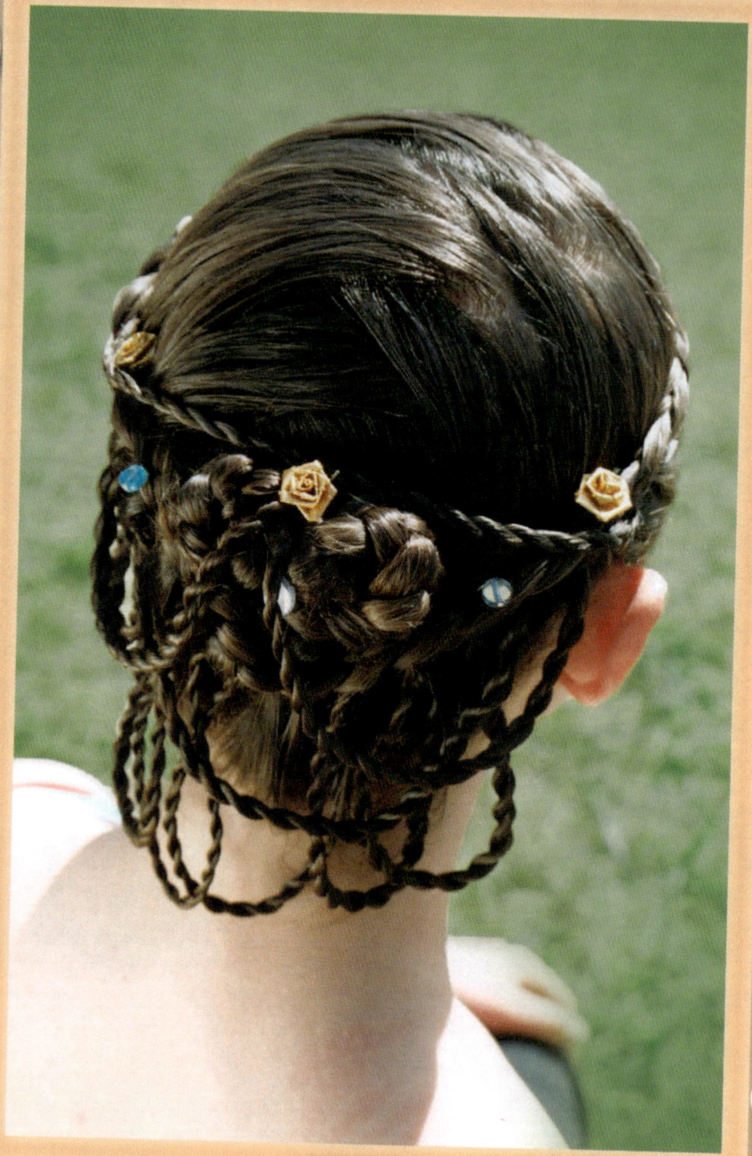

As you traverse more complicated forms, you will find your skills improving and the compliments you recieve more rewarding.

Forms

Gather like this!

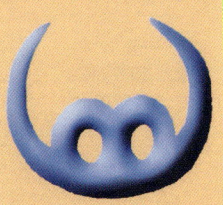

Braiding icon for the next eight pages.

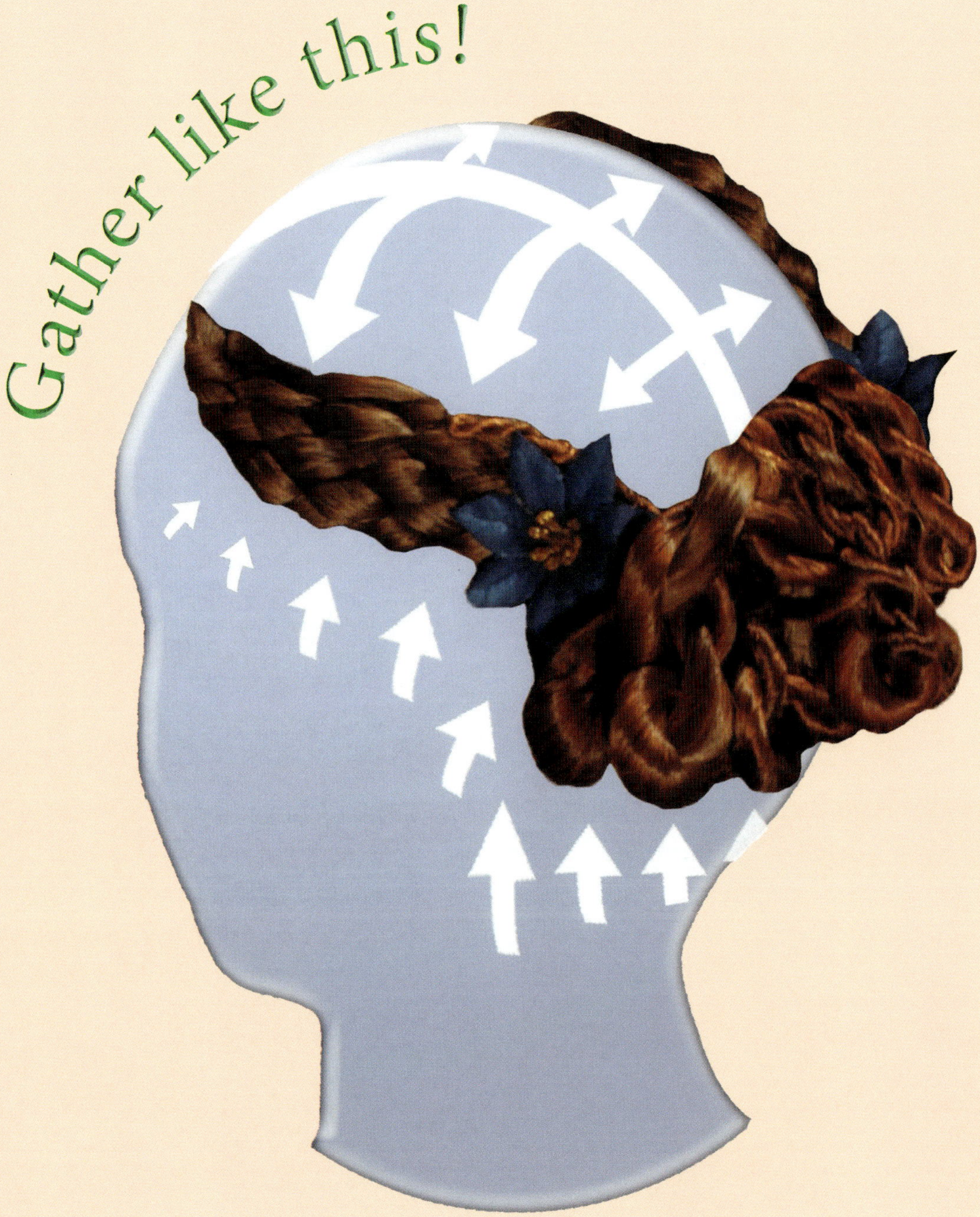

Another form that allows your creativity some elbow room with the part down the center. Keep in mind the bun is the key factor in this form. Bun size is determined by the amount of hair placed in said bun.

The Classic Form

Forms   397

Basic Classic

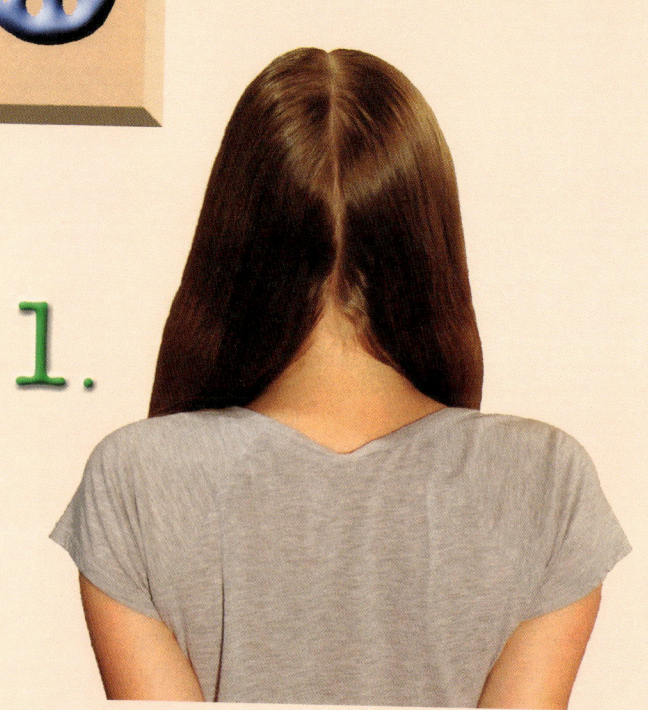

1. Part down the middle.

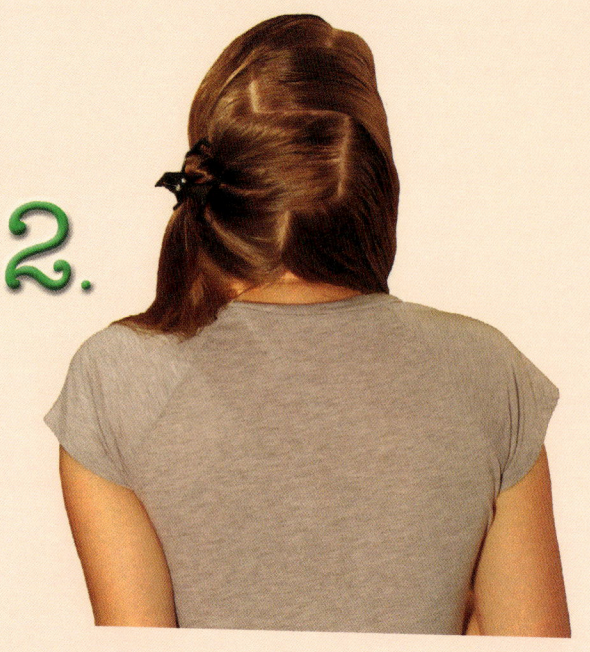

2. I am using a square part to add some fun to the form. This is a three-strand dutch merged into a two-strand rope for the bun.

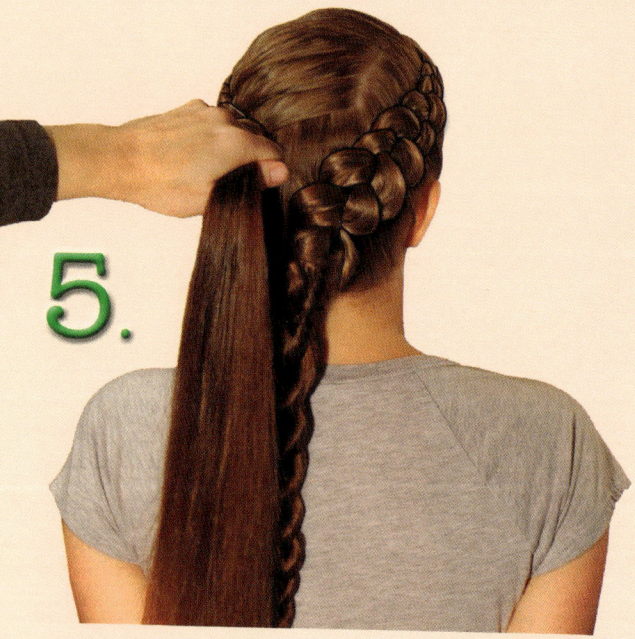

5. Braid around the side of the head and finishing at the back.

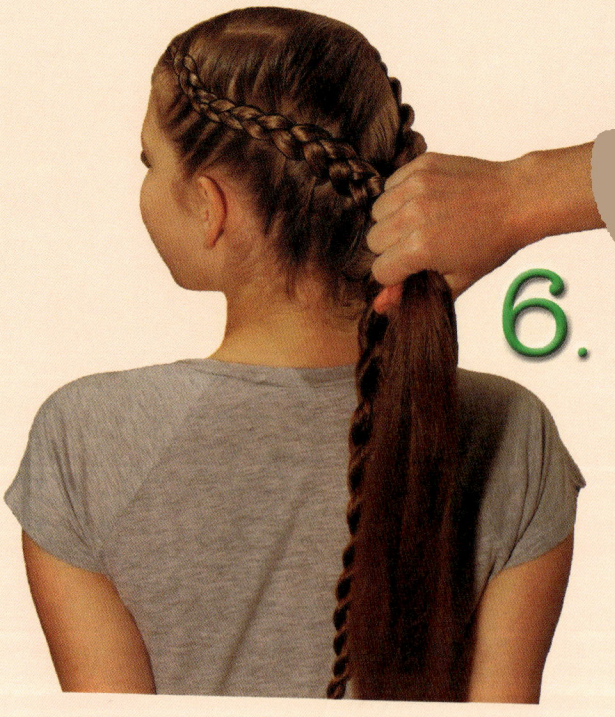

6. Whether you aim high or low for the bun, placement effects the over all look of the style. Bear that in mind as you traverse the head.

Basic Classic

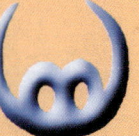

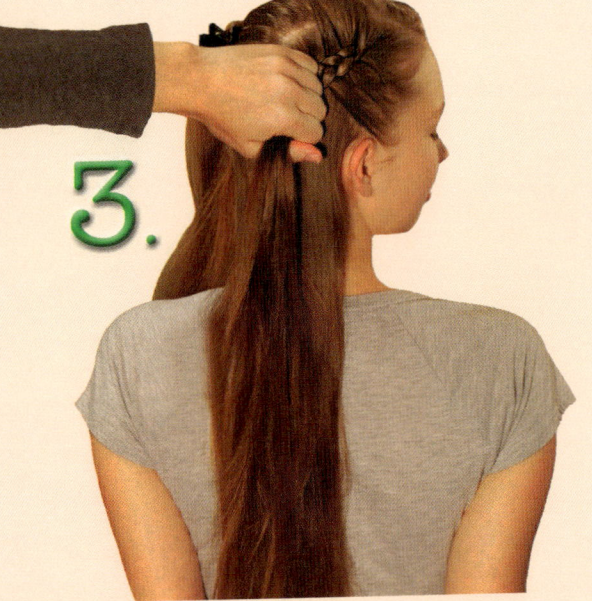

Braid to the back of the head from each side.

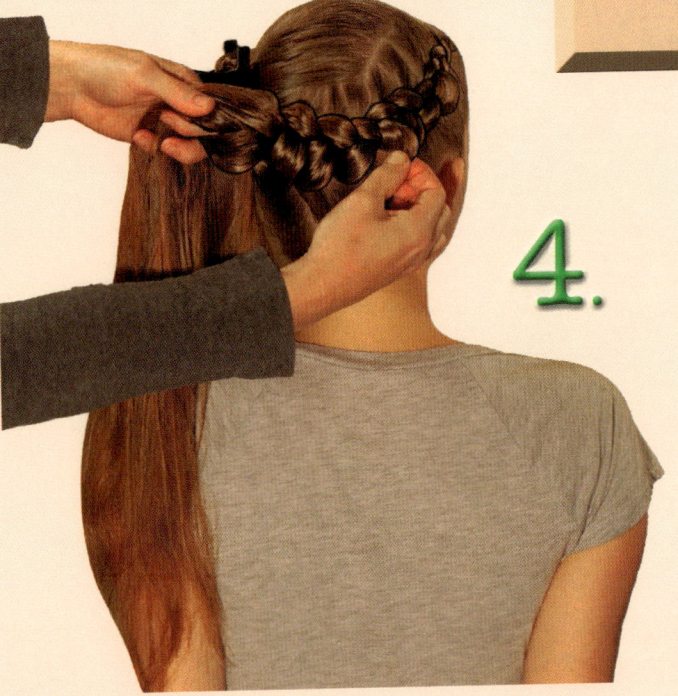

To acheive the bulk look in the braid, pull and tug on each bump of the braid before finishing the tails.

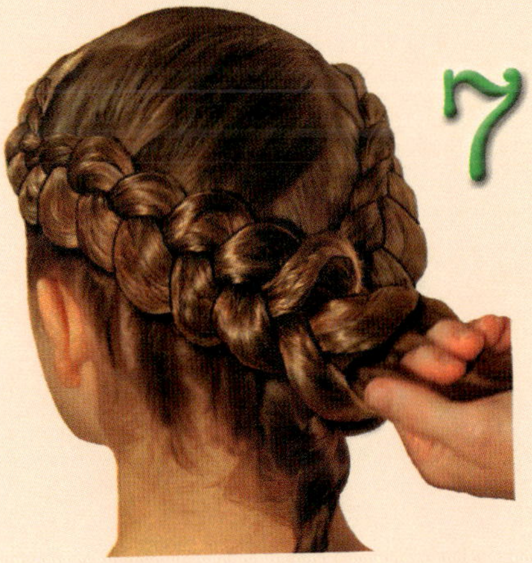

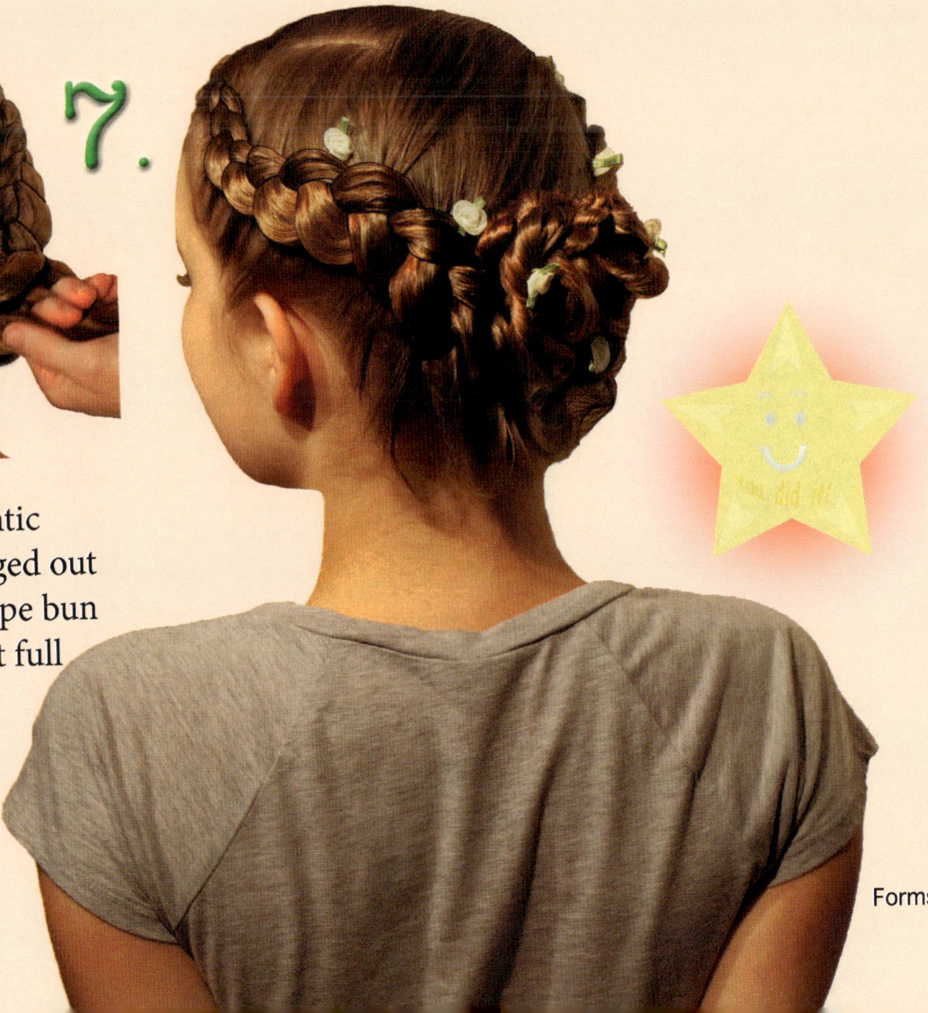

I enjoy the romantic soft look of a tugged out braid. And the rope bun continues the soft full look of the style.

Forms

Accented Classic

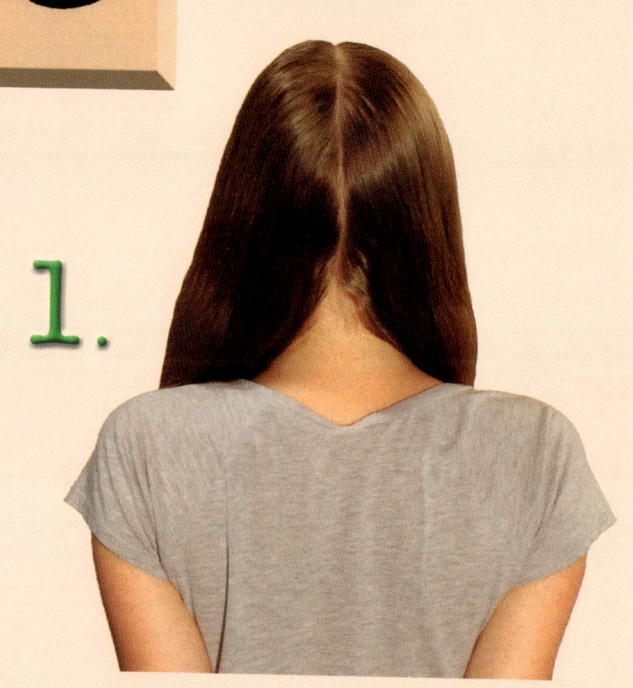

1. Part down the middle.

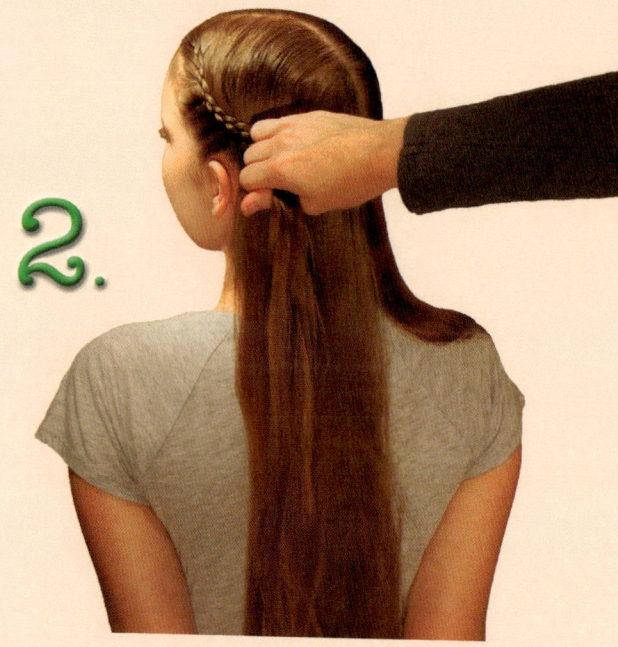

2. Choose the number of strands you will braid with. This is four-strand plait. The braid and form will be done feather loose to create a draped effect in back. The accent is a heart from loose hair.

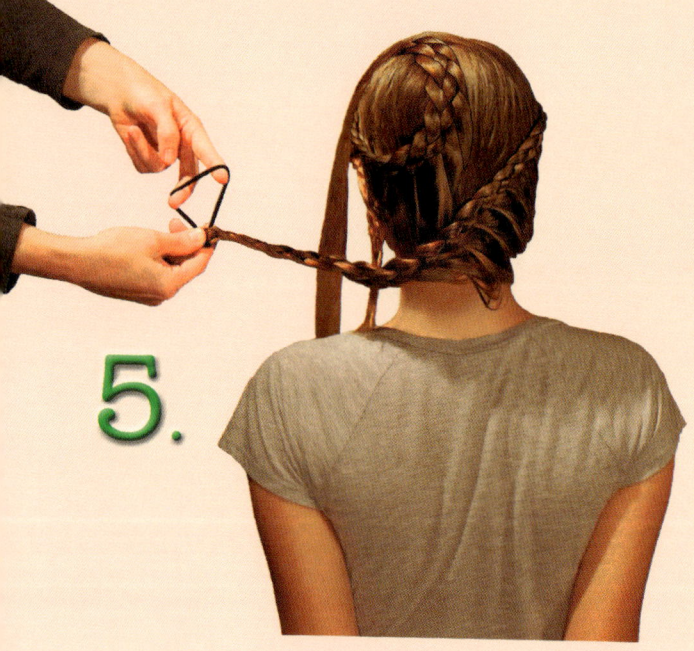

5. Pin the bun to create the style effect you are going for. I used large bobby pins to get this look. Hairspray kept the drape from having a mind of its own.

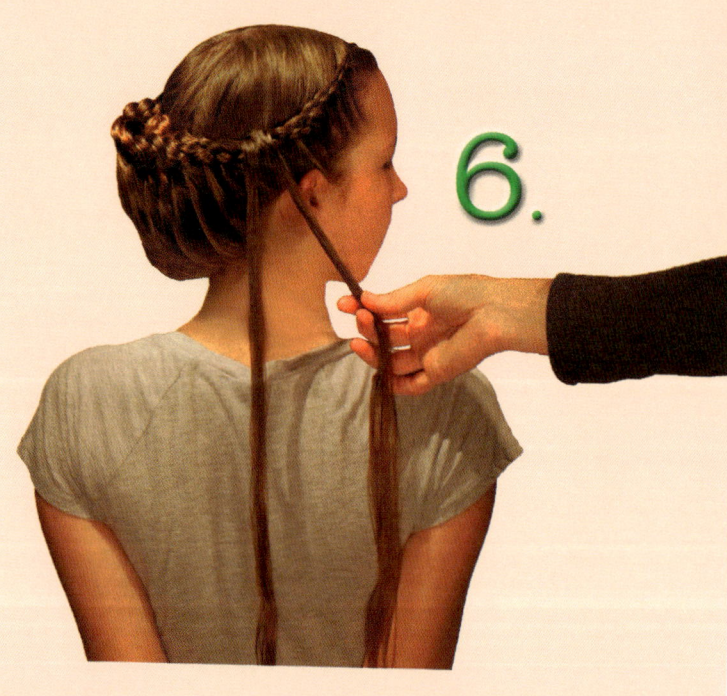

6. The heart accent is created with two strands twisted in opposite directions.

Accented Classic

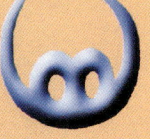

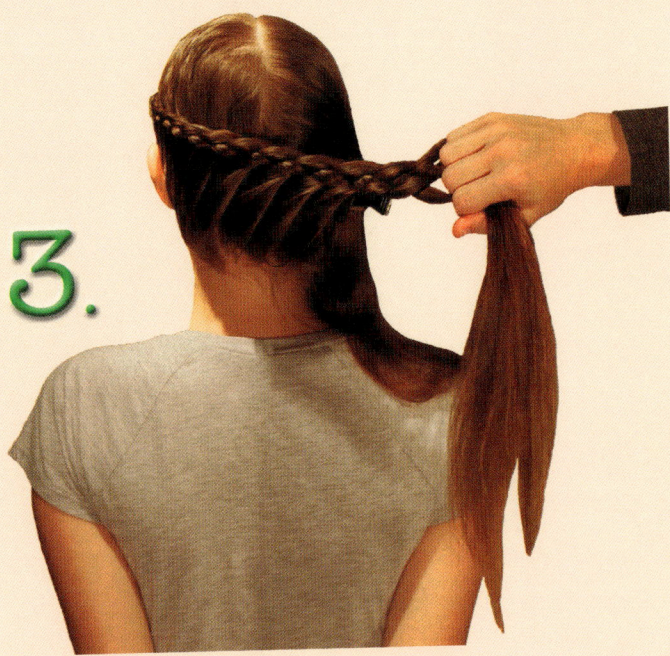

3. Braid to the back of the head from each side. End each braid where you wish to place the bun.

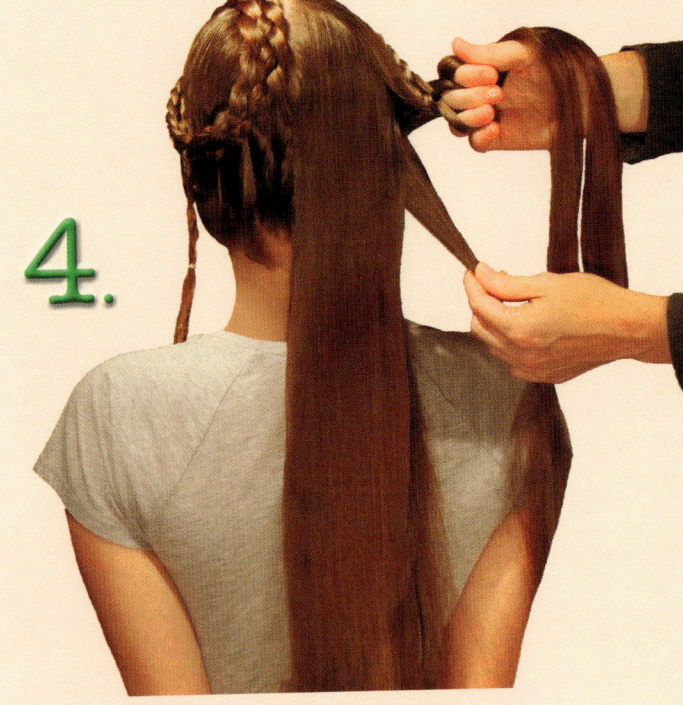

4. Take accents from the desired location.

7. Bend in the shape of a heart and rubber banded at the bottom of the heart. I used a latchhook to hide the ends of the tail.

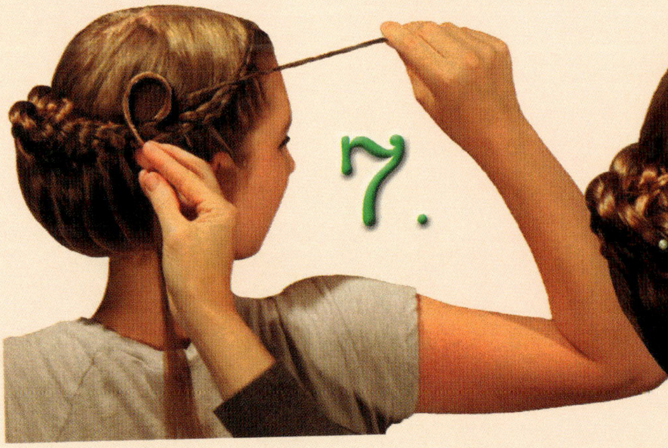

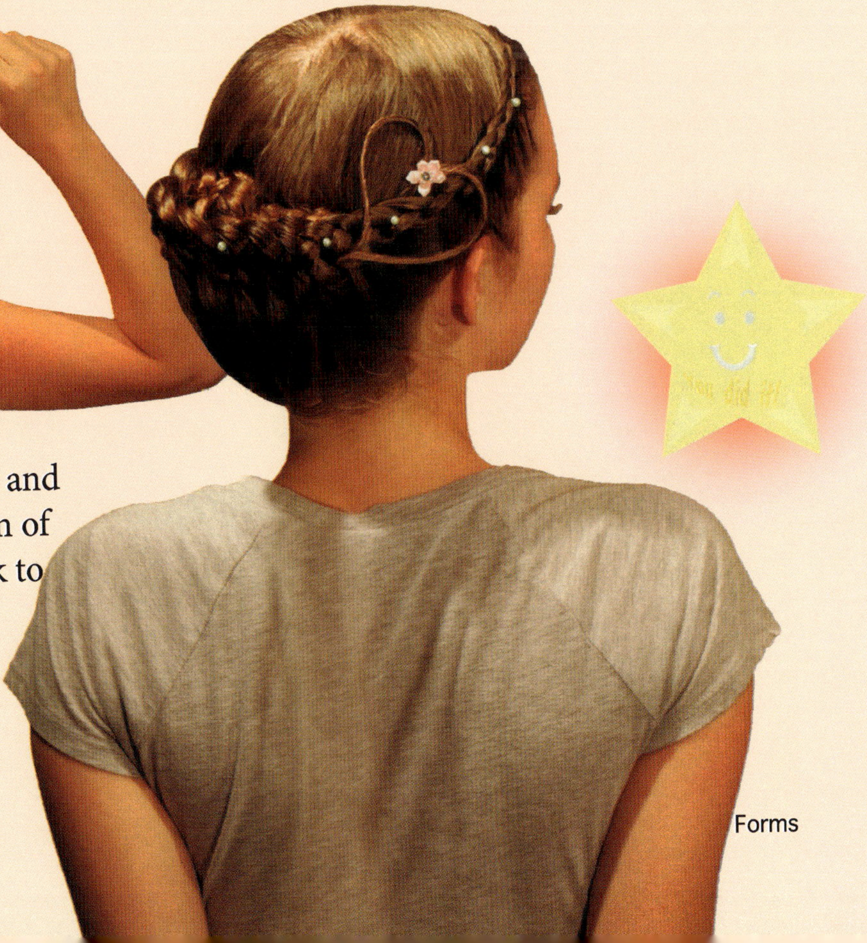

Classic Cascade

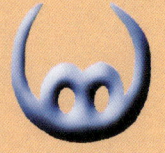

1.

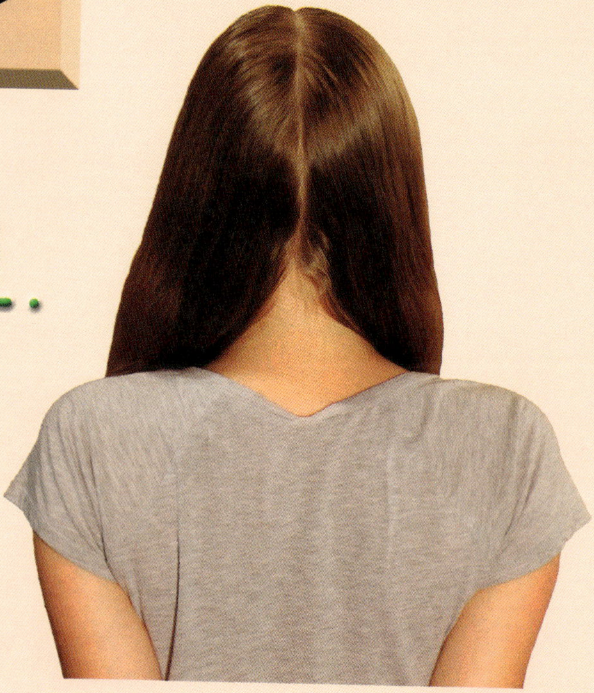

Part down the middle.

2.

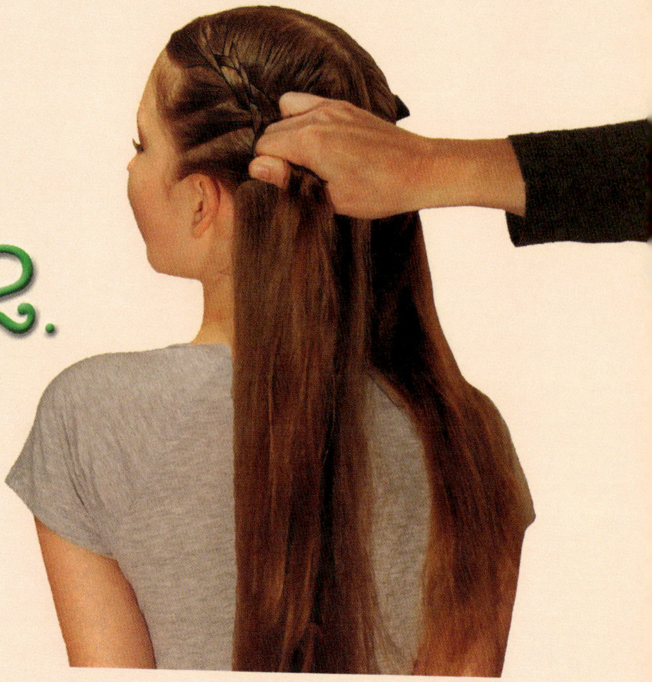

Choose the number of strands you will work with. This is four-strand round. Braid to the back of the head from each side and end each side where you wish to place the bun.

5.

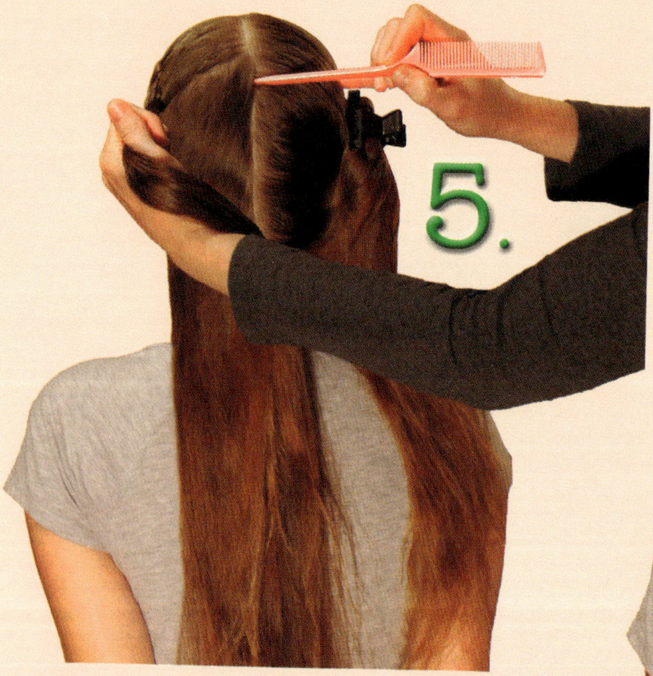

6.

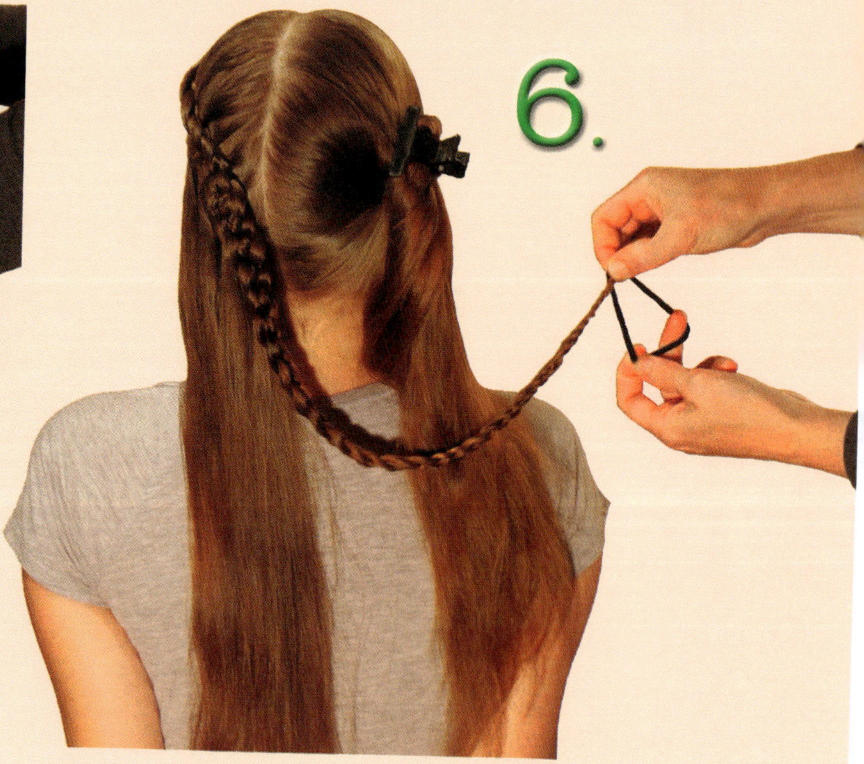

Classic Cascade

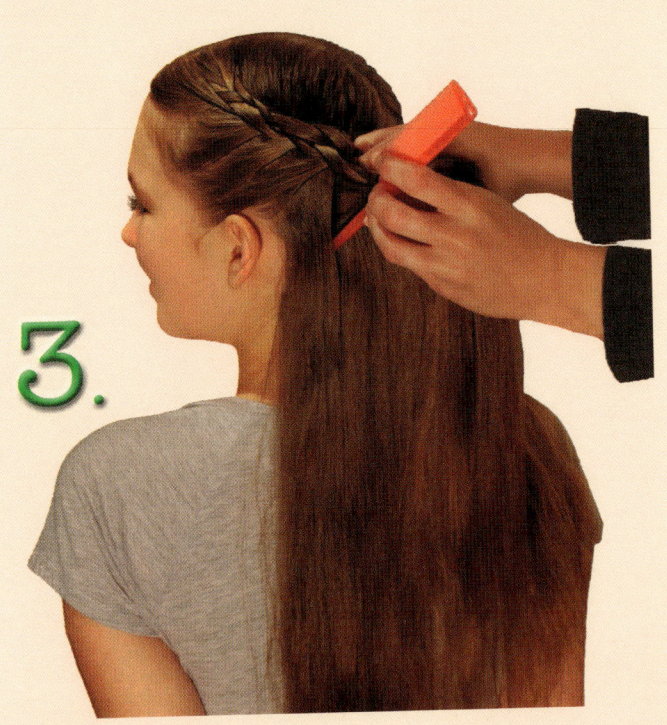

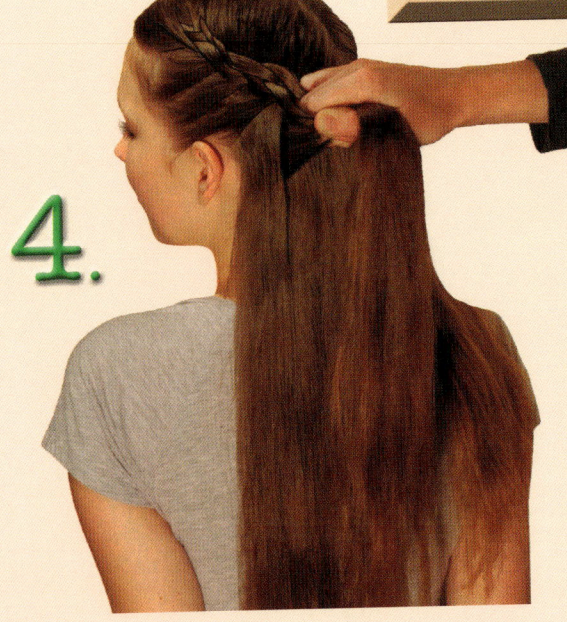

If you sliver small gathers into the braid from the cascade across the back you get a much sturdier version of the form.

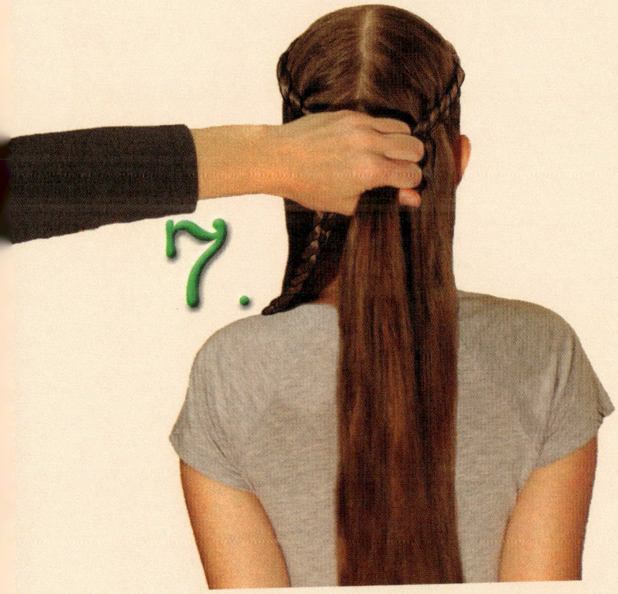

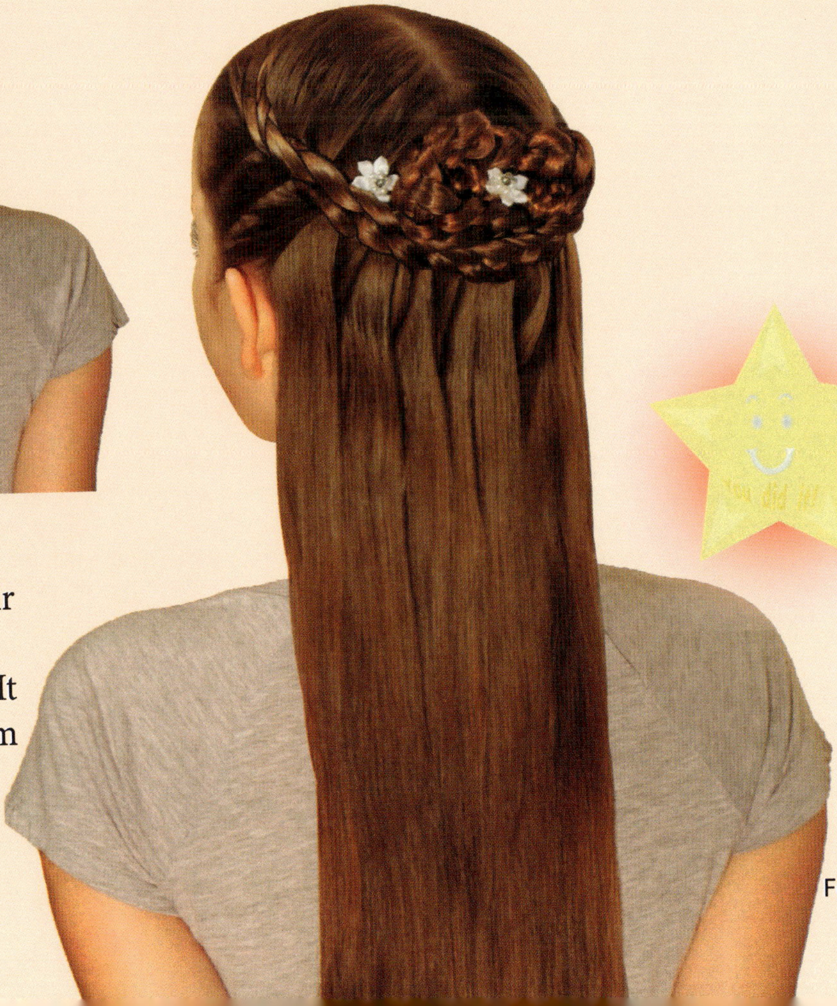

Cascades showcase the length of your hair and provide shelter from wind and cold. It also keeps a style from looking too severe around the face.

Accented Classic Cascade

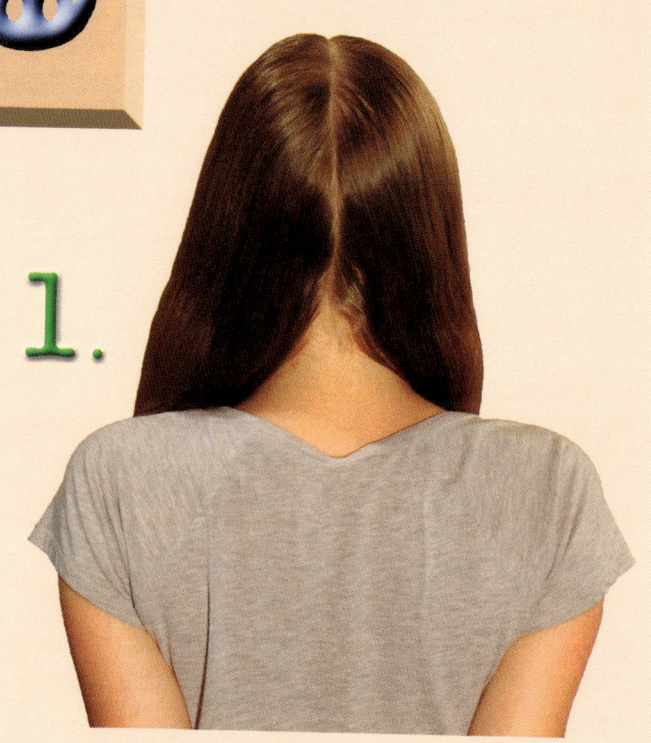

1.

Part down the middle.

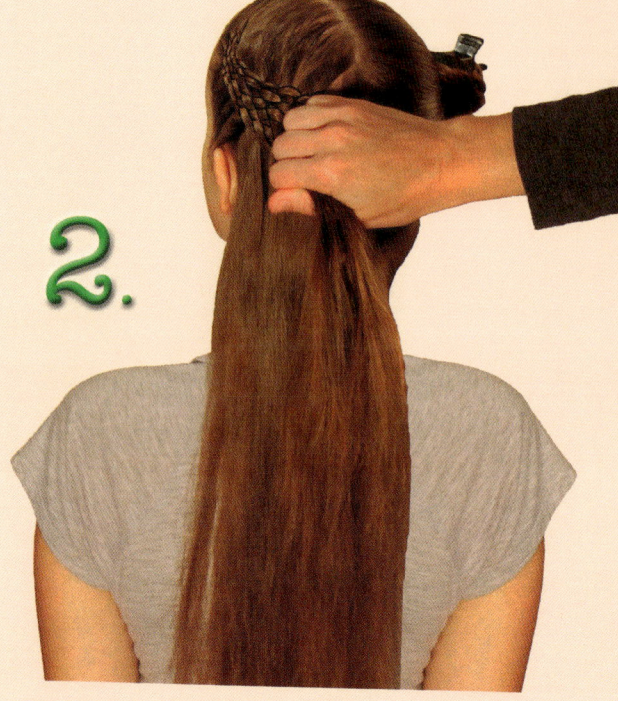

2.

Choose the number of strands you will work with. This is nine-strands. The accents are mini one-strand twists. Braid your way to the back of the head from each side ending where you wish to place the bun.

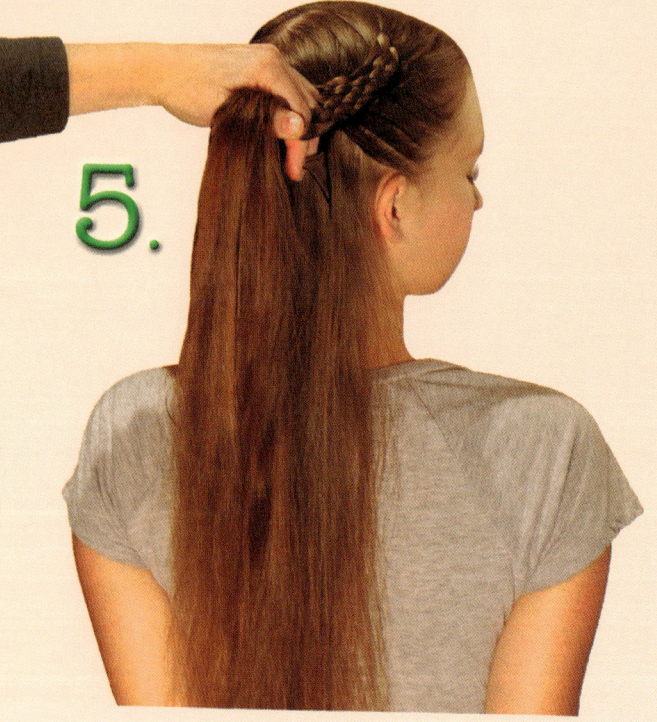

5.

The braids sit where a crown would sit. They follow the curvature of the head and end in back in a bun or accents.

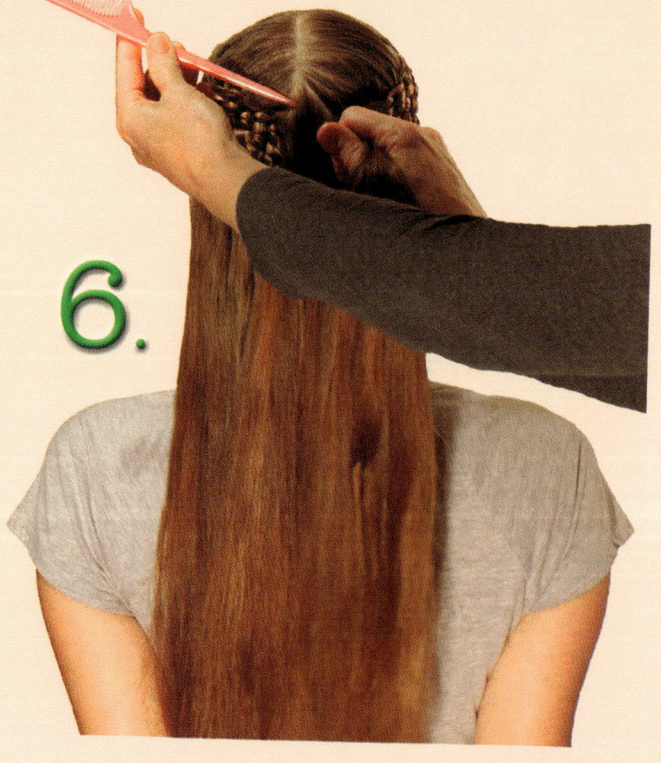

6.

404 www.findingbraids.com

Accented Classic Cascade

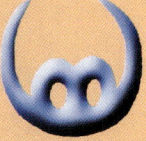

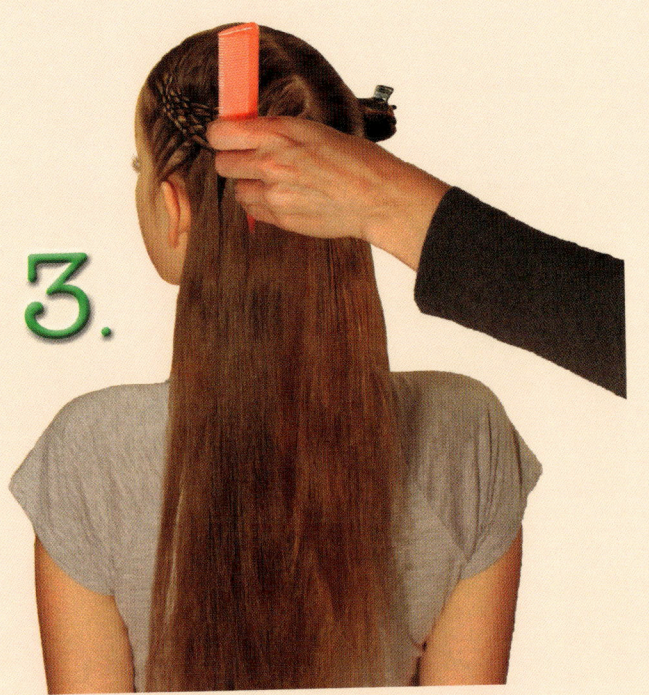

3.

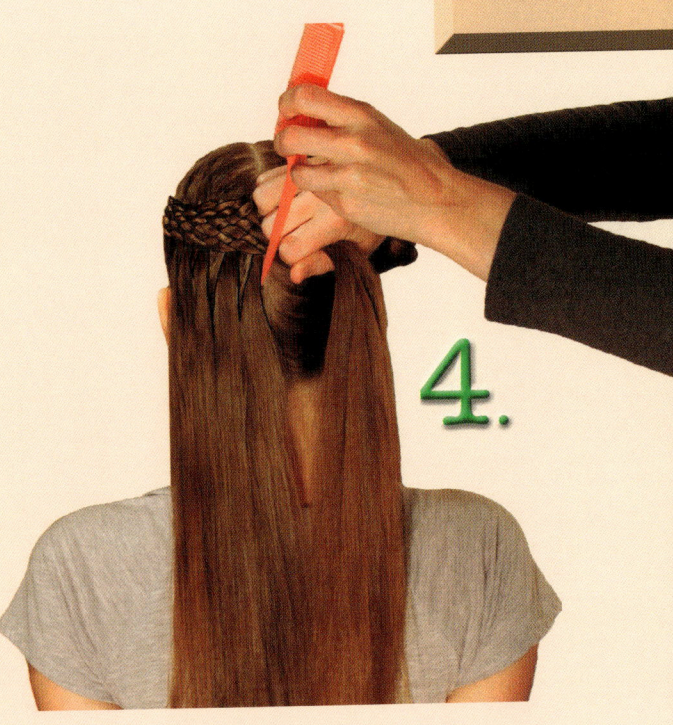

4.

Sliver small gathers into the braid from the cascade.

7.

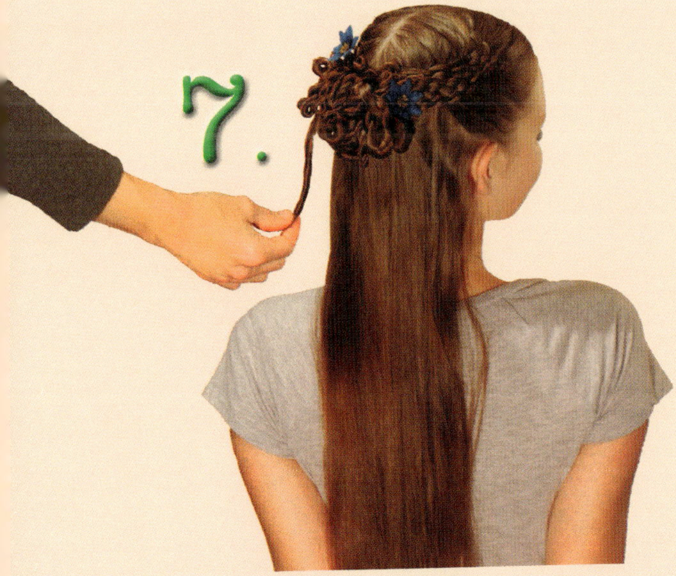

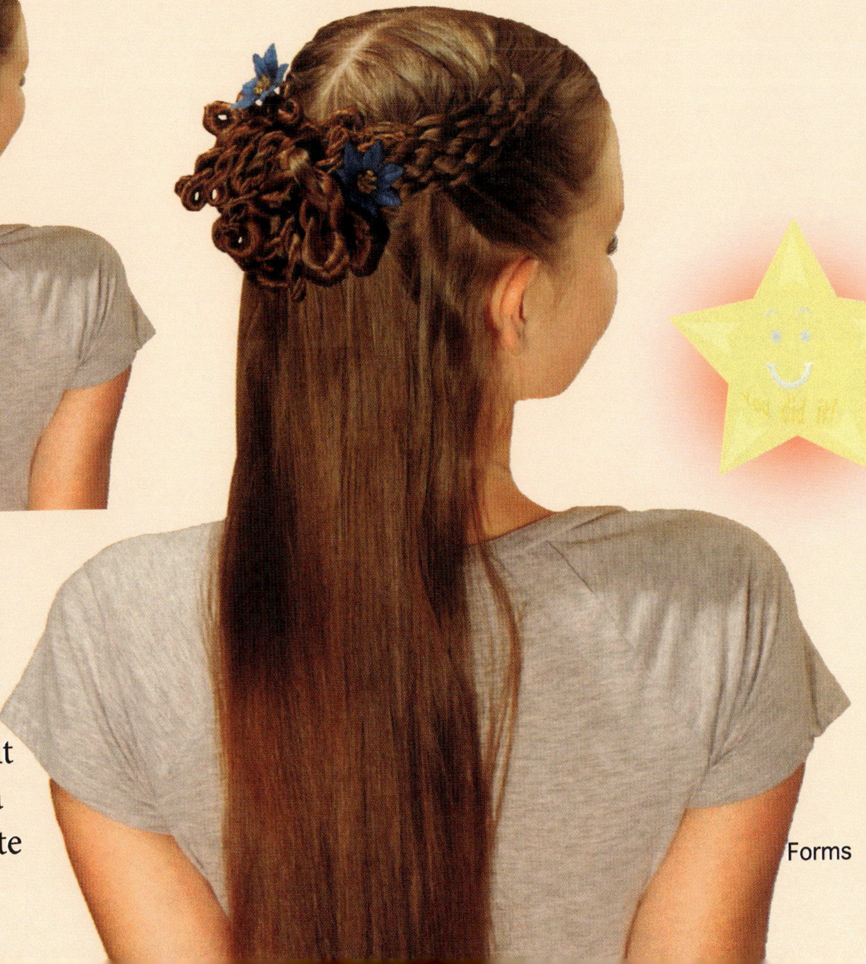

I chose to use the hair from the tails to create a bunch of accents. There is no bun, I tied the hair once and bobby pinned it secure, then twisted up a lot of mini twists to create this fun accent.

Forms 405

Forms

Notes

Examples of Classics

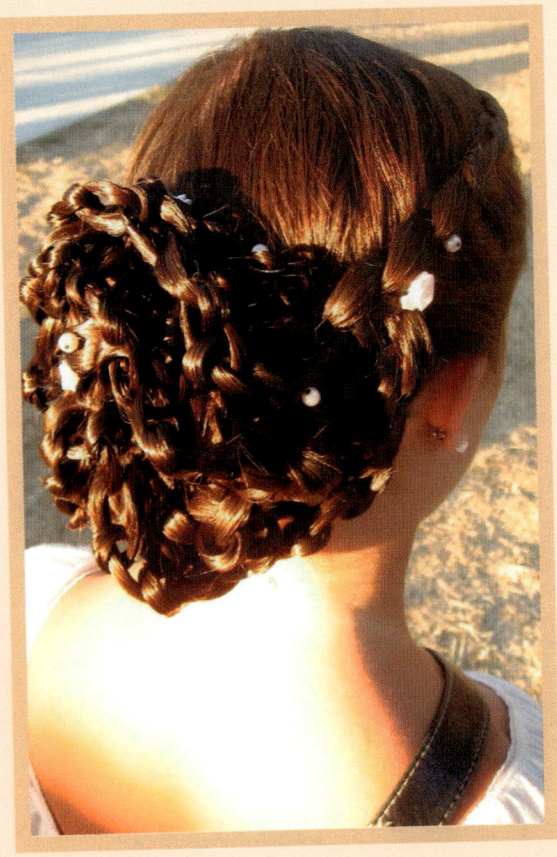
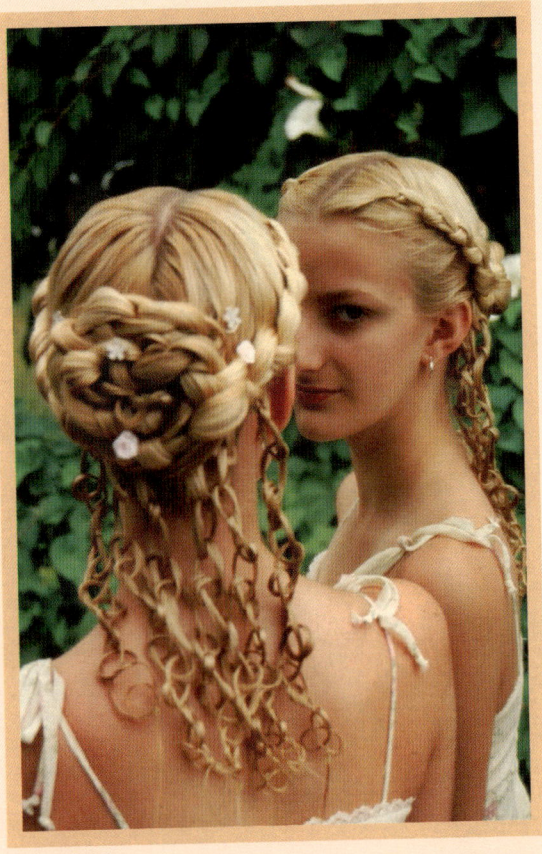
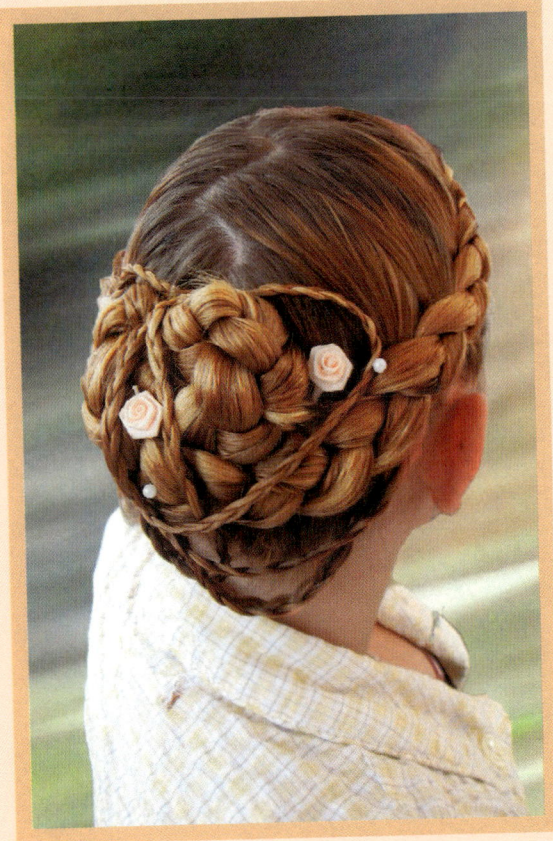
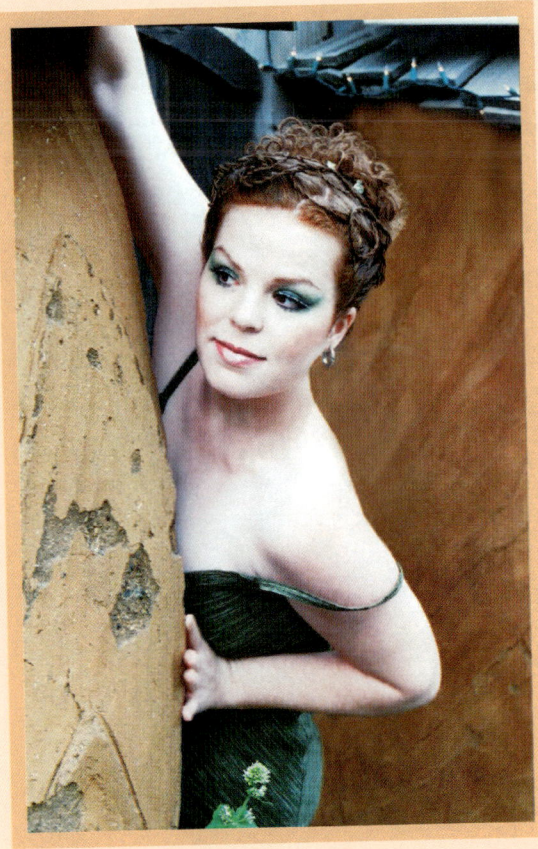

Visit my website to see more examples of Classics

Forms

TEARDROP

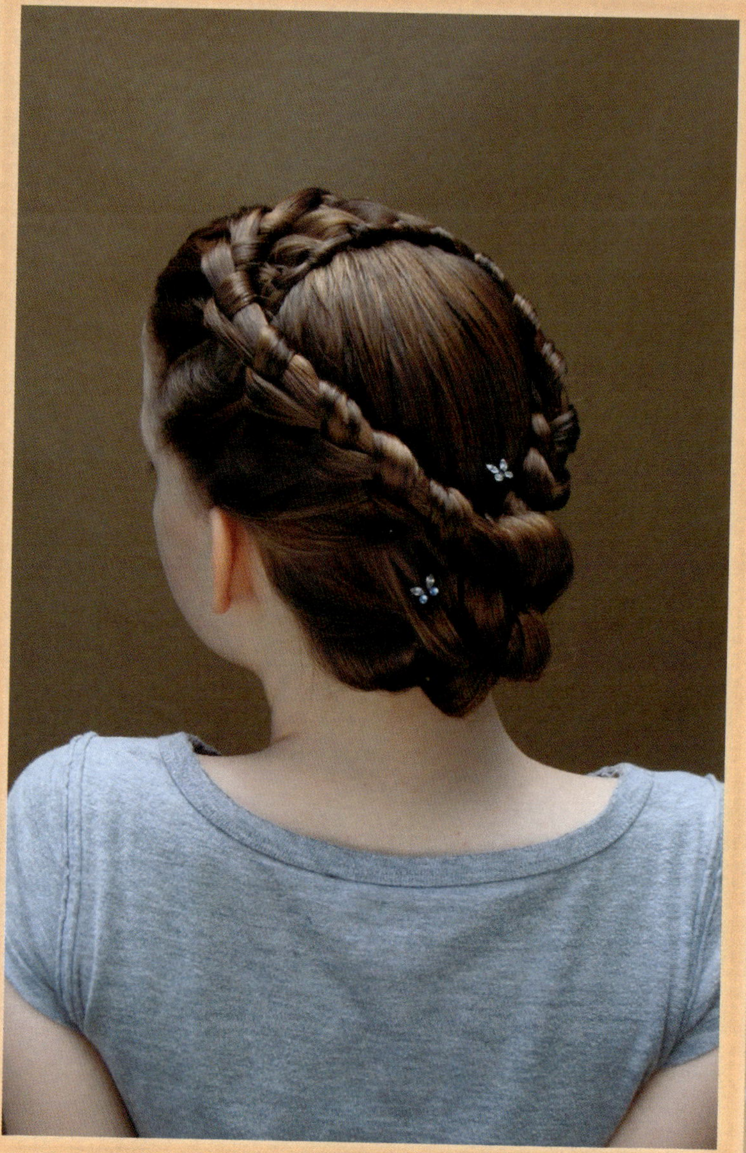

The soft full look of this form is appealing for so many reasons. Lacking a part, this is ideal for thinner hair.

Forms

Gather like this!

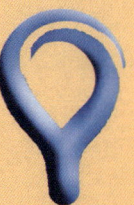

Braiding icon for the next eight pages.

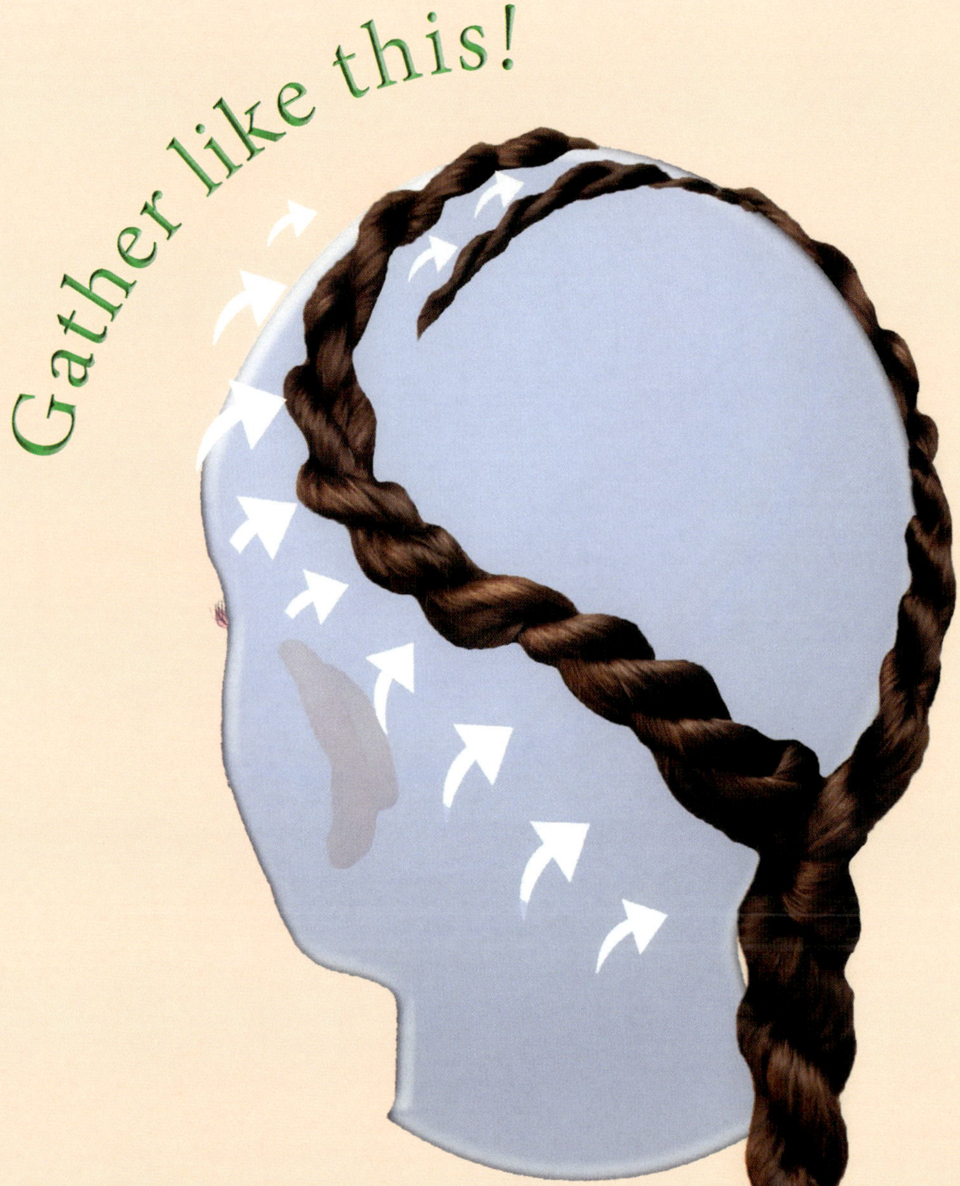

You can achieve a balance with this style if you braid the back half of the form first and then return and braid the front half of the form. Calculate the amount of hair you take into each gather to end with a symetrical style.

The **Teardrop** Form

Basic Teardrop

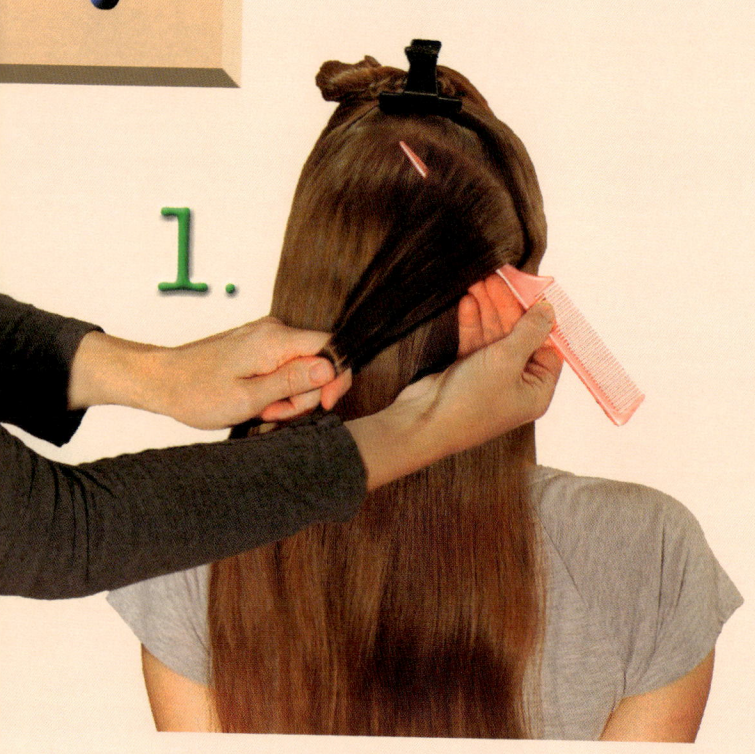

1. Secure the headband portion of hair in front. Start at an ear from behind the headband placement. Braid from ear to ear.

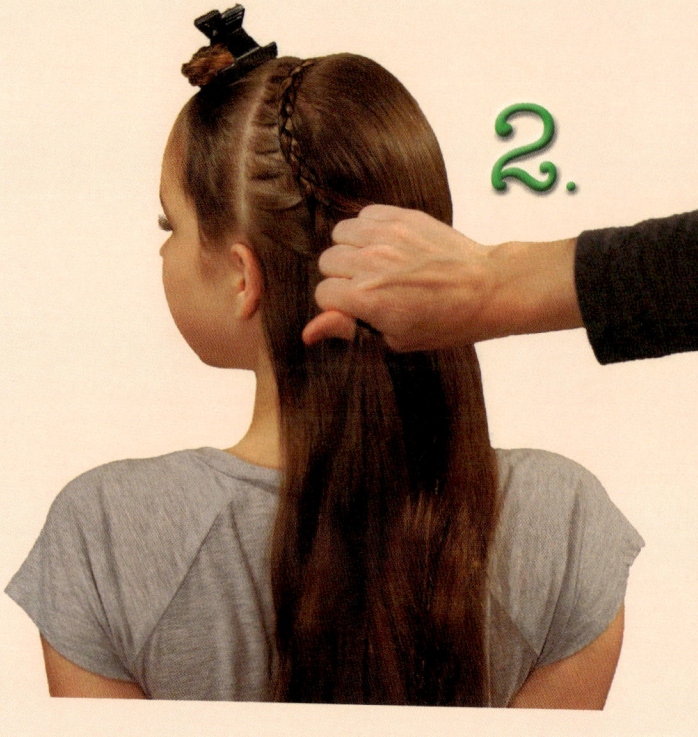

2. Clip off the braid so you can braid the other side.

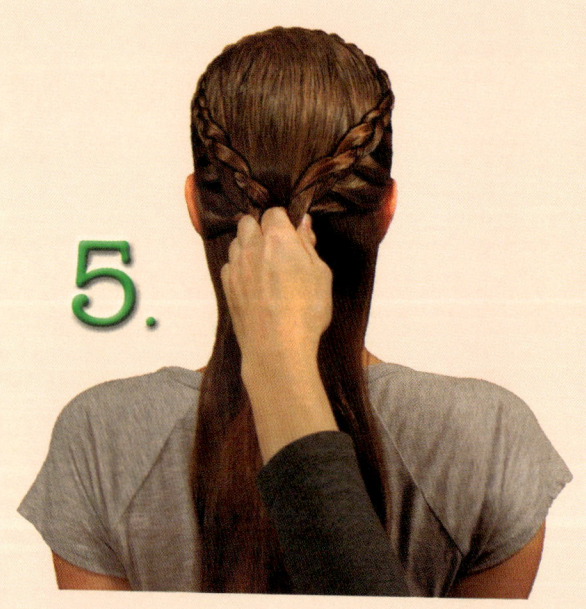

5.

6. Merge the tails at the back of the head and continue braiding down the back to the ends of the hair.

Basic Teardrop

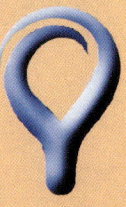

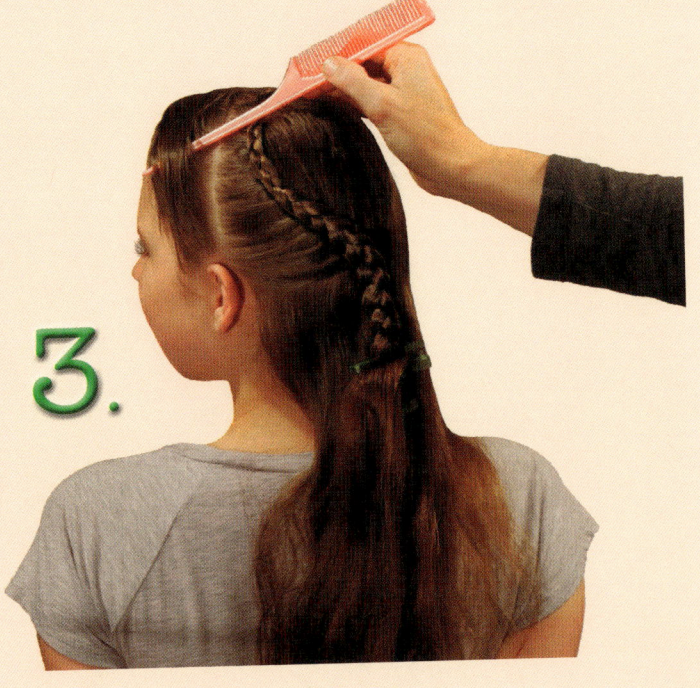

3. Braid from ear to ear, then around to the back of the head.

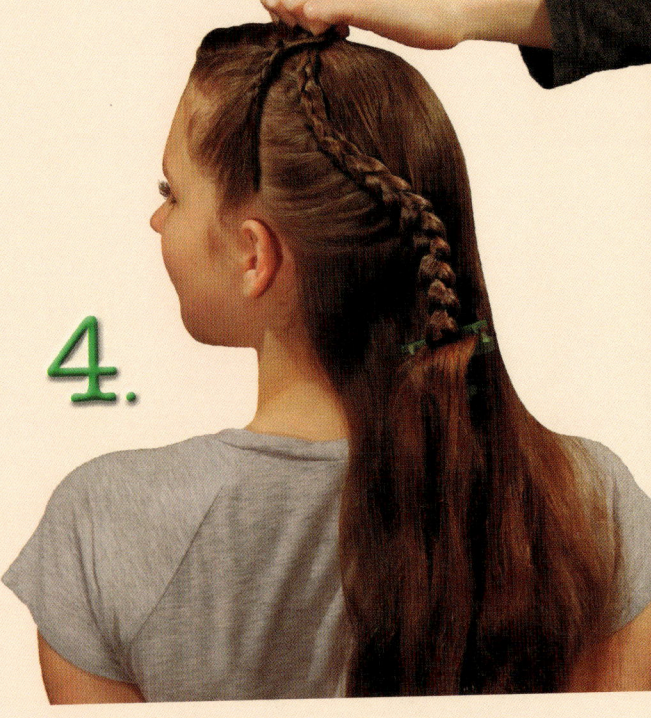

4. This is a three-strand merged into a two-strand herringbone.

7.

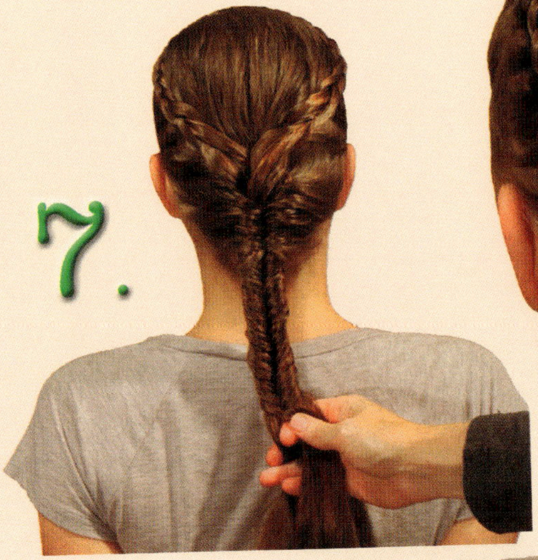

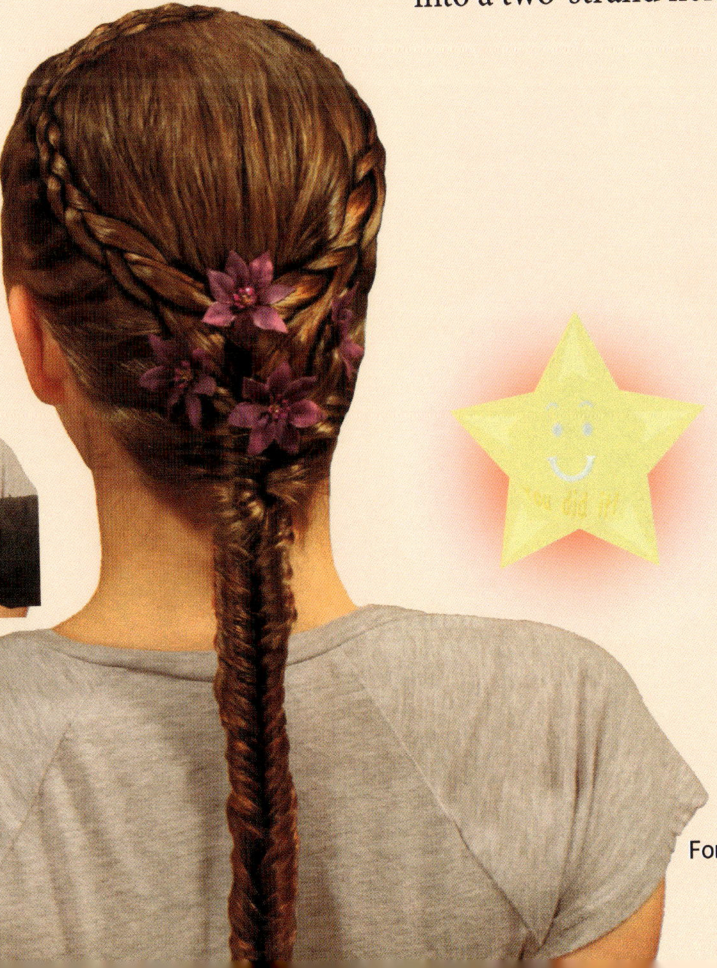

Forms 411

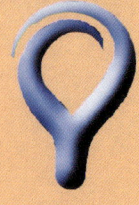

Accented Teardrop

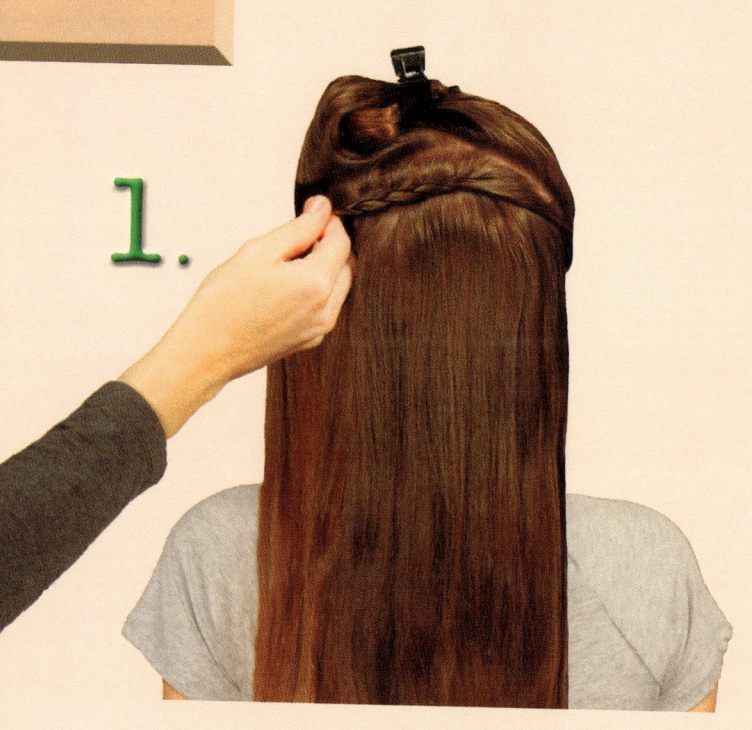

1. Secure the headband portion of hair in front. Start at an ear from behind the headband placement. Braid from ear to ear.

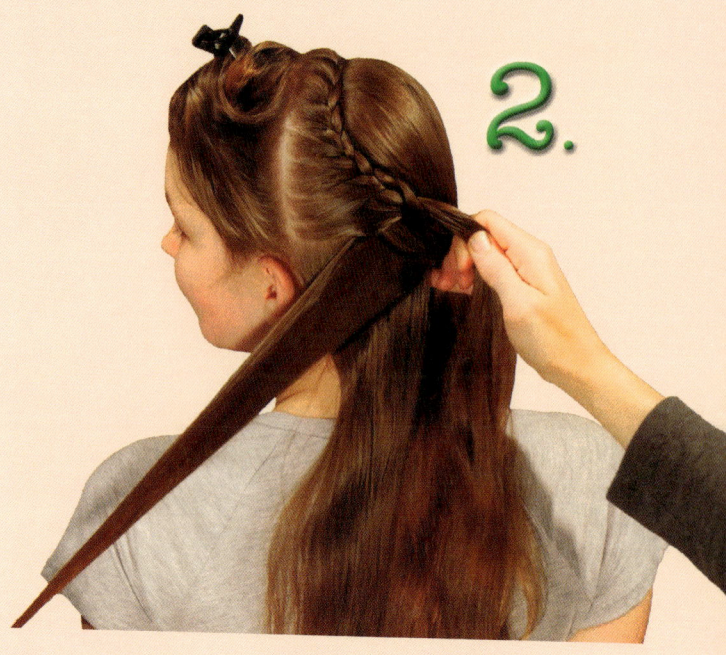

2. Take accent from desired locations while you braid. Clip off the braid behind the ear so you can braid the other side.

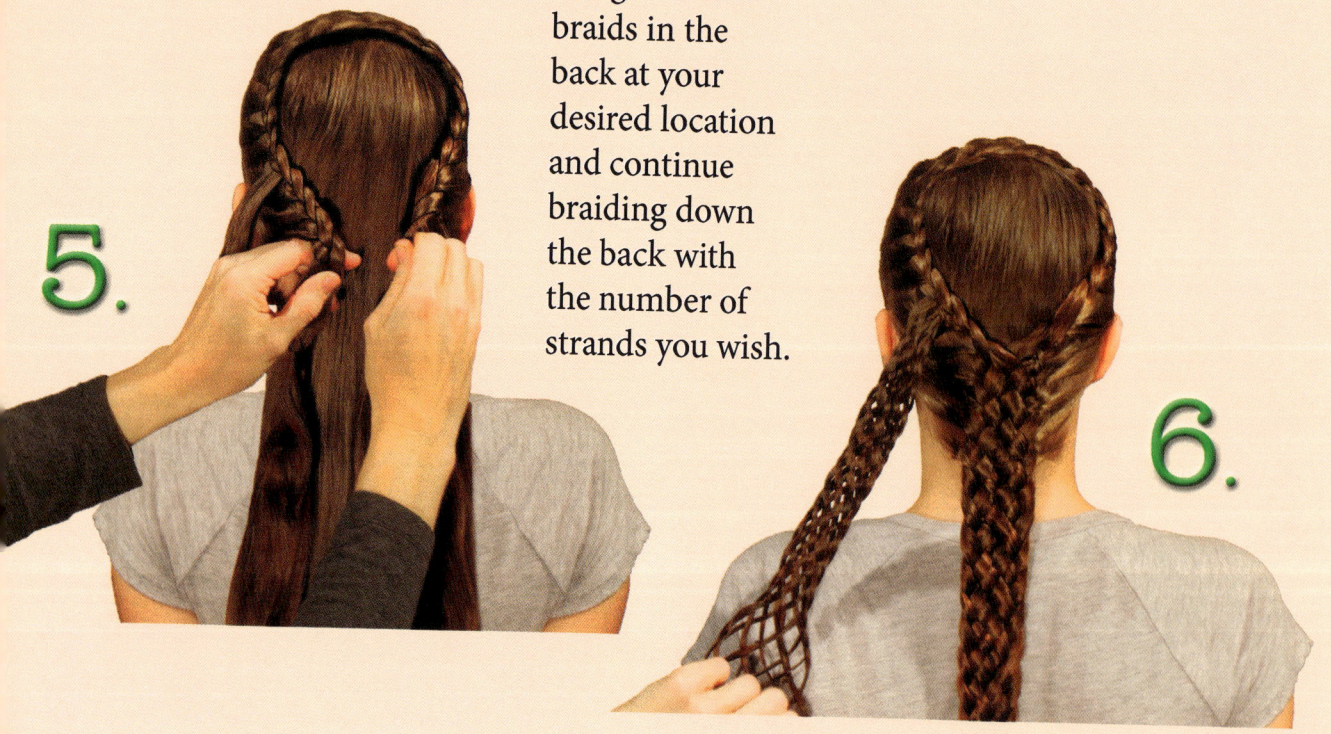

5. Merge the two braids in the back at your desired location and continue braiding down the back with the number of strands you wish.

6. Remember you can mix odd and even strand braids.

www.findingbraids.com

Accented Teardrop

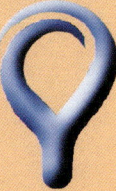

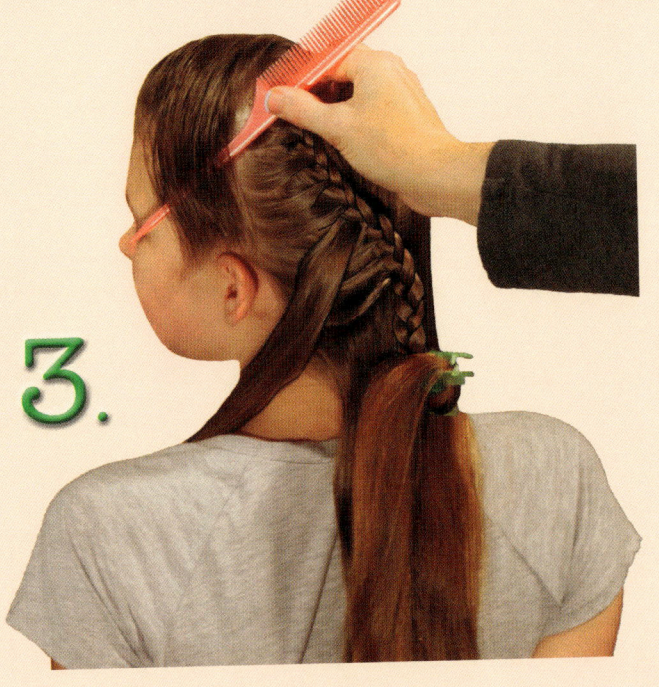

3. Braid from ear to ear, then around to the back of the head.

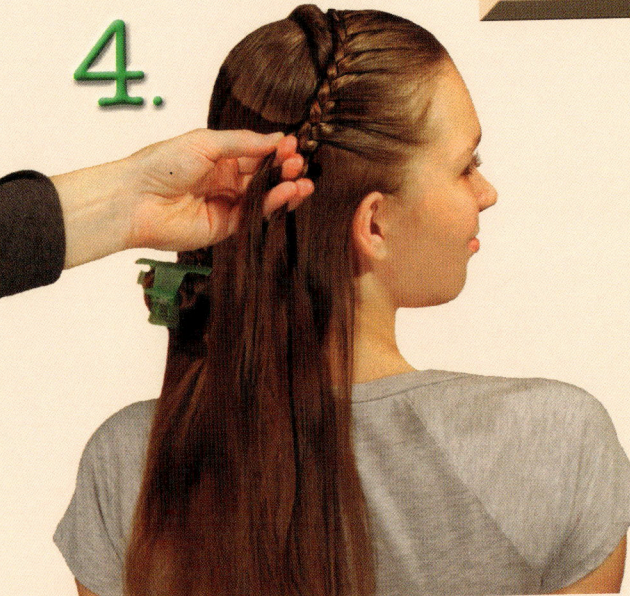

4. This is a three-strand merged into a seven-strand with a mini nine-strand braid for an accent.

7. Use your accent strand to create the accent of your choice and place that accent in a manner that finishes your style.

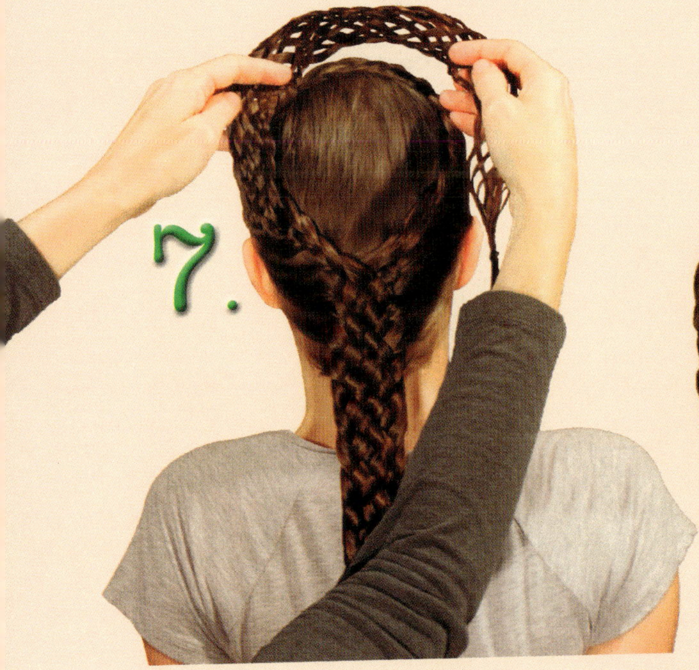

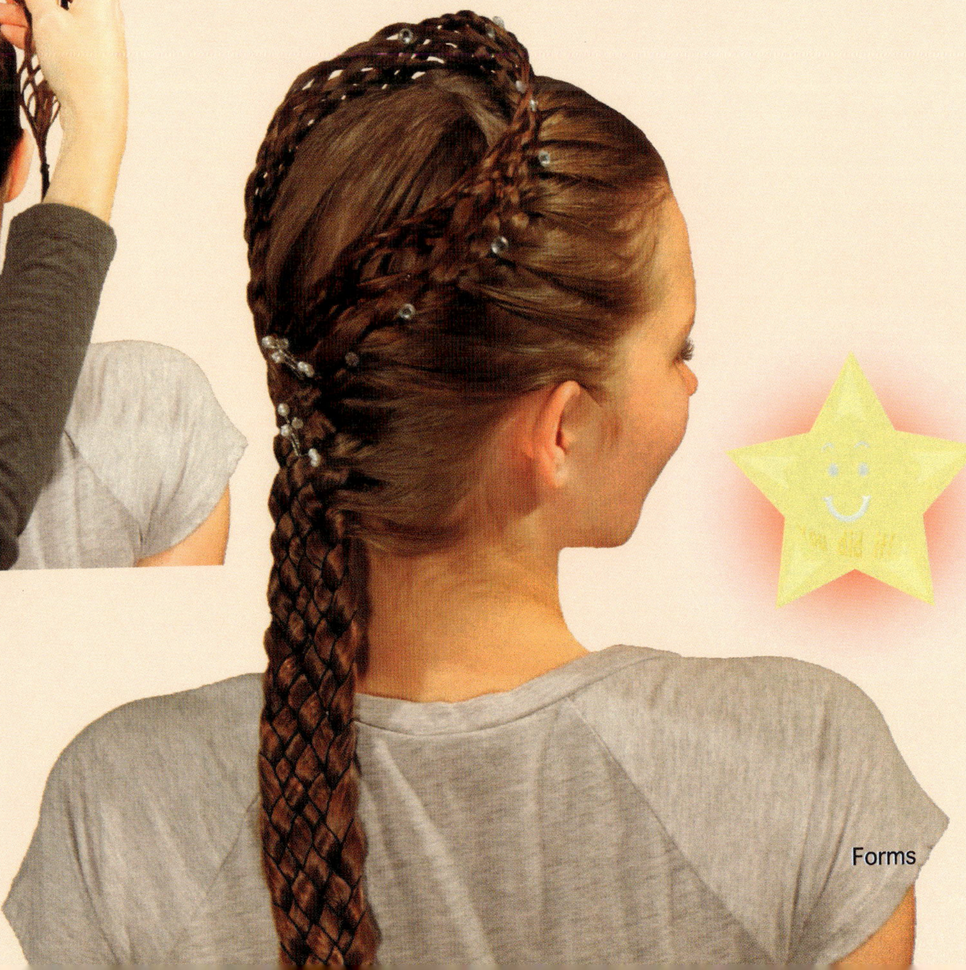

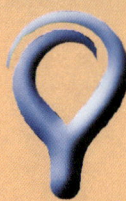

Teardrop Cascade

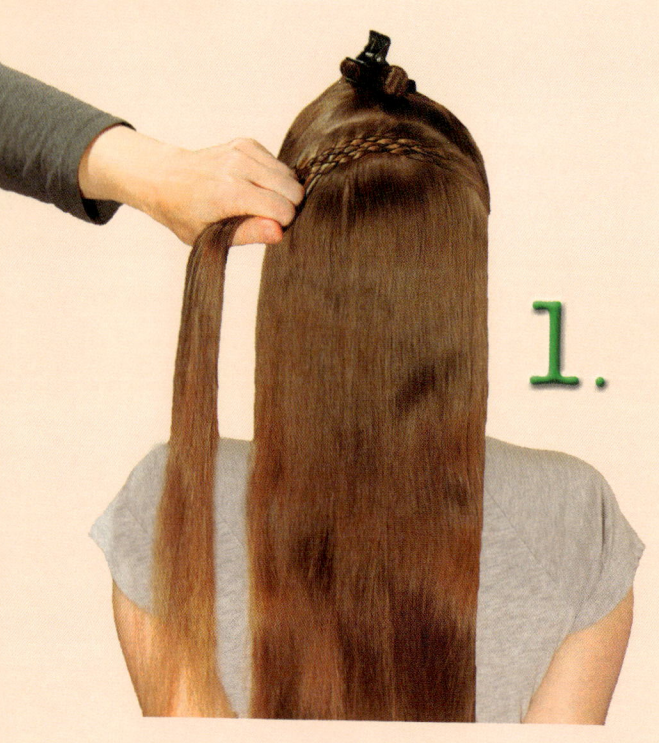

1. Secure the headband portion of hair in front. Start at an ear from behind the headband placement. Braid from ear to ear.

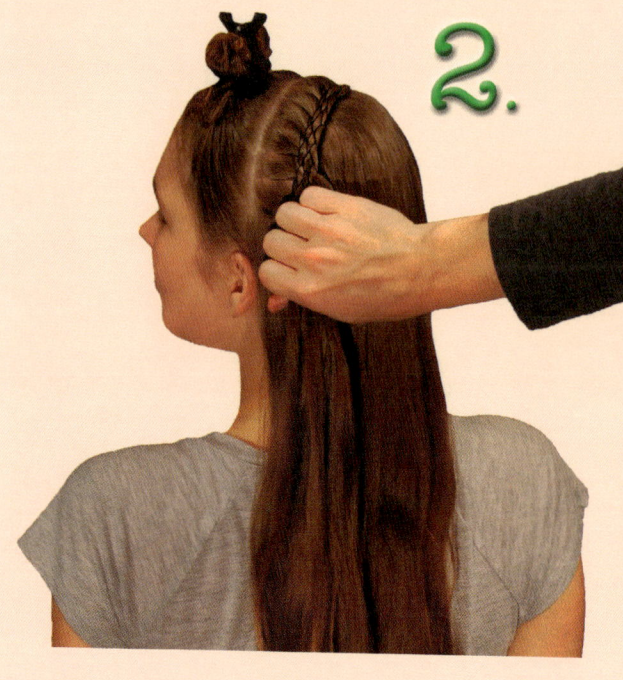

2. This is a five-strand merged into a five-strand. The back half of the hair is not braided and is left down as a cascade.

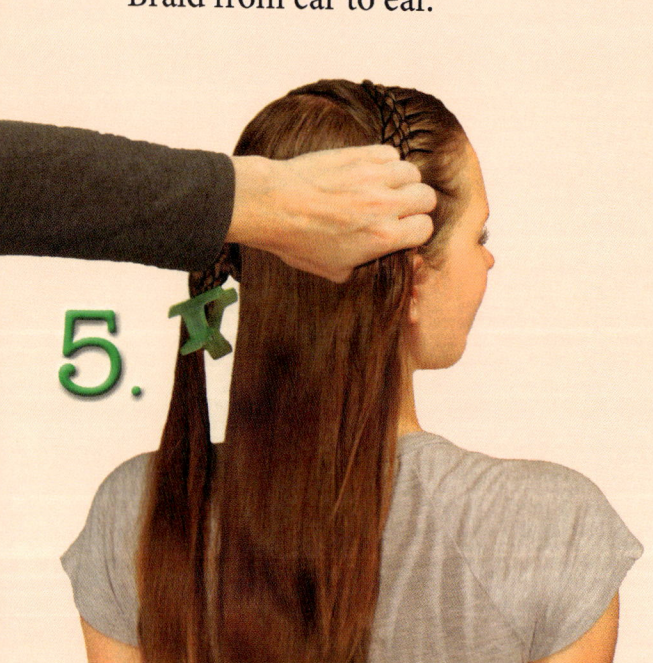

5.

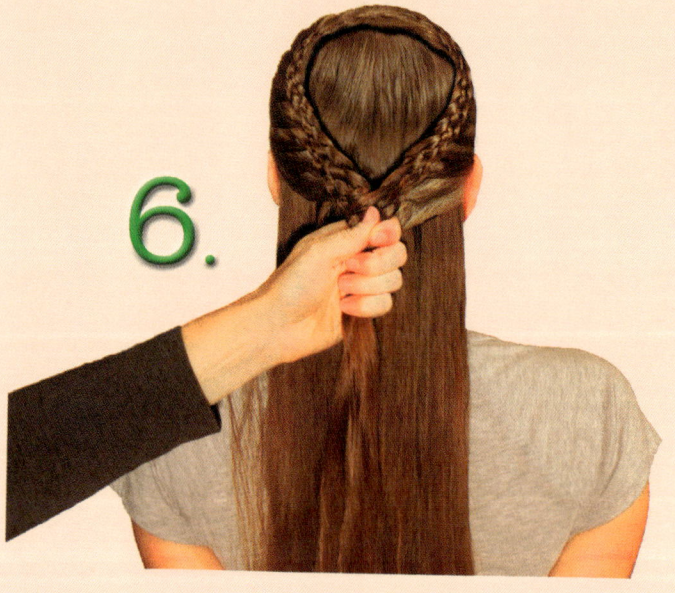

6. Merge the two braids in the back of the head at the desired location and decide what to do with the tail. It may be braided all the way down or left as a pony tail.

414   www.findingbraids.com

Teardrop Cascade

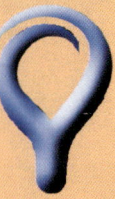

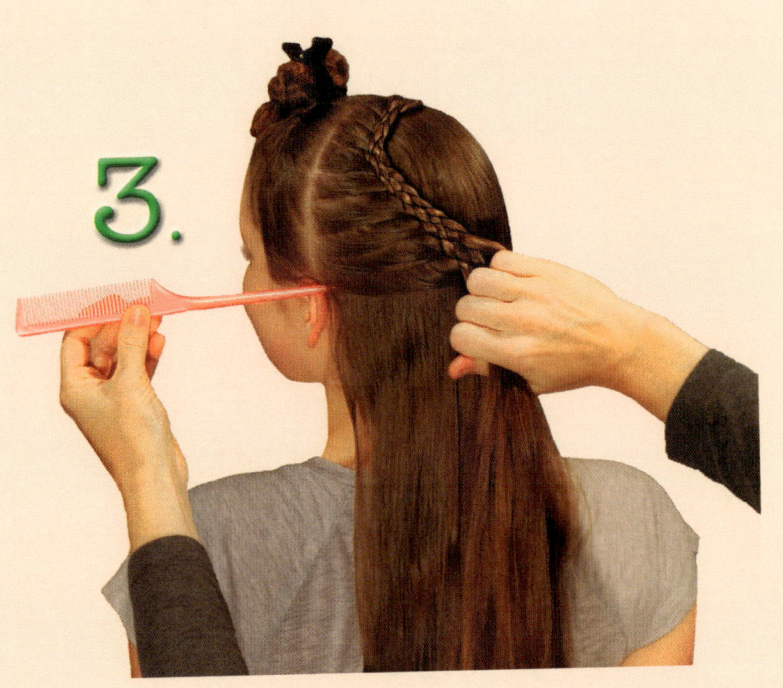

Clip off the braid so you can braid the other side.

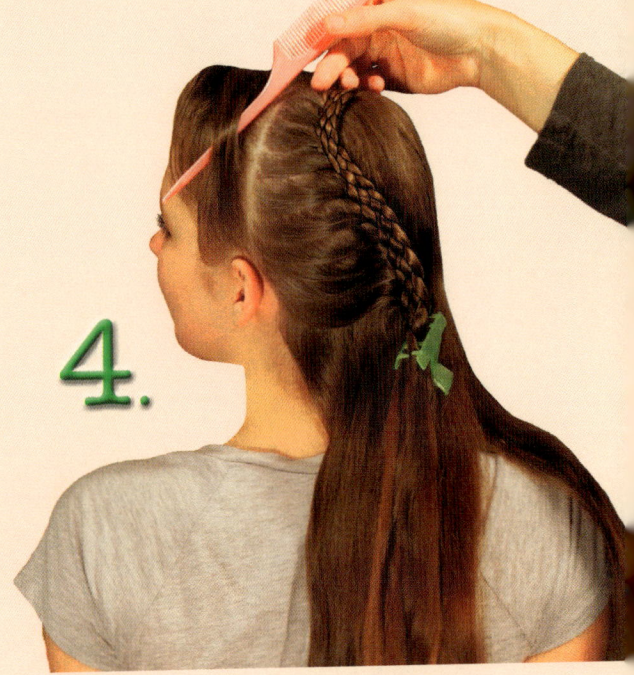

Braid from ear to ear, then around to the back of the head.

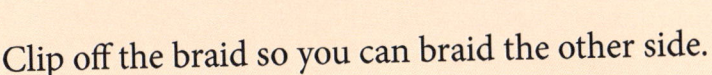

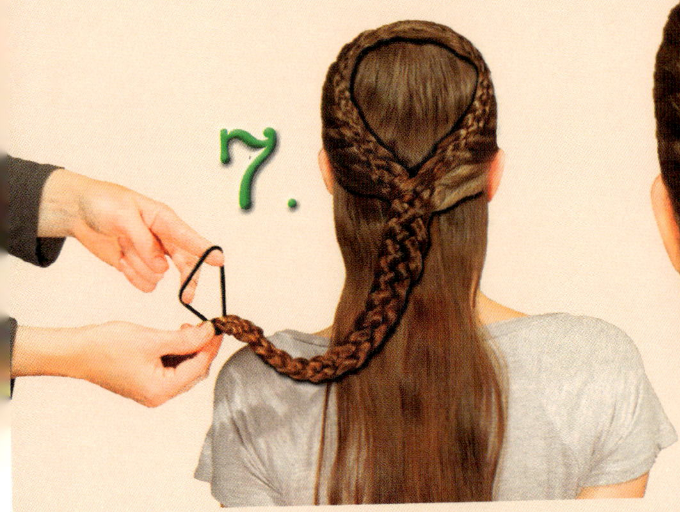

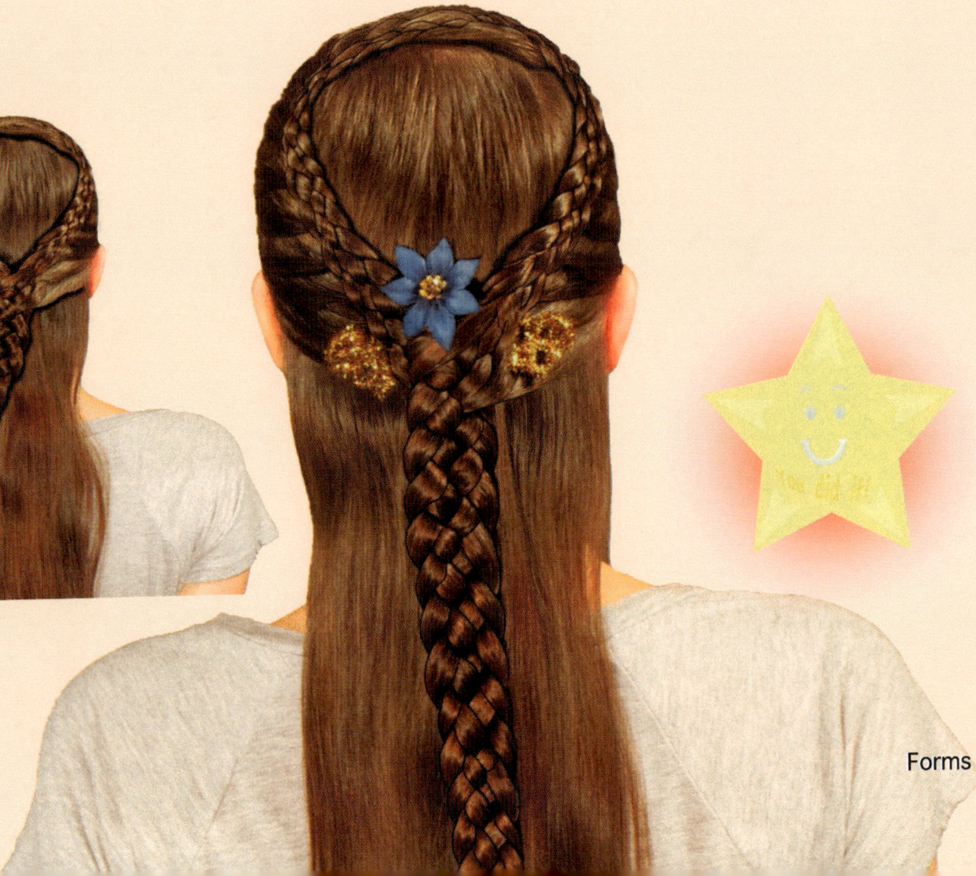

Accented Teardrop Cascade

This is a one-strand pretzel merged into a one-strand pretzel and the accents are also mini one-strand pretzels. The accents are taken from the cascade.

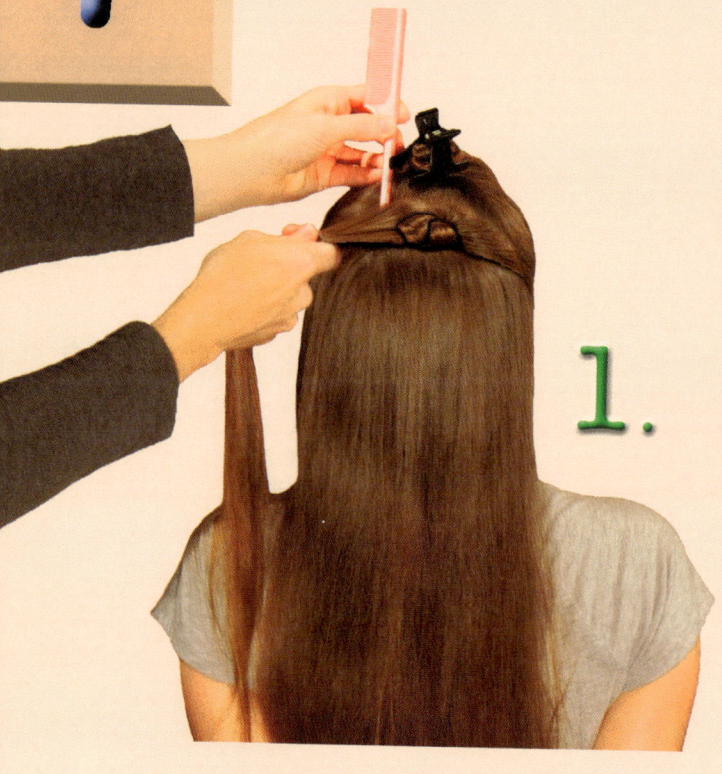

1.

Secure the headband portion of hair in front. Start at an ear from behind the headband placement. Braid from ear to ear.

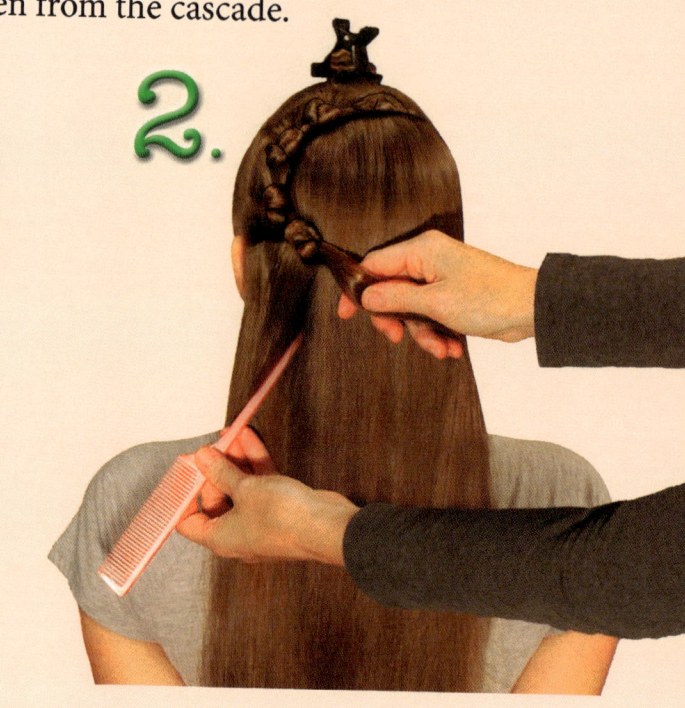

2.

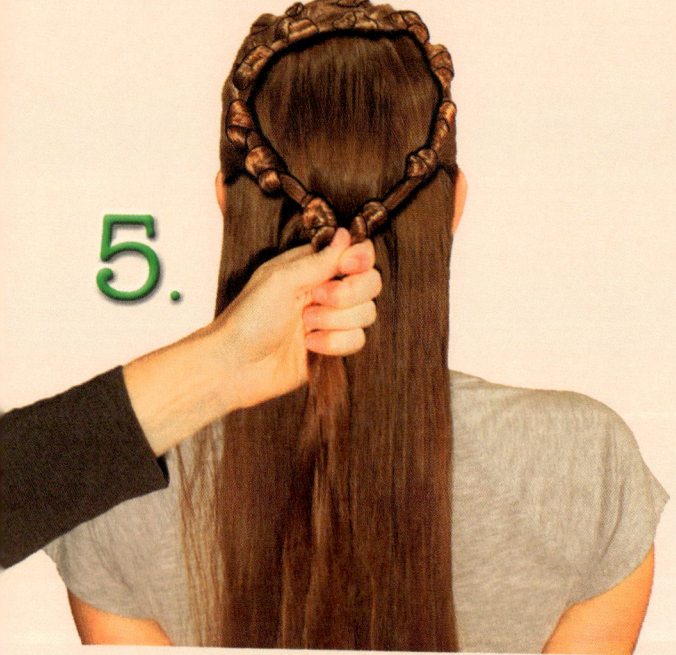

5.

Merge the two braids in the desired location.

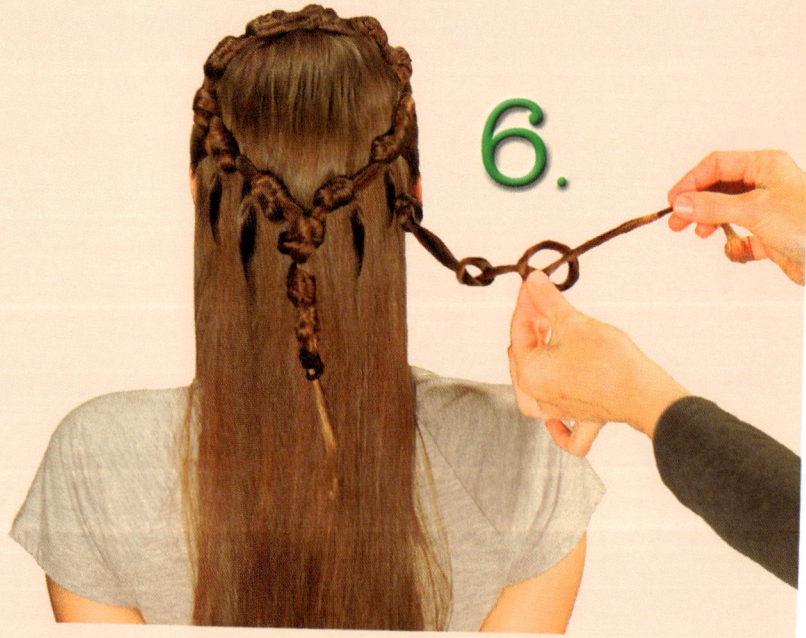

6.

Create your accents and place them in the manner that finishes your style.

416   www.findingbraids.com

Accented Teardrop Cascade

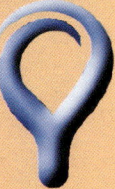

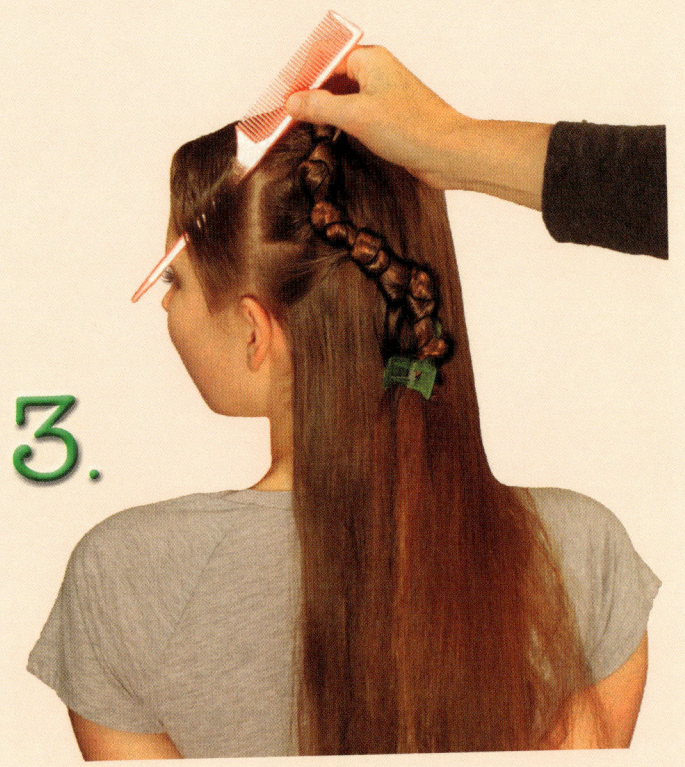

3.

Clip off the braid behind the ear so you can braid the other side.

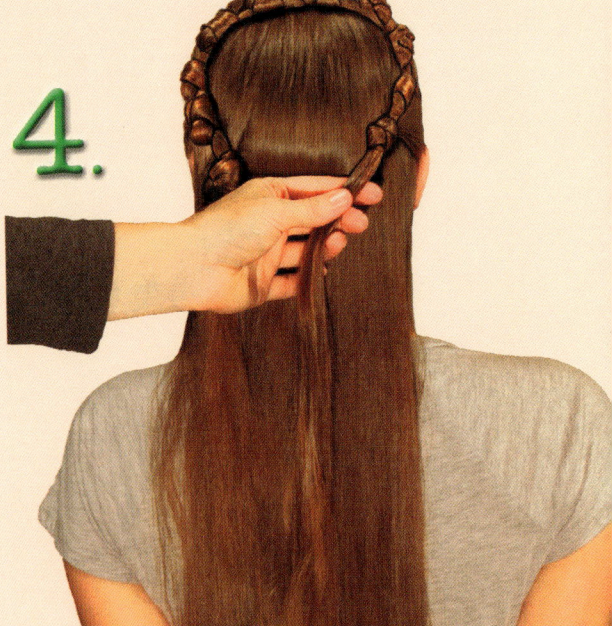

4.

Braid from ear to ear, then around to the back of the head.

7.

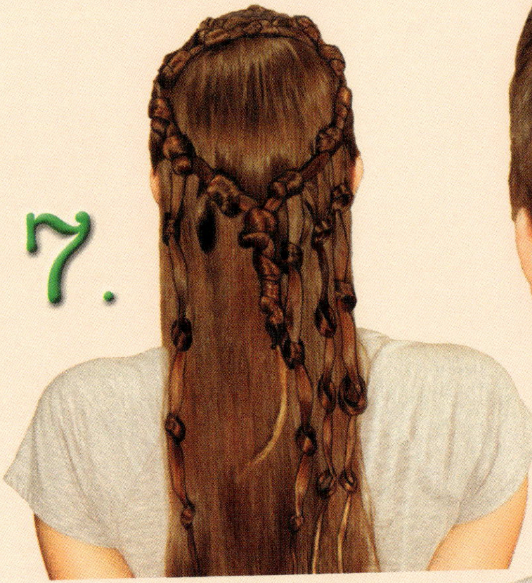

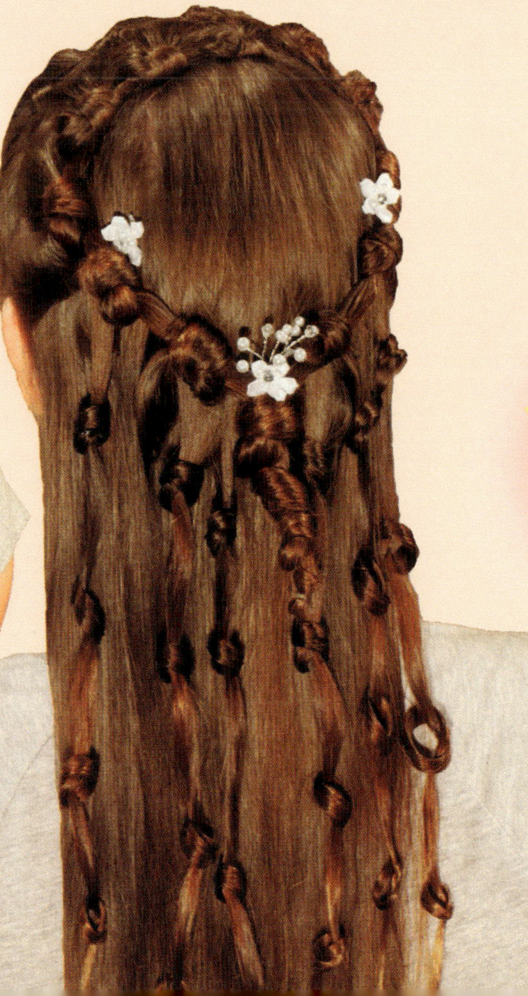

Forms 417

Forms

Notes

Examples of Teardrops

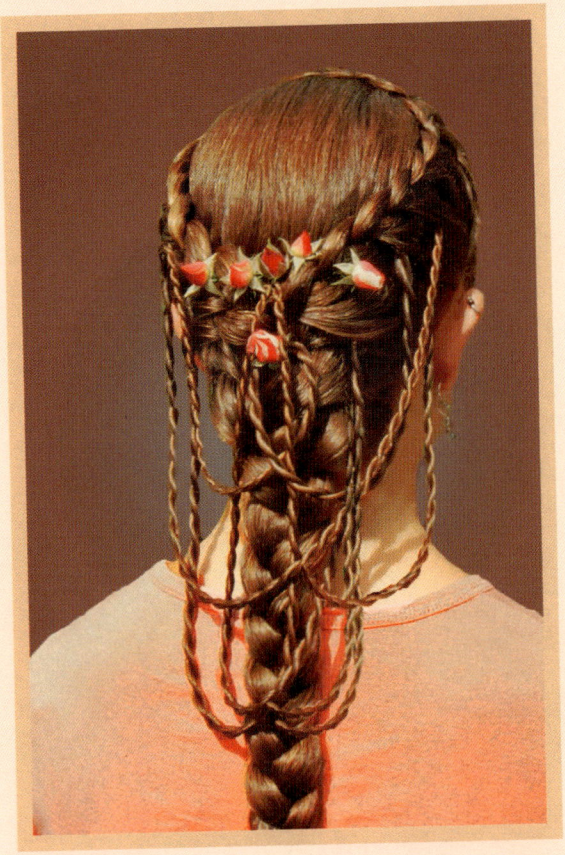
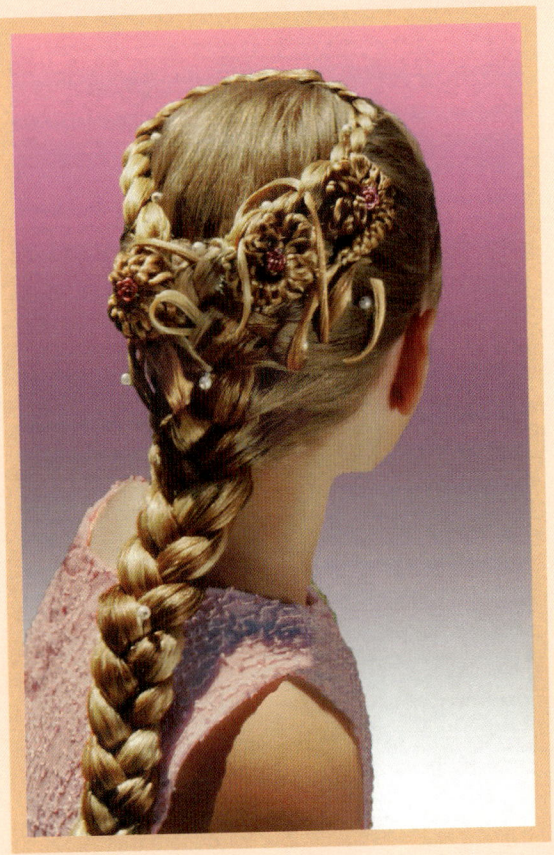
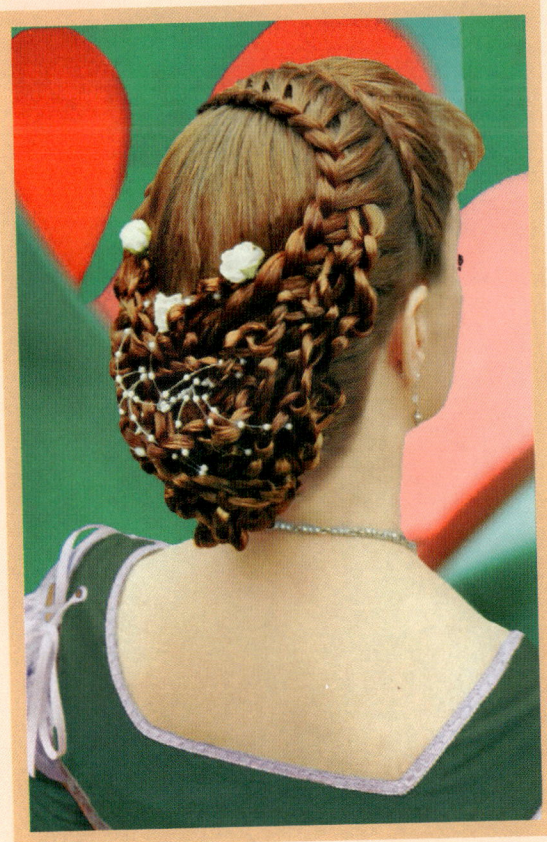
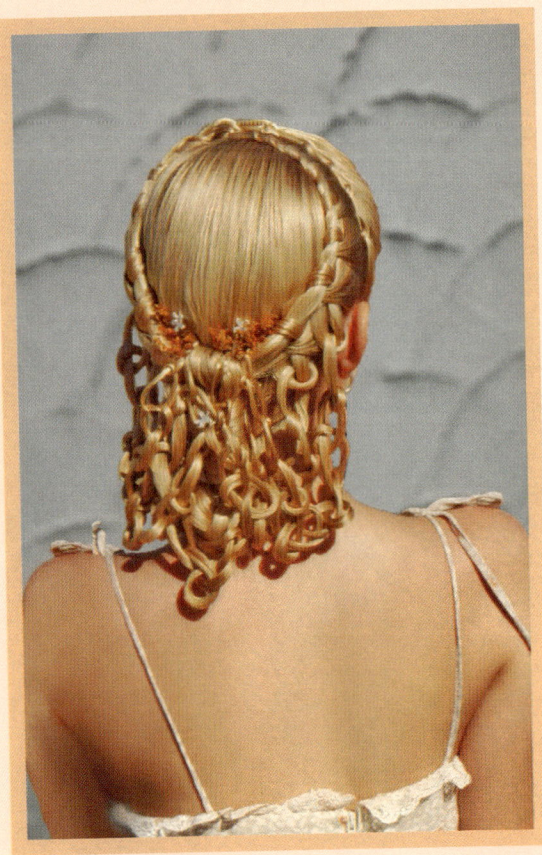

Visit my website to see more examples of Teardrops

Forms

F R I N G E

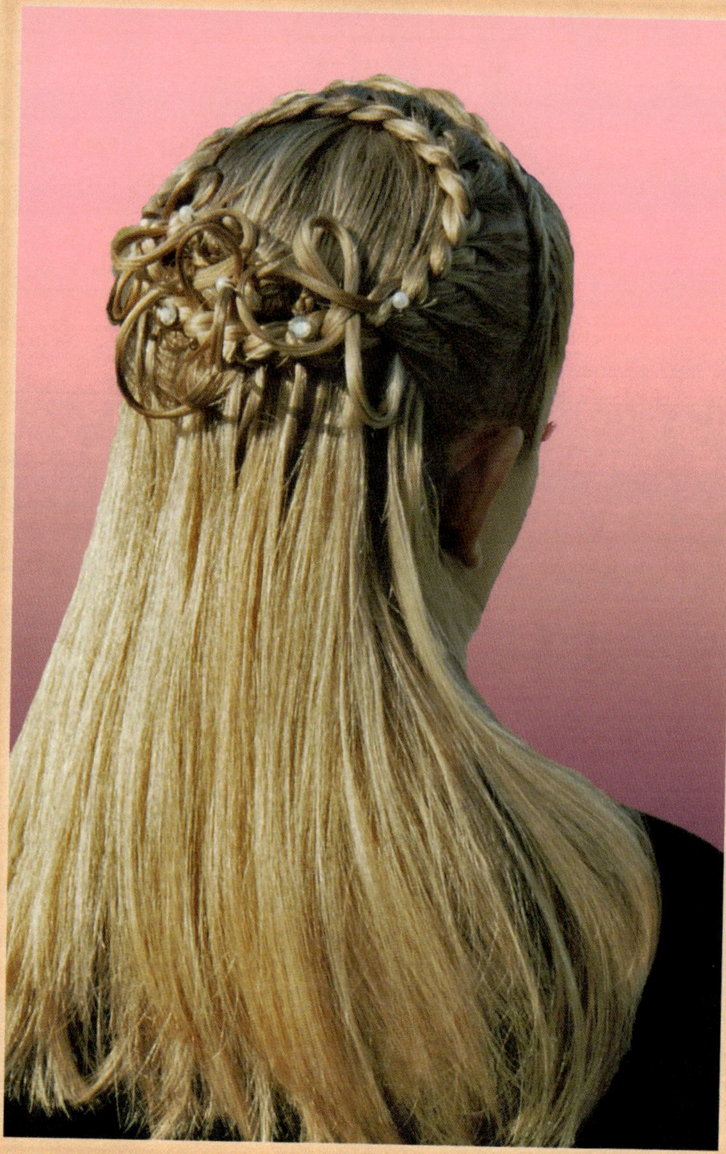

Hairstyles refine the ensemble specifically chosen for your event. The sweep of each gather matching the material and design of your outfit and occasion.

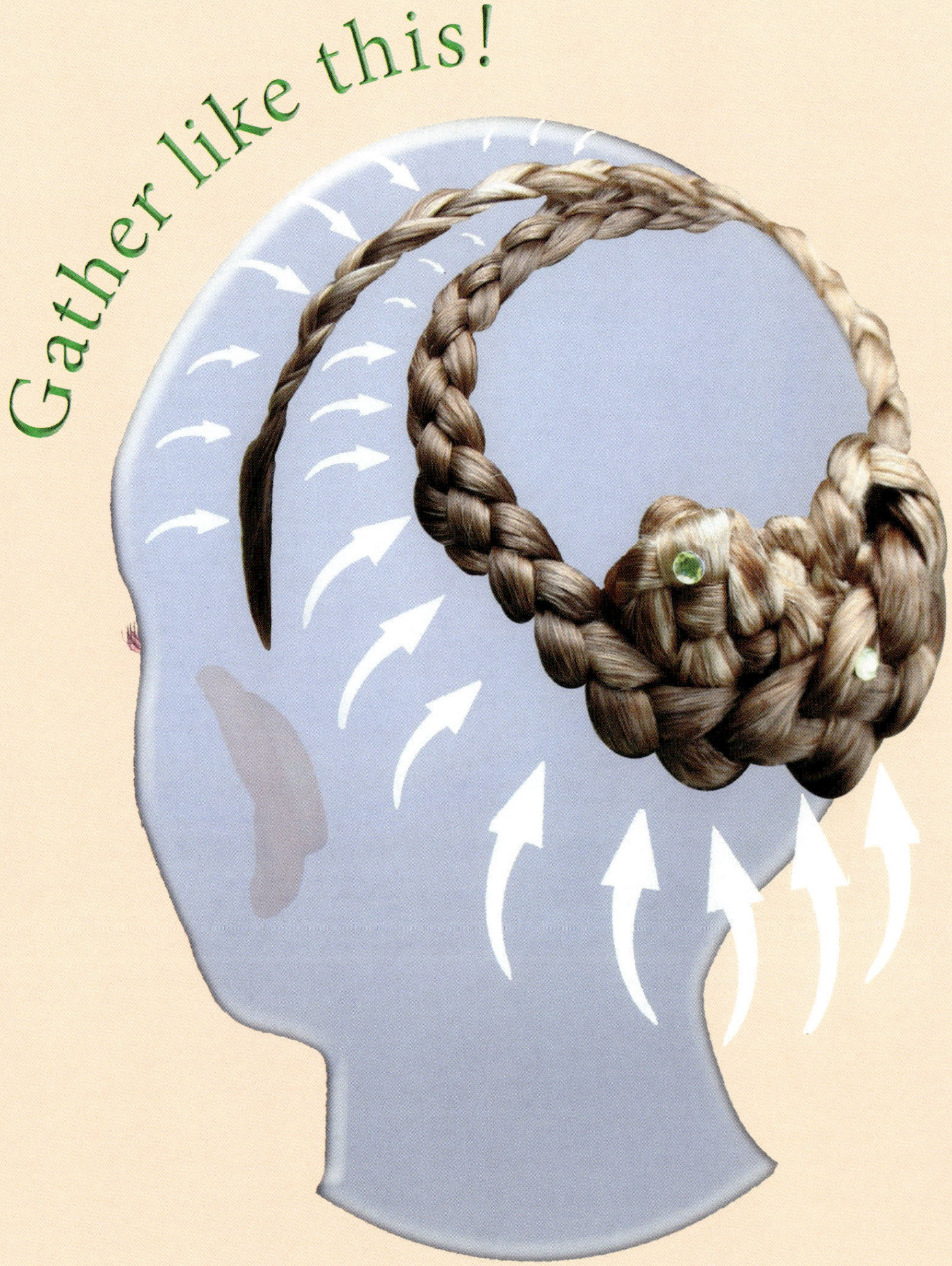

Forms

Gather like this!

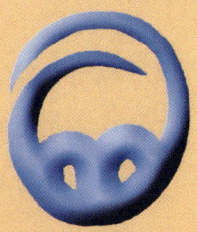

Braiding icon for the next eight pages.

The crisscross in front and back of this form lend a spiral motion. Spellbinding passersby with its charm. The style may not be worth the attention you receive. Who am I kidding, we love the attention.

The **Fringe** Form

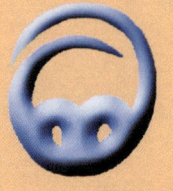

Basic Fringe

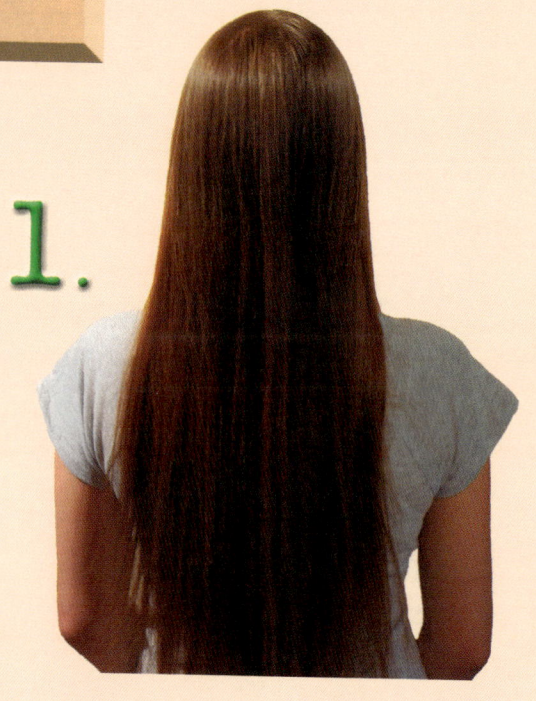

1. Begin with clean, brushed hair.

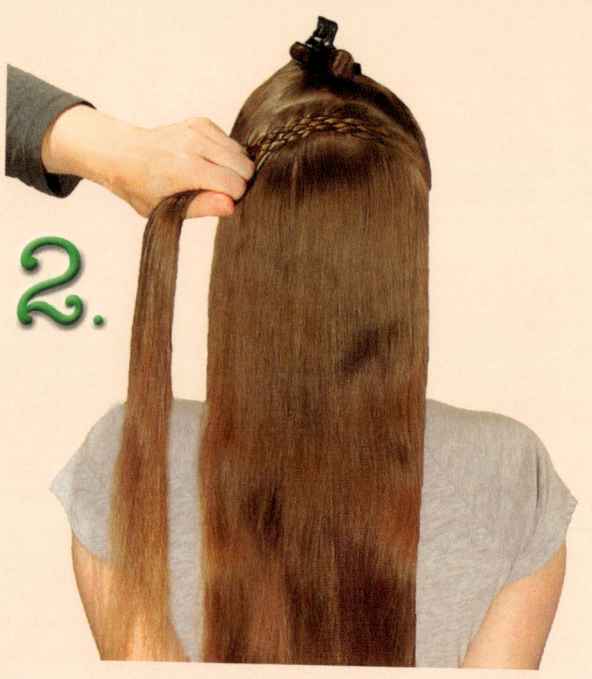

2. Secure the headband portion of hair in front. Start at an ear from behind the headband placement. Braid from ear to ear. This is a seven-strand.

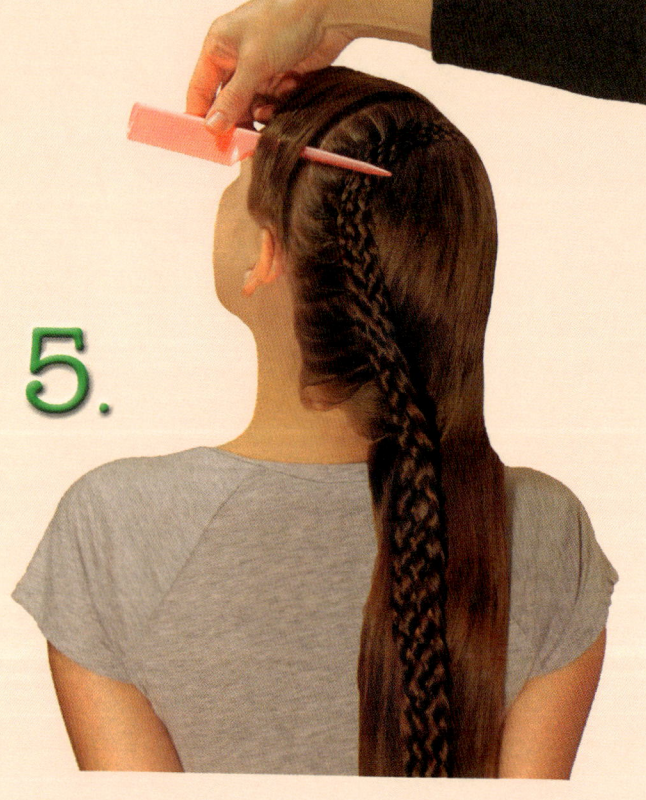

5.

6. Proceed the same on the other side.

422 www.findingbraids.com

Basic Fringe

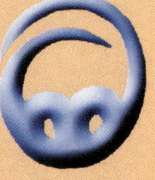

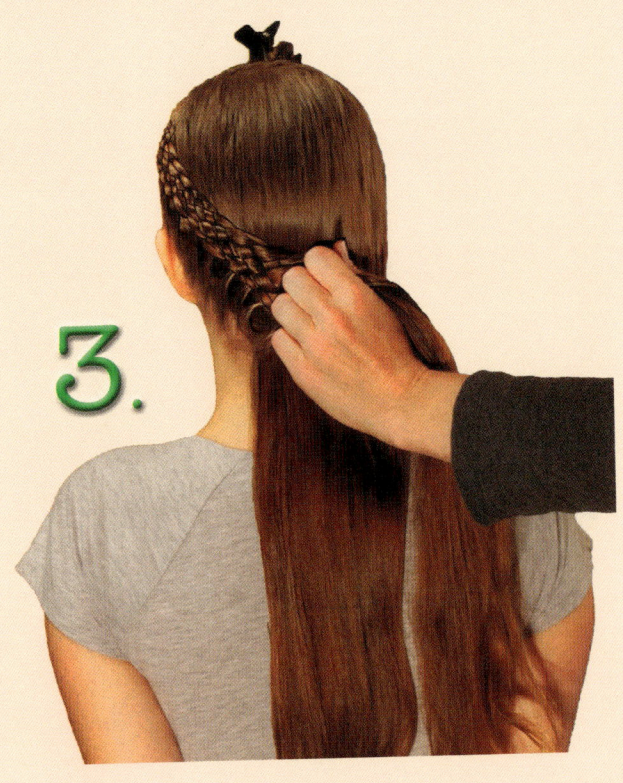

3. Continue all the way around to the back of the head to where the bun will be placed.

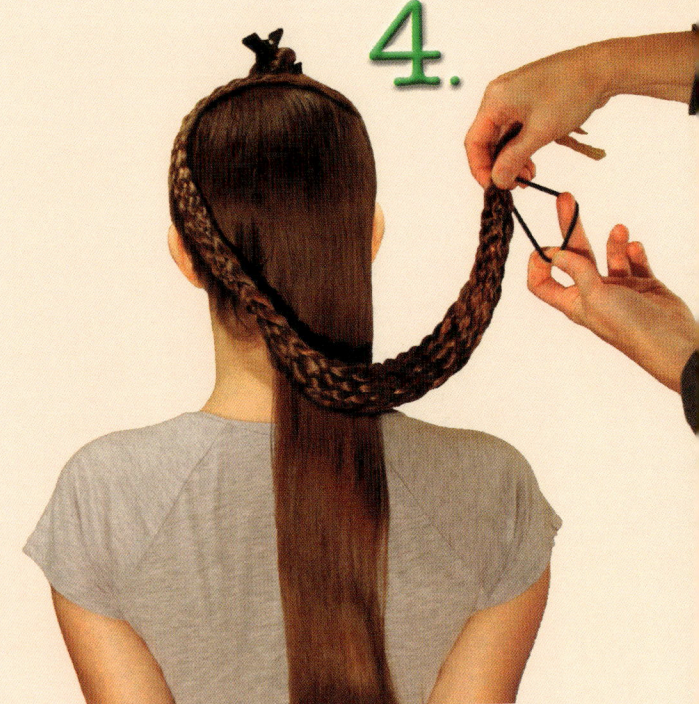

4. Finish braiding the tail and band the end.

7. Design a stunning bun and pin it securely in place.

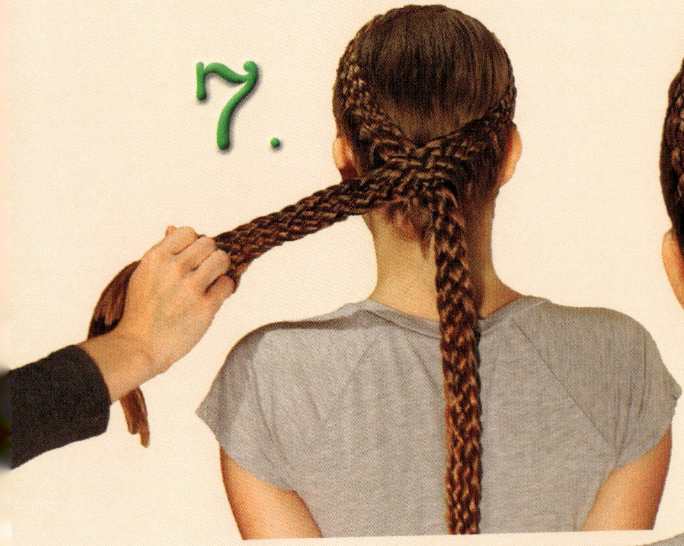

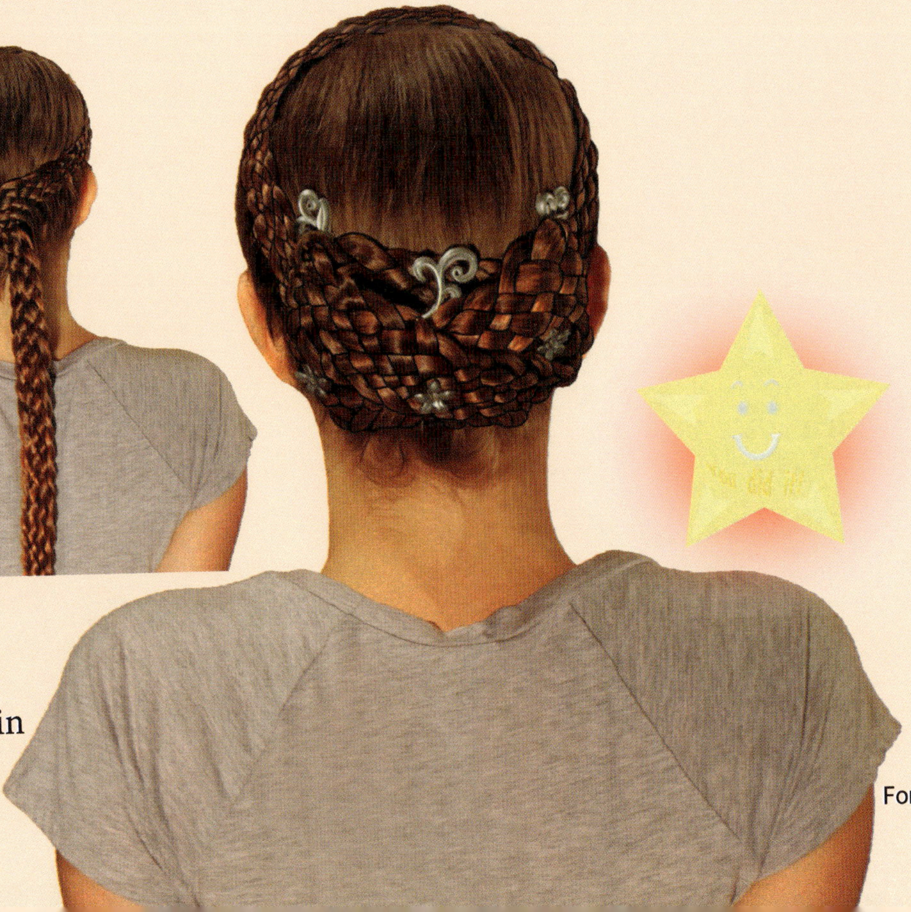

Forms 423

Accented Fringe

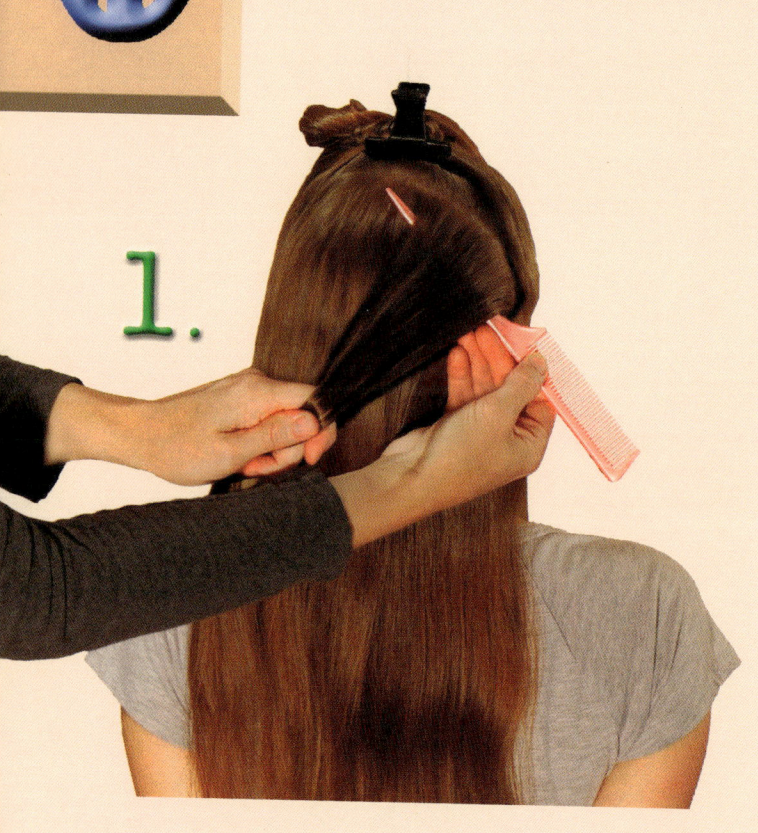

1. Secure the headband portion of hair in front. Start at an ear from behind the headband placement. Braid from ear to ear.

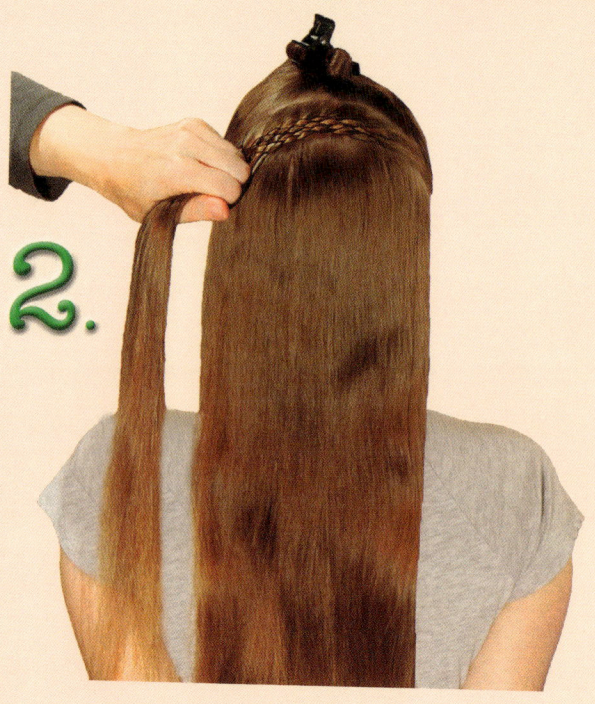

2. Continue all the way around to the back of the head to where the bun will be placed. This is a five-strand french.

5. Half of the accents here will come from the tails. I use a bun to create bulk and some of the tails to create curls to pin to that bulk.

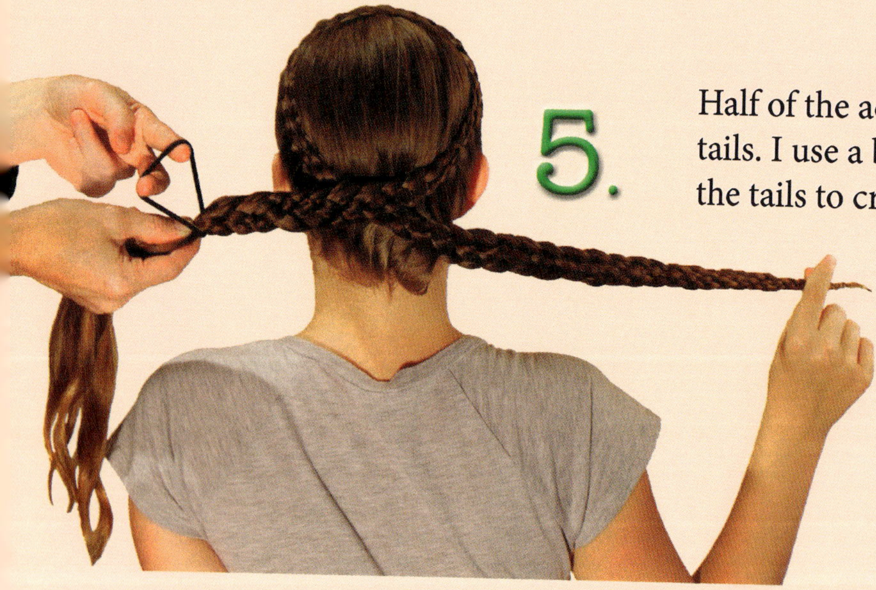

6.

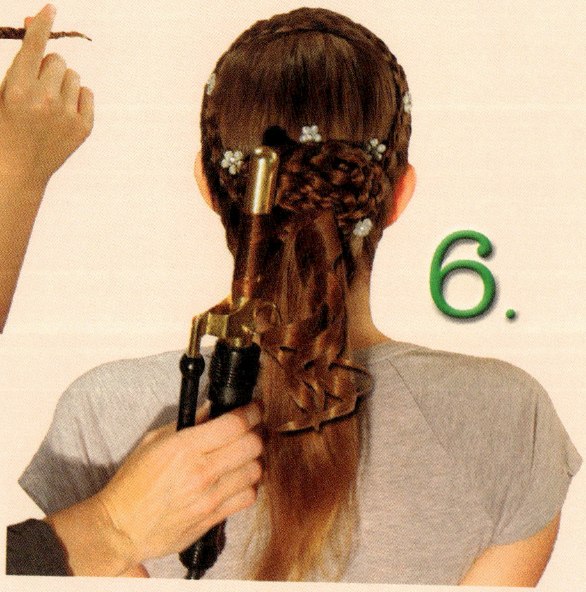

www.findingbraids.com

Accented Fringe

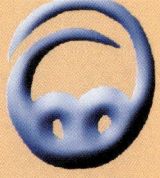

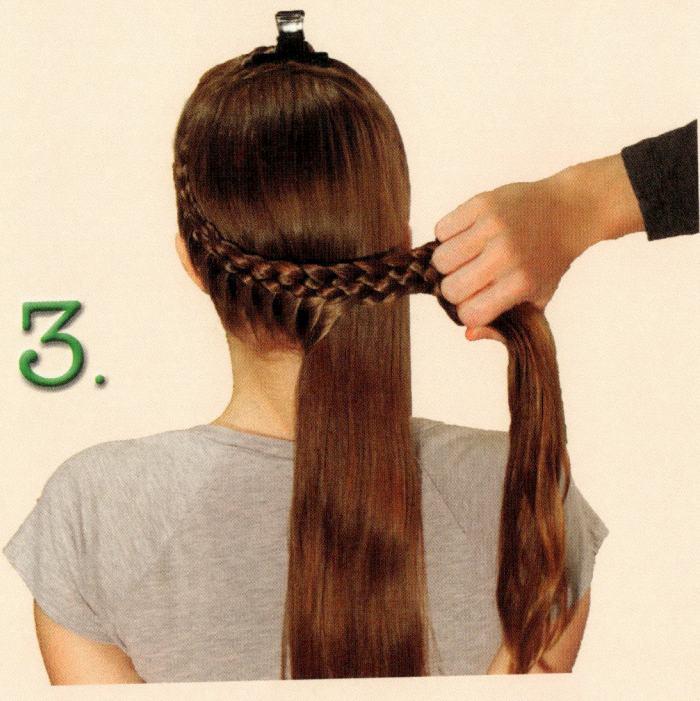

3. Finish braiding the tail and band the end.

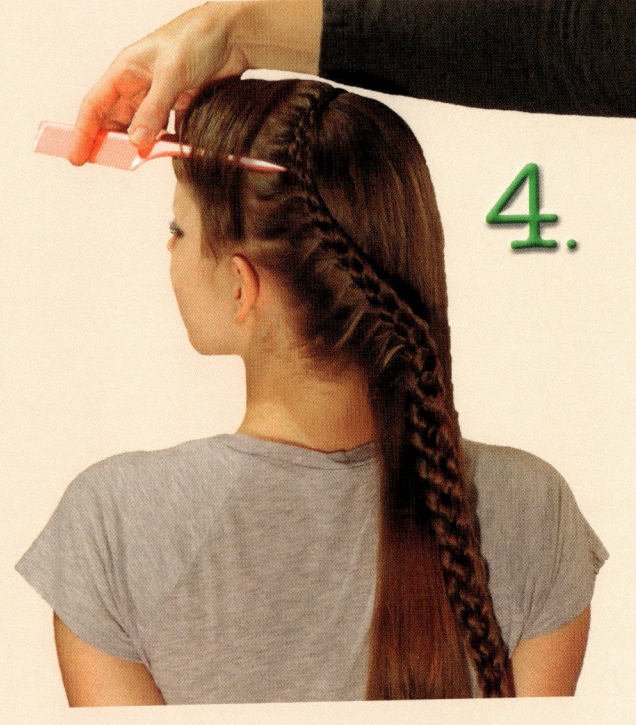

4. Proceed the same on the other side.

The other half of the accents are from fake hair that match her hair. I use a latchhook to weave the fake hair into curls, entwined with the real curls.

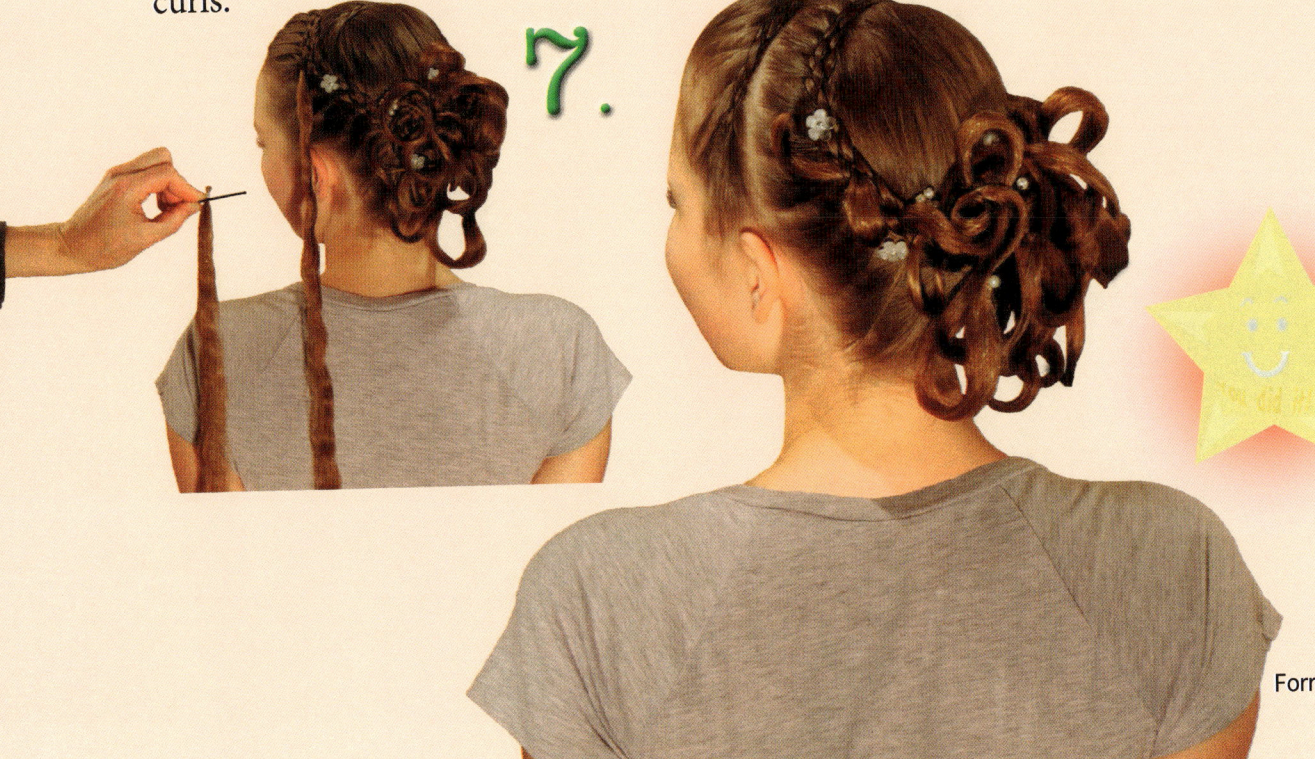

7.

Forms 425

Fringe Cascade

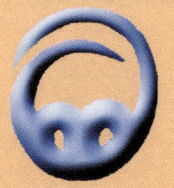

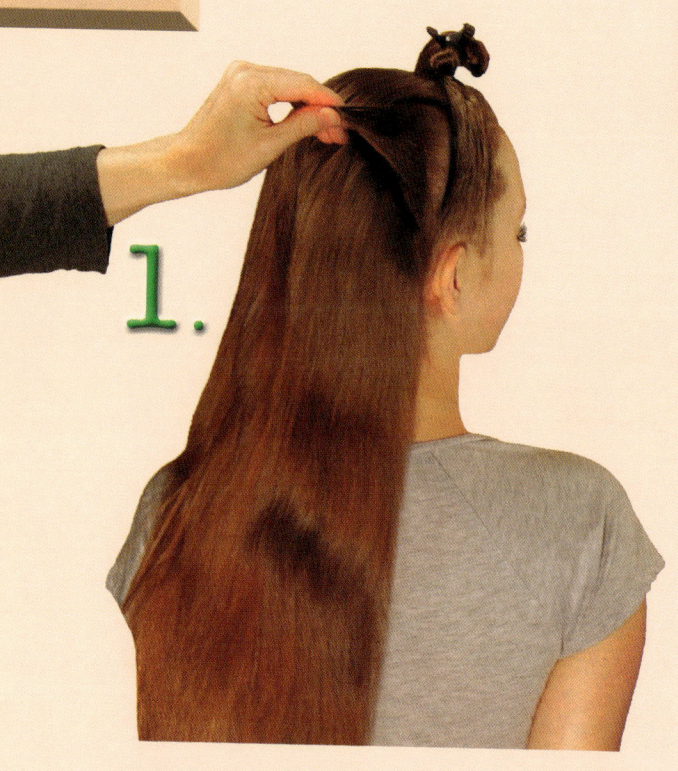

1. Secure the headband portion of hair in front. Start at an ear from behind the headband placement. Braid from ear to ear.

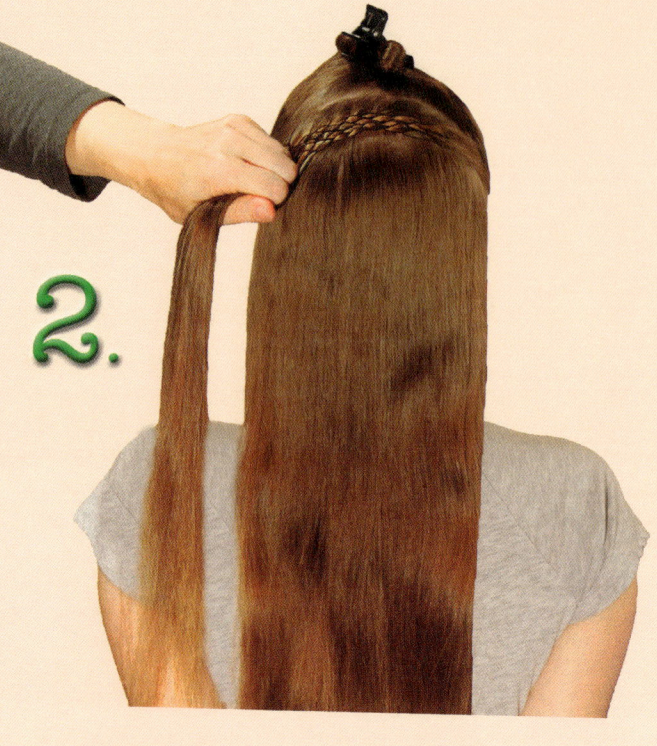

2. Continue all the way around to the back of the head to where the bun will be placed. Make sure you cascade from behind the ear to the back of the head.

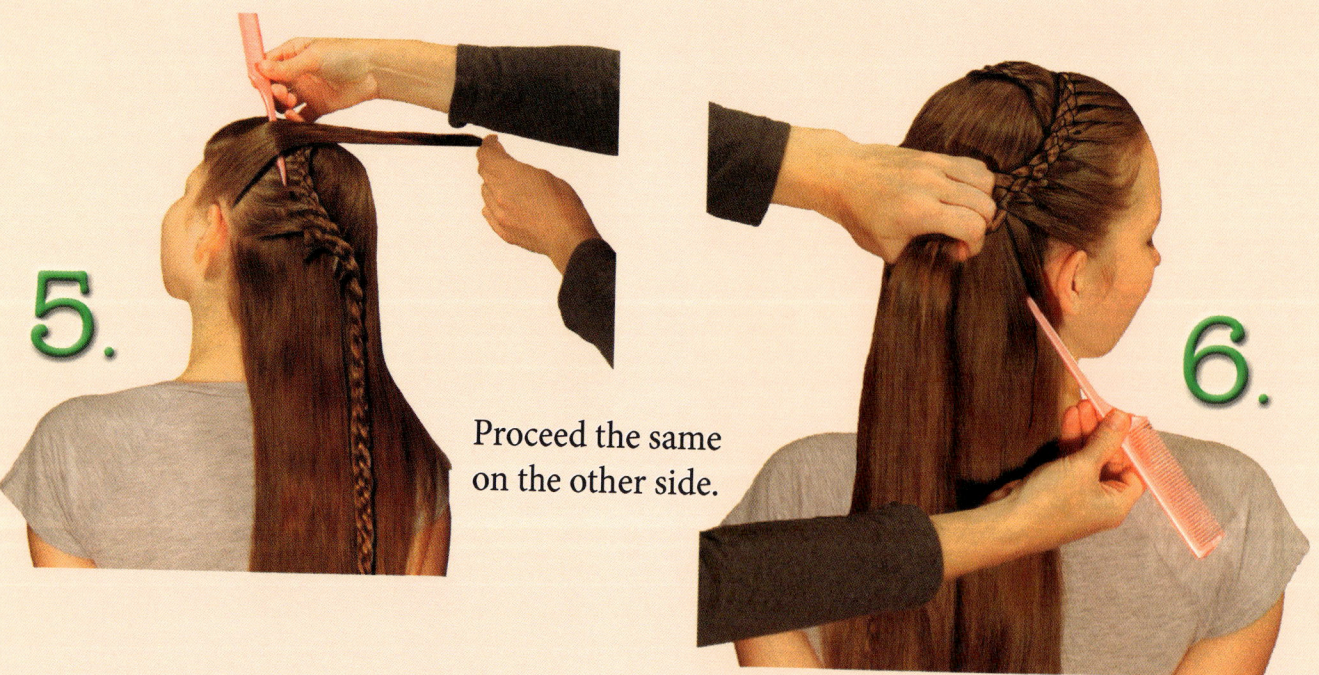

5.

Proceed the same on the other side.

6.

426 www.findingbraids.com

Fringe Cascade

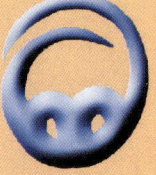

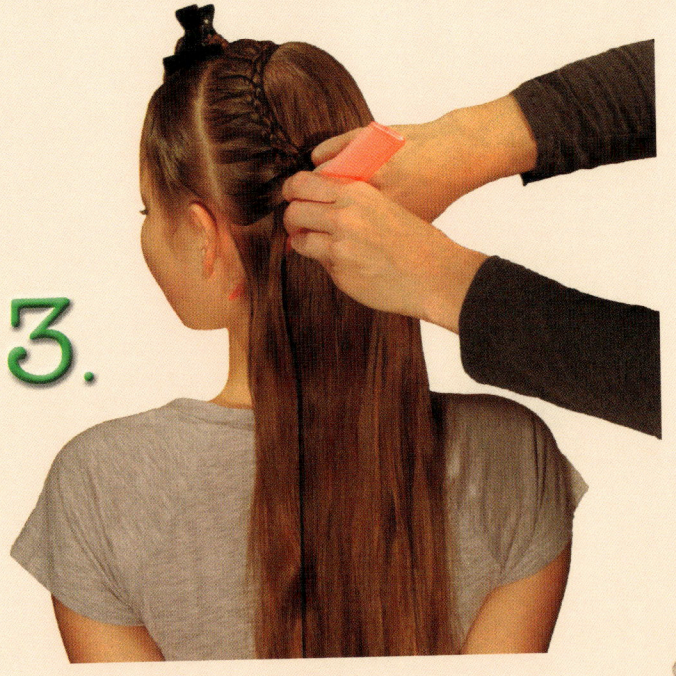

3.

To cascade the back, only take up a sliver of each gather. Leave most of each gather down and not braided. This is a four-strand french lace.

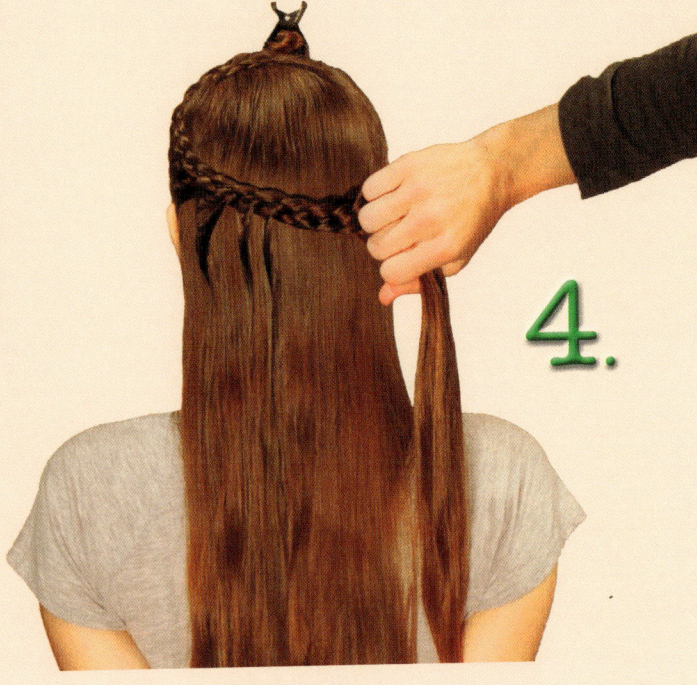

4.

Finish braiding the tail and band the end.

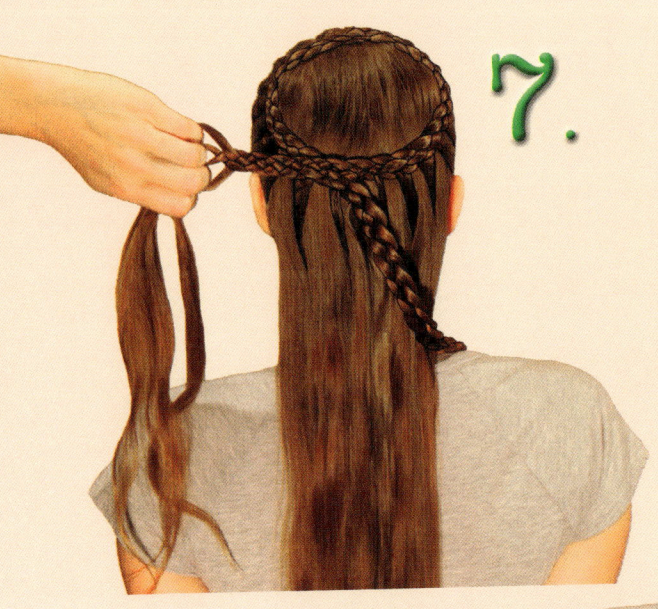

7.

Design a stunning bun and pin it securely in place.

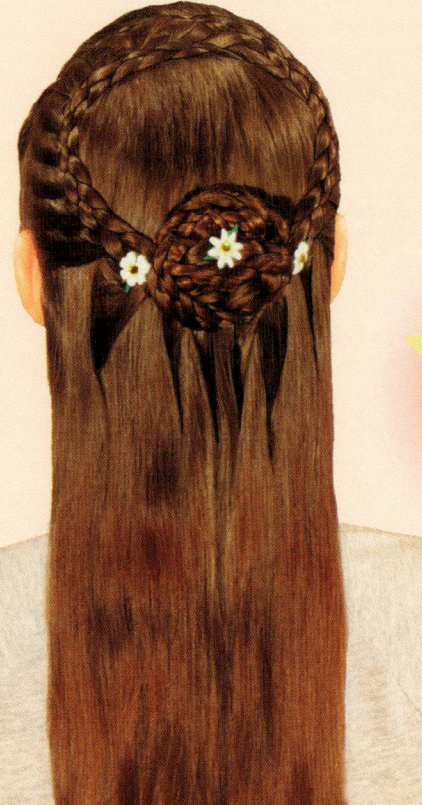

Forms 427

Accented Fringe Cascade

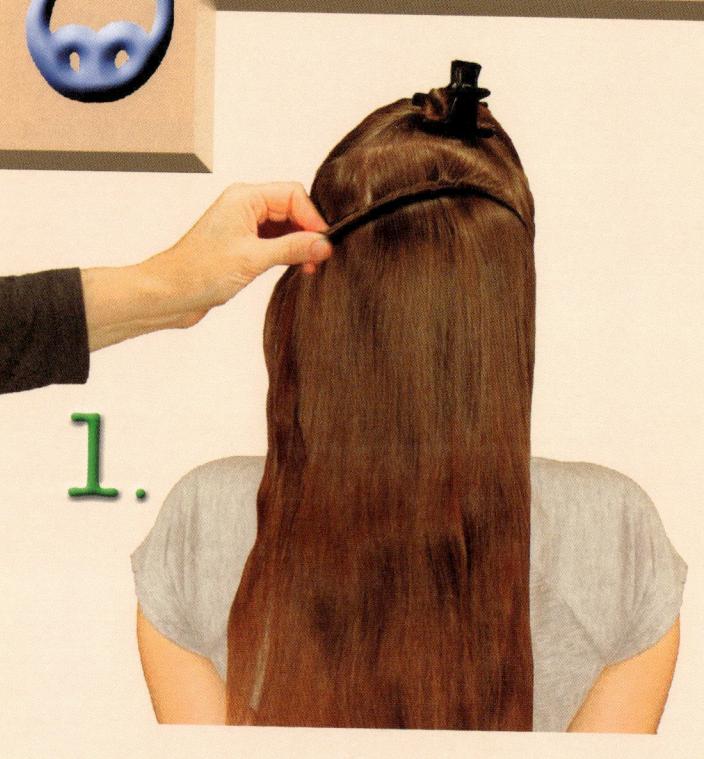

1.

Secure the headband portion of hair in front. Start at an ear from behind the headband placement. Braid from ear to ear.

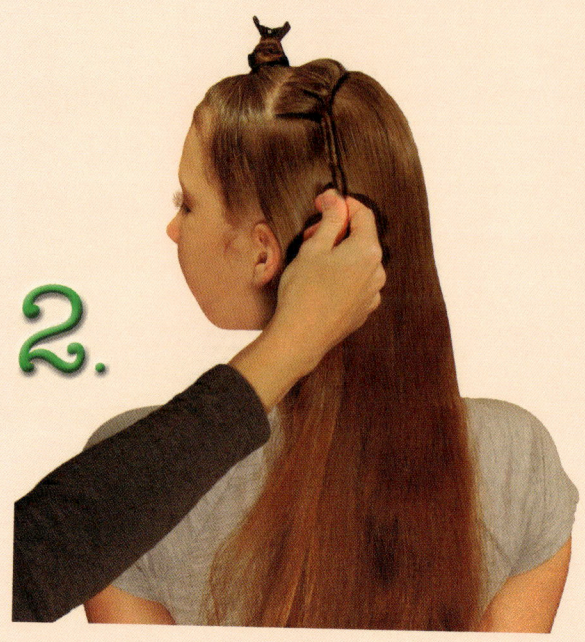

2.

Continue all the way around to the back of the head to where the bun will be placed. Make sure you cascade from behind the ear to the back of the head.

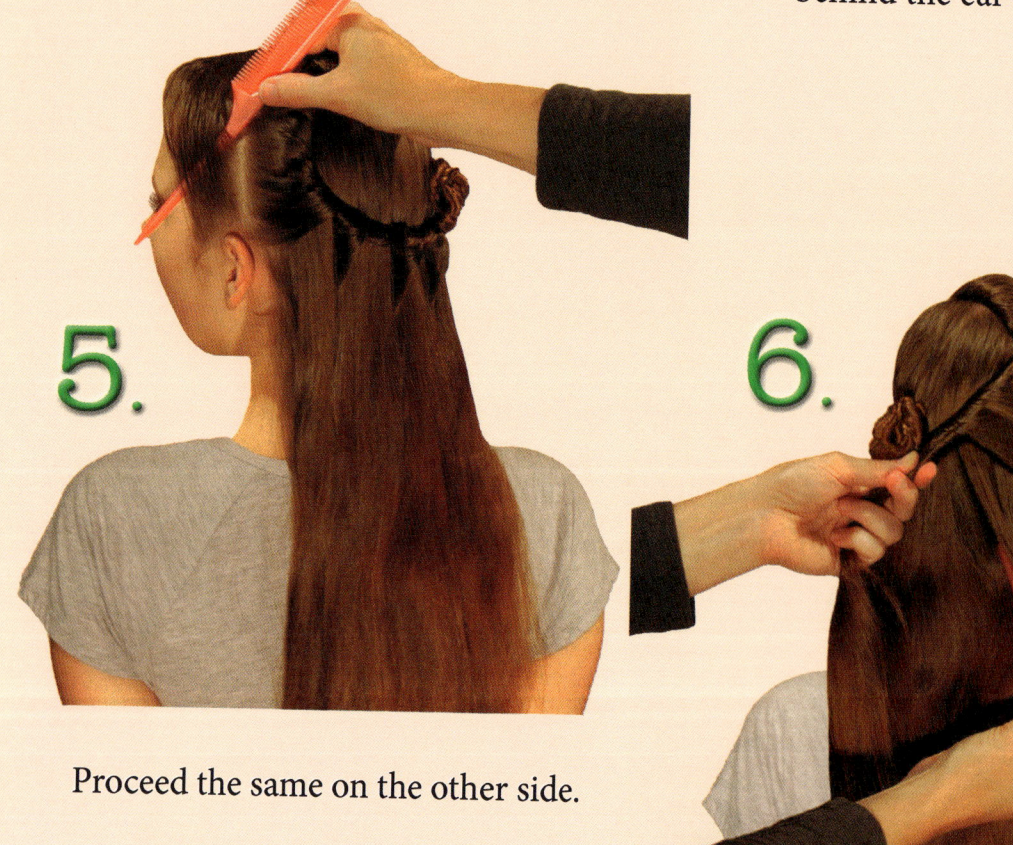

5.

Proceed the same on the other side.

6.

Accented Fringe Cascade

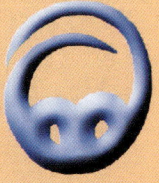

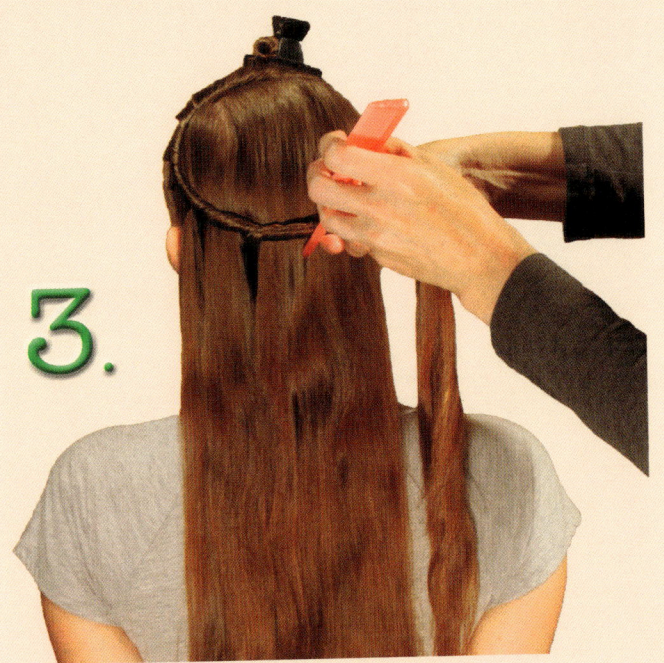

3. Finish braiding the tail and band the end. This is a one-strand twist with beads as an accent.

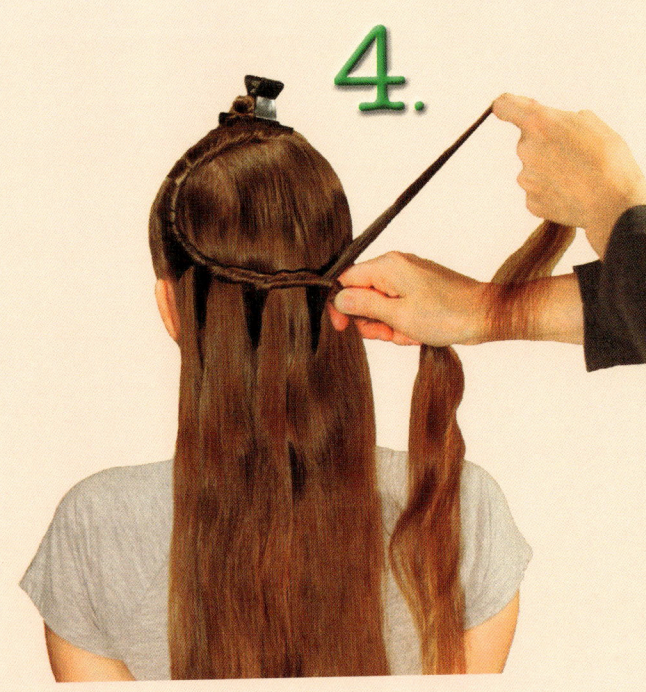

4.

7.

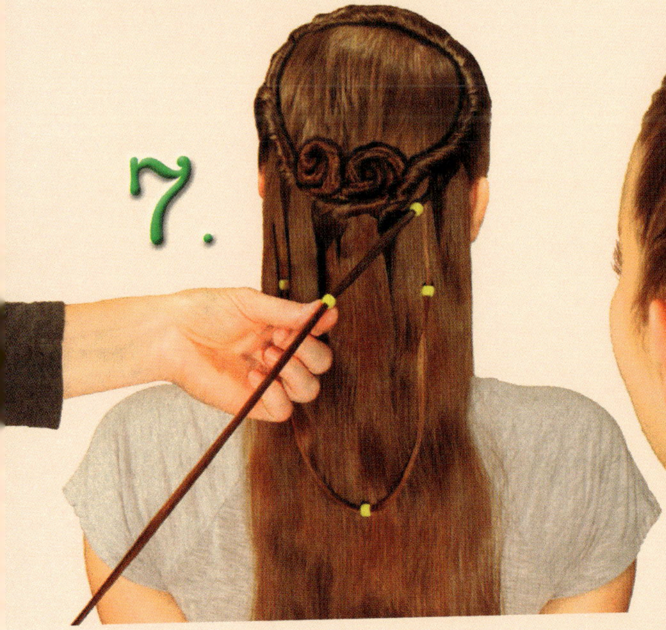

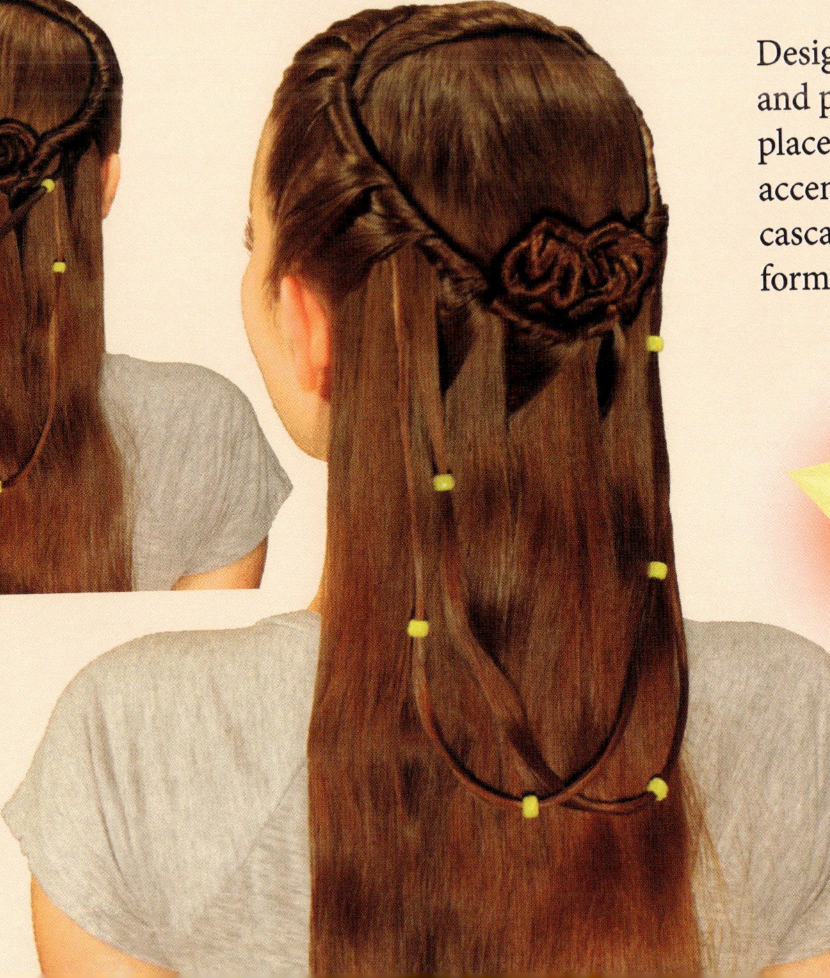

Design a stunning bun and pin it securely in place. I have taken the accent strands from the cascade portion of the form.

Forms 429

Forms

Examples of Fringes

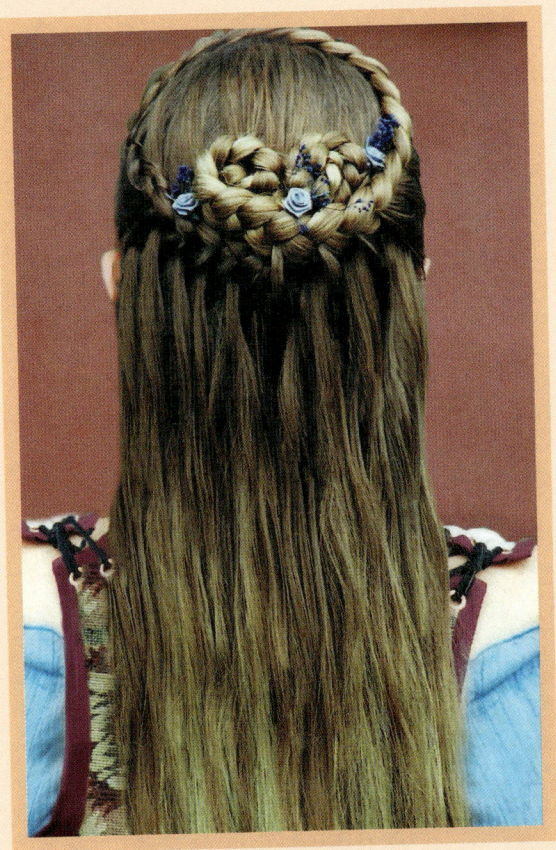
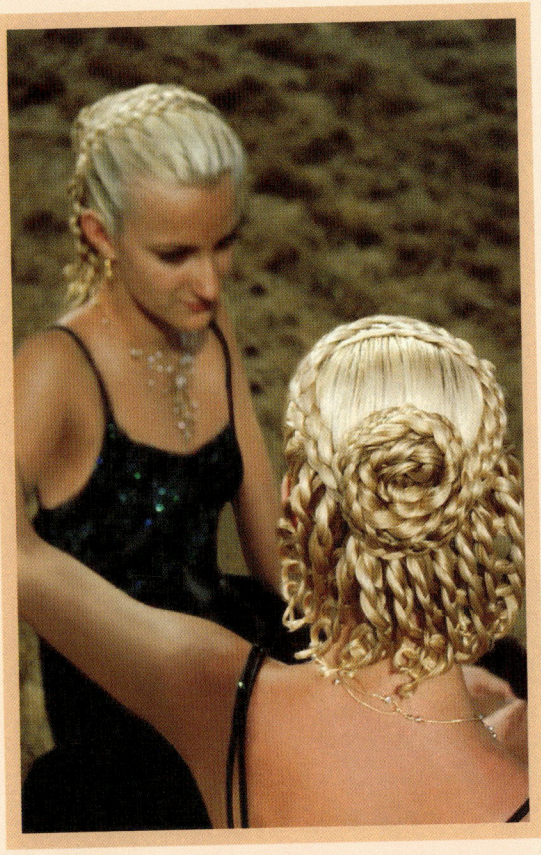
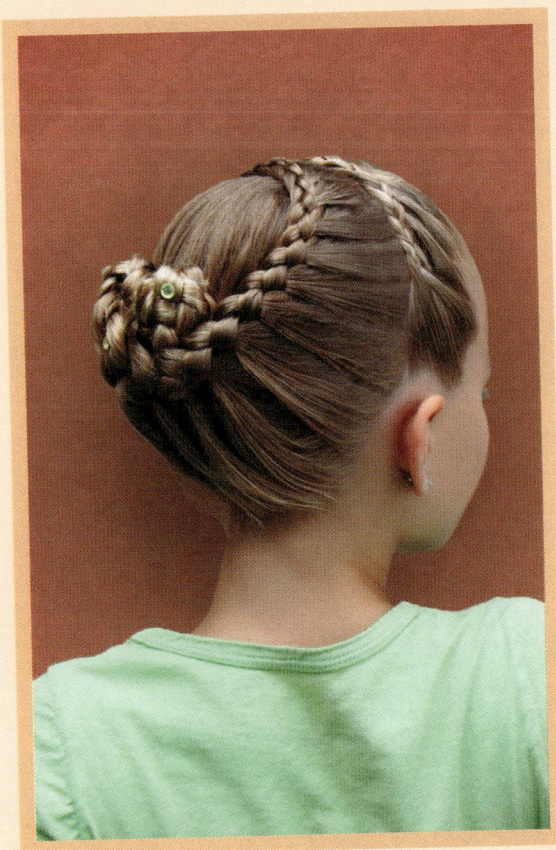
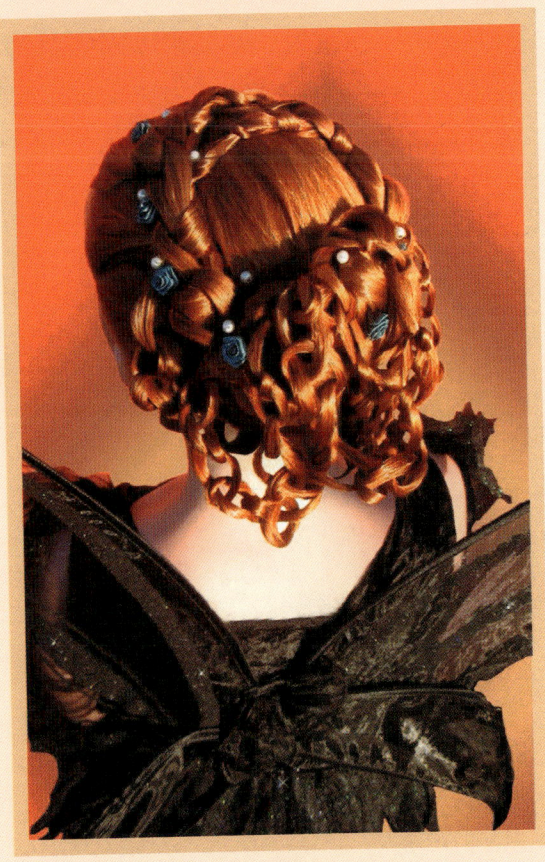

Visit my website to see more examples of Fringes

Forms

CROWN

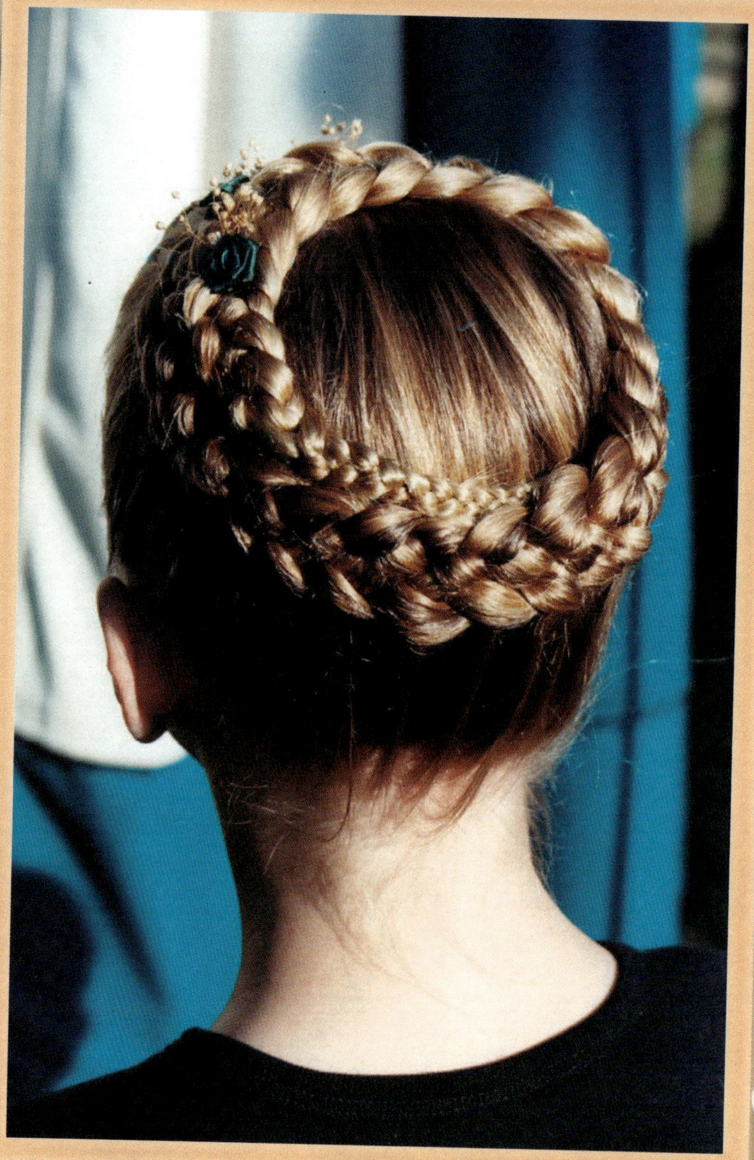

Hairstyles tell your story. They highlight your mood and inform the world who you are. Find the styles that flatter your features.

Forms

Gather like this!

Braiding icon for the next eight pages.

The crown sits atop the head with intention. It is smooth in the center while being gathered from all around the outside. Add flowers and it becomes a garland. Add jewels and it transforms into a decadent crown.

The **Crown** Form

Forms   433

Basic Crown

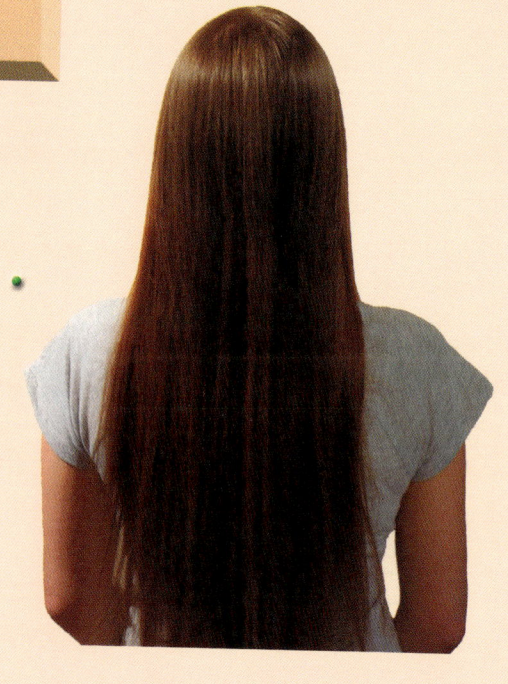

1. Begin with clean, brushed hair.

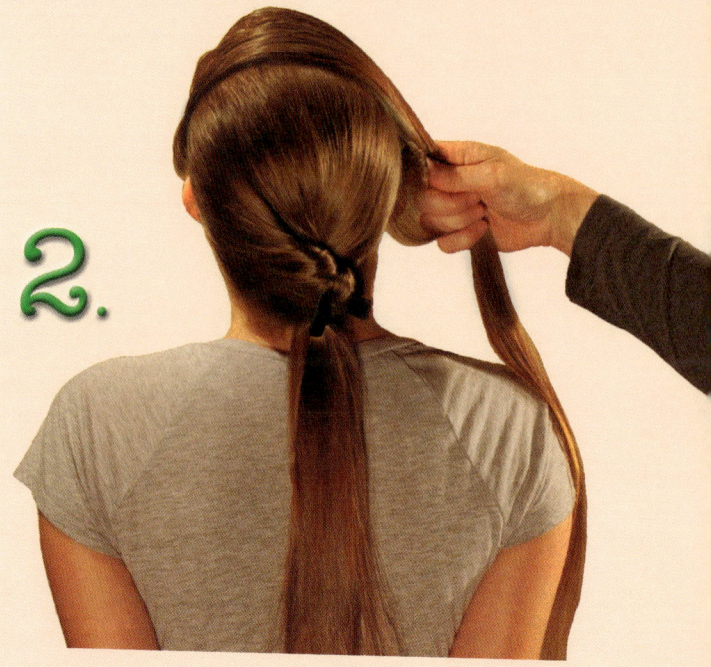

2. Seperate the headband portion of the hair and comb it in the direction you will be braiding.

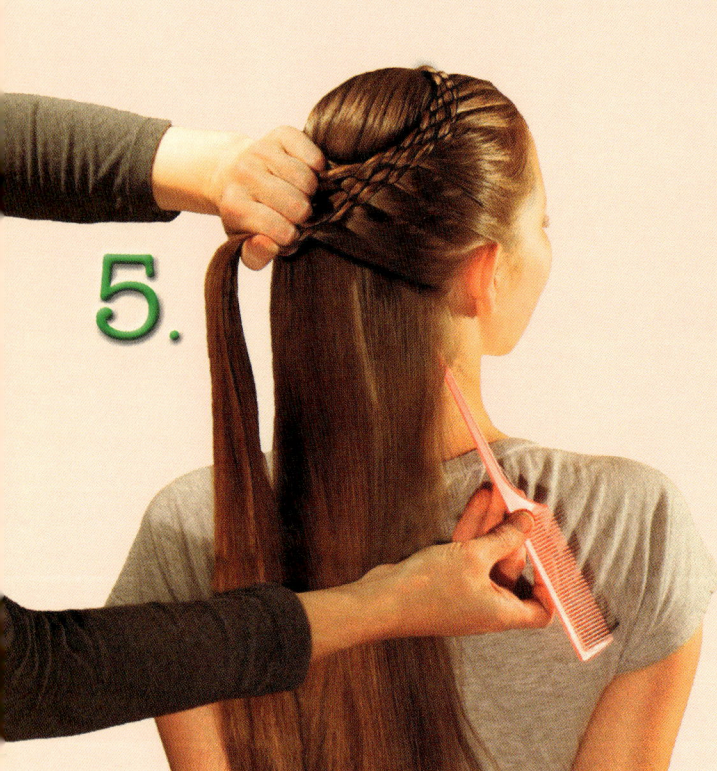

5. Continue braiding the rest of the way around the head.

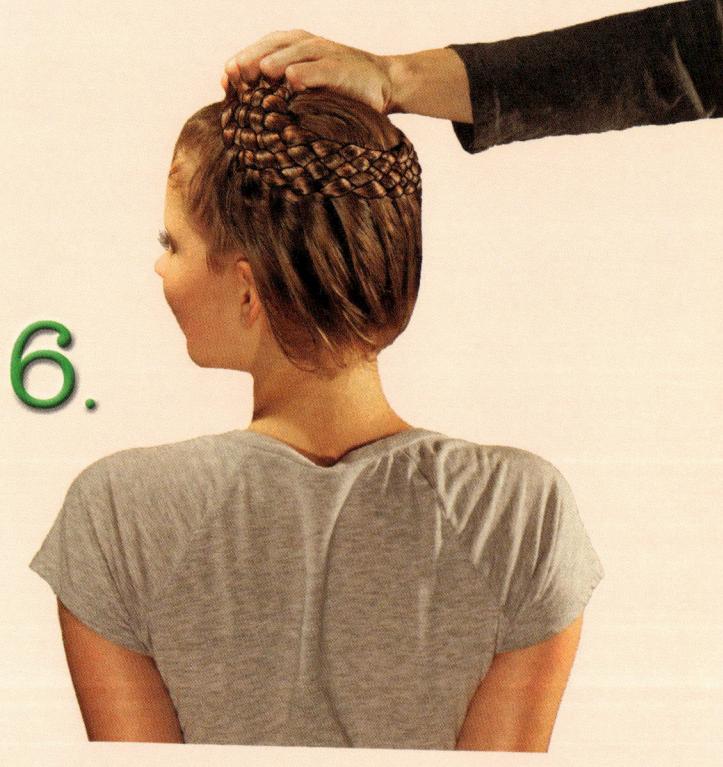

6. Finish the last gather where you took the first section to begin the braid. Close the seam and pin in place.

434   www.findingbraids.com

Basic Crown

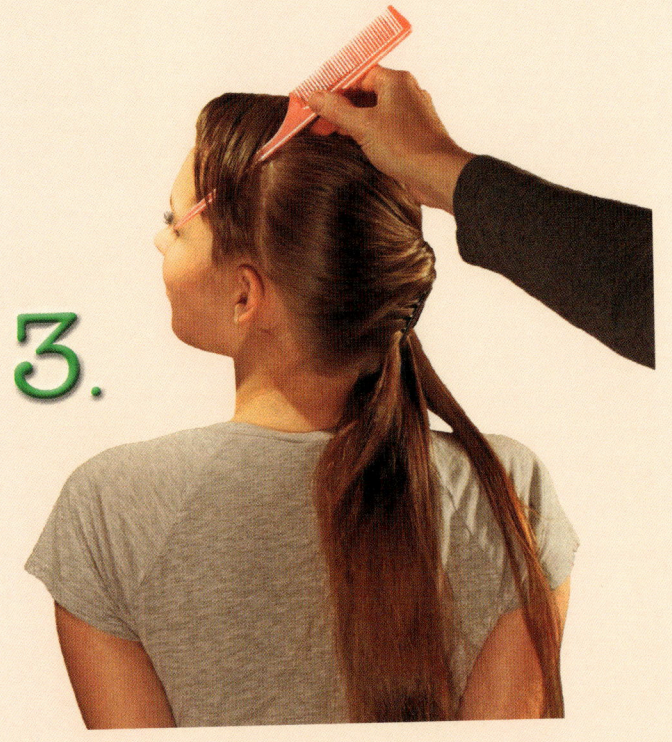

3. Braid from ear to ear. This is a nine-strand.

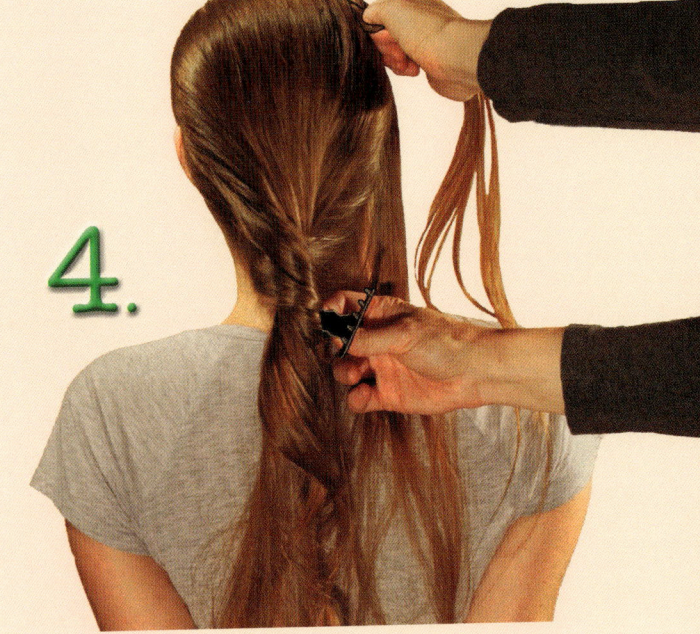

4. Let down the back of the hair upon reaching the opposite ear.

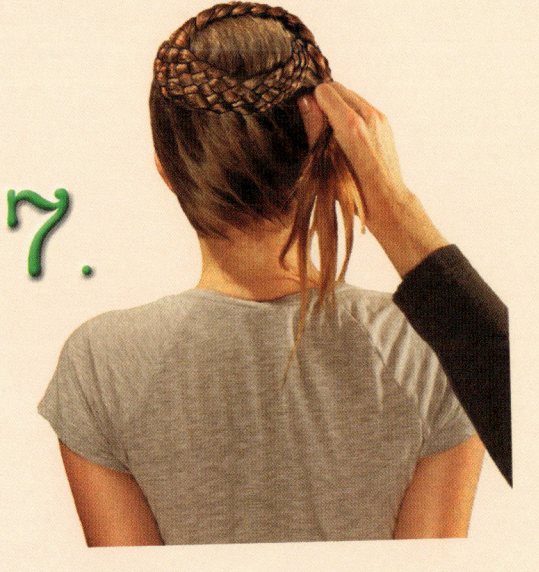

7. Make the crown as narrow or as wide as you wish. It can be made as tight or loose as you desire.

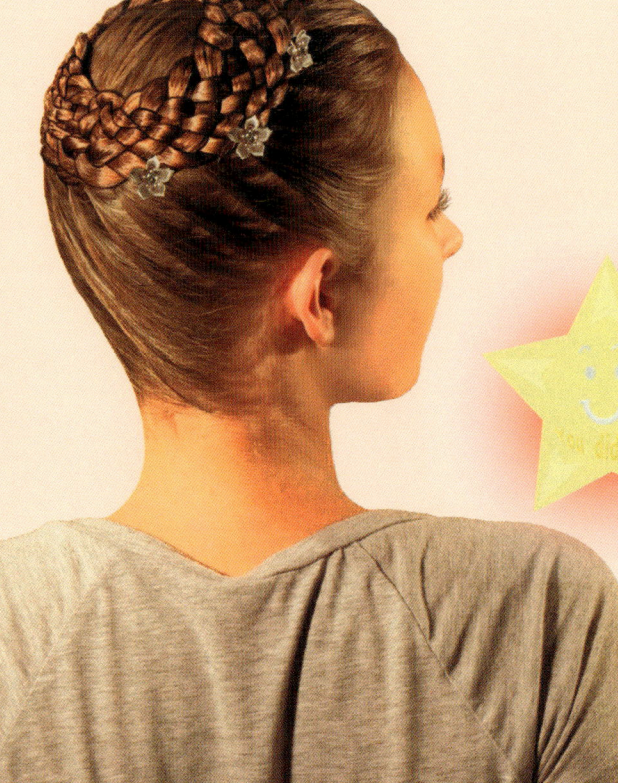

Accented Crown

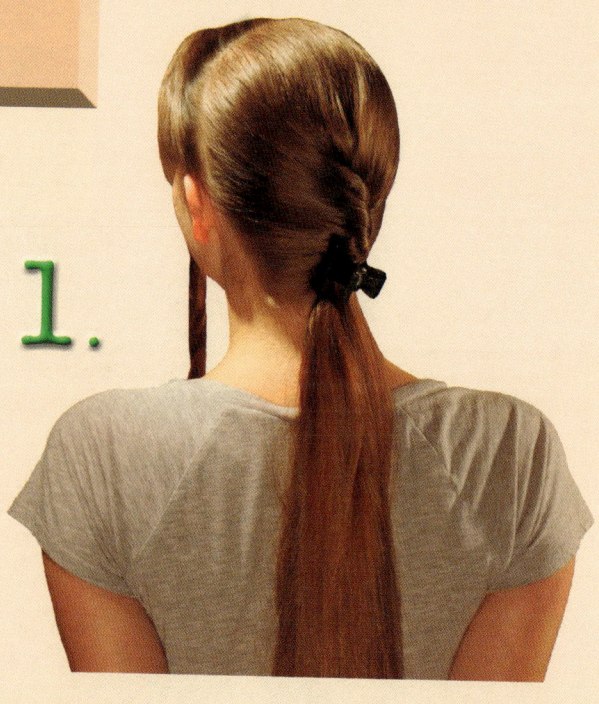

1. Seperate the headband portion of the hair and comb it in the direction you will be braiding.

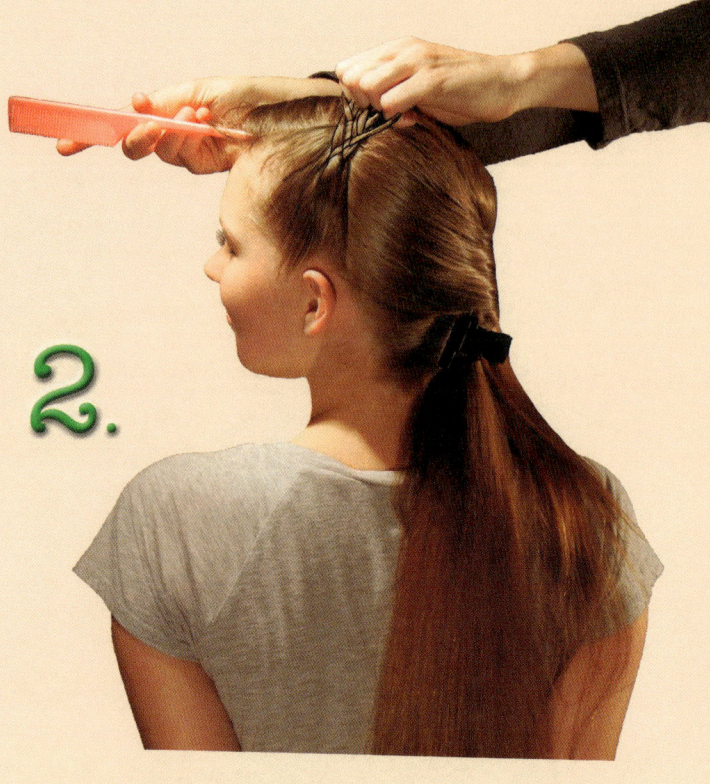

2. Choose the number of strands you will be braiding with. This is a five-strand.

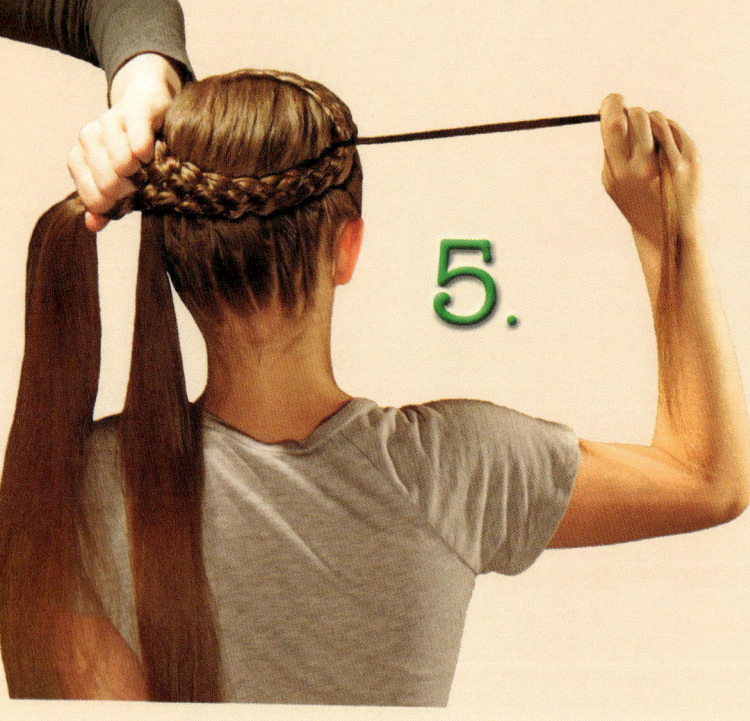

5. Continue braiding the rest of the way around the head.

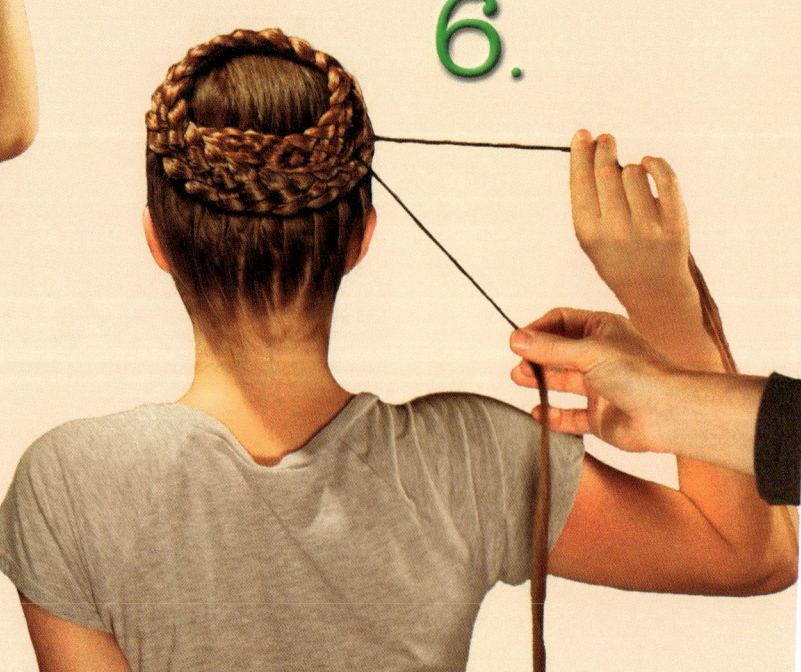

6.

Accented Crown

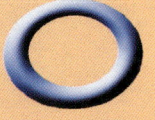

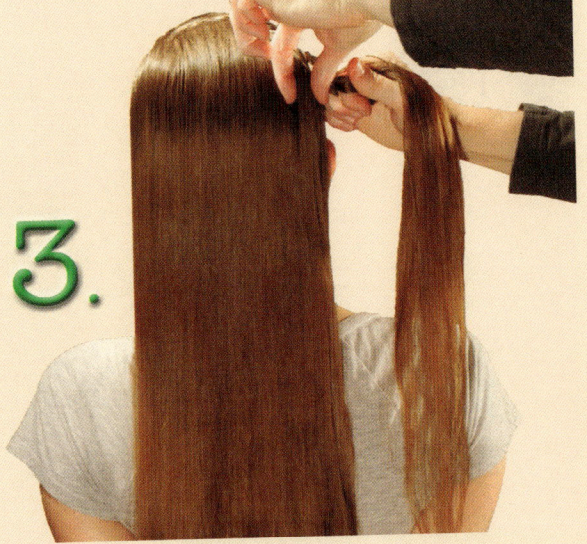

Take out accent strands as you need them to be able to complete your style.

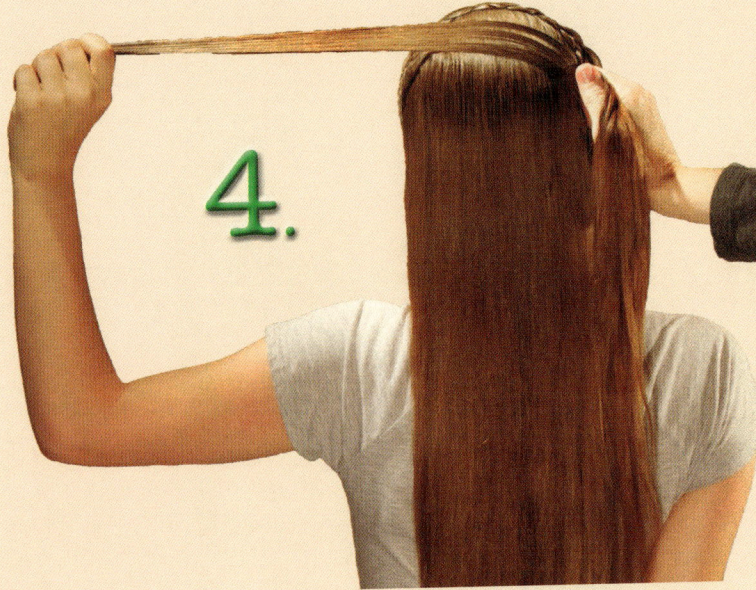

3. Braid from ear to ear. Let down the back of the hair upon reaching the opposite ear.

7. 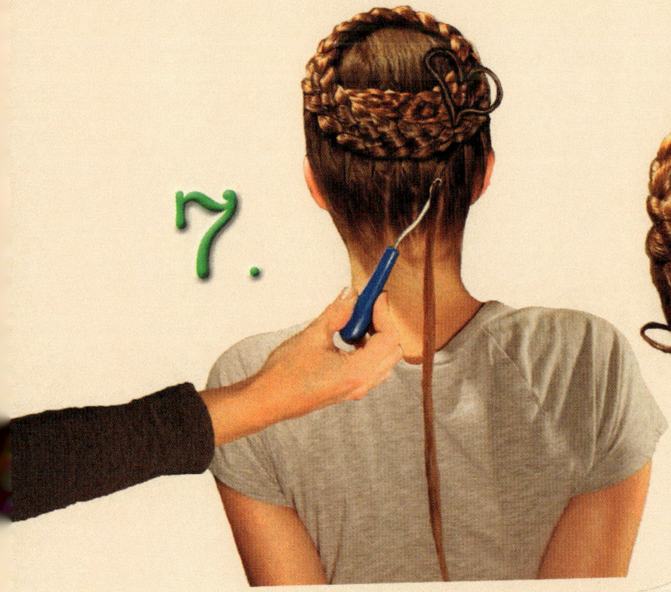 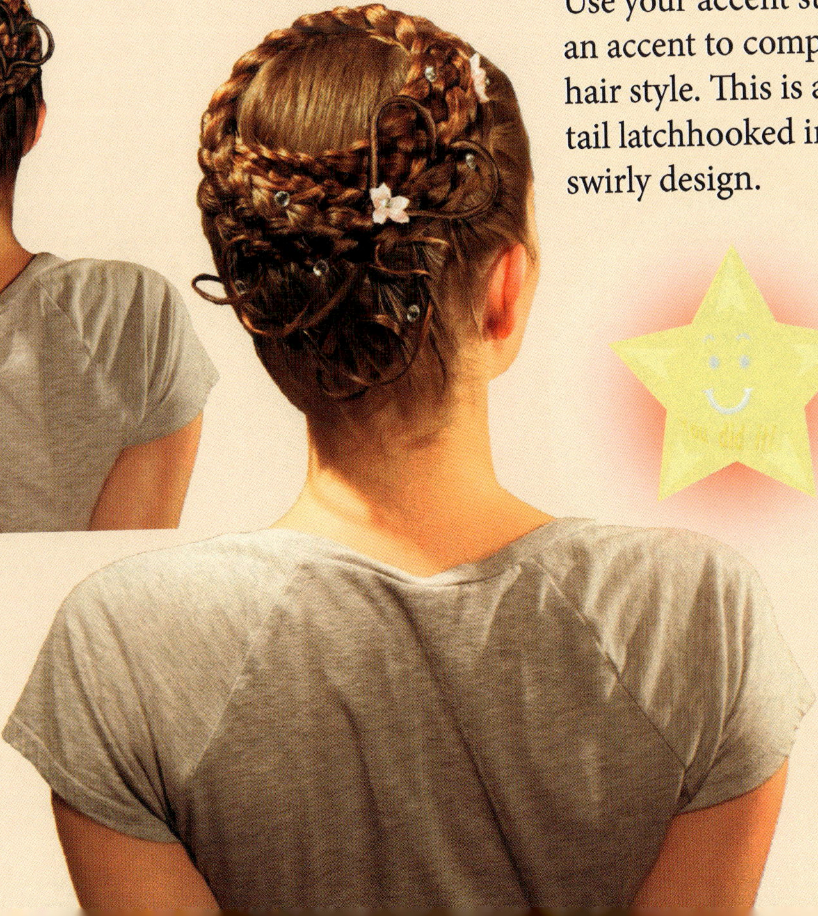 Use your accent strand to create an accent to compliment your hair style. This is a heart with the tail latchhooked into a beautiful swirly design.

Forms 437

Crown Cascade

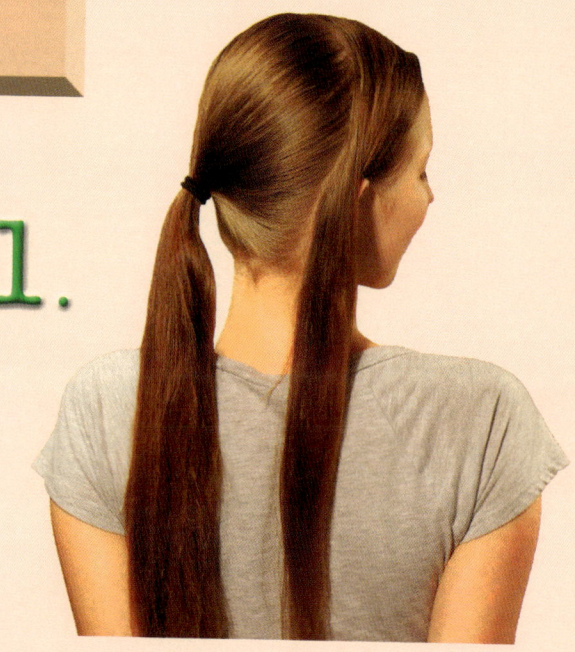

1.

Seperate the headband portion of the hair and comb it in the direction you will be braiding.

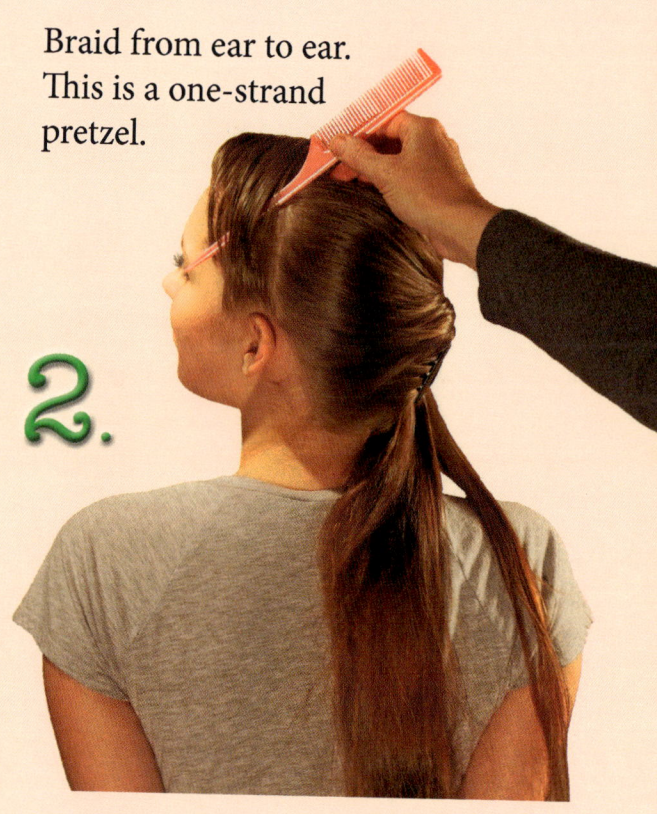

Braid from ear to ear. This is a one-strand pretzel.

2.

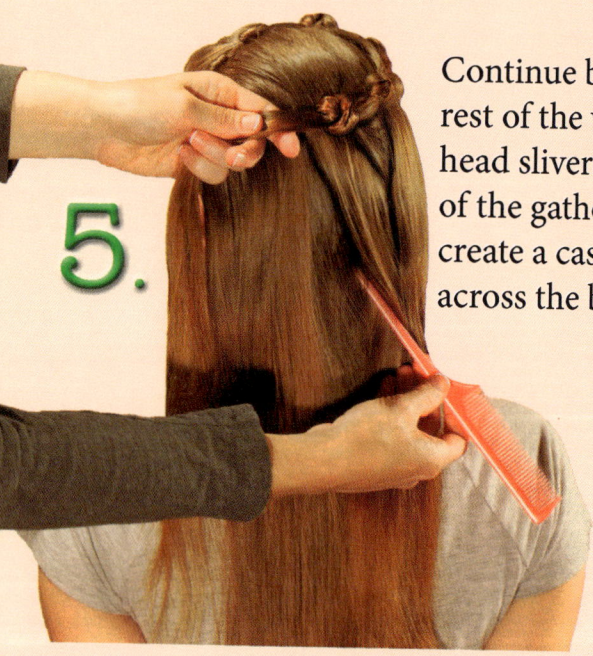

5.

Continue braiding the rest of the way around the head slivering up portions of the gathers in back to create a cascade effect across the back.

6.

Crown Cascade

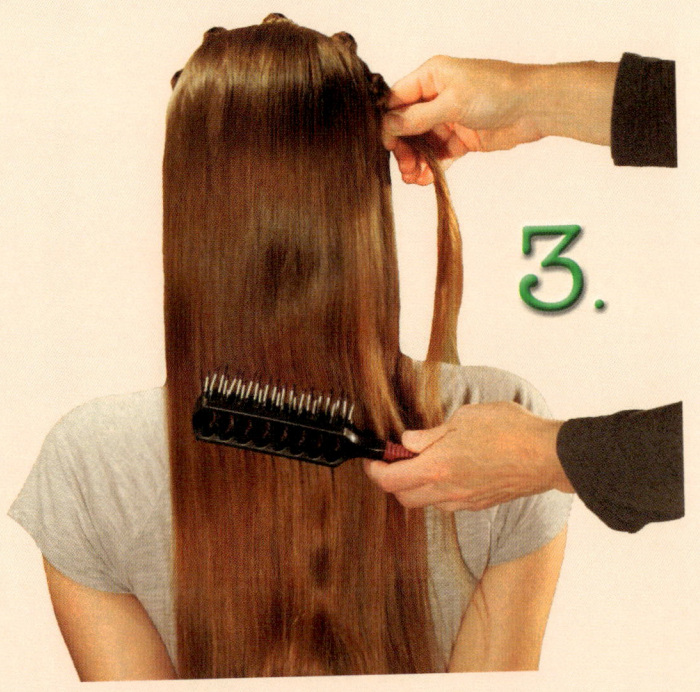

3.

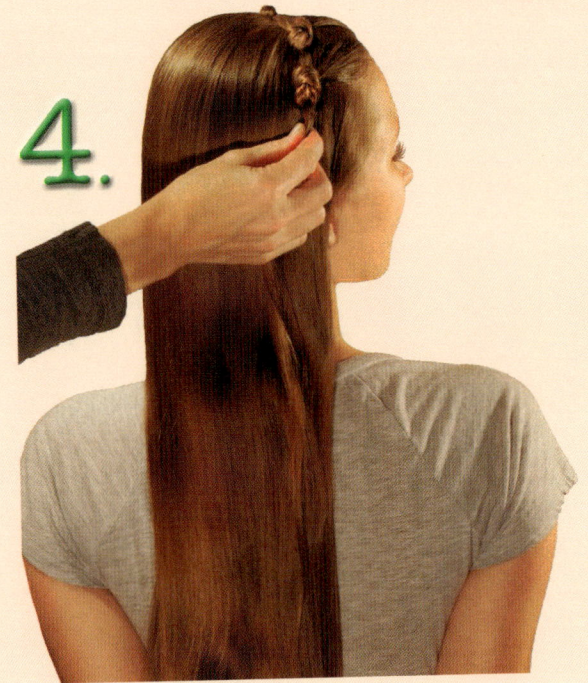

4.

Let down the back of the hair upon reaching the opposite ear.

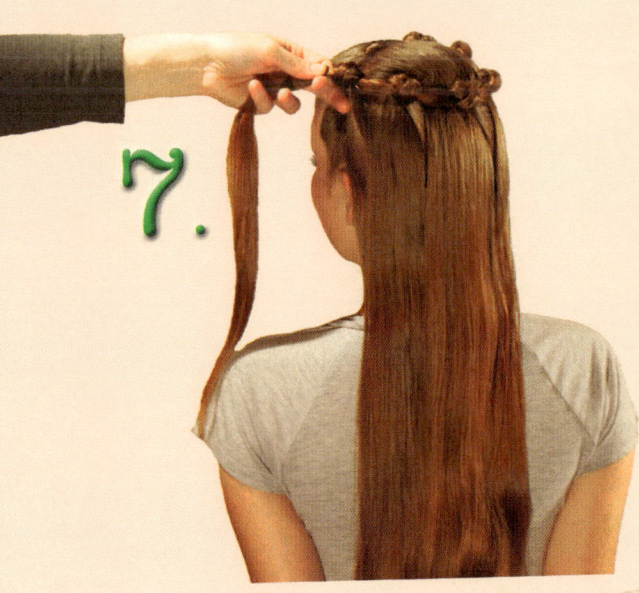

7.

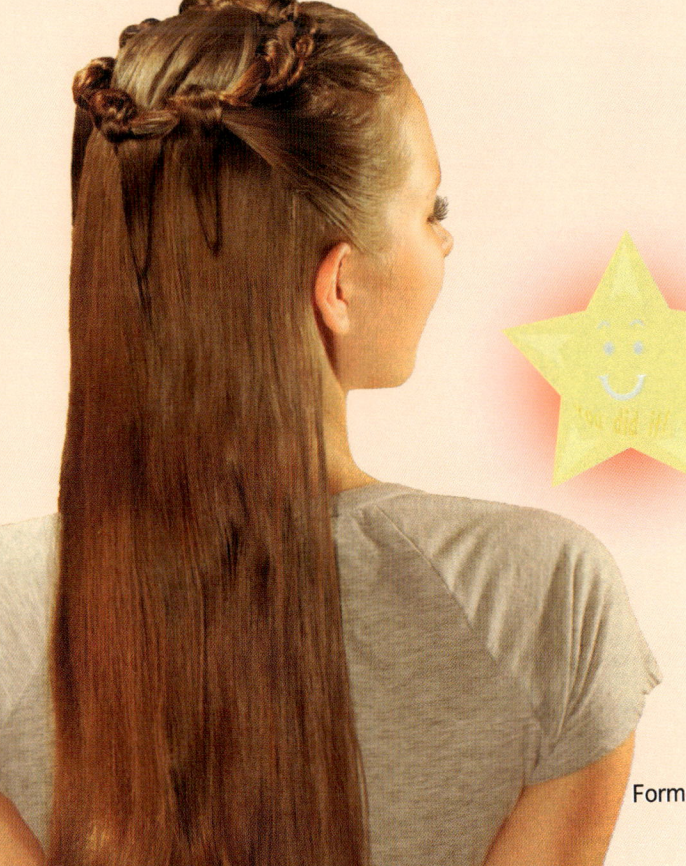

Finish the last gather where you took the first section to begin the braid. Close the seam and pin in place.

Forms 439

Accented Crown Cascade

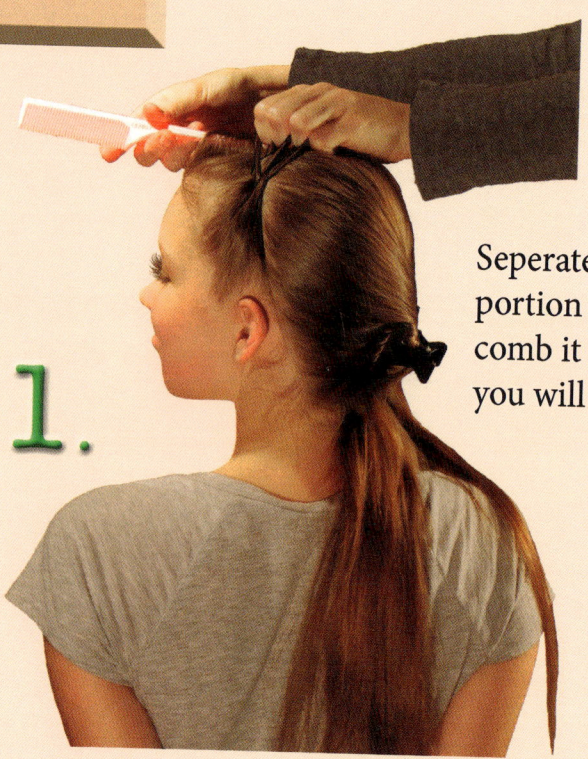

1.

Seperate the headband portion of the hair and comb it in the direction you will be braiding.

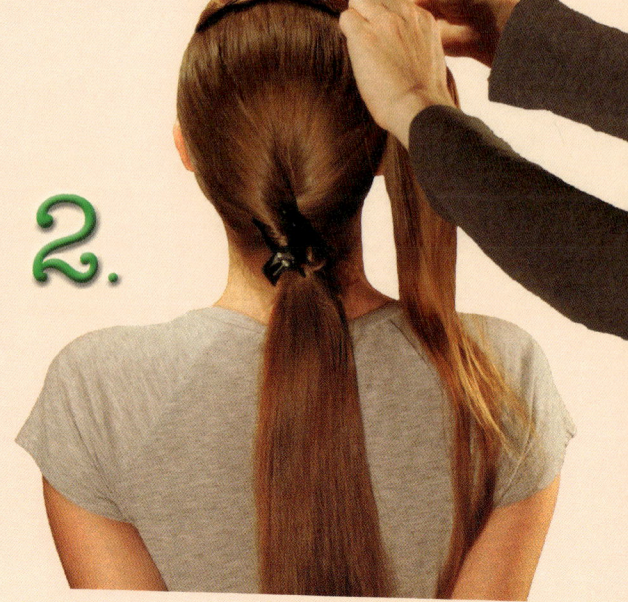

2.

Braid from ear to ear. This is a four-strand round with bead accents.

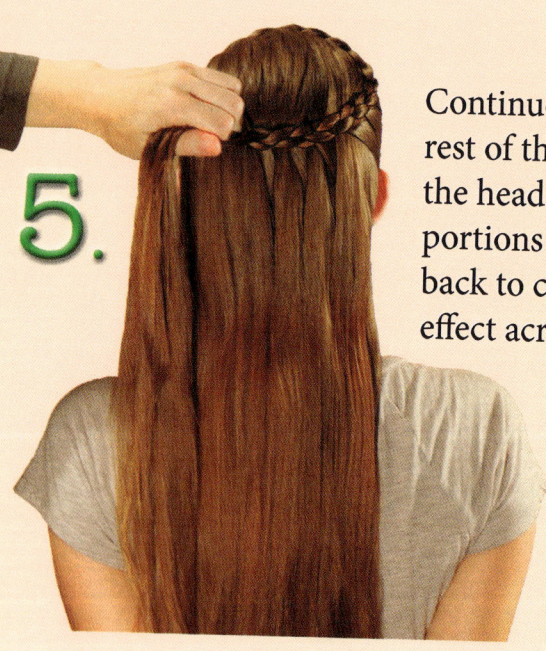

5.

Continue braiding the rest of the way around the head slivering up portions of the gathers in back to create a cascade effect across the back.

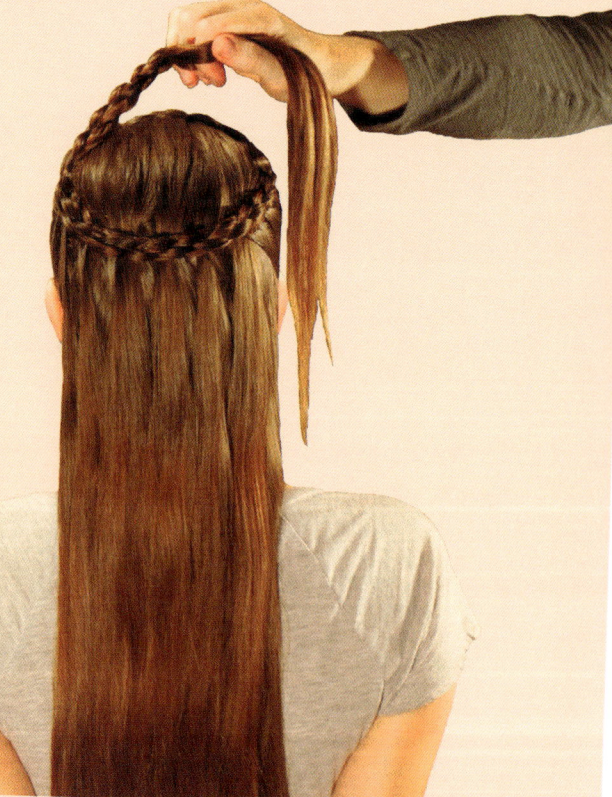

6.

Finish the last gather where you took the first section to begin the braid. Close the seam and pin in place.

Accented Crown Cascade

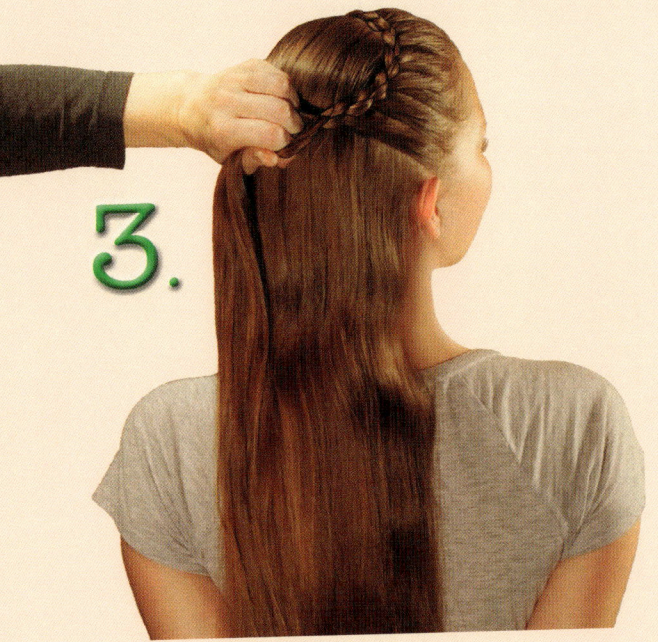

3.

Let down the back of the hair upon reaching the opposite ear.

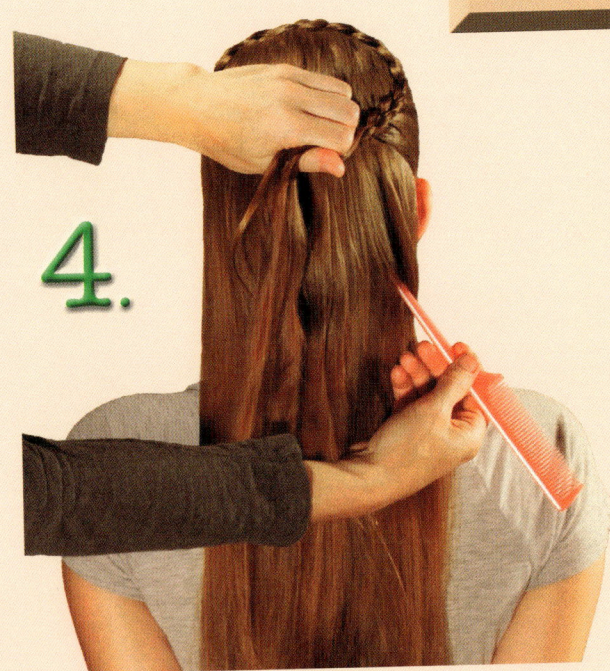

4.

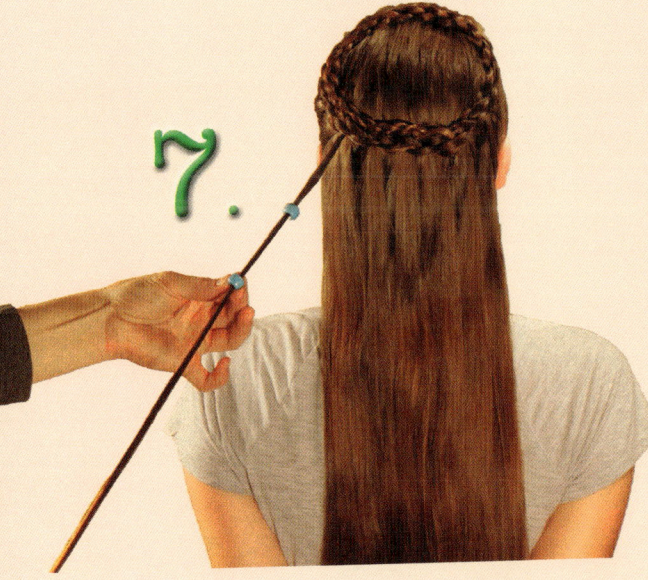

7.

I am taking accent strands from the cascade portion of the form. Create accents to compliment your style.

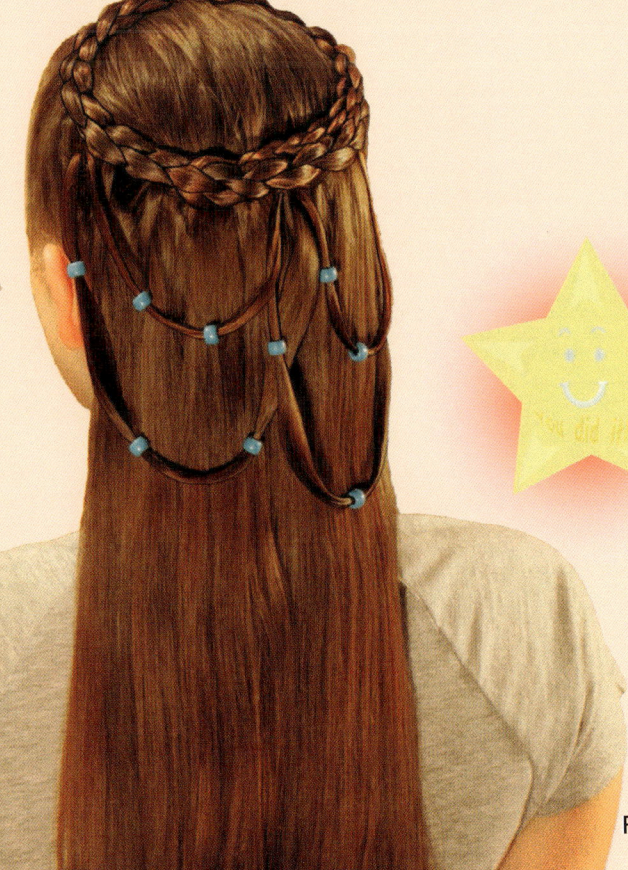

Forms 441

Forms

Notes

Examples of Crowns

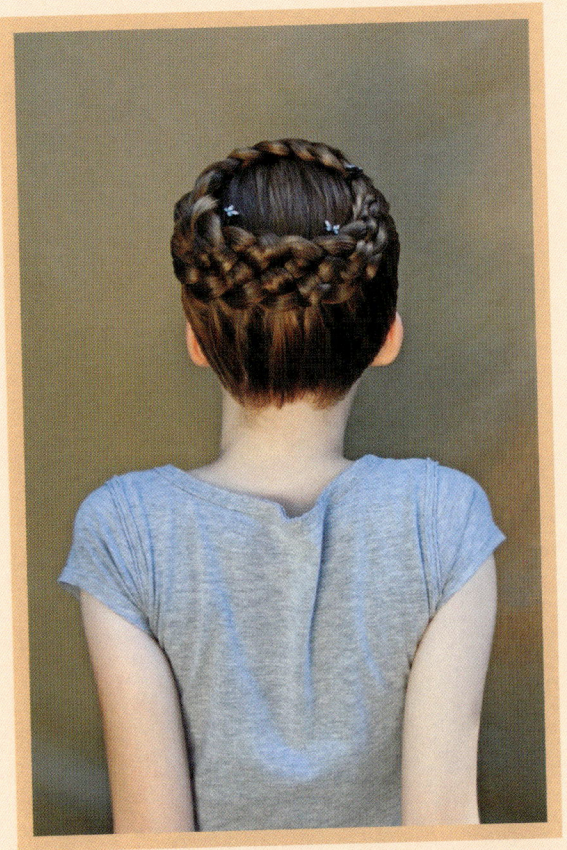
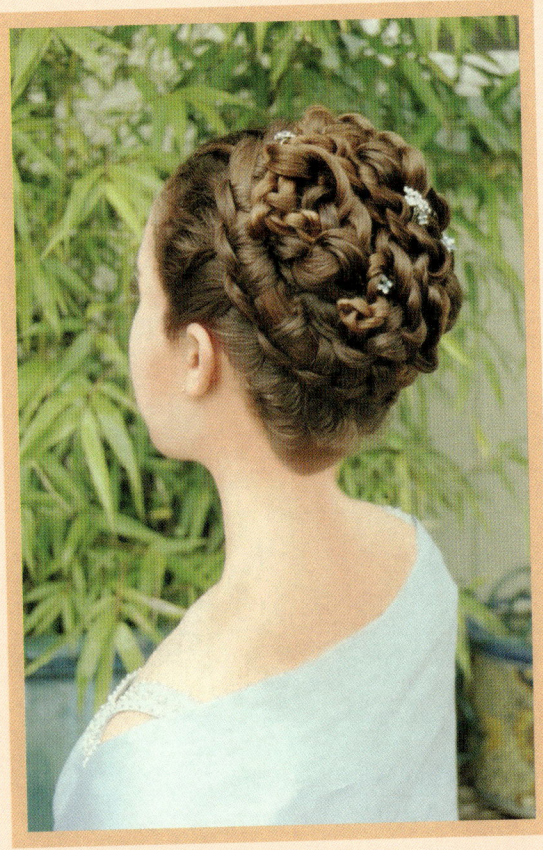
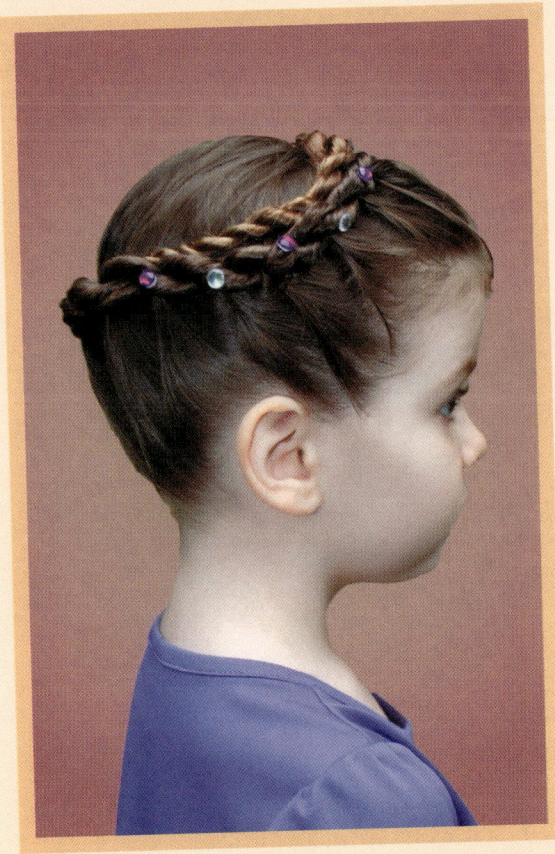
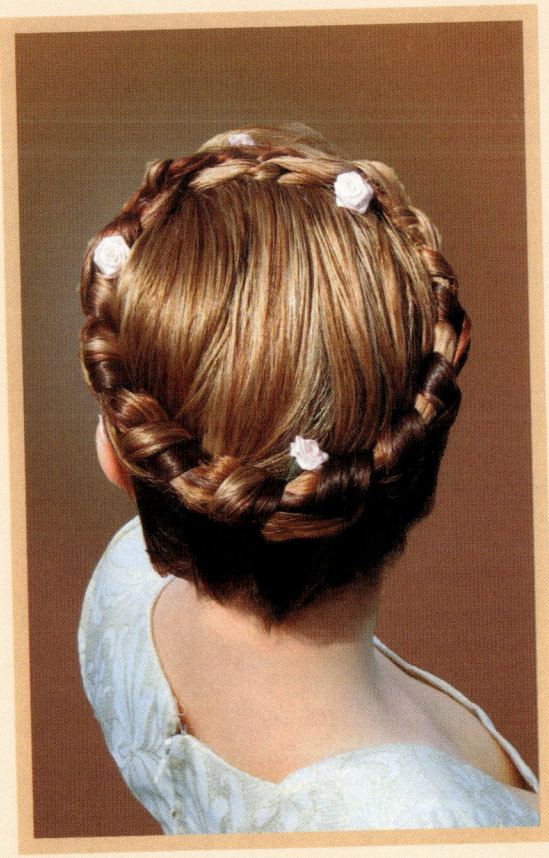

Visit my website to see more examples of Crowns

Forms

HALO

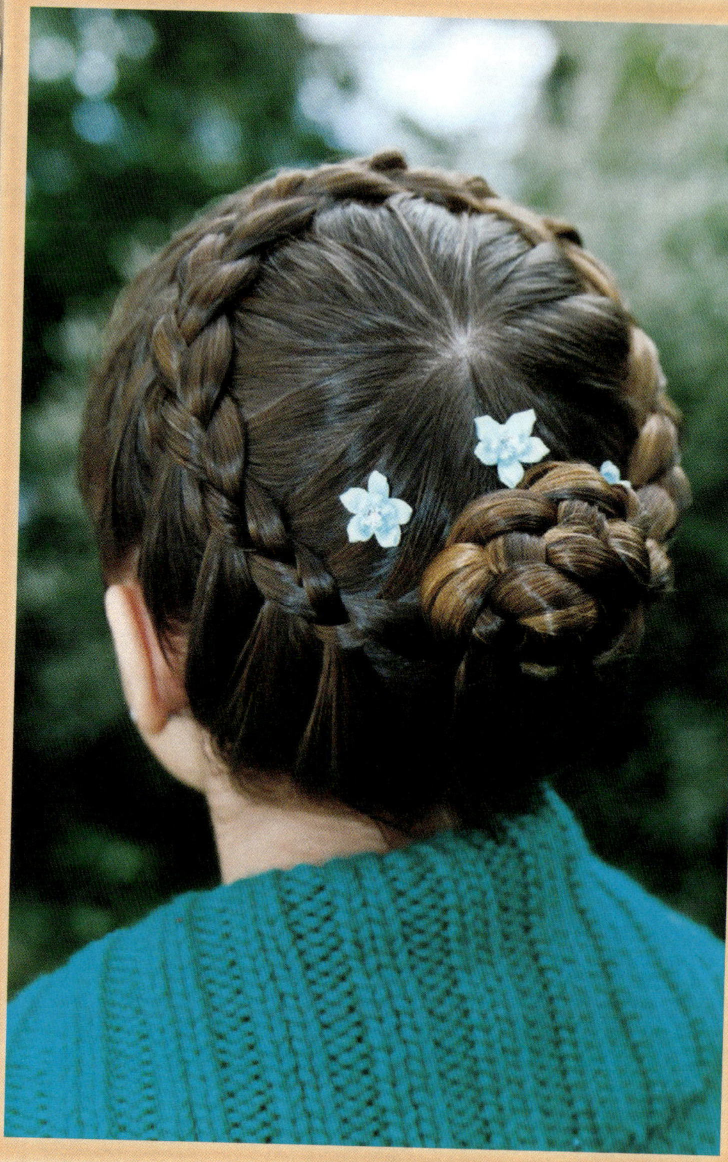

Sweet braids to celebrate all seasons. A pretty dress is all this form needs to brighten any celebration. Very similar to the crown, this has a distinct star pattern inside the circle. You may think it needs to be stitch gathered but it can be lace gathered and still achieve the same effect. Although the lace gather is more difficult it offers many unusual options to play with.

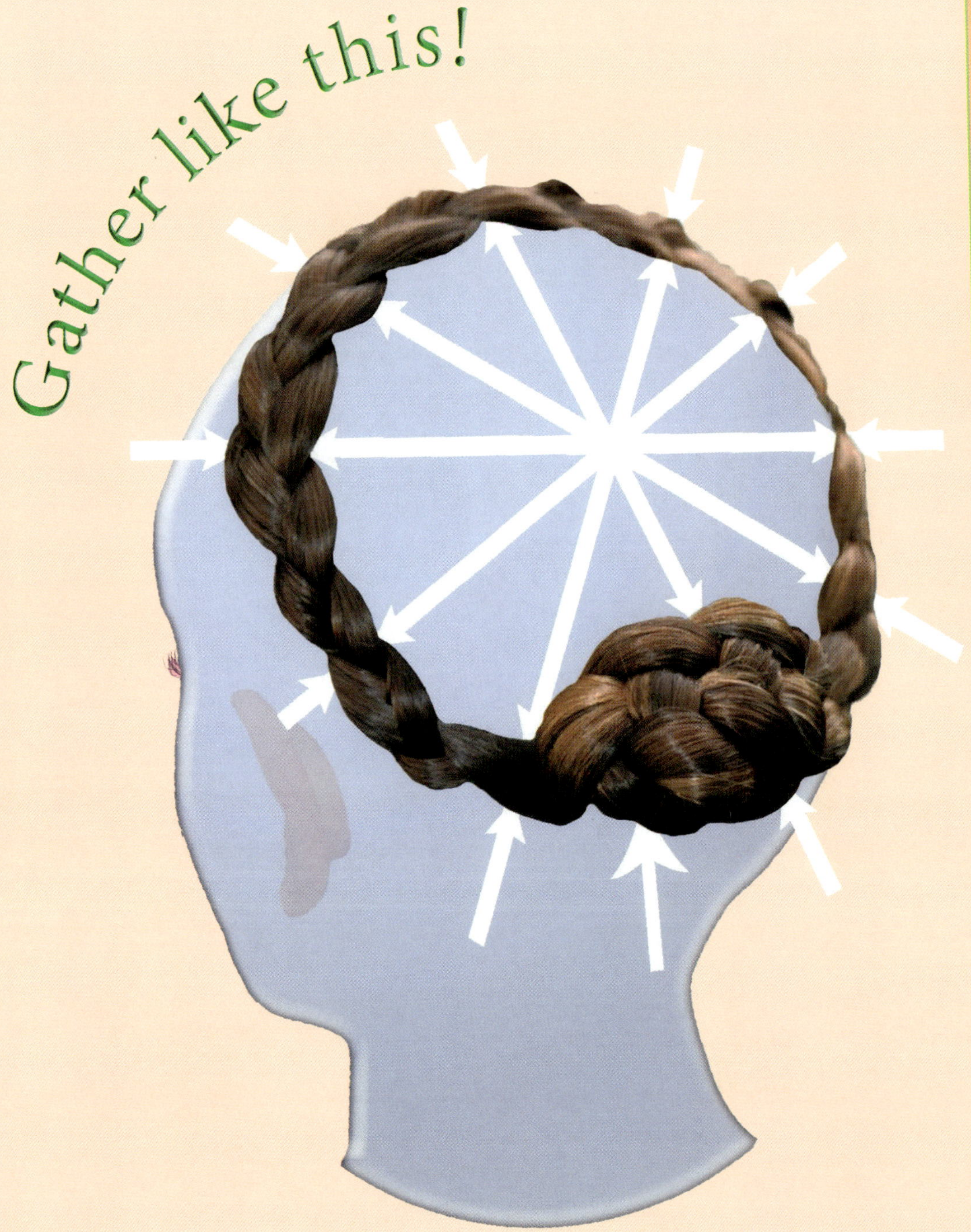

Forms

Gather like this!

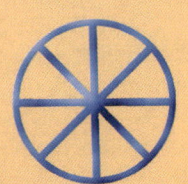

Braiding icon for the next eight pages.

Specific sectioning creates this finished "starburst" pattern. Just like cutting pieces of a pie, you will gather in a pie graph pattern around the head. Focus on a single strand of hair in the center and you will get it to look like a sun instead of a line down the middle in a parted form.

The 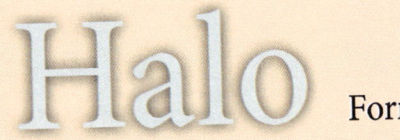 Form

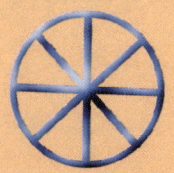

Basic Halo

1.

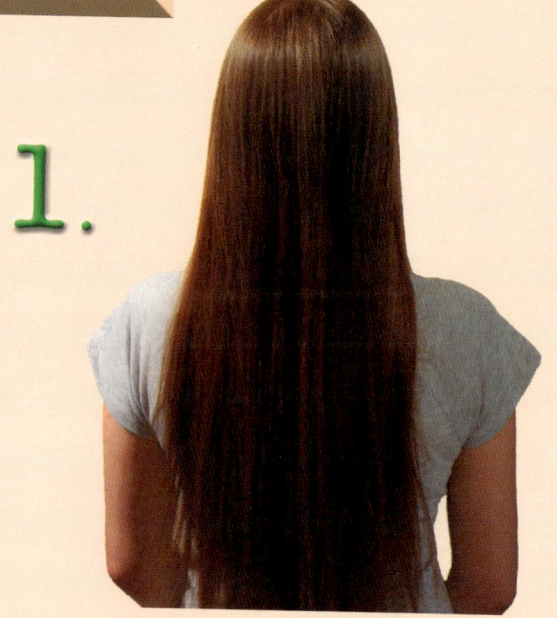

Begin with clean, brushed hair.

2.

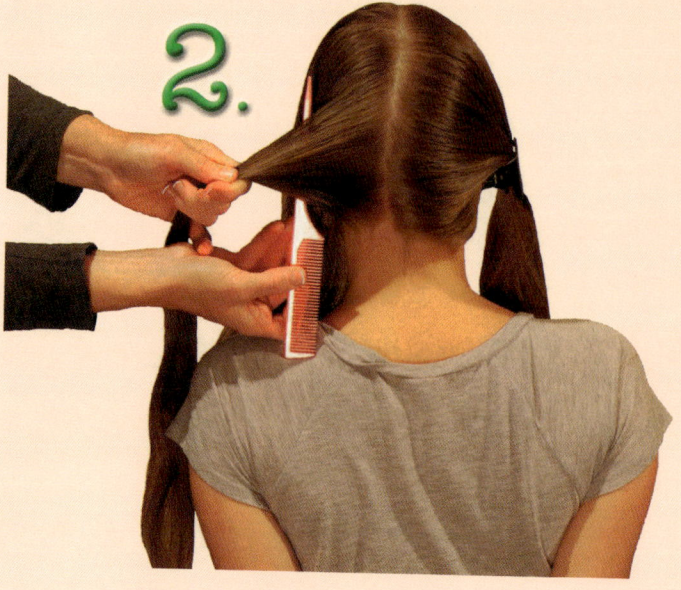

Part down the middle. Clip off one side. Take a section from the top center of the head parting down towards the nape of the neck creating a pie slice about an inch wide at the base.

5.

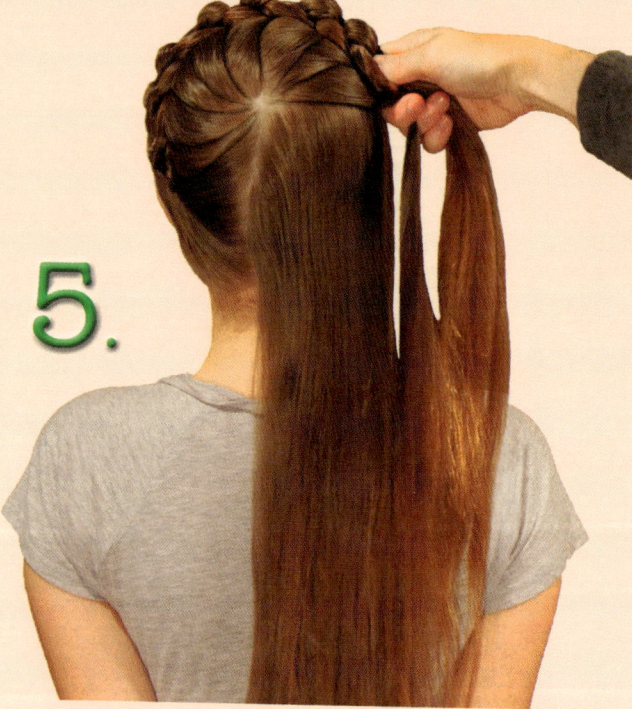

The outside gathers should line up with the inside gathers all pointing towards the center.

6.

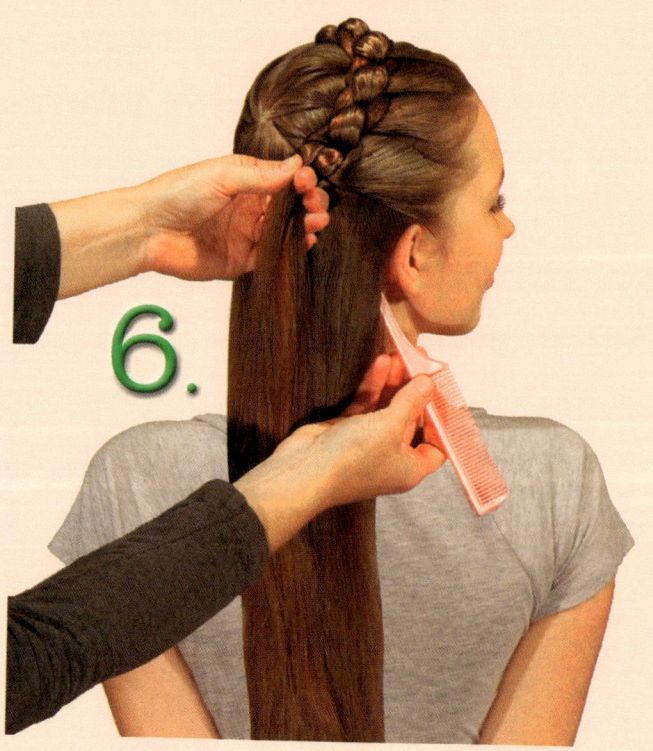

446   www.findingbraids.com

Basic Halo

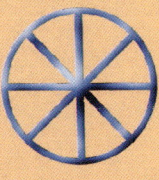

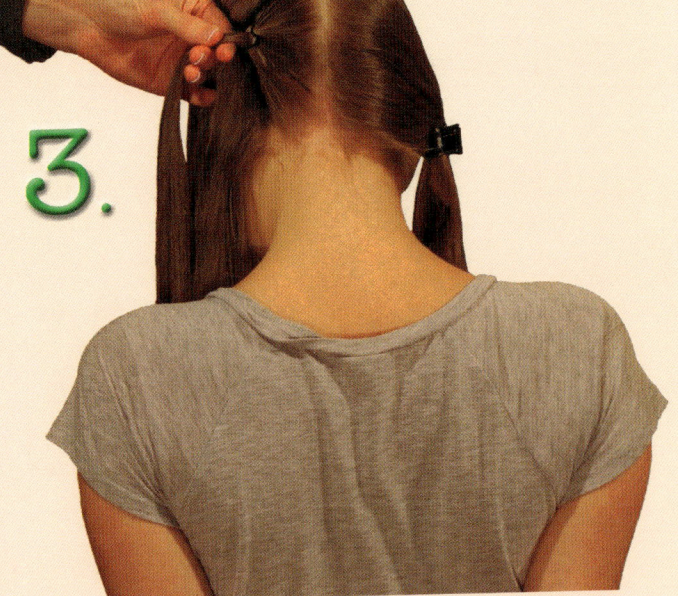

3. Choose the number of strands you will braid with. This is a two-strand knot. Braid and walk around the person in a complete circle. Gather in the shape of a pie chart.

4.

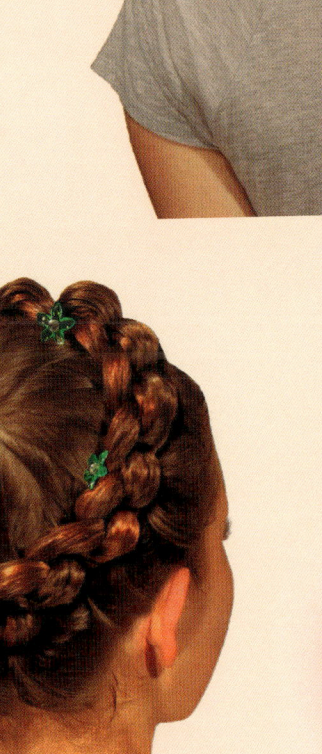

7. Finish the braid where you started and close the seam. Pin the tail to the halo or make a bun.

Forms 447

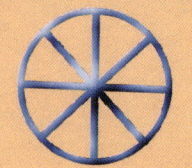

Accented Halo

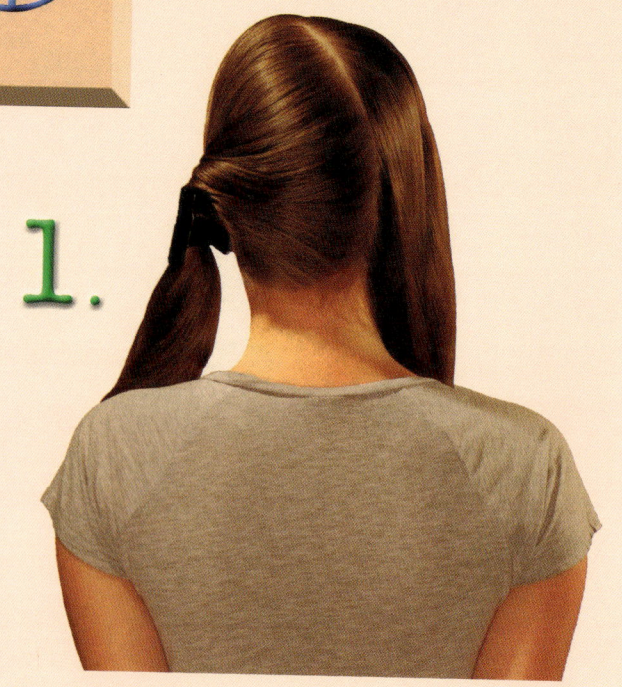

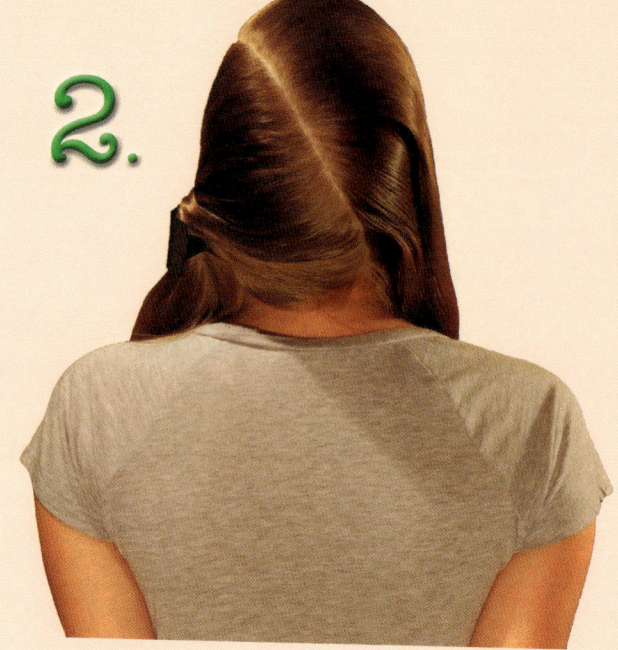

1. Part down the middle. Clip off one side.

2. Take a section from the top center of the head parting down towards the nape of the neck creating a pie slice about an inch wide at the base. Choose the number of strands you will braid with.

Take your accent strands out as you need them. The outside gathers should line up with the inside gathers all pointing towards the center.

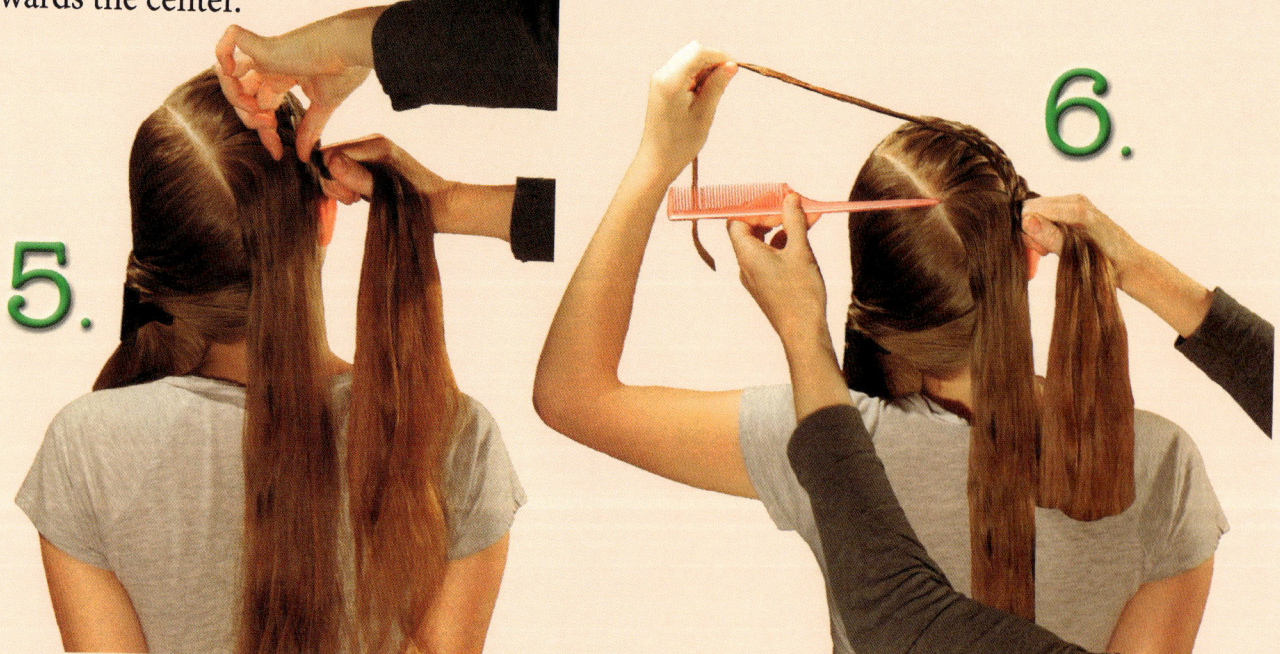

448   www.findingbraids.com

Accented Halo

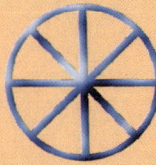

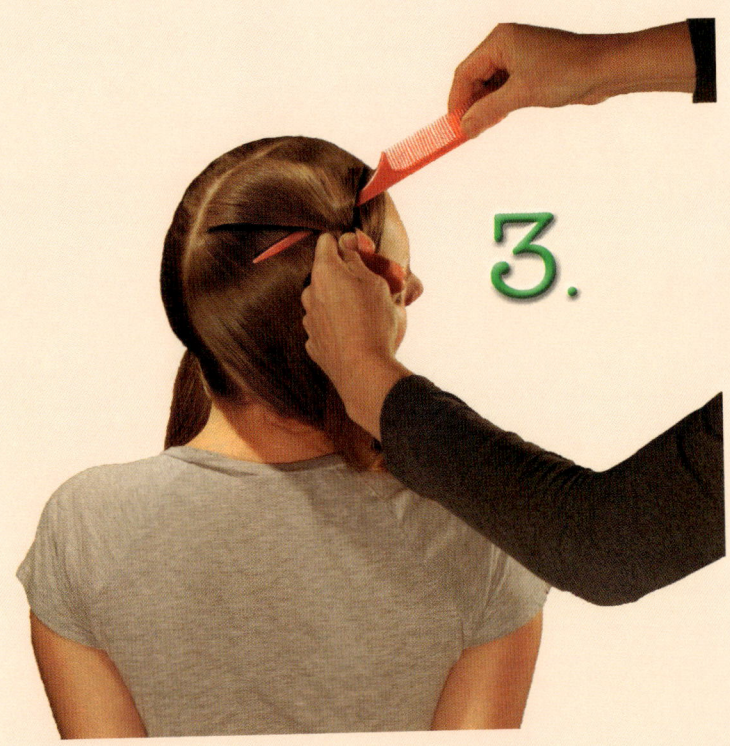

3. Take a section from the top center of the head parting towards the middle center of the head creating a pie slice about an inch wide near the face.

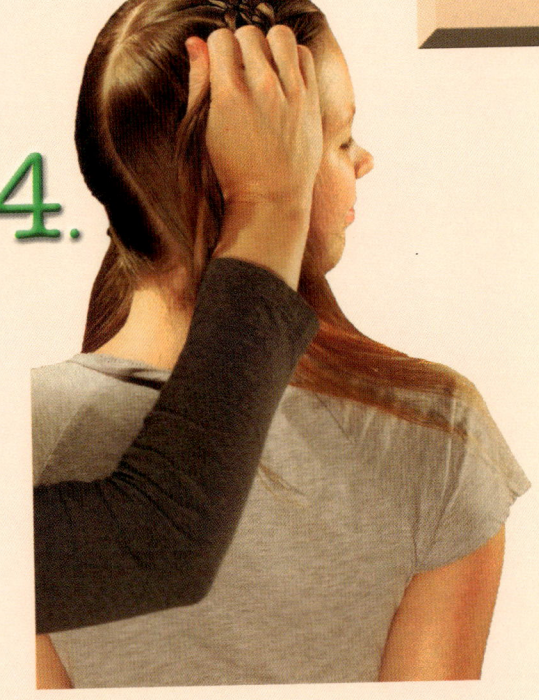

4. This is a nine-strand. Braid and walk around the person in a complete circle.

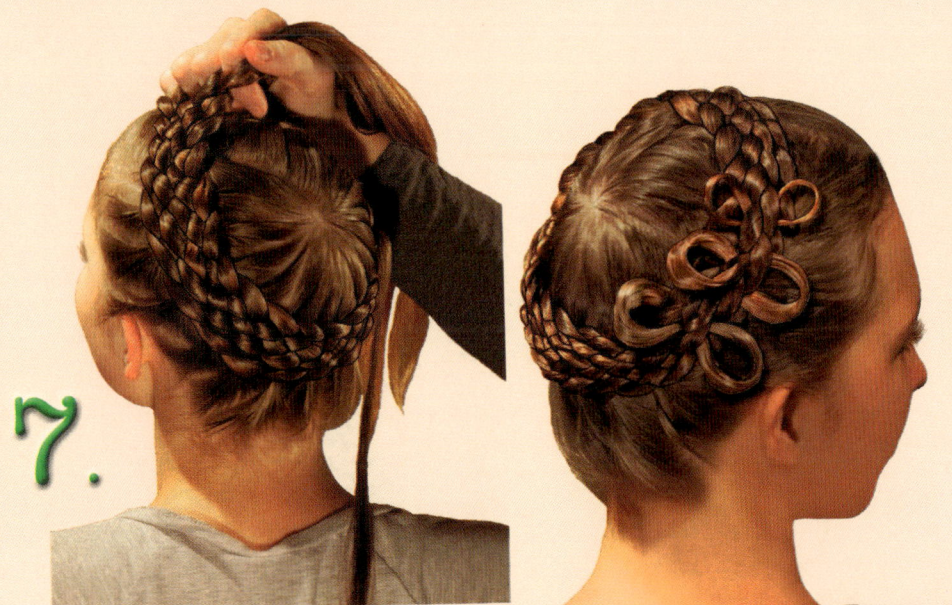

7. Finish the braid where you started and close the seam. Pin the tail to the halo or make a bun. Create your accents with the strands left out. This is loose hair latchhooked into bows.

Forms 449

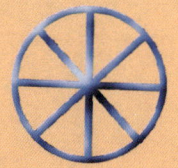
Halo Cascade

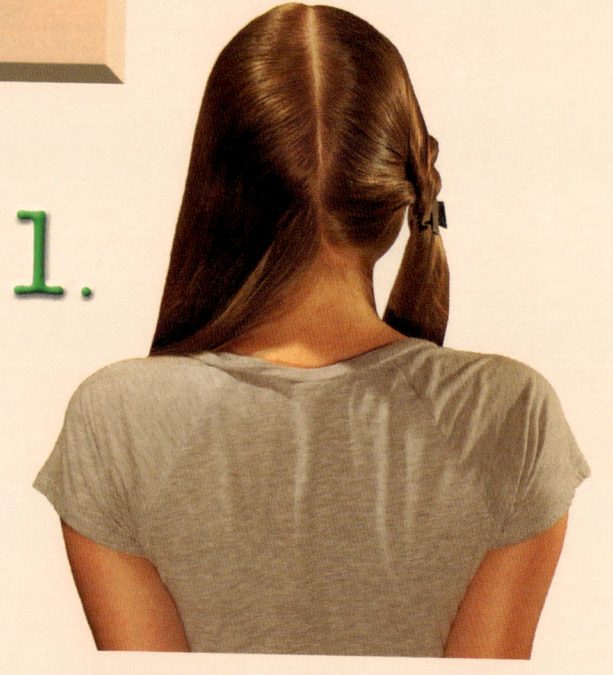

1. Part down the middle. Clip off one side.

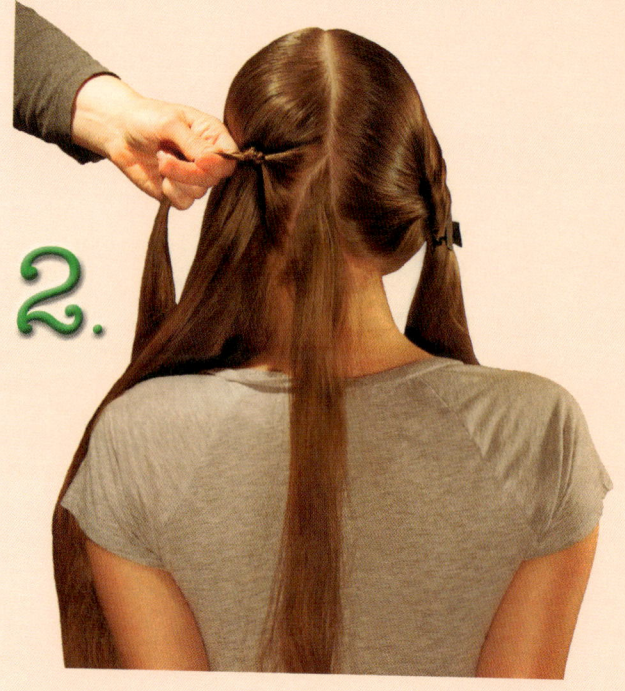

2. Part down the middle. Clip off one side. Take a section from the top center of the head parting down towards the nape of the neck creating a pie slice about an inch wide at the base. Choose the number of strands you will braid with.

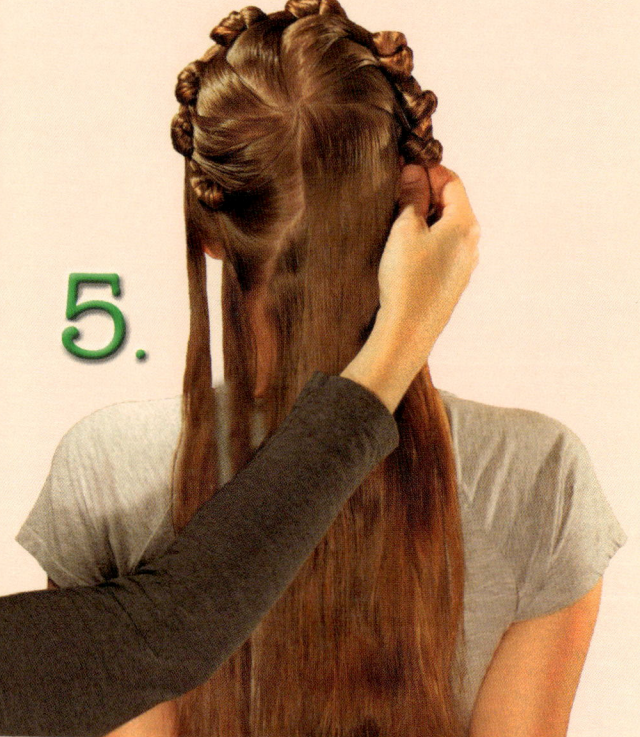

5. The outside gathers should line up with the inside gathers all pointing towards the center.

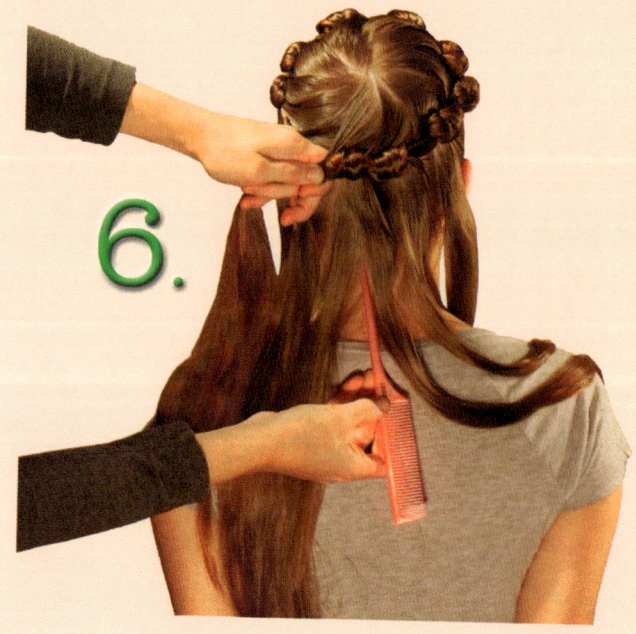

6.

450   www.findingbraids.com

Halo Cascade

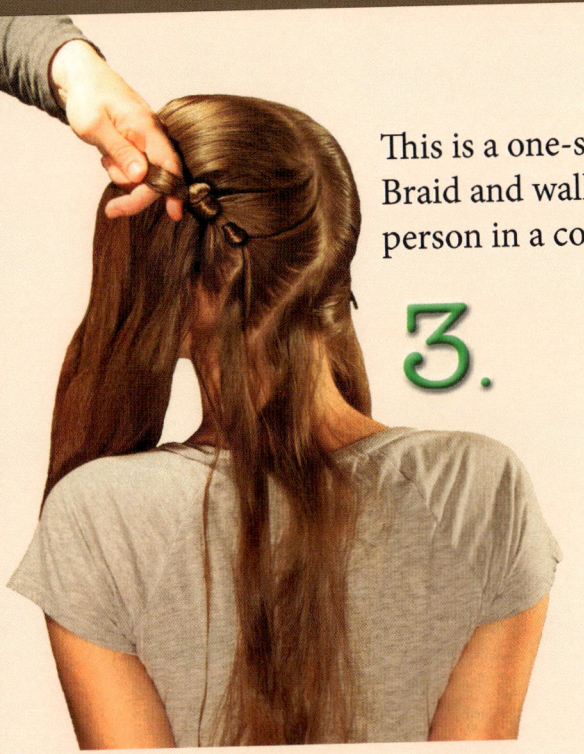

This is a one-strand pretzel. Braid and walk around the person in a complete circle.

3.

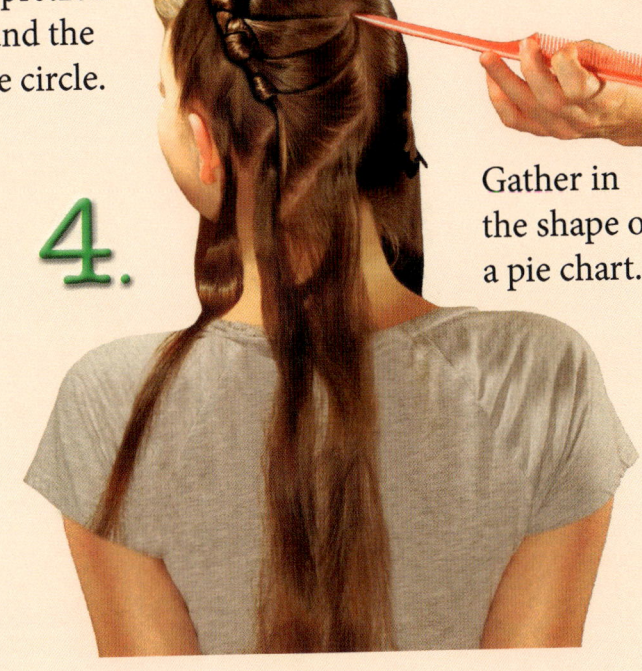

4.

Gather in the shape of a pie chart.

When gathering behind the ear to cascade, remember to leave out most of each gather.

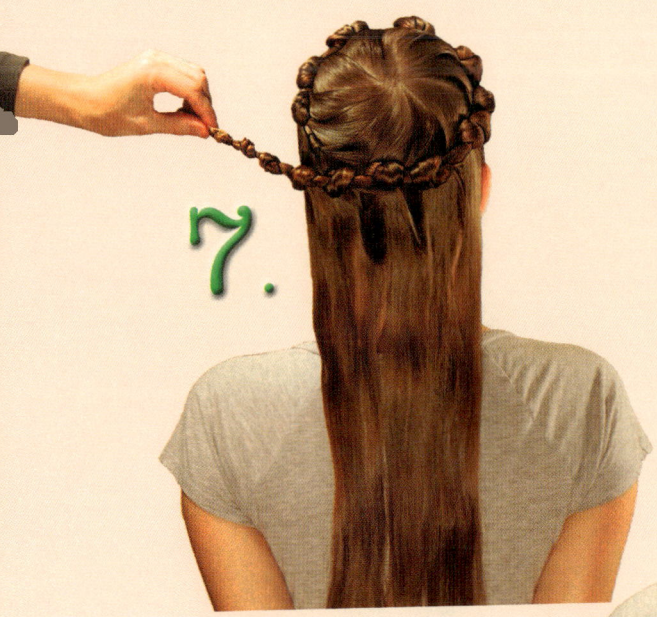

7.

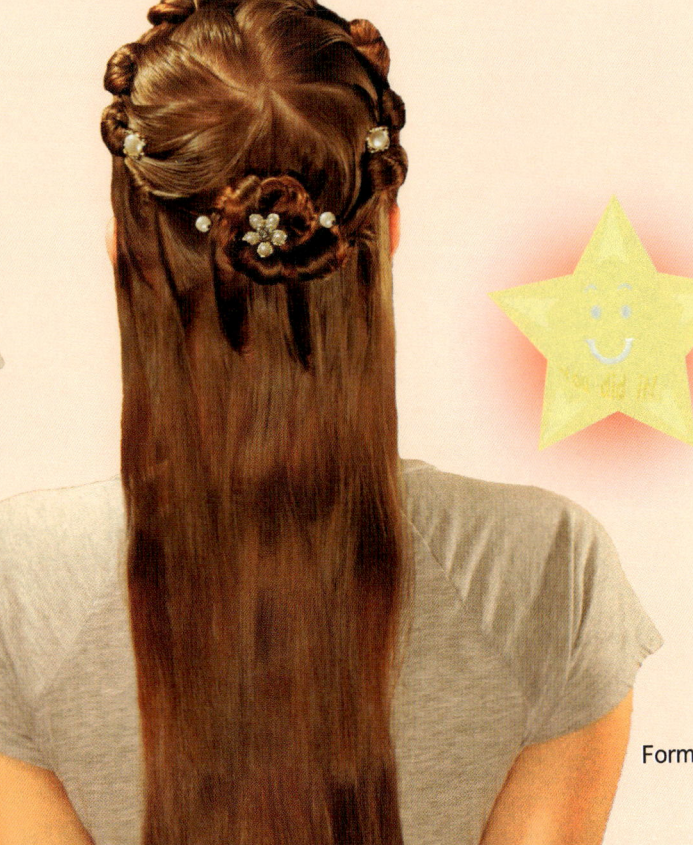

Finish the braid where you started and close the seam. Pin the tail to the halo or make a bun.

Forms 451

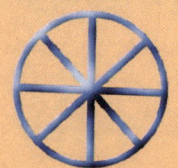

Accented Halo Cascade

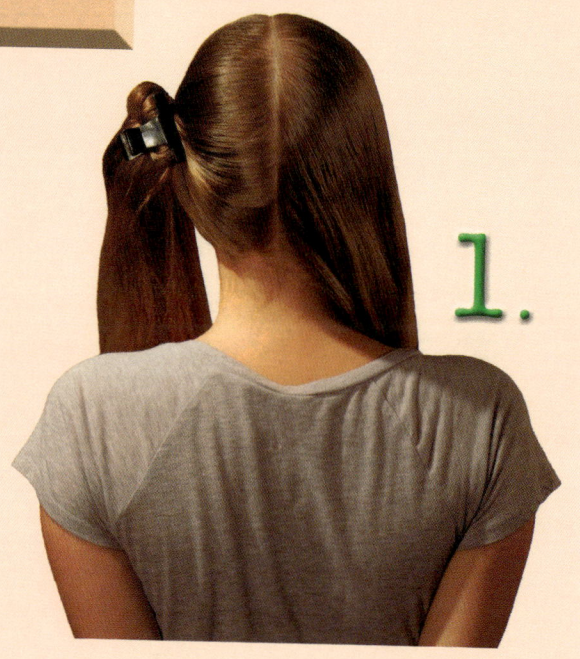

1. Part down the middle. Clip off one side.

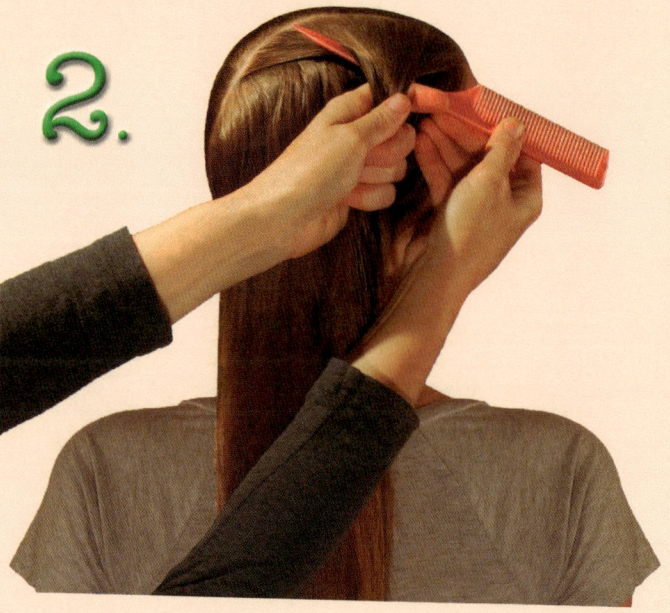

2. Part down the middle. Clip off one side. Take a section from the top center of the head parting down towards the nape of the neck creating a pie slice about an inch wide at the base. Choose the number of strands you will braid with.

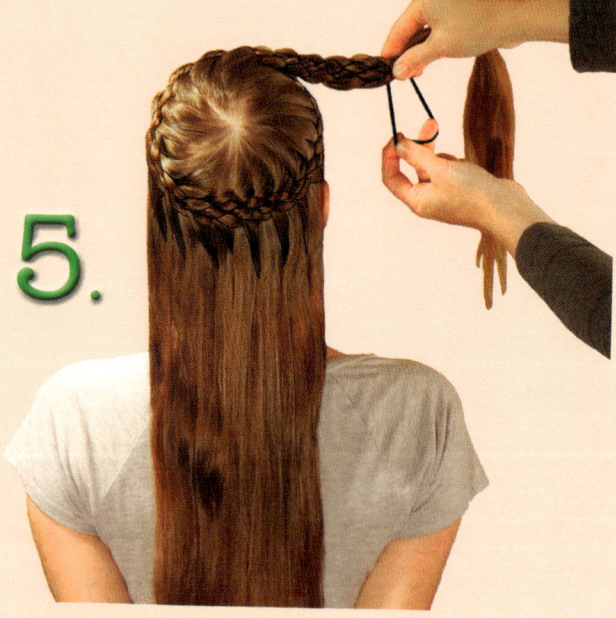

5. The outside gathers should line up with the inside gathers all pointing towards the center.

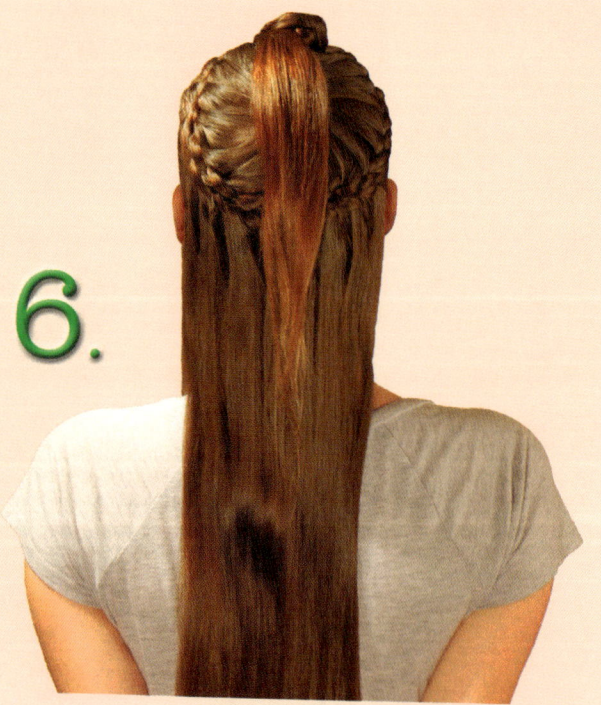

6.

452   www.findingbraids.com

Accented Halo Cascade

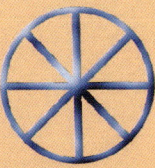

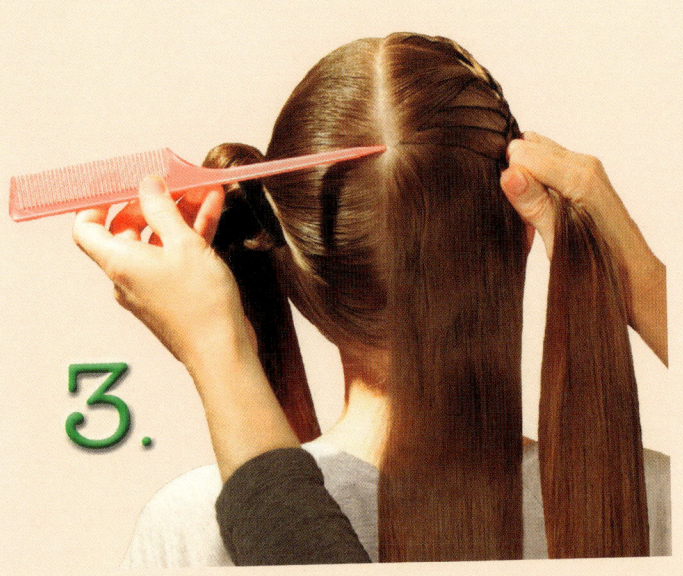

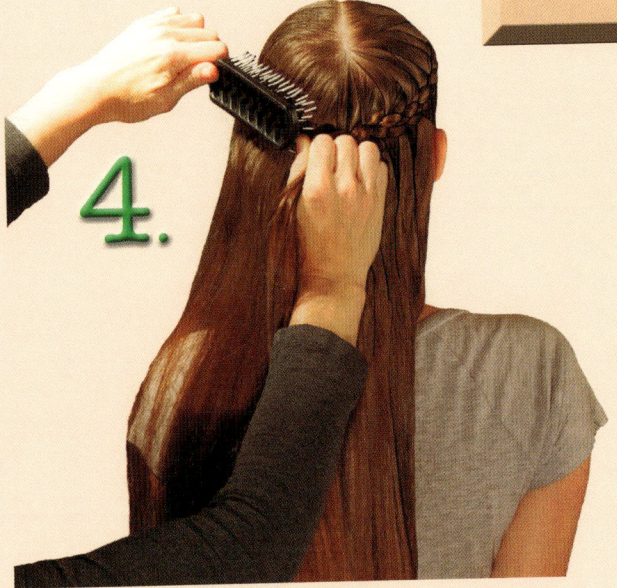

This is a five-strand. Braid and walk around the person in a complete circle. Gather in the shape of a pie chart.

This is a cascade; so, only take a sliver of each gather behind the ears leaving most of the hair down.

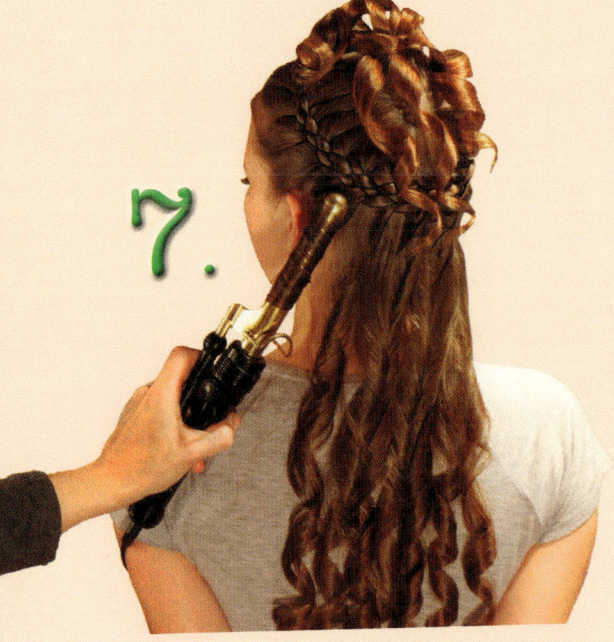

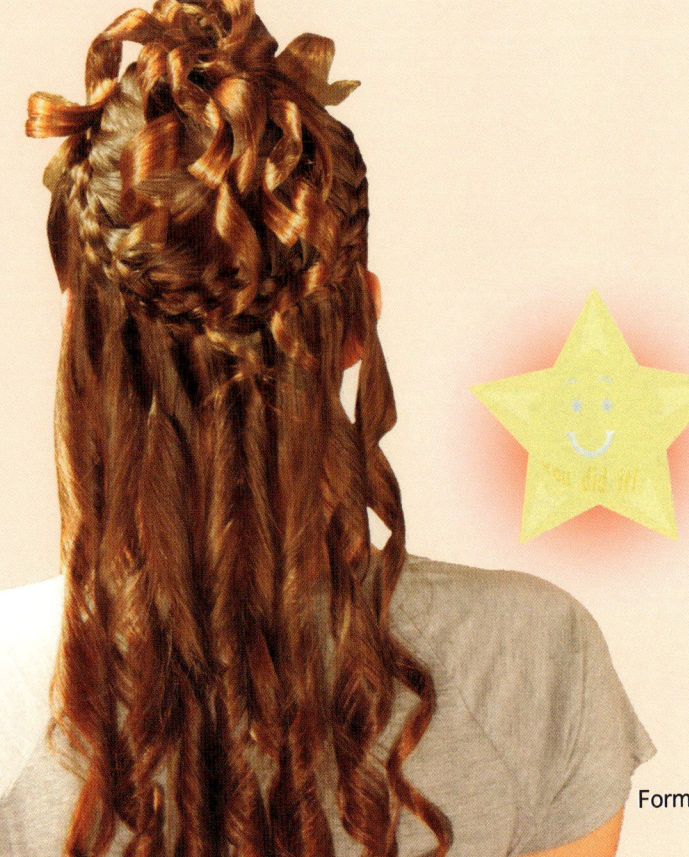

Finish the braid where you started and close the seam. Pin the tail to the halo or make a bun. I am creating the accents with the unbraided tail and the cascade.

Forms 453

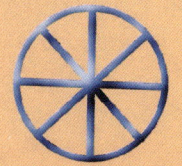

Fake Halo

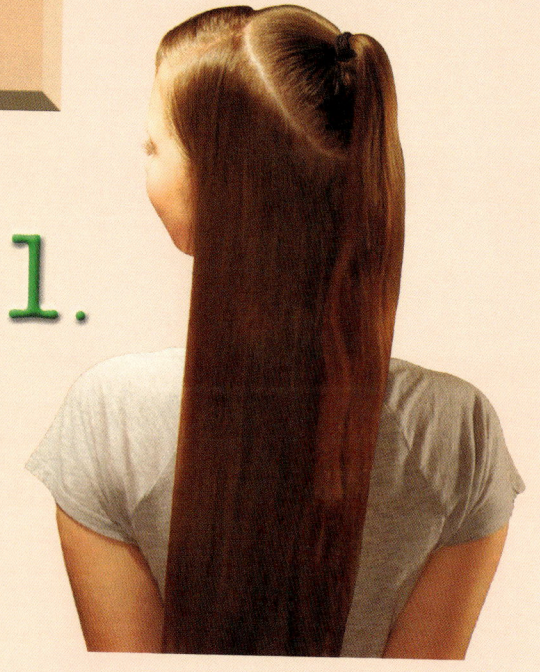

1. Reminiscent of the circle form, pony tail out the center hair. Tilt the persons head forward, chin down and spread out the hair around them.

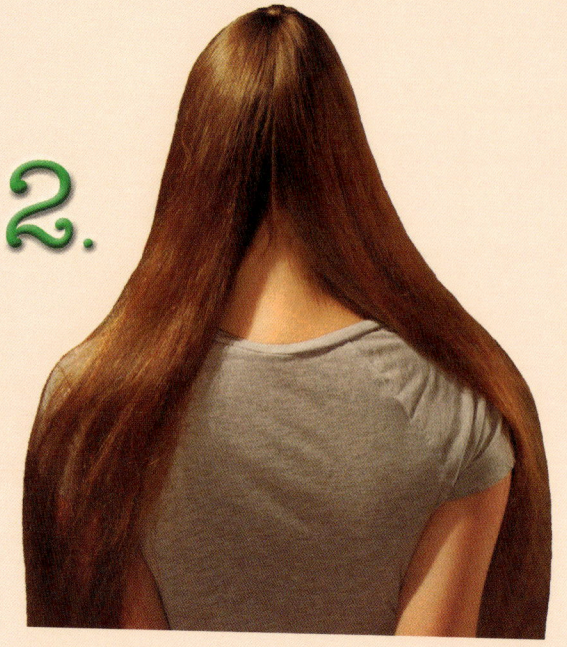

2. Choose the number of strands you will braid with. This is a three-strand. Braid and walk around the person in a complete circle. Gather in the shape of a pie chart.

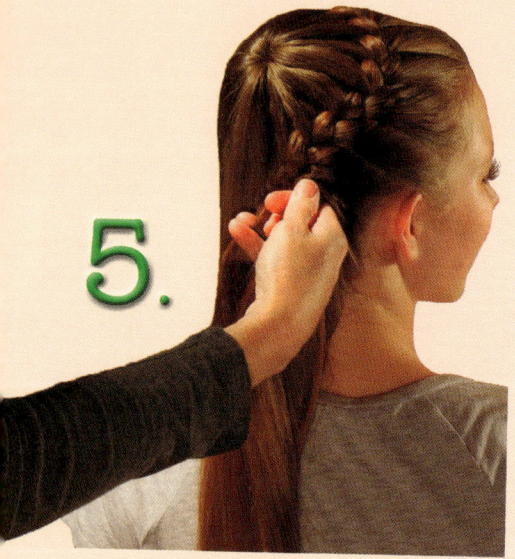

5. The outside gathers should line up with the inside gathers all pointing towards the center.

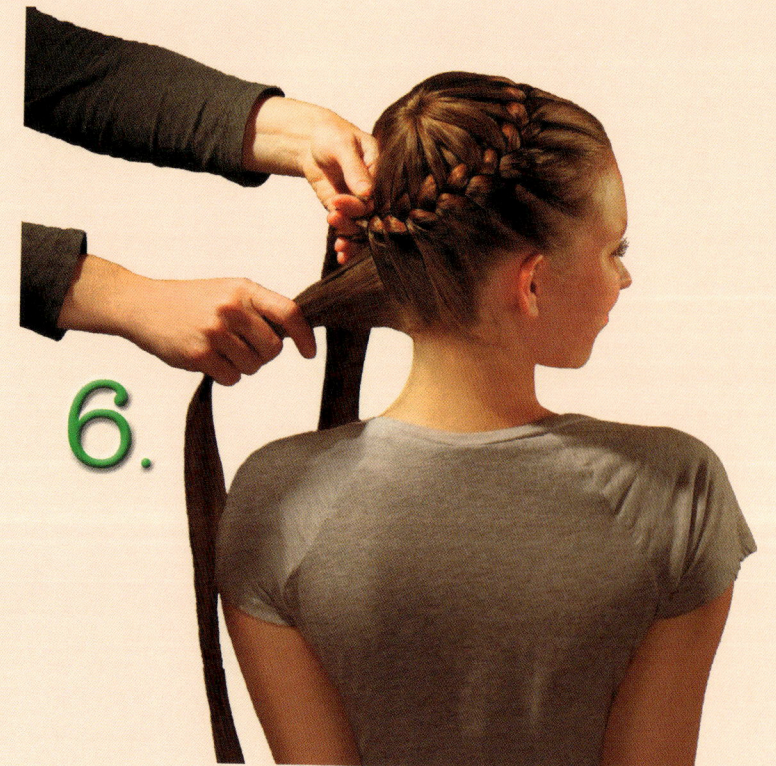

454   www.findingbraids.com

Fake Halo

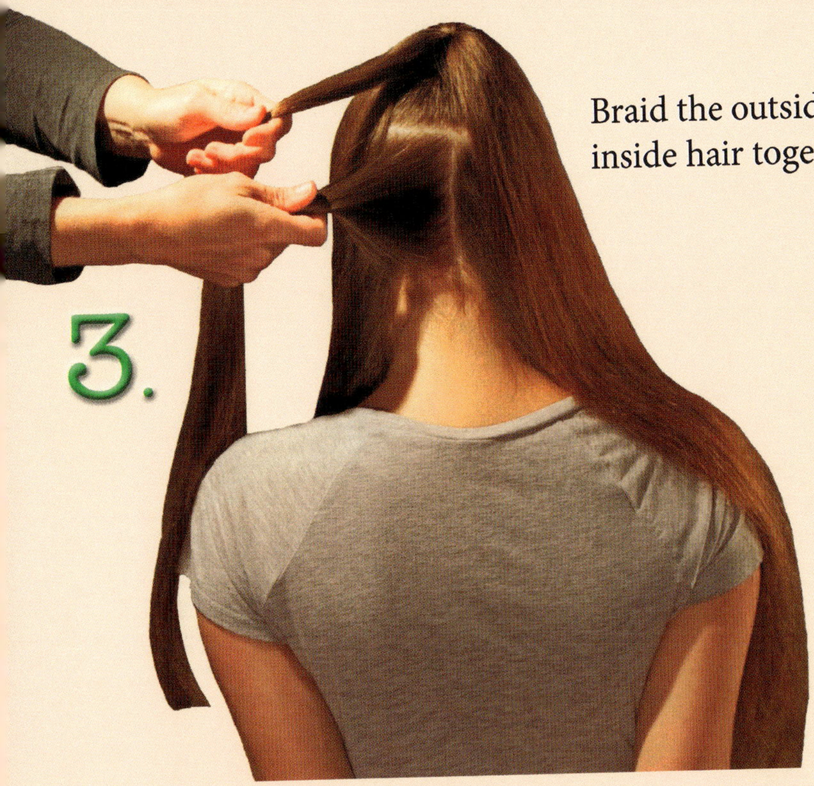

3. Braid the outside and inside hair together.

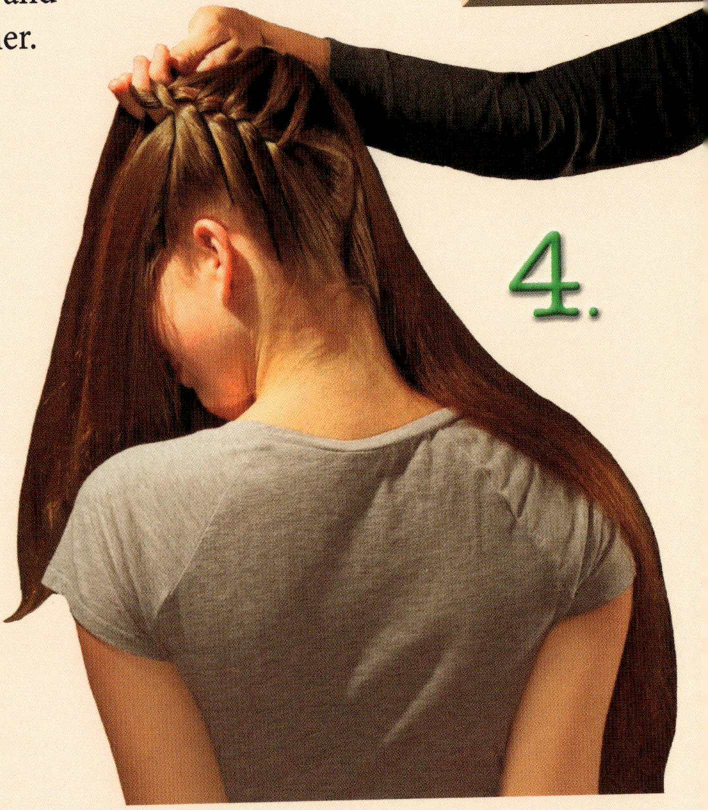

4.

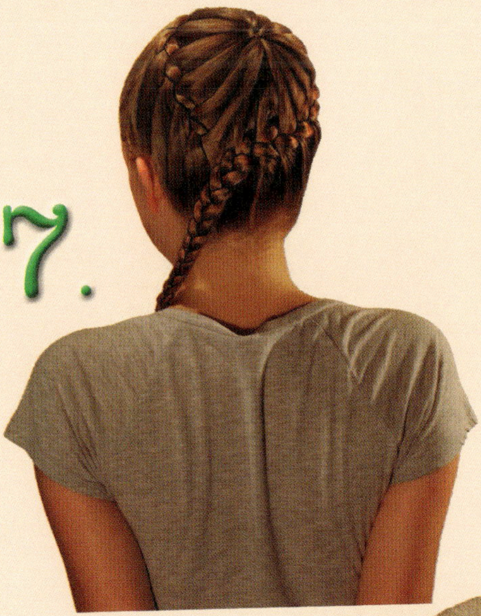

7. Finish the braid where you started and close the seam. Pin the tail to the halo or make a bun.

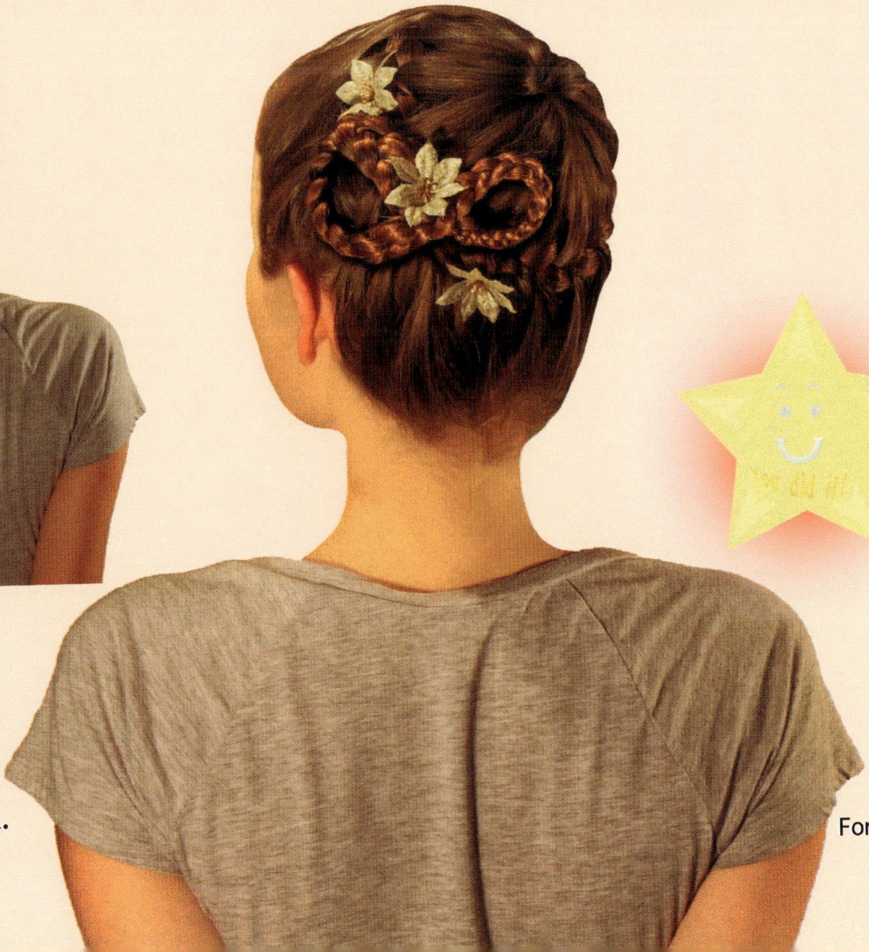

Forms 455

Forms

Notes

Examples of Halos

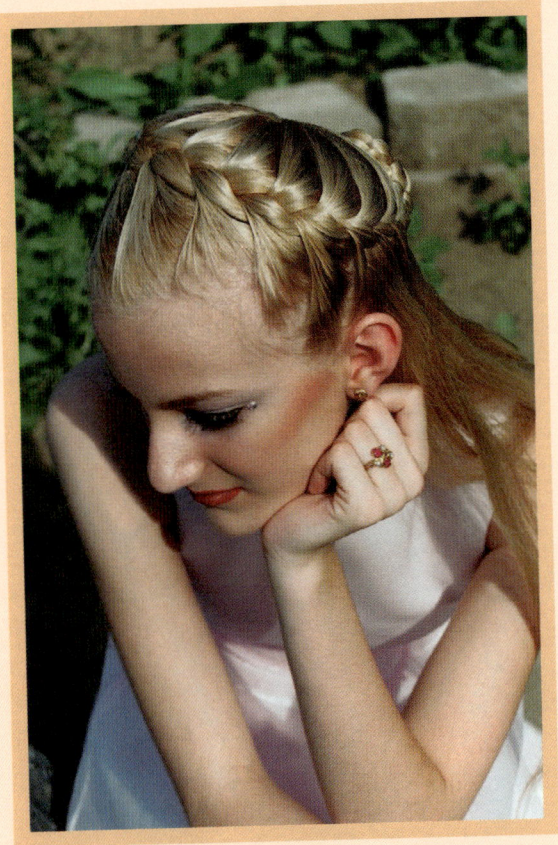
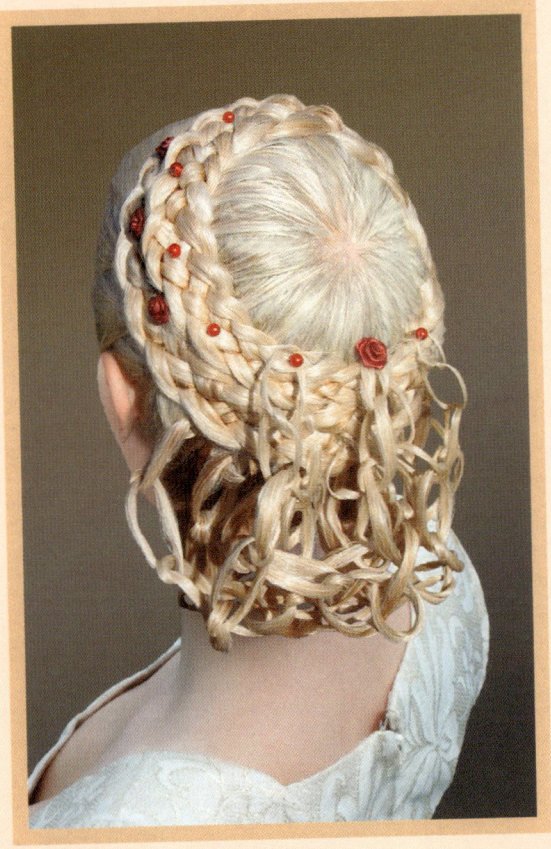
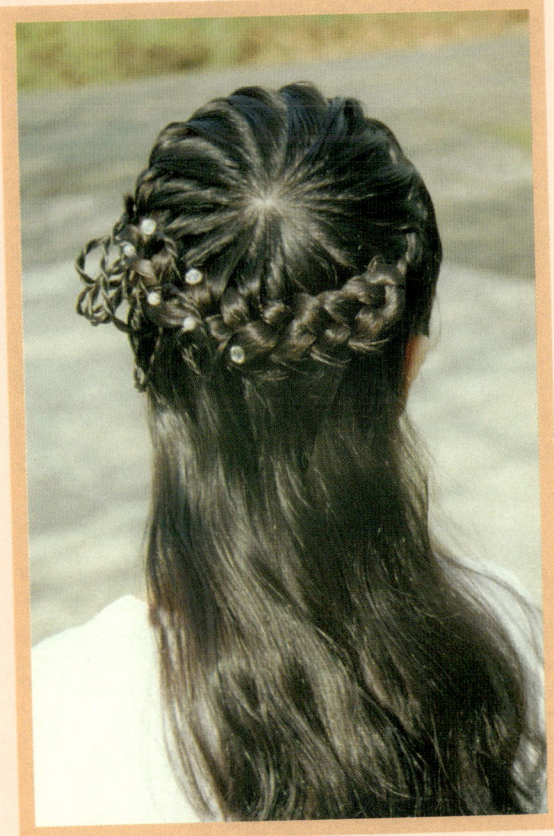
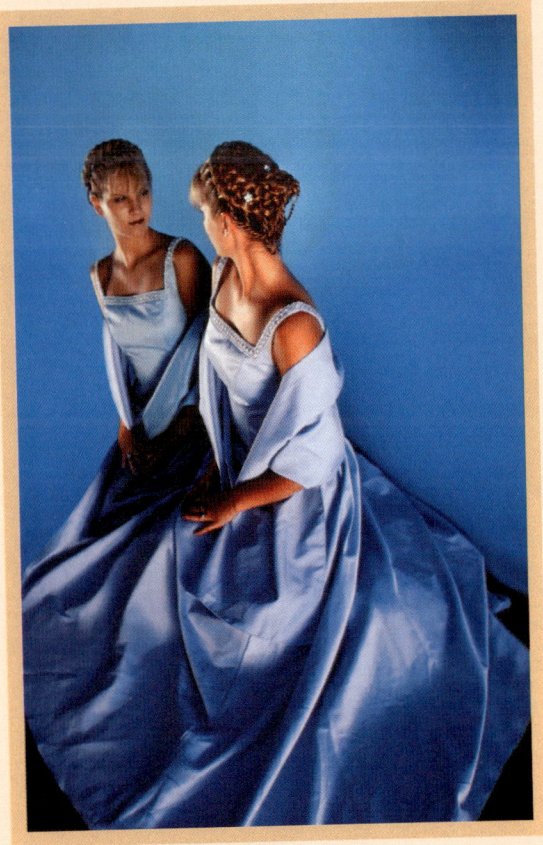

Visit my website to see more examples of Halos

Forms

HEART

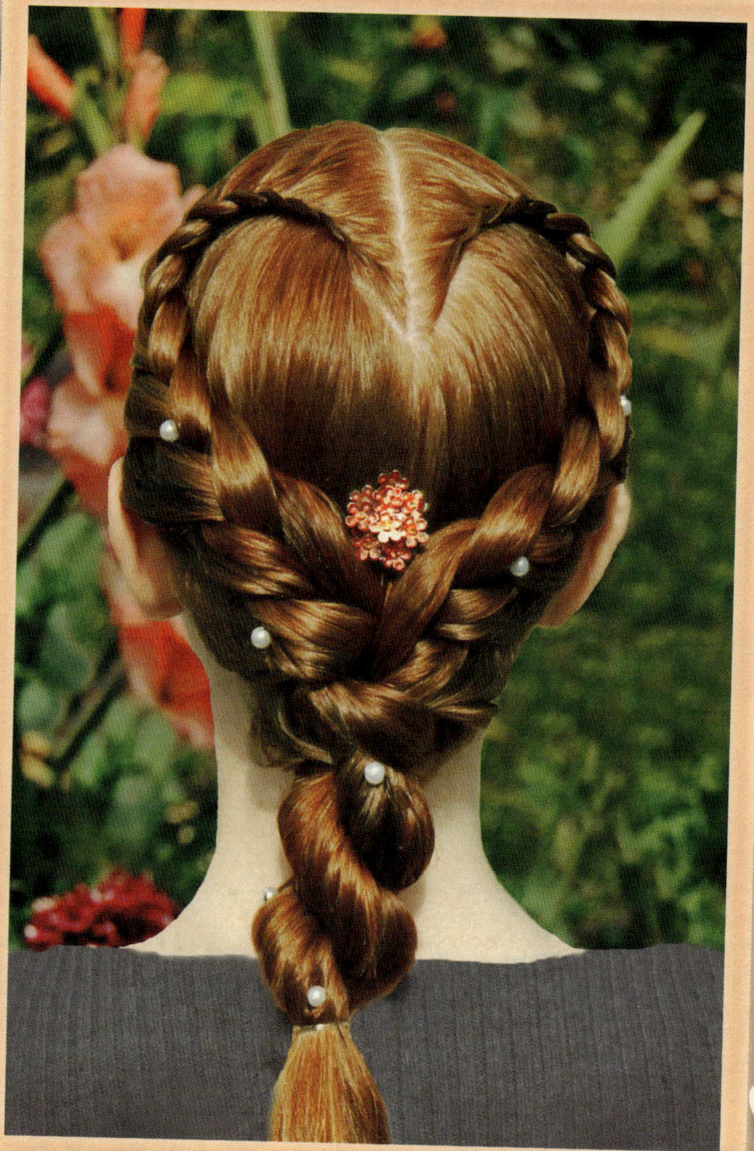

A romantic statement made with your whole being. Integrate your thoughts into your look.

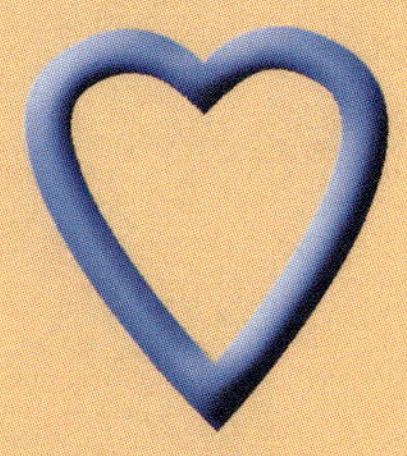

Forms

Gather like this!

Braiding icon for the next eight pages.

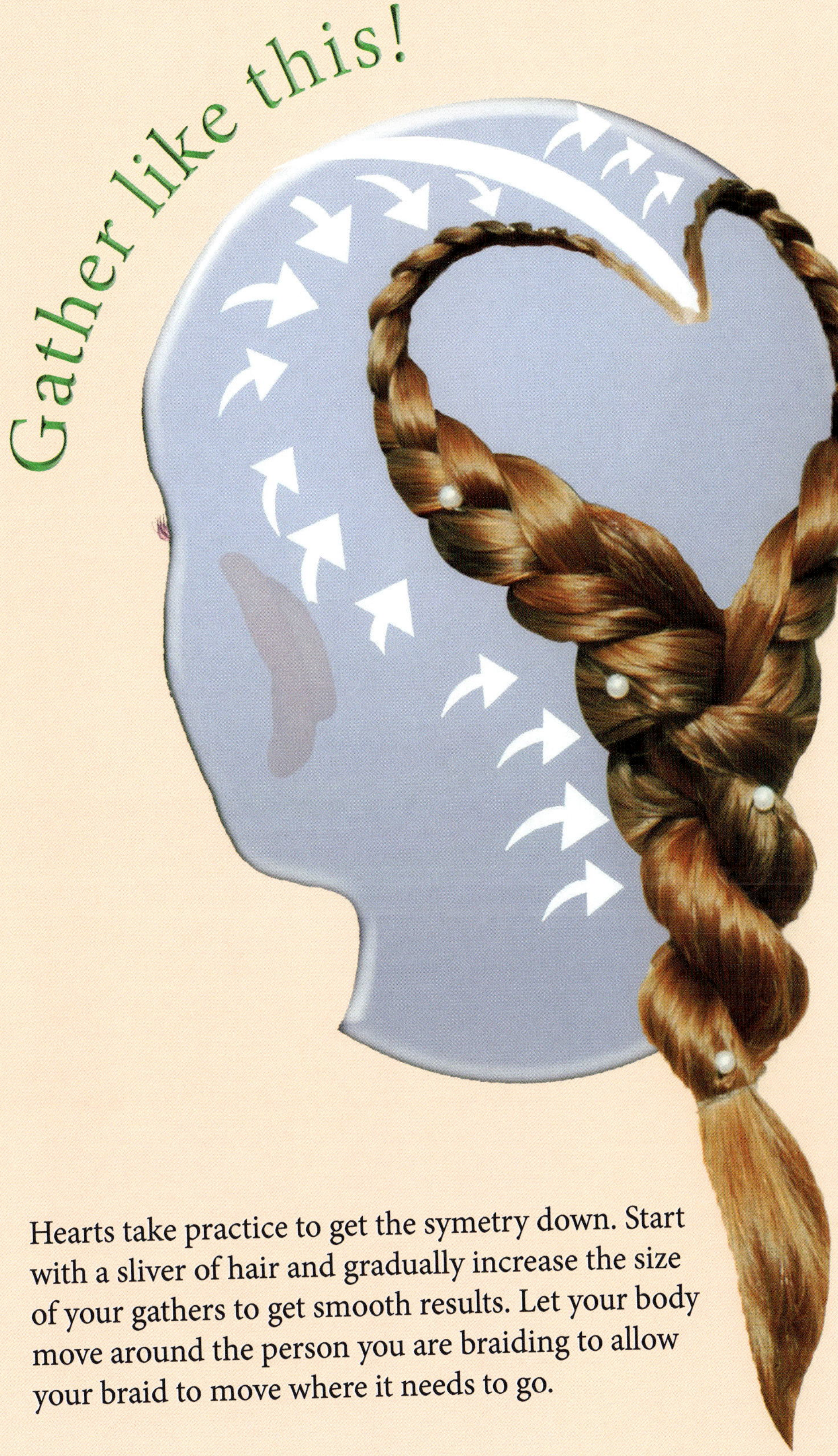

Hearts take practice to get the symetry down. Start with a sliver of hair and gradually increase the size of your gathers to get smooth results. Let your body move around the person you are braiding to allow your braid to move where it needs to go.

The **Heart** Form

Basic Heart

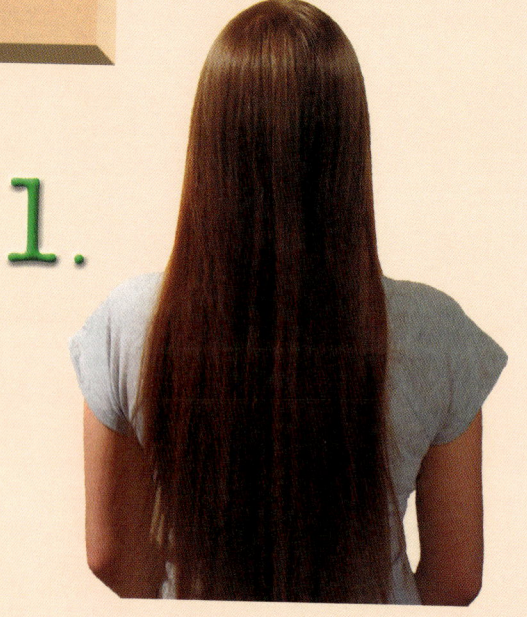

1. Begin with clean, brushed hair.

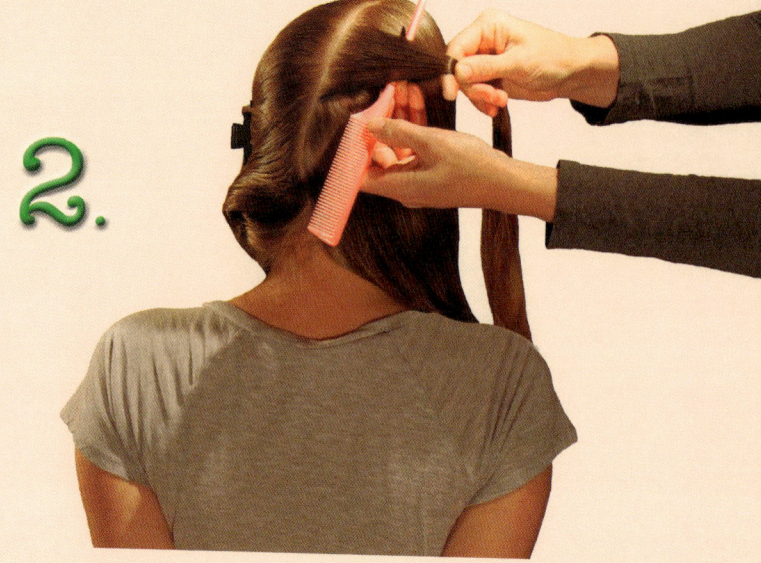

2. Part down the middle. Clip off one side. Take a section from the center-most point out about two inches.

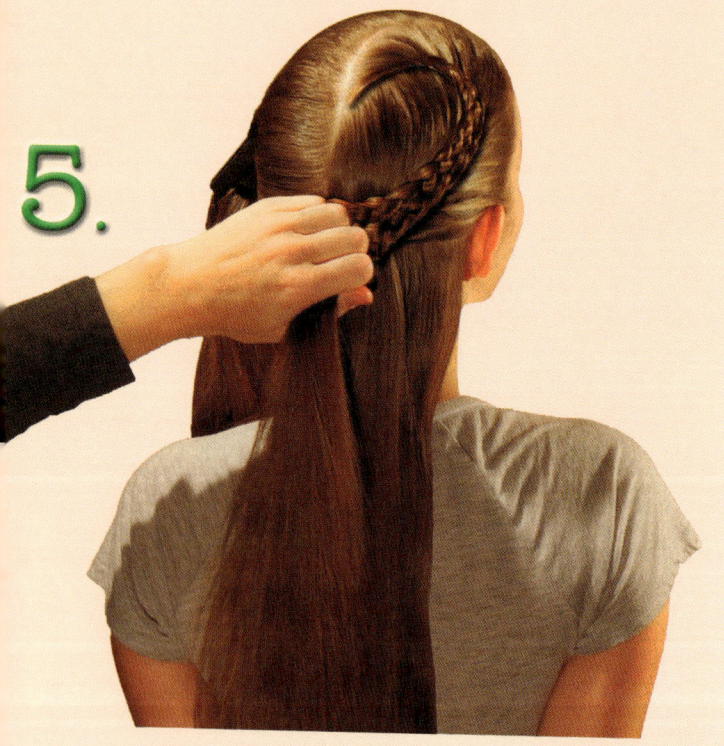

5. Gather in the shape of a heart.

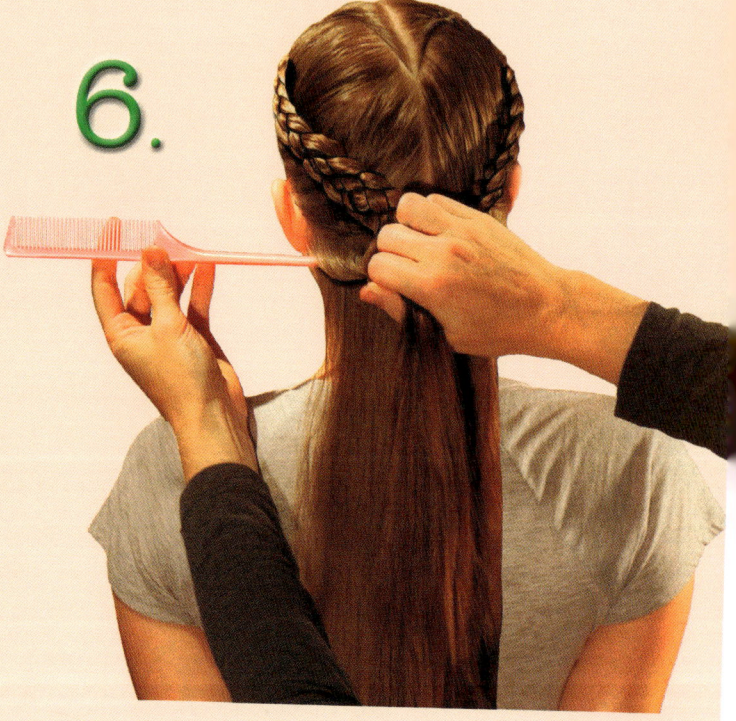

6. Merge the two braids in a pleasing spot in the back of the head. High or low is up to you and where you choose to navigate to.

Basic Heart

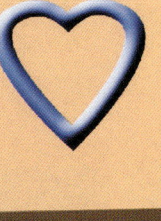

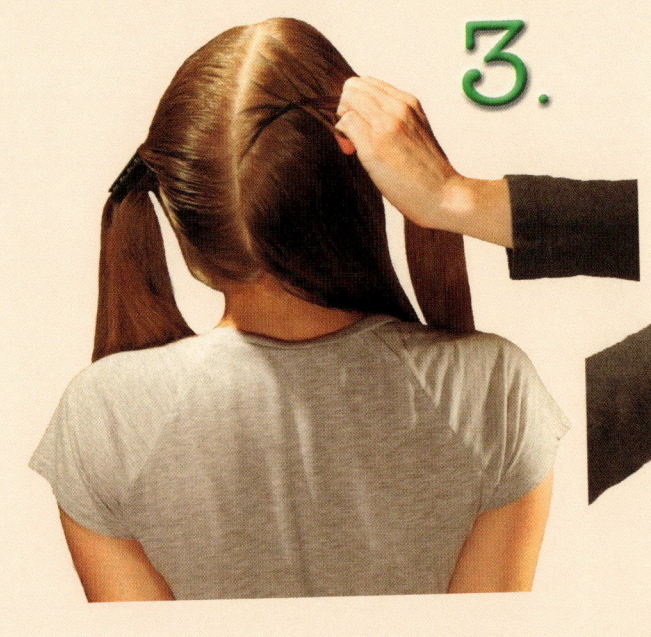

Choose the number of strands you will braid with.

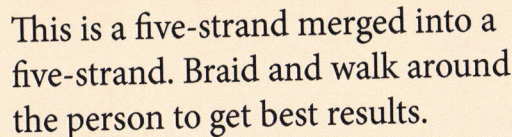

This is a five-strand merged into a five-strand. Braid and walk around the person to get best results.

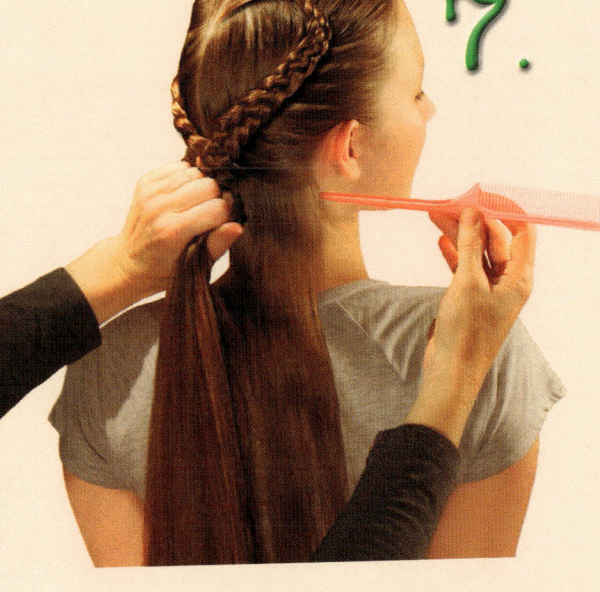

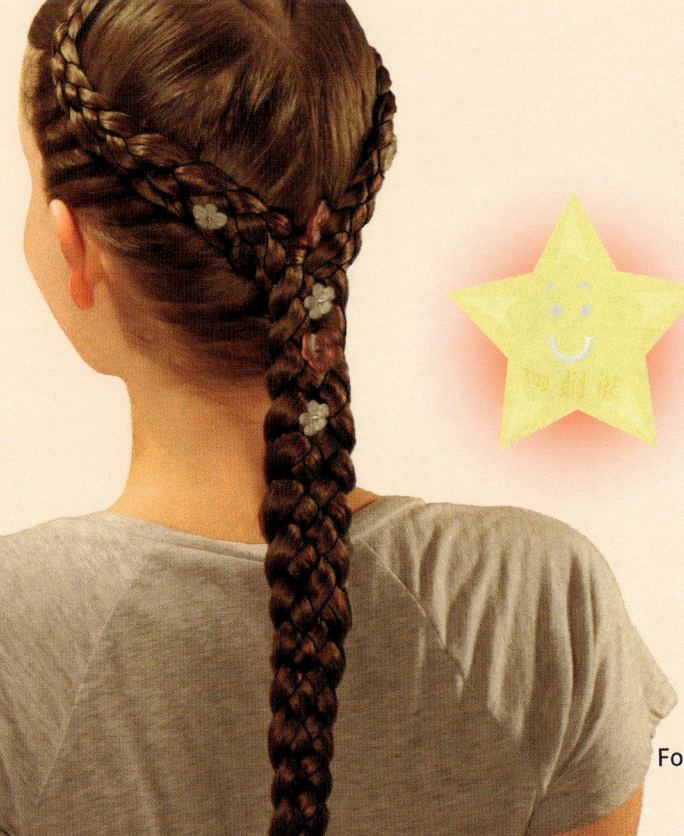

Continue braiding down the back of the head to the ends of the hair. Finish the tail with the same number of strands or mix it up and use a different number.

Accented Heart

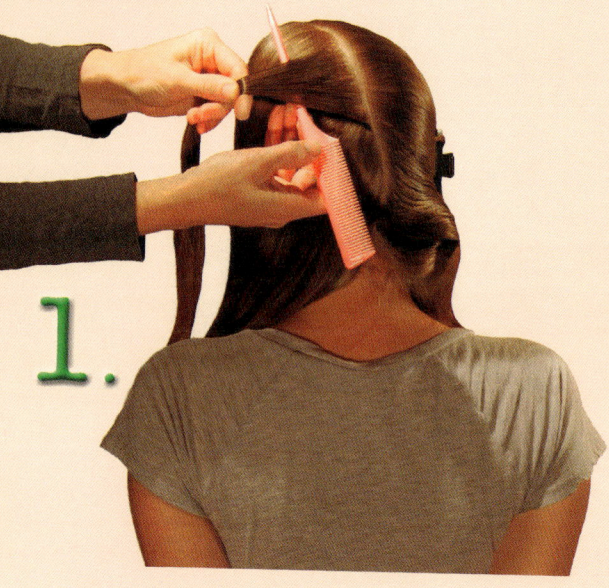

1. Part down the middle. Clip off one side. Take a section from the centermost point out about two inches.

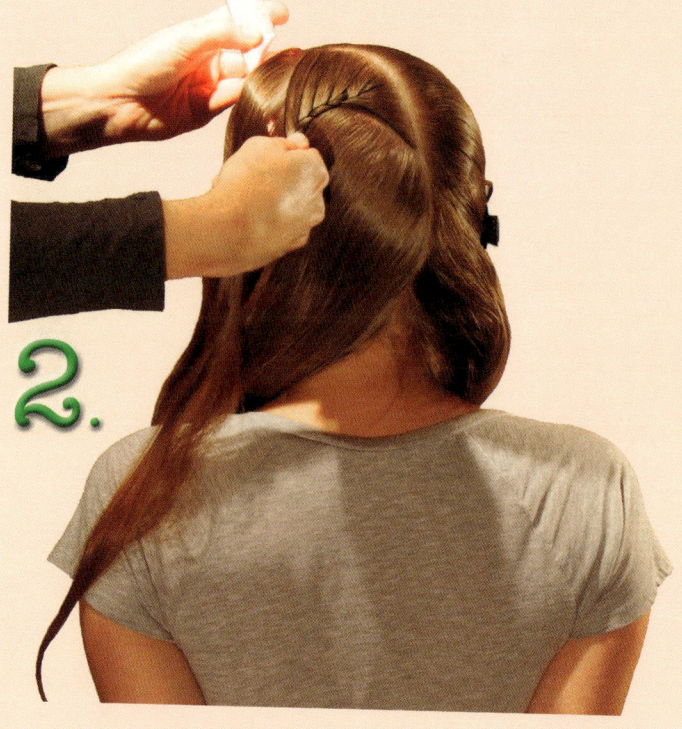

2. Choose the number of strands you will braid with. Braid towards their face a few passes and then make your way to the back of the head.

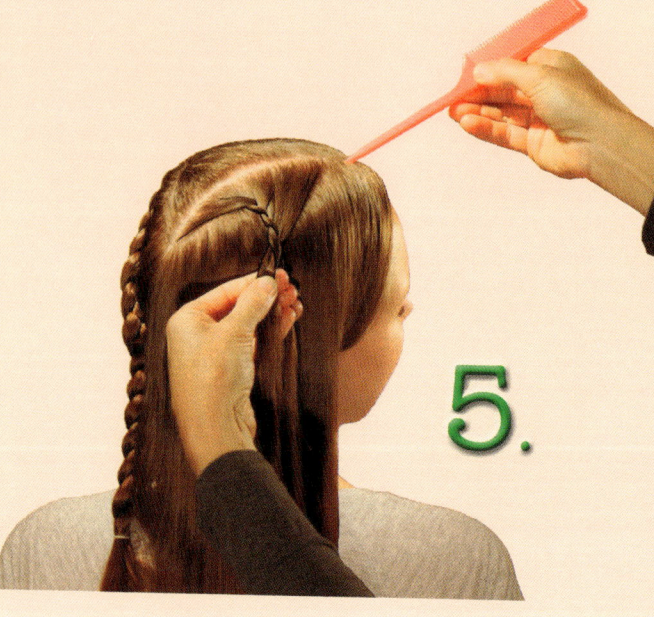

5. Repeat on the opposite side.

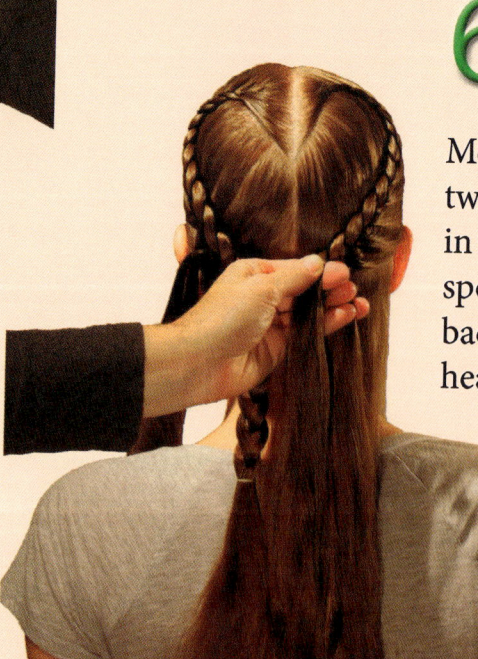

6. Merge the two braids in a pleasing spot in the back of the head.

Accented Heart

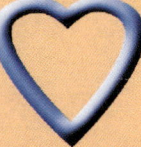

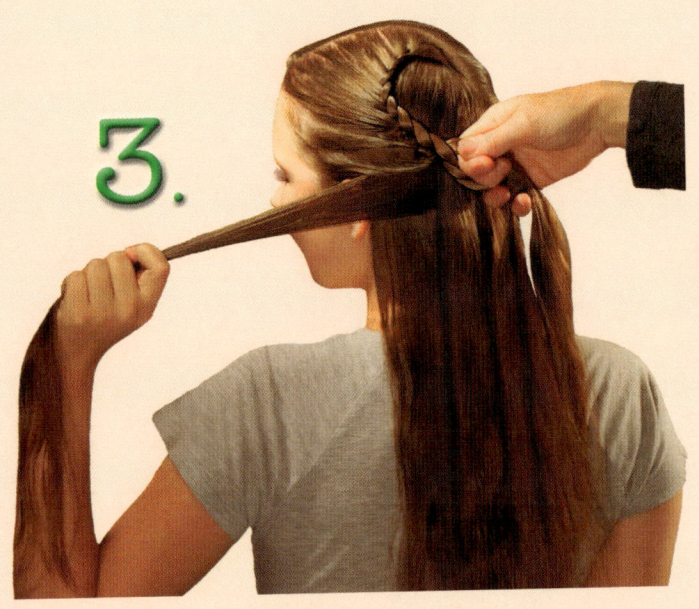

3.

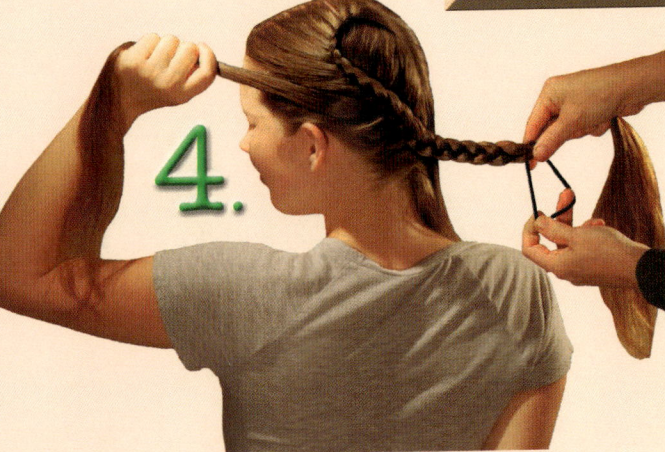

4.

Gather in the shape of a heart.

This is a three-strand merged into a ponytail. Take out strands for your accents as needed for your style.

Continue braiding down the back.

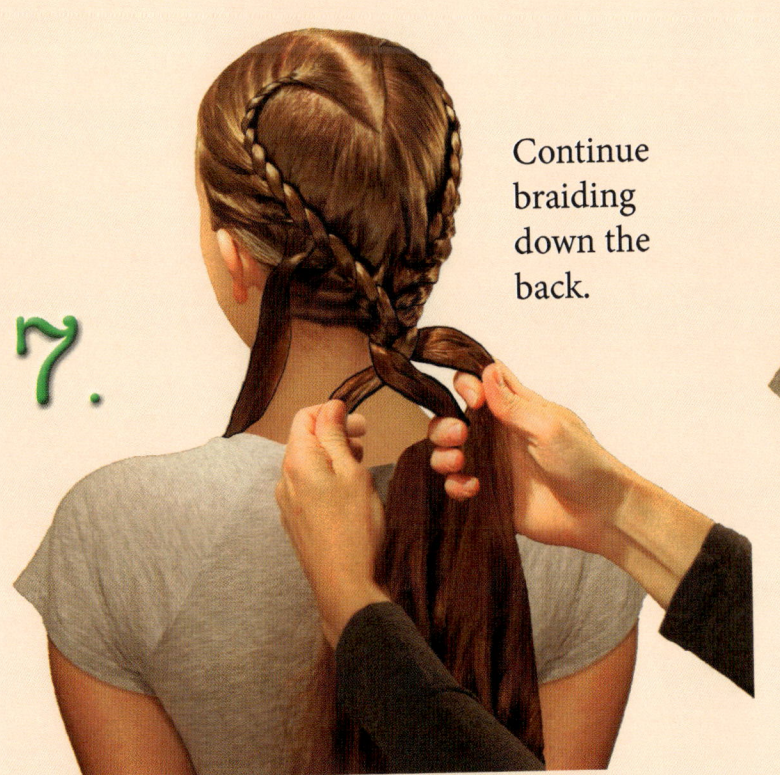

7.

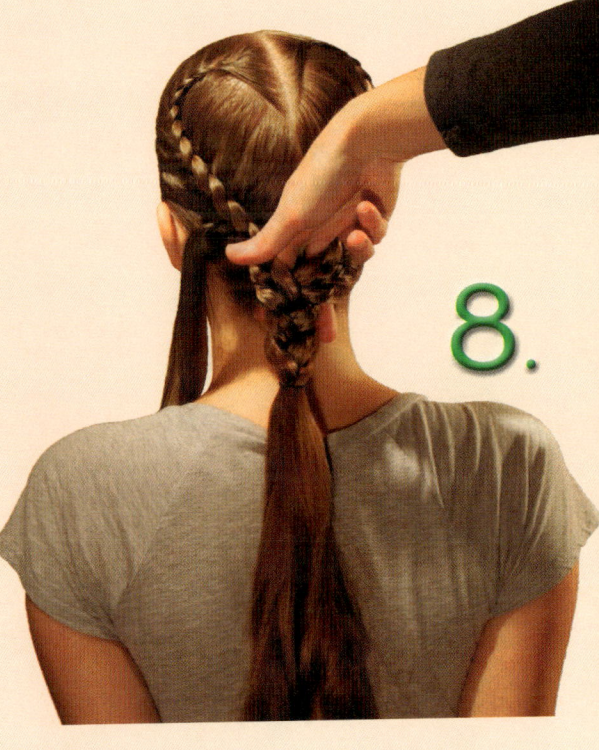

8.

Pull the pony tail up through the bottom of the form to create a lifted pony tail of loose hair.

Forms   463

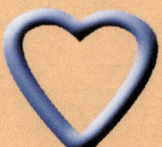

Accented Heart

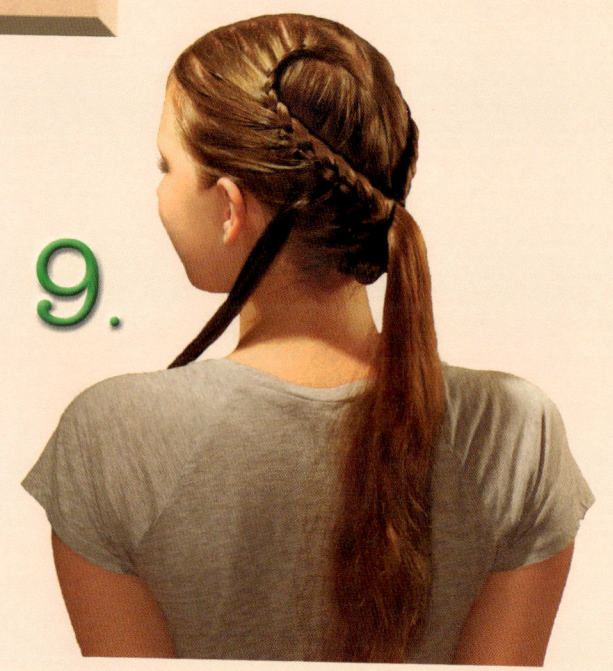

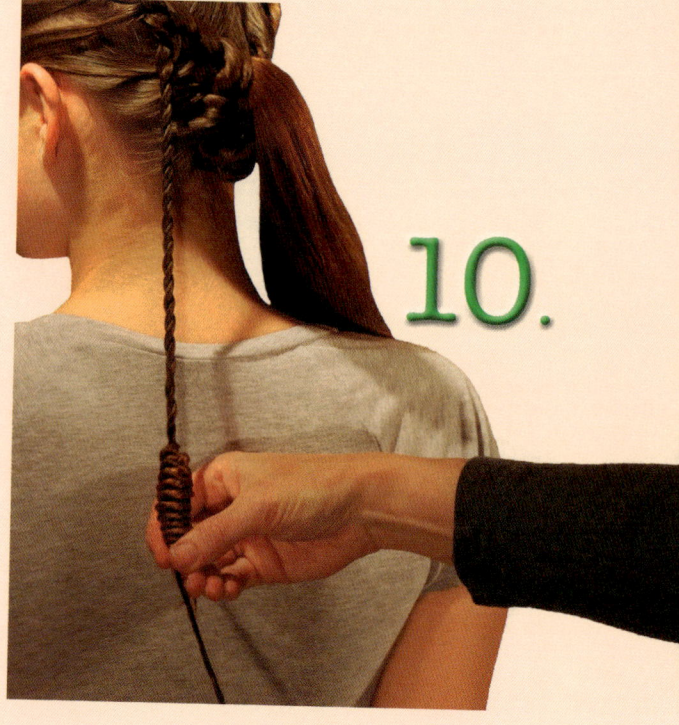

Choose an accent for your accent strand. Here we are making a push-up with two-strand rope.

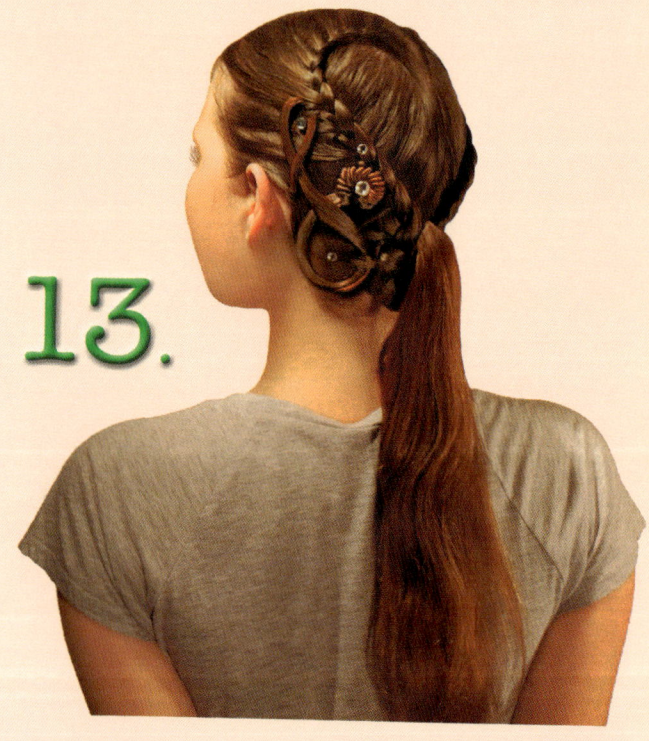

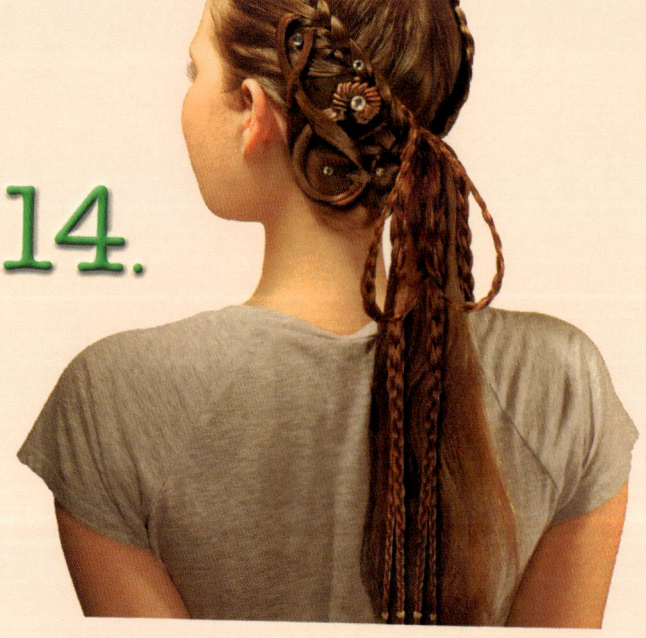

Create many accents with the unbraided tail of the form. I use mini three-strands.

Accented Heart

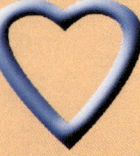

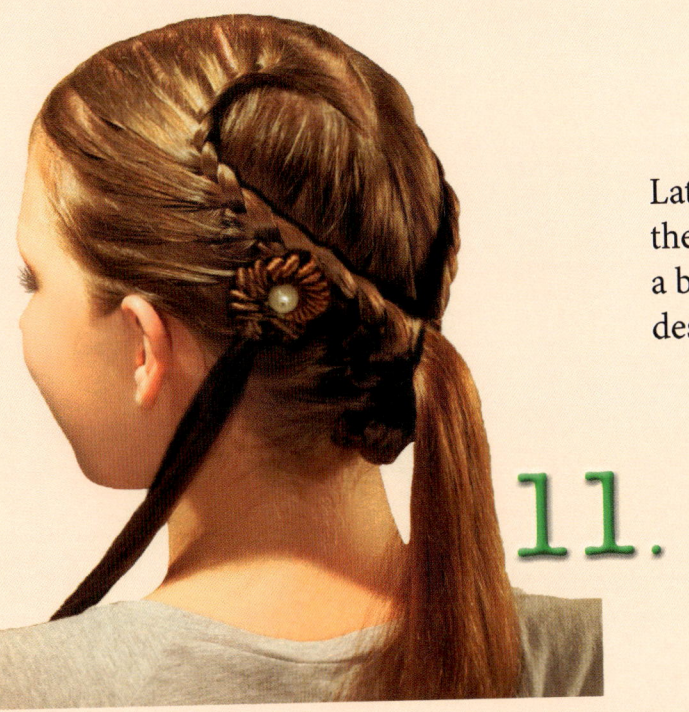

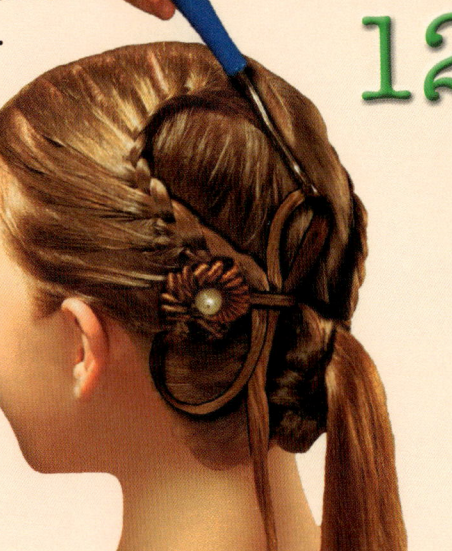

Latchhook the tail into a beautiful design.

Create a flower by pinning the end of the push-up to the beginning of the push-up and adding a sparkle decoration.

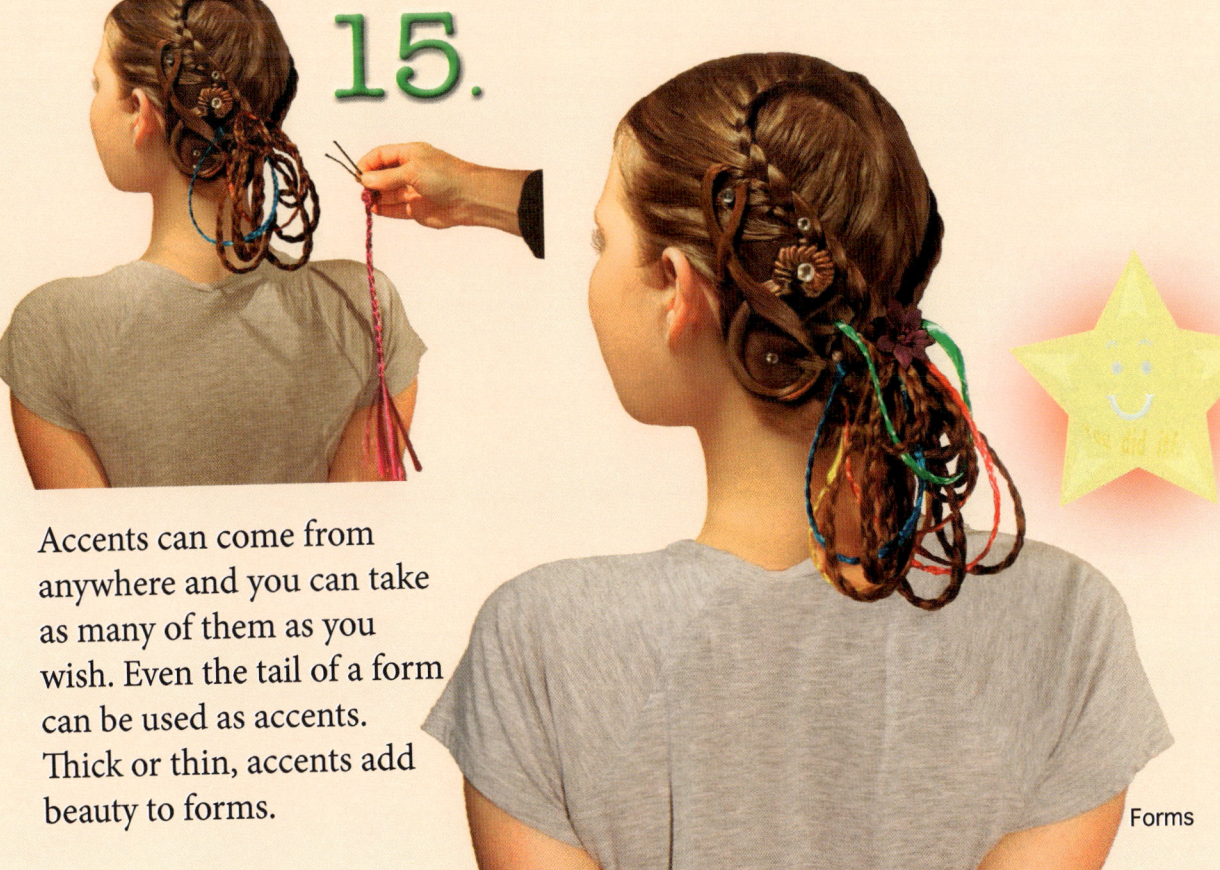

Accents can come from anywhere and you can take as many of them as you wish. Even the tail of a form can be used as accents. Thick or thin, accents add beauty to forms.

Heart Cascade

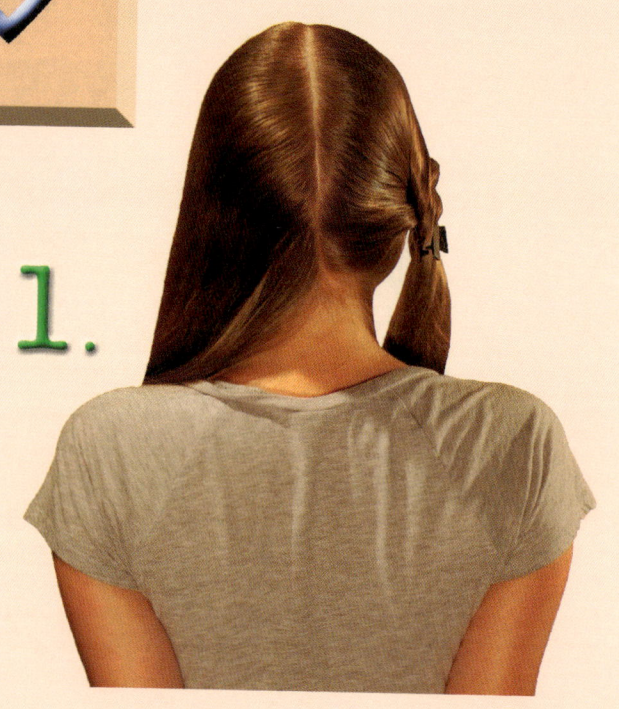

1.

Part down the middle. Clip off one side.

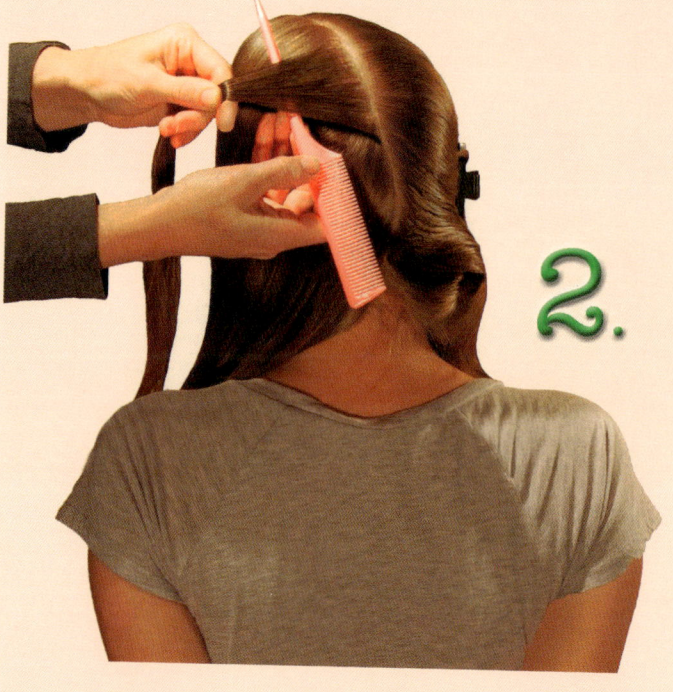

2.

Take a section from the centermost point out about two inches.

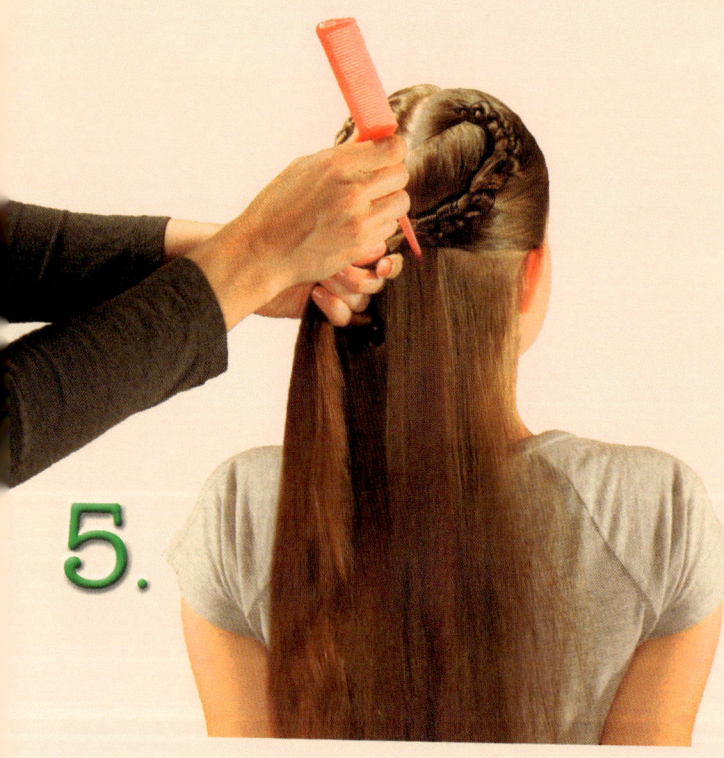

5.

Repeat on the other side.

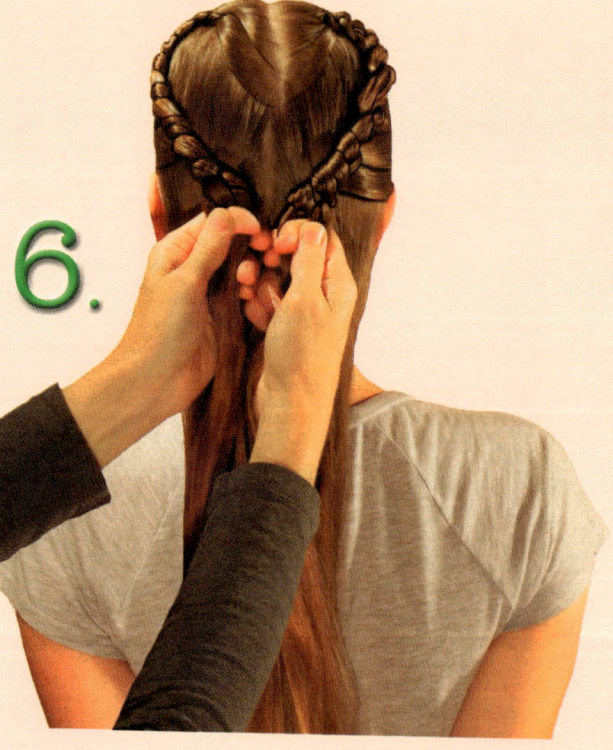

6.

Merge the two braids in a pleasing spot in the back of the head.

Heart Cascade

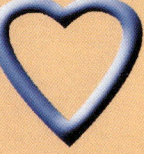

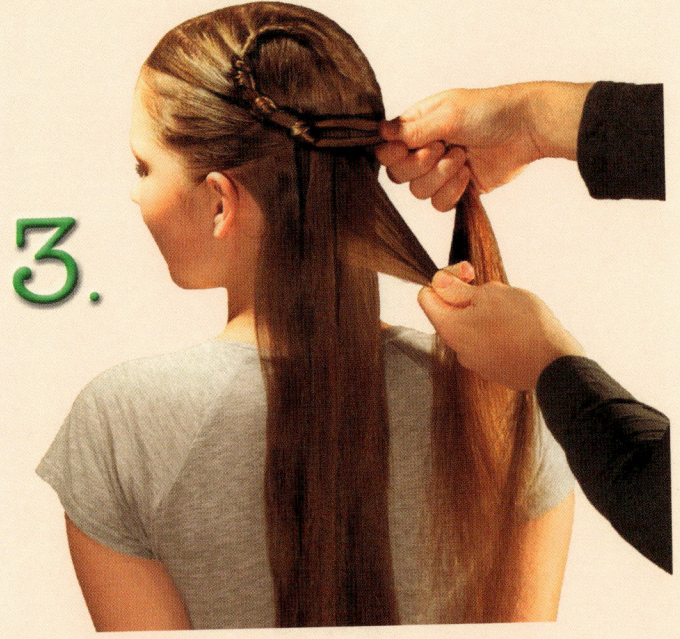

3.

This is a two-strand knot merged into a four-strand round. To cascade this form, sliver up a small portion of each gather to add into the braid leaving most of each gather left down behind the ears.

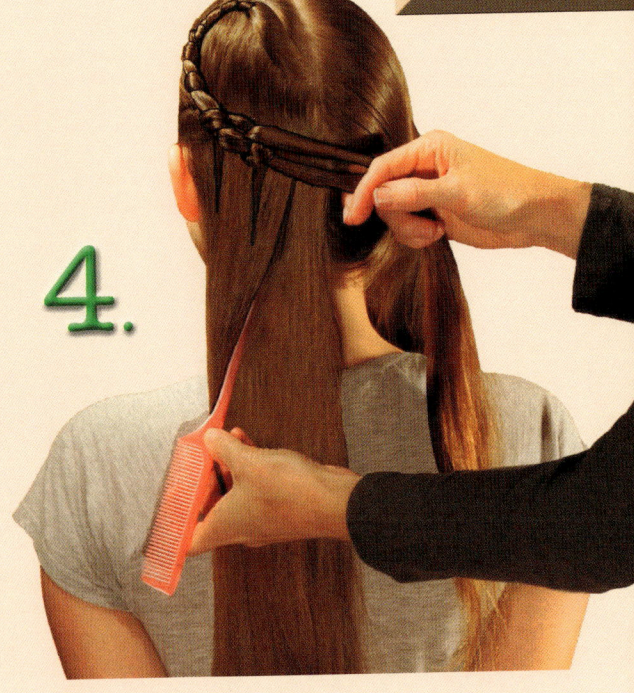

4.

Gather in the shape of a heart.

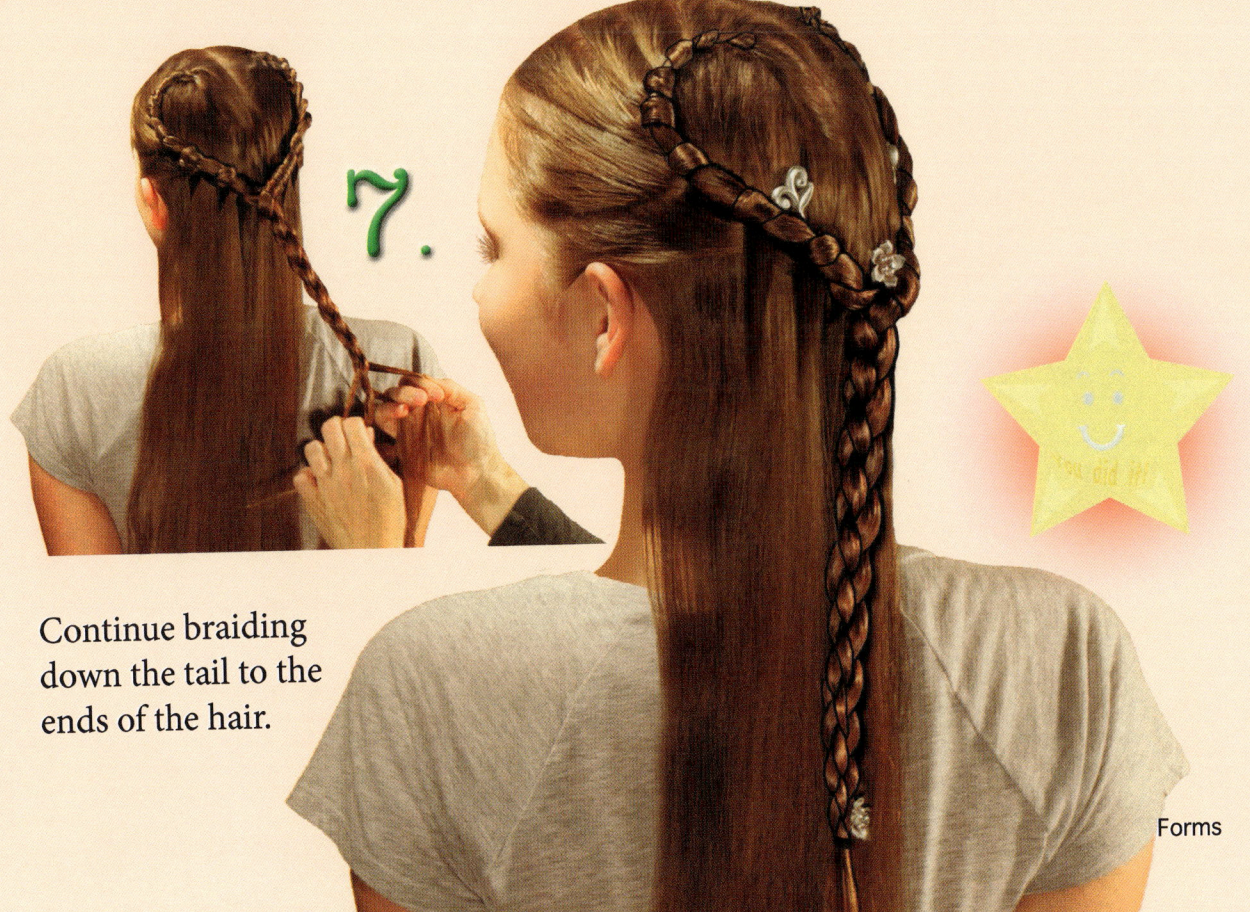

7.

Continue braiding down the tail to the ends of the hair.

Forms 467

Accented Heart Cascade

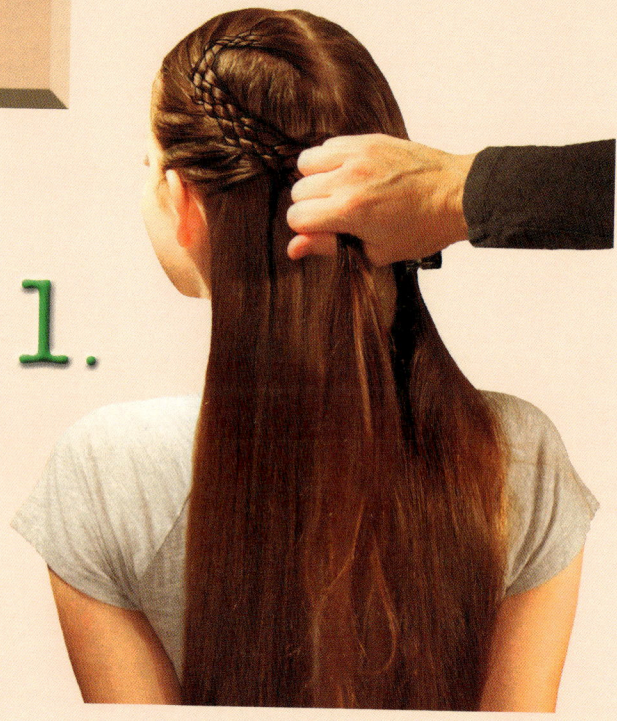

1\. Braid your heart form on one side.

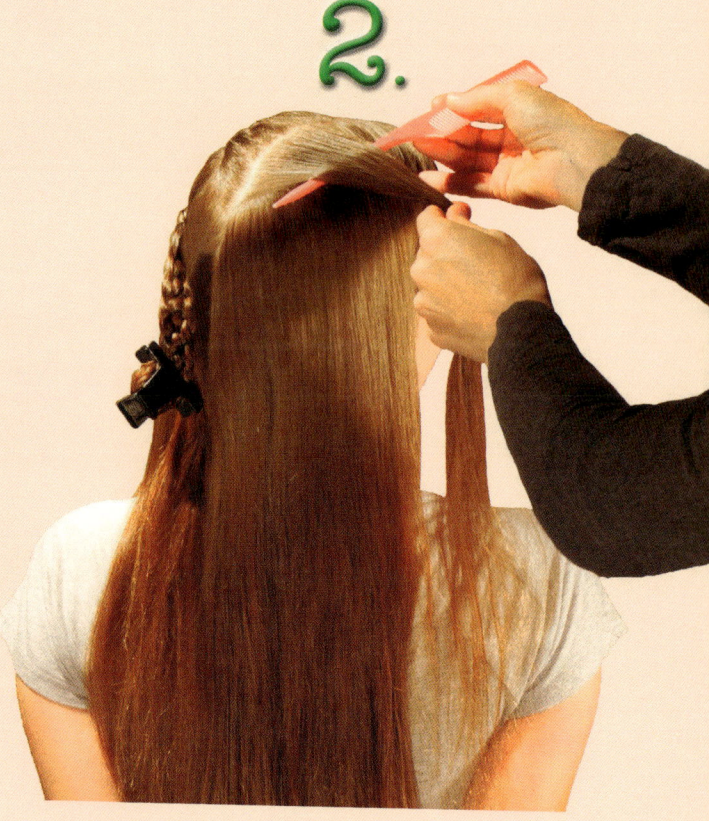

2\. On the other side take a section from the center most point.

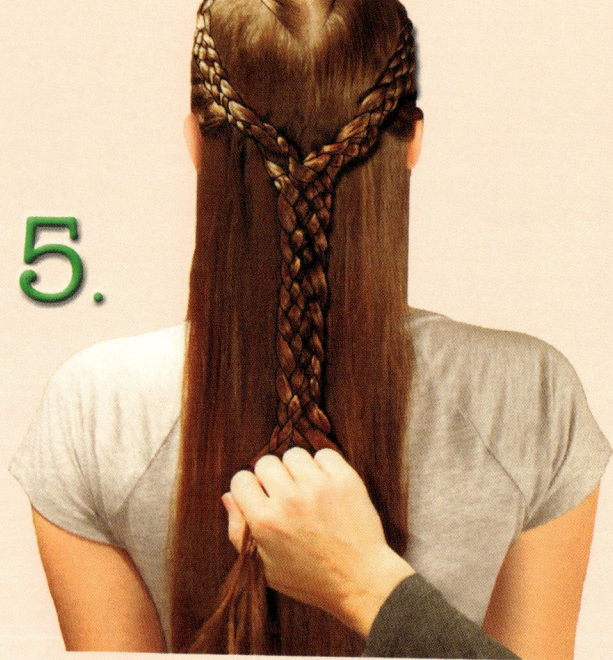

5\. Continue braiding down the tail to the ends of the hair.

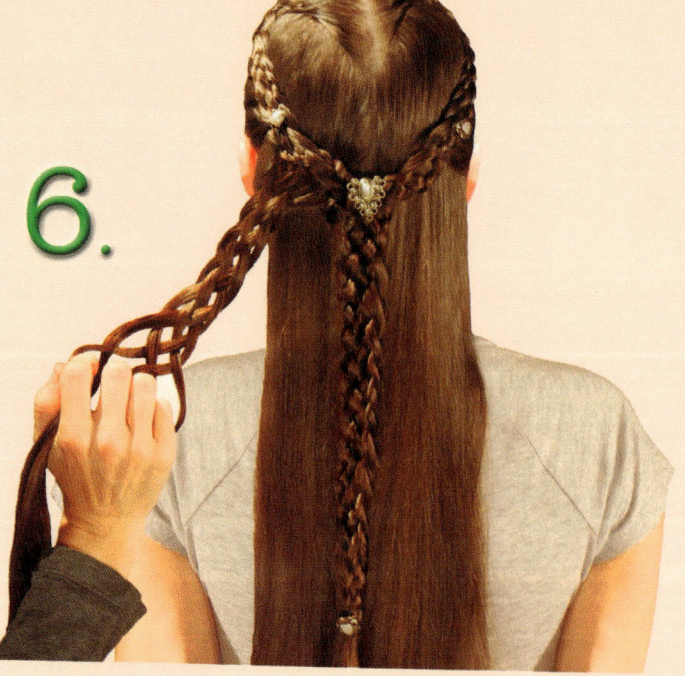

6\. Choose an accent for your accent strand. Here we are making a mini five-strand.

468   www.findingbraids.com

Accented Heart Cascade

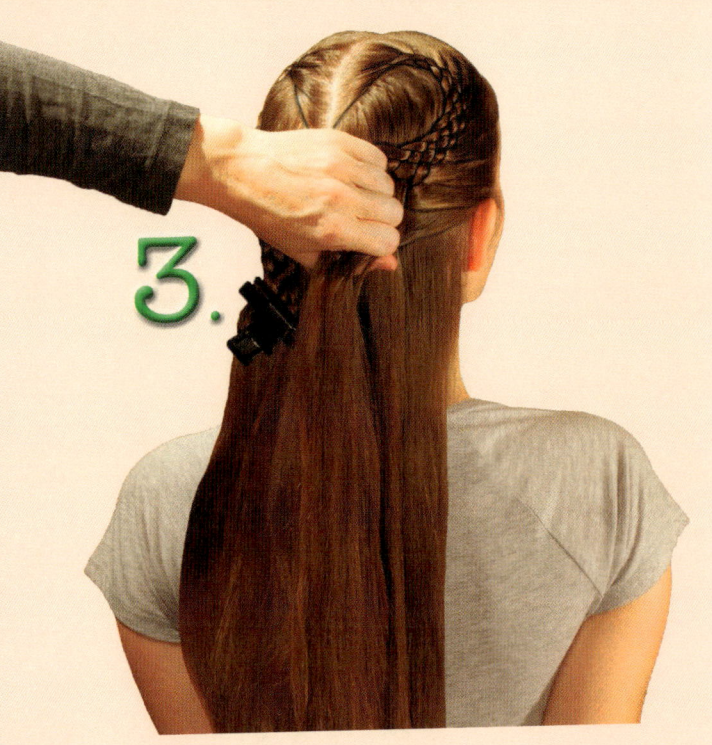

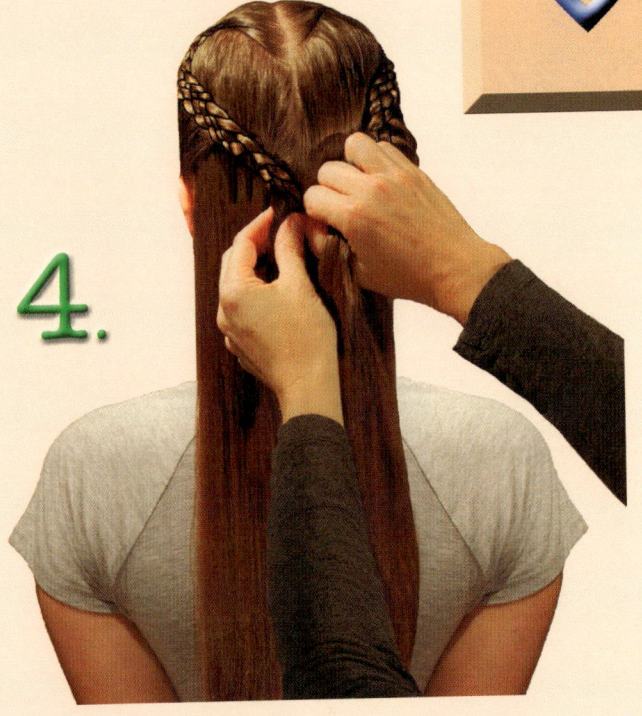

3. This is a five-strand merged into a five-strand with a mini five-strand accent. To cascade this form, sliver up a small portion of each gather to add into the braid leaving most of each gather left down behind the ears.

4. Merge the two braids in a pleasing spot in the back of the head.

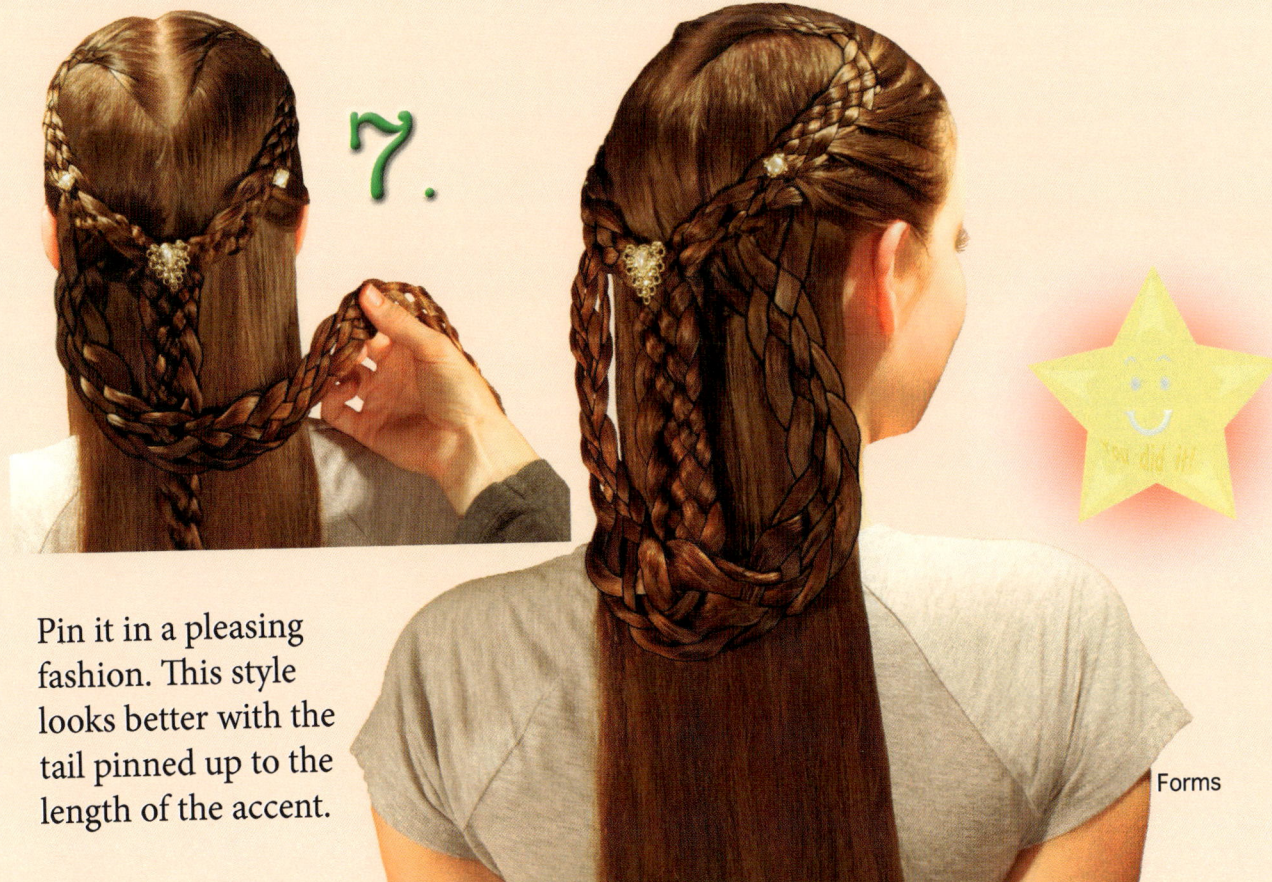

7. Pin it in a pleasing fashion. This style looks better with the tail pinned up to the length of the accent.

Forms

Forms

Notes

Examples of Hearts

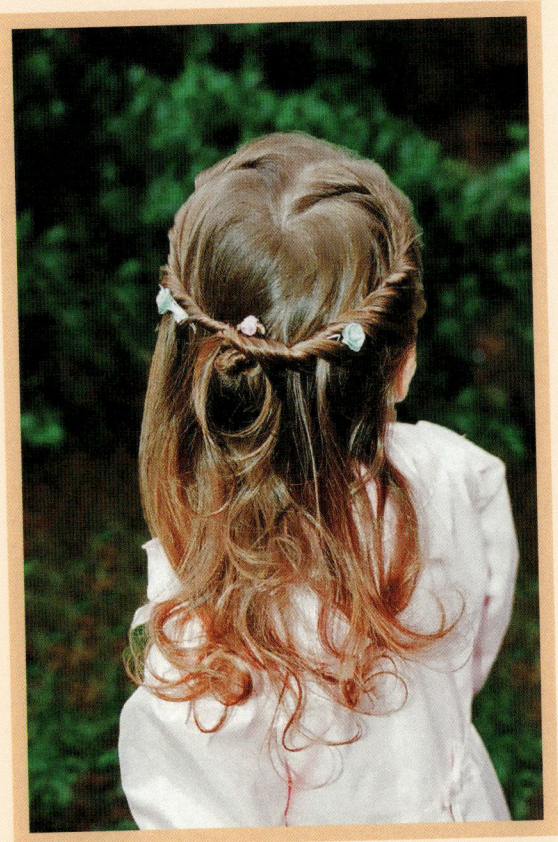
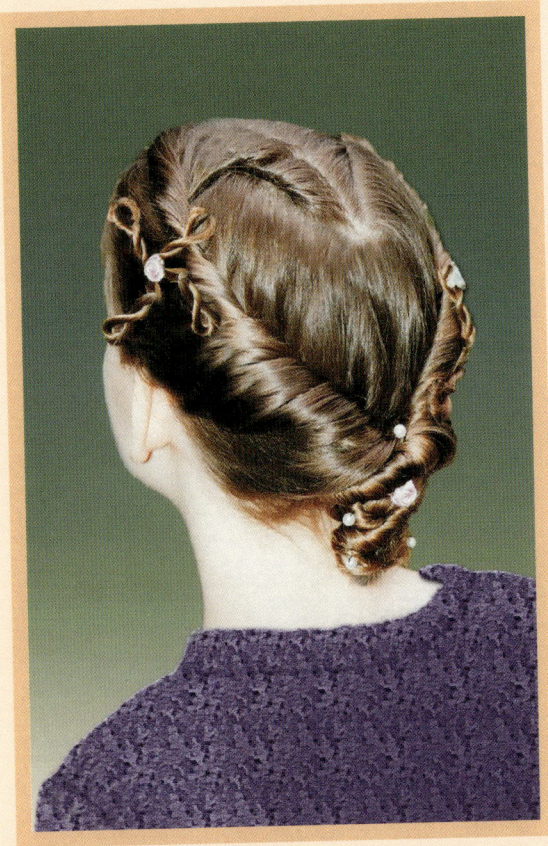
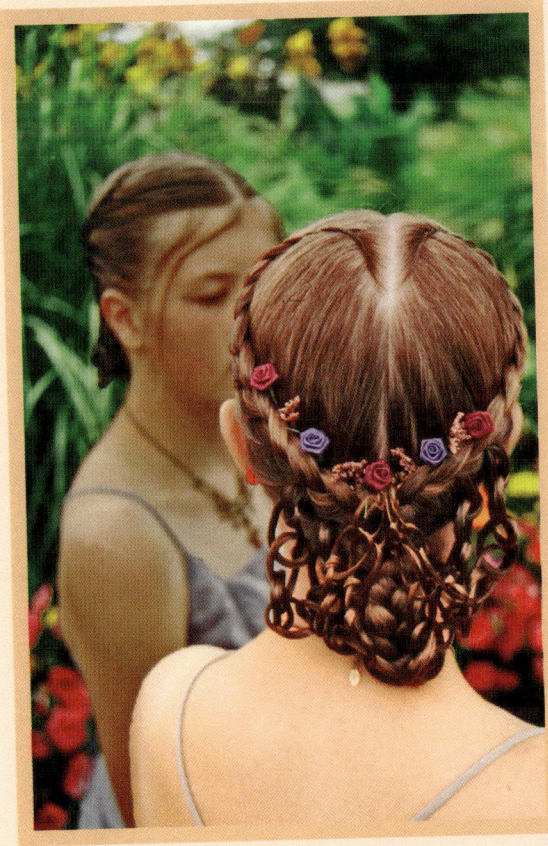
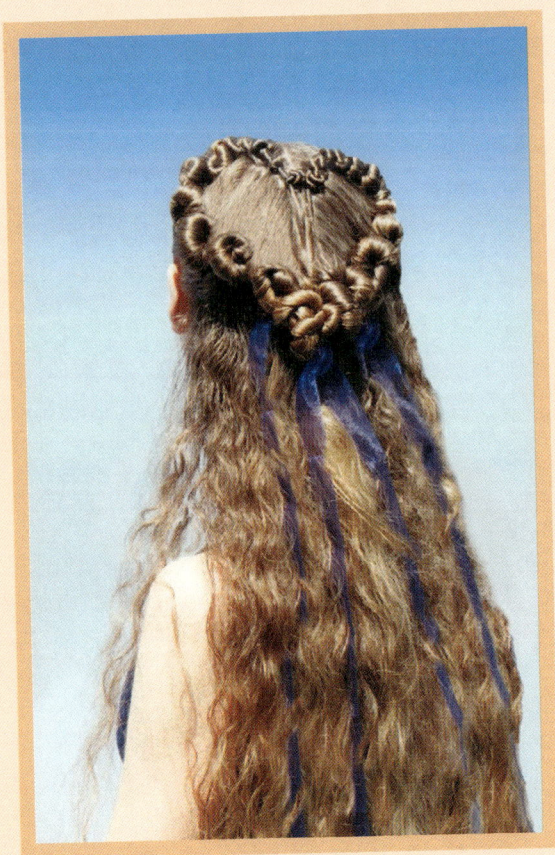

Visit my website to see more examples of Hearts

Variations within each form

Form Variations

Creativity with hairstyles is where the fun comes in

This book has many forms (even specific styles) to imitate. Don't stop there, mix and match them, use pieces of them, blend them together and add your own ideas to them. I will use this single as my only example on this page, after that you can search through the example pages in the book to see what I mean and to get more great ideas. This is one variation for one form. The single is usually done up right. To shake it up a bit, do it upside down.

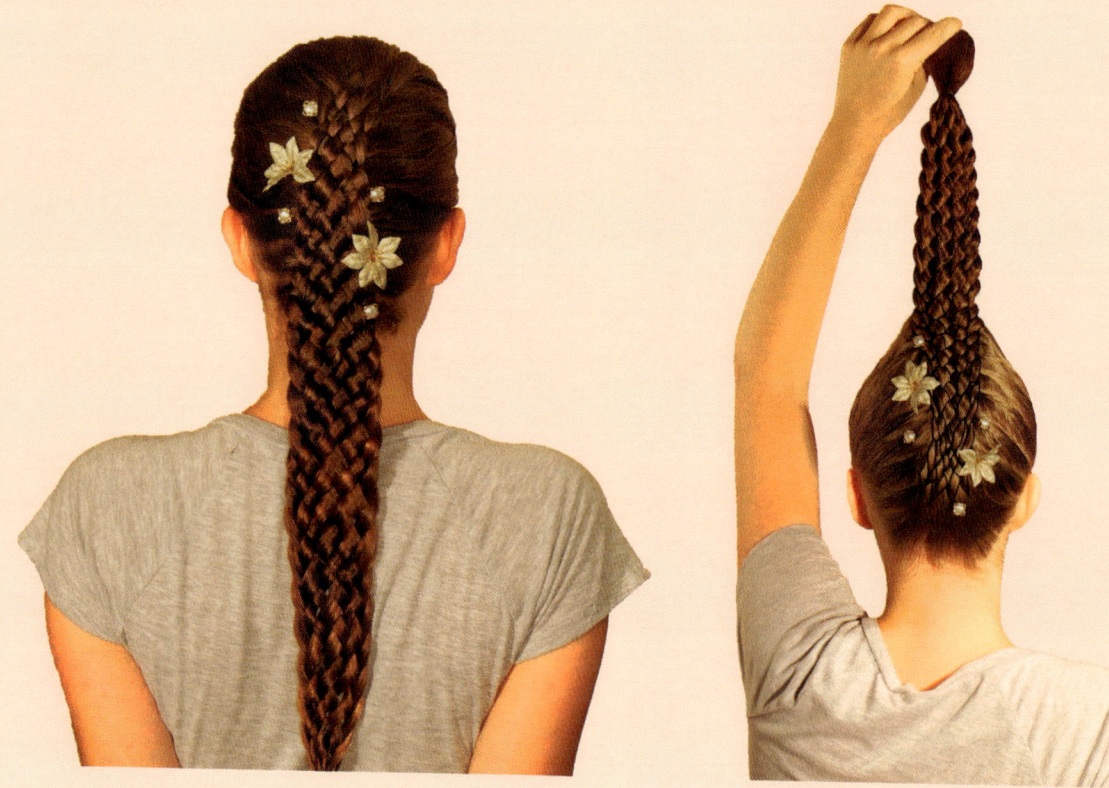

Other forms invite creativity like the double can be done in an 'X'. A crown can continuously spiral inward to create a dizzying effect. And tails provide endless opportunity for original hairstyles, even for beginners.

Form Variations

Something I have not spoken about yet is length, thickness and texture of hair.

There is a ratio of hair qualities that can create the perfect braid. This ratio changes with every hairstyle. That's why I talk my clients into subtle to major changes when they pick out a style.

Let's pretend you will only braid one persons hair for the rest of your life, and you purchased this book to do that hair in five thousand different styles. What you would find is that only some of the styles work well. The limits will come from that persons hair length, thickness and texture. (cowlicks also come into play)

Tail, headband, double and halos work well with all combinations of hair. Why? Long hair does not hinder these forms. Thick hair does not get in the way with these forms. Short hair still fits into these forms. Thin hair does not restrict these forms. As long as your willing to use an appropriate number of strands for specific hair with these forms, you will have stellar results. Like if the hair is thin, don't use nine-strands.

Fringe, teardrop, crown, and hearts work well with medium length and medium to thin hair. These forms are more delicate forms. They do not respond well to long thick hair. However long thin hair can be okay. Except the fringe because of the bun. I like to add more accents and or cascade the form if the client wants the form but has thicker hair.

Circle, single, classic and junctions love the long thick hair. Bring it on. These sturdy forms can take the most blessed of hair. Just beware the bun size on the classic in relation to hair quantity. Lots of hair = lots of bun.

Some people are under the impression that wavy or curly hair is hard to braid. That may be true for people who have not practiced on that type of hair. If I only braid thin whispy hair, than that is the type of hair that is easy for me to work with. I personally find that curly hair will hold a braid very well during sleep. The hair hugs itself in place for days.

Chapter Three

Tools useful for executing accents.

- Tail Comb
- Water Spray Bottle
- Hair Product
- Tiny Rubber Bands
- Bobby Pins
- Latch Hook
- Beads
- Ribbon
- Curling Iron
- Flat Iron

Chapter Three ~ Accents

An accent is a piece of hair left out during the braiding process, to decorate the form.

Accent hair can come from:
* Underneath the braid
* The braid itself
* A random spot
* The cascade
* Fake hair

From under the braid!

From the cascade!

From a braid strand!

Random spots on the head!

Add in fake hair!

If it can be done on short hair it can be done on long hair
but
not necessarily the other way around.

SHORT and LONG HAIR
Beads
Fluff
Loose
Mini
Pretzel
Ribbon

LONG HAIR ONLY
Crochet
Headdress
Leafing
Push-ups

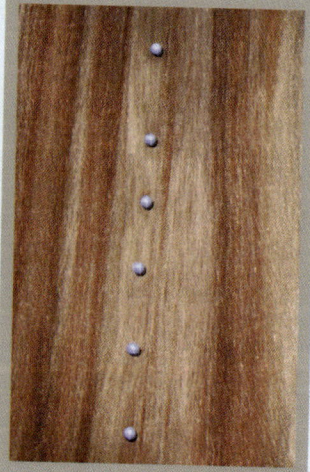
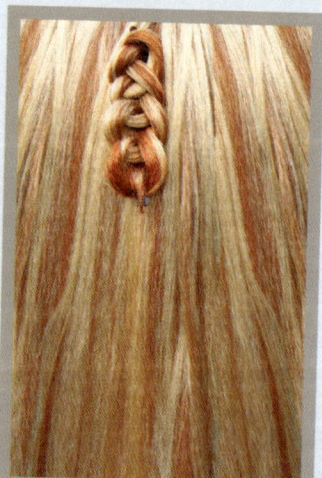

If you would know the road ahead, ask someone who has traveled it.
– Saying (Chinese)

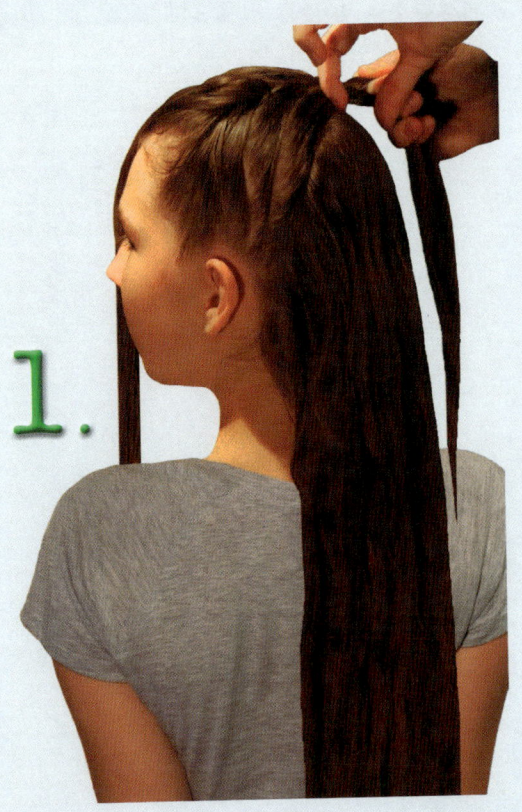

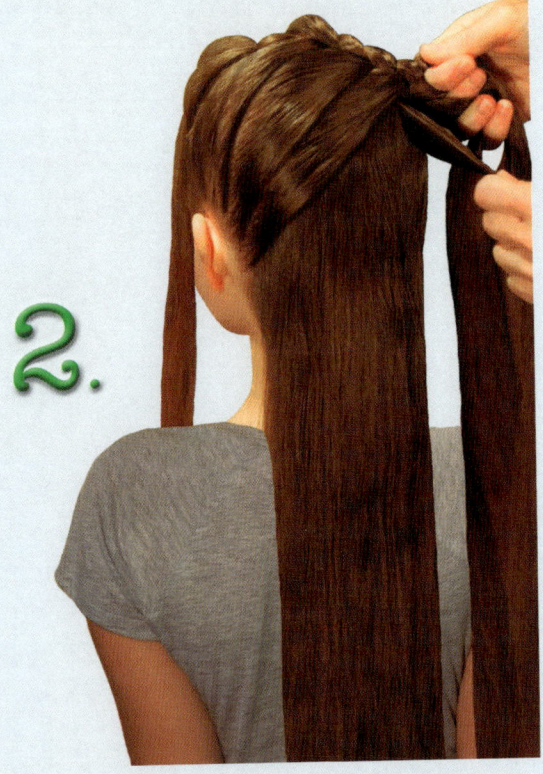

The photographs show an accent being taken from underneath the braid. This makes its origins undetectable. They can also come from half of a strand of the braid itself or the cascade or a random spot on the person's head. Any hair will do. Even fake hair added to the style as an accent will do. The fake hair can be natural or neon.

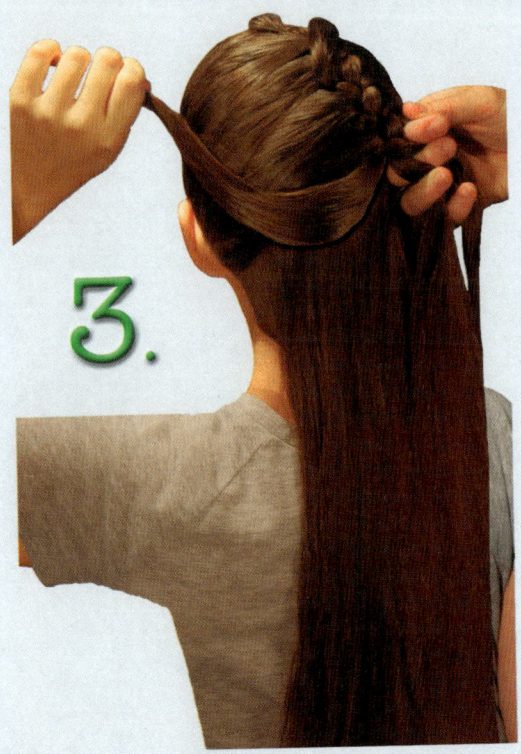

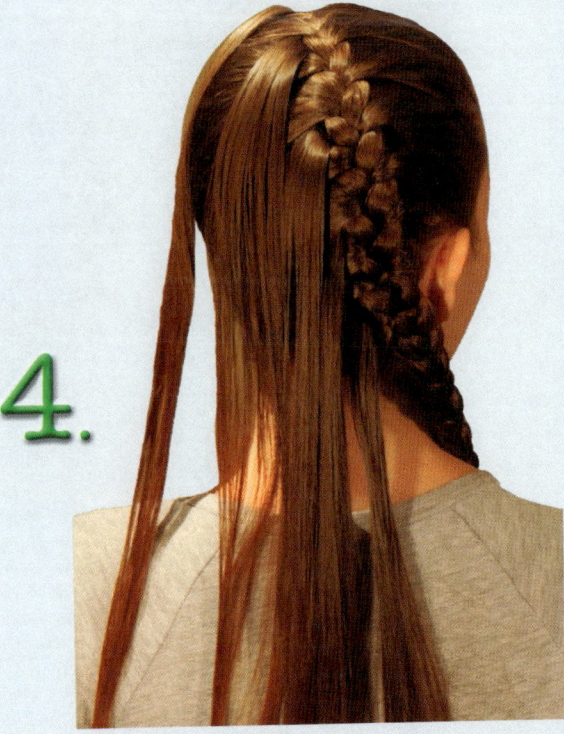

Accents

Beads

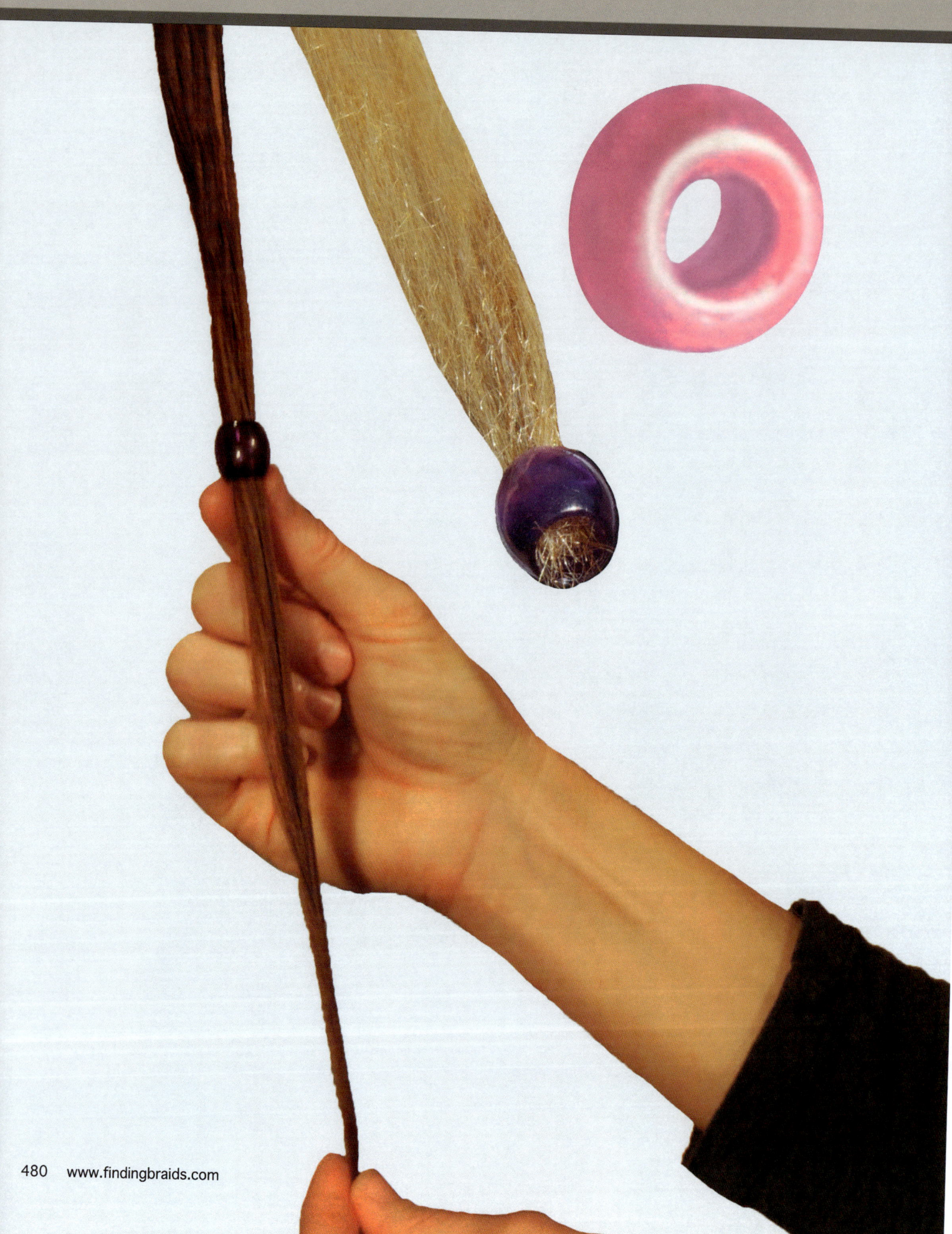

Examples with Beads

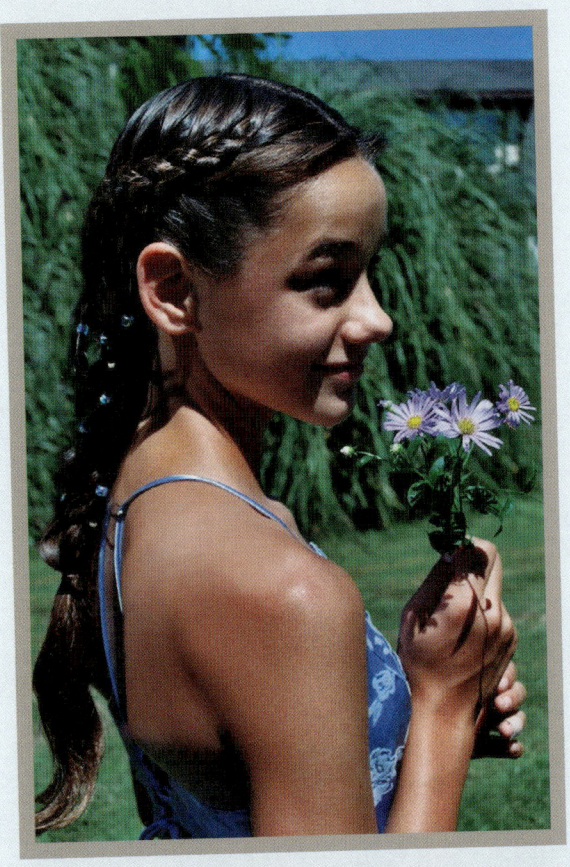
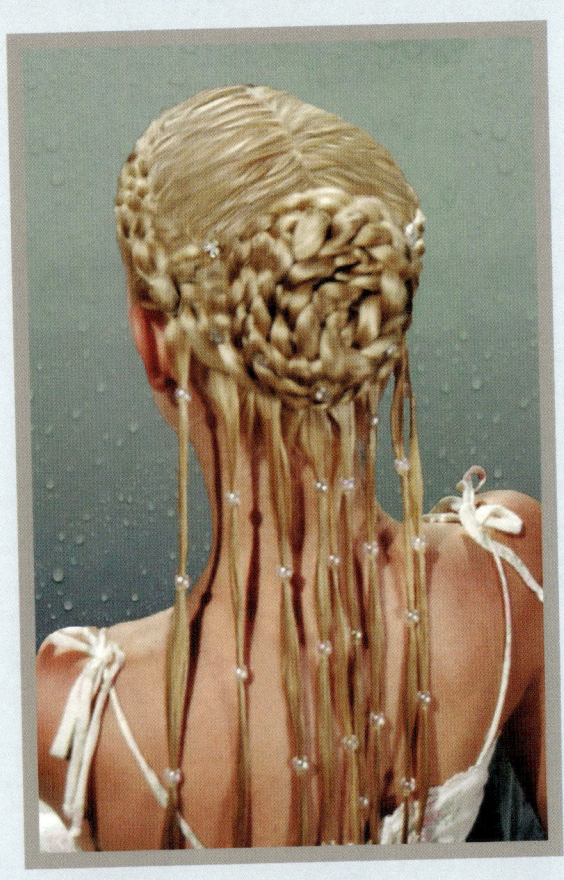
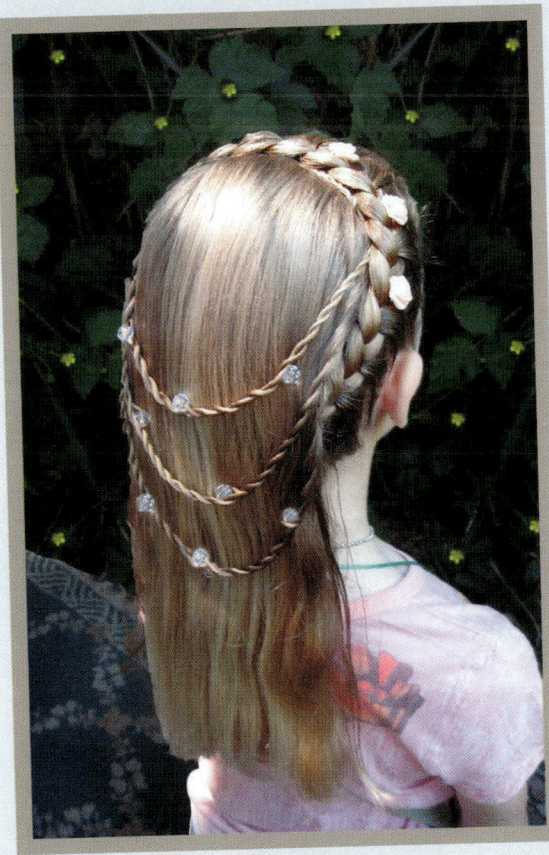
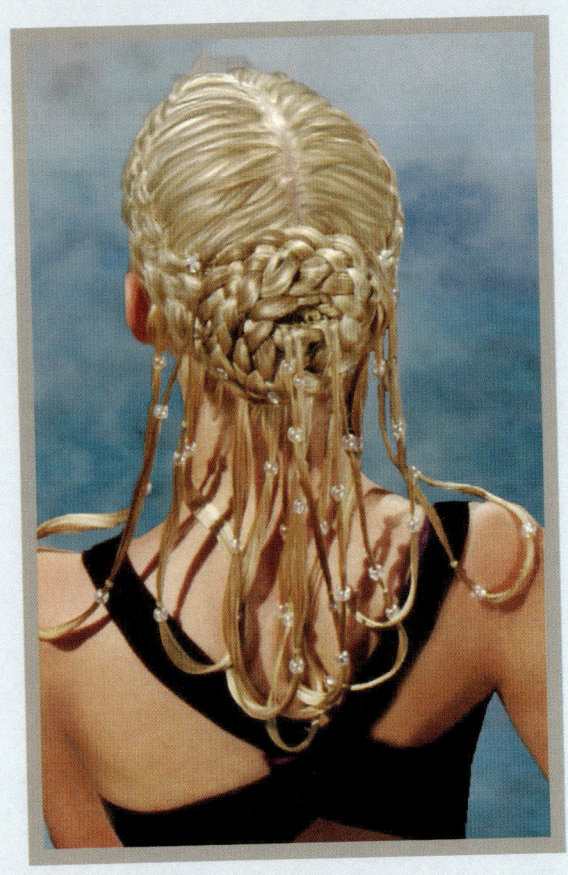

Visit my website to see more examples of Beads

Accents

Finger Crochet

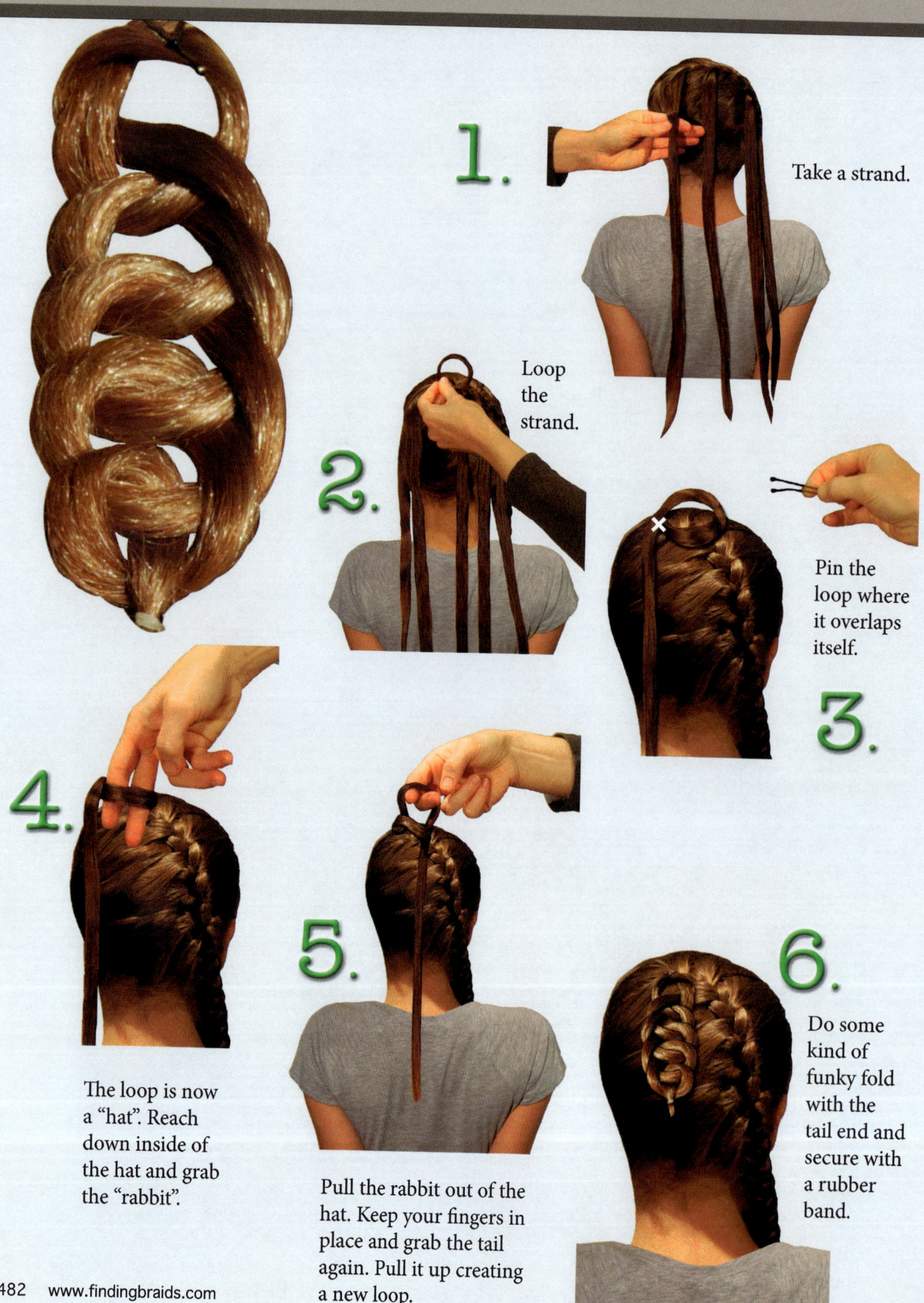

1. Take a strand.
2. Loop the strand.
3. Pin the loop where it overlaps itself.
4. The loop is now a "hat". Reach down inside of the hat and grab the "rabbit".
5. Pull the rabbit out of the hat. Keep your fingers in place and grab the tail again. Pull it up creating a new loop.
6. Do some kind of funky fold with the tail end and secure with a rubber band.

Examples with Finger Crochet

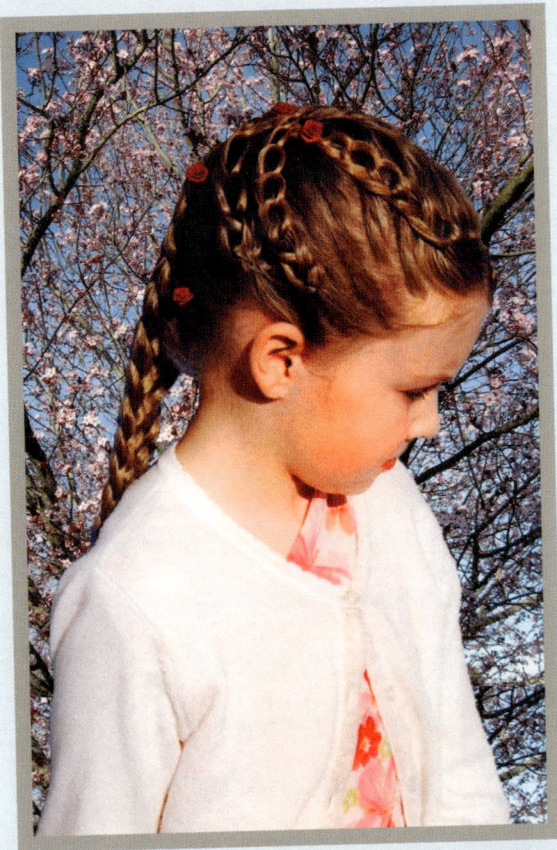
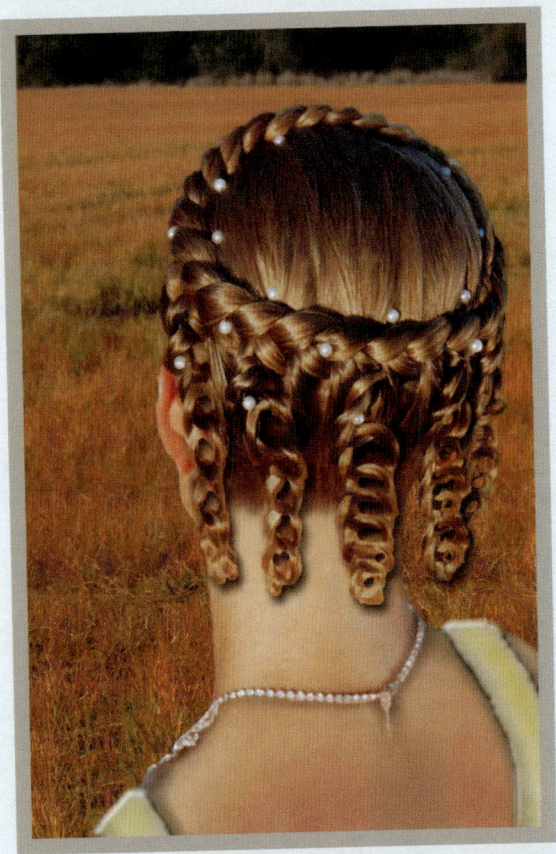
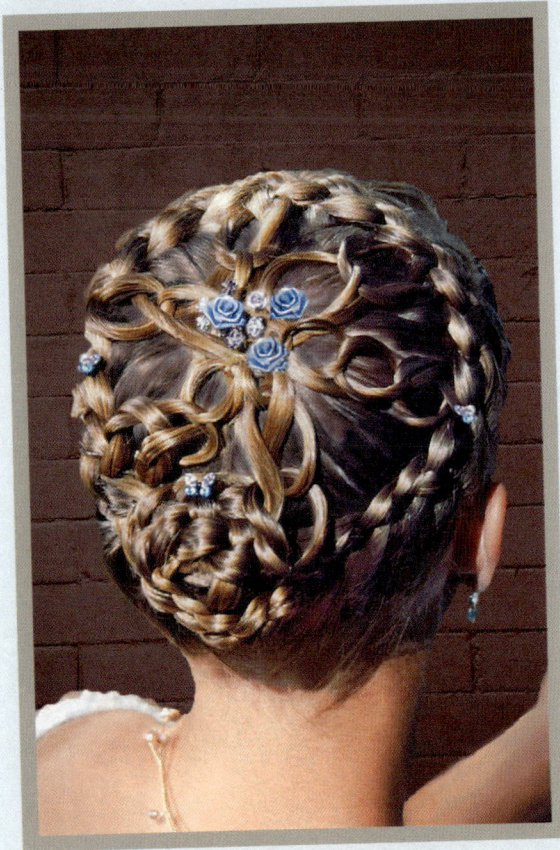
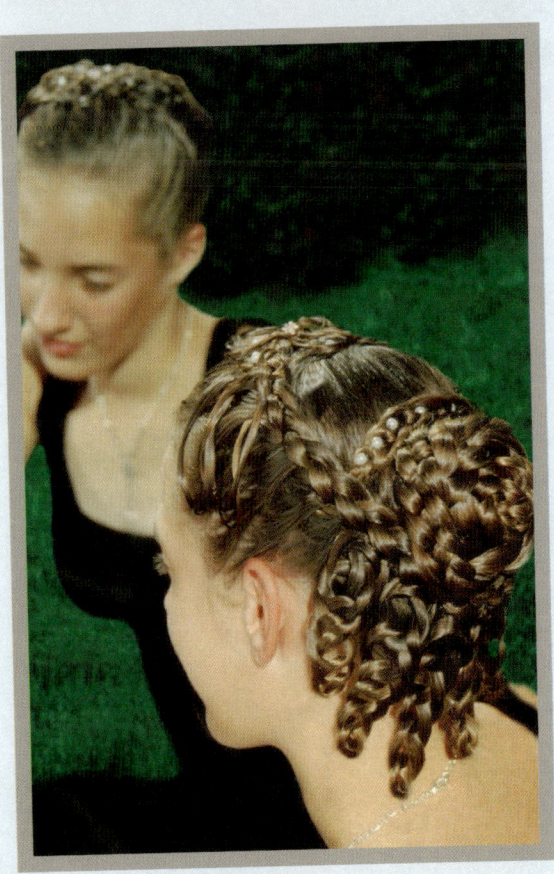

Visit my website to see more examples of Finger Crochet

Fluff

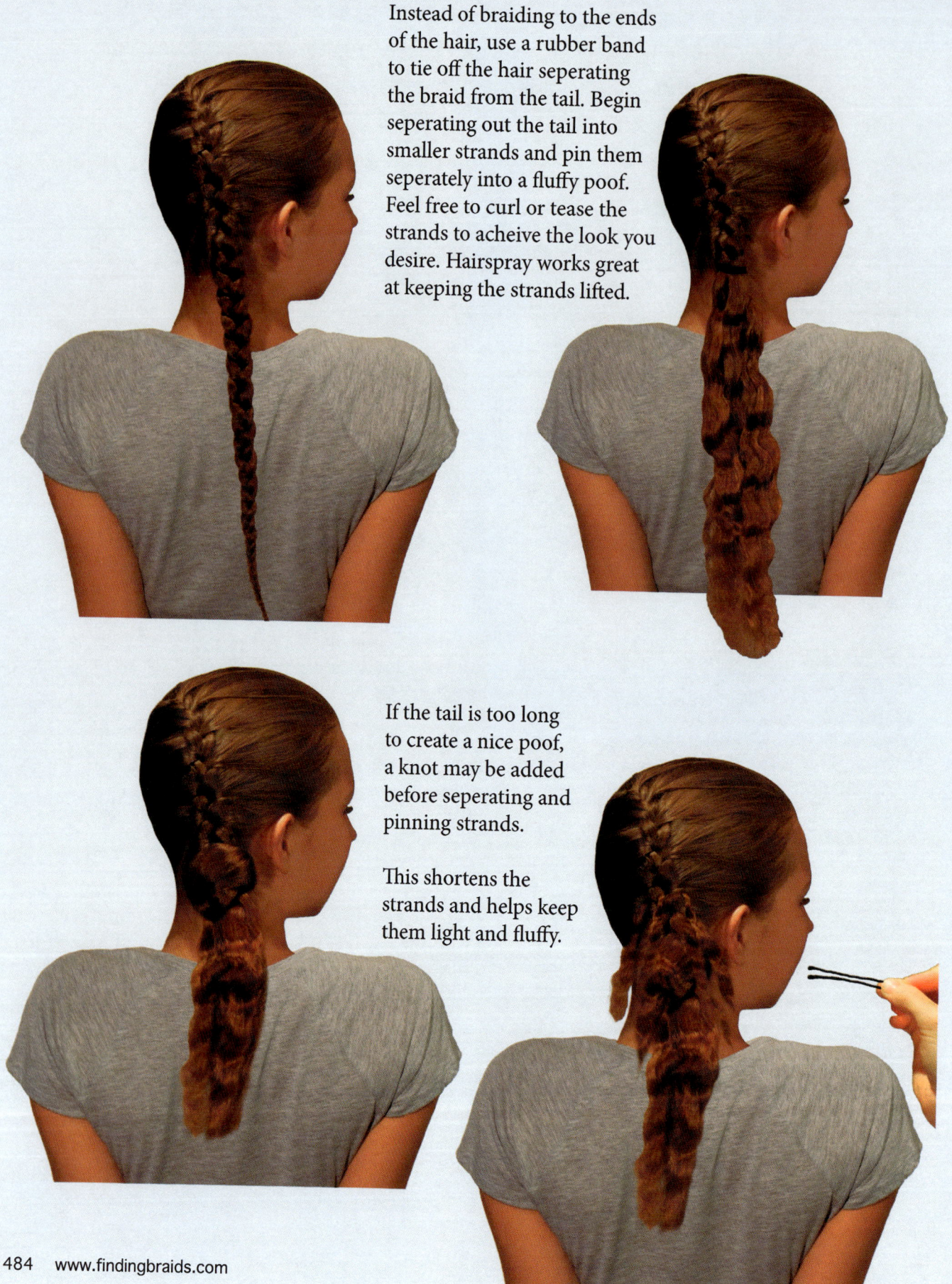

Instead of braiding to the ends of the hair, use a rubber band to tie off the hair seperating the braid from the tail. Begin seperating out the tail into smaller strands and pin them seperately into a fluffy poof. Feel free to curl or tease the strands to acheive the look you desire. Hairspray works great at keeping the strands lifted.

If the tail is too long to create a nice poof, a knot may be added before seperating and pinning strands.

This shortens the strands and helps keep them light and fluffy.

Examples with Fluff

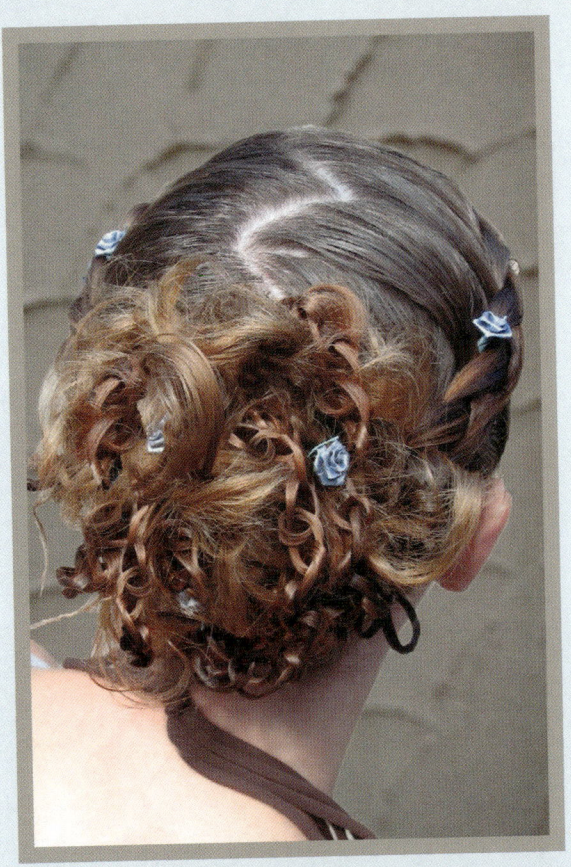
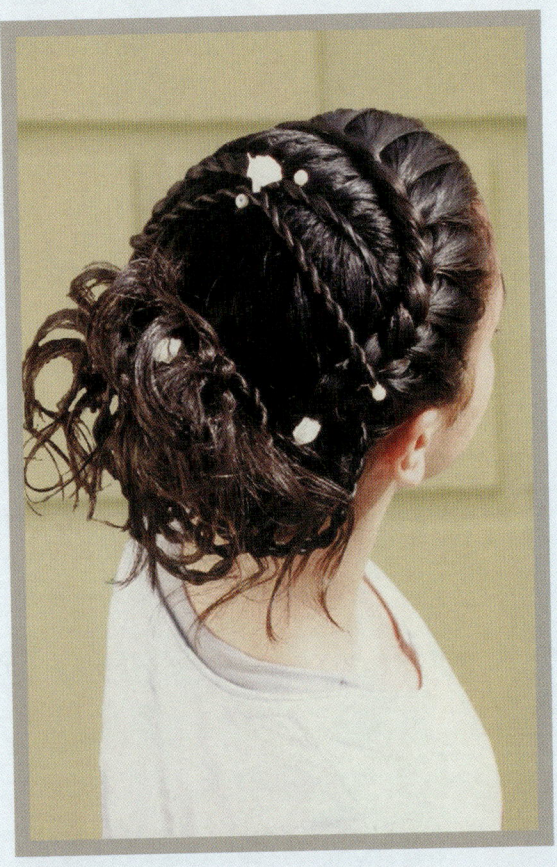
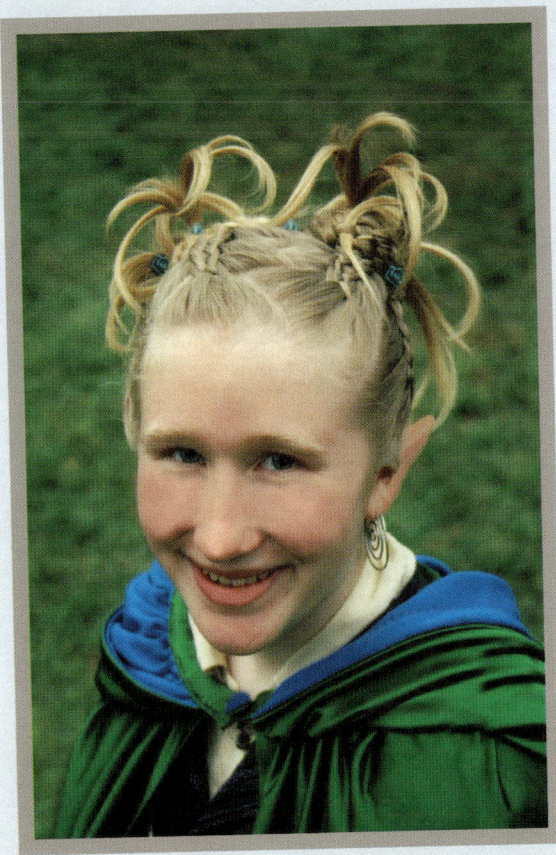
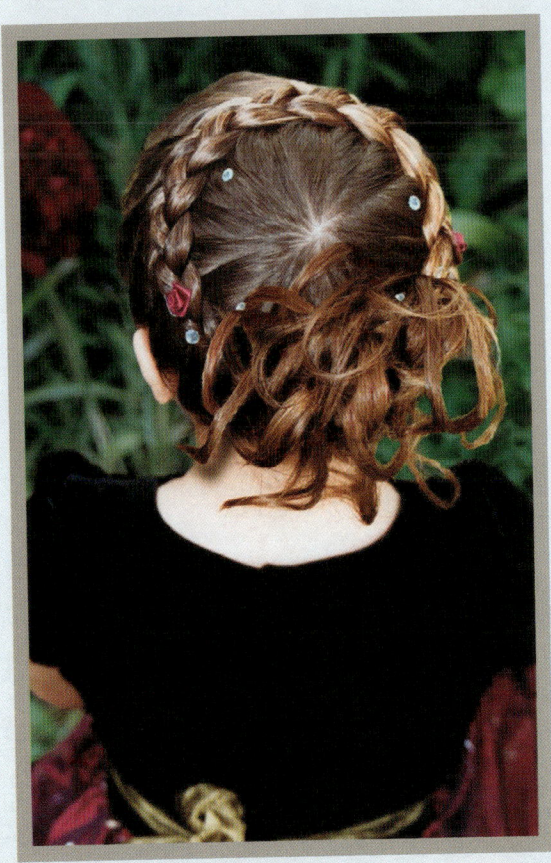

Visit my website to see more examples of Fluff

Headdress

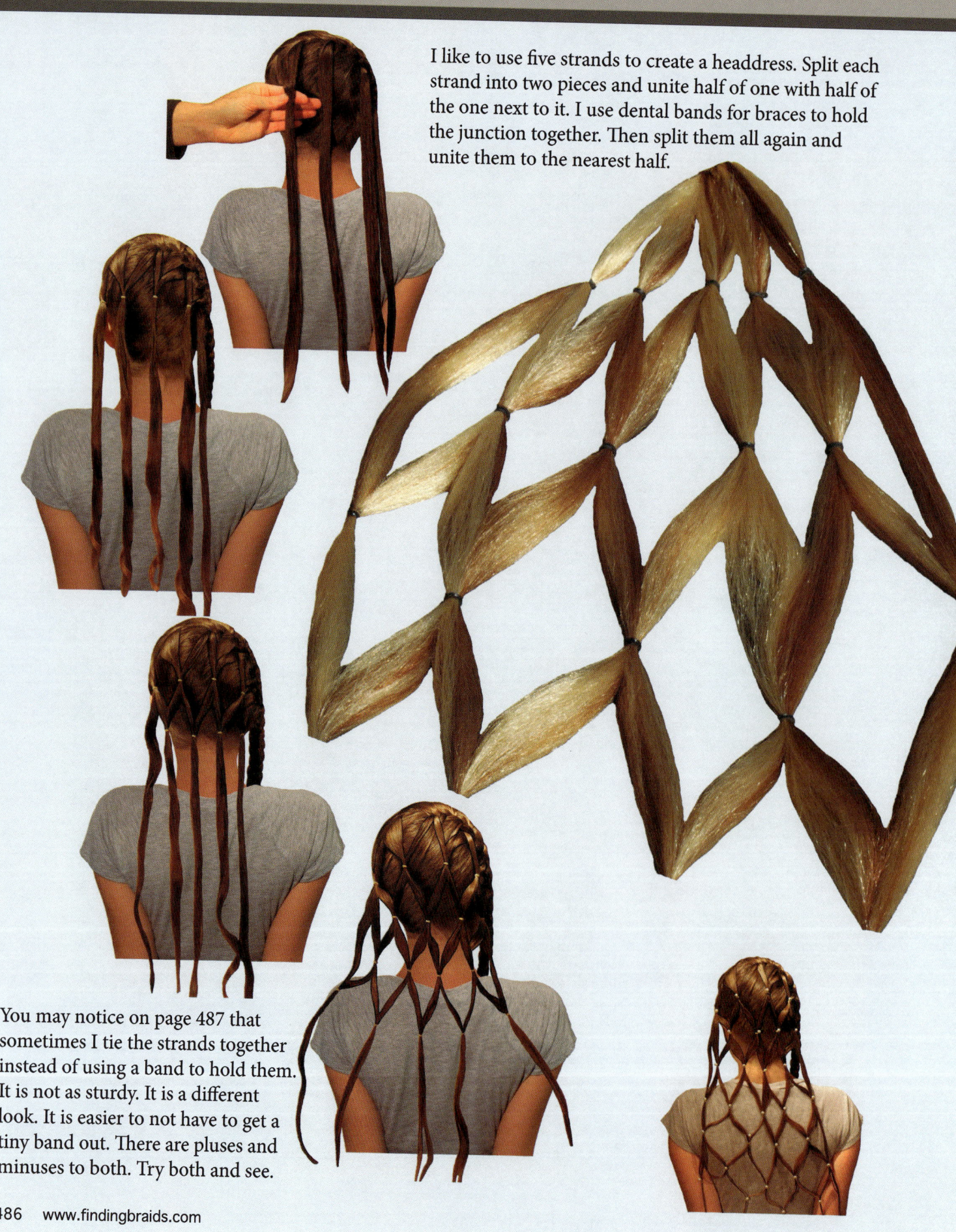

I like to use five strands to create a headdress. Split each strand into two pieces and unite half of one with half of the one next to it. I use dental bands for braces to hold the junction together. Then split them all again and unite them to the nearest half.

You may notice on page 487 that sometimes I tie the strands together instead of using a band to hold them. It is not as sturdy. It is a different look. It is easier to not have to get a tiny band out. There are pluses and minuses to both. Try both and see.

Examples with Headdress

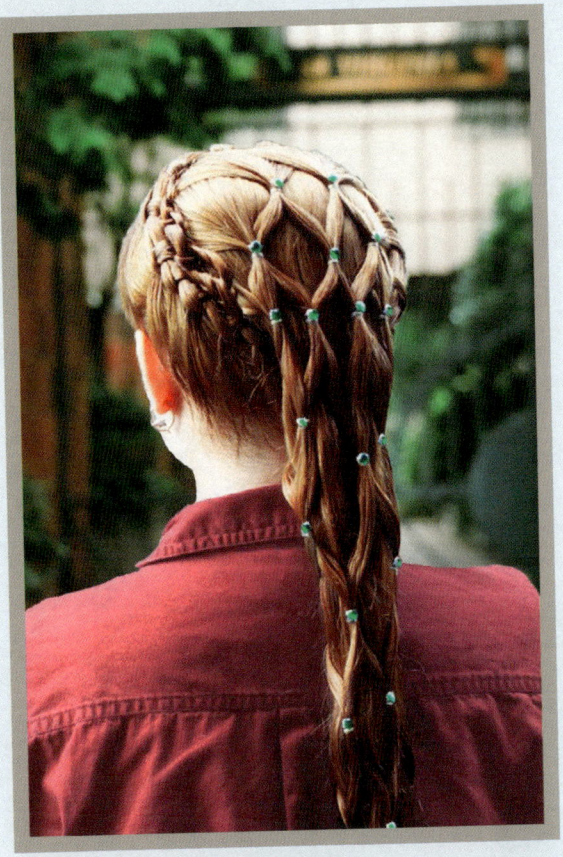
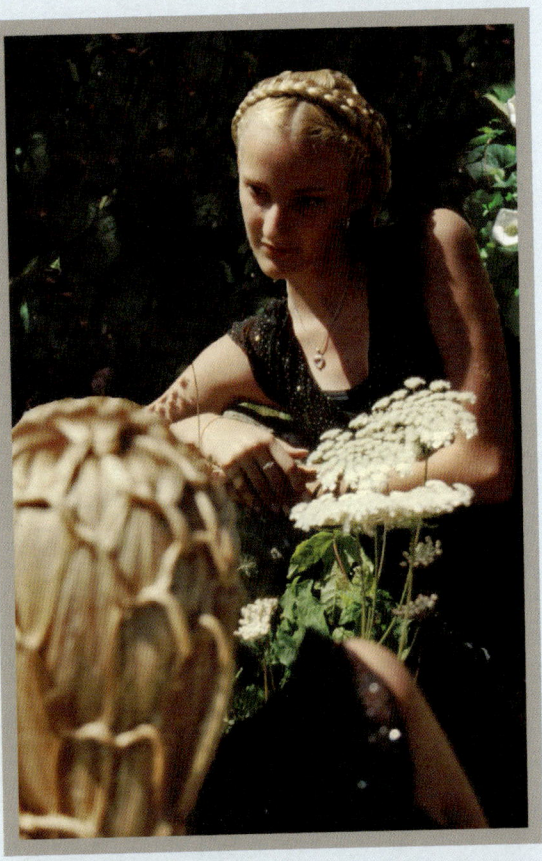
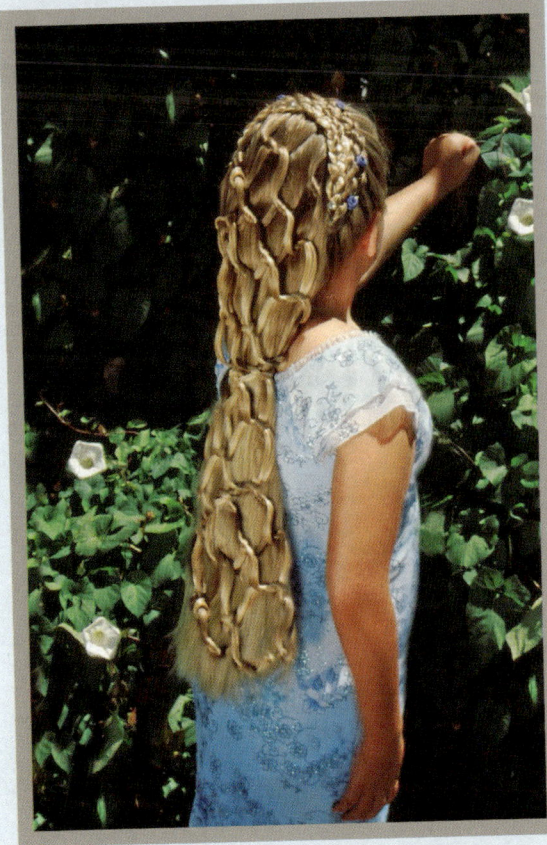
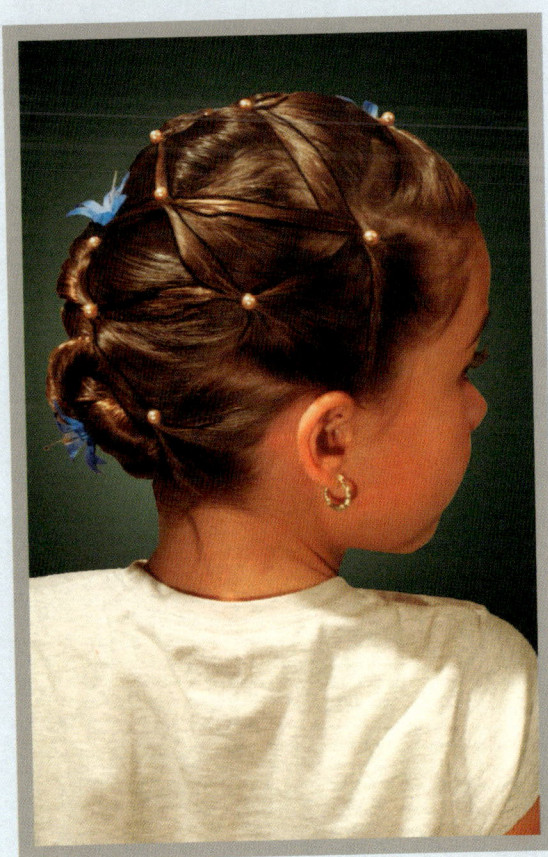

Visit my website to see more examples of the Headdress

Leafing

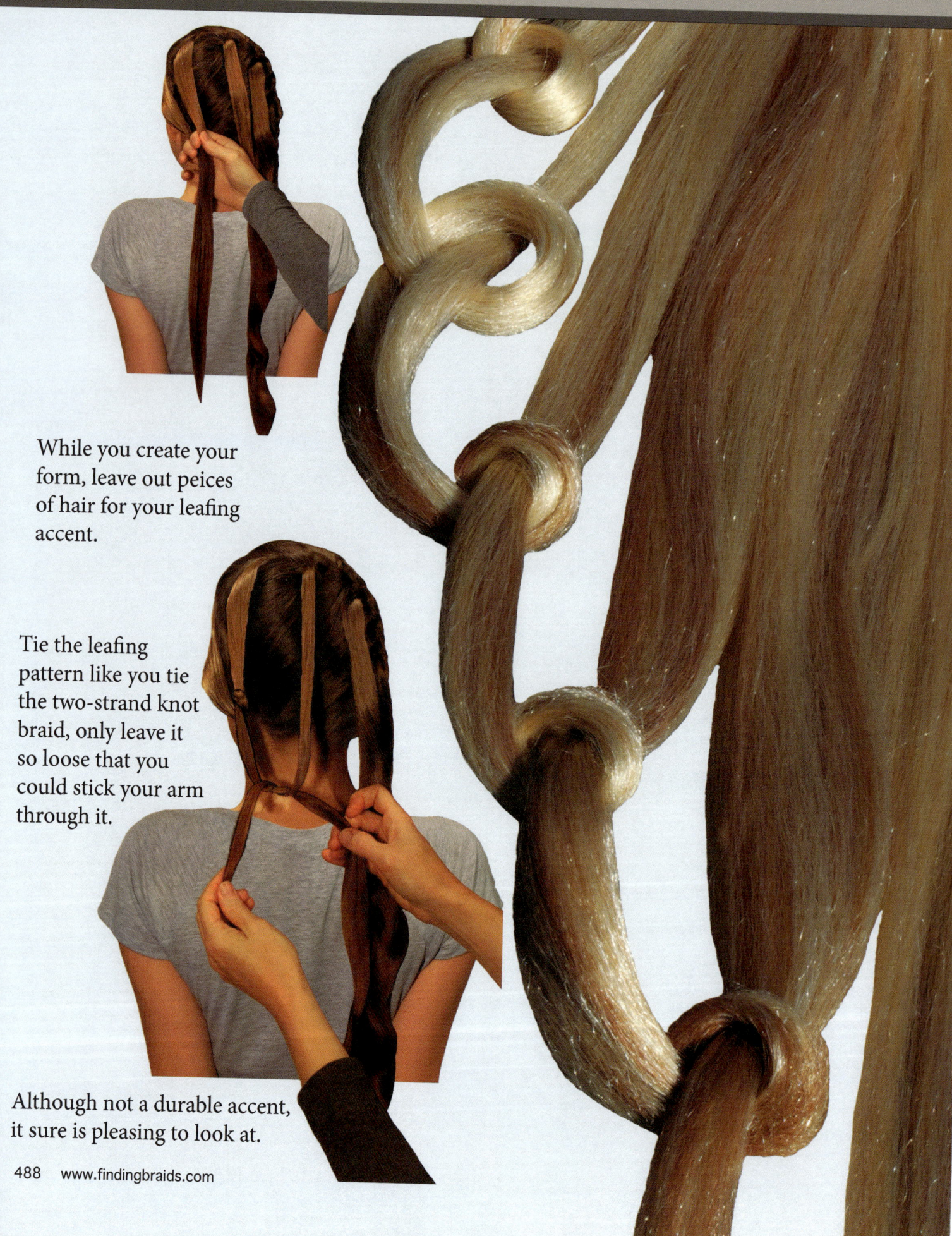

While you create your form, leave out peices of hair for your leafing accent.

Tie the leafing pattern like you tie the two-strand knot braid, only leave it so loose that you could stick your arm through it.

Although not a durable accent, it sure is pleasing to look at.

www.findingbraids.com

Examples with Leafing

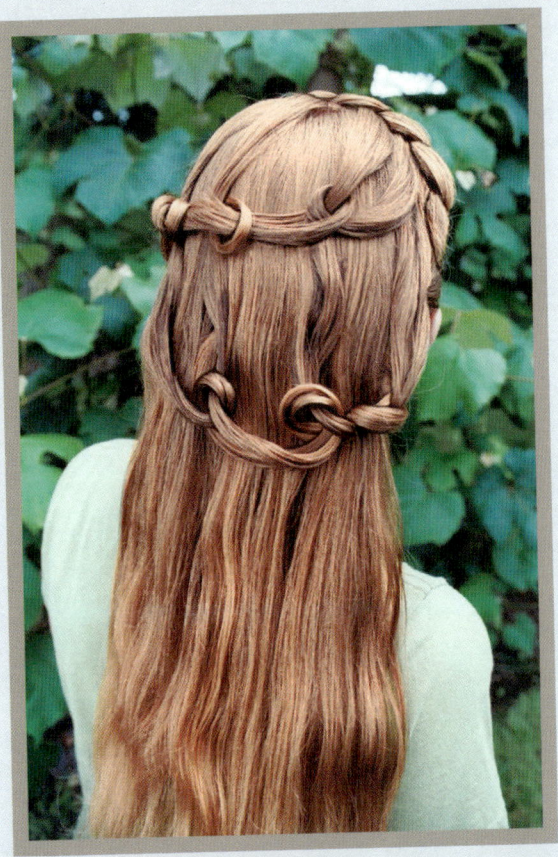
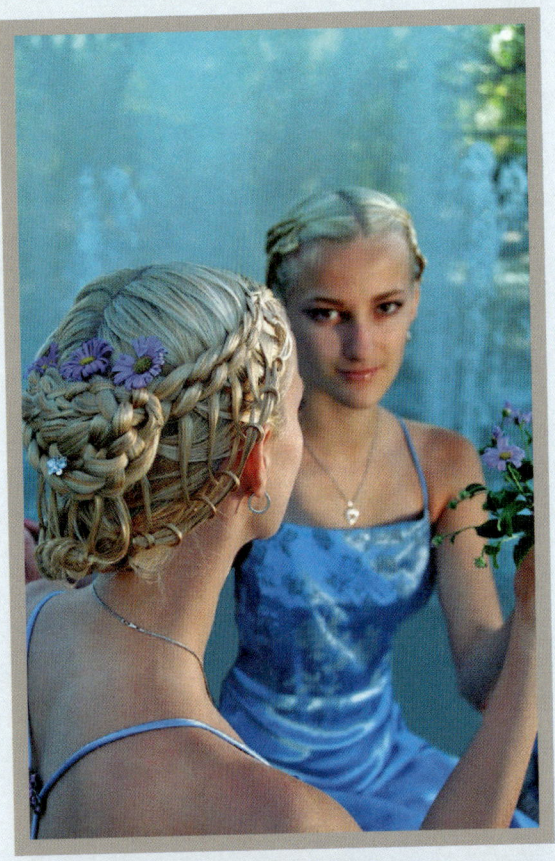
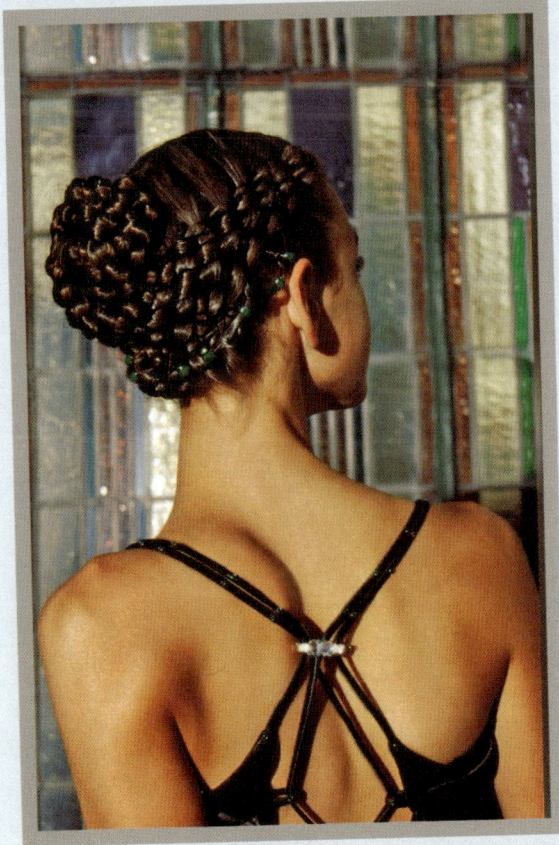
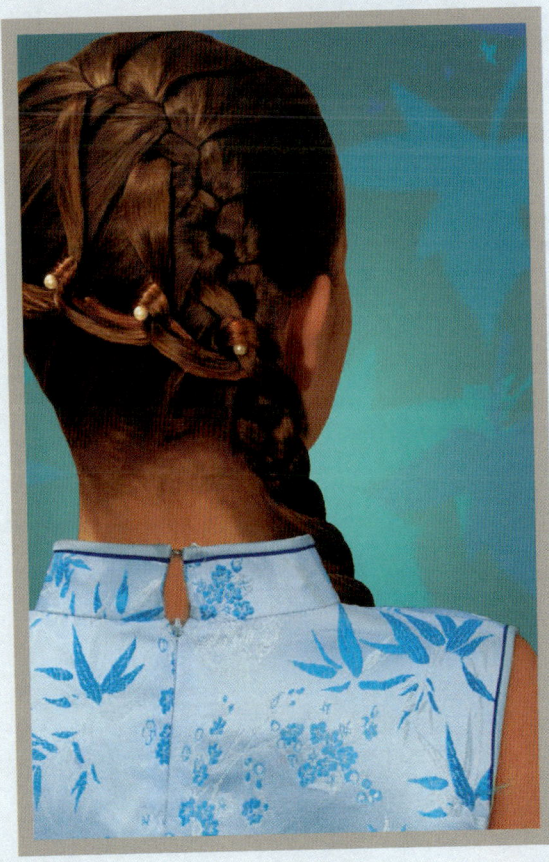

Visit my website to see more examples of Leafing

Loose strands of hair

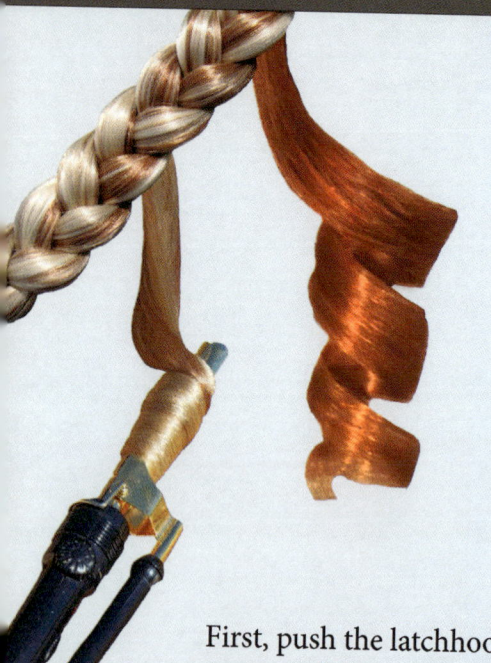

Latchhooks are an essential tool for your creations with loose hair. Add some fake hair, a curling iron and you have an arsenal of tools to make big time magic.

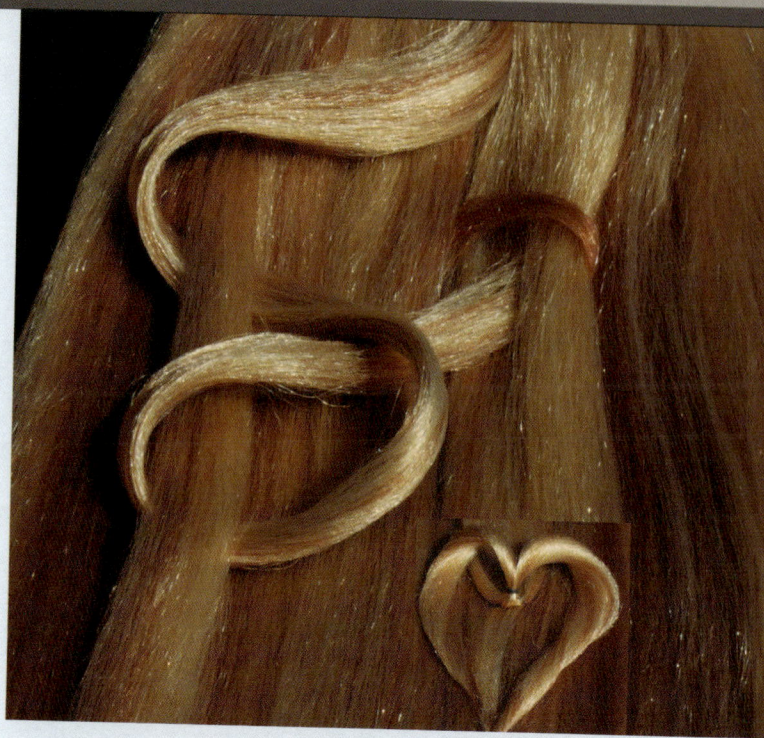

First, push the latchhook through some restrained hair and grab some loose hair. Second, pull the loose hair as much as you need to get the look your going for. Third, continue until the style is finished.

One link at the back of the book shows how to do a celtic knot. The language is spanish, but the hand motions are universal.

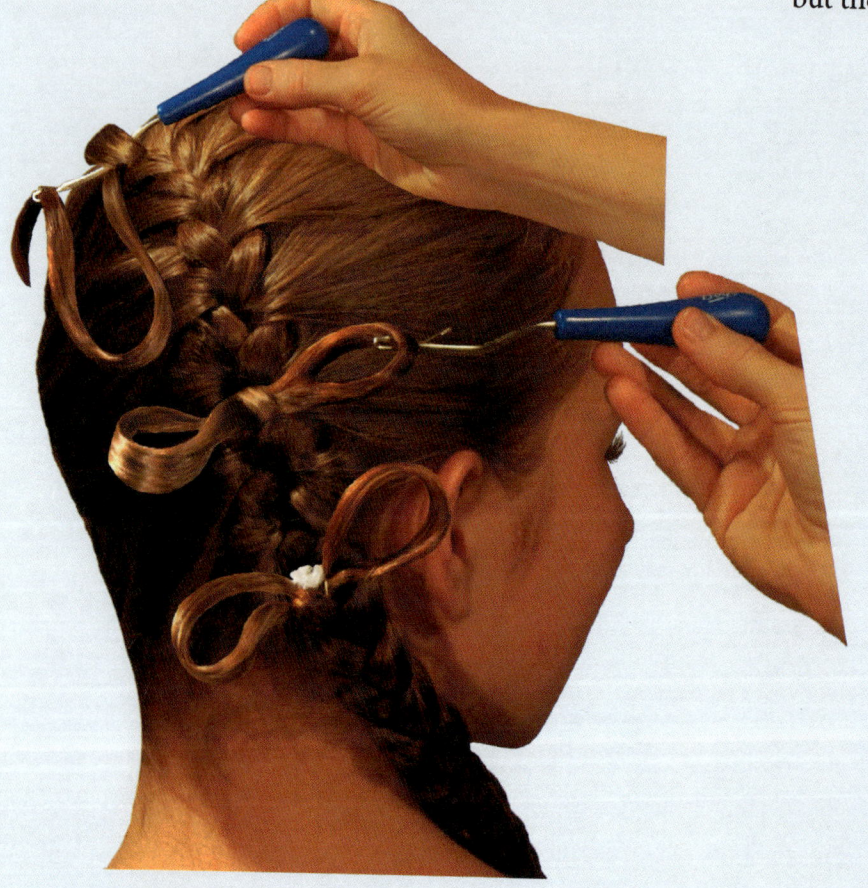

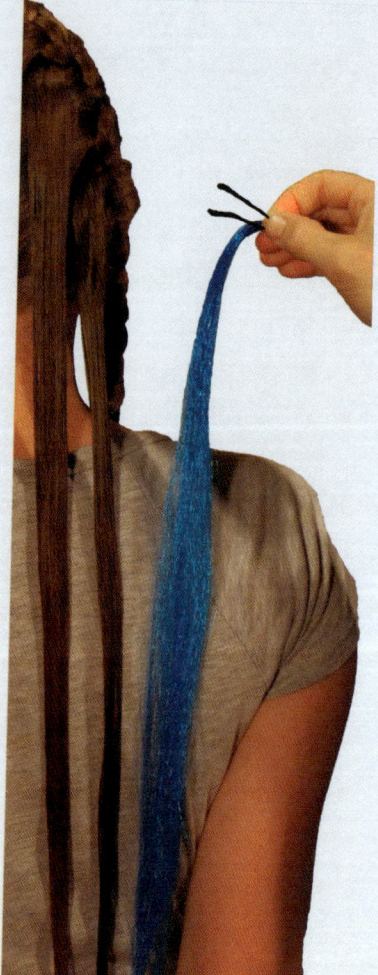

www.findingbraids.com

Examples with Loose strands of hair

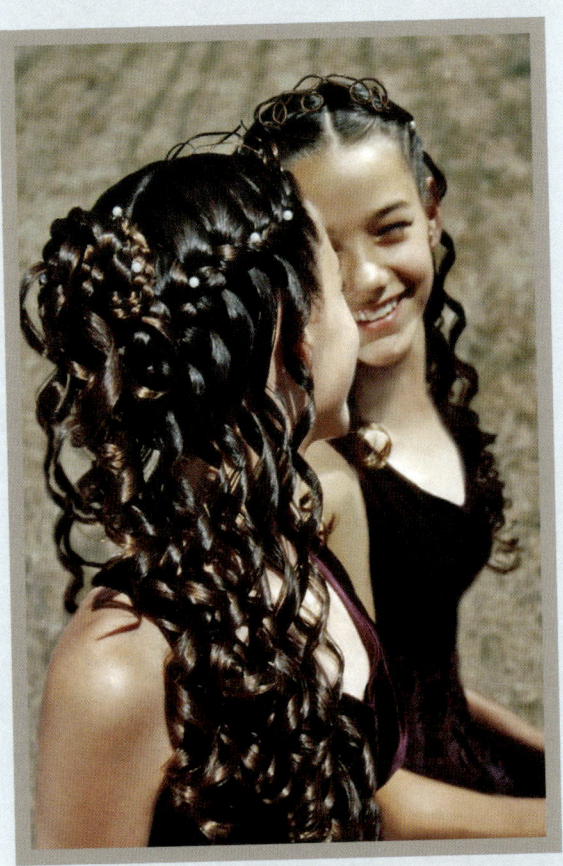
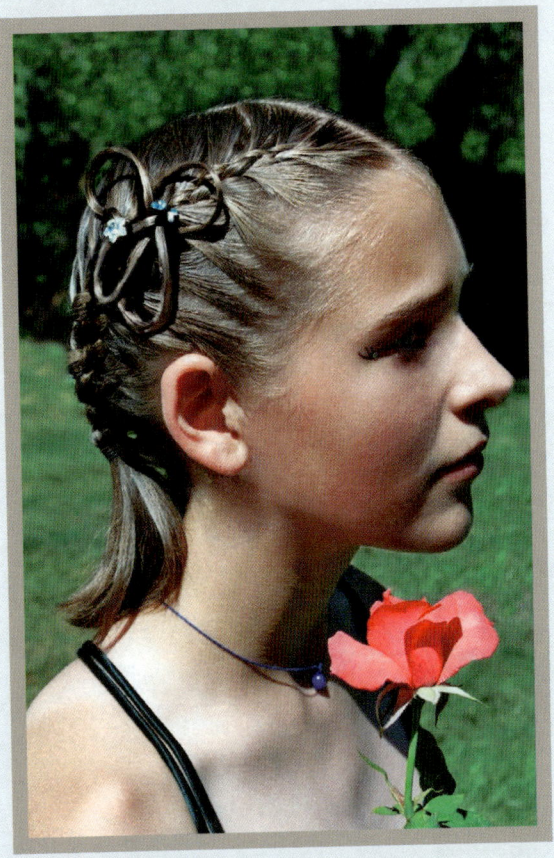
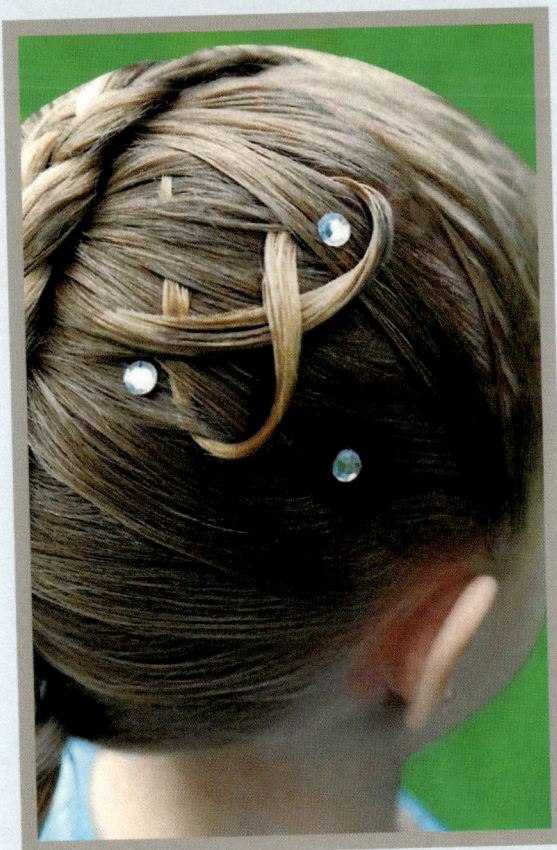
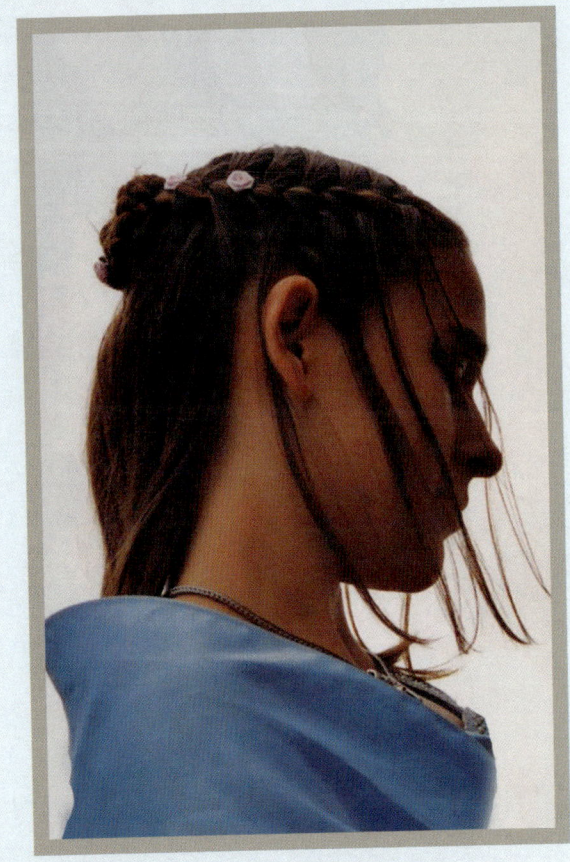

Visit my website to see more examples of Loose strands of hair Accents

Mini braids

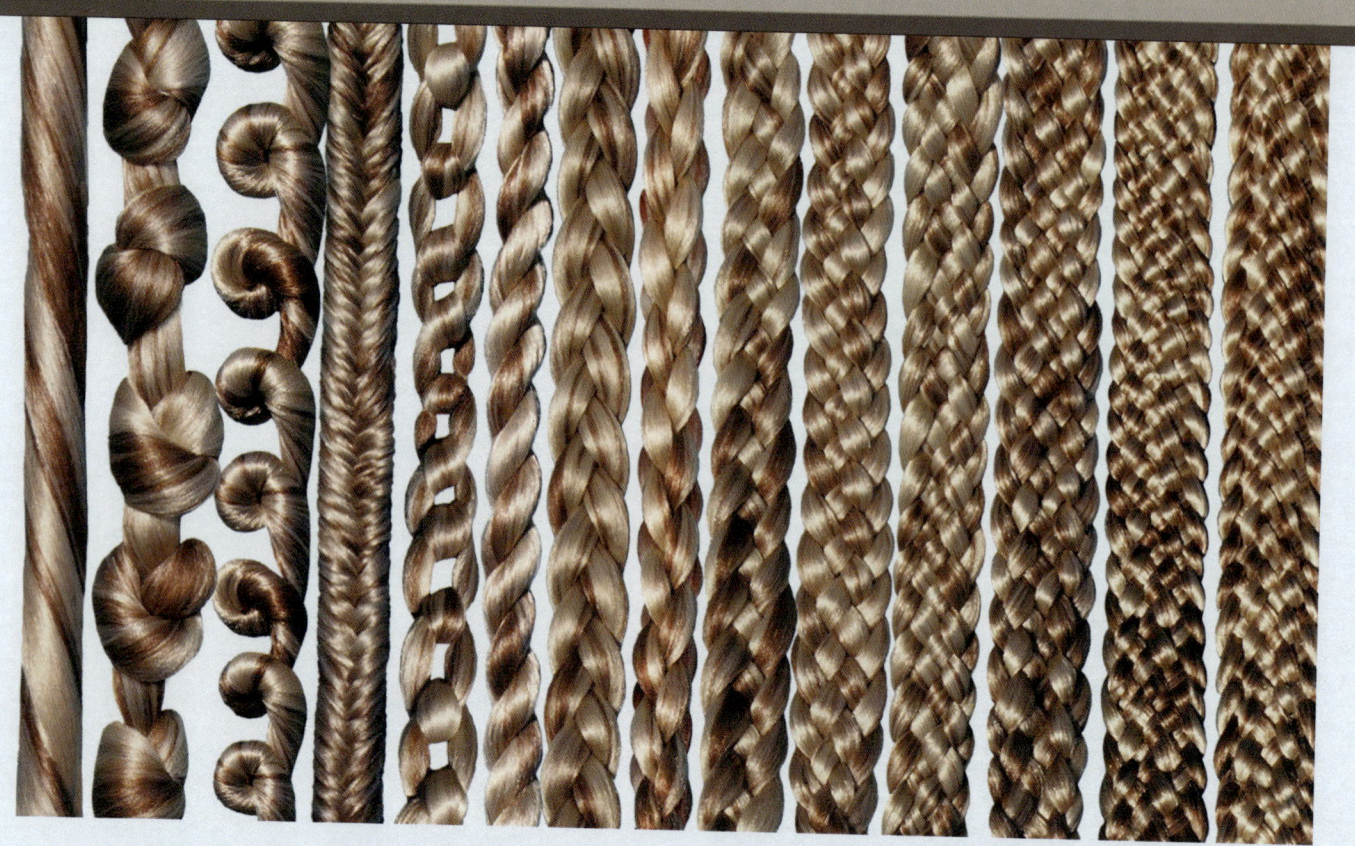

See chapter one to create mini versions of any braid. Use a three-strand braid to create any form, then use mini three-strand braids to accent the form. Or mix and match the form braid with a different number of mini braid. My son likes to use a variety of mini braids to accent his forms. Creativity is the only way to find what pleases you or the person you are braiding.

Take photos of what you do even if you think it looks terrible. There is a photo in this book that I thought was ridiculous until I saw the same thing a few years later splashed all over the internet, so I found my photo and it is proving to be useful after all. During the making of this book I did something that I would never do otherwise. I used a mini nine-strand braid as an accent. I had no idea what I was going to do with it; I was winging it and being creative. It worked. I love the photo. When you dare to try something new, nice surprises will follow.

The mini accent braids can be done tight or super crazy loose. Remember that hairspray or gel help when getting funky with the styling. Do not let this book limit your braiding ideas. Search the world over for new input and incorporate them into your hairstyling palette.

Examples with Mini braids

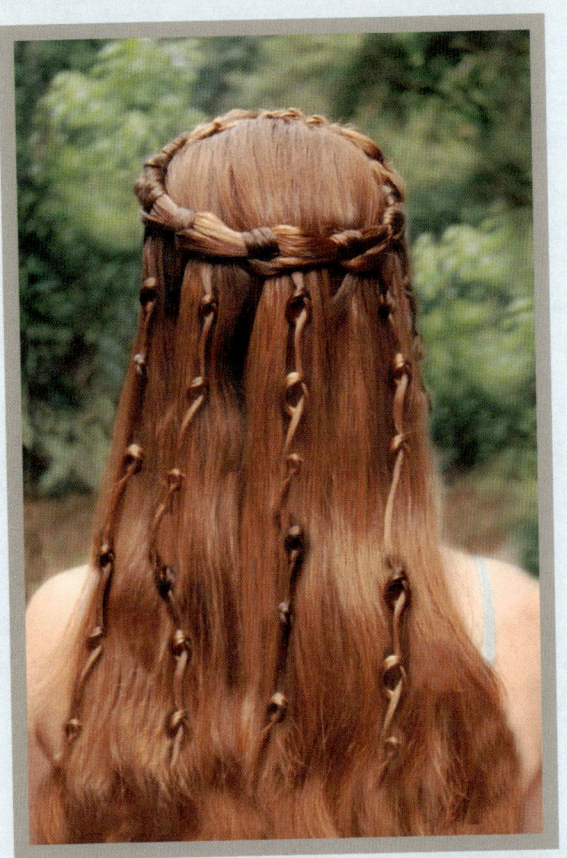
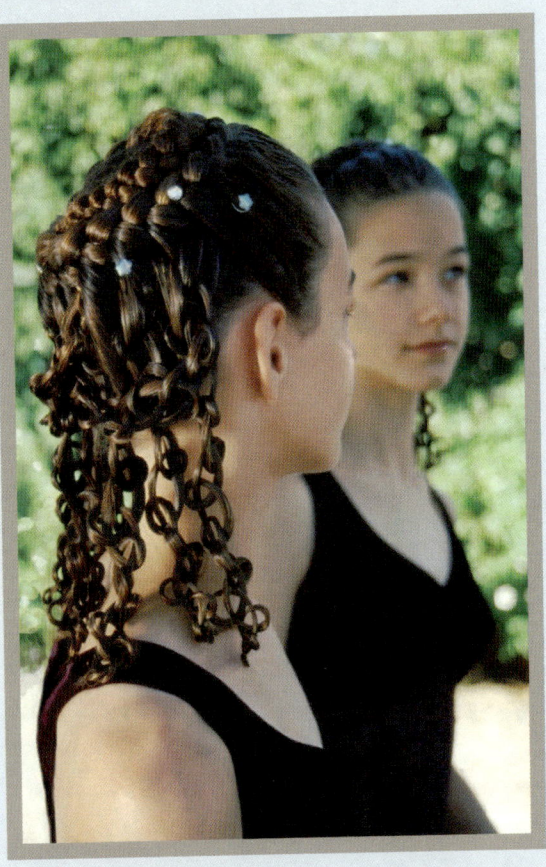
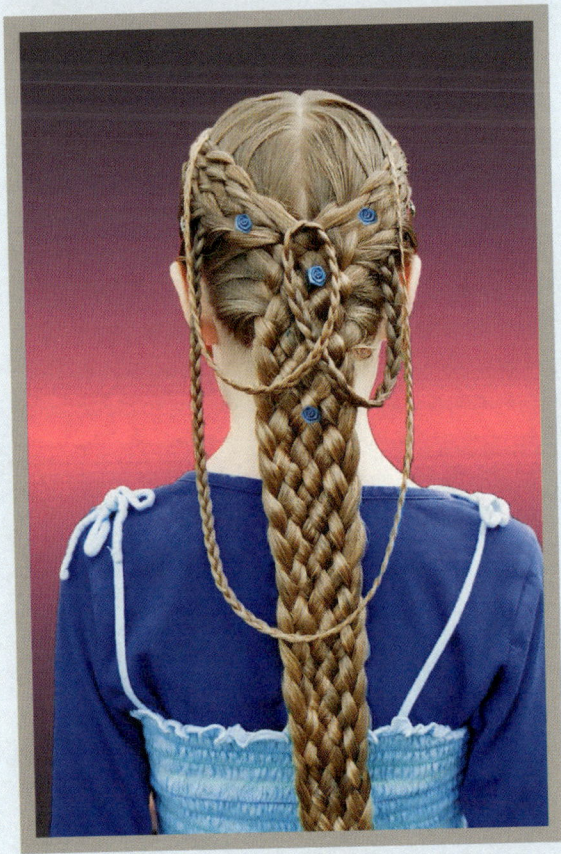
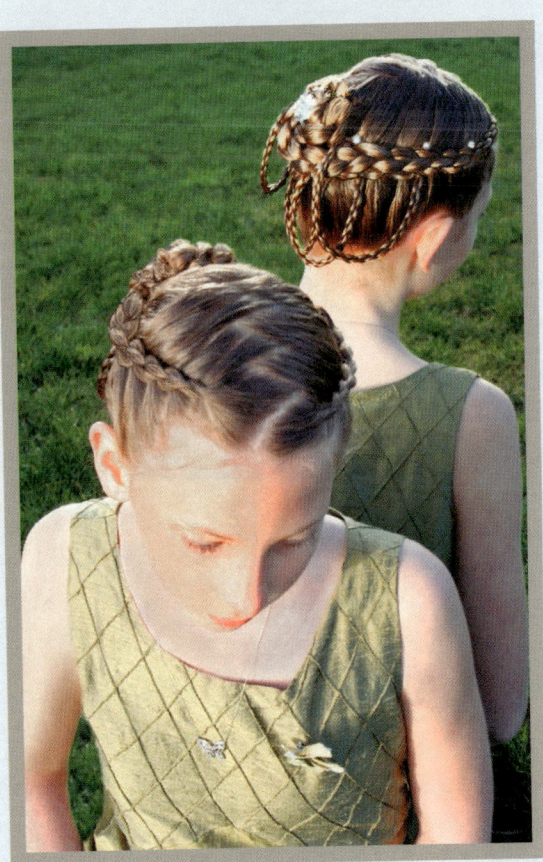

Visit my website to see more examples of Mini braids

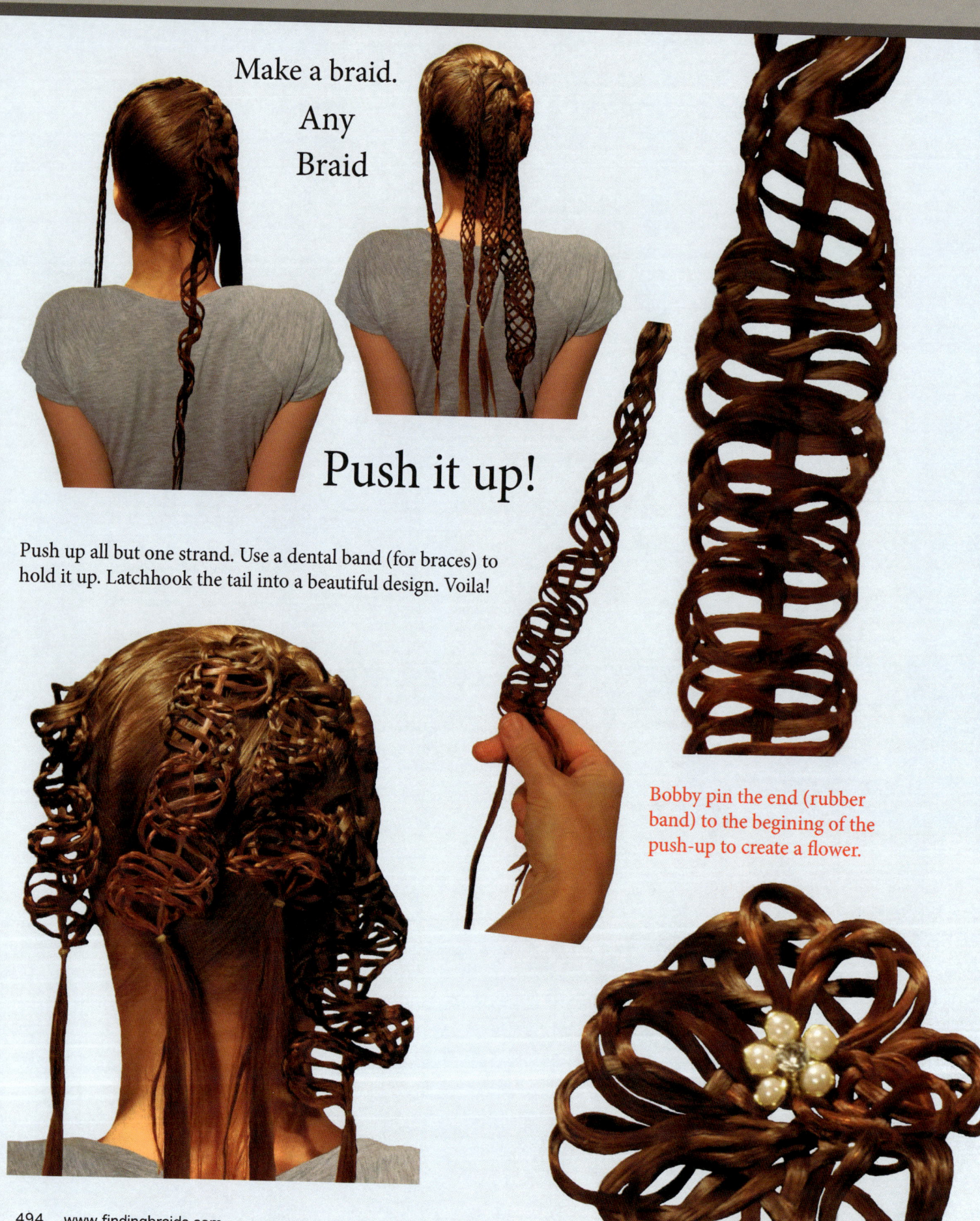

Examples with Push-ups

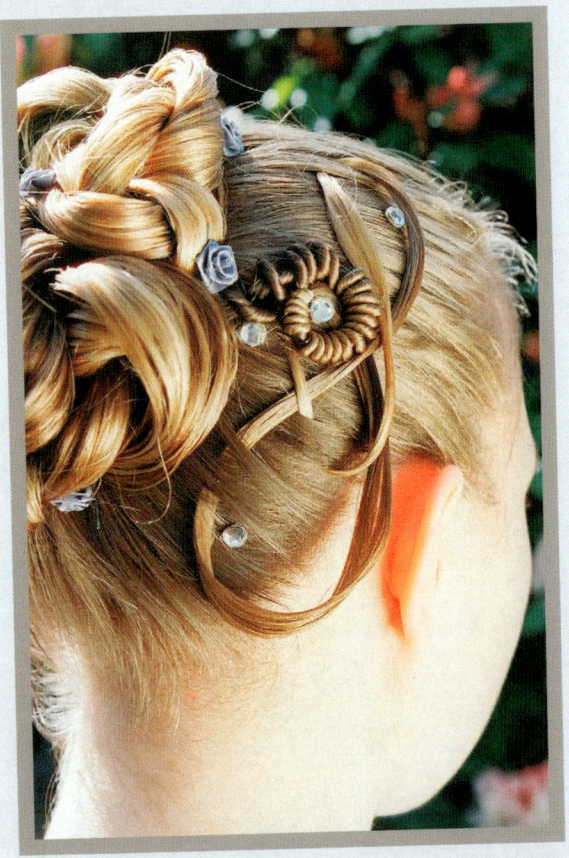
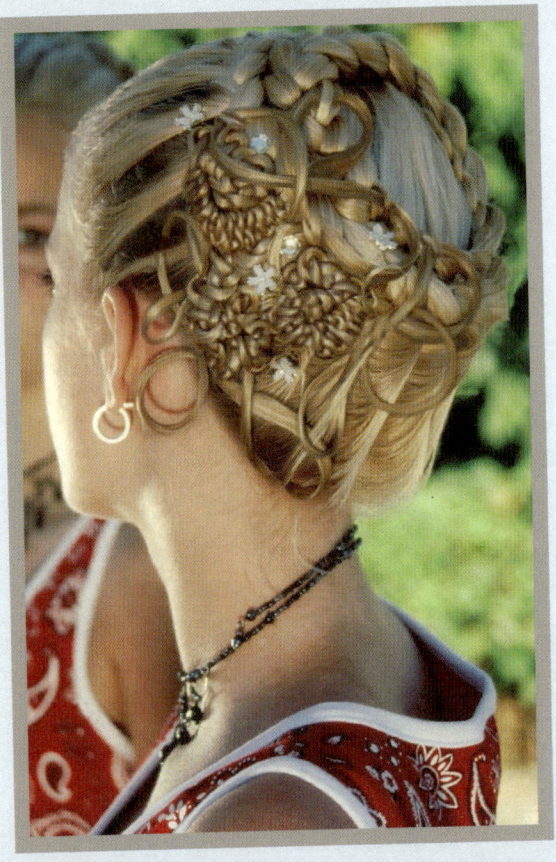
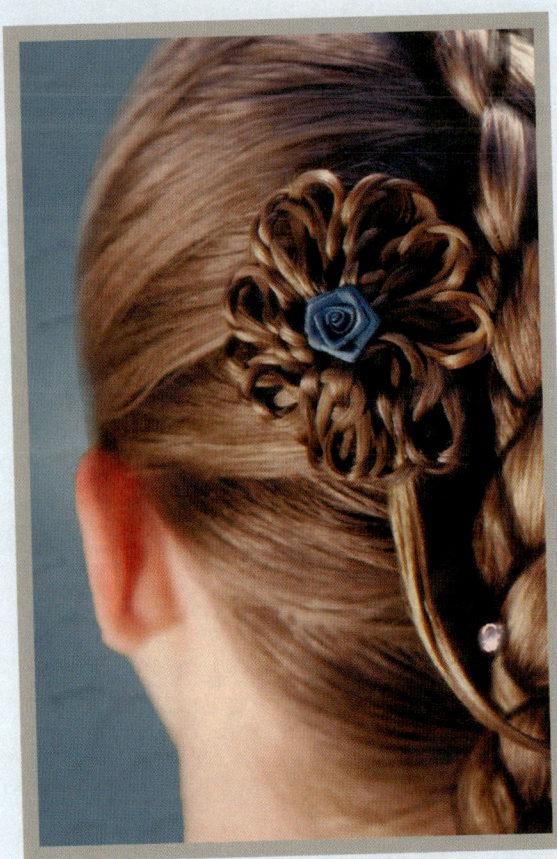
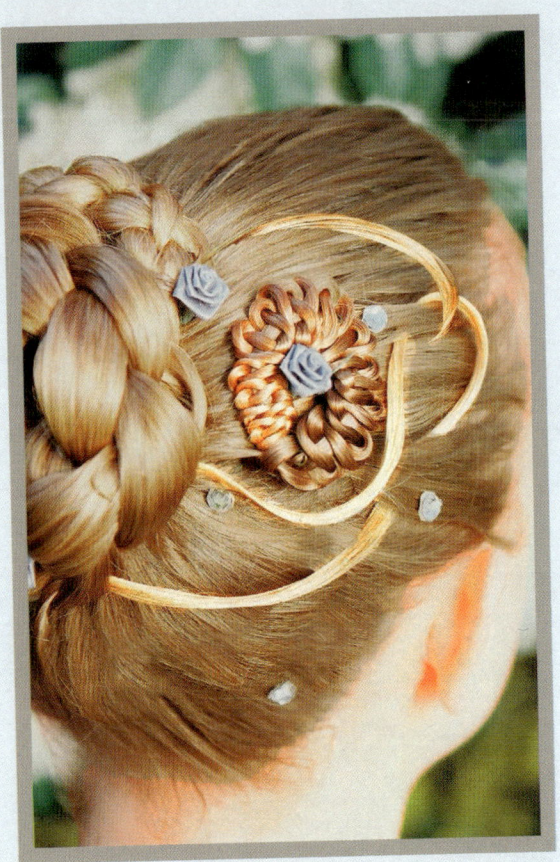

Visit my website to see more examples of Push-ups

Ribbon

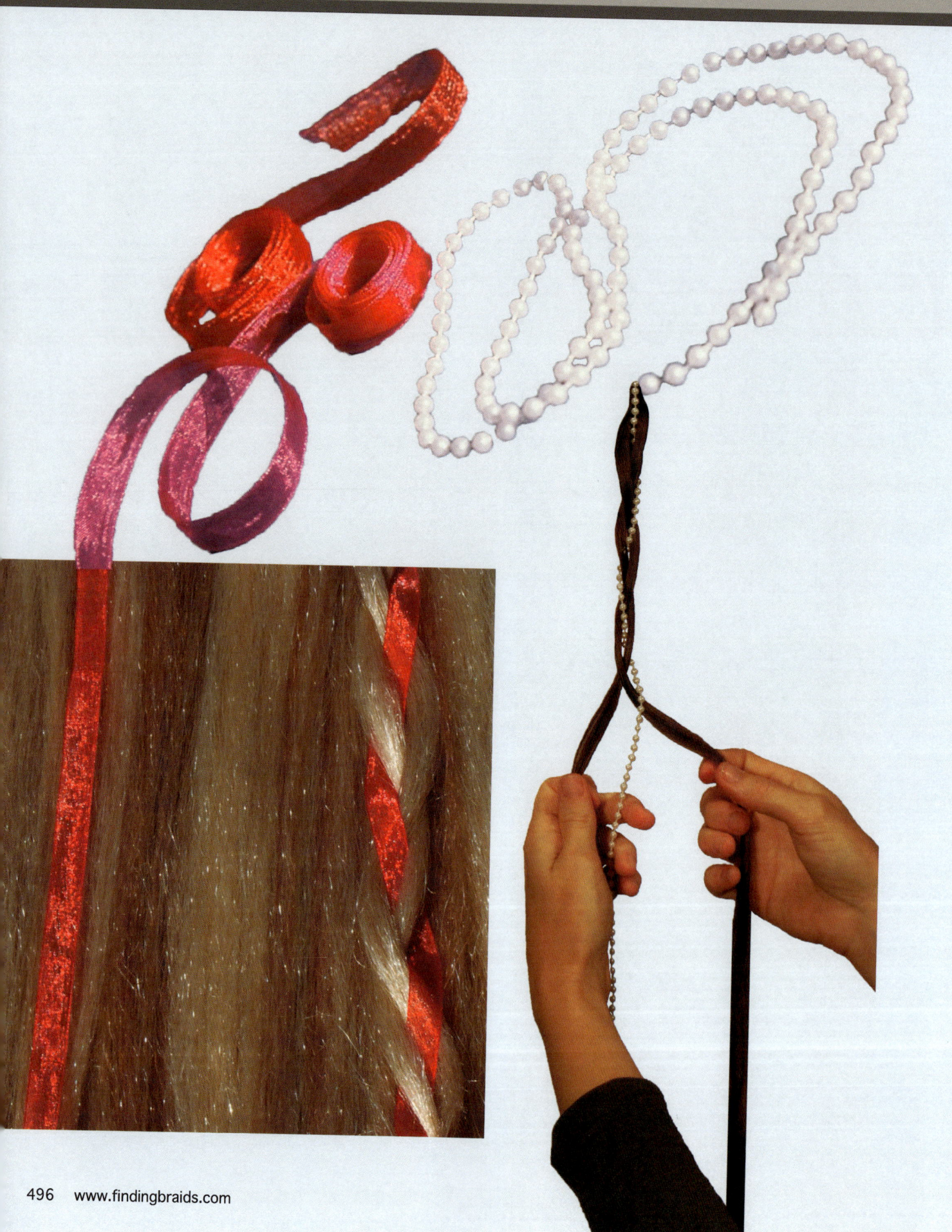

Examples with Ribbon

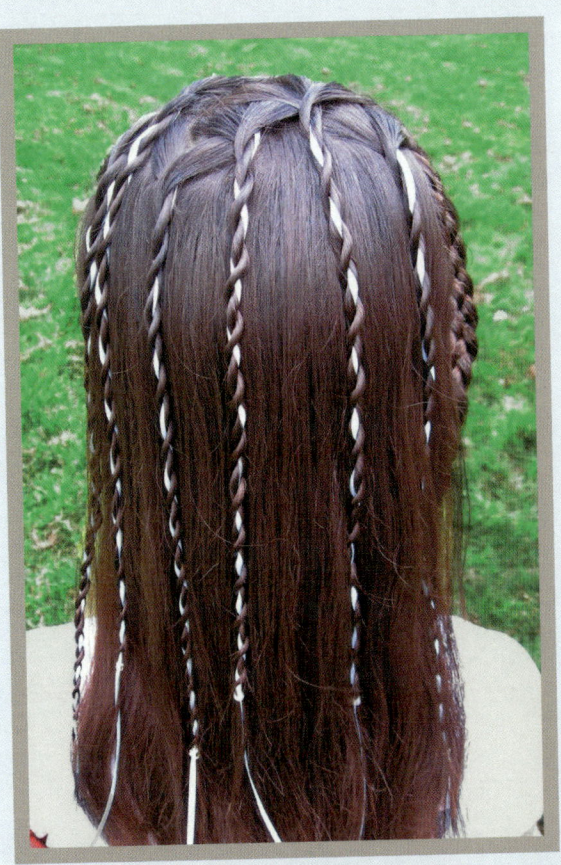
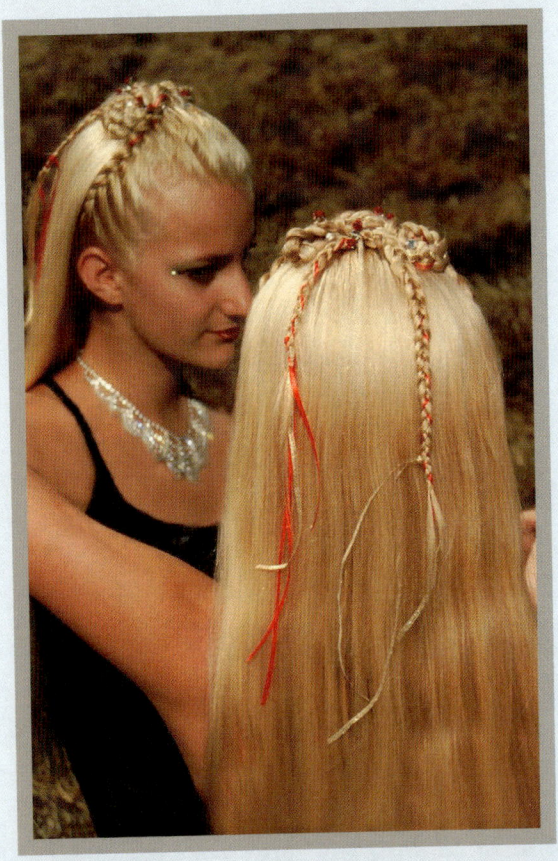
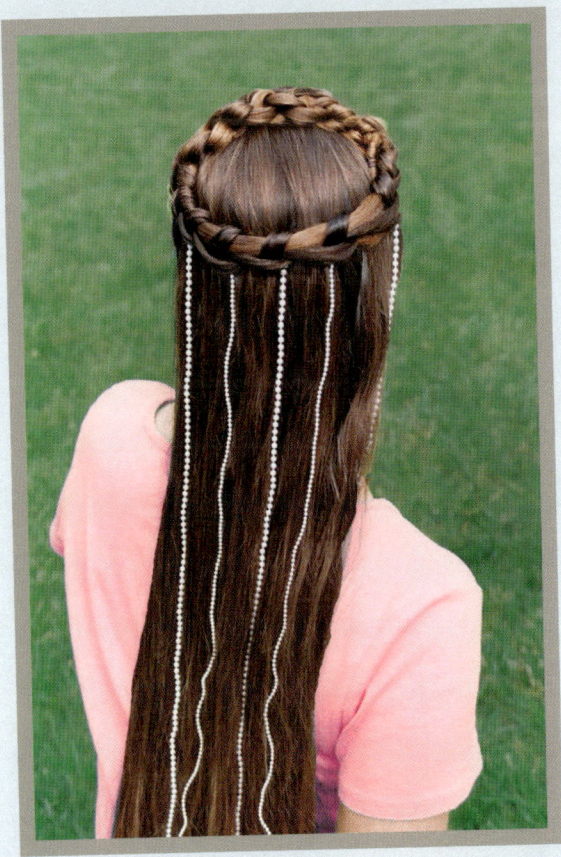
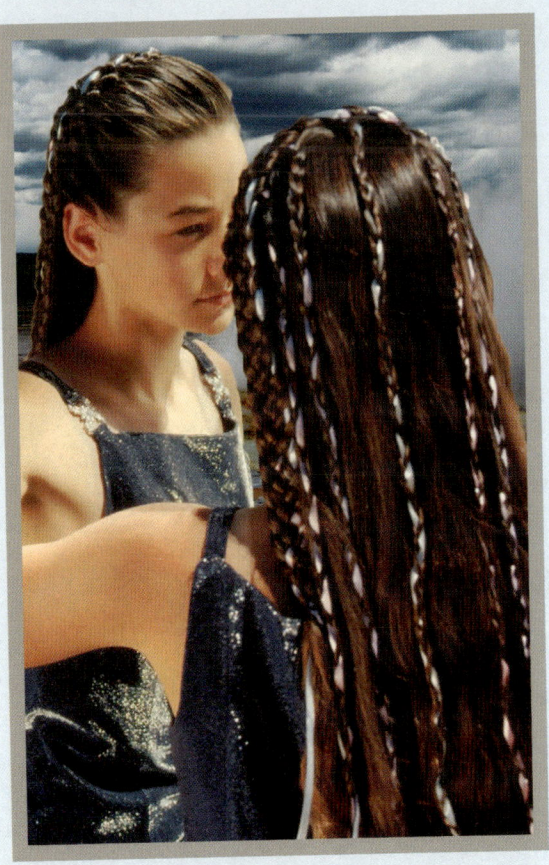

Visit my website to see more examples of Ribbon

References/Links

Gerald Edelman, <u>Bright Air, Brilliant Fire: On the Matter of the Mind</u>.
Robert Sylwester, "What the Biology of the Brain Tells Us About Learning,"
Renate and Geoffrey Caine, <u>Making Connections: Teaching and the Human Brain</u>.
Bobbi Deporter, <u>Quantum Learning</u>,
Lorenzen Huber, gerontology curriculum coordinator for Indiana University's Center on Aging and Aged. "Brain Teasers: Engage your mind in fun new ways."
www.theosociety.org
Educational Technology & Society
Robert Leamnson, Ph D
(http://www.umassd.edu/cas/biology/leamnson/learning.doc)

www.findingbraids.com

frenchbraidsbytwistedsisters.com

www.martinparsons.com

www.aquage.com

http://www.patrick-cameron.com

http://www.youtube.com/raychelnorberg

http://www.youtube.com/ViriYueMoon

http://www.youtube.com/lilithedarkmoon

http://www.youtube.com/womenbeauty1

http://www.youtube.com/cinthiatruong

At one point I owned twenty six books on how to braid. After ten years, I only refer back to these. I highly recommend the first four.

<u>Braids and more</u>, by Andrea Jeffery, 1991

<u>Braids and updos</u>, by Jamie Rines Jones, 1996

<u>Trenzas Plaits 2</u>, by Susana Burgos, 2002

<u>Great braids</u>, by Thomas Hardy, 1997

<u>The complete book of braids</u>, by Linda Shields Ksiazek, 1991

<u>Braids</u>, by Mary Beth Janssen-Fleischman, 1994

Biography

Melanie Mundy was my first mentor. She is the most meticulous braider I have ever met. I was blessed to have had her as a teacher.

During the years I lived in Oregon I attended cosmetology school to get my barber's license. I came across a hairdresser named Martin Parsons. For months, I sat in front of my television absorbing all of his videos. The man is brilliant.

The magic of the Aquage Team caught my attention. I trained with them, carefully learning all I could. Luis Alvarez is a genius.

After digesting and blending this knowledge I now do unique hairstyles for my clients.

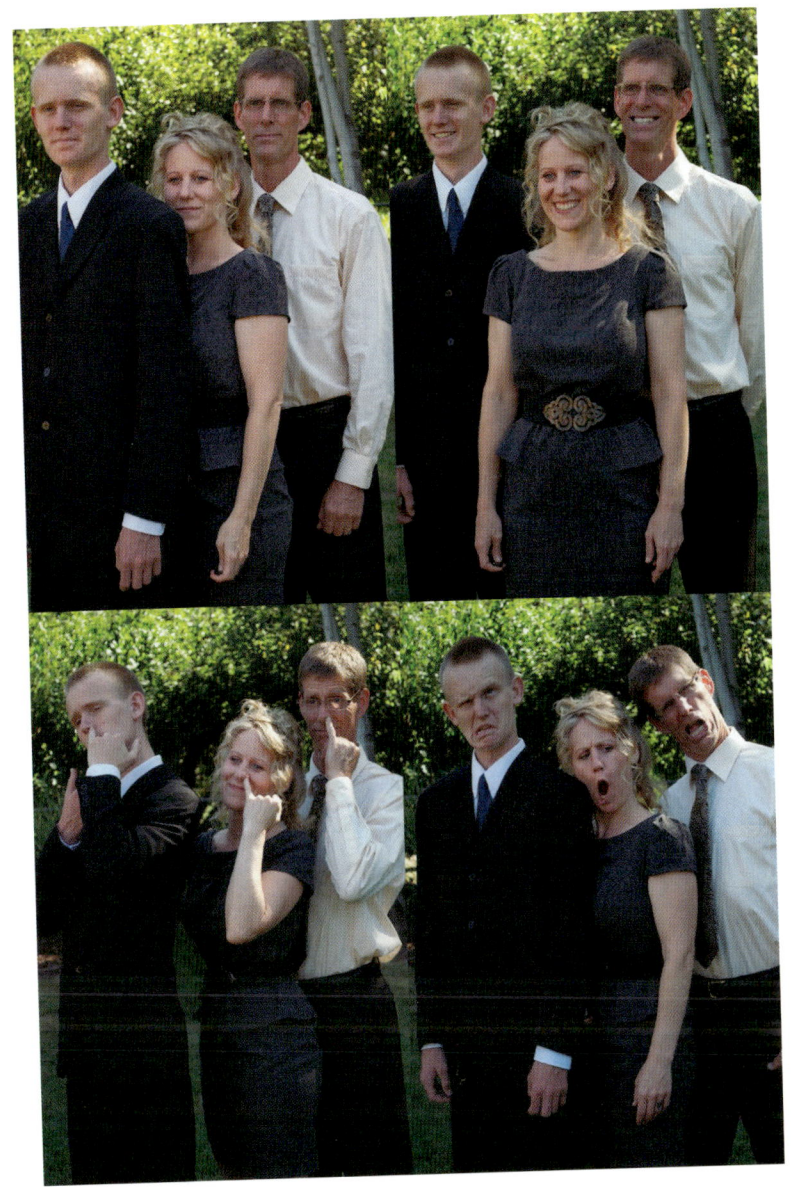

I enjoy volunteering my skill to local community events. My favorites in the past have been high school plays, community theaters, girl scout troops, fashion shows, and giving back to the beauty schools. I taught classes at the community college in Corvallis. Gift certificates make it easy for me to donate to local fundraisers.

My work is a happy work. I love what I do. It never crossed my mind that I would be a hair stylist when I grew up. When I wa a kid I wanted to be a ballerina and when I was a teenager I wanted to be a geologist. Now, I am a happy hair artist.

Made in the USA
San Bernardino, CA
06 December 2013